CLINICAL MANAGEMENT OF RENAL TUMORS

CLINICAL MANAGEMENT OF RENAL TUMORS

Edited by

RONALD M. BUKOWSKI, MD

Taussig Cancer Center, Cleveland Clinic Foundation, Cleveland, OH

and

ANDREW C. NOVICK, MD

Glickman Urological and Kidney Institute, Cleveland Clinic Foundation, Cleveland, OH

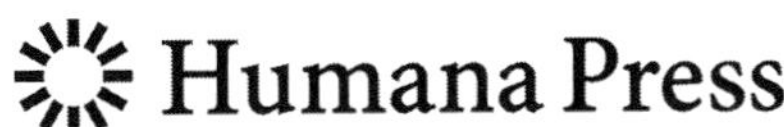

Humana Press

Editors
Ronald M. Bukowski, MD
Taussig Cancer Center
Cleveland Clinic Foundation
Cleveland, OH, USA

Andrew C. Novick, MD
Glickman Urological and Kidney Institute
Cleveland Clinic Foundation
Cleveland, OH, USA

ISBN: 978-1-58829-251-3   e-ISBN: 978-1-60327-149-3
DOI: 10.1007/978-1-60327-149-3

Library of Congress Control Number: 2007932995

Cover illustration: Both images from Chapter 4, "Pathology of Renal Cell Carcinomas," by Ming Zhou. Background art derived from Figure 2. Inset photo derived from Figure 1.

Printed on acid-free paper

9 8 7 6 5 4 3 2 1

springer.com

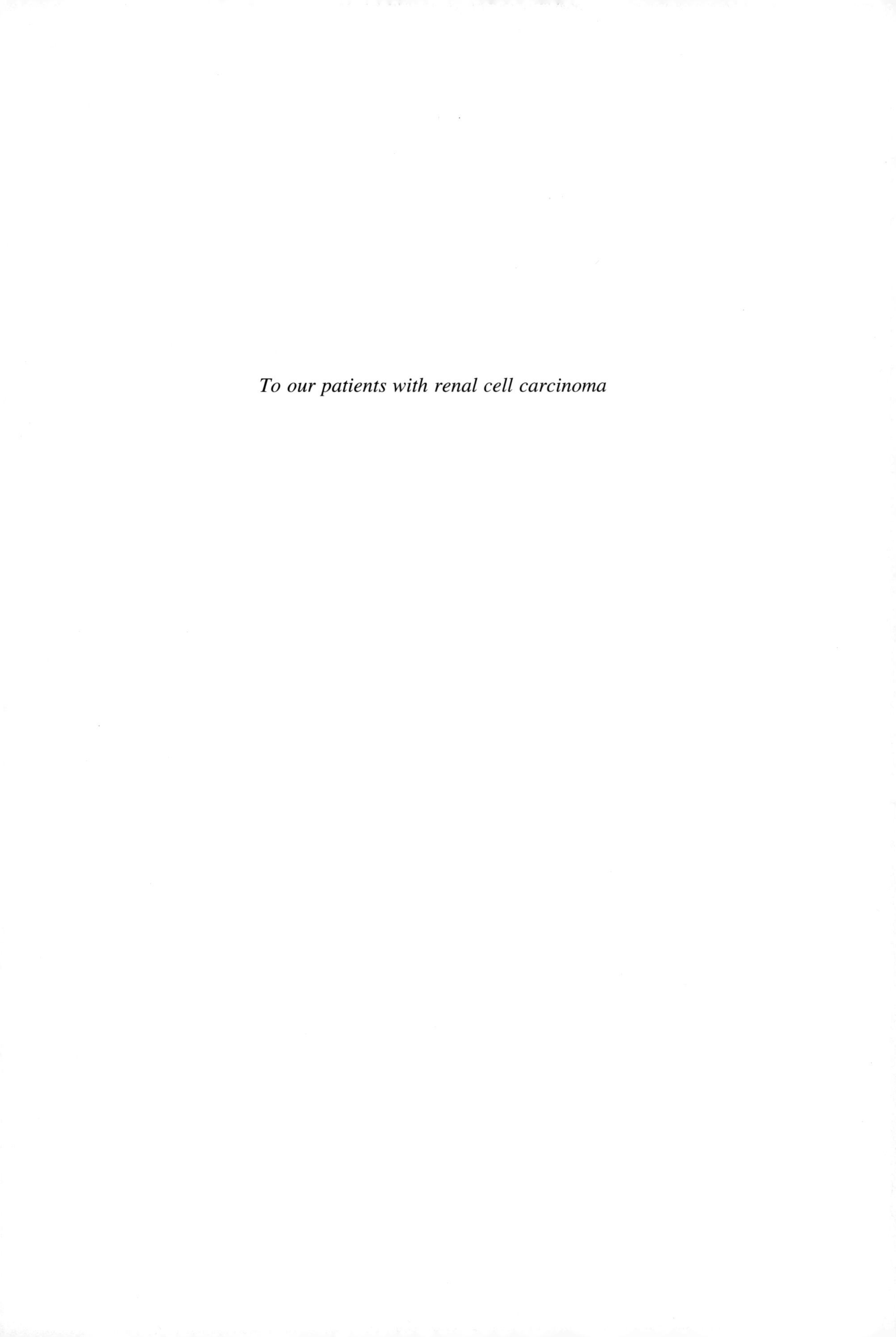

To our patients with renal cell carcinoma

Preface

Renal cancer accounts for 3% of all malignant tumors. An estimated 39,000 new cases and 13,000 deaths were predicted for 2006. Carcinomas arising from the renal epithelium account for approximately 85% of renal tumors. The major risk factors include smoking (responsible for 24% to 30% of all cases of renal cell carcinoma [RCC]), obesity, and various environmental and occupational factors. Presentation varies, with most patients having a solitary lesion and 33% presenting with locally advanced or metastatic disease. An additional 20% to 40% of surgically resected patients may ultimately develop metastatic disease. Advances in imaging and techniques have increased the percent of patients who have renal masses discovered incidentally, but a significant percent of patients still present with surgically unresectable disease. We now recognize the importance of histology in predicting the biologic characteristics and clinical behavior of renal cancers.

Clear cell renal carcinoma is the most common type of renal cancer, accounting for approximately 70% of renal epithelial malignancies and arising from the proximal convoluted tubule. Papillary renal cancer is the second most common type, comprising 10% to 15% of renal tumors. Understanding histologic subtypes and associated gene alterations has provided the opportunity to develop targeted therapeutic agents.

Patients with the von Hippel–Lindau (VHL) syndrome and RCC have provided a unique opportunity to study the development of clear cell tumors and their genetic characteristics. In sporadic renal cancer, both the maternal and paternal VHL alleles are inactivated by acquired mutations, whereas in the VHL syndrome the first mutation is inherited. Loss of VHL function may be responsible for approximately 60% of cases of sporadic clear cell renal carcinomas.

The VHL protein is the product of the VHL gene, functions as a tumor suppressor gene, and is responsible for ubiquination of hypoxia-inducible factor α (HIF-α) and its subsequent degradation. In conditions of hypoxia or abnormal VHL function, HIF-α accumulates and activates the transcription of a variety of hypoxia-inducible genes, including vascular endothelial growth factor (VEGF) and platelet-derived growth factor β (PDGF-β). Blocking the VEGF pathway and the function of HIF-α, therefore, are currently the major therapeutic strategies for treatment of advanced renal cancer, replacing immunotherapy utilizing cytokines such as interferon and interleukin-2 (IL-2). A series of new agents such as sunitinib, sorafenib, temsirolimus, and bevacizumab are now being utilized in patients with advanced clear cell carcinoma.

Major advances in the surgical management of renal tumors have also occurred over the last 10 to 15 years. The type of surgical intervention is determined by tumor size, location, and involvement of the inferior vena cava (IVC), and includes nephrectomy and partial (nephron-sparing) nephrectomy performed through an open abdominal or laparoscopic procedure. Partial nephrectomy preserves long-term renal function for patients with tumors smaller than 4 cm, and radical nephrectomy remains the treatment of choice for tumors 4 cm or larger or multiple lesions when the opposite kidney is normal. Partial nephrectomy is also indicated for patients who have a solitary kidney, bilateral renal masses, or severe renal insufficiency. Laparoscopic procedures for complete or partial nephrectomy are emerging minimally invasive procedures with shorter hospitalization, decreased narcotic use, and a more rapid convalescence.

In conclusion, the treatment paradigms for patients with localized and advanced renal cell carcinoma have changed dramatically in the last 5 to 10 years. Surgical advances are now mirrored by the dramatic changes in therapy available for metastatic disease. The chapters in *Clinical Management of Renal Tumors* provide an update for urologists, medical oncologists, and researchers who are interested in this malignancy.

Ronald M. Bukowski, MD
Andrew C. Novick, MD

CONTENTS

Preface .... **vii**

Contributors .... **xiii**

List of Color Plates .... **xvii**

1   Renal Cell Carcinoma: *Background* **1**
    Ronald M. Bukowski and Andrew C. Novick

2   Imaging of Renal Cell Carcinoma **9**
    Brian R. Herts

3   The Role of Percutaneous Imaging-Guided Biopsy in the Diagnosis
    and Management of Renal Masses **43**
    Brian R. Herts and Stuart G. Silverman

4   Pathology of Renal Cell Carcinomas **55**
    Ming Zhou

5   Epidemiology of Renal Tumors **73**
    Jeffrey S. Montgomery and David P. Wood

6   Molecular Genetics in Inherited Renal Cell Carcinoma: Identification
    of Targets in the Hereditary Syndromes **97**
    Nadeem Dhanani, Cathy Vocke, Gennady Bratslavsky,
    and W. Marston Linehan

7   T-Cell Unresponsiveness in Renal Cell Carcinoma Patients **115**
    James H. Finke and Mahesh Goel

8   Renal Cell Carcinoma: *Clinical Presentation and Diagnosis* **131**
    Venkatesh Krishnamurthi

9   Clinical and Pathologic Staging of Renal Cell Carcinoma **145**
    Alison M. Lake, Cara Cimmino, James E. Montie,
    and Khaled S. Hafez

10   Active Surveillance of Localized Renal Tumors **159**
    Paul L. Crispen, Sameer N. Chawla, and Robert G. Uzzo

11   Radical Nephrectomy **177**
    Benjamin I. Chung, and John A. Libertino

12   Laparoscopic Radical Nephrectomy **195**
    Benjamin I. Chung, Jose R. Colombo, Jr., and Inderbir S. Gill

13   Open Nephron-Sparing Surgery for Renal Cell Carcinoma **205**
    Andrew C. Novick

14 Minimally Invasive Nephron-Sparing Surgery for Renal Tumors:
Laparoscopic Partial Nephrectomy and Probe Ablative Treatments .. **219**
Monish Aron, Georges-Pascal Haber, and Inderbir S. Gill

15 The Role of Angioinfarction in the Management of Renal Tumors **247**
Bryan T. Kansas, Paul L. Crispen, and Robert G. Uzzo

16 Surveillance Strategies Following Curative Therapy for
Localized Renal Cell Carcinoma **265**
Vitaly Margulis, Surena F. Matin, and Christopher G. Wood

17 Local Recurrence of Renal Cell Carcinoma: *Management* **275**
Brian K. McNeil and Steven C. Campbell

18 Adjuvant Therapy of Renal Cell Carcinoma...................... **293**
Ronald M. Bukowski

19 Prognostic Factors for Survival in Metastatic Renal Cell Carcinoma **307**
Paul J. Elson

20 Functional Imaging of Renal Cell Carcinoma **323**
Navneet S. Majhail and Ronald M. Bukowski

21 Nephrectomy in Patients with Metastatic Renal Cell Carcinoma:
Clinical and Biologic Effects **335**
Bradley G. Orris and Robert C. Flanigan

22 Spontaneous Regression of Renal Cell Carcinoma and the Role
of Prognostic Factors **355**
Tim Oliver, Tom Powles, Vinod Nargund, and Dan Berney

23 Systemic Therapy for Metastatic Renal Cell Carcinoma: *Cytokines* **367**
Thomas E. Hutson

24 Chemotherapy for Metastatic Clear-Cell Renal Cell Carcinoma **385**
James O. Jin and Walter M. Stadler

25 Signal Transduction Inhibitors in Renal Cell Carcinoma **399**
*Ellen A. Ronnen, Saby George, Ronald M. Bukowski,
and Robert J. Motzer*

26 Pulmonary Metastases in Patients with Advanced Renal Cell Carcinoma:
Role of Metastasectomy **415**
Sudish Murthy

27 Management of Skeletal Metastases in Renal Cell
Carcinoma Patients **421**
Michael J. Joyce

28 Renal Cell Carcinoma Metastatic to the Pancreas:
Clinical and Therapeutic Aspects **461**
Ahmed Al-Hazzouri, Brian R. Herts, and Ronald M. Bukowski

29 Intracranial Renal Cell Cancer Metastasis **481**
Kene Ugokwe and Steven A. Toms

30 Role of Radiation Therapy in Advanced Renal Cell Carcinoma **497**
Arul Mahadevan

31 Palliation in Renal Cancer **507**
Mellar P. Davis

32 Management of Patients with Pathologic Variants of Renal Cell
Carcinoma: *Papillary, Collecting Duct, Medullary and Chromophobe
Carcinoma, and Sarcomatoid Differentiation* **529**
Vladimir Hugec and Janice P. Dutcher

33 Renal Cell Carcinoma in Patients with End-Stage Renal Disease **545**
John C. Rabets and David A. Goldfarb

34 Management of Renal Adenomas and Oncocytomas **555**
Igor Frank and Michael L. Blute

35 Renal Angiomyolipoma: *Diagnosis and Management* **565**
Surena F. Matin, Pheroze Tamboli, and Christopher G. Wood

36 Transitional Cell Carcinoma of the Renal Pelvis: *Management* **587**
Jorge A. Garcia and Robert Dreicer

37 Wilms' Tumor in Children and Adults **599**
Jonathan H. Ross

38 Rare Malignancies of the Kidney: *Evaluation and Management* **617**
Kristian R. Novakovic and Steven C. Campbell

Index **637**

Contributors

AHMED AL-HAZZOURI, MD, *Taussig Cancer Center, Cleveland Clinic Foundation, Cleveland, OH*

MONISH ARON, MD, *Glickman Urological and Kidney Institute, Cleveland Clinic Foundation, Cleveland, OH*

DAN BERNEY, MD, *Department of Medical Oncology, Royal Marsden, St. Bartholomew's Hospital, London, England*

MICHAEL L. BLUTE, MD, *Department of Urology, Mayo Clinic, Rochester, MN*

GENNADY BRATSLAVSKY, MD, *National Cancer Institute, Bethesda, MD*

RONALD M. BUKOWSKI, MD, *Taussig Cancer Center, Cleveland Clinic Foundation, Cleveland, OH*

STEVEN C. CAMPBELL, MD, PHD, *Department of Urology, Cleveland Clinic Foundation, Cleveland, OH*

SAMEER N. CHAWLA, MD, *Department of Surgical Oncology, Fox Chase Cancer Center, Philadelphia, PA*

BENJAMIN I. CHUNG, MD, *Glickman Urological and Kidney Institute, Cleveland Clinic Foundation, Cleveland, OH*

CARA CIMMINO, MD, *Department of Urology, University of Michigan, Ann Arbor, MI*

JOSE R. COLOMBO, JR., MD, *Glickman Urological and Kidney Institute, Cleveland Clinic Foundation, Cleveland, OH*

PAUL L. CRISPEN, MD, *Department of Urology, Fox Chase Cancer Center, Philadelphia, PA*

MELLAR P. DAVIS, MD, FCCP, *The Harry R. Horvitz Center for Palliative Medicine, Taussig Cancer Center, Cleveland Clinic Foundation, Cleveland, OH*

NADEEM DHANANI, MD, *National Cancer Institute, Bethesda, MD*

ROBERT DREICER, MD, *Department of Hematology/Oncology and the Glickman Urological and Kidney Institute, Cleveland Clinic Foundation, Cleveland, OH*

JANICE P. DUTCHER, MD, *Our Lady of Mercy Medical Center, Comprehensive Cancer Center, Bronx, NY*

PAUL J. ELSON, SCD, *Taussig Cancer Center, Cleveland Clinic Foundation, Cleveland, OH*

JAMES H. FINKE, PHD, *Department of Immunology, Cleveland Clinic Foundation, Cleveland, OH*

ROBERT C. FLANIGAN, MD, *Department of Urology, Loyola University Medical Center, Maywood, IL*

IGOR FRANK, MD, *Department of Urology, Mayo Clinic, Rochester, MN*

JORGE A. GARCIA, MD, *Department of Hematology/Oncology and the Glickman Urological and Kidney Institute, Cleveland Clinic Foundation, Cleveland, OH*

SABY GEORGE, MD, *Taussig Cancer Center, Cleveland Clinic Foundation, Cleveland, OH*

INDERBIR S. GILL, MD, *Glickman Urological and Kidney Institute, Cleveland Clinic Foundation, Cleveland, OH*

MAHESH GOEL, MD, *Glickman Urological and Kidney Institute, Cleveland Clinic Foundation, Cleveland, OH*

DAVID A. GOLDFARB, MD, *Glickman Urological and Kidney Institute, Cleveland Clinic Foundation, Cleveland, OH*

GEORGES-PASCAL HABER, MD, *Glickman Urological and Kidney Institute, Cleveland Clinic Foundation, Cleveland, OH*

KHALED S. HAFEZ, MD, *Department of Urology, University of Michigan, Ann Arbor, MI*

BRIAN R. HERTS, MD, *Department of Radiology, Cleveland Clinic Foundation, Cleveland, OH*

VLADIMIR HUGEC, MD, *Our Lady of Mercy Medical Center, Comprehensive Cancer Center, Bronx, NY*

THOMAS E. HUTSON, DO, PHARMD, *Sammons Cancer Center, Baylor University Medical Center, Dallas, TX*

JAMES O. JIN, MD, PhD, *Department of Medicine, University of Chicago, Chicago, IL*

MICHAEL J. JOYCE, MD, *Department of Orthopedic Surgery, Cleveland Clinic Foundation, Cleveland, OH*

BRYAN T. KANSAS, MD, *Department of Urology, Fox Chase Cancer Center, Philadelphia, PA*

VENKATESH KRISHNAMURTHI, MD, *Glickman Urological and Kidney Institute, Cleveland Clinic Foundation, Cleveland, OH*

ALISON M. LAKE, MD, *Department of Urology, University of Michigan, Ann Arbor, MI*

JOHN A. LIBERTINO, MD, *Department of Urology, Lahey Clinic, Burlington, MA*

W. MARSTON LINEHAN, MD, *National Cancer Institute, Bethesda, MD*

ARUL MAHADEVAN, MD, FRCS, *Department of Radiation Oncology, Cleveland Clinic Foundation, Cleveland, OH*

NAVNEET S. MAJHAIL, MD, *Taussig Cancer Center, Cleveland Clinic Foundation, Cleveland, OH*

VITALY MARGULIS, MD, *Department of Urology, MD Anderson Cancer Center, Houston, TX*

SURENA F. MATIN, MD, *Department of Urology, MD Anderson Cancer Center, Houston, TX*

BRIAN K. MCNEIL, MD, *Department of Urology, Loyola University Medical Center, Maywood, IL*

JEFFREY S. MONTGOMERY, MD, *Department of Urology, University of Michigan, Ann Arbor, MI*

JAMES E. MONTIE, MD, *Department of Urology, University of Michigan, Ann Arbor, MI*

ROBERT J. MOTZER, MD, *Department of Medicine, Memorial Sloan-Kettering Cancer Center, New York, NY*

SUDISH MURTHY, MD, PhD, FACS, FCCP, *Department of Thoracic and Cardiovascular Surgery, Cleveland Clinic Foundation, Cleveland, OH*

VINOD NARGUND, MD, *Department of Medical Oncology, Royal Marsden,*
  St. Bartholomew's Hospital, London, England

KRISTIAN R. NOVAKOVIC, MD, *Department of Urology, Loyola University Medical*
  Center, Maywood, IL

ANDREW C. NOVICK, MD, *Glickman Urological and Kidney Institute, Cleveland*
  Clinic Foundation, Cleveland, OH

TIM OLIVER, MD, *Department of Medical Oncology, Royal Marsden,*
  St. Bartholomew's Hospital, Medical School, Rahere, West Smithfield,
  London, England

BRADLEY G. ORRIS, MD, *Department of Urology, Loyola University Medical Center,*
  Maywood, IL

TOM POWLES, MD, *Department of Medical Oncology, Royal Marsden,*
  St. Bartholomew's Hospital, London, England

JOHN C. RABETS, MD, *Glickman Urological and Kidney Institute, Cleveland Clinic*
  Foundation, Cleveland, OH

ELLEN A. RONNEN, MD, *Department of Medicine, Memorial Sloan-Kettering Cancer*
  Center, New York, NY

JONATHAN H. ROSS, MD, *Glickman Urological and Kidney Institute, Cleveland Clinic*
  Foundation, Cleveland, OH

STUART G. SILVERMAN, MD, *Department of Radiology, Brigham and Women's*
  Hospital, Boston, MA

WALTER M. STADLER, MD, *Department of Medicine, University of Chicago,*
  Chicago, IL

PHEROZE TAMBOLI, MD, *Department of Pathology, MD Anderson Cancer Center,*
  Houston, TX

STEVEN A. TOMS, MD, MPH, *Department of Neurological Surgery, Brain Tumor*
  Institute, Cleveland Clinic Foundation, Cleveland, OH

KENE UGOKWE, MD, *Department of Neurological Surgery, Brain Tumor Institute,*
  Cleveland Clinic Foundation, Cleveland, OH

ROBERT G. UZZO, MD, *Department of Urologic Oncology, Fox Chase Cancer Center,*
  Philadelphia, PA

CATHY VOCKE, PhD, *National Cancer Institute, Bethesda, MD*

CHRISTOPHER G. WOOD, MD, *Department of Urology, MD Anderson Cancer Center,*
  Houston, TX

DAVID P. WOOD, MD, *Department of Urology, University of Michigan,*
  Ann Arbor, MI

MING ZHOU, MD, PhD, *Department of Anatomic Pathology, Cleveland Clinic*
  Foundation, Cleveland, OH

LIST OF COLOR PLATES

The images listed below appear in the color insert following page 334.

Color Plate 1.   *Fig. 2, Chapter 4:* (**A**) Papillary renal cell carcinoma (PRCC) has a pseudocapsule and extensive hemorrhage and necrosis. It is composed of papillae covered by a single layer of tumor cells with scant cytoplasm. (**B**) The fibrovascular cores are expanded with foamy histiocytes.
Fig. 3, Chapter 4: (**A**) Renal cell carcinoma, chromophobe type (ChRCC) forms a circumscribed, nonencapsulated mass with a homogeneous light brown cut surface. (**B**) The large and polygonal tumor cells have finely reticulated cytoplasm, prominent cell border, and irregular nuclei with perinuclear clearing.

Color Plate 2.   *Fig. 1, Chapter 6:* Phenotypic manifestations of von Hippel-Lindau (VHL). Renal masses are common in VHL patients. (**A**) Computed tomography (CT) scans of a VHL patient demonstrating characteristic bilateral multifocal renal lesions consisting of simple and complex cysts as well as enhancing solid masses. (**B**) Gross specimen removed from a VHL patient showing classic multiple golden-yellow tumors. (**C**) Hematoxylin and eosin (H&E) stain of a classic clear cell renal carcinoma found in patients with VHL. (**D**) In addition to renal manifestations, VHL affects organs systems throughout the body. (From Linehan WM, et al. Genetic Basis of Cancer of the Kidney: Disease-Specific Approaches to Therapy. 2004.)

Color Plate 3.   *Fig. 2, Chapter 6:* Manifestations and genetics of hereditary papillary renal cancer (HPRC). Patients with HPRC primarily develop bilateral multifocal renal masses. (**A**) Abdominal CT demonstrates HPRC tumors with characteristic poor enhancement on contrasted study that may frequently be mistaken for simple cysts. The tumors are best seen on late phase images of a contrast CT. Low (**B**) and high (**C**) power H&E stain of type I papillary renal cell carcinoma (RCC) seen in patients with HPRC. (**D**) Fluorescence in situ hybridization (FISH) using a MET probe demonstrating trisomy of chromosome 7 (red signal) in papillary type 1 RCC compared with chromosome 11 serving as control (green signal).

(From Schmidt et al. Early Onset Hereditary Papillary Renal Carcinoma: Germline Missense Mutations in the Tyrocine Kinase Domain of the MET Proto-Oncogene. 2004.)

Color Plate 4. *Fig. 6, Chapter 6: VHL* gene mutation, downstream effects, and molecular targeting of the VHL pathway. **(A)** With a *VHL* gene mutation, the VHL complex is disrupted and allows for accumulation of HIF with subsequent activation of downstream pathways for angiogenesis, glucose transport, and growth. **(B)** Inhibition of over-accumulated HIF and prevention of downstream activation with a small molecule is one of the strategies for molecular targeting of the VHL/HIF pathway. **(C)** New tyrosine kinase inhibitors as well as direct vascular endothelial growth factor (VEGF) and platelet-derived growth factor (PDGF) receptor blockers are examples of downstream targeting. EGFR, epidermal growth factor receptor; TGF, transforming growth factor. (From Linehan WM et al. Genetic Basis of Cancer of the Kidney: Disease-Specific Approaches to Therapy. 2004.)

Renal Cell Carcinoma: *Background*

Ronald M. Bukowski and Andrew C. Novick

KEYWORDS

RENAL CELL CARCINOMA

Renal cancer accounts for 2 to 3% of all malignant tumors. An estimated 39,000 new cases and 13,000 deaths were predicted for 2006.[1] Renal cancer is diagnosed in patients ranging from 40 to 70 years of age, with a male predominance of 1.6 to 1.0.[1] A comparison of 43,685 cases of renal cancer diagnosed in the period 1973 to 1985 with those diagnosed from 1986 to 1998 (Surveillance, Epidemiology, and End Results [SEER] database) demonstrated a marginal increase in the proportion of localized cancers and a decrease in advanced cases in the latter group. The differences were not significant, and importantly, overall survival was not improved.[2] While increased imaging and laboratory testing may generally explain the increased incidence, other factors may play a role.[2]

Risk factors include smoking (responsible for 24% to 30% of all cases of renal cell carcinoma [RCC]), obesity, sedentary lifestyle, environmental and occupational factors (asbestos, cadmium, polycyclic hydrocarbons, solvents), and long-term use of diuretics or phenacetin-containing analgesics.[1] Patients with end-stage renal disease undergoing dialysis, particularly those with cystic disease, are also more likely to develop RCC than the general population.

Renal cell carcinomas arising from the renal epithelium account for approximately 85% percent of renal tumors.[3] Presentation varies, with most presenting with a solitary lesion, less than 4% presenting with bilateral renal masses, and 33% presenting with locally advanced or metastatic disease.[4] Additionally, 20% to 40% of surgically resected patients may ultimately develop metastatic disease. Historically, patients presented with the classic triad of symptoms including flank pain, hematuria, and a palpable abdominal mass, but currently, increasing numbers of individuals are being diagnosed when asymptomatic with an incidental renal mass found. Advances in imaging and techniques have increased the percent of patients who are eligible for surgical intervention, but a significant number of patients still present with surgically unresectable disease.[4]

Patients with advanced disease may present with symptoms produced by the tumor or resulting from chemical abnormalities, or paraneoplastic syndromes associated with

From: *Clinical Management of Renal Tumors*
Edited by: R.M. Bukowski and A.C. Novick © Humana Press Inc., Totowa, NJ

the neoplasm. Common sites for metastasis include lung, bone, lymph nodes, adrenal gland, liver, soft tissue, and brain.

HISTOLOGY

The importance of histology in predicting the biologic characteristics and clinical behavior of renal cancers was recognized in the last decade. Renal cell carcinoma represents a group of histologic subtypes with unique morphologic and genetic characteristics. The Heidelberg classification of renal cell tumors was developed to subdivide renal cell tumors into benign and malignant subtypes with associated genetic alterations.[5]

Clear cell renal carcinoma is the most common type of renal cancer, accounting for approximately 70% of renal epithelial malignancies and arising from the proximal convoluted tubule. Papillary renal cancer is the second most common type, comprising 10% to 15% of renal tumors. Understanding histologic subtypes and associated gene alterations has provided the opportunity to develop targeted therapeutic agents.

VON HIPPEL-LINDAU (VHL) SYNDROME

Patients with the VHL syndrome provided researchers a unique opportunity to study the development of clear cell tumors and their genetic characteristics. In sporadic renal cancer, both the maternal and paternal VHL alleles are inactivated by acquired mutations whereas in the VHL syndrome the first mutation is inherited. Loss of VHL function may be responsible for approximately 60% of cases of sporadic clear-cell renal carcinomas.[6]

The VHL protein is the product of the *VHL* gene, functions as a tumor suppressor gene, and is responsible for ubiquitination of hypoxia-inducible factor α (HIF-α), tagging it for degradation.[3,6] In conditions of hypoxia or abnormal VHL function, HIF-α accumulates and activates the transcription of a variety of hypoxia-inducible genes. These include vascular endothelial growth factor (VEGF), platelet-derived growth factor β (PDGF-β), transforming growth factor α (TGF-α), and erythropoietin (EPO). The *VHL* gene may enable this process to be controlled through suppressing angiogenesis, but loss of the *VHL* gene or its function leads to increased secretion of VEGF and PDGF and appears to produce the vascular phenotype associated with this tumor. Blocking VEGF and thus the function of HIF-α is currently the major therapeutic strategy for treatment of advanced renal cancer, replacing immunotherapy with the cytokines interferon and interleukin-2 (IL-2).

SURGICAL MANAGEMENT OF RENAL CELL CARCINOMA

The management of renal cancer is based on the stage at diagnosis, the sites of metastatic disease, and the patient characteristics, including comorbid diseases and functional status. Surgical intervention is determined by tumor size, location, and involvement of the inferior vena cava (IVC), and includes nephrectomy and partial (nephron-sparing) nephrectomy performed through an open abdominal or laparoscopic procedure. Careful case selection allows for surgical resection of renal tumors with vena caval tumor extension and limited metastatic disease using a flank, transperitoneal, transabdominal, or retroperitoneal approach.[4] Partial nephrectomy preserves long-term renal function for patients with tumors <4 cm, and radical nephrectomy remains the treatment of choice for tumors ≥4 cm or multiple lesions when the opposite kidney is normal.[7] Partial nephrectomy is also indicated for patients who have a solitary kidney, bilateral renal masses, or severe renal insufficiency.[8] Laparoscopic procedures for complete or partial nephrectomy are emerging minimally invasive procedures with shorter hospitalization, decreased narcotic use, a more rapid convalescence, with continued efforts to improve operative techniques including reduction of warm renal ischemia time, renal hemorrhage, and urinary leakage.[9]

Cytoreductive nephrectomy may provide survival and palliative advantages, and should be considered for patients presenting with synchronous metastatic renal cancer based on the potential for spontaneous regression of metastatic disease (primarily lung metastasis), but understanding that the primary tumor rarely responds to systemic disease. Studies have demonstrated that cytoreductive nephrectomy followed by interferon-alfa-2b therapy can delay time to progression and improve survival for patients with metastatic renal cancer.[10]

Three approaches for patients with localized renal tumors are currently employed: (1) active surveillance, especially in the older patient; (2) partial nephrectomy; and (3) radical nephrectomy. The latter remains the most commonly performed procedure for patients with localized renal cell carcinoma, and the major story in recent years has been the incorporation or development of laparoscopic nephrectomy as a standard of care for selected patients, namely those who have T1 or T2 renal tumors. The study by Kavoussi et al.[11] demonstrates the long-term efficacy of laparoscopic radical nephrectomy. In this study, open and laparoscopic nephrectomy for T1 to T2 cancers was compared. At a median follow-up in excess of 6 years, 5-year and 10-year cancer-specific survival appears to be similar. For patients with locally advanced disease (T3a and T3b tumors) and those requiring lymphadenectomy, the open technique remains the standard of care.

Currently, increasing numbers of patients are being seen who are candidates for nephron-sparing approaches. Data suggest that the stage I tumors are smaller and are being detected at an earlier stage, increasing the number of patients eligible for nephron-sparing surgery. However, partial nephrectomy is still being performed on a limited number of these cases. A study from the University of Michigan,[12] looking at the percentage of surgically treated patients undergoing partial nephrectomy, shows that only 12.3% had this procedure, suggesting nephron-sparing surgery is still underutilized.

Clinically, preservation of renal function remains an important issue. The patients considered for partial nephrectomy are those with a tumor less than 4 cm in size. In patients with occult multicentric tumors, partial nephrectomy is not optimal, but the incidence of occult multicentric tumors is much less with smaller and with low stage tumors. This observation has led to modification of the American Joint Committee on Cancer (AJCC) tumor, node, metastasis (TNM) staging system where patients with T1 tumors are now subdivided into those with T1a versus T1b; the aim here is to delineate those patients, namely those with T1a tumors, who are most suitable for an elective partial nephrectomy with a normal opposite kidney.

The indications for elective partial nephrectomy may be changing, with recent reports suggesting partial nephrectomy in patients with T1b tumors (4 to 7 cm in size) is an option.[13] The experience at the Cleveland Clinic confirms these findings.

The importance of elective partial nephrectomy is related to functional and quality of life advantages associated with preservation of renal tissue, even in the presence of a normal contralateral kidney. Patients with small remnant kidneys and reduced renal function are prone to developing hyperfiltration, renal injury, and remnant kidney nephropathy. The risk of this problem is directly related to the amount of remaining renal tissue and develops over an extended period. Histologically, focal segmental glomerulosclerosis develops, and is characterized by proteinuria.

Open partial nephrectomy is the gold standard, and is associated with the largest experience and longest follow-up. More than 2500 open partial nephrectomies have been performed at the Cleveland Clinic with long-term results in 1231 patients treated prior to 2002. This experience, along with that of many other centers, has shown that preservation of renal function can be achieved in a very high percentage of these cases, with excellent 10-year survival comparable to that obtained with a total nephrectomy. In patients with localized, sporadic renal cell cancer, recurrent malignancy develops in under 10% of treated cases. A new era of minimally invasive nephron-sparing surgery is now being explored.

A retrospective review of Cleveland Clinic data in 1049 patients who underwent either a laparoscopic or an open partial nephrectomy for a single, localized, sporadic, suspected renal cancer that was less than 7 cm in size was conducted. There were 595 open and 454 laparoscopic procedures. Patients were not matched, and it is not surprising that there were more high-risk patients in the open group, more with comorbid disease, more with symptomatic tumors, many more with solitary kidneys, more with impaired renal function, more with T1b tumors, and more with central tumors.

Laparoscopic surgery was associated with about 1 hour less of operating time, but longer renal ischemia time. There were a small number of cases in the laparoscopic group that converted to radical nephrectomy, and a small number converted to open surgery, differences that were not significant. The major finding in the study is that while both approaches were successful in the majority of cases, there was an increase in postoperative urologic or renal morbidity with the laparoscopic approach. There were twice as many renal or urologic complications. Most notable among these was postoperative hemorrhage, which occurred in 5.7% of patients in the laparoscopic group, and only 2% in the open group. There was no significant difference in the incidence of urinary fistulas. A few kidneys were lost in the laparoscopic group, but this was not significant. Another major difference was in the need for a subsequent procedure generally to treat a complication. That occurred about twice as commonly in the laparoscopic group as in the open group. A diagnosis of renal cancer was made in 84% of patients in the open group and only 73% in the laparoscopic group, probably based on tumor size. There was no significant difference in positive surgical margin rate or in very early 3-year cancer-specific outcome. Cancer was less likely to be detected with the laparoscopic surgery, and postoperative urological complications, hemorrhage in particular, and the need for a subsequent procedure were respectively two, three, and four times more likely to occur with laparoscopic surgery.

Both of these approaches are successful and effective. For a T1 tumor, the laparoscopic approach can yield functional and short-term oncologic outcomes that appear equivalent to the open technique associated with longer ischemia time and more postoperative complications. The open approach remains the standard for more complex tumors.

Patients with a single small peripheral tumor, particularly older individuals with comorbid disease, may be less than ideal candidates for an open or laparoscopic partial nephrectomy. Patients who have undergone a previous renal operation or have developed a local recurrence after a partial nephrectomy are high-risk surgical candidates, as are individuals with severe azotemia, where any form of major intervention on the kidney may result in a need for dialysis. Ablation may be a safer approach, but the overall utility of these approaches remains to be fully defined.

Control of tumor margins during ablation procedures is at times uncertain. An example is the use of radiofrequency ablation, during which the extent of tumor destruction is difficult to quantitate, in contrast to partial nephrectomy. In this latter case, tissue margins, stage, and grade can be determined. Studies with these forms of ablation currently utilized indirect techniques such as imaging to infer a successful outcome.

A small group of 60 patients with small tumors have been treated with laparoscopic renal cryoablation, and have been followed for 5 years or more at the Cleveland Clinic. Their median follow-up is 6 years. So far the recurrence rate has been relatively low and the cancer specific-survival rate is acceptable. With cryoablation we have a technique for monitoring intraoperative tumor destruction. This has been studied in preclinical models before we applied it to patients, and it involves the use of intraoperative ultrasound, and distinguishes cryoablation from other techniques.

When considering minimally invasive nephron-sparing surgery, two options are available: laparoscopic partial nephrectomy and tumor ablation. The morbidity with laparoscopic partial nephrectomy is somewhat higher. Renal function is equally well preserved with both, but the greater amount of oncologic information that we obtain and the greater oncologic efficacy with laparoscopic partial nephrectomy today is a major advantage over ablative approaches. When nephron-sparing therapy for renal cancer is considered, open partial nephrectomy is the gold standard based on the established long-term efficacy. Laparoscopic partial nephrectomy in the hands of skilled surgeons is applicable for selected patients, but there remain significant technical limitations; tumor ablation approaches still need to be considered investigational pending longer term outcome data.

SYSTEMIC THERAPY: METASTATIC DISEASE

Immunotherapy consisting of IL-2 and interferon-α (IFN-α) has been the standard approach for systemic treatment of metastatic renal cell carcinoma, in addition to clinical trials investigating new agents. Responses were best with high-dose intravenous IL-2 (21%) compared to low-dose intravenous IL-2 (11%) and subcutaneous IL-2 (10%), although no survival advantage was observed.[14] Similar response rates were reported comparing high-dose IL-2 (23.2%) versus subcutaneous IL-2 plus IFN-α (9.9%) and no survival advantage.[15] The high-dose IL-2 regimens have been associated with complete durable remissions in 5% to 7% of treated subjects.[14,15]

Interferon-α has been established as the standard comparative treatment arm for phase 3 clinical trials of new agents for the treatment of metastatic renal cancer. Several randomized trials have demonstrated improvement in medial survival for treated patients,[16] and in a retrospective review a median overall survival (OS) of 13.1 months and a median time to progression (TTP) of 4.7 months for IFN-α patients was noted.[17]

Retrospective analysis of untreated and previously treated patients with metastatic renal cancer has identified clinical characteristics that can be used to categorize patients into groups with differences in prognosis. For previously untreated patients, an initial prognostic model was developed, which has been validated and expanded. Five clinical characteristics were identified and validated at the Cleveland Clinic.[17,18] These prognostic criteria have been utilized in phase 3 clinical trials of sorafenib, sunitinib, temsirolimus (CCI-779), and bevacizumab.

The cloning of the VHL tumor suppressor gene and the elucidation of its role in upregulating growth factors associated with angiogenesis are recent discoveries that have provided insights into RCC biology, as well as defining a series of potential targets for novel therapeutic approaches. Renal cell carcinoma is a highly vascularized tumor; therefore, controlling its vascularity by targeting angiogenic factors could theoretically control its growth and survival. Several isoforms of VEGF and its receptors (VEGFR) have been identified; VEGF-A, VEGFR-1, and VEGFR-2 were found to be overexpressed in RCC compared to normal renal tissue, and VEGFR-2 is believed to be the major receptor mediating the angiogenic effects of VEGF.[19] When VEGF binds to the extracellular domain of its receptor, it induces tyrosine autophosphorylation and downstream effects that include tumor-associated angiogenesis, endothelial cell proliferation, migration, and survival. During the past 5 years a number of agents inhibiting the VEGF pathway have been investigated in advanced RCC patients, and a series of these have clearly demonstrable clinical benefits such as significant increases in progression free survival (PFS) and overall survival.

Both sorafenib and sunitinib were first studied and shown to have activity in cytokine refractory patients as second-line therapy. The Food and Drug Administration (FDA) label for both describes efficacy for the treatment of "advanced kidney cancer." Given the lack of efficacy and the toxicity associated with interleukin-2 and interferons, sorafenib and sunitinib will be widely used as initial therapy. Randomized trials with these agents have compared their efficacy to first-line cytokine therapy. A randomized phase 3 trial of sunitinib compared to IFN-α accrued 750 patients, and demonstrated improvement in progression-free survival (primary end point) and preliminarily, in overall survival.[20] Efficacy and safety data for sorafenib in treatment-naive patients have been assessed in a randomized phase 2 trial, which accrued 190 patients.[21] The data from this study have not been analyzed as yet. A phase 3 trial comparing CCI-779 with or without IFN-α to IFN-α in poor-risk patients demonstrated a survival advantage for patients receiving monotherapy.[22] In the absence of randomized studies directly comparing these agents in similar patient populations, treatment recommendations are problematic. Finally, several phase 2 randomized trials suggest bevacizumab has significant activity in metastatic RCC,[23,24] and a preliminary report of a phase 3 trial comparing IFN-α with or without bevacizumab suggests a significant increase in PFS[25] associated with administration of this VEGF inhibitor.

Based on the efficacy (overall response rate, PFS, and survival) observed in the randomized phase 3 trial, sunitinib is an accepted standard for therapy and can be offered to patients as initial therapy. An acceptable alternative is sorafenib, but the supporting data are in cytokine refractory patients, with only limited data available in untreated patients. Studies with CCI-779 were performed in poor-risk patients. Data in good- and intermediate-risk patients should be obtained to permit preliminary comparisons with the other targeted agents. It is likely results seen in various subgroups will mirror those currently available; however, current recommendations rely on available data. The data with bevacizumab remain very preliminary, but clearly will add another active agent to the list of those available to treat this disease. As with all new treatment options, multiple questions remain to be answered. These include duration of therapy, the importance of stable disease and percent tumor reduction, the issue of sequential therapy, and the use of combination therapy.

Finally, several trials are now in progress to assess the role of targeted therapy in the adjuvant setting. One randomized phase 3 adjuvant trial compared sorafenib to a placebo, and a second National Cancer Institute (NCI)-sponsored phase 3 trial compared sorafenib and sunitinib to a placebo. Data from both trials will not be available for 5 to 10 years. Unless the results of one or both of these trials demonstrates a benefit in relapse-free or overall survival, the standard of care remains observation alone following nephrectomy for localized RCC.

CONCLUSION

The treatment paradigm for patients with localized and advanced renal cell carcinoma has changed dramatically in the last 5 to 10 years. Surgical advances are now mirrored by the dramatic changes in therapy available for metastatic disease. The chapters in this text provide an update for urologists, medical oncologists, and researchers interested in this tumor.

REFERENCES

1. American Cancer Society. Cancer Facts and Figures 2006. Atlanta, GA: American Cancer Society, 2006.
2. Hock LM, Lynch J, Balaji KC. Increasing incidence of all stages of kidney cancer in the last 2 decades in the United States: of Surveillance, Epidemiology and End Results program data. J Urol 2002;167:57–60.
3. Cohen HT, McGovern FJ. Renal-cell carcinoma. N Engl J Med 2005;353:2477–2490.
4. Russo P. Renal cell carcinoma: presentation, staging, and surgical treatment. Semin Oncol 2000;27:160–176.
5. Kovacs G, Akhtar M, Beckwith BJ, et al. The Heidelberg classification of renal cell tumours. J Pathol 1997;183:131–133.
6. Kim WY, Kaelin WG. The Role of VHL gene mutation in Human Cancer. J Clin Oncol 2004;22:4991–5004.
7. Novick AC. Nephron-sparing surgery for renal cell carcinoma. Annu Rev Med 2002;53:393–407.
8. Linehan WM, Vasselli J, Srinivasan R, et al. Genetic basis of cancer of the kidney: disease-specific approaches to therapy. Clin Can Res 2004;10:6282s–6289s.
9. Gill IS. Minimally invasive nephron-sparing surgery. Urol Clin North Am 2003;30:551–579.
10. Flanigan RC, Mickisch G, Sylvester R, et al. Cytoreductive nephrectomy in patients with metastatic renal cancer: a combined analysis. J Urol 2004;171:1071–1076.
11. Permpongkosol S, Chan DY, Link RE, Sroka M, Allaf M, Varkarakis I, Lima G, Jarrett TW, Kavoussi LR. Long-term survival analysis after laparoscopic radical nephrectomy. J Urol 2005;174:1222–1225.
12. Hollenbeck BK, Taub DA, Miller DC, Dunn RL, Wei JT. National utilization trends of partial nephrectomy for renal cell carcinoma: a case of underutilization. Urology 2006;67:254–259.
13. Leibovich BC, Blute ML, Cheville, Lohse CM, Weaver AL, Zincke H. Nephron sparing surgery for appropriately selected renal cell carcinoma between 4 and 7 cm results in outcome similar to radical nephrectomy. J Urol 2004;171:1066–1070.
14. Yang JC, Sherry RM, Steinberg SM, et al. Randomized study of high-dose and low-dose interleukin-2 in patients with metastatic renal cancer. J Clin Oncol 2003;21:3127–3132.

15. McDermott DF, Regan MM, Clark JI, et al. Randomized phase III trial of high-dose interleukin-2 versus subcutaneous interleukin-2 and interferon in patients with metastatic renal cell carcinoma. J Clin Oncol 2005;23:133–141.
16. Medical Research Council and Collaborators. Interferon alfa and survival in metastatic renal carcinoma: early results of a randomized controlled trial. Lancet 1999;353:14–17.
17. Motzer RJ, Bacik J, Murphy BA, et al. Interferon-alfa as a comparative treatment for clinical trials of new therapies against advanced renal cell carcinoma. J Clin Oncol 2002;20:289–296.
18. Mekhail TM, Abou-Jawde RM, BouMerhi G, et al. Validation and extension of the Memorial Sloan-Kettering prognostic factors model for survival in patients with previously untreated metastatic renal cell carcinoma. J Clin Oncol 2005;23:832–841.
19. Ferrara N, Gerber HP, LeCouter J. The biology of VEGF and its receptors. Nat Med 2003;9(6): 669–676.
20. Motzer RJ, Hutson TE, Tomczak P, et al. Phase III randomized trial of sunitinib malate (SU 11248) versus interferon-alfa (IFN-a) as first-line systemic therapy for patients with metastatic renal cell carcinoma (mRCC). J Clin Oncol 2006;24(18S, pt II):930s.
21. Escudier B, Szczylik C, Demkow T, et al. Randomized phase II trial of the multi-kinase inhibitor sorafenib versus interferon (IFN) in treatment-naïve patients with metastatic renal cell carcinoma (mRCC). J Clin Oncol 2006;24 (18S pt I):217s.
22. Hudes GR, Carducci M, Tomczak P, et al., A phase III, randomized, 3–arm study of temsirolimus (TEMSR) or interferon-alpha (IFN) or the combination of TEMSR + IFN in the treatment of first-line, poor-risk patients with advanced renal cell carcinoma (adv RCC). J Clin Oncol 2006;24(18S pt II):930s.
23. Yang JC, Haworth L, Sherry RM, et al. A randomized trial of bevacizumab, an anti-vascular endothelial growth factor antibody, for metastatic renal cancer. N Engl J Med 2003;349(5):427–434.
24. Bukowski R, Kabbinavar F, Figlin RA, et al. Bevacizumab with or without erlotinib in metastatic renal cell carcinoma (RCC). J Clin Oncol 2006;24(18S pt I):222s.
25. Genentech Press Release. www.gene.com.

2
Imaging of Renal Cell Carcinoma

Brian R. Herts

KEYWORDS

COMPUTED TOMOGRAPHY
MAGNETIC RESONANCE
ULTRASOUND
SURGICAL PLANNING
RENAL CELL CARCINOMA

ABSTRACT

Imaging of renal neoplasms is performed with computed tomography, magnetic resonance, and ultrasound to detect disease, characterize lesions, stage primary renal neoplasms, and provide surgical planning information. Imaging is also used to distinguish between benign and malignant disease and between surgical and nonsurgical disease. Computed tomography (CT) and magnetic resonance (MR) exams of renal cell carcinoma should be designed to maximize identification of prognostic factors as well as staging features: size, extension outside the renal capsule and fascia, lymphadenopathy, renal vein invasion, and metastatic disease.

INTRODUCTION

Renal cell carcinoma (RCC) accounts for approximately 3% of new cancer diagnoses and 3% of deaths from cancer annually.[1] Nearly 36,000 new cases are diagnosed each year. Fortunately, with the common use of cross-sectional imaging, there has been a significant shift in the type of RCCs being identified; more tumors are asymptomatic and these asymptomatic tumors are more frequently lower stage and lower grade tumors with a better prognosis.[2–5] Goals for the imaging of renal neoplasms are to detect disease, to characterize lesions, to stage primary renal neoplasms, and to provide surgical planning information. Imaging is also performed to distinguish between benign and malignant disease and between surgical and nonsurgical disease. Ideally, imaging would be able to distinguish between primary renal cell carcinoma and benign primary tumors of the kidneys, and between primary and secondary renal tumors, such as metastatic lung cancer and lymphoma.

The most important prognostic factors for RCC include histologic grade, cell type, patient age, performance status, number and location of metastases, and time to appear-

From: *Clinical Management of Renal Tumors*
Edited by: R.M. Bukowski and A.C. Novick © Humana Press Inc., Totowa, NJ

ance of metastases.[6–8] Imaging of RCC, therefore, should be designed to maximize identification of prognostic factors as well as staging features, including tumor size and tumor extension outside the renal capsule and outside Gerota's and Zuckerkandl's fascia. Imaging should also be designed to detect pathologically enlarged lymph nodes and renal vein invasion, as well as metastatic disease, either at the time of presentation or on follow-up imaging.[9]

Renal masses have a varied appearance on imaging with a complexity that has resulted in a large body of literature. With the rapid improvements in imaging over the last decade, much of the recent literature has redefined or reversed many of the initial concepts in the imaging of renal masses. This chapter addresses imaging of renal cell carcinoma as it relates to the detection of RCC and the characterization and differential diagnoses of renal masses. It also reviews the detection of factors relevant for treatment and prognosis, such as tumor size and staging, with an assessment of lymphadenopathy, renal vein tumor thrombus, adrenal gland involvement, and metastatic disease. Imaging features of the different cell types of primary RCC are also reviewed. While most RCC is sporadic, solid and cystic renal neoplasms are associated with several syndromes; these are covered elsewhere in this book and thus will not be addressed here.

THE VARIOUS APPEARANCES OF RENAL LESIONS AT IMAGING

Renal lesions can be solid, cystic, infiltrating, or vascular. Renal cell carcinoma can be solid, cystic, or infiltrating; however, many other types of renal pathology can have a similarly varied appearance. Lesion detection and characterization are dependent on the size and cell type of lesion, the blood supply, neovascularity, and the type(s) of tissue in the lesion. The diagnosis and management of renal lesions is highly dependent on the imaging features, due to the high prevalence of RCC in solid and complex cystic renal lesions.[10]

Solid Lesions

The typical appearance of RCC is a heterogeneous, enhancing solid mass following contrast[11] (Figure 2.1). While the majority of RCCs are solid, space-occupying mass lesions, some RCCs are infiltrating or complex cystic mass lesions. Clear cell, papillary, and chromophobe RCC subtypes are all solid on computed tomography (CT), ultrasound (US), and magnetic resonance (MR). Unfortunately, both benign (e.g., oncocytoma, angiomyolipoma) and malignant (e.g., some transitional cell carcinoma and metastatic disease) lesions are also solid, space-occupying lesions.

Cystic and Complex Cystic Renal Lesions

Renal cell carcinoma can have a cystic histologic growth pattern. Cystic RCC can be unilocular, multilocular, or necrotic, or RCC can develop within the wall of an otherwise benign cyst.[12] Renal epithelial cysts are common, and many individuals have these and other benign renal cysts. Benign cysts typically contain simple serous fluid, but they can also contain fluid with a high protein content, hemorrhage, or infection, making the differentiation between a simple cyst and cystic RCC difficult.[13,14] Different classification schemes have been proposed to help stratify the likelihood of malignancy of a cystic lesion; one such classification system that is used by both radiologists and urologists was originally described in 1986 by Bosniak and has since been modified. Bosniak[15–18] originally proposed four categories, with increasing likelihood of malignancy, and this has been modified more recently to include a fifth category.

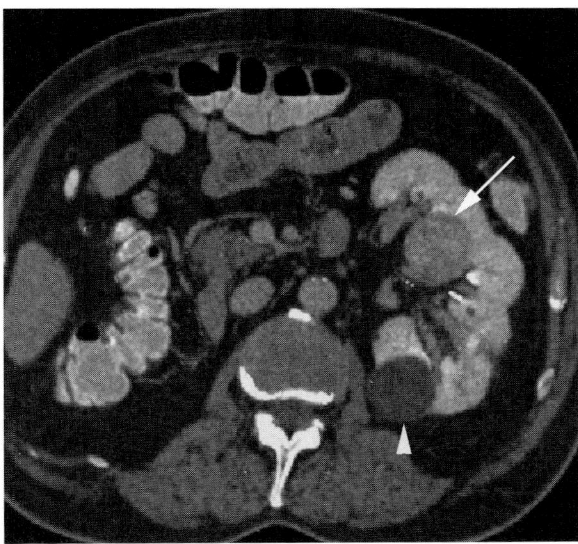

Figure 2.1. Solid renal mass (arrow) and simple renal cyst (arrowhead) in the same kidney. Most renal cell carcinomas are solid space-occupying lesions that demonstrate intermediate to high soft tissue density enhancing after intravenous (IV) contrast media.

Category I cysts are simple unilocular cysts, either round or oval, with a thin, non-calcified wall. These cysts contain simple serous fluid measuring less than 10 to 20 Hounsfield units (HU) at CT, and have MR signal characteristics of simple fluid (low signal on T1- and high signal on T2-weighted imaging sequences). There is no solid, soft tissue density in the lesion or enhancement after IV contrast.

Category II cysts are minimally complicated cysts either with high-density fluid due to a high protein content or hemorrhage within the cysts (higher than 20 HU density, a "hyperdense" cyst), or are multilocular with a few septations or thin peripheral calcifications. Category II cysts do not demonstrate enhancement after IV contrast and are almost always benign.[19,20] Contrast is needed to distinguish between a hyperdense cyst and a homogeneous solid renal neoplasm. Both lesions may look similar on pre- or postcontrast scans, but the hyperdense cyst will not enhance after contrast, where the homogeneous solid renal neoplasm will enhance. Category II cysts have a less than 15% change of malignancy in most studies using the Bosniak criteria and, therefore, are often followed to document stability over time.

Category IIF cysts are complex lesions with multiple septations or calcifications that have a more benign appearance. Calcifications, which were once felt to be a potential sign of malignancy, are now considered less important.[17]

Category III cysts are complicated cystic lesions that have some features suggesting malignancy—multiple septations, thick or irregular rim—or heterogeneity suggesting necrosis. Category III cysts have an approximately 50% to 60% chance of being a cystic RCC according to published studies.[19,21] Typically, these lesions are explored; although controversial, aspiration biopsy can also be performed to diagnose malignancy.

Category IV cysts contain solid, soft tissue enhancing elements seen either within the cyst or as part of a complex cystic mass. These lesions are almost always cystic RCC and should be treated as such (Figures 2.2 and 2.3).

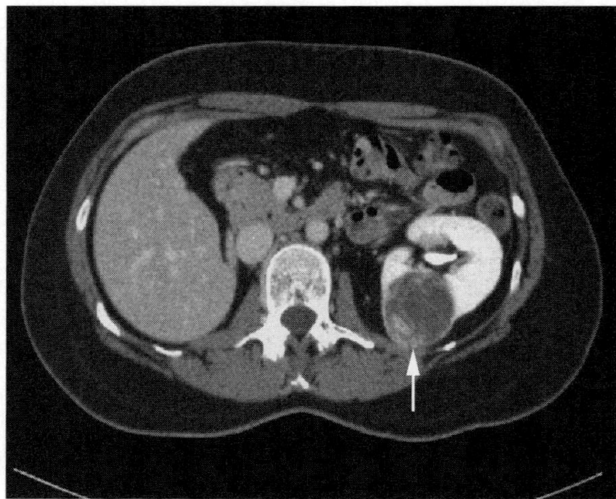

Figure 2.2. Cystic necrotic renal cell carcinoma on computed tomography (CT) (arrow). This renal cell carcinoma has a nonenhancing low attenuation component that was necrosis at pathology. The lack of enhancement in necrosis mimics a cystic lesion.

Management guidelines are based on this stratification, but of course every patient should be treated individually. In general, category I lesions do not need further evaluation; category II lesions, if larger than 3 cm or irregular, and category IIF lesions should be followed for interval growth or change, which suggest malignancy; category III lesions should be explored or resected; and category IV lesions should be appropriately treated as presumed RCC. Biopsy of indeterminate cystic renal masses can also be performed. It is important to note that the Bosniak criteria are guidelines for describing and managing cystic renal masses. Other factors, including risk factors for RCC, a

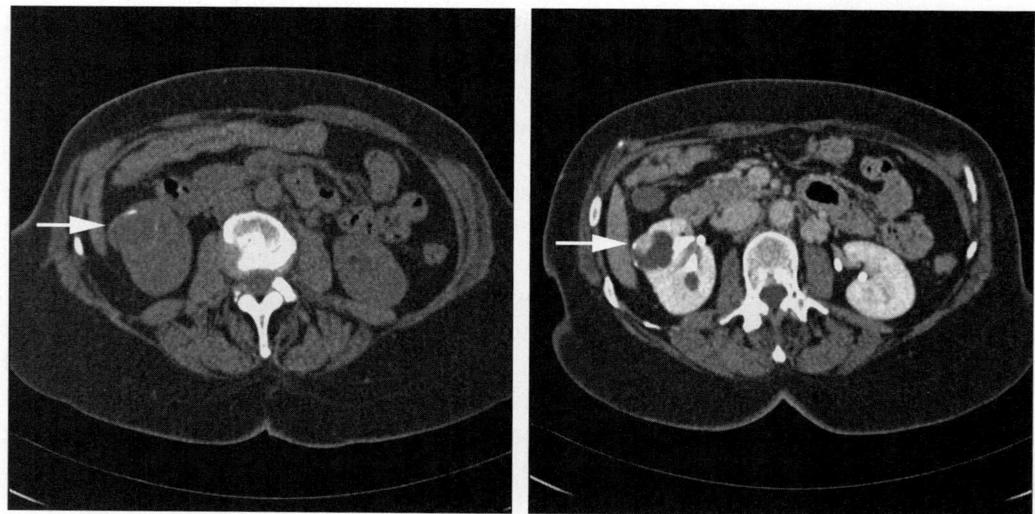

Figure 2.3. Complex cystic renal cell carcinoma (arrow) at unenhanced (A) and contrast-enhanced CT (B). This renal cell carcinoma has calcifications seen on the unenhanced image (A), and both a low attenuation cystic nonenhancing component and a higher attenuation enhancing soft tissue component. This lesion meets criteria for a Bosniak IV cyst (cystic renal cell carcinoma).

genetic disorder that predisposes the individual to cystic renal tumors, age, and comorbid conditions should influence any management decision.

Infiltrating Renal Lesions

While many renal tumors exhibit radial growth patterns with a space-occupying mass and some cystic growth patterns, RCC can infiltrate within the renal parenchyma along the interstitium[22] (Figure 2.4). In these instances, the renal contour is maintained but the involved portion of the kidney is typically enlarged. Infiltrating tumors encase rather than displace the vasculature and collecting system. On CT, infiltrating lesions are poorly marginated areas of relatively decreased enhancement reflecting the disruption of the normal tubular concentration of contrast. On ultrasound, these are often isoechoic, severely limiting sonographic detection. Only occasionally are infiltrating renal lesions slightly hypoechoic or hyperechoic in relation to the normal renal parenchyma.

Several other tumors demonstrate an infiltrating pattern at imaging.[22] Transitional cell carcinoma (TCC) of the kidney comprises 90% of urothelial tumors; squamous cell carcinoma comprises most of the rest. While typically a slow-growing papillary tumor, TCC of the kidney is occasionally high grade with an infiltrating appearance centrally located in the kidney or in the renal pelvic sinus.

Primary renal non-Hodgkin's lymphoma (NHL) can arise in the renal parenchyma or renal hilar lymph nodes. Extranodal lymphoma is more common with Hodgkin's than with non-Hodgkin's lymphoma. Perinephric confluent tissue is more suggestive of NHL than RCC. In general, however, renal involvement in lymphoma is associated with systemic disease. At CT and MR, renal lymphoma is typically hypovascular with multiple solid or infiltrating masses.[23]

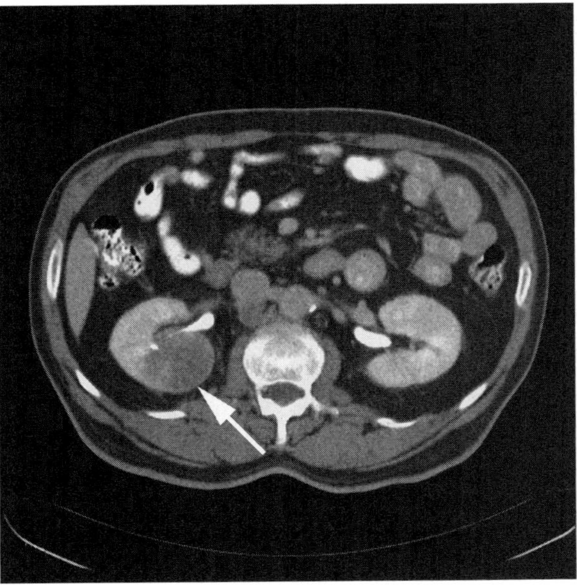

Figure 2.4. Infiltrating renal cell carcinoma (RCC) on CT. This renal cell carcinoma (arrow) enlarges the posterior segment of the kidney and is poorly marginated. Infiltrative RCCs are typically more aggressive than solid lesions. Less than 5% to 10% of renal cell carcinomas demonstrate an infiltrative growth pattern at CT.

Leukemia is always infiltrating, typically enlarging the kidneys.[24] Metastatic disease to the kidneys presents with multiple, bilateral, poorly marginated solid lesions that can occasionally demonstrate an infiltrative pattern.[25,26]

Some noncancerous conditions can demonstrate an infiltrating pattern at imaging, and it is vitally important to recognize these entities. Acute pyelonephritis demonstrates a striated nephrogram on CT early after contrast and a dense parenchyma staining on delayed CT due to clearance failure of concentrated contrast. This should be distinguishable from tumor infiltration, and a history of fever, flank pain, and pyuria should certainly suggest pyelonephritis. Chronic infection can result in xanthogranulomatous pyelonephritis (XGP). In XGP, below-water attenuation regions are due to lipid-laden macrophages associated with chronic inflammation and typically are seen in conjunction with a staghorn calculus.

Infiltrating tumors are often associated with a more aggressive behavior than solid or cystic tumors, and can be either an uncommon appearance of common tumors, such as primary renal cell adenocarcinoma, lymphoma, or metastatic disease, or a more common appearance of uncommon tumors, such as collecting duct or medullary RCC.

Vascular Lesions

Vascular lesions of the kidney include renal artery aneurysms (Figure 2.5), renal arteriovenous malformations (AVMs), and renal arteriovenous fistulas. The addition of a corticomedullary phase to renal imaging can help distinguish renal vascular lesions from solid renal masses. On contrast-enhanced CT and MR, renal artery aneurysms demonstrate only arterial blood flow similar to the renal artery. Renal AVMs appear

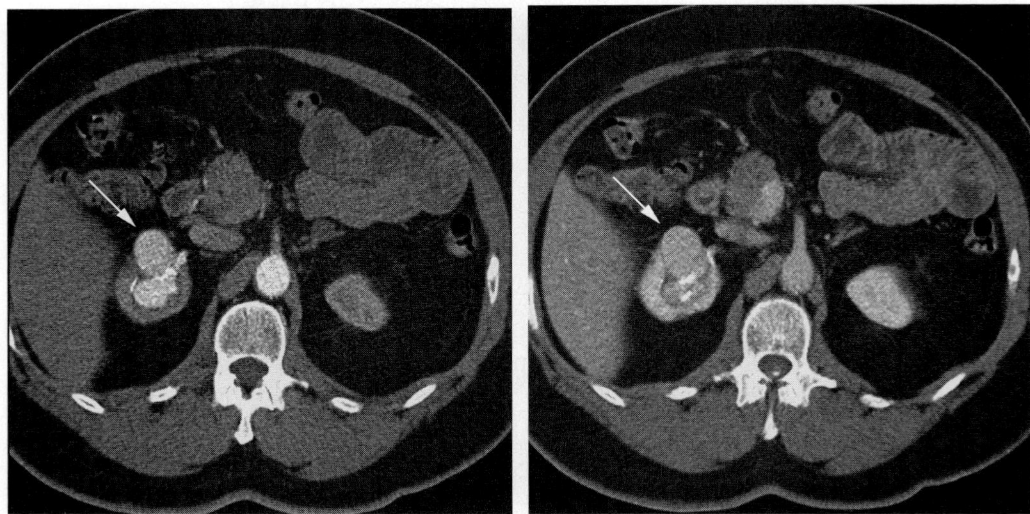

A   B

Figure 2.5. Renal artery aneurysm on corticomedullary phase (A) and nephrographic phase CT (B). The lesion is soft tissue density mimicking a renal tumor on the nephrographic phase (B, arrow), but markedly hyperdense similar to the aorta on the corticomedullary phase (A, arrow). Vascular renal lesions are typically homogeneous attenuation with density that follows the aorta or renal vein on both the corticomedullary and nephrographic phase scans. This enhancement pattern helps distinguish these lesions from renal cell carcinoma.

similar to renal tumors and not cysts because of enhancement after contrast media caused by contrast pooling in the bloodstream. These malformations have a cirsoid appearance[27] and are typically recognized because at CT they appear as homogeneous lesions with density similar to the vasculature, at ultrasound they demonstrate color flow or pulse Doppler signal, and at MR they exhibit flow enhancement or signal void.[27,28]

Renal AVMs are significantly less common than primary or secondary renal tumors. Patients with renal AVMs often present with gross or microscopic hematuria,[29] and AVMs have been mistaken for RCC. Renal arteriovenous fistulas are usually post-traumatic, often described after penetrating trauma and after biopsy in renal transplants.[30,31]

PRIMARY IMAGING METHODS FOR THE DETECTION OF RENAL CELL CARCINOMA

Detection of renal lesions on US is dependent on either a contour abnormality or a difference in echogenicity between the lesion and normal parenchyma. Detection of renal lesions on CT and MR is possible because of a difference in density or signal intensity from the normal renal parenchyma. This occurs not only because the kidneys filter contrast, but also because contrast is concentrated within the collecting tubules as water is reabsorbed. Normal renal parenchyma becomes denser at CT and has higher signal on T1-weighted MR as contrast is concentrated. The degree of contrast concentration is dependent on the normal function of nephrons. The degree of contrast excretion and concentration is also dependent on the volume and concentration of contrast given.[32] Neither cysts nor renal tumors concentrate contrast. Therefore, the kidneys should be imaged at peak concentration of contrast with the highest contrast load to maximize detection of renal lesions. Unfortunately, for patients with impaired renal function the risk of contrast-induced nephropathy is increased while detection and characterization of renal masses are decreased.

ULTRASOUND

Ultrasound, CT, and MR can all be used to image renal lesions, and each has different advantages and disadvantages. Ultrasound is ideal for distinguishing between cystic and solid renal masses.[33] Ultrasound is not considered the best test for the detection and characterization of renal tumors because small renal tumors are often isoechoic and because detection of fat within a lesion to identify angiomyolipoma (AML) is less sensitive with US than with other cross-sectional imaging. However, renal tumors that are large, contour-deforming, or partially cystic can be detected sonographically (Figures 2.6 and 2.7). On ultrasound, RCC can be hypoechoic, isoechoic, or hyperechoic. Calcifications in renal lesions can obscure tumors because of acoustic shadowing. Advantages of renal ultrasound include the noninvasive nature of the exam without use of contrast agents or radiation. Lack of contrast eliminates the potential nephrotoxicity of iodinated agents.

Ultrasound is performed with a 3- to 6-MHz transducer, and images are obtained through each kidney in both the axial and longitudinal planes. Tissue harmonic imaging can be used to increase the sensitivity of US for renal masses. Cysts appear as round or oval, and anechoic structures appear with a thin or imperceptible wall. Solid and

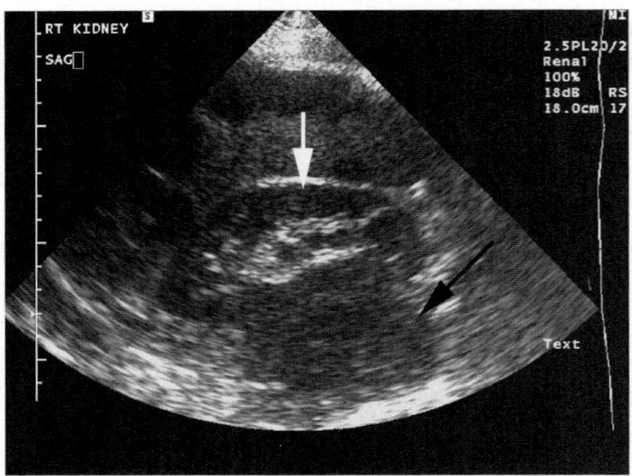

Figure 2.6. Renal cell carcinoma (RCC) on ultrasound. This large RCC (black arrow) is relatively easy to detect by ultrasound because it deforms the contour of the kidney. It is also mildly hyperechoic to the normal renal parenchyma (white arrow). Renal cell carcinoma can be hypo-, iso-, or hyperechoic at ultrasound.

complex cystic masses either deform the renal contour or are distinguished from the normal renal parenchyma by a difference in echogenicity. The sensitivity of US for the detection of RCC is dependent on the size of the lesion. Ultrasound is insensitive for small tumors. Ultrasound has also been used to screen for RCC in a select patient population, although ultrasound is not a recommended screening exam in the United States.[34,35]

Kitamura et al.[36] compared color flow Doppler (CFD) US to contrast-enhanced CT for the detection of renal tumors. In that study, 91% of clear cell carcinomas seen at CT were identifiable as hypervascular lesions on CFD US. However, there was no additional benefit gained by using CFD US. The sensitivity of US for the detection of renal tumors may improve with IV contrast agents for US, in one study increasing sen-

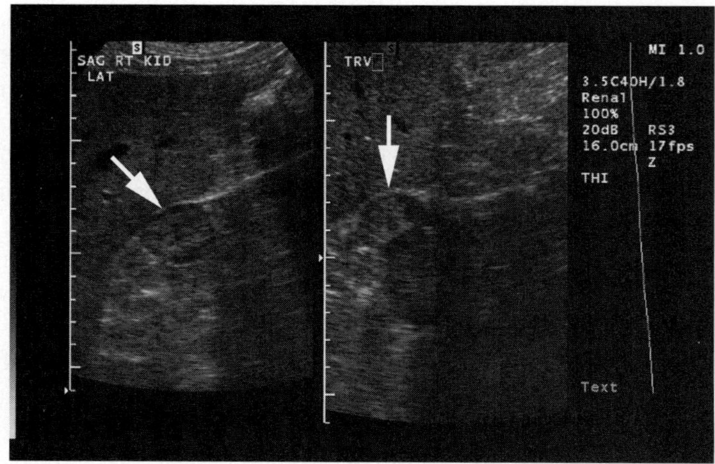

Figure 2.7. Small renal cell carcinoma on ultrasound. This lesion (arrows) is only 2 cm in diameter but was detected because of the increased echogenicity.

sitivity to 97% compared with 70% for gray scale US.[37] Ultrasound contrast agents are available for use with Doppler US systems but are not in general usage. The administration of contrast eliminates the main advantage of ultrasound by making it minimally invasive instead of noninvasive.

COMPUTED TOMOGRAPHY

Computed tomography is the gold standard for the detection and characterization of renal masses. The sensitivity of CT for the detection of RCC is 88% to 100%. Any CT of the kidneys must include pre- and postcontrast imaging for both the increased detection of renal masses and the characterization of renal lesions. The optimal time to image the kidney is during peak concentration: 90 to 150 seconds after the initiation of a bolus of 100 to 150 mL of contrast. This is termed the nephrographic or parenchymal phase. Solid renal tumors contain a blood supply and, thus, enhance after contrast. The more vascular renal tumors are clear cell RCC, AVM, AML, and oncocytoma.

After a standard dose of intravenous (IV) contrast, most RCCs, the majority of which are clear cell carcinomas, enhance more than 120 HU on CT[38]; some tumors, such as papillary and chromophobe carcinomas, are much less vascular.[39] Because of image noise and correction factors used for reconstructing CT images, an increase in 10 HU density between unenhanced CT and nephrographic phase (NP) CT is typically considered evidence for enhancement; such a lesion is then considered solid with a blood supply. One caveat is that with the detection of smaller lesions there is more variability in the HU density due to partial-volume averaging; an apparent increase in density of 15 HU has been reported for small intrarenal cysts. This is termed pseudoenhancement and is discussed briefly below.

Multiphase Scanning

A three-phase CT scan is considered the optimal technique for detecting and characterizing renal masses, as well as staging RCC. This includes an unenhanced scan, a vascular or corticomedullary phase (CMP) scan, and a tubular or NP scan (Figure 2.8). Several studies have shown that the NP is the most sensitive for the detection of renal tumors, although in one study more lesions are seen when a combination of unenhanced, CMP, and NP scans is used.[40–45]

The CMP is useful for assessing the renal vasculature.[40,41,46] The enhancement seen on the CMP can also be useful for characterizing lesions and, in one case report an RCC that was seen only on the CMP.[38] However, when used alone, the CMP can result in missed lesions and a false-positive diagnosis of medullary lesions.[45,47]

Delayed Computed Tomography

With the widespread use of cross-sectional imaging, many renal masses are found on CT and MR scans performed only with IV contrast. When renal lesions are small and homogeneous, any lesion seen on a postcontrast exam could be a renal neoplasm or a hyperdense (hemorrhagic or proteinaceous) cyst. As such, these patients are typically brought back to the department for a dedicated three-phase renal CT, adding time, cost, and inconvenience for the patient. Therefore, when it is feasible, some authors recommend performing a delayed CT scan to determine if a lesion decreases in

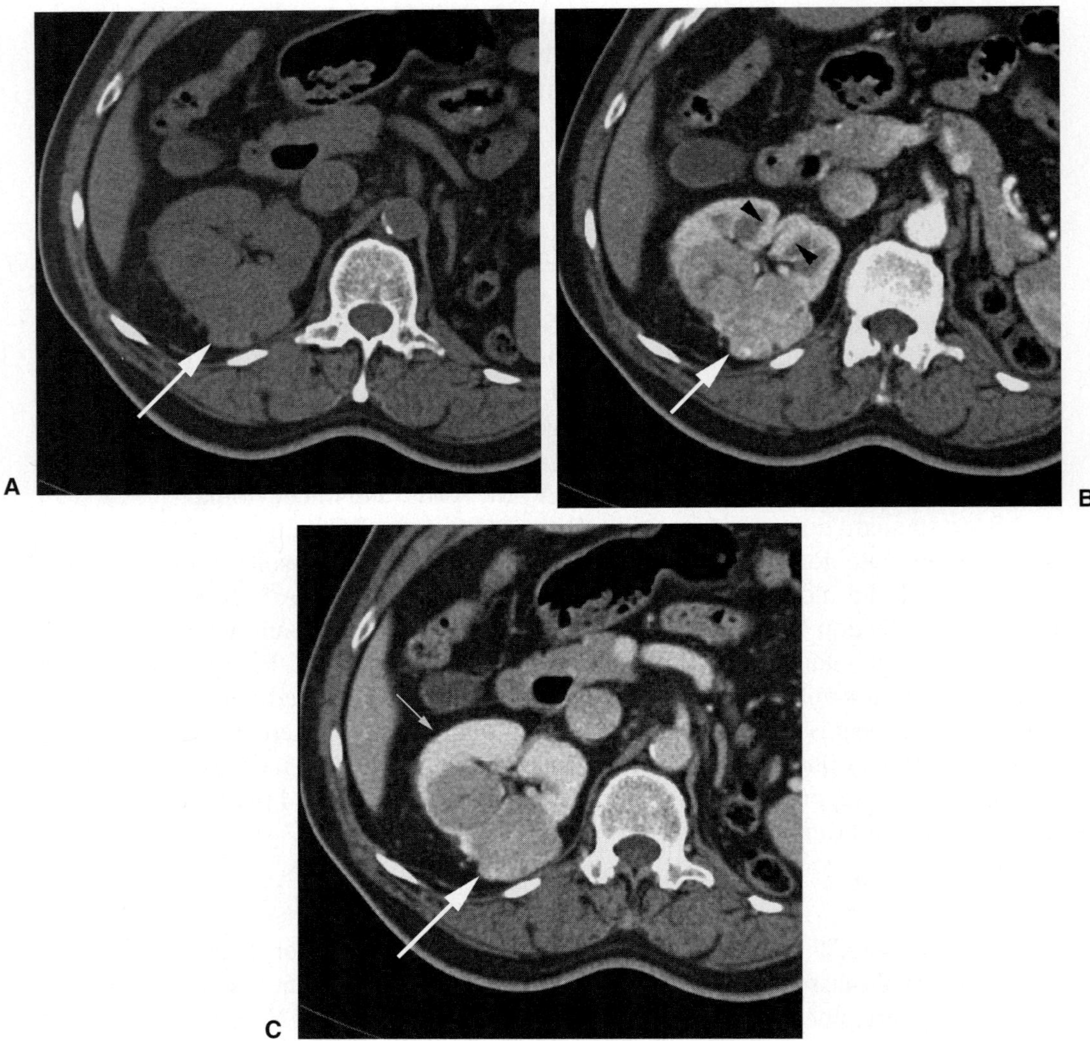

Figure 2.8. Three-phase renal CT scan of renal cell carcinoma (white arrow). (A) Unenhanced scan phase: the unenhanced normal renal parenchyma is approximately 30 to 35 Hounsfield units (HU). (B) Corticomedullary phase: this scan phase occurs at approximately 30 to 35 seconds after the bolus of IV contrast media. During the corticomedullary phase, the cortex is brightly enhanced due to the high vascularity, and the renal medulla is only mildly enhanced, resulting in sharp corticomedullary differentiation (black arrowheads). (C) Nephrographic phase. During this phase, contrast concentrated by the nephrons accounts for the renal parenchyma density, and the renal parenchyma (thin arrow) enhances homogeneously.

attenuation with time; a decrease in 10 HU after an approximately 15-minute delay is highly accurate for identifying solid renal tumors.[48,49]

Pseudoenhancement

The improved spatial resolution of CT allows the detection of many lesions less than 1 cm that are difficult to characterize accurately due to volume averaging. In one study, more than 95% of cysts demonstrated a change in attenuation value less than 10 HU,

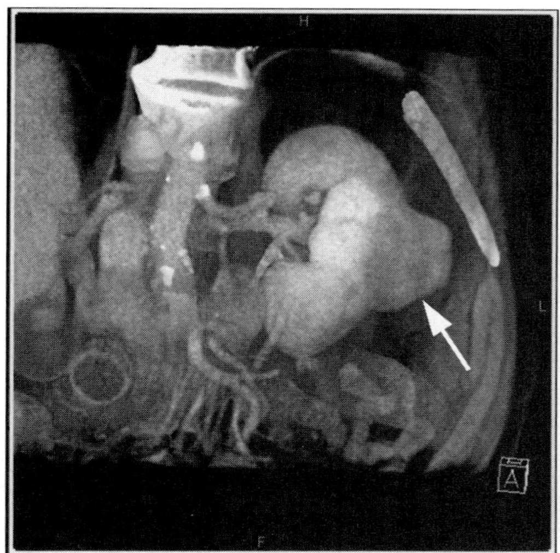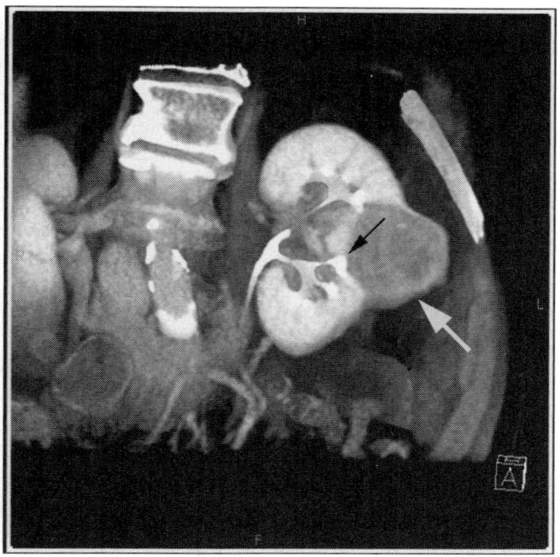

Figure 2.9. Three-dimensional volume rendered imaging for surgical planning. Imaging can now provide surgical planning information in addition to lesion characterization and staging. The tumor (arrow) position is seen both in relationship to the entire kidney (A) and in relationship to the collection system (B, black arrow) by using a cutting plane to "dissect" into the kidney (B).

and most less than 8 HU.[50] However, some true cysts, because of small size and technical factors related to volume averaging and reconstruction algorithms for helical CT, can have a measurable increase of more than 10 HU after contrast. This technical phenomenon is termed "pseudoenhancement." One needs to take the lesion size and location into consideration when using change in attenuation value to characterize renal lesions.[51,52]

Surgical Planning

With the introduction of multidetector high-speed CT scanners, high-resolution MR imaging, and three-dimensional (3D) postprocessing imaging software, surgical planning can now be performed using CT and MR.[53–58] These 3D images provide a detailed depiction of the renal vasculature, including accessory and branch vessels, the renal tumor position and depth of extension, the collecting system, adrenal gland, and lymphadenopathy (Figure 2.9). Surgical planning for renal cancer with CT and MR imaging is growing rapidly; however, full discussion of the techniques and utility of 3D rendering is beyond the scope of this chapter.

MAGNETIC RESONANCE IMAGING

Magnetic resonance can also be used to characterize and stage RCC and is the test of choice in patients with contrast allergies. At clinical doses, gadolinium-based MR contrast agents do not appear to have any direct nephrotoxic effects.[59] However, there is evolving data regarding a link between gadolinium contrast agents and nephrogenic systemic sclerosis in patients with severe chronic kidney disease; therefore contrast-enhanced MR should be used with caution in these patients. Magnetic resonance is also used to attempt characterization of indeterminate lesions at CT; MR is more contrast-sensitive than CT.

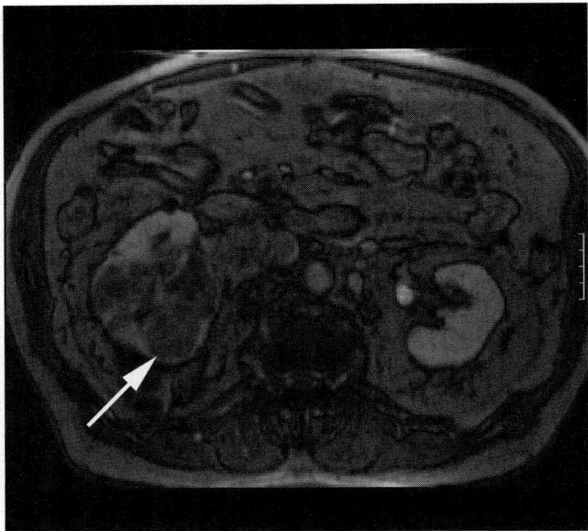

Figure 2.10. Magnetic resonance of renal cell carcinoma. Renal cell carcinoma (arrow) is typically low signal on fat-saturated T1-weighted images relative to the normal renal parenchyma following IV gadolinium.

Similar to CT, MR imaging must be performed before and after contrast. T1-weighted imaging (T1WI), usually with a fat-saturation breath-hold sequence, is performed before contrast and after contrast during several phases, both axial and coronal planes.[60,61] Before contrast, T2-weighted imaging (T2WI) is performed to characterize cysts, and in- and out-of-phase imaging and imaging with and without fat-saturation is performed to assess for fat within the lesion. Magnetic resonance is highly sensitive for renal tumors, approaching 100%, and has some advantages over CT for the characterization of subcentimeter cysts. A major drawback of MR is the limitation in determining enhancement criteria following contrast. Signal intensity in MR is based on a relative scale, not on absolute density, as is the Hounsfield unit scale.[62] Therefore, most authors recommend a subtraction between pre- and postcontrast MR exams to eliminate the subjectivity of determining enhancement after contrast on MR (Figure 2.10). A threshold of 15% increase in signal intensity has also been advocated to identify enhancement in renal tumors.[63,64] Magnetic resonance identification of calcium in renal lesions is limited because calcium appears as a signal void.

The sensitivity for the detection of RCC is reported to be as high as 88% to 100% for CT and 78% to 100% for MR.[65–68] In direct comparison studies, the sensitivity for detecting renal tumors is similar between MR and CT, and both are more sensitive than ultrasound.[65,66]

IMAGING APPEARANCES OF THE DIFFERENT TYPES OF PRIMARY RENAL NEOPLASMS

Primary Renal Cell Carcinoma

CLEAR CELL RENAL CELL CARCINOMA: 70% TO 80%

Renal cell neoplasms can be classified as clear cell, granular cell, sarcomatoid adeno-carcinoma, chromophobe, papillary, collecting duct, medullary, mixed cell types, or

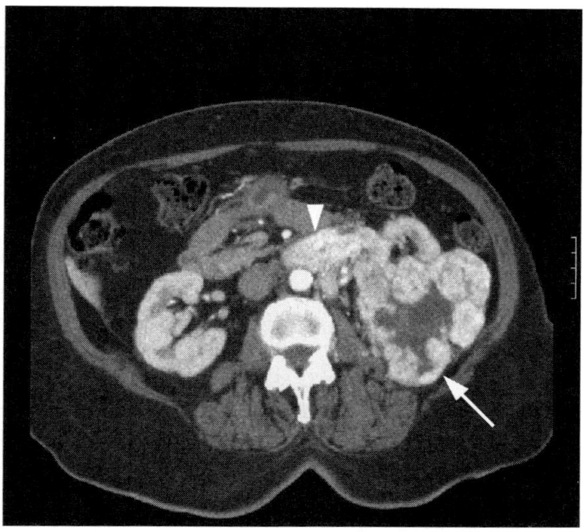

Figure 2.11. Clear-cell renal cell carcinoma (CCRCC) on CT. Clear-cell RCC is typically hypervascular with heterogeneous peripheral enhancement (arrow) on contrast-enhanced CT. Clear-cell RCC usually enhances more than 120 HU after iodinated IV contrast media. This is in stark contrast to hypovascular lesions such as papillary renal cell carcinoma (see Figure 2.13). Renal vein tumor thrombus is also seen (arrowhead).

adenocarcinoma not specified; or as oncocytoma, small cell carcinoma, juxtaglomerular tumor, or carcinoid.[69–71]

Since there are differences in prognosis between the different cell types of RCC, it is worth reviewing the more common descriptions of each cell type at imaging. Clear cell carcinoma, the most common cell type, accounts for 70% to 80% of all RCC. Clear cell carcinomas are typically hypervascular on CT, with enhancement more avid than that displayed by other subtypes.[38,72,73] A hypervascular pattern is present in nearly 50% of clear cell carcinomas, compared to approximately 15% of papillary and 4% of chromophobe subtypes. On MR, clear-cell renal cell carcinoma (CCRCC) is typically isointense on T1WI and isointense to hyperintense on T2WI.[74] Clear cell carcinomas are commonly more aggressive tumors than other cell types, and they directly involve and invade the renal collecting system.[75] Clear cell carcinoma also has heterogeneous peripheral enhancement more frequently than papillary and chromophobe RCC[72] (Figures 2.11 and 2.12).

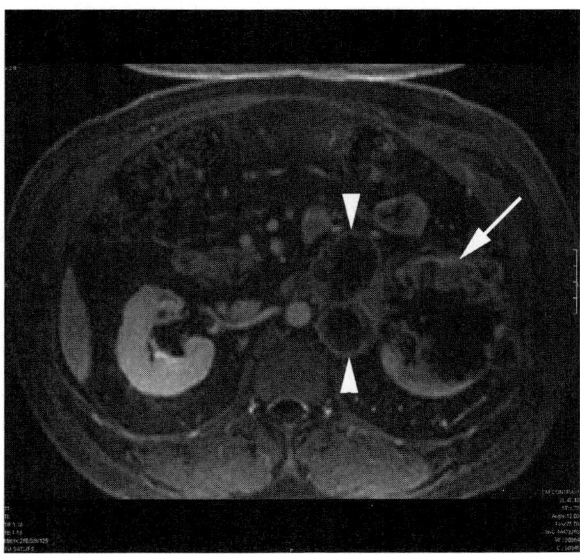

Figure 2.12. Clear-cell renal cell carcinoma (CCRCC) on magnetic resonance (MR). As with CT (Figure 2.11), on MR clear-cell RCC typically has heterogeneous enhancement along the periphery (arrow). Retroperitoneal adenopathy is present (arrowheads).

The degree of enhancement is significantly different among the clear cell, papillary, and chromophobe subtypes in the corticomedullary and excretory phases.[73] Cystic degeneration is also more common in the clear cell subtype than in the other subtypes regardless of tumor size. The chromophobe subtype shows homogeneous enhancement in 75% of cases in comparison to 45% and 65% of clear cell and papillary subtypes. Calcification occurs equally, in 21% to 25% of clear cell, papillary, and chromophobe subtypes.

Overall, enhancement is the most valuable parameter used to differentiate the subtypes of RCC. The degree of, or presence or absence of, cystic degeneration, vascularity, and enhancement patterns can serve a supplemental role in differentiating RCC subtypes.

PAPILLARY RENAL CELL CARCINOMA: 10% TO 15%

Papillary renal cell carcinoma (PRCC) accounts for 10% to 15% of RCCs.[76,77] It typically has a lower stage and better prognosis than CCRCC. Papillary RCC can be bilateral and multiple.[78] On CT, PRCC is typically a hypovascular solid mass[39,79] (Figure 2.13). Relative enhancement less than 25% of the normal parenchyma of the CMP and NP significantly increases the likelihood of a tumor being a papillary subtype. Conversely, tumors that enhance more than 25% of the enhancement of the normal renal parenchyma are rarely PRCC.[39] Papillary RCC rarely invades the collecting system.[75] On MR, PRCC can be hemorrhagic, leading to heterogeneous signal intensity on T1WI and decreased signal intensity on T2WI.[74] There are no reports of specific sonographic features of PRCC. There are histologic descriptions of two different types of PRCC: those with small basophilic cells (PRCC1) and those with eosinophilic cells (PRCC2).[80] These carry different prognoses, with overall survival being worse for the PRCC2 type. There are no reports of imaging describing either of the subtypes of PRCC.

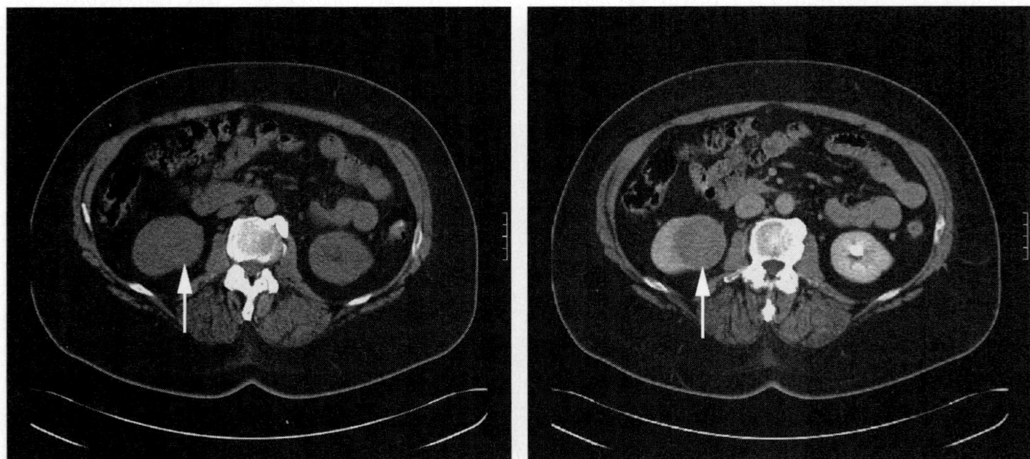

A   B

Figure 2.13. Papillary renal cell carcinoma (PRCC). Papillary RCC (arrow) can be isodense to slightly hyperdense to normal renal parenchyma on unenhanced CT (A), and homogeneously hypodense to kidney on the nephrographic phase after contrast (B). Papillary RCC is typically hypovascular, in distinction to typically hypervascular lesions such as clear cell renal cell carcinoma (Figure 2.11).

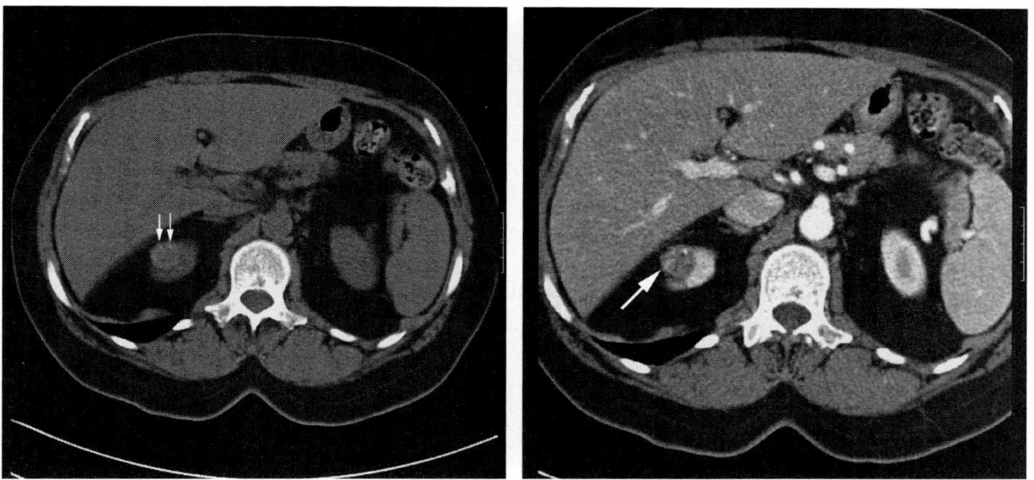

Figure 2.14. Chromophobe renal cell carcinoma (RCC). This chromophobe RCC is slightly hyperdense to normal renal parenchyma on unenhanced CT (A) and contains small flecks of calcium (small arrows). After contrast (B), the lesion (arrow) is hypodense and hypovascular, similar to papillary RCC.

CHROMOPHOBE RENAL CELL CARCINOMA: 5%

The chromophobe subtype accounts for only a small percentage of RCC.[81] Chromophobe RCC is typically hypovascular at CT, similar to PRCC[72] (Figure 2.14). In one study of 11 patients with the chromophobe cell type, there was a spoke-like enhancement pattern with a central stellate form.[82] This can be seen with chromophobe RCC and oncocytoma and thus is not specific for either tumor.

COLLECTING/BELLINI DUCT CARCINOMA: 1% TO 2%

Collecting duct carcinomas are uncommon, occurring as 1% to 2% of all RCC. These are also referred to as Bellini duct carcinomas. Histologically, these are characterized by a tubular or tubulopapillary infiltrative growth pattern, which is reflected in the CT appearance. Collecting-duct RCC (CDRCC) are medullary and infiltrating in the central sinus and only rarely reported in the renal cortex.[83–86] Metastases are more common at presentation than other RCC, occurring in 35% to 40% of patients.[83,86] When bone metastases occur, they are frequently osteoblastic, unlike metastases from CCRCC, which are osteolytic.[83] At CT and at angiography, CDRCC are hypovascular tumors.[86]

In one study reporting 11 cases of CDRCC, the vast majority of CDRCCs were hyperechoic on ultrasound and hyperintense on T2WI on MR. The differential diagnosis of CDRCC includes infiltrating type of TCC, squamous cell carcinoma of the renal pelvis, and NHL.[87]

SARCOMATOID RENAL CELL CARCINOMA: 1% TO 2%

Sarcomatoid RCC is a highly aggressive primary renal tumor, and as such typically has an infiltrating appearance on imaging; the vast majority are symptomatic at presentation.[88] Renal sarcoma and sarcomatoid RCC should be considered when there is an extensively infiltrating tumor with extension into the perinephric space and adjacent organs. The differential diagnosis of sarcomatoid RCC includes other infiltrating tumors such as TCC, NHL, fibrosarcoma, and leiomyosarcoma.[89]

MEDULLARY CARCINOMA

Medullary carcinoma is often considered a distinct entity, but may be an aggressive form of CDRCC in younger patients. Medullary renal carcinoma has been associated with sickle cell trait but not sickle cell disease. As with CDRCC, medullary RCC is typically infiltrating and aggressive with centrally located tumors. Medullary carcinoma can demonstrate necrosis and hemorrhage.[22,87]

JUXTAGLOMERULAR TUMORS

Few specific imaging details are available regarding juxtaglomerular tumors. In one report these tumors were described as small and hypovascular.[90] Different from the majority of RCCs that are asymptomatic and currently discovered incidentally, juxtaglomerular tumors are often associated with hypertension and hypokalemia due to the production of renin or renin analogues, which activate the renin-angiotensin systems.[90]

Other Primary and Secondary Renal Neoplasms

ONCOCYTOMA

Stellate central scars on CT and MR and spoke-wheel enhancement on angiography have both been described as imaging features suggestive of renal oncocytoma. However, the presence or absence of such features is neither sensitive nor specific. Oncocytoma is hypervascular, similar to clear cell carcinoma, and homogeneous in attenuation (Figure 2.15), but CT cannot reliably distinguish between RCC and oncocytoma.[91] No specific descriptions of oncocytoma have been reported with MR and US. Furthermore, it was not previously possible to diagnose oncocytoma on biopsy reliably. The histopathologic features of oncocytoma allowing differentiation from RCC on biopsy have been described only in the last decade.[92,93]

BENIGN CYSTIC NEPHROMA

Also referred to a multilocular cystic nephroma (CN), these lesions have a complicated cystic appearance with multiple septations (Figure 2.16). Typically there are no soft tissue masses within the lesion. Patients with benign CN have a bimodal distribution, often occurring in younger males or older females. The diagnosis can be suggested by a typical round or oval appearance and multiple thin septations, but these findings are not specific. Benign CN can also prolapse or project into the renal pelvis.

METASTATIC DISEASE

Metastatic disease to the kidneys is particularly common with lung and breast carcinoma, melanoma, and lymphoma.[26,94] Metastatic disease to the kidneys is usually multiple and bilateral. When there is a history of a nonrenal primary tumor, as many as 50% to 85% of solitary renal masses are metastatic disease.[25,95] Conversely, nearly 90% of patients with pathologically proven metastatic disease to the kidney have a history of a primary malignancy.[26]

RENAL LYMPHOMA

Renal lymphoma can be primary, involving the renal or perirenal lymphatics, or secondary, with lymphadenopathy. On CT and MR, lymphoma can be either solid or infiltrating[23,96] (Figures 2.17 and 2.18). Renal lymphoma should be considered when there is splenomegaly, bulky retroperitoneal or mesenteric lymphadenopathy, and organ

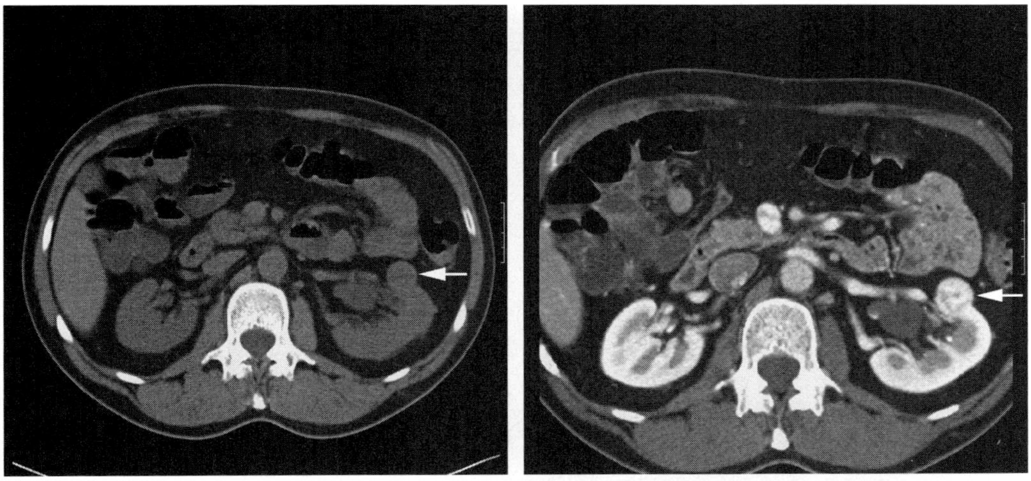

Figure 2.15. Oncocytoma. Unenhanced (A), corticomedullary phase (B), and nephrographic phase (C) CT scans show a small homogeneous hypervascular mass (arrow) exophytic from the left kidney. Oncocytomas are often homogeneous and hypervascular, and are essentially indistinguishable from clear cell renal cell carcinoma.

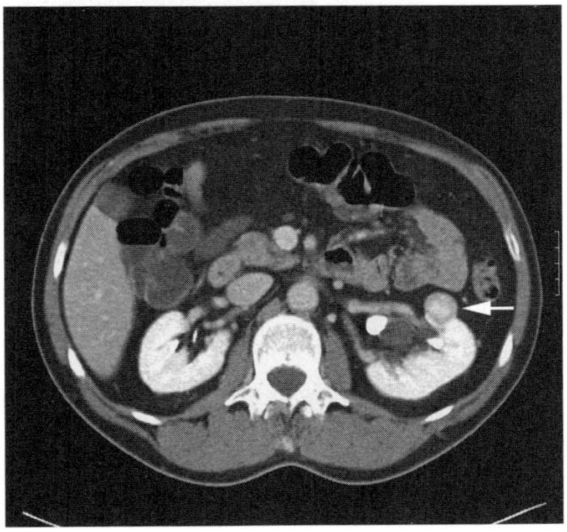

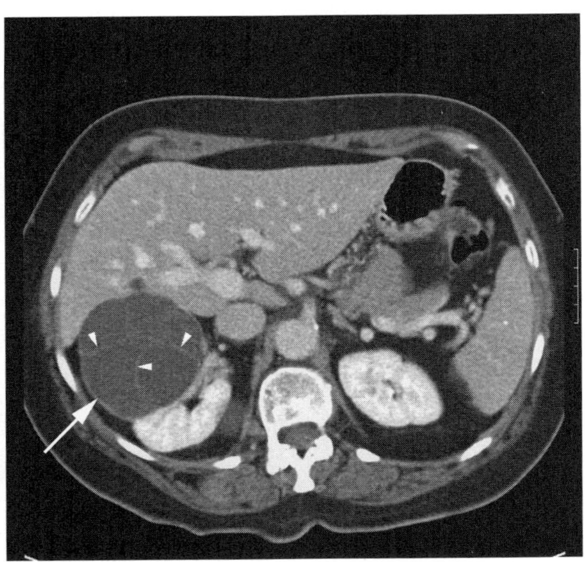

Figure 2.16. Benign cystic nephroma (arrow). This benign lesion contains several septations (arrowheads) and therefore would be classified as a Bosniak III cyst.

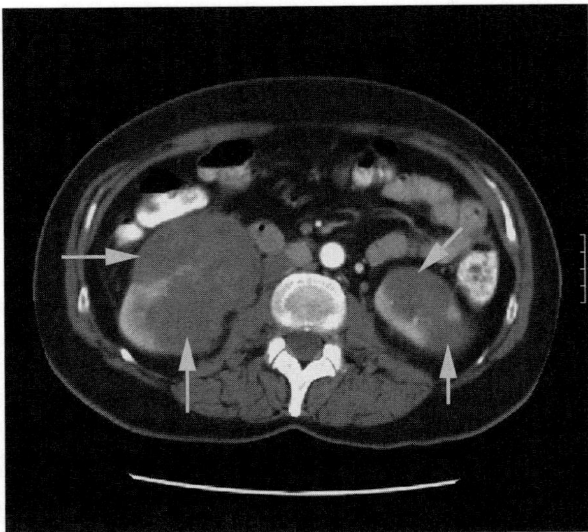

Figure 2.17. Renal lymphoma on CT. Contrast-enhanced CT shows multiple homogeneous hypodense masses (arrows) typical of renal involvement by lymphoma.

involvement such as bowel involvement, which is not typical of RCC. Biopsy should be considered to differentiate lymphoma from RCC when there are imaging findings suggesting lymphoma or a history of lymphoma.

PAPILLARY AND METANEPHRIC ADENOMAS

Papillary and metanephric adenomas are uncommon tumors of the renal tubular epithelium, all less than 5 mm at pathology.[97] There are no reports in the radiologic or urologic literature discussing imaging features of these uncommon tumors.

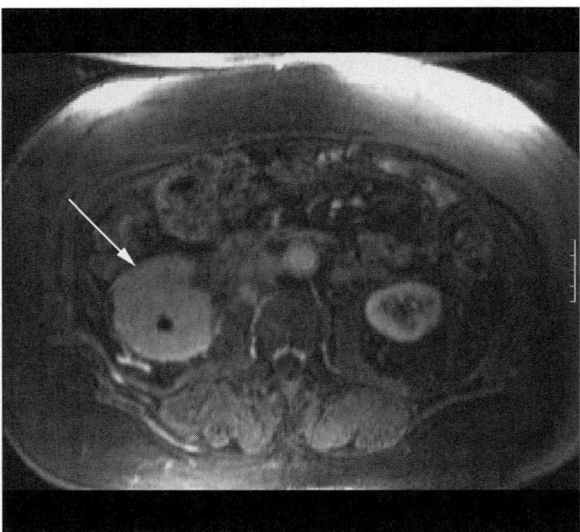

Figure 2.18. Renal lymphoma on MR. T1-weighted fat-suppressed MR with contrast shows lymphoma infiltrating the lower pole of the right kidney (arrow).

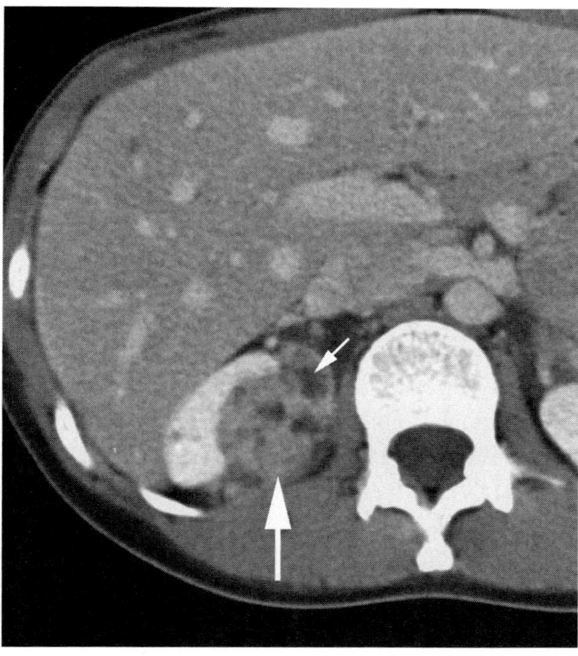

Figure 2.19. Angiomyolipoma (AML). Contrast-enhanced CT scan shows a 4-cm right renal mass (large arrow) with multiple fat-density components (small arrow) diagnostic of AML.

ANGIOMYOLIPOMA AND OTHER FAT-CONTAINING RENAL TUMORS

Angiomyolipoma (AML) is a benign renal hamartoma containing lipomatous, smooth muscle, and vascular tissue. Most AML have macroscopic fat associated with the lipomatous elements (Figure 2.19); however, there have been several recent descriptions of AML with minimal fat not identified preoperatively at CT. This represents a normal variation in the expression of the different cell types. Angiomyolipoma with minimal fat is radiographically similar to RCC at CT. Kim et al.[98] described prolonged enhancement and homogeneous enhancement in AML with minimal fat as opposed to such enhancement in RCC. Both findings together have a 91% positive predictive value (PPV) for AML. When calcification is seen in a lesion with no or minimal fat, this is most likely RCC and not AML.[99,100] On ultrasound, AML are generally smaller and more frequently hyperechoic; shadowing from a renal lesion is also more suggestive of AML than RCC.[101] Two cases reporting fat density within an RCC showed tumoral necrosis and empty lipid vacuoles with xanthoma cells and cholesterol clefts, and not true fat, within the specimen.[102,103]

Exophytic AML can usually be differentiated from a retroperitoneal or renal capsular liposarcoma by the presence of a renal parenchyma defect, large blood vessels, aneurysms, or varices.[104,105]

Infections Simulating Renal Masses

ACUTE FOCAL BACTERIAL NEPHRITIS/RENAL ABSCESS

Pyelonephritis can be diffuse but can also be focal, mimicking a renal neoplasm. A striated nephrogram and a history of fever, chills, or an elevated white blood cell count suggest acute focal bacterial nephritis (AFBN) rather than a renal tumor, especially in younger patients in whom tumors are much less common. Acute focal bacterial nephritis and infected cysts can evolve into renal abscesses. Renal abscesses are typically thick-walled unilocular cystic lesions surrounded by a patchy, diminished nephrogram in the adjacent parenchyma due to edema. Renal abscess should be differentiated from RCC because it is typically treated conservatively with IV antibiotics, with or without aspiration and drainage of the infected fluid.

STAGING OF RENAL CELL CARCINOMA BY COMPUTED TOMOGRAPHY AND MAGNETIC RESONANCE

Accuracy of Imaging for Staging

The tumor, node, metastasis (TNM) and Robson criteria are both used for staging RCC.[106–111] The criteria have been revised, with the 1997 criteria better demonstrating the probability of survival between stage I and stage II disease.[112] The overall accuracy for CT and MR for staging RCC is similar.[113–118] Magnetic resonance is 78% to 98% accurate for staging.[66,67,119] There was no difference between overall CT and MR accuracy in one study,[67] and MR demonstrated higher accuracy than CT in another.[66] Magnetic resonance was better than CT for stage II disease and worse than CT for stage IV disease.[120]

The major limitation of imaging for staging is identifying tumors that have spread beyond the renal capsule, the presence of which increases the stage from T1 or T2 to T3 by the TNM system, or stage 1 to stage 2 by Robson's staging. Criteria such as a discrete nodule or thickening of a septum, either greater than 3 mm, in the perinephric space are neither sensitive nor specific for spread beyond the renal capsule (Figure 2.20). Most studies demonstrate understaging by CT, which is acceptable in that it offers

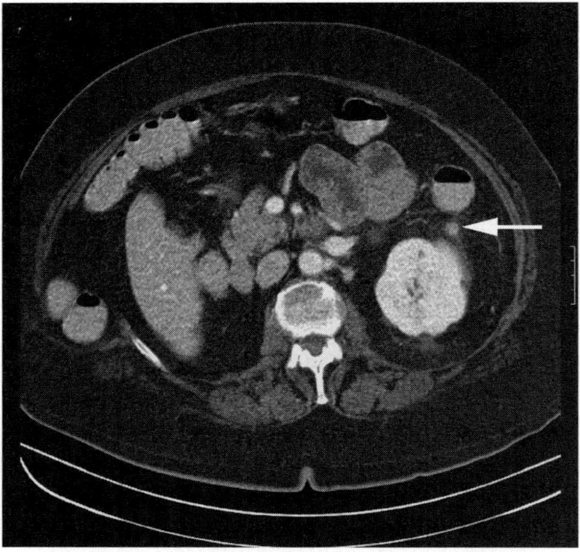

Figure 2.20. Extracapsular extension of renal cell carcinoma. Contrast-enhanced CT scan shows a 3-mm nodule in the perinephric space (arrow) in this patient with a left renal cell carcinoma (not shown). The sensitivity of CT for extracapsular extension is low, but discrete nodules such as this are highly suggestive.

the patient the better prognosis. This understaging by CT does not affect the overall prognosis; patients with clinical stage T1 disease and pathologic stage T1 disease were compared to patients with clinical stage T1 disease and pathologic stage T3 disease. There was no statistically significant difference in 5-year survival between the groups.[121]

Ultrasound is not generally recommended for staging. Ultrasound is inferior to CT and MR in large part because of poor lymph node visibility.[120] Ultrasound may be accurate for assessing renal vein involvement and can be used as an adjunct to CT or MR if equivocal or limited in any way.

The mode of presentation is a significant factor in the overall stage of RCC. Most RCCs are now incidentally discovered as asymptomatic tumors identified on imaging performed for other reasons. These incidentally detected tumors are often smaller and lower stage than symptomatic RCC.[122,123]

Renal Central Sinus Invasion and Urothelial Invasion

While not included in the Robson or TNM staging system, invasion of the central sinus fat may have significant prognostic indications, similar to extension outside the renal capsule.[124] Urothelial invasion has also been suggested as an added criterion for staging, as it was associated with a worse prognosis in one series.[75] In this study, patients with pathologically determined T2 tumors with urothelial invasion did worse than patients with T2 tumors without urothelial invasion.

Tumor Size

Final pathologic tumor size is an important prognostic staging criterion in the TNM staging system. In general, there has been excellent correlation between CT size and pathologic size with correlation coefficients 0.90 to 0.95.[125,126] Smaller tumors are overestimated by CT.[125] No other factors in that study affected the difference between CT and pathologic size. Clear cell tumors were smaller at pathology than CT; in one study of RCC greater than 4 cm, 22 CCRCCs were overestimated by more than 1 cm by CT.[127] Larger tumors may be underestimated by CT.

Several studies have compared clinical tumor (CT) size with pathologic size.[125–127] Factors that might create a difference between CT and pathologic size include orientation of the tumor such that the longest axis is not in the axial plane or, with multidetector-row CT, in an orthogonal plane. Another factor is lack of blood within the tumor at pathology, which may account for why the more vascular CCRCC has a larger size discrepancy than hypovascular RCC.

Pelvic and Chest Computed Tomography

Pelvic CT is probably not needed for the initial staging evaluation of RCC. There are few significant findings.[128,129] For expected low-stage disease with small primary tumors, a normal chest x-ray will likely suffice for pulmonary staging[130]; for larger tumors and patients with extensive regional disease or pulmonary symptoms, chest CT is indicated. Pulmonary metastases typically appear as lobular masses of varying size (Figure 2.21). Mediastinal lymphadenopathy is more common with more extensive pulmonary metastatic disease (Figure 2.22).

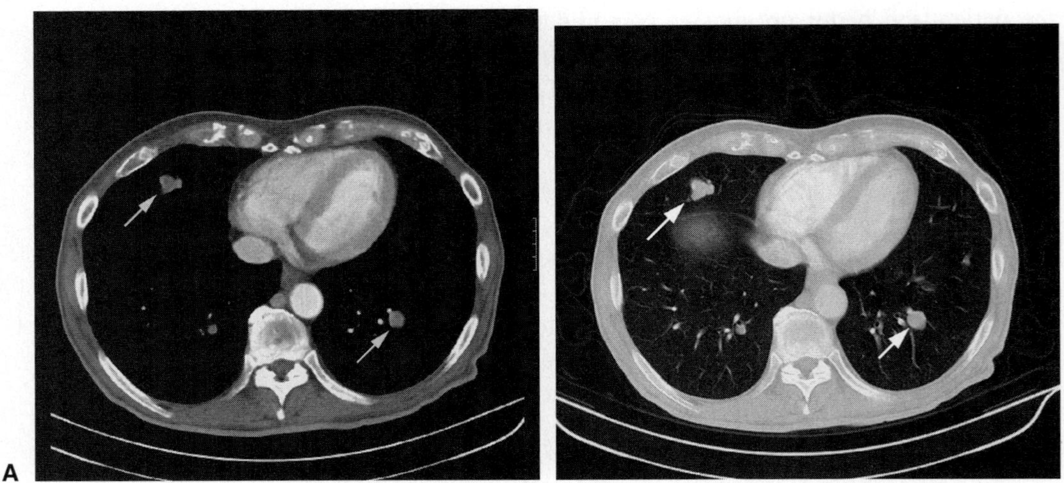

Figure 2.21. Pulmonary metastases from renal cell carcinoma. Soft tissue (A) and lung (B) windows from a chest CT shows two small lobular soft tissue density masses (arrows).

Lymphadenopathy

Both CT and MR are highly sensitive for metastatic lymphadenopathy using a criterion of 1 cm short-axis diameter. Computed tomography sensitivity for lymph node involvement is 89% to 100%.[66,114] The appearance of lymph node metastases often mimics that of the primary tumor, such that lymph node metastases from CCRCC are frequently hypervascular (Figures 2.22 and 2.23).

Adrenal Gland Involvement

Adrenal gland involvement by RCC is uncommon, particularly so in the modern era with earlier presentation, smaller and lower grade tumors, and asymptomatic, incidental

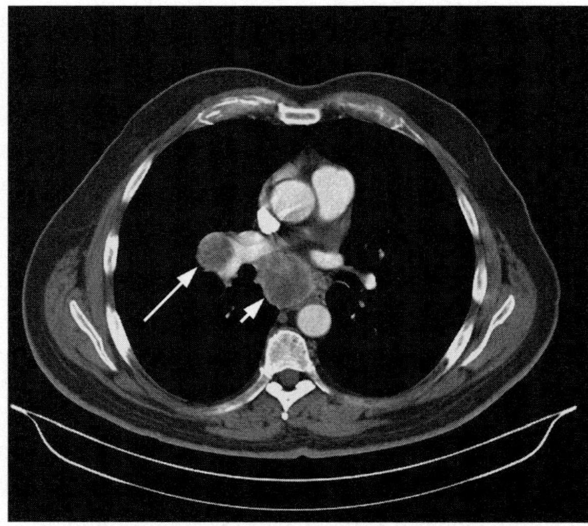

Figure 2.22. Right hilar and mediastinal metastasis from renal cell carcinoma. Soft tissue window of a chest CT shows a mass in the right hilum (long arrow) and a subcarinal mass (short arrow).

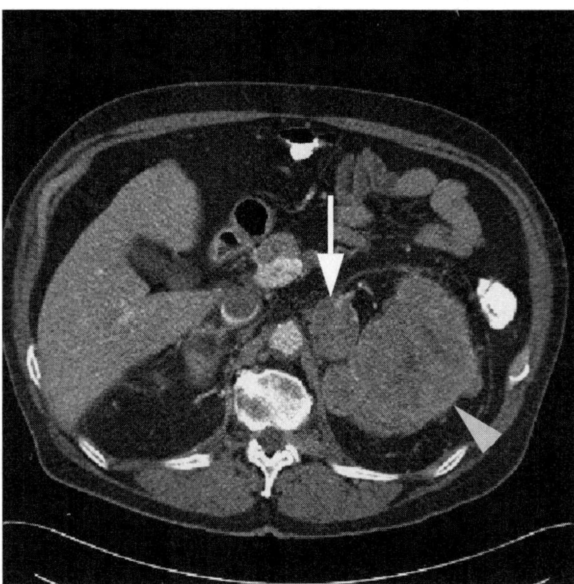

Figure 2.23. Retroperitoneal adenopathy from renal cell carcinoma on CT. Unenhanced CT shows an enlarged lymph node (arrow) 2 cm in short-axis diameter in a patient with renal cell carcinoma (arrowhead). Lymph nodes are considered pathologically enlarged when the short-axis diameter is greater than 1 cm, but even smaller lymph nodes with vascular patterns of enhancement mimicking the primary tumor usually contain metastatic disease.

presentation.[131] In one series, adrenal gland involvement ranged from less than 1% in early, low-stage disease to 8% in advanced disease.[132] Computed tomography has a reported 94% to 100% negative predictive value for adrenal involvement.[131,133,134] To restate, when the CT demonstrates a normal ipsilateral adrenal gland, the gland is almost certainly not involved. Moreover, when the adrenal is not seen or a renal mass obscures visualization, the adrenal gland is still only involved in a small percentage of cases.[134] Positive predictive value of CT for adrenal involvement is low, only 11% to 26%.

When there is a discrete nodule, unenhanced CT or MR with in- and out-of-phase imaging can be used to distinguish between lipid-rich adenomas and metastatic disease; performing a bolus and delayed phase scan at 10 to 15 minutes and calculating washout can further increase the sensitivity for adrenal adenomas by identifying lipid-poor adenomas.[135,136]

Renal Vein and Inferior Vena Cava Tumor

The identification of renal vein invasion or tumor thrombus and its cephalad extent into the inferior vena cava (IVC) are critical for proper staging of RCC.[137] Briefly, level I tumor thrombus extends only within the renal vein, or into the renal vein and IVC within 2 cm of the renal vein ostia; level II extends within the IVC more than 2 cm from the renal vein ostia but not into the intrahepatic IVC; level III extends into the intrahepatic IVC but not above the hepatic veins; and level IV extends above the hepatic veins including into the right atrium (Figures 2.24 to 2.27). The presence of renal vein invasion not only increases the stage of what may otherwise have been a stage I or II tumor to stage III, but it also directly affects surgical management.[137–139] The level of extension

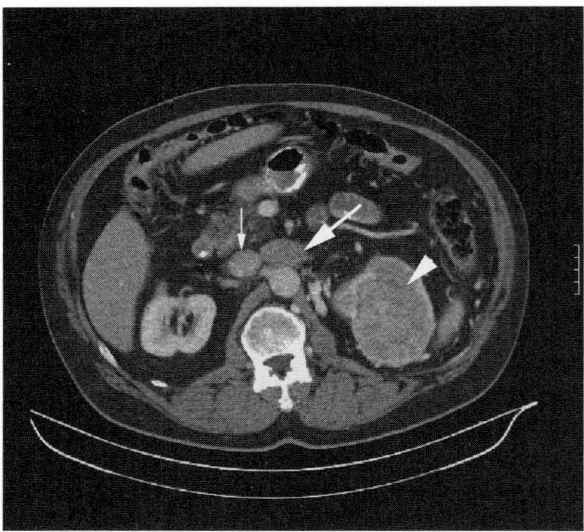

Figure 2.24. Level I renal vein tumor thrombus. Axial CT image shows a left lower pole renal cell carcinoma (arrowhead) and tumor enlarging the left renal vein (arrow), but no extension into the inferior vena cava (IVC) (thin arrow).

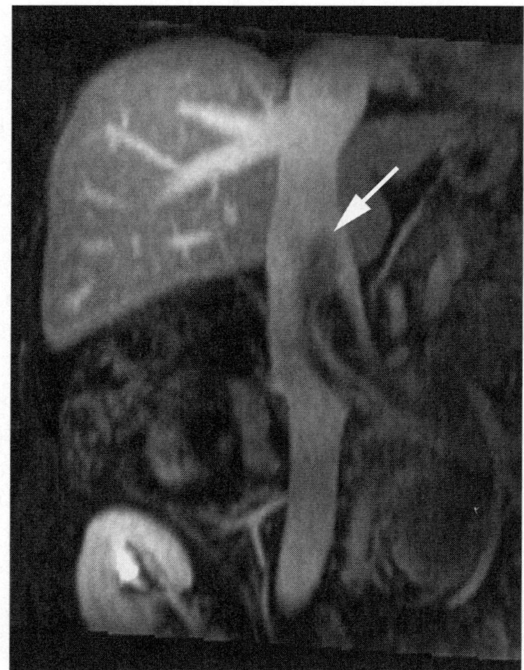

Figure 2.25. Level II renal vein tumor thrombus. Coronal contrast-enhanced MR scan showing tumor thrombus (arrow) extending within the intrahepatic IVC terminating just below the intrahepatic portion.

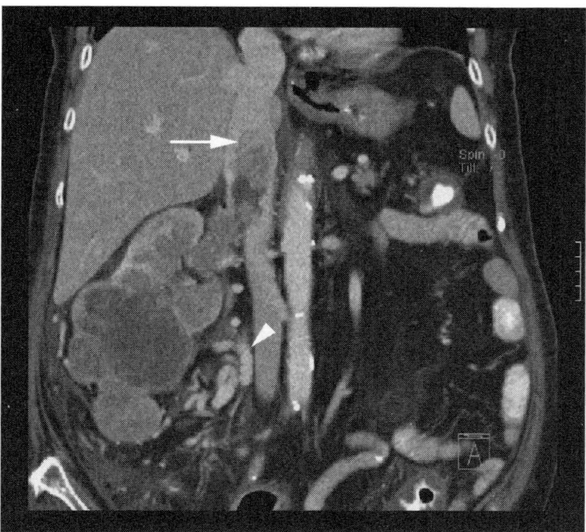

Figure 2.26. Level III renal vein tumor thrombus. Coronal reformation contrast-enhanced CT scan showing tumor thrombus extending within the intrahepatic IVC (arrow) terminating below the hepatic veins. Small collateral vessels are seen in the retroperitoneum from the IVC tumor thrombus (arrowhead).

of tumor thrombus within the IVC can be evaluated by transesophageal echo, ultrasound, MR, and CT. Magnetic resonance has excellent sensitivity and specificity for renal vein involvement: 90% to 100%.[140–144] Earlier reports noted that CT was not as sensitive as MR[66,114,140,143]; however, with the use of state-of-the-art multidetector CT (MDCT) with multiphase and multiplanar imaging, CT at 87% is essentially equivalent to MR sensitivity.[115,142]

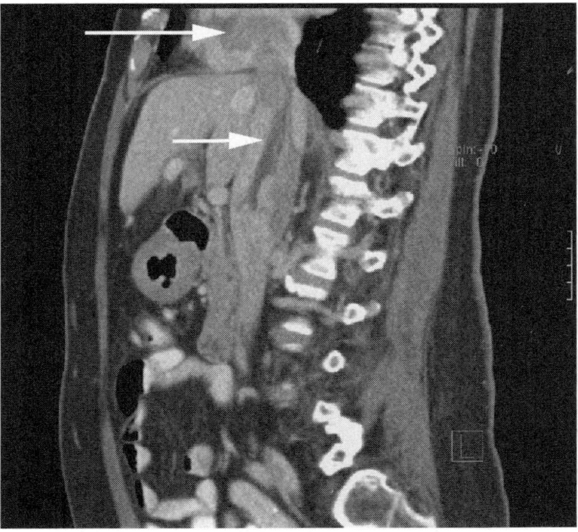

Figure 2.27. Level IV renal vein tumor thrombus. Sagittal reformation of a contrast-enhanced CT scan showing tumor thrombus extending within the intrahepatic IVC and into the right atrium (arrows).

Ultrasound can also be used to assess renal vein and IVC involvement, but is frequently technically indeterminate.[142] Ultrasound with CFD in experienced hands nearly matches the sensitivity of CT, but is not recommended for staging for the reasons described earlier. Inferior vena cava diameter has also been used to assess direct invasion into the vessel wall; Gohji et al.[145] reported that there was 100% PPV for IVC wall invasion in patients with IVC diameter greater than 40 mm. If there is equivocation of CT and MR, MR is recommended by most authors as the best means of detecting and staging renal vein and IVC involvement.[138,140,142,143]

Metastatic Disease

Up to 30% of patients with a new diagnosis of RCC can have metastasis at presentation.[146] Renal cell carcinoma can metastasize almost anywhere, but lung, brain, and bone are the most common sites. The appearance of the metastasis, whether hypervascular, hypovascular, or cystic, typically resembles the primary lesion. Lung metastases typically appear at chest x-ray or CT as multiple round pulmonary nodules of varying size, and are from hematogenous spread.[130] Bone lesions tend to be expansile and osteolytic (Figures 2.28 and 2.29). Patients with metastatic RCC may have spread to the liver, adrenal glands, and soft tissue; and now pancreas metastases are more commonly recognized due to improvements in scanning techniques[147,148] (Figures 2.30 to 2.33). Peritoneal carcinomatosis has also been reported.[149]

Nuclear Grade

Computed tomography has not been able to predict nuclear grade reliably in the absence of other factors such as small tumor size.[150] Increased tumor size is in general

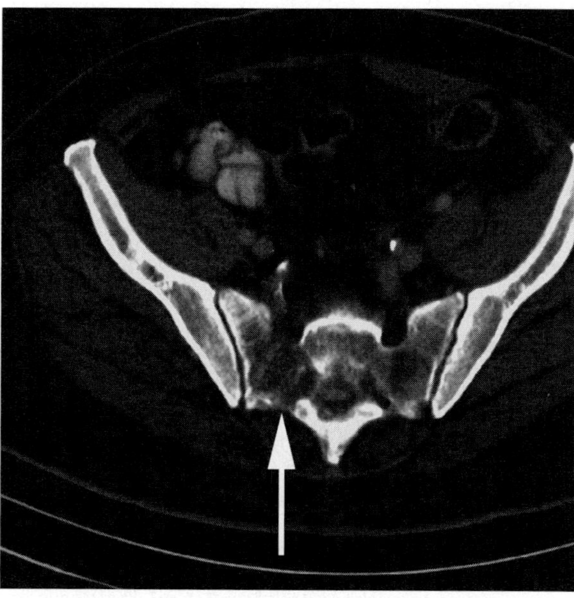

Figure 2.28. Metastatic renal cell carcinoma to bone. Bone window from a CT scan of the pelvis shows a lytic metastasis in the right sacrum (arrow).

Figure 2.29. Metastatic renal cell carcinoma to bone. Bone window from a CT scan of the pelvis shows a large destructive mass in the left iliac wing (arrows) with central necrosis.

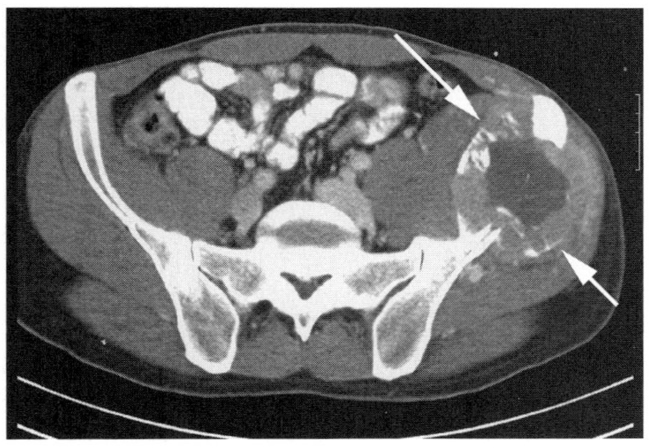

Figure 2.30. Metastatic renal cell carcinoma to the liver on CT. Contrast-enhanced CT scan shows multiple low attenuation liver masses (arrows).

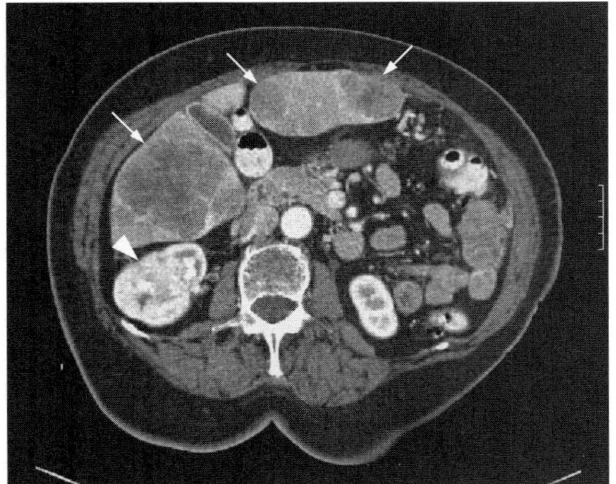

Figure 2.31. Metastatic renal cell carcinoma to the pancreas on MR. A low signal mass (large arrow) from metastatic renal cell carcinoma is present in the body of the pancreas. This results in pancreatic duct dilation (small arrow).

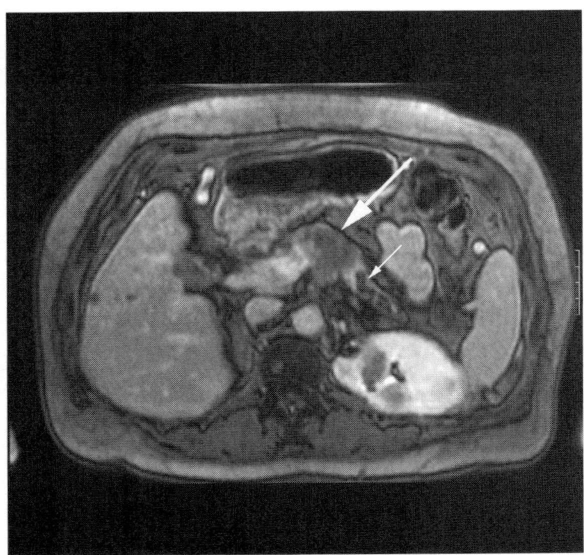

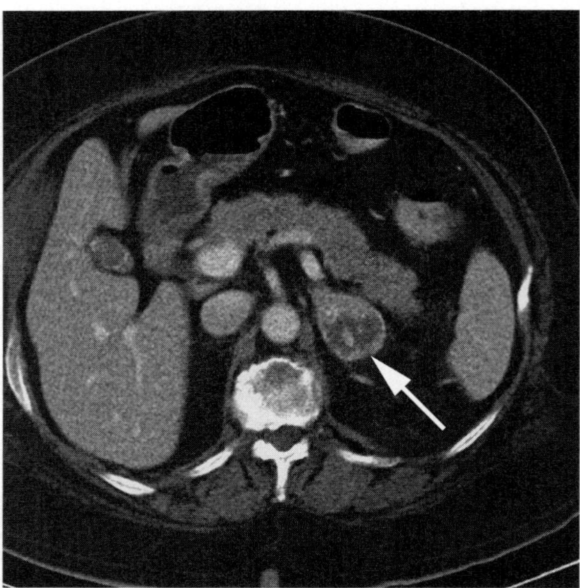

Figure 2.32. Metastatic renal cell carcinoma to the adrenal gland on CT. Contrast-enhanced CT scan of the abdomen shows a heterogeneously enhancing left adrenal mass (arrow) from metastatic renal cell carcinoma.

associated with higher nuclear grade; only 2.3% of tumors less than 1 cm were high grade compared to 58% of tumors greater than 7 cm.[151] If nuclear grade would effect therapeutic decisions, the determination of nuclear grade could be accomplished by percutaneous imaging-guided biopsy; there is a high concordance rate between nuclear grade on percutaneous biopsy and histologic specimens.[152]

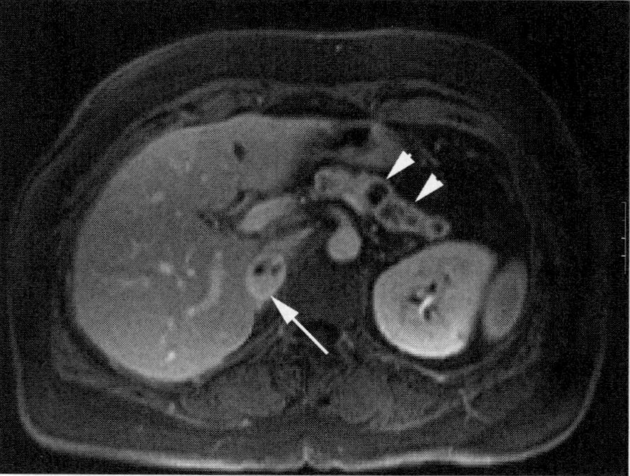

Figure 2.33. Metastatic renal cell carcinoma to the pancreas and adrenal gland on MR. This patient with renal cell carcinoma has both a solid enhancing adrenal mass (arrow) and a cystic pancreatic tail metastasis (arrowheads).

CONCLUSION

Computed tomography and MR examinations performed with and without IV contrast are both excellent imaging modalities for the diagnosis and staging of renal cell carcinoma. Ultrasound can also detect renal tumors, but more often plays an adjunct role in the characterization of renal lesions. Clear-cell renal cell carcinoma, oncocytoma, and AML are the most vascular of the renal primary tumors; AML can usually be distinguished from other tumors based on the presence of fat within the lesion. Papillary and chromophobe renal cell carcinoma are typically hypovascular and less aggressive tumors. Infiltrative lesions, such as medullary carcinoma and TCC, are usually more aggressive tumors. Each of the imaging modalities have distinct advantages and disadvantages, but CT, because of its ready availability, ease of use, and accuracy, is the primary imaging modality for diagnosis and staging of RCC. Magnetic resonance has accuracy similar to CT, and even surpasses CT for staging in some areas; but MR is often reserved for patients with lesions indeterminate at CT, an allergy to iodinated contrast or mild renal insufficiency.

ACKNOWLEDGMENT

I would especially like to thank Sylvia Zavatchen for her invaluable editorial assistance in the preparation of this chapter.

REFERENCES

1. Jemal A, Murray T, Samuels A, et al. Cancer statistics. CA Cancer J Clin 2003;53:5–26.
2. Jayson M, Sanders H. Increased incidence of serendipitously discovered renal cell carcinoma. Urology 1998;51:203–205.
3. Luciani LG, Cestari R, Tallarigo C. Incidental renal cell carcinoma-age and stage characterization and clinical implications: study of 1092 patients (1982–1997). Urology 2000;56:58–62.
4. Smith SJ, Bosniak MA, Megibow AJ, Hulnick Dh, Horri SC, Ragavendra BN. Renal cell carcinoma: earlier discovery and increased detection. Radiology 1989;170:699–703.
5. Breatheau D, Lechevallier E, Eghazarian C, et al. Prognostic significance of incidental renal cell carcinoma. Eur Urol 1995;27:319–323.
6. Mejean A, Oudard S, Thiounn N. Prognostic factors of renal cell carcinoma. J Urol 2003;169: 821–827.
7. Fuhrman SA, Lasky LC, Limas C. Prognostic significance of morphologic parameters in renal cell carcinoma. Am J Surg Pathol 1982;6:655–663.
8. Bostwick DG, Murphy GP. Diagnosis and prognosis of renal cell carcinoma: highlights from an international consensus workshop. Semin Urol Oncol 1998;16:46–52.
9. Heidenreich A, Ravery V. Preoperative imaging in renal cell cancer. World J Urol 2004;22: 307–315.
10. Wolf JS Jr. Evaluation and management of solid and cystic renal masses. J Urol 1998;159: 1120–1133.
11. Zagoria RJ, Wolfman NT, Karstaedt N, Hinn GC, Dyer RB, Chen YM. CT features of renal cell carcinoma with emphasis on relation to tumor size. Invest Radiol 1990;25:261.
12. Yamashita Y, Watanabe O, Miyazaki T, et al. Cystic renal cell carcinoma; imaging findings with pathologic correlation. Acta Radiol 1994;35:19–24.
13. Curry NS. Atypical cystic renal masses. Abdom Imaging 1998;23:230–236.
14. Eble JN, Bonsib SM. Extensively cystic renal neoplasms: cystic nephroma, cystic partially differentiated nephroblastoma, multilocular cystic renal cell carcinoma, and cystic hamartoma of the renal pelvis. Semin Diagn Pathol 1998;15:2–20.
15. Bosniak MA. The current radiological approach to renal cysts. Radiology 1986;158:1–10.
16. Bosniak MA. Difficulties in classifying cystic lesions of the kidney. Urol Radiol 1991;13:91–93.

17. Israel GM, Bosniak MA. Calcification in cystic renal masses: is it important in diagnosis? Radiology 2003;226:47–52.
18. Israel GM, Hindman N, Bosniak MA. Evaluation of cystic renal masses: comparison of CT and MR using the Bosniak classification system. Radiology 2004;231:365–371.
19. Siegel CL, Fisher AJ, Bennett HF. Interobserver variability in determining enhancement of renal masses on helical CT. AJR 1999;172:1207–1212.
20. Wilson TE, Doelle EA, Cohan RH, et al. Cystic renal masses: a reevaluation of the usefulness of the Bosniak classification system. Acad Radiol 1996;3:564–570.
21. Harishinghani MG, Maher MM, Gervais DA, et al. Incidence of malignancy in complex cystic renal masses (Bosniak III): should biopsy precede surgery. AJR 2003;180:755–758.
22. Pickhardt PJ, Lonergan GJ, Davis CJ, et al. Infiltrative renal lesions: radiologic-pathologic correlation. Radiographics 2000;20:215–243.
23. Cohan RH, Dunnick NR, Leder RA. Computed tomography of renal lymphoma. J Comput Assist Tomogr 1990;14:933–938.
24. Araki T. Leukemic involvement of the kidney in children: CT features. J Comput Assist Tomogr 1982;6:781–784.
25. Mitnick JS, Bosniak MA, Rothberg M. Metastatic neoplasm to the kidney studied by computed tomography and sonography. J Comput Assist Tomogr 1985;9:43–49.
26. Gattuso P, Ramzy I, Truong LD, et al. Utilization of fine-needle aspiration in the diagnosis of metastatic tumors to the kidney. Diagn Cytopathol 1999;21:35–38.
27. Honda H, Onitsuka H, Naitou S, et al. Renal arteriovenous malformations: CT features. J Comput Assist Tomogr 1991;15:261–264.
28. King BF, Hattery RR. Case of the day. Ultrasound. Congenital cirsoid renal arteriovenous malformation (AVM) involving the lower pole of the right kidney. Radiographics 1990;10:1101–1104.
29. Vasavada SP, Manion S, Flanigan RC, et al. Renal arteriovenous malformations masquerading as renal cell carcinoma. Urology 1995;46:716–721.
30. Morton MJ, Charboneau JW. Arteriovenous fistula after biopsy of renal transplant: detection and monitoring with color flow and duplex ultrasonography. Mayo Clin Proc 1989;64:531–534.
31. Middleton WD, Kellman GM, Melson GL, et al. Postbiopsy renal transplant arteriovenous fistulas: color Doppler US characteristics. Radiology 1989;171:253–257.
32. Israel GM, Bosniak MA. Renal imaging for diagnosis and staging of renal cell carcinoma. Urol Clin North Am 2003;30:499–514.
33. Helenon O, Correas JM, Balleyquier C, et al. Ultrasound of renal tumors. Eur Radiol 2001;11:1890–1901.
34. Mihara S, Kuroda K, Yoshioka R, et al. Early detection of renal cell carcinoma by ultrasonographic screening—based on 13 years screening in exam. Ultrasound Med Biol 1999;25:1033–1039.
35. Tosaka A, Ohya K, Yamada K, et al. Incidence and properties of renal masses and asymptomatic renal cell carcinoma detected by abdominal ultrasonography. J Urol 1990;144:1097–1099.
36. Kitamura H, Fujimoto H, Tobisu K, et al. Dynamic computed Tomography and color Doppler ultrasound of renal parenchymal neoplasms: correlation with histopathological findings. Jpn J Cln Oncol 2004;34:78–81.
37. Park BK, Kim SH, Choi HJ. Characterization of renal cell carcinoma using agent detection imaging: comparison with gray-scale ultrasound. Korean J Radiol 2005;6:173–178.
38. Jinzaki M, Tanimoto A, Mukai M, et al. Double-phase helical CT of small renal parenchymal neoplasms: correlation with pathological findings and tumor angiogenesis. J Comput Assist Tomogr 2000;24:835–842.
39. Herts BR, Coll DM, Novick AC, et al. Enhancement characteristics of papillary renal neoplasms revealed on triphasic helical CT of the kidneys. AJR 2002;178:367–372.
40. Kopka L, Fischer U, Zoeller G, et al. Dual-phase helical CT of the kidney: value of the corticomedullary and nephrographic phase for evaluation of renal lesions and preoperative staging of renal cell carcinoma. AJR 1997;169:1573–1578.
41. Kauczor HU, Schwickert HC, Schweden F, et al. Bolus-enhanced renal spiral CT: techniques, diagnostic value and drawbacks. Eur J Radiol 1994;18:153–157.
42. Garant M, Bonaldi VM, Taourel P, et al. Enhancement patterns of renal masses during multiphase helical CT acquisitions. Abdom Imaging 1998;23:431–436.
43. Cohan RH, Sherman LS, Korobkin M, et al. Renal masses: assessment of corticomedullary-phase and nephrographic-phase CT scans. Radiology 1995;196:445–451.

44. Birnbaum BA, Jacobs JE, Ramchandani P. Multiphasic renal CT: comparison of renal mass enhancement during the corticomedullary and nephrographic phases. Radiology 1996;200:753–758.
45. Szolar DH, Kammerhuber F, Altziebler S, et al. Multiphasic helical CT of the kidney: increased conspicuity for detection and characterization of small (<3–cm) renal masses. Radiology 1997;202:211–217.
46. Herts BR, Coll DM, Lieber ML, et al. Triphasic helical CT of the kidneys: contribution of vascular phase scanning in patients before urologic surgery. AJR 1999;1273–1277.
47. Herts BR, Einstein DM, Paushter DM. Spiral CT of the abdomen: artifacts and potential pitfalls. AJR 1993;161:1185–1190.
48. Macari M, Bosniak MA. Delayed CT to evaluate renal masses incidentally discovered at contrast-enhanced CT: demonstration of vascularity with deenhancement. Radiology 1999;213:674–680.
49. Voci SL, Gottlieb RH, Fultz PJ, et al. Delayed computed tomographic characterization of renal masses: a preliminary experience. Abdom Imaging 2000;25:317–321.
50. Chung EP, Herts BR, Linnell G, et al. Analysis of changes in attenuation of proven renal cysts on different scanning phases of triphasic MDCT. AJR 2004;182:405–410.
51. Coulam CH, Sheafor DH, Leder RA, et al. Evaluation of pseudoenhancement of renal cysts during contrast-enhanced CT. AJR 2000;174:493–498.
52. Maki DD, Birnbaum BA, Chakraborty DP, et al. Renal cyst pseudoenhancement: beam-hardening effects on CT numbers. Radiology 1999;213:468–472.
53. Coll DM, Uzzo RG, Herts BR, et al. 3–dimensional volume rendered computerized Tomography for preoperative evaluation and intraoperative treatment of patients undergoing nephron sparing surgery. J Urol 1999;161:1097–1102.
54. Coll DM, Herts BR, Davros WJ, et al. Preoperative use of 3D volume rendering to demonstrate renal tumors and renal anatomy. RadioGraphics 2000;20:431–438.
55. Choyke PL, Walther MM, Wagner JR, et al. Renal cancer: preoperative evaluation with dual-phase three-dimensional MR angiography. Radiology 1997;205:767–771.
56. Catalano C, Fraioli F, Laghi A, et al. High-resolution multidetector CT in the preoperative evaluation of patients with renal cell carcinoma. AJR 2003;180:1271–1277.
57. Sheth S, Scatarige JC, Horton KM, et al. Current concepts in the diagnosis and management of renal cell carcinoma: role of multidetector CT and three-dimensional CT. RadioGraphics 2001;21: S237–254.
58. Wunderlich H, Reichelt O, Schubert R, et al. Preoperative simulation of partial nephrectomy with three-dimensional computed tomography. BJU Int 2000;86:777–781.
59. Rofsky NM, Weinreb JC, Bosniak MA, et al. Renal lesion characterization with gadolinium-enhanced MR imaging: efficacy and safety in patients with renal insufficiency. Radiology 1991;180:85–89.
60. Kramer LA. Magnetic resonance imaging of renal masses. World J Urol 1998;16:22–28.
61. Narumi Y, Hricak H, Presti JC Jr, et al. MR imaging of renal cell carcinoma. Abdom Imaging 1997;22:216–225.
62. Ho VB, Allen SF, Hood MN, et al. Renal masses: quantitative assessment of enhancement with dynamic MR imaging. Radiology 2002;224;695–700.
63. Hecht EM, Israel GM, Krinsky GA, et al. Renal masses: quantitative analysis of enhancement with signal intensity measurements versus qualitative analysis of enhancement with image subtraction for diagnosing malignancy at MR imaging. Radiology 2004;232:373–378.
64. Ho VB, Choyke PL. MR evaluation of solid renal masses. MRI Clin North Am 2004;12:413–427.
65. Walter C, Kruessell M, Gindele A, et al. Imaging of renal lesions: evaluation of fast MRI and helical CT. Br J Radiol 2003;76:696–703.
66. Semelka RC, Shoenut JP, Magro CM, et al. Renal cancer staging: comparison of contrast-enhanced CT and Gadolinium-enhanced fat-suppressed spin-echo and gradient-echo MR imaging. J MRI 1993;3:597–602.
67. Hallscheidt PJ, Bock M, Riedasch G, et al. Diagnostic accuracy of staging renal cell carcinoma using multidetector-row computed tomography and magnetic resonance imaging. J Comput Assist Tomogr 2004;28:333–339.
68. Pretorius ES, Wickstrom L, Siegelman ES. MR imaging of renal neoplasms. MRI Clin North Am 2000;8:813–836.
69. Weiss LM, Gelb AB, Medeiros LJ. Adult renal epithelial neoplasms. Am J Clin Pathol 1995;103:624–635.

70. Bostwick DG, Eble JN. Diagnosis and classification of renal cell carcinoma. Urol Clin North Am 1999;26:627–635.
71. Zisman A, Chao DH, Pantuck AJ, et al. Unclassified renal cell carcinoma: clinical features and prognostic impact of a new histological subtype. J Urol 2002;168:950–955.
72. Kim JK, Kim TK, Ahn HJ, Kim CS, Kim KR, Cho KS. Differentiation of subtypes of renal cell carcinoma on helical CT scans. AJR 2002;178:1499–1506.
73. Sheir KZ, El-Azab M, Mosbah A, et al. Differentiation of renal cell carcinoma subtypes by multislice computerized tomography. J Urol 2005;174:451–455.
74. Shinmoto H, Yuasa Y, Tanimoto A, et al. Small renal cell carcinoma: MRI with pathological correlation. J MRI 1998;8:690–694.
75. Uzzo RG, Cherullo EE, Myles J, et al. Renal cell carcinoma invading the urinary collecting system: implications for staging. J Urol 2002;167:2392–2396.
76. Delahunt B, Eble JN. Papillary renal cell carcinoma: a clinicopathologic and immunohistochemical study of 105 cases. Mod Pathol 1997;10:537–544.
77. Lager DJ, Huston BJ, Timmerman TG, Bonsib SM. Papillary renal tumors. Cancer 1995;76:669.
78. Onishi T, Ohishi Y, Goto H, et al. Papillary renal cell carcinoma: clinicopathological characteristics and evaluation of prognosis in 42 patients. BJU Int 1999;83:937–943.
79. Ruppert-Kohlmayr AJ, Uggowitzer M, Meissnitzer T, et al. Differentiation of renal clear cell carcinoma and renal papillary carcinoma using quantitative CT enhancement parameters. AJR 2004;183:1387–1391.
80. Mejean A, Hopirtean V, Bazin JP, et al. Prognostic factors for the survival of patients with papillary renal cell carcinoma: meaning of histologic typing and multifocality. J Urol 2003;170:764–767.
81. Megumi Y, Nishimura K. Chromophobe renal cell carcinoma. Urol Int 1998;61:172–174.
82. Kondo T, Nakazawa H, Sakai F, et al. Spoke-wheel-like enhancement as an important imaging finding of chromophobe cell renal carcinoma: a retrospective analysis on computed tomography and magnetic resonance imaging studies. Int J Urol 2004;11:817–824.
83. Srigley JR, Eble JN. Collecting duct carcinoma of kidney. Semin Diagn Pathol 1998;15:54–67.
84. Fukuya T, Honda H, Goto K, et al. Computed tomographic findings of Bellini duct carcinoma of the kidney. J Comput Assist Tomogr 1996;20:399–403.
85. Gurocak S, Sozen S, Akyurek N, et al. Cortically located collecting duct carcinoma. Urology 2005;65:1226.
86. Pickhardt PJ, Siegel CL, McLarney JK. Collecting duct carcinoma of the kidney: are imaging findings suggestive of the diagnosis? AJR 2001;176:627–633.
87. Pickhardt PJ. Collecting duct carcinoma arising in a solitary kidney: imaging findings. Clin Imaging 1999;23:115–118.
88. Mian BM, Bhadkamkar NJ, Slaton JW, et al. Prognostic factors and survival of patients with sarcomatoid renal cell carcinoma. Urology 2002;167:65–70.
89. Staelens L, Van Poppel H, Vanuytsel L, et al. Sarcomatoid renal cell carcinoma: case report and review of the literature. Acta Urol Belg 1997;65:39–42.
90. Tanabe A, Naruse M, Ogawa T, et al. Dynamic computed tomography is useful in the differential diagnosis of juxtaglomerular cell tumor and renal cell carcinoma. Hypertens Res 2001;24:331–336.
91. Davidson AJ, Hayes WJ, Hartman DS, et al. Renal oncocytoma and carcinoma: failure of differentiation with CT. Radiology 1993;186:693–696.
92. Wiatrowska BA, Zakowski MF. Fine-needle aspiration biopsy of chromophobe renal cell carcinoma and oncocytoma: comparison of cytomorphologic features. Cancer 1999;87:161–167.
93. Liu J, Fanning CV. Can renal oncocytomas be distinguished from renal cell carcinoma on fine-needle aspiration specimens? A study of conventional smears in conjunction with ancillary studies. Cancer 2001;93:390–397.
94. Bracken RB, Chica G, Johnson DE, et al. Secondary renal neoplasms: an autopsy study. South Med J 1979;72:806–807.
95. Wood BJ, Khan MA, McGovern F, et al. Imaging guided biopsy of renal masses: indications, accuracy and impact on clinical management. J Urol 1999;161:1470–1474.
96. Sheeran SR, Sussman SK. Renal lymphoma: spectrum of CT findings and potential mimics. AJR 1998;171:1067–1072.
97. Grignon DJ, Eble JN. Papillary and metanephric adenomas of the kidney. Semin Diagn Pathol 1998;15:41–53.
98. Kim JK, Park SY, Shon JH, et al. Angiomyolipoma with minimal fat: differentiation from renal cell carcinoma at biphasic helical CT. Radiology 2004;230:677–684.

99. Schuster TG, Ferguson MR, Baker DE, et al. Papillary renal cell carcinoma containing fat without calcification mimicking angiomyolipoma on CT. AJR 2004;183:1402–1404.
100. Hammadeh MY, Thomas K, Philp T, et al. Renal cell carcinoma containing fat mimicking angiomyolipoma: demonstration with CT scan and histopathology. Eur Radiol 1998;8:228–229.
101. Siegel CL, Middleton WD, Teefey SA, et al. Angiomyolipoma and renal cell carcinoma: US differentiation. Radiology 1996;198:789–793.
102. Roy C, Tuchman C, Linder V, et al. Renal cell carcinoma with a fatty component mimicking angiomyolipoma at CT. Br J Radiol 1998;71:977–979.
103. Radin DR, Chandrasoma P. CT demonstration of fat density in renal cell carcinoma. Acta Radiol 1992;33:365–367.
104. Wang LJ, Wong YC, Chen CJ, et al. Computerized Tomography characteristics that differentiate angiomyolipomas from liposarcomas in the perinephric space. J Urol 2002;167:490–493.
105. Israel GM, Bosniak MA, Slywotzky CM, et al. CT differentiation of large exophytic angiomyolipomas and perirenal liposarcomas. AJR 2002;179:769–773.
106. Robson CJ, Churchill BM, Anderson W, et al. The results of radical nephrectomy for renal cell carcinoma. J Urol 1969;101:297.
107. Fleming ID, et al., editors. American Joint Committee on Cancer (AJCC). AJCC Manual for Staging of Cancer, 5th ed. Philadelphia: Lippincott-Raven, 1997:231–234.
108. Gettman MT, Blute ML, Spotts B, et al. Pathologic staging of renal cell carcinoma. Cancer 2001;91:354–361.
109. Guinan P, Sobin LH, Algaba F, et al. TNM staging of renal cell carcinoma. Cancer 1997; 80:992–993.
110. Sobin LH, Wittekind Ch, eds. International Union Against Cancer (UICC). TNM Classification of Malignant Tumors, 5th ed. New York: UICC, 1997:180–182.
111. Tsui KH, Shvarts O, Smith R, et al. Prognostic indicators for renal cell carcinoma: a multivariate analysis of 643 patients using the revised 1997 TNM staging system. J Urol 200;163:1090–1095.
112. Javidan J, Strciker HJ, Tamboli P, et al. Prognostic significance of the 1997 TNM classification of renal cell carcinoma. J Urol 2000;162:1277–1281.
113. Dinney CP, Awad SA, Gajewski J, et al. Analysis of imaging modalities, staging systems, and prognostic indicators for renal cell carcinoma. Urology 1992;39:122–129.
114. Constantinides C, Recker F, Bruehlmann W, et al. Accuracy of magnetic resonance imaging compared to computerized tomography and selective renal Angiography in preoperatively staging renal cell carcinoma. Urol Int 1991;47:181–185.
115. Bechtold RE, Zagoria RJ. Imaging approach to staging of renal cell carcinoma. Urol Clin North Am 1997; 24:507–522.
116. Johnson CD, Dunnick NR, Cohan RH, et al. Renal adenocarcinoma: CT staging of 100 tumors. AJR 1987;148:59–63.
117. Cronan JJ, Zeman RK, Rosenfeld AT. Comparison of computerized tomography, ultrasound and angiography in staging renal cell carcinoma. J Urol 1982;127:712–714.
118. Prati GF, Saggin P, Boschiero L, et al. Small renal-cell carcinomas: clinical and imaging features. Urol Int 1993;51:19–22.
119. Hricak H, Thoeni RF, Carroll PR, et al. Detection and staging of renal neoplasms: a reassessment of MR imaging. Radiology 1988;166:643–649.
120. Zagoria RJ, Bechtold RE, Dyer RB. Staging of renal adenocarcinoma: role of various imaging procedures. AJR 1995;164:363–370.
121. Roberts WW, Bhayani J, Allaf ME, et al. Pathological stage does not alter the prognosis for renal lesions determined to be stage T1 by computerized tomography. Urology 2005;173:713–715.
122. Ozen H, Colowick A, Freiha FS. Incidentally discovered solid renal masses: what are they? Br J Urol 1993:72:274–276.
123. Siow WY, Yip SK, Ng LG, et al. Renal cell carcinoma: incidental detection and pathological staging. J R Coll Surg Edinb 2000;45:291–295.
124. Thompson RH, Leibovich BC, Cheville JC, et al. Is renal sinus fat invasion the same as perinephric fat invasion for a renal cell carcinoma? J Urol 2005;174:1218–1221.
125. Irani J, Humbert M, Lecocq B, et al. Renal tumor size: comparison between computed tomography and surgical measurements. Eur Urol 2001;39:300–303.
126. Yaycioglu O, Rutman MP, Balasubramaniam M, et al. Clinical and pathologic tumor size in renal cell carcinoma; difference, correlation, and analysis of influencing factors. Urology 2002:60:33–38.

127. Herr HW, Lee CT, Sharma S, et al. Radiographic versus pathologic size of renal tumors: implications for partial nephrectomy. Urology 2001;58:157–160.
128. Khaitan A, Gupta NP, Hemal AK, et al. Is there a need for pelvic CT scan in cases of renal cell carcinoma? Int Urol Nephrol 2002;33;13–15.
129. Fielding JR, Aliabadi N, Renshaw AA, et al. Staging of 119 patients with renal cell carcinoma: the yield and cost-effectiveness of pelvic CT. AJR 1999;172:1721–1723.
130. Lim DJ, Carter F. Computerized tomography in the preoperative staging for pulmonary metastases in patients with renal cell carcinoma, J Urol 1993;150:1112–1114.
131. Tsui KH, Shvarts O, Barbaric Z, et al. Is adrenalectomy a necessary component of radical nephrectomy? UCLA experience with 511 radical nephrectomies. J Urol 2000;163:437–441.
132. Tsui KH, Shvarts O, Smith RB, Figlin R, DeKernion JB, Belldegrun A. Renal cell carcinoma: prognostic significance of incidentally detected tumors. J Urology 2000;163:426–430.
133. Sawai Y, Kinochi T, Mano M, et al. Ipsilateral adrenal involvement from renal cell carcinoma: retrospective study of the predictive value of computed tomography. Urology 2002;59:28–31.
134. Gill IS, McClennan BL, Kerbi K, et al. Adrenal involvement from renal cell carcinoma: predictive value of computerized tomography. J Urol 1994;154:1082–1085.
135. Hamrahian AH, Ioachimescu AG, Remer EM, et al. Clinical utility of noncontrast computed tomography attenuation value (Hounsfield units) to differentiate adrenal adenomas/hyperplasias from nonadenomas: Cleveland Clinic Experience. J Clin Endocr Metab 2005;90:871–877.
136. Israel GM, Korobkin M, Wang C, et al. Comparison of unenhanced CT and chemical shift MRI in evaluating lipid-rich adrenal adenomas. AJR 2004;183:215–219.
137. Hatcher PA, Anderson EE, Paulson DF, et al. Surgical management and prognosis of renal cell carcinoma invading the vena cava. J Urol 1991;145:20–24.
138. Oto A, Herts BR, Remer EM, Novick AC. Inferior vena cava tumor thrombus in renal cell carcinoma: staging by MR imaging and impact on surgical treatment. AJR 1998; 171:1619–1624.
139. Gupta NP, Ansari MD, Khaitan A, et al. Impact of imaging and thrombus level in management of renal cell carcinoma extending to veins. Urol Int 2004;72:129–134.
140. Glazer A, Novick AC. Preoperative transesophageal echocardiography for assessment of venal caval tumor thrombi: a comparative study with venacavography and magnetic resonance imaging. Urology 1997;49:32–34.
141. Lawrentschuk N, Gani J, Riordan R, et al. Multidetector computed tomography vs. magnetic resonance imaging for defining the upper limit of tumour thrombus in renal cell carcinoma: a study and review. BJU Int 2005;96:291–295.
142. Kallman DA, King BF, Hattery RR, et al. Renal vein and inferior vena cava tumor thrombus in renal cell carcinoma: CT, US, MRI and venacavography. J Comput Assist Tomogr 1992;16:240–247.
143. Goldfarb DA, Novick AC, Lorig R, et al. Magnetic resonance imaging for assessment of vena cava tumor thrombi: a comparative study with venacavography and computerized tomography scanning. J Urol 1990;144:1100–1103.
144. Hockley NM, Foster RS, Bihrle R, et al. Use of magnetic resonance imaging to determine surgical approach to renal cell carcinoma with vena caval extension. Urology 1990;36:55–60.
145. Gohji K, Yamashita C, Ueno K, et al. Preoperative computerized Tomography detection of extensive invasion of the inferior vena cava by renal cell carcinoma: possible indication for resection with partial cardiopulmonary bypass and patch grafting. J Urol 1997;152:1993–1996.
146. Motzer RJ, Bander NH, Nanus DM. Medical progress: renal cell carcinoma. N Engl J Med 1996;335:865.
147. Ghavamian R, Klein KA, Stephens DH, et al. Renal cell carcinoma metastatic to the pancreas: clinical and radiographic features. Mayo Clin Proc 2000;75:581–585.
148. Ng CS, Loyer EM, Iyer RB, et al. Metastases to the pancreas from renal cell carcinoma: findings on three-phase contrast-enhanced helical CT. AJR 1999;172:1555–1559.
149. Tartar VM, Heiken JP, McClennan BL. Renal cell carcinoma presenting with diffuse peritoneal metastases: CT findings. J Comput Assist Tomogr 1991;15:450–453.
150. Birnbaum BA, Bosniak MA, Krinsky GA, Cheng D, Waisman J, Ambrosino MM. Renal cell carcinoma: correlation of CT findings with nuclear morphologic grading in 100 tumors. Abdom Imaging 1994;19:262–266.
151. Frank I, Blute ML, Cheville, et al. Solid renal tumors: an analysis of pathological features related to tumor size. J Urol 2003;170:2217–2220.
152. Kelley CM, Cohen MB, Raab SS. Utility of fine-needle aspiration biopsy in solid renal masses. Diagn Cytopathol 1996;14:14–19.

3

The Role of Percutaneous Imaging-Guided Biopsy in the Diagnosis and Management of Renal Masses

Brian R. Herts and Stuart G. Silverman

KEYWORDS

> IMAGING-GUIDED BIOPSY
> RENAL CELL CARCINOMA
> COMPUTED TOMOGRAPHY
> ULTRASOUND
> FINE-NEEDLE ASPIRATION BIOPSY

ABSTRACT

This chapter reviews the role of percutaneous imaging-guided biopsy of renal masses in the diagnosis and management of renal tumors. Percutaneous imaging-guided biopsy of renal masses is a safe, accurate, and lower-cost alternative to surgical biopsy. It can be performed in an outpatient setting and is frequently all that is necessary to establish a diagnosis and effect patient management. Percutaneous biopsy is largely used to differentiate primary renal neoplasms from renal tumors not treated surgically, such as metastatic disease and lymphoma. Percutaneous biopsy is also used to differentiate primary neoplasms from benign renal lesions and to establish a diagnosis of renal cell carcinoma in those patients with widespread metastatic disease or with contraindications to surgery.

Percutaneous imaging-guided biopsy of many abdominal and pelvic masses is a safe, accurate, and lower-cost alternative to open or laparoscopic surgical biopsy and can be performed in an outpatient setting.[1–7] Percutaneous biopsy is frequently all that is necessary to establish a diagnosis and affect patient management.[8–10]

Historically, however, percutaneous biopsy of renal masses has not been as common as percutaneous biopsies of other abdominal masses. Most renal lesions are masses larger than 3 cm, tumors that have a high likelihood of being renal cell carcinoma (RCC). In such cases a negative biopsy would most likely be due to sampling error; and therefore, surgery would still be indicated, negating the need for preoperative

From: *Clinical Management of Renal Tumors*
Edited by: R.M. Bukowski and A.C. Novick © Humana Press Inc., Totowa, NJ

biopsy. Currently, biopsy of a renal mass is not often necessary because of the high sensitivity and specificity of noninvasive cross-sectional imaging, computed tomography (CT), ultrasound (US), and magnetic resonance imaging (MRI) for differentiating between many benign and malignant renal lesions. Percutaneous biopsy of renal masses may not be used because of a lack of familiarity with indications for its use by urologists, radiologists, and oncologists compounded by, until recently, few detailed descriptions of the cytologic features of renal tumors.[11]

Current trends in the diagnosis and management of RCC have created interest in redefining the role for percutaneous biopsy of renal masses; in the last few years there have been several reports regarding the role of percutaneous imaging-guided biopsy in the diagnosis of renal masses, including an assessment of its costs.[9,12–19] Furthermore, the widespread use of CT, MRI, and US has resulted in an increase in the detection of small, less than 3 cm, asymptomatic renal tumors. These incidentally detected tumors are often low-grade, low-stage, slow-growing RCCs, and asymptomatic tumors carry a better prognosis than their symptomatic counterparts.[20–26] Moreover, although these small, incidentally detected masses are often RCCs, a substantial percentage of these masses are benign and a specific diagnosis cannot always be made noninvasively. Cytologic differentiation between benign and malignant etiologies has traditionally been difficult; however, several reports suggest that a specific tissue diagnosis is possible in many cases.[17,27–30] Although there are reports suggesting that percutaneous biopsy may not be sufficient to determine patient management, most reports in the last 8 years on the role of percutaneous fine-needle aspiration and core needle biopsy in the evaluation of renal masses have been favorable.[16,18,28]

Another reason for renewed interest in percutaneous biopsy for the diagnosis of renal masses is the early success of nephron-sparing procedures, including partial nephrectomy and percutaneous ablative therapies (both cryoablation and radiofrequency ablation). In patients with small, low-grade tumors, the nephron-sparing treatments rival that of radical and total nephrectomy.[31–33] While percutaneous biopsy does not usually play a role prior to total nephrectomy, it does play a role in the preoperative evaluation of patients with tumors prior to nephron-sparing procedures; it documents malignancy before treatment.[34] Biopsy is uniquely important prior to percutaneous ablative therapy because there is no other means of confirming the tissue diagnosis.[34]

Principally, percutaneous biopsy is used to differentiate primary renal malignancies from benign renal lesions and from those renal tumors not treated surgically, such as metastatic disease and lymphoma. Another important role biopsy plays is to establish a diagnosis of RCC when a definitive diagnosis is required preoperatively in patients with widespread metastatic disease or with a strong contraindication to surgery.

This chapter reviews the current indications, relative contraindications, and prevailing techniques for percutaneous imaging-guided biopsy of renal masses, whether it is for obtaining cytologic specimens by fine-needle aspiration (FNA) or fine-needle capillary (FNC) (nonaspiration) techniques, or for obtaining histologic specimens by core needle biopsy. The techniques and potential complications of percutaneous imaging-guided biopsy, as well as the sensitivity, specificity, and accuracy of biopsy specimens, are reviewed. Except for direct references to cytologic and histologic sampling, the term *percutaneous biopsy* refers to FNA, FNC, and core biopsy. The imaging techniques and differential diagnoses of renal masses are beyond the scope of this chapter.

INDICATIONS AND RELATIVE CONTRAINDICATIONS

Prior to the introduction of US, CT, and MRI over the last two and a half decades, renal cyst aspiration and angiography were used with a moderate degree of accuracy to characterize masses identified on intravenous urography (IVU).[35] However, with the high diagnostic accuracy available with US, CT, and MRI for the identification of both benign and malignant diseases, there is little indication to use percutaneous biopsy to confirm many radiographically benign lesions: simple cysts, benign complicated cysts, and angiomyolipomas demonstrating fat at CT. Conversely, when a renal mass has typical imaging features of RCC, a positive or negative biopsy will not alter surgical management. In these cases a percutaneous biopsy is not necessary. Furthermore, cyst aspiration is not recommended to confirm a simple cyst since cyst aspiration can be falsely negative even in the presence of mural tumors within a cyst.

There are several indications for percutaneous biopsy of renal masses (Table 3.1). In general, percutaneous biopsy can and should be used to differentiate benign from malignant disease, and surgical from nonsurgical disease.[9,12] Renal cell carcinoma can appear as a solid, complex cystic, or infiltrating lesion on cross-sectional imaging. Based on the appearance, the differential diagnosis may include transitional cell carcinoma, oncocytoma, metastatic disease, juxtaglomerular tumor, lymphoma, angiomyolipoma, focal bacterial nephritis, renal abscess, and renal sarcoma.[36]

Percutaneous imaging-guided biopsy is indicated to differentiate metastatic disease, lymphoma, or renal abscess from primary RCC. This is because treatment is nonsurgical in the case of metastatic disease, lymphoma, and renal abscess, and surgical for primary RCC.[2,4,9,20,37,38] The medical history will often give some indication as to how strongly some of these differential possibilities should be considered, but the history may be insufficient to establish a firm diagnosis.

Metastatic disease to the kidneys is particularly common with lung carcinoma and lymphoma, but can also be seen with pancreatic carcinoma, malignant melanoma, and hepatocellular carcinoma.[39] Wood et al.[9] reported that when there was a history of a nonrenal primary, 50% of renal masses were metastatic disease. Although metastatic

Table 3.1.
Established indications and relative contraindications for percutaneous biopsy of renal masses

Established indications	To distinguish between a primary renal cell carcinoma and metastasis in patients with an extrarenal primary malignancy
	To establish a diagnosis of renal cell carcinoma or another primary tumor in a patient with disseminated metastases or an unresectable tumor
	To establish a diagnosis of benign or malignant disease in patients with relative contraindications to surgery
	To establish and document a diagnosis before percutaneous ablative therapies
	To investigate an infectious cause
Relative contraindications	Imaging suggestive of transitional cell carcinoma
	Uncorrectable bleeding diathesis
	Lack of a safe access route

disease to the kidneys is more often multiple and bilateral, in another study 85% of patients with a solitary renal mass and an extrarenal primary malignancy had metastatic disease to the kidneys; 15% had RCC as a second primary malignancy.[40] Gattuso et al.[39] reported that 89% of the patients with metastatic disease to the kidney had a history of a primary malignancy. In patients with a history of lymphoma, or secondary evidence of lymphoma such as splenomegaly or massive or distant lymphadenopathy, a small solitary renal mass may be lymphoma rather than a primary RCC. Biopsy, therefore, is indicated to distinguish between lymphoma and RCC, again distinguishing between nonsurgical and surgical management of disease.[9,27]

Another important indication for percutaneous biopsy is to establish a tissue diagnosis of a renal mass in those patients with disseminated metastatic disease, unresectable renal tumors, or other contraindications to surgical intervention.[10,37] In patients with disseminated metastases from a previously undiagnosed primary tumor, or in patients with unresectable RCC, percutaneous biopsy can document a primary renal tumor or metastatic disease to the kidney. In many patients with metastatic disease, biopsy of the renal mass is the most direct, safest, and least invasive route.

Percutaneous biopsy is also indicated in patients with medical contraindications to surgery because documentation of benign disease would obviate surgery and confirmation of malignant disease might influence treatment plans regarding underlying illnesses. Similarly, percutaneous biopsy may be useful in documenting benign lesions when complex cystic renal lesions are indeterminate radiographically, avoiding unnecessary surgery.[41] However, this is not universally accepted because of the potential for a falsely negative biopsy.[42] Finally, percutaneous biopsy can also provide an accurate diagnosis of a small, low-grade primary RCC, allowing for imaging surveillance without surgical intervention; close interval follow-up has been advocated as an option to surgery when tumors are small and slow-growing.[24]

A potential advantage of performing percutaneous biopsy before surgical therapy is to identify the nuclear grade of an RCC. Although the accuracy and sensitivity of CT and MRI for the diagnosis of RCC is quite high, the accuracy of CT for predicting nuclear grade is poor.[25,43] Since survival rates for RCC inversely correlate with both the stage and nuclear grade of the tumor, preoperative knowledge of the nuclear grade may influence the decision between total nephrectomy and nephron-sparing surgery. Elective nephron-sparing surgery may not be indicated for high-grade tumors. Unfortunately, reports of accuracy of FNA biopsy for predicting nuclear grade are mixed.[27,44–46]

Relative Contraindications

Percutaneous biopsy is generally not indicated in a patient without a history of a primary malignancy when a renal lesion appears radiographically as a typical solid or complex cystic RCC.[36,47] This is especially true for patients in whom the tumor is not suited for nephron-sparing surgery. In this situation, if patients are to undergo total nephrectomy, there is little to be gained by percutaneous biopsy; since there is a high likelihood that the renal lesion is RCC, a negative biopsy is more than likely to be a false negative due to sampling error.

Suspected transitional cell carcinoma (TCC) is a relative contraindication to percutaneous biopsy, although biopsy can establish a diagnosis.[48] Since urine cytology is noninvasive and ureteroscopy and biopsy are minimally invasive means to establish a diagnosis of TCC, a diagnosis can frequently be made without increasing the potential for tumor seeding outside the urothelial tract.[49] Transitional cell carcinoma is thought to have a higher propensity for seeding due to the high incidence of multiplicity in the urinary tract.

Other contraindications to percutaneous biopsy include relative contraindications common to all percutaneous abdominal biopsies, including uncorrectable bleeding disorders and lack of safe access.[6,10]

TECHNIQUES

Preprocedural Hemostatic Evaluation

Self-limited, clinically insignificant bleeding from the kidney following a renal mass biopsy or renal parenchymal biopsy is fairly common,[19] but hemorrhage that warrants treatment is rare. The risk of bleeding is increased for any procedure with abnormal coagulation factors, however. The most appropriate and cost-effective means of performing a meaningful hemostatic screening evaluation prior to percutaneous biopsy and other minor but invasive procedures is not truly known; however, most authors agree on the need for a thorough screening history of bleeding problems.[50] A detailed history regarding medications, specifically warfarin, heparin, aspirin, and nonsteroidal antiinflammatory medications, is also advised.[50] Recommended preprocedural testing includes an evaluation of primary and secondary hemostasis. Primary hemostasis, specifically platelet plugging, can be evaluated by platelet count or bleeding time. Secondary hemostasis, the formation of fibrin, is usually evaluated by prothrombin time (PT) and partial thromboplastin time (PTT). The ratio of PT to a control, the international normalized ratio (INR), is used at many institutions instead of the PT.

The risks of percutaneous procedures are categorized into two groups: minor procedures (paracentesis, thoracentesis, cyst aspiration) with minimal risks of significant complications, and invasive procedures (catheter placements, percutaneous biopsies) with small but defined risks.[50] Silverman and colleagues[50] recommend different preprocedural screening tests determined by the medical bleeding history and the procedure planned. Percutaneous biopsy of a renal mass is an invasive procedure with small but defined risks. In a patient with a normal bleeding history, the screening evaluation includes PT or INR, PTT, and platelets. This evaluation measures both primary and secondary hemostatic mechanisms. One might argue that since some minor surgical procedures are performed without laboratory testing in healthy patients, laboratory evaluation is not necessary for minor invasive radiologic procedures. However, while intraoperative hemostasis can be achieved during minor surgical procedures, it cannot be achieved during percutaneous procedures.

In patients with an abnormal bleeding history, a thorough evaluation of bleeding parameters is recommended; PT, PTT, platelet count, INR, and bleeding time are suggested.[50] Further laboratory evaluation may be necessary including clotting factor assays and thrombin time. In a patient with abnormal bleeding parameters, it may be best to obtain a formal hematology consultation to determine the appropriate screening tests and the clinical significance of any abnormal test results.

Aspirin should be stopped 5 to 7 days prior to the procedure, or 3 to 4 days if taken infrequently. Warfarin and heparin should also be stopped prior to the procedure; the common practice is to convert patients on warfarin to heparin and then stop the heparin 4 to 6 hours prior to the procedure.

At our institutions, INR, PTT, and platelet count are obtained prior to most invasive procedures. An INR <1.5, a platelet count >50,000 U/ml to 60,000 U/ml, and a normal PTT are considered acceptable parameters within which to proceed. *As always, when requesting or forgoing specific laboratory evaluations of hemostasis, one must treat each patient on an individual basis, taking into account the medical history, the indications for the biopsy, and the technical difficulty of the procedure before proceeding with a biopsy.*

Imaging-Guided Procedure Techniques

During the procedure, patients are usually administered intravenous (IV) sedation, with the goal of achieving a moderate degree of conscious sedation (wherein the patient remains responsive); deep sedation is not usually necessary, and may be detrimental since the patient must be able to suspend respiration intermittently during the procedure. Percutaneous imaging-guided biopsies of renal masses are performed using CT, US, or MRI; fluoroscopically guided renal biopsies are now historical. In Europe and Japan, percutaneous biopsy of renal masses are more often performed using US guidance, while in the United States percutaneous biopsy is performed using ultrasound or CT guidance.[4,38] This difference is because of the greater availability of ultrasound relative to CT in European and Asian countries, which is not a factor in the United States. The choice among CT, US, and MRI should be made on the basis of lesion size, accessibility, and ability to visualize the lesion, as well as user familiarity and preference. The accuracy of CT-guided biopsy approaches 90%,[28] similar to that of US-guided biopsy.[28,51]

The general method of performing CT- and US-guided biopsies is similar, but there are relative advantages and disadvantages to each. Computed tomography has a higher sensitivity than US for detection and visualization of renal masses, but CT-guided procedures may be more expensive and time-consuming.[10] Iodinated contrast material may be needed during CT-guided biopsies to help identify the tumor since renal masses are often isodense on unenhanced CT scans. As a result, CT may be of limited use in patients with renal insufficiency. Ultrasound has the advantage of real-time imaging allowing the operator to compensate for patients who have difficulty suspending respiration. However, a major limitation to the use of US guidance is that small and isoechoic renal masses are often not visualized sonographically. Another limitation to the use of US for guidance is a limited ability to visualize the route of access to ensure that pleural space and bowel are not transgressed. In general, the shortest route that does not traverse bowel or solid organs, e.g., lung, liver, spleen, kidney, or renal hilus, is preferred.

Patients can be placed in a supine, prone, or decubitus position as necessary to provide the best access for any imaging-guided procedure. Computed tomography–fluoroscopy (real-time CT visualization) is now available to image the location of the needle during its placement. With a posterior approach in the prone position, the lung may be interposed in the access route increasing the risk of pneumothorax. This is more common for upper pole than lower pole lesions.[52] Decubitus positioning with the affected side down can be used to minimize the risk of pneumothorax.

Ultrasound-guided biopsies are performed either "free-hand" or with a needle-guide attached to the transducer. The free-hand method allows independent movement of both the sampling needle and the transducer in order to visualize needle placement. This can be more difficult for an inexperienced operator but with experience it is a more flexible technique. The needle guide is used in conjunction with the transducer and identifies a path for the needle at angles specific to the guide. This allows for direct placement and visualization of the sampling needle along a specified path.

Many different sizes and types of biopsy needles are available, including beveled-edge needles and serrated-tip needles for aspiration and capillary technique procedures, as well as mechanical and automated spring-loaded cutting devices for core biopsies. In general, fine-needle sizes (19 to 25 gauge) are used to biopsy renal masses because the risk of bleeding is less than with large-gauge needles (less than 19 gauge).[53] For obtaining adequate specimens, the size and type of needle used are less important than the proper use of the needle and the experience of the user.

At our institutions, a cytologist or cytotechnologist evaluates aspirates during the biopsy to determine if there is adequate cellularity. If initial aspirates are insufficient for diagnosis, larger gauge needles can be used. If rapid evaluation of cytologic specimens is not available to confirm if the specimen contains adequate cellularity, two passes are often sufficient to obtain a specimen and have been reported successful in 97% of patients.[38] In addition to cytology or histologic evaluation, specimens should be sent for Gram stain, fungal stain, acid-fast bacilli stain, and culture if there is clinical suspicion for infection, including tuberculosis.

POTENTIAL COMPLICATIONS

The major complications of percutaneous biopsy are bleeding, pneumothorax, and tumor seeding (TS) along the needle tract; bleeding is cited as the most frequent complication.[2] In one study of percutaneous imaging-guided renal biopsies, the rate of significant complications was 6%, although only one of 51 patients in that series required transfusion for persistent excessive hematuria.[4] Mild bleeding is common; there was CT evidence of perinephric hemorrhage reported in approximately 90% of patients in a series of 200 percutaneous renal biopsies.[54] When a patient develops signs or symptoms suggesting hemorrhage after a biopsy, CT is usually recommended because it is more sensitive and accurate than US for the detection of perinephric hemorrhage.[54] Gross hematuria occurs in 5% of patients but is usually self-limited and resolves in 3 days.[2] Persistent gross hematuria may be due to an arteriovenous fistula or large vessel laceration and should be treated appropriately.

As noted, pneumothorax may occur particularly when using the posterior approach for upper pole lesions. When a patient lies prone for a renal biopsy, the posterior segments of the lower lobes of both lungs can expand into the access route. This is seen in up to 30% of patients.[52] Angling from below the ribs, placing the patient in a decubitus position (affected side down), injecting sterile normal saline to increase the paraspinal window, or performing the biopsy in expiration may all minimize or eliminate the amount of lung traversed to access the lesion.

Probably the most controversial complication of percutaneous biopsy is TS along the needle tract. In a large review of percutaneous biopsy of abdominal masses, TS occurred in less than 0.01% of cases.[1] Tumor seeding occurred most frequently with biopsies of pancreatic cancer; only three cases of TS originated from biopsy of RCC. Most cases of TS presented within 2 to 6 months of the procedure, with only one case presenting 5 years after the biopsy. There is no indication that the size of the needle is related to the tendency to seed; in five case reports, a variety of different needle types were used.[40,55–58] Tumor seeding may occur more frequently with aspiration needles than with cutting needles.[1]

There are several case reports of TS from percutaneous biopsies of renal tumors,[49,55–58] but there is no large series specifically devoted to TS from renal mass biopsy; furthermore, there have been no peer-reviewed published case reports or series regarding needle tract seeding from percutaneous biopsy of renal tumors in the last several years. There is no consensus as to the importance of the risk of TS; conclusions vary in case reports, probably reflecting author bias. For example, in one report the authors specifically write that biopsy is contraindicated for the diagnosis of solid renal masses due to the risk of TS.[55] In another report the authors suggest that the role of biopsy be limited to the confirmation of benign disease because of the risk of TS. Still another group writes that biopsy should be used only for equivocal noninvasive imaging.[49,58]

Although TS from a percutaneous biopsy of a renal mass is rare, a route for the biopsy that avoids traversing the liver, spleen, and bowel should be used whenever possible. This should make any recurrent tumor simpler to detect and easier to treat. In our opinion, the risk of TS should not be considered a contraindication to biopsy whenever there is an appropriate indication.

Infection is an uncommon complication, easily treatable, and is not usually discussed in reviews. Infection can be introduced into the cutaneous or subcutaneous tissues, or the biopsied organ.[1,2] Death from a percutaneous needle biopsy is rare but is a potential complication of any procedure. Deaths are extremely uncommon without significant comorbid conditions; in a large survey of complications following abdominal mass biopsies, the death rate from percutaneous biopsy was less than 0.1%.[1] The mortality rate from renal mass biopsy is likely to be considerably below this rate.

SENSITIVITY, SPECIFICITY, AND ACCURACY OF PERCUTANEOUS BIOPSY

A variety of renal tumors can be diagnosed accurately by percutaneous biopsy, including renal adenocarcinoma, sarcomatoid renal cell carcinoma,[59] TCC, angiomyolipoma,[60,61] leiomyosarcoma,[62] lymphoma,[63] multilocular cystic nephroma,[64] and metastatic carcinoma.[39] More recently, several studies have reported on the ability of biopsy to distinguish between renal oncocytoma and RCC, including the chromophobe subtype.[65–69] These studies conclude that oncocytoma can now reliably be differentiated from low-grade RCC and chromophobe RCC. Previously, this had not been the case, but may now be possible due to improvements in cytologic analysis, specimen retrieval, and more detailed descriptions of the cytologic features of each.[69] This is important because imaging cannot yet reliably be used to differentiate between oncocytoma and RCC.[70]

There are several reports of sensitivity, specificity, and positive and negative predictive values for imaging-guided and non–imaging-guided renal mass biopsies.[4,11,37,38,71–76] (Table 3.2) When imaging was used, there was a wide variation in imaging-guided techniques, with biopsies performed using fluoroscopy, US, and CT guidance. Many different needle sizes and types were also used. Overall, the sensitivity of cytology (biopsy with FNA or FNC) for the diagnosis of renal tumors is 80% to 90%, and for histology 70% to 92%. The specificity is reported to be 80% to 100% for cytology and as high as 100% for histology. Positive and negative predictive values for both cytology and histology are 90% to 95%, with an accuracy of 87% to 93%.[4,11,37,38,71–76]

Table 3.2.
Reported test characteristics for diagnosis of renal masses by
percutaneous imaging-guided biopsy

	Overall range reported
Sensitivity	70–92%
Specificity	83–100%
Positive predictive value	90–95%
Negative predictive value	87–93%

Note: Combined from references 4, 10, 36, 37, and 69–74.

False-positive diagnoses of malignancy have been reported with multiloculated cystic nephroma,[77] angiomyolipoma,[71,73] and chronic pyelonephritis.[71,72] However, these reports are all from 18 years ago or longer, and may reflect old cytologic diagnostic criteria. One group reported a higher false-positive rate for cytology compared with histology.[75] In general, the specificity and accuracy for cytology is high, but ultimately dependent upon the skills of cytologists and their familiarity with the cytologic features of the disease processes. False-negative diagnoses are most often due to insufficient specimens, which are often bloody aspirates. In one series, a sarcomatoid renal cell cancer was misdiagnosed as xanthogranulomatous pyelonephritis.[11]

The reliability of tumor grading from cytologic and histologic specimens has also been reported.[44,45] In one series, 76% of specimens were graded correctly; the remaining 24% were incorrectly graded by only one grade. Variable grades were also seen within the same tumor in 25% of cases.[44] There is a high concordance rate between nuclear grade assessed with percutaneous biopsy specimens and nuclear grade assessed with pathologic specimens.[45,46]

CONCLUSION

Percutaneous imaging-guided biopsy of renal masses is both safe and accurate. Oncologists, urologists, and radiologists should all be familiar with the role of percutaneous biopsy, including the indications, relative contraindications, techniques, risks, and potential complications. Percutaneous imaging-guided biopsy is best reserved for diagnosis of suspected metastatic disease to the kidneys, for diagnosis before ablative therapies, for diagnosis of a RCC in patients with unresectable tumors or disseminated metastases, and for diagnosis of renal lymphoma. Percutaneous biopsy is also indicated if there is clinical evidence of infection, or if there are contraindications to surgical intervention. In all of these situations, the results of percutaneous imaging-guided biopsy will impact the care of the patient.

REFERENCES

1. Smith EH. Complications of percutaneous abdominal fine-needle biopsy. Radiology 1991; 178:253–258.
2. Vassiliades VG, Bernardino ME. Percutaneous renal and adrenal biopsies. Cardiovasc Intervent Radiol 1991;14:50–54.
3. Welch TJ, Sheedy PF 2nd, Johnson CD, et al. CT-guided biopsy: prospective analysis of 1,000 procedures. Radiology 1989;171:493–496.

4. Nadel L, Baumgartner BR, Bernardino ME. Percutaneous renal biopsies: accuracy, safety, and indications. Urol Radiol 1986;8:67–71.
5. Dunnick NR, Leder RA, Rouxbidoux MA. Percutaneous biopsy of the kidney and adrenal gland. Urol Radiol 1990;12:125–129.
6. Charboneau JW, Reading CC, Welch TJ. CT and sonographically guided needle biopsy: current techniques and new innovations. AJR 1990;154:1–10.
7. Silverman SG, Deuson TE, Kane N, et al. Percutaneous abdominal biopsy: cost-identification analysis. Radiology 1998;206:429–435.
8. Bree RL, Jafri SZ, Schwab RE, et al. Abdominal fine needle aspiration biopsies with CT and ultrasound guidance: techniques, results and clinical implications. Comput Radiol 1984;8:9–15.
9. Wood BJ, Khan MA, McGovern F, et al. Imaging guided biopsy of renal masses: indications, accuracy and impact on clinical management. J Urol 1999;161:1470–1474.
10. Gazelle GS, Haaga JR. Guided percutaneous biopsies of intraabdominal lesions. AJR 1989;153:929–935.
11. Murphy WM, Zambroni BR, Emerson LD, et al. Aspiration biopsy of the kidney. Cancer 1985;56:200–205.
12. Hara I, Miyake H, Hara S, et al. Role of percutaneous image-guided biopsy in the evaluation of renal masses. Urol Int 2001;67:199–201.
13. Richter F, Kasabian NG, Irwin RJ Jr., et al. Accuracy of diagnosis by guided biopsy of renal mass lesions classified indeterminate by imaging studies. Urology 2000;55:348–352.
14. Nguyen GK, Akin MR. Fine needle aspiration cytology of the kidney, renal pelvis, and adrenal. Clin Lab Med 1998;18:429–459.
15. Phillips MD, Silverman SG, Cibas ES, et al. Negative predictive value of imaging-guided abdominal biopsy results: cytologic classifications and implications for patient management. AJR 1998; 171:693–696.
16. Brierly RD, Thomas PJ, Harrison NW, et al. Evaluation of fine-needle aspiration cytology for renal masses. BJU Int 2000;85:14–18.
17. Lang EK, Macchia RJ, Gayle B, et al. CT-guided biopsy of indeterminate renal cystic masses (Bosniak 3 and 2F): accuracy and impact on clinical management. Eur Radiol 2002;12:2518–2524.
18. Dechet CB, Zincke H, Sebo TJ, et al. Prospective analysis of computerized tomography and needle biopsy with permanent sectioning to determine the nature of solid renal masses in adults. J Urol 2003;169:71–74.
19. Campbell SC, Novick AC, Herts BR, et al. Prospective evaluation of fine needle aspiration of small, solid renal masses: accuracy and morbidity. Urology 1997;50:25–29.
20. Curry N. Small renal masses (lesions smaller than 3 cm): imaging evaluation and management. AJR 1995;164:355–362.
21. Smith SJ, Bosniak MA, Megibow AJ. Renal cell carcinoma: earlier discovery and increased detection. Radiology 1989;170:699–703.
22. Thompson IM, Peek M. Improvement in survival of patients with renal cell carcinoma—the role of the serendipitously detected tumor. J Urol 1988;140:487–490.
23. Breatheau D, Lechevallier E, Eghazarian C, et al. Prognostic significance of incidental renal cell carcinoma. Eur Urol 1995;27:319–323.
24. Birnbaum BA, Bosniak MA, Megibow AJ, et al: Observations on the growth of renal neoplasms. Radiology 1990;176:695–701.
25. Birnbaum BA, Bosniak MA, Krinsky GA, et al. Renal Cell Carcinoma: correlation of CT findings with nuclear morphologic grading in 100 tumors. Abdom Imaging 1994;19:262–266.
26. Frank I, Blute ML, Cheville JC, et al. Solid renal tumors: an analysis of pathological features related to tumor size. J Urol 2003;170:2217–2220.
27. Neuzillet Y, Lechevallier E, Andre M, et al. Accuracy and clinical role of fine needle percutaneous biopsy with computerized tomography guidance of small (less than 4.0 cm) renal masses. J Urol 2004;171:1802–1805.
28. Caoili EM, Bude RO, Higgins EJ, et al. Evaluation of sonographically guided percutaneous core biopsy of renal masses. AJR 2002;179:373–378.
29. Lechevallier E, Andre M, Barriol D, et al. Fine-needle percutaneous biopsy of renal masses with helical CT guidance. Radiology 2000;216:506–510.
30. Zardawi IM. Renal fine needle aspiration cytology. Acta Cytol 1999;43:184–190.
31. Novick AC, Streem S, Montie JE, et al. Conservative surgery for renal cell carcinoma: a single-center experience with 100 patients. J Urol 1989;141:835–839.

32. Provet J, Tessler A, Brown J, et al. Partial nephrectomy for renal cell carcinoma: indications, results and implications. J Urol 1991;145:472–476.

33. Thrasher JB, Robertson JE, Paulson DE. Expanding indications for conservative renal surgery in renal cell carcinoma. Urology 1994;43:160–168.

34. Tuncali K, van Sonnenberg E, Shankar S, et al. Evaluation of patients referred for percutaneous ablation of renal tumors: importance of a preprocedural diagnosis. AJR 2004;183:575–582.

35. Sandler CM, Houston GK, Hall JT, et al. Guided cyst puncture and aspiration. Radiol Clin North Am 1986;24:527–537.

36. Bosniak M. The small (≤3.0 cm) renal parenchymal tumor: detection, diagnosis, and controversies. Radiology 1991;179:307–317.

37. Niceforo J, Coughlin B. Diagnosis of renal cell carcinoma: value of fine-needle aspiration cytology in patients with metastases or contraindications to nephrectomy. AJR 1993;161:1303–1305.

38. Cristallini EG, Paganelli C, Bolis GB. Role of fine-needle aspiration biopsy in the assessment of renal masses. Diagn Cytopathol 1991;7:32–35.

39. Gattuso P, Ramzy I, Truong LD, et al. Utilization of fine-needle aspiration in the diagnosis of metastatic tumors to the kidney. Diagn Cytopathol 1999;21:35–38.

40. Mitnick JS, Bosniak MA, Rothberg M. Metastatic neoplasm to the kidney studied by computed tomography and sonography. J Comput Assist Tomogr 1985;9:43–49.

41. Harishingani MG, Maher MM, Gervais DA, et al. Incidence of malignancy in complex cystic masses (Bosniak category III): should imaging-guided biopsy precede surgery? AJR 2003;180:755–758.

42. Bosniak MA. Should we biopsy complex cystic renal masses (Bosniak III)? AJR 2003; 181:1425–1426.

43. Nurmi M, Tyrkko J, Puntala P, et al. Reliability of aspiration biopsy cytology in the grading of renal adenocarcinoma. Scand J Urol Nephrol 1984;18:151–156.

44. Cajulis RS, Katz RL, Dekmezian R, El-Naggar A. Fine needle aspiration biopsy of renal cell carcinoma: cytologic parameters and their concordance with histology and flow cytometric data. Acta Cytol 1993;37:367–372.

45. Zagoria R, Bechtold R, Dyer R. Staging of renal adenocarcinoma: role of various imaging procedures. AJR 1995;164:363–370.

46. Kelley CM, Cohen MB, Raab SS. Utility of fine-needle aspiration biopsy in solid renal masses. Diagn Cytopathol 1996;14:14–19.

47. Bosniak MA. The current radiological approach to renal cysts. Radiology 1986;58:1–10.

48. Santamaria M, Jauregui I, Urtasun F, et al. Fine needle aspiration biopsy in urothelial carcinoma of the renal pelvis. Acta Cytol 1995;39:443–448.

49. Gibbons RP, Bush WH, Burnett LL. Needle tract seeding following aspiration of renal cell carcinoma. J Urol 1977;118:865–867.

50. Silverman SG, Mueller PR, Pfister RC. Hemostatic evaluation before abdominal interventions: an overview and proposal. AJR 1990;154:233–238.

51. Johnson PT, Nazarian LN, Feld RI, et al. Sonographically guided renal mass biopsy: indications and efficacy. J Ultrasound Med 2001;20:749–753.

52. Hopper KD, Yakes WF. The posterior intercostal approach for percutaneous renal procedures: risk of puncturing the lung, spleen and liver as determined by CT. AJR 1990;54:115–117.

53. Gazelle GS, Haaga JR, Rowland DY. Effect of needle gauge, level of anticoagulation, and target organ on bleeding associated with aspiration biopsy. Radiology 1992;83:509–513.

54. Ralls PW, Barakos JA, Kaptein EM, et al. Renal biopsy-related hemorrhage: frequency and comparison of CT and sonography. J Comput Assist Tomogr 1987;11:1031–1034.

55. Wehle MJ, Grabstald H. Contraindications to needle aspiration of a solid renal mass: tumor dissemination by renal needle aspiration. J Urol 1986;136:446–448.

56. Slywotzky C, Maya M. Needle tract seeding of transitional cell carcinoma following fine-needle aspiration of a renal mass. Abdom Imaging 1994;19:174–176.

57. Shenoy PD, Lakhkar BN, Ghosh MK, et al. Cutaneous seeding of renal carcinoma by Chiba needle aspiration biopsy. Acta Radiol 1991;32:50–52.

58. Kiser GC, Totonchy M, Barry JM. Needle tract seeding after percutaneous renal adenocarcinoma aspiration. J Urol 1986;136:1292–1293.

59. Auger M, Katz Rl, Sella A, et al. Fine-needle aspiration cytology of sarcomatoid renal cell carcinoma: a morphologic and immunocytochemical study of 15 cases. Diagn Cytopathol 1996;14:14–19.

60. Sant GR, Ayers DK, Bankoff MS, et al. Fine needle aspiration biopsy in the diagnosis of renal angiomyolipoma. J Urol 1990;143:999–1001.

61. Bonzanini M, Pea M, Martignoni G, et al. Preoperative diagnosis of renal angiomyolipoma: fine-needle aspiration cytology and immunocytochemical characterization. Pathology 1994;26:170–175.

62. Villanueva RR, Nguyen-Ho P, Nguyen GK. Leiomyosarcoma of the kidney: report of a case diagnosed by fine needle aspiration cytology and electron microscopy. Acta Cytol 1994;38:568–572.

63. Truong LD, Caraway N, Ngo T, et al. Renal Lymphoma. The diagnostic and therapeutic roles of fine-needle aspiration. Am J Clin Pathol 2001;115:18–31.

64. Clark SP, Kung IT, Tang SK. Fine-needle aspiration of cystic nephroma (multi-locular cyst of the kidney). Diagnostic Cytopathol 1992;8:349–351.

65. Renshaw AA, Lee KR, Madge R, et al. Accuracy of fine-needle aspiration in distinguishing subtypes of renal cell carcinoma. Acta Cytol 1997;41:987–994.

66. Granter SR, Renshaw AA. Fine-needle aspiration of chromophobe renal cell carcinoma. Cancer 1997;81:122–128.

67. Akhtar M, Ali MA. Aspiration of chromophobe cell carcinoma of the kidney. Diagn Cytopathol 1995;13:287–294.

68. Wiatrowska BA, Zakowski MF. Fine-needle aspiration biopsy of chromophobe renal cell carcinoma and oncocytoma: comparison of cytomorphologic features. Cancer 1999;87:161–167.

69. Liu J, Fanning CV. Can renal oncocytomas be distinguished from renal cell carcinoma on fine-needle aspiration specimens? A study of conventional smears in conjunction with ancillary studies. Cancer 2001;93:390–397.

70. Davidson AJ, Hayes WJ, Hartman DS, et al. Renal oncocytoma and carcinoma: failure of differentiation with CT. Radiology 1993;186:693–696.

71. Leiman G. Audit of fine needle aspiration cytology of 120 renal lesions. Cytopathology 1990;1:65–72.

72. Helm CW, Burwood RJ, Harrison NW, et al. Aspiration cytology of solid renal tumours. Br J Urol 1983;55:249–253.

73. Orell SR, Langlois SL, Marshall VR. Fine needle aspiration cytology in the diagnosis of solid renal and adrenal masses. Scand J Urol Nephrol 1985;19:211–216.

74. Juul N, Torp-Pedersen S, Gronvall S, et al. Ultrasonically guided fine needle aspiration biopsy of renal masses. J Urol 1985;133:579–581.

75. Torp-Pedersen S, Juul N, Larsen T, et al. US-Guided fine needle biopsy of solid renal masses—comparison of histology and cytology. Scand J Urol Nephrol Suppl 1991;137:41–43.

76. Abe M, Saitoh M. Selective renal tumour biopsy under ultrasonic guidance. Br J Urol 1992;70:7–11.

77. Pilotti S, Rilke F, Alasio L, et al. The role of fine needle aspiration in the assessment of renal masses. Acta Cytol 1988;32:1–10.

4   Pathology of Renal Cell Carcinomas

Ming Zhou

KEYWORDS

RENAL CELL CARCINOMA
CLEAR-CELL RENAL CELL CARCINOMA
PAPILLARY RENAL CELL CARCINOMA
CHROMOPHOBE RENAL CELL CARCINOMA
COLLECTING-DUCT RENAL CELL CARCINOMA
Xp11.2/TFE3 RENAL CELL CARCINOMA
RENAL ONCOCYTOMA
WHO CLASSIFICATION
PATHOLOGY
CYTOGENETICS
PROGNOSIS

ABSTRACT

A wide range of neoplasms can occur in the kidney. Renal cell neoplasms, a group of heterogeneous tumors arising from the renal tubular epithelium, represent over 90% of all the tumors in adult kidneys. These tumors have characteristic pathologic, cytogenetic, and molecular characteristics, and biologic behavior and therapeutic outcomes. The 2004 World Health Organization classification of renal tumors represent the most updated classification system based on histomorphology and genetics. Pathologic examination of the renal cell carcinoma specimens is critical because it not only renders diagnosis, but also provides information important for prognosis and therapeutic decisions. In addition, tumor tissues could be procured for clinical trials and experimental studies. Furthermore, pathologists could allocate any redundant tumor tissues not required for diagnosis to basic research programs. Pathologists, urologists, and other clinicians play equally important roles in the optimal handling and processing of renal cell carcinoma specimens.

A wide array of tumors has been described in the kidney. Renal cell carcinoma (RCC), a group of heterogeneous tumors arising from the epithelium of the renal tubules, accounts for over 90% of all malignancies in adult kidneys. These tumors have unique pathologic, cytogenetic, and molecular characteristics. They also have distinct biologic behavior, clinical manifestation, and therapeutic response.

From: *Clinical Management of Renal Tumors*
Edited by: R.M. Bukowski and A.C. Novick © Humana Press Inc., Totowa, NJ

Table 4.1.
**2004 World Health Organization (WHO) classification of
renal cell neoplasms**

Renal cell carcinoma
    Clear-cell renal cell carcinoma
    Multilocular cystic clear-cell renal cell carcinoma
    Papillary renal cell carcinoma
    Chromophobe renal cell carcinoma
    Carcinoma of the collecting ducts of Bellini
    Renal medullary carcinoma
    Xp11 translocation carcinomas
    Carcinoma associated with neuroblastoma
    Mucinous tubular and spindle cell carcinoma
    Renal cell carcinoma, unclassified
Papillary adenoma/renal cortical adenoma
Oncocytoma

HISTOLOGIC CLASSIFICATION OF RENAL CELL CARCINOMA

The current classification, published by the World Health Organization (WHO) in 2004 (Table 4.1),[1] is based on histomorphology, presumptive histogenic origin, and cytogenetic and molecular characteristics of the renal tumors. The genetic criterion has also been incorporated into this classification. Although this classification is still based primarily on histomorphology, it has been recognized that different histologic subtypes of RCC have characteristic cytogenetic and molecular changes. For example, RCC associated with Xp11.2 translocation is a group of RCCs with chromosomal translocations involving the *TFE3* gene on chromosome Xp11.2. Although morphologically it may overlap with clear cell or papillary RCCs, it has been defined as a distinct clinico-pathologic entity based on this characteristic genetic change.[2] It is hoped that in the future, a classification based on the molecular and genetic characteristics of the different subtypes of RCC will provide not only more accurate pathologic classification, but also better prognostic and therapeutic information and may help design more specific, genetically based therapeutic strategies.

HISTOLOGIC SUBTYPES OF RENAL CELL CARCINOMA

Renal Cell Carcinoma, Clear Cell Type

CLINICAL FEATURES

Clear-cell renal cell carcinoma (CCRCC) is the most common histologic subtype, accounting for 60% to 70% of all renal cell neoplasms. Its peak incidence is in the 6th and 7th decades of life. The disease predominantly affects men, with a male to female ratio of 2:1.[3] The majority of CCRCC arises sporadically, with <5% of the cases presenting as part of the inherited cancer syndromes,[4] including von Hippel–Lindau syndrome, tuberous sclerosis, Birt-Hogg-Dubé syndrome, and constitutional chromosomal 3 translocation syndrome. In general, familial CCRCC presents at a younger age and is more likely to be multifocal and bilateral.

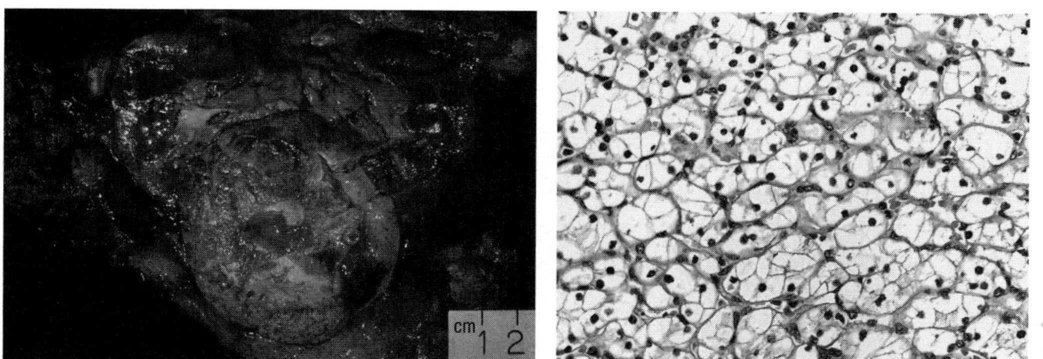

Figure 4.1. (A) Clear-cell renal cell carcinoma (CCRCC) forms a mass with distinctive yellow or light orange color. Hemorrhage and cystic changes are common. (B) It is composed of compact nests of tumor cells with clear cytoplasm separated by delicate vasculature.

PATHOLOGY

Both kidneys are affected equally.[5] Multicentricity or bilaterality occur in <5% of cases in sporadic CCRCC, but they are more often associated with inherited cancer syndromes. Most CCRCC presents as a well-circumscribed, nonencapsulated mass with hemorrhage, necrosis, cystic degeneration, and calcification. It is characteristically golden yellow due to rich lipid content of the tumor cells (Figure 4.1A).

Microscopically tumor cells have clear cytoplasm due to the rich cytoplasmic lipid and glycogen that is lost during the processing of the tissue and preparation of slides (Figure 4.1B),[5] although high-grade CCRCC often has more eosinophilic and granular cytoplasm. It contains a regular network of thin-walled blood vessels, a distinct and consistent feature that is diagnostically quite helpful. Indicative of a worse prognosis, sarcomatoid differentiation is found in about 5% of the cases.[6] Rhabdoid cells with large eccentric nuclei, macronucleoli, and prominent acidophilic globular cytoplasm are occasionally seen and are thought to be associated with worse prognosis.[7] Although some RCCs with "granular" cytoplasm are now classified as CCRCC, many are of other histologic subtypes. Therefore, "granular cell RCC" is not considered as a specific subtype. The term is antiquated and its use is discouraged.

MOLECULAR GENETICS

Chromosome 3p alterations have been detected in the vast majority of sporadic CCRCCs.[8–10] At least three different regions on 3p are implicated, including 3p25-6, which harbors, among others, *von Hippel-Lindau (VHL)* gene, 3p21-22 (including *RASSF1A* and *DRR1*), and 3p11-12 (*FHIT*). Duplication of 5q22~qter is the second most common cytogenetic finding and may be associated with more favorable prognosis. Other cytogenetic alterations affect 6q, 8p, 9, 11q, 14q, 17p, 18q, and 19p.[11]

Mutations in the *VHL* gene have been found in 22% to 71% of sporadic CCRCCs.[12,13] Inactivation of *VHL* gene by promoter hypermethylation is seen in another 20% of cases. Together, inactivation of both VHL alleles by different mechanisms occur in >70% of sporadic CCRCCs. Therefore, it seems that inactivation of the *VHL* gene plays a critical role in the development of CCRCC, even in nonfamilial cases.

The VHL protein plays a critical role in the so-called hypoxia inducible pathway.[14] Mutations in the *VHL* gene abolish the function of the VHL protein and result in overexpression of many hypoxia inducible genes, including genes in angiogenesis (vascular endothelial growth factor [VEGF]), cell growth (platelet-derived growth factor β [PDGF-β], and transforming growth factor α [TGF-α]), glucose transporter 1 (GLUT-1), acid and base balance carbonic anhydrase IX (CA IX), and red cell production (erythropoietin). Uncontrolled expression of these genes contributes to the tumorigenesis and many clinical manifestations of CCRCC. Many clinical trials are targeting several of these genes, including VEGF and TGF-α, using small molecule inhibitors of tyrosine kinase, such as sorafenib and sunitinib, in the treatment of advanced-stage CCRCC.[15]

Multilocular Cystic Renal Cell Carcinoma

Multilocular cystic renal cell carcinoma is a rare subset of CCRCC, accounting for 5% of CCRCC and is associated with an excellent clinical outcome.[16,17] These tumors form well-circumscribed, entirely cystic masses. Microscopically they contain variably sized cysts that are lined with a single layer, and occasionally several layers, of attenuated flat or plump clear cells. No expansile cellular nodules are allowed. The nuclei almost always are small with dense chromatin. If strict diagnostic criteria are applied, multilocular cystic RCC has a very favorable prognosis. No local or distant metastasis has been documented after complete surgical removal.

Renal Cell Carcinoma, Papillary Type

CLINICAL FEATURES

Papillary renal cell carcinoma (PRCC) accounts for 10% to 15% of RCCs.[3] The gender and age distribution is similar to that of CCRCC. Papillary renal cell carcinoma has a better prognosis than CCRCC, with a 5-year survival approaching 90%.

PATHOLOGY

Grossly PRCC presents as a well-circumscribed mass with a pseudocapsule, foci of hemorrhage, and necrosis (Figure 4.2A). Bilateral and multifocal tumors are more common in PRCC than in other RCCs. Microscopically, PRCC has variable proportions of papillae, tubulopapillae, and tubules. The papillae characteristically contain delicate fibrovascular cores expanded with foamy histiocytes (Figure 4.2B). Necrosis, hemorrhage, hemosiderin deposition in tumor cells, macrophages, and stromal cells are common. Psammomatous calcification is also common.

Two types of PRCC are recognized based on the histomorphology.[18] Accounting for about two thirds of PRCC, type I contains papillae that are lined with single layer of tumor cells with scant pale cytoplasm and low-grade nuclei. In contrast, type II tumor cells have abundant eosinophilic cytoplasm and large pseudostratified nuclei with prominent nucleoli. Type I PRCC has a better prognosis than type II PRCC.

MOLECULAR GENETICS

Chromosomal gain, including tri- or tetrasomy 7 and 17, and loss of Y chromosome are the most common cytogenetic changes observed in PRCC and its presumptive precursor lesion, papillary adenoma.[8,19] After acquiring additional cytogenetic changes, such as trisomy 12, 16, and 20, papillary adenomas develop into PRCC.[20] Loss of heterozygosity (LOH) at 9p13 is associated with shorter survival.[21] Type I and II PRCC possess distinct genetic features, with 7p and 17p gains more commonly seen in

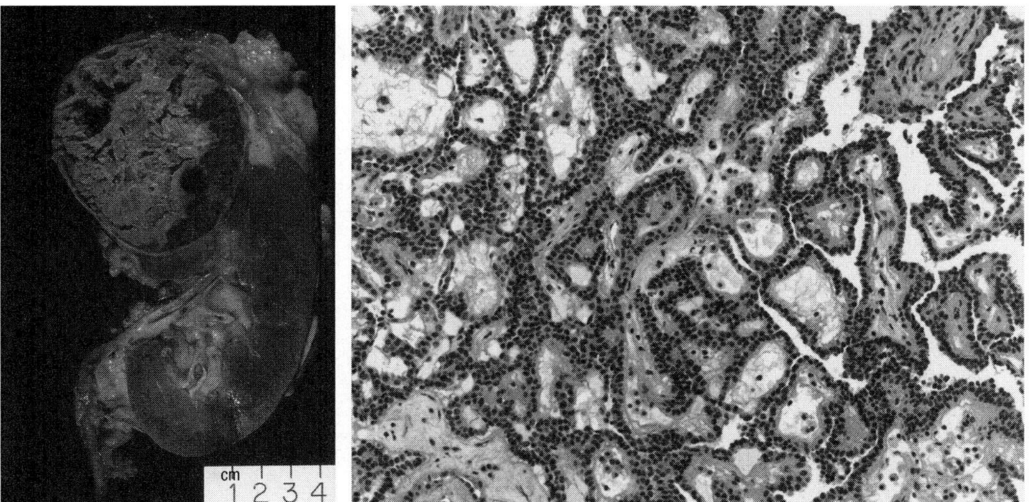

Figure 4.2. (A) Papillary renal cell carcinoma (PRCC) has a pseudocapsule and extensive hemorrhage and necrosis. (B) It is composed of papillae covered by a single layer of tumor cells with scant cytoplasm. The fibrovascular cores are expanded with foamy histiocytes. (To view this figure in color, see the insert.)

type I PRCC.[22] Patterns of allelic imbalance are also distinct between type I and II PRCC.[23]

Occasionally, PRCC occurs in the setting of inherited cancer syndromes, including hereditary papillary renal cell carcinoma syndrome (HPRCC) and hereditary leiomyomatosis renal cell carcinoma (HLRCC).[4] Hereditary papillary renal cell carcinoma is associated with a germline mutation in the tyrosine kinase domain of the *c-met* proto-oncogene[24] on chromosome 7q31 and develops RCC of type I histologic features. However, sporadic PRCC infrequently has c-*met* mutations.

Hereditary leiomyomatosis and renal cell carcinoma is an autosomal dominant disease and contains mutations in the fumarate hydratase *(FH)* gene on chromosome 17. Patients are at risk for cutaneous and uterine leiomyomas and PRCC with type II histology.[25] *FH* is a key regulator of the Krebs cycle. A recent study demonstrated that inactivation of *FH* also correlated with hypoxia-inducible factor (HIF) overexpression and potentially dysregulated hypoxia inducible pathway.[26]

Renal Cell Carcinoma, Chromophobe Type

CLINICAL FEATURES

Renal cell carcinoma, chromophobe type (ChRCC) accounts for approximately 5% of RCCs.[3] The prognosis is significantly better than for CCRCC, with mortality less than 10%. Most cases are sporadic, although rare familial cases are associated with Birt-Hogg-Dubé syndrome.[4]

PATHOLOGY

Renal cell carcinoma, chromophobe type is usually a solitary, circumscribed, and nonencapsulated mass with a homogeneous light brown cut surface (Figure 4.3A). The

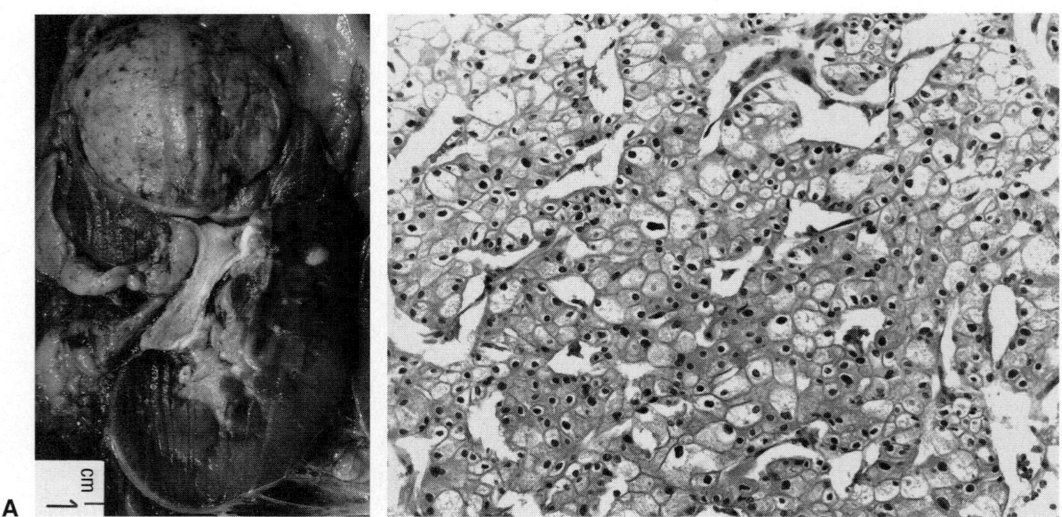

Figure 4.3. (A) Renal cell carcinoma, chromophobe type (ChRCC) forms a circumscribed, nonencapsulated mass with a homogeneous light brown cut surface. (B) The large and polygonal tumor cells have finely reticulated cytoplasm, prominent cell border, and irregular nuclei with perinuclear clearing. (To view this figure in color, see the insert.)

tumor cells are large and polygonal and have finely reticulated cytoplasm due to numerous cytoplasmic microvesicles, prominent cell border resembling plant cells, and irregular, often wrinkled, nuclei with perinuclear clearing (Figure 4.3B). A ChRCC with these features represents the so-called classic type. Other cases of ChRCC are composed predominantly of tumor cells with intensely eosinophilic cytoplasm, hence termed "eosinophilic" variant.[27] These cases should be distinguished from renal oncocytoma, a benign renal neoplasm with similar, sometimes overlapping histology. The distinction can usually be made based on histologic examination, although immunohistochemistry or cytogenetic studies may be required in difficult cases. One such test is Hale's colloidal iron stain, which highlights the mucopolysaccharide content of microvesicles of tumor cells in ChRCC, but is negative in other neoplasms.[28]

MOLECULAR GENETICS

Renal cell carcinoma, chromophobe type shows extensive chromosomal loss, most commonly involving chromosomes 1, 2, 6, 10, 13, 17, and 21.[8] Occasionally, ChRCC can occur in Birt-Hogg-Dubé syndrome, an autosomal dominant disorder characterized by benign skin tumors (fibrofolliculomas, trichodiscomas of hair follicles, and skin tags), renal epithelial neoplasms, and spontaneous pneumothorax. Renal neoplasms are often multifocal and bilateral and present in the form of hybrid oncocytic tumors with features of both ChRCC and oncocytoma, ChRCC, oncocytomas, CCRCC, and occasionally PRCC. *BHD*, the gene implicated in the syndrome, encodes a potential tumor suppressor gene folliculin on 17p11.2.[29] *BHD* mutations are rarely found in sporadic ChRCC or renal oncocytoma.

Carcinoma of the Collecting Duct of Bellini

CLINICAL FEATURES

Carcinoma of the collecting duct of Bellini is an aggressive malignant neoplasm postulated to arise from the principal cells of the collecting duct of Bellini. It is rare, comprising <1% of RCCs. It has a poor prognosis, with metastasis at presentation in many patients, and two thirds of patients succumb to the disease within 2 years of the diagnosis.[30]

PATHOLOGY

Collecting duct carcinoma arises in the central region of the kidney and appears firm, gray-white, with infiltrative borders. The origin within the renal pyramid may be observed for small tumors and is also supported by dysplastic changes involving adjacent collecting duct epithelium. Secondary extension into the cortex may occur, especially in large tumors. Tumor cells form complex and angulated tubules or tubulopapillary structures embedded in a remarkably desmoplastic stroma (Figure 4.4A). Cytologically they are highly atypical with marked nuclear pleomorphism, vesicular chromatin prominent nucleoli, and frequent mitosis.

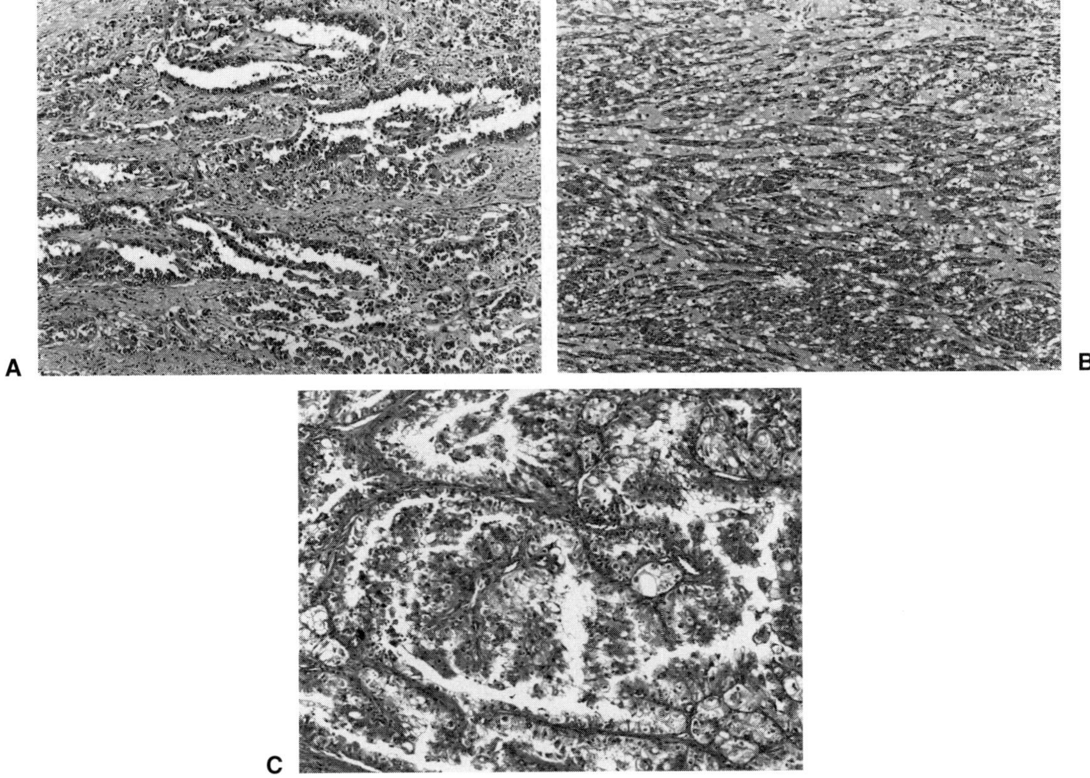

Figure 4.4. (A) Collecting duct renal cell carcinoma consists of high-grade tumor cells forming complex and angulated tubules or tubulopapillary structures embedded in a remarkably desmoplastic stroma. (B) Mucinous tubular and spindle cell carcinoma is composed of elongated cords and collapsed tubules with slit-like spaces embedded in a lightly basophilic myxoid stroma. (C) ASPL-TFE3 renal cell carcinoma with t(X;17)(p11.2;q25) consists of nested to pseudopapillary structures lined tumor cells with abundant clear, sometimes eosinophilic, cytoplasm.

MOLECULAR GENETICS

Only very limited genetic data of collecting duct carcinoma are available.[31] Loss of heterozygosity has been observed on chromosomes 1q, 6p, 8p, 13q, and 21q. Her2/neu amplification has also been documented.

Renal Medullary Carcinoma

CLINICAL FEATURES

Medullary carcinoma of the kidney is an extremely rare and highly aggressive renal tumor of renal medulla.[32,33] It almost exclusively affects patients with sickle cell hemoglobinopathies (almost always sickle cell trait). The patients are young, between age 10 and 20, and have a male to female ratio of 2:1. The tumor is believed to originate from the collecting ducts, but is distinct from the collecting duct carcinomas.

PATHOLOGY

Renal medullary carcinoma appears as a poorly circumscribed, centrally located, gray-white mass with hemorrhage and necrosis grossly. It often extends into the perihilar adipose tissue. Microscopically it resembles collecting duct carcinoma with high-grade tumor cells arranged in solid sheets or more commonly reticular growth pattern with microcystic or "yolk sac–like" appearance. The tumor cells are embedded in a desmoplastic stroma and are infiltrated by neutrophils and lymphocytes. Sickle red blood cells are readily recognized.

Other Newly Described Renal Cell Carcinomas

Several new entities of renal cell carcinomas have been described recently. Mucinous tubular and spindle cell carcinoma is a low-grade tumor of possible distal nephron or loop of Henle origin.[34,35] It affects patients in a wide age range of 17 to 82 years (mean 53) and has a female predominance (female to male ratio of 4:1). As its name implies, the tumor is composed of elongated cords and collapsed tubules with slit-like spaces embedded in a lightly basophilic myxoid background (Figure 4.4B). The tumor cells are usually spherical or oval with scant cytoplasm and low-grade nuclear features. The prognosis seems favorable, with the majority of the patients free of disease after surgical resection. A few cases showed chromosomal losses involving chromosomes 1, 4, 6, 8, 13, and 14, and gains involving 7, 11, 16, and 17. However, 3p alteration and trisomy 7 and 17 have not been reported.[35,36]

Renal cell carcinoma associated with Xp11.2 translocation/*TFE3* gene fusion is defined by chromosomal translocation involving the *TFE3* gene on chromosome Xp11.2, resulting in overexpression of the TFE3 protein.[2,37] The translocation partner genes include *PRCC* on 1q21, *ASPL* on 17q26, *PSL* on 1p34, and *NonO* on Xq12. These carcinomas typically affect children and young adults. Although RCC accounts for <5% of pediatric renal tumors, Xp11.2-associated RCCs make up a significant proportion of these cases. The RCC involving *ASPL-TFE3* translocation characteristically present at an advanced stage and also with lymph node metastasis.[38] The morphology varies with different chromosomal translocations; however, the most distinctive histologic feature is papillary structures lined with clear cells (Figure 4.4C). The diagnosis can be confirmed by positive nuclear immunostain for *TFE3*.

Rarely, RCC affects the long-term survivors of neuroblastoma.[39] All affected children were diagnosed with neuroblastoma at 2 years of age or younger, and the majority had advanced stage neuroblastoma. Renal cell carcinoma was diagnosed at ages ranging from 5 to 14 years and occurred after a period of 3 to 11.5 years (average 9 years) following the neuroblastoma diagnosis. Morphologically, many of these tumors are typical CCRCC. However, some tumors have solid and papillary architecture with oncocytoid cells.

Renal Cell Carcinoma, Unclassified Type

Two to five percent of RCCs do not fit into any of the entities in the 2004 WHO classification and therefore are termed renal cell carcinoma, unclassified type. It is a diagnostic category rather than a distinct biologic entity. Since unclassified RCCs comprise a heterogeneous group of tumors with little in common, they share no common clinical, morphologic, or genetic features. These cases often have poorer clinical outcomes.[40]

Papillary Adenoma

CLINICAL FEATURES

By definition, papillary adenomas are benign epithelial neoplasm of papillary or tubular architecture, <5 mm in size, and have low-grade nuclei. They are the most common renal cell neoplasm, and frequently are incidental findings in nephrectomy and autopsy specimens. Its incidence increases with age and also in patients on long-term dialysis, with acquired renal cystic disease or in scarred kidneys in patients with chronic pyelonephritis or renal vascular disease.

PATHOLOGY

Papillary adenomas appear as a well-circumscribed, yellow or white nodule in the renal cortex. They have a papillary, tubular, or tubulopapillary architecture, similar to PRCC.[41] The cells lining those structures have uniform small nuclei and inconspicuous nucleoli similar to Fuhrman grade 1 or 2 nuclei.

MOLECULAR GENETICS

The earliest genetic changes observed in papillary adenomas are combined trisomy 7 and 17, and loss of chromosome Y, changes that are also present in PRCC.[20] Additional genetic alterations have been reported as they evolve. Therefore, papillary adenoma is postulated to be the precursor to PRCC.

Renal Oncocytoma

CLINICAL FEATURES

Renal oncocytoma accounts for 5% of renal cell neoplasms; they occur in a wide age range, with a peak incidence in the 7th decade of life. Most cases are sporadic, although familial cases have been reported in association with Birt-Hogg-Dubé syndrome and familial renal oncocytoma syndrome.[4]

PATHOLOGY

Oncocytomas are typically solitary, well-circumscribed, nonencapsulated tumors with homogeneous cut surface and a characteristic mahogany-brown color (Figure 4.5A).[5] A central stellate scar is seen in one third of the cases, and is more common in larger tumors.

Renal oncocytoma is characterized by bright eosinophilic cells with a nested, micro-acinar or microcystic pattern associated with a loose hypocellular and hyalinized stroma (Figure 4.5B). The tumor cells, also called oncocytes, are uniform, round to polygonal,

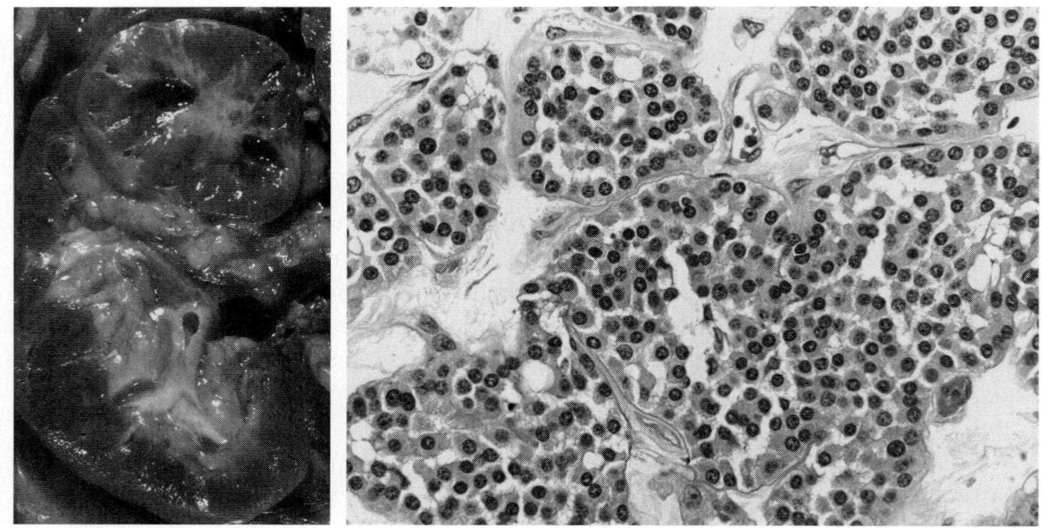

Figure 4.5. (A) Renal oncocytoma forms solitary, well-circumscribed, nonencapsulated mass with homogeneous mahogany-brown cut surface and a central scar. (B) It consists of bright eosinophilic cells nested in a loose stroma. The tumor cells are uniform, round to polygonal, with granular eosinophilic cytoplasm and regular round nuclei with evenly dispersed chromatin.

with granular eosinophilic, mitochondria-rich cytoplasm, and regular round nuclei. Renal oncocytoma presents with evenly dispersed chromatin. Mitoses are rare or absent. Occasionally, oncocytes with scant granular cytoplasm, high nuclear to cytoplasmic ratio, and clusters of hyperchromatic and pleomorphic nuclei are also present. Extension of oncocytoma into the perinephric fat, or rarely into vascular space, is well documented and does not appear to adversely affect the prognosis.

When multiple oncocytomas are present, along with oncocytic change in renal tubules, oncocyte-lined microcysts, and clusters of neoplastic oncocytes among renal tubules, the term *oncocytosis* is applied.[42] It is often seen in Birt-Hogg-Dubé syndrome.[43]

MOLECULAR GENETICS

Most oncocytomas are composed of a mixed population of cells with normal and abnormal karyotypes.[44] Some cases display loss of chromosomes 1 and 14.[45] Occasionally, t(5; 11) is observed.[46]

HISTOLOGIC PROGNOSTIC FACTORS FOR RENAL CELL CARCINOMA

Prognosis of RCCs is influenced by many clinical, pathologic, and molecular factors. The pathologic parameters include histologic subtypes, tumor size, nuclear grade, sarcomatoid differentiation, tumor necrosis, vascular invasion, and status of surgical margins. Many of these parameters have been incorporated into the American Joint Committee on Cancer (AJCC) tumor, node, metastasis (TNM) staging for RCC. Recently, several outcome prediction models have been designed to incorporate all the clinical and pathologic parameters that are independently predictive of outcomes, and to accurately stratify patients into clinically significant prognostic groups.

Histologic Subtypes

Many studies have shown differing survival among patients with different subtypes of RCC.[3,47] Histologic subtypes often correlate with TNM stages and other pathologic parameters. Clear-cell renal cell carcinoma usually demonstrates worse pathologic features than PRCC and ChRCC, including larger tumor size, higher Fuhrman nuclear grade, pathologic tumor stage, and the likelihood of developing distant metastasis. By univariate analysis, most studies found that CCRCC fares worse than PRCC and ChRCC. In a recent study by Cheville et al.,[3] the 5- and 10-year cancer-specific survival are 68.9% and 60.3% for CCRCC, 90.1% and 81.9% for PRCC, and 88.1% and 83.3% for ChRCC. By multivariate analysis, however, the histologic subtypes have not been found to be independent predictors of the clinical outcomes. Nevertheless, histologic classification of RCC is still clinically important, since different subtypes may exhibit diverse therapeutic response. For example, Upton et al.[48] found 20% of CCRCC responded to interleukin-2–based therapy in contrast to 6% of response in non-CCRCC.

Fuhrman Nuclear Grading

Fuhrman grading system, the most widely used grading system for RCC, is based on the nuclear size, irregularity of the nuclear membrane, and nucleolar prominence, and is categorized into grades 1 to 4. Grade 1 and 2 may be grouped together as low grade since the two are not significantly different in prognosis.[49] Furthermore, grouping Fuhrman grades into low grade (grade 1 and 2) and high grade (grade 3 and 4) can improve the interobserver agreement and still preserve its prognostic significance.[50]

Most studies have confirmed that Fuhrman nuclear grade is an independent prognostic predictor for CCRCC and RCC not otherwise specified.[3,40] However, its prognostic significance for PRCC and ChRCC remains controversial. For PRCC, Fuhrman nuclear grade correlates with clinical outcomes in univariate analysis; however, there is no significant correlation in multivariate analysis. Only a few studies addressed the prognostic significance of Fuhrman nuclear grade in ChRCC using univariate analysis.

Sarcomatoid Differentiation

Sarcomatoid differentiation can arise in any subtype of RCC.[6] Therefore, sarcomatoid RCC is not considered as a distinct subtype of RCC by current WHO classification; rather, it is thought to represent transformation to a higher grade RCC, and the classification of such RCCs should be based on the identification of the coexisting RCC components. Sarcomatoid differentiation is present in 1% to 6.5% of RCCs. Histologically, the sarcomatoid component ranges from malignant spindle cells to those resembling leiomyosarcoma, fibrosarcoma, angiosarcoma, rhabdomyosarcoma, and other sarcomas. Sarcomatoid differentiation is considered an adverse pathologic parameter and is graded as Fuhrman nuclear grade 4.[6,51] Renal cell carcinoma with sarcomatoid differentiation often presents as high-stage and high-grade disease with frequent distant metastasis. Even a small sarcomatoid component confers a worse prognosis. Univariate analysis found that sarcomatoid differentiation significantly affects the survival adversely.

Tumor Necrosis

Histologically confirmed tumor necrosis is strongly associated with adverse clinical outcomes both in uni- and multivariate analysis.[3,40] In a Mayo Clinic study, histologic necrosis is associated with twice the risk of death from RCC compared to those without necrosis. Lam et al.[52] also reported that the presence and extent of histologic necrosis in RCC were independent predictors of survival in localized but not metastatic cases. However, tumor necrosis is not prognostically useful for PRCC since it is commonly observed in this tumor.[53]

Invasion of the Urinary Collecting System

Involvement of the collecting system, including renal calyces, pelvis, and ureter, occurs most frequently in high-stage and high-grade RCC. Therefore, Uzzo et al.[54] found that collecting system invasion did not portend a worse prognosis in high-stage (T3 or higher) tumor, whereas it was an adverse pathologic feature in low-stage RCC. Another study found that collecting system invasion provides independent prognostic significance, associated with 1.4-fold greater risk of death compared to those without collecting system invasion.[55] However, Terrone et al.'s[56] study did not confirm the independent prognostic value of the involvement of the collecting system, although such a finding was associated with worse prognosis in the univariate analysis.

Microvascular Invasion

Microvascular invasion, defined as the vascular invasion identified only by microscopic examination, is detected in 13.6% to 44.6% of RCC, and is more common in RCC of higher stage and nuclear grade, and larger size. Its presence is associated with worse prognosis and higher likelihood of disease recurrence in univariate analyses, although such findings are not confirmed in multivariate analysis.[57,58]

Completeness of Tumor Resection

Positive renal parenchymal margin in nephron-sparing surgery indicates incomplete resection of RCC and is associated with poor prognosis.[59,60] However, the width of the margins does not seem to correlate with prognosis as long as the surgical margins are free of tumor.[60]

American Joint Committee on Cancer's Tumor, Node, and Metastasis Staging System

For RCC, purely anatomic staging systems have historically served as the best prognostic tools. The AJCC TNM staging system, most recently updated in 2002 (Table 4.2), incorporates the pathologic parameters of the primary tumor, regional lymph nodes, and distant metastasis, and provides the most significant prognostic values for RCC. A recent study by Frank et al.[61] showed that the 2002 TNM classification is significantly associated with death from RCC, with a stepwise decrease in survival rates with each increase in the primary tumor stage. When combined with lymph node status and distant metastasis, the predictive ability of TNM staging is further improved.

However, the TNM staging has constantly been the subject of debate. One of the contentious issues is the optimal tumor size breakpoint. The current pT staging divides the T1 tumors into T1a (≤ 4 cm) and T1b (>4 cm and ≤ 7 cm), since the T1a tumors have significantly better prognosis than T1b tumors and are amenable to nephron-sparing

Table 4.2.
Tumor, node, metastasis (TNM) classification of renal cell carcinoma

T: Primary tumor

TX Primary tumor cannot be assessed

T0 No evidence of primary tumor

T1 Tumor 7 cm or less in greatest dimension, limited to the kidney
T1a Tumor 4 cm or less
T1b Tumor more than 4 cm but not more than 7 cm

T2 Tumor more than 7 cm in greatest dimension, limited to the kidney
T3 Tumor extends into major veins or directly invades adrenal gland or perinephric tissues but not beyond Gerota fascia
T3a Tumor directly invades adrenal gland or perinephric tissues but not beyond Gerota fascia

T3b Tumor grossly extends into renal vein(s) or vena cava or its wall below diaphragm

T3c Tumor grossly extends into vena cava or its wall above diaphragm
T4 Tumor directly invades beyond Gerota fascia

N: Regional lymph nodes
NX Regional lymph nodes cannot be assessed
N0 No regional lymph node metastasis
N1 Metastasis in a single regional lymph node
N2 Metastasis in more than one regional lymph node

M: Distant metastasis
MX Distant metastasis cannot be assessed
M0 No distant metastasis

M1 Distant metastasis

Stage grouping

Stage I	T1	N0	M0
Stage II	T2	N0	M0
Stage III	T3	N0	M0
	T1,T2,T3	N1	M0
Stage IV	T4	N0,N1	M0
	Any T	N2	M0
	Any T	Any N	M1

surgery.[62] However, other studies failed to show statistically significant difference in survival between T1b and T2 tumors.[63] While these studies disagree over the exact size (4 to 5.5 cm), they all agree that the cutoff size to discriminate T1 and T2 tumors needs to be modified.[62–66]

Invasion of the ipsilateral adrenal glands is grouped together with perinephric invasion as T3a. However, several studies have challenged this classification.[67,68] Compared to RCCs with only perinephric fat invasion, RCCs with invasion of adrenal glands are more likely to have higher grade, lymph node involvement, and distant metastases. The cancer-specific survival is the same as for a T4 tumor. In addition, these patients have poor response to interleukin-2 therapy. Therefore, these studies advocate reclassifying T3a RCC with direct adrenal invasion as T4.

Comprehensive Outcome Prediction Models

Other clinical and pathologic parameters have been proven to be independent prognostic predictors. Several comprehensive outcome prediction models have been developed utilizing TNM stage, histologic subtypes, tumor size, nuclear grade, presence of tumor necrosis, and Eastern Cooperative Oncology Group (ECOG) performance status.[69–73] These different outcome prediction models promise to improve upon the TNM staging system and provide more discriminating power for predicting survival, metastasis, and pattern of recurrence. Therefore, they may be useful for patient counseling, surveillance, and identification of high-risk patients for adjuvant therapy.

HANDLING AND REPORTING OF RENAL CELL CARCINOMA SPECIMENS

The handling of RCC specimens by pathologists is critical because the pathologic examination not only renders diagnoses, but also provides important information for prognosis and therapeutic decisions. In addition, tumor tissues could be procured for clinical trials and experimental studies. Furthermore, pathologists could allocate any redundant tumor tissues not required for diagnosis to basic research programs. Several protocols have been published on this subject.

Urologists and other clinicians play equally important roles in the optimal handling and processing of RCC specimens. Urologists should try to preserve the anatomic structures of the nephrectomy specimen. If for any reason the perinephric fat has to be separated from the kidney, it should be oriented and the zone of tumor contact should be indicated. Should a lymphadenectomy be performed, it should be submitted in a separate container. If the lymphadenectomy is not separated from the perihilar tissue, the information should be communicated to pathologists. The specimen should be sent to the pathology service fresh without fixative in a sterile fashion immediately after it is removed from the patient. Fix the specimen in formalin only if the delivery of the specimen is expected to be delayed, or no molecular or cytogenetic studies are anticipated. The importance of the availability of fresh tumor tissue for molecular and cytogenetic studies could not be overemphasized. Approximately 2% to 5% of renal tumors remain unclassified using the current WHO classification. Molecular and genetic approaches offer the only hope that these unclassified RCCs would be classifiable based on genetic and molecular features.

We recently implemented a protocol at Cleveland Clinic. All the resection specimens that contain renal tumors are delivered to pathology service fresh. Pathologists perform gross and frozen section examination of the specimens. Any tumor with unusual histology is sent for cytogenetic studies. Using this approach, we have identified one Xp11.2 translocation-associated RCC in the first 6 months. In addition, several difficult papillary RCC cases were confirmed by the cytogenetic studies.

Clinical information is also critical and should accompany the surgical specimens. Previous medical history, including prior renal tumors, and family history are extremely important for identifying familial RCC cases. Awareness of such history will prompt pathologists to preserve fresh tumor tissues for molecular and genetic study and order additional tests to work up the case.

REFERENCES

1. Eble J, Sauter G, Epstein J, et al. Tumours of the Urinary System and Male Genital Organs. Lyon, France: IAPC Press, 2004:9–88.
2. Argani P, Ladanyi M. Translocation carcinomas of the kidney. Clin Lab Med 2005;25(2):363–378.
3. Cheville JC, Lohse CM, Zincke H, et al. Comparisons of outcome and prognostic features among histologic subtypes of renal cell carcinoma. Am J Surg Pathol 2003;27(5):612–624.

4. Cohen D, Zhou M. Molecular genetics of familial renal cell carcinoma syndromes. Clin Lab Med 2005;25(2):259–277.

5. Murphy W, Grignon D, Perlman E. Tumors of the Kidney, Bladder, and Related Urinary Structures. Washington, DC: American Registry of Pathology, 2004.

6. de Peralta-Venturina M, Moch H, Amin M, et al. Sarcomatoid differentiation in renal cell carcinoma: a study of 101 cases. Am J Surg Pathol 2001;25(3):275–284.

7. Gokden N, Nappi O, Swanson PE, et al. Renal cell carcinoma with rhabdoid features. Am J Surg Pathol 2000;24(10):1329–1338.

8. Hoglund M, Gisselsson D, Soller M, et al. Dissecting karyotypic patterns in renal cell carcinoma: an analysis of the accumulated cytogenetic data. Cancer Genet Cytogenet 2004;153(1):1–9.

9. Linehan WM, Vasselli J, Srinivasan R, et al. Genetic basis of cancer of the kidney: disease-specific approaches to therapy. Clin Cancer Res 2004;10(18 pt 2):6282S–6289S.

10. Strefford JC, Stasevich I, Lane TM, et al. A combination of molecular cytogenetic analyses reveals complex genetic alterations in conventional renal cell carcinoma. Cancer Genet Cytogenet 2005;159(1):1–9.

11. Jones TD, Eble JN, Cheng L. Application of molecular diagnostic techniques to renal epithelial neoplasms. Clin Lab Med 2005;25(2):279–303.

12. Banks RE, Tirukonda P, Taylor C, et al. Genetic and epigenetic analysis of von Hippel-Lindau (VHL) gene alterations and relationship with clinical variables in sporadic renal cancer. Cancer Res 2006;66(4):2000–2011.

13. Gimenez-Bachs JM, Salinas-Sanchez AS, Sanchez-Sanchez F, et al. Determination of VHL gene mutations in sporadic renal cell carcinoma. Eur Urol 2006;49(6):1051–1057.

14. Kim W, Kaelin WG Jr. The von Hippel-Lindau tumor suppressor protein: new insights into oxygen sensing and cancer. Curr Opin Genet Dev 2003;13(1):55–60.

15. Rathmell WK, Wright TM, Rini BI. Molecularly targeted therapy in renal cell carcinoma. Expert Rev Anticancer Ther 2005;5(6):1031–1040.

16. Suzigan S, Lopez-Beltran A, Montironi R, et al. Multilocular cystic renal cell carcinoma: a report of 45 cases of a kidney tumor of low malignant potential. Am J Clin Pathol 2006;125(2):217–222.

17. Nassir A, Jollimore J, Gupta R, et al. Multilocular cystic renal cell carcinoma: a series of 12 cases and review of the literature. Urology 2002;60(3):421–427.

18. Delahunt B, Eble JN, McCredie MR, et al. Morphologic typing of papillary renal cell carcinoma: comparison of growth kinetics and patient survival in 66 cases. Hum Pathol 2001;32(6):590–595.

19. Brunelli M, Eble JN, Zhang S, et al. Gains of chromosomes 7, 17, 12, 16, and 20 and loss of Y occur early in the evolution of papillary renal cell neoplasia: a fluorescent in situ hybridization study. Mod Pathol 2003;16(10):1053–1059.

20. Kovacs G, Fuzesi L, Emanual E, et al. Cytogenetics of papillary renal cell tumors. Genes Chromosomes Cancer 1991;3(4):249–255.

21. Schraml P, Muller D, Bednar R, et al. Allelic loss at the D9S171 locus on chromosome 9p13 is associated with progression of papillary renal cell carcinoma. J Pathol 2000;190(4):457–461.

22. Jiang F, Richter J, Schraml P, et al. Chromosomal imbalances in papillary renal cell carcinoma: genetic differences between histological subtypes. Am J Pathol 1998;153(5):1467–1473.

23. Sanders ME, Mick R, Tomaszewski JE, et al. Unique patterns of allelic imbalance distinguish type 1 from type 2 sporadic papillary renal cell carcinoma. Am J Pathol 2002;161(3):997–1005.

24. Schmidt L, Duh FM, Chen F, et al. Germline and somatic mutations in the tyrosine kinase domain of the MET proto-oncogene in papillary renal carcinomas. Nat Genet 1997;16(1):68–73.

25. Launonen V, Vierimaa O, Kiuru M, et al. Inherited susceptibility to uterine leiomyomas and renal cell cancer. Proc Natl Acad Sci U S A 2001;98(6):3387–3392.

26. Isaacs JS, Jung YJ, Mole DR, et al. HIF overexpression correlates with biallelic loss of fumarate hydratase in renal cancer: novel role of fumarate in regulation of HIF stability. Cancer Cell 2005;8(2):143–153.

27. Thoenes W, Storkel S, Rumpelt HJ, et al. Chromophobe cell renal carcinoma and its variants—a report on 32 cases. J Pathol 1988;155(4):277–287.

28. Tickoo SK, Amin MB, Zarbo RJ. Colloidal iron staining in renal epithelial neoplasms, including chromophobe renal cell carcinoma: emphasis on technique and patterns of staining. Am J Surg Pathol 1998;22(4):419–424.

29. Nickerson ML, Warren MB, Toro JR, et al. Mutations in a novel gene lead to kidney tumors, lung wall defects, and benign tumors of the hair follicle in patients with the Birt-Hogg-Dube syndrome. Cancer Cell 2002;2(2):157–164.

30. Srigley JR, Eble JN. Collecting duct carcinoma of kidney. Semin Diagn Pathol 1998;15(1):54–67.
31. Antonelli A, Portesi E, Cozzoli A, et al. The collecting duct carcinoma of the kidney: a cytogenetical study. Eur Urol 2003;43(6):680–685.
32. Avery RA, Harris JE, Davis CJ Jr, et al. Renal medullary carcinoma: clinical and therapeutic aspects of a newly described tumor. Cancer 1996;78(1):128–132.
33. Davis CJ Jr, Mostofi FK, Sesterhenn IA. Renal medullary carcinoma. The seventh sickle cell nephropathy. Am J Surg Pathol 1995;19(1):1–11.
34. Parwani AV, Husain AN, Epstein JI, et al. Low-grade myxoid renal epithelial neoplasms with distal nephron differentiation. Hum Pathol 2001;32(5):506–512.
35. Rakozy C, Schmahl GE, Bogner S, et al. Low-grade tubular-mucinous renal neoplasms: morphologic, immunohistochemical, and genetic features. Mod Pathol 2002;15(11):1162–1171.
36. Ferlicot S, Allory Y, Comperat E, et al. Mucinous tubular and spindle cell carcinoma: a report of 15 cases and a review of the literature. Virchows Arch 2005;447(6):978–983.
37. Argani P, Ladanyi M. Distinctive neoplasms characterised by specific chromosomal translocations comprise a significant proportion of paediatric renal cell carcinomas. Pathology 2003;35(6):492–498.
38. Argani P, Antonescu CR, Illei PB, et al. Primary renal neoplasms with the ASPL-TFE3 gene fusion of alveolar soft part sarcoma: a distinctive tumor entity previously included among renal cell carcinomas of children and adolescents. Am J Pathol 2001;159(1):179–192.
39. Medeiros LJ, Palmedo G, Krigman HR, et al. Oncocytoid renal cell carcinoma after neuroblastoma: a report of four cases of a distinct clinicopathologic entity. Am J Surg Pathol 1999;23(7):772–780.
40. Amin MB, Tamboli P, Javidan J, et al. Prognostic impact of histologic subtyping of adult renal epithelial neoplasms: an experience of 405 cases. Am J Surg Pathol 2002;26(3):281–291.
41. Grignon DJ, Eble JN. Papillary and metanephric adenomas of the kidney. Semin Diagn Pathol 1998;15(1):41–53.
42. Tickoo SK, Reuter VE, Amin MB, et al. Renal oncocytosis: a morphologic study of fourteen cases. Am J Surg Pathol 1999;23(9):1094–1101.
43. Pavlovich CP, Walther MM, Eyler RA, et al. Renal tumors in the Birt-Hogg-Dube syndrome. Am J Surg Pathol 2002;26(12):1542–1552.
44. Lindgren V, Paner GP, Omeroglu A, et al. Cytogenetic analysis of a series of 13 renal oncocytomas. J Urol 2004;171(2 pt 1):602–604.
45. Presti JC Jr, Moch H, Reuter VE, et al. Comparative genomic hybridization for genetic analysis of renal oncocytomas. Genes Chromosomes Cancer 1996;17(4):199–204.
46. Sinke RJ, Dijkhuizen T, Janssen B, et al. Fine mapping of the human renal oncocytoma-associated translocation (5;11)(q35;q13) breakpoint. Cancer Genet Cytogenet 1997;96(2):95–101.
47. Patard JJ, Leray E, Rioux-Leclercq N, et al. Prognostic value of histologic subtypes in renal cell carcinoma: a multicenter experience. J Clin Oncol 2005;23(12):2763–2771.
48. Upton MP, Parker RA, Youmans A, et al. Histologic predictors of renal cell carcinoma response to interleukin-2–based therapy. J Immunother 2005;28(5):488–495.
49. Ficarra V, Novara G, Galfano A, et al. Application of TNM 2002 version, in localized renal cell carcinoma: is it able to predict different cancer-specific survival probability? Urology 2004;63(6):1050–1054.
50. Lang H, Lindner V, de Fromont M, et al. Multicenter determination of optimal interobserver agreement using the Fuhrman grading system for renal cell carcinoma: assessment of 241 patients with >15-year follow-up. Cancer 2005;103(3):625–629.
51. Moch H, Gasser T, Amin MB, et al. Prognostic utility of the recently recommended histologic classification and revised TNM staging system of renal cell carcinoma: a Swiss experience with 588 tumors. Cancer 2000;89(3):604–614.
52. Lam JS, Shvarts O, Said JW, et al. Clinicopathologic and molecular correlations of necrosis in the primary tumor of patients with renal cell carcinoma. Cancer 2005;103(12):2517–2525.
53. Amin MB, Crotty TB, Tickoo SK, et al. Renal oncocytoma: a reappraisal of morphologic features with clinicopathologic findings in 80 cases. Am J Surg Pathol 1997;21(1):1–12.
54. Uzzo RG, Cherullo EE, Myles J, et al. Renal cell carcinoma invading the urinary collecting system: implications for staging. J Urol 2002;167(6):2392–2396.
55. Palapattu GS, Pantuck AJ, Dorey F, et al. Collecting system invasion in renal cell carcinoma: impact on prognosis and future staging strategies. J Urol 2003;170(3):768–772; discussion 772.
56. Terrone C, Cracco C, Guercio S, et al. Prognostic value of the involvement of the urinary collecting system in renal cell carcinoma. Eur Urol 2004;46(4):472–476.

57. Goncalves PD, Srougi M, Dall'lio MF, et al. Low clinical stage renal cell carcinoma: relevance of microvascular tumor invasion as a prognostic parameter. J Urol 2004;172(2):470–474.
58. Ishimura T, Sakai I, Hara I, et al. Microscopic venous invasion in renal cell carcinoma as a predictor of recurrence after radical surgery. Int J Urol 2004;11(5):264–268.
59. Castilla EA, Liou LS, Abrahams NA, et al. Prognostic importance of resection margin width after nephron-sparing surgery for renal cell carcinoma. Urology 2002;60(6):993–997.
60. Sutherland SE, Resnick MI, Maclennan GT, et al. Does the size of the surgical margin in partial nephrectomy for renal cell cancer really matter? J Urol 2002;167(1):61–64.
61. Frank I, et al. Independent validation of the 2002 American Joint Committee on cancer primary tumor classification for renal cell carcinoma using a large, single institution cohort. J Urol 2005;173(6): 1889–1892.
62. Hafez KS, Fergany AF, Novick AC. Nephron sparing surgery for localized renal cell carcinoma: impact of tumor size on patient survival, tumor recurrence and TNM staging. J Urol 1999;162(6):1930–1933.
63. Ficarra V, et al. Application of TNM 2002 version, in localized renal cell carcinoma: is it able to predict different cancer-specific survival probability? Urology 2004;63(6):1050–1054.
64. Lau WK, et al. Prognostic features of pathologic stage T1 renal cell carcinoma after radical nephrectomy. Urology 2002;59(4):532–537.
65. Zisman A, et al. Reevaluation of the 1997 TNM classification for renal cell carcinoma: T1 and T2 cutoff point at 4.5 rather than 7cm better correlates with clinical outcome. J Urol 2001;166(1): 54–58.
66. Cheville JC, et al. Stage pT1 conventional (clear cell) renal cell carcinoma: pathological features associated with cancer specific survival. J Urol 2001;166(2):453–456.
67. Han KR, et al. TNM T3a renal cell carcinoma: adrenal gland involvement is not the same as renal fat invasion. J Urol 2003;169(3):899–903; discussion 903–904.
68. Thompson RH, et al. Should direct ipsilateral adrenal invasion from renal cell carcinoma be classified as pT3a? J Urol 2005;173(3):918–921.
69. Elson PJ, Witte RS, Trump DL. Prognostic factors for survival in patients with recurrent or metastatic renal cell carcinoma. Cancer Res 1988;48(24 pt 1):7310–7313.
70. Motzer RJ, et al. Survival and prognostic stratification of 670 patients with advanced renal cell carcinoma. J Clin Oncol 1999;17(8):2530–2540.
71. Frank I, et al. An outcome prediction model for patients with clear cell renal cell carcinoma treated with radical nephrectomy based on tumor stage, size, grade and necrosis: the SSIGN score. J Urol 2002;168(6):2395–2400.
72. Zisman A, et al. Improved prognostication of renal cell carcinoma using an integrated staging system. J Clin Oncol 2001;19(6):1649–1657.
73. Kattan MW, et al. A postoperative prognostic nomogram for renal cell carcinoma. J Urol 2001; 166(1):63–67.

5
Epidemiology of Renal Tumors

Jeffrey S. Montgomery and David P. Wood

KEYWORDS

KIDNEY NEOPLASMS
EPIDEMIOLOGY
RISK FACTORS
INCIDENCE
MORTALITY
TOBACCO
DIET
OBESITY
OCCUPATIONS

ABSTRACT

Renal parenchymal cancer is the third most common genitourinary malignancy, and over 36,000 Americans are diagnosed with this disease yearly. This chapter discusses the United States and worldwide incidences and mortality rates for renal tumors, presents the specific details for classification of both benign and malignant renal neoplasms, and discusses the adult renal neoplasia syndromes. Data regarding specific risk factors for renal cancer, including family history, tobacco, diet, obesity, physical activity, urinary tract pathology, general medical conditions, occupational exposures, analgesic use, and reproductive factors, are included.

INCIDENCE AND MORTALITY

Renal cell carcinoma (RCC) accounts for 2% to 3% of all cancers.[1] Overall, the kidney is the third most common site of cancer formation in the urinary tract following the prostate and bladder, respectively.[2] The majority of the national and world cancer databases report renal parenchymal tumors together with renal pelvis urothelial tumors. Since RCC accounts for 80% to 85% of malignant kidney tumors,[1] these databases can be used to approximate the rates of RCC incidence and mortality.

United States Patterns

In 2005 it was estimated that there were over 36,000 incident cases of kidney cancer in the United States, and over 12,600 people died from this disease.[2] According to the

From: *Clinical Management of Renal Tumors*
Edited by: R.M. Bukowski and A.C. Novick © Humana Press Inc., Totowa, NJ

most recent data from the Surveillance, Epidemiology, and End Results (SEER) database, the overall incidence of renal cancers in the U.S. from 1997 to 2001 was 11.3 (all rates per 100,000 people, adjusted for a standard year 2000 U.S. population), with a rate of 15.7 for men and 7.8 for women.[3] The overall mortality rate was 4.2, with rates of 6.1 and 2.8 for men and women, respectively, and the 5-year survival rate was 63.9%.[3] From 1995 to 2000, the distribution of renal tumors varied little among blacks and whites, with 52% of tumors being local at diagnosis, 21% regional, 22% distant, and 32.7% unstaged overall (Table 5.1). The 5-year survival rates were lower for all stages in blacks as compared to the total, although the 5-year survival for all groups improved by nearly 20% comparing the 1974–1976 time period with 1995–2000. The

Table 5.1.

Surveillance, Epidemiology, and End Results (SEER) renal parenchymal and renal pelvis tumor data, stratified by race

	All races			Whites			Blacks		
	Total	Male	Female	Total	Male	Female	Total	Male	Female
Median age at diagnosis, 1997–2001	65.0	65.0	67.0	66.0	65.0	68.0	61.0	61.0	62.0
Median age at death, 1997–2001	71.0	69.0	74.0	71.0	70.0	74.0	67.0	65.0	70.0
5-year survival rate (%)									
1974–1976	51.6	51.0	52.6	51.7	50.9	52.9	49.2	50.2	47.4
1977–1979	51.0	51.2	50.8	51.0	51.5	50.2	51.8	44.7	60.9
1980–1982	51.7	52.1	51.1	51.1	51.9	49.8	56.3	53.8	60.2
1983–1985	55.7	56.5	54.3	55.8	56.8	54.2	55.0	54.1	56.4
1986–1988	57.0	57.4	56.3	57.6	58.2	56.7	53.6	52.2	55.5
1989–1991	60.1	60.7	59.2	60.8	61.9	59.2	58.1	55.1	62.3
1992–1994	62.5	62.1	63.0	63.1	62.9	63.4	60.0	58.3	62.3
1995–2000	63.9	63.9	63.9	63.9	64.1	63.6	63.5	63.5	63.5
Survival by stage, 1995–2000 (%)									
Localized	91.1	91.4	90.6	91.7	91.7	91.8	87.7	89.7	85.5
Regional	59.1	60.7	56.4	58.9	60.8	55.8	58.7	61.9	54.3
Distant	9.3	9.3	9.2	9.1	9.2	8.7	9.2	8.4	9.9
Unstaged	32.7	35.0	30.1	33.3	38.3	26.9	21.2	12.8	33.6
Stage distribution, 1995–2000 (%)									
Localized	52	51	54	52	51	53	57	56	59
Regional	21	22	19	21	22	20	16	16	16
Distant	22	22	21	22	22	21	19	21	18
Unstaged	6	5	7	6	5	7	8	7	8

5-year survival for all stages has increased from 36% in the early 1960s to 63.9% in 2000.[3,4] According to a study of over 1000 patients using the revised 1997 tumor, node, metastasis (TNM) RCC staging system,[5] the 10-year cause-specific survival rate for stages T1, T2, T3a, T3b, and T3c tumors was 91%, 70%, 53%, 42%, and 43%, respectively.[6]

From 1999 to 2001, the lifetime risk of being diagnosed with a renal tumor was approximately 1.49% for men and 0.9% for women, with a 0.57% and 0.34% lifetime chance of dying from this disease in men and women, respectively.[3] According to SEER, the prevalence of kidney cancers as of January 1, 2001, was 211,000 cases.[3] In total, 75.4% of these tumors occur in people over 55 years old, with the highest rate in the 70- to 84-year age group[3] (Figure 5.1). In 2001, it is estimated that 188,700 years of life were lost to renal cancer, averaging 15.6 years per person diagnosed with the disease.[3]

Coincident with the increased use of computed tomography (CT) imaging, the incidence of RCC is rising. Chow et al.[7] compared the time periods of 1975–1977 and 1993–1995 in the SEER database and found that the greatest increase in RCC incidence occurred in localized tumors, rising annually by 3.8% in white men, 4.7% in white women, 5.0% in black men, and 5.6% among black women.[7] Overall, from 1973 to 1998, the annual percent increases in localized, regional, and distant renal tumors in the SEER database were 3.7%, 1.9%, and 0.68%, respectively.[8] Although there has been a statistically significant increase in the incidence of all stages of renal cancer with time, there has been no significant change in the distribution of renal tumors stages at diagnosis, indicating a lack of stage migration with time.[8] From 1992 to 2001, the incidence of renal cancers increased annually overall by 1.4 per 100,000 in men and 1.5 per

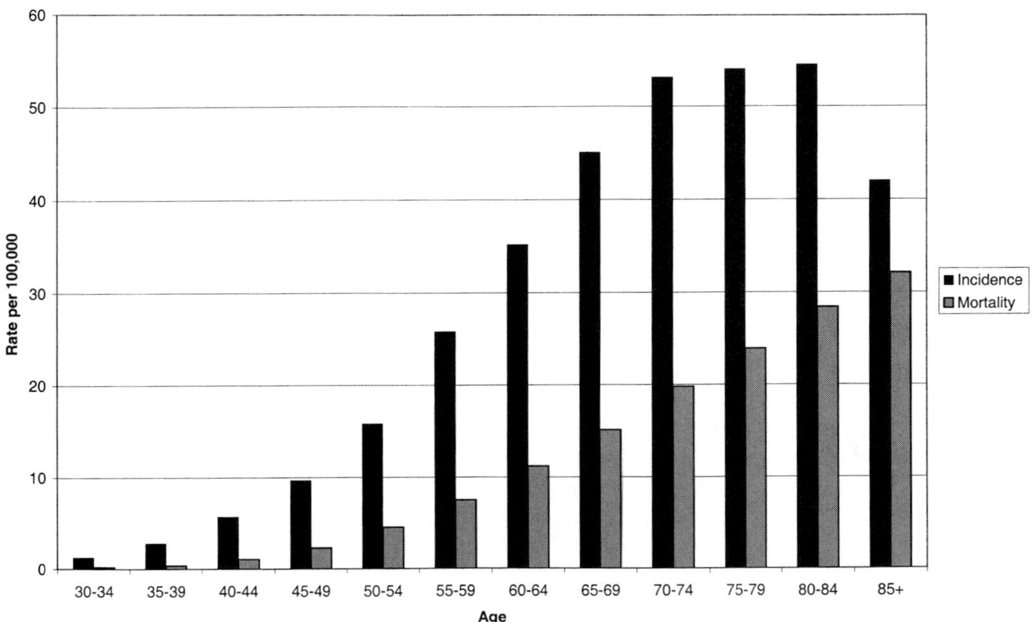

Figure 5.1. United States kidney and renal pelvis cancer incidence and mortality rates by age. (From Surveillance, Epidemiology, and End Results [SEER] database, 2002.)

100,000 in women and 1.5 per 100,000 in people <65 years old and 1.3 per 100,000 in people ≥65 years old.[3] The incidence from 1975 to 2001 steadily increased in all race groups, with the incidence in blacks surpassing the incidence in whites in the mid-1980s[3] (Figure 5.2). The annual mortality rate for all races from 1992 to 2001 fell by 0.2 per 100,000, but there were increases in mortality in blacks (0.2), Asians (1.0), and nonwhite Hispanics (0.4), with the most significant increase in Asian women (1.6).[3] Currently, there are no definitive explanations for why RCC incidence and mortality have risen at a greater rate in blacks than in whites.

With the increased use of abdominal imaging, the majority of renal tumors are incidentally diagnosed, asymptomatic at diagnosis, small, and present at an early stage.[8] In fact, 25% to 30% of all renal tumors are now incidentally diagnosed.[9] Despite this, the rates for diagnosing renal tumors with regional extension and distant metastasis increased from 1975 to 1995, but at a lower rate than localized disease.[7] Even though the majority of tumors discovered incidentally on CT scan are confined to the kidney, the mortality rate for kidney cancer has risen between 1975 and 1995, with a more rapid increase among blacks than whites.[7] Though RCC is incidentally diagnosed at a higher rate with the advent of modern imaging techniques, the fact that both the diagnosis of advanced stage disease and the mortality rate for renal cancers has steadily increased indicates that the detection of presymptomatic tumors alone cannot fully explain the rising incidence of RCC. It has been shown that 20% of tumors 4 cm or smaller are benign as compared to 17% of tumors 4 to 7 cm, and 0% of tumors >7 cm in diameter.[10] It seems that small, localized, incidentally discovered tumors may tend to be less aggressive and contribute little to the overall progression and mortality of the disease. The steady increase in localized, regional, and distant renal tumors over the last three decades

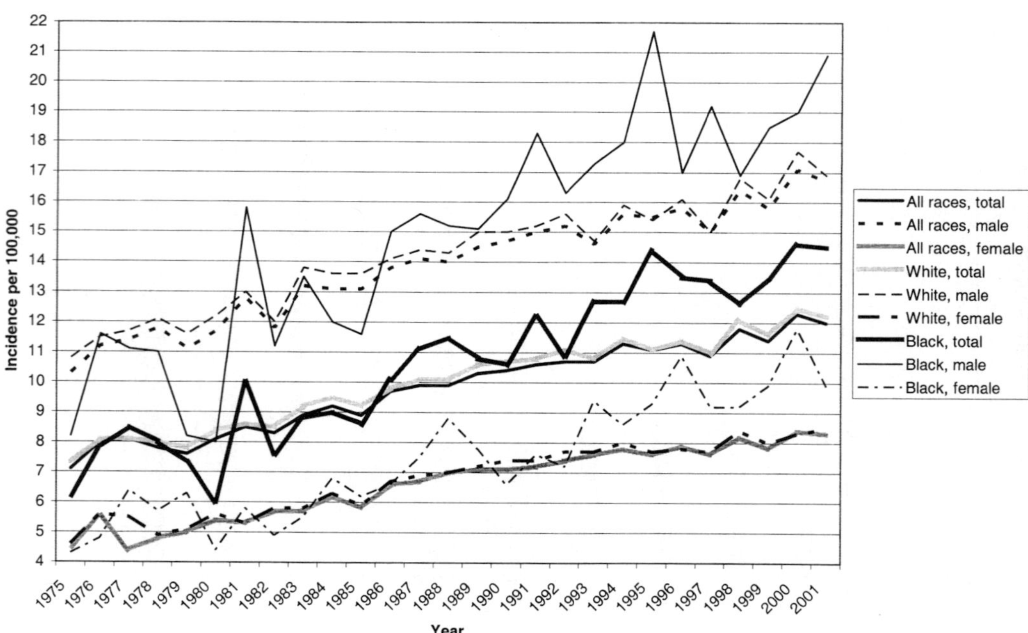

Figure 5.2. Change in United States kidney and renal pelvis cancer incidence from 1975 to 2001, stratified by race. (From Surveillance, Epidemiology, and End Results [SEER] database, 2002.)

indicates that factors other than greater use of abdominal imaging are contributing to the increasing incidence of this disease.

International Patterns

In 2002, over 200,000 kidney cancers were diagnosed worldwide, and over 100,000 people died from this disease.[11] The incidence of RCC varies among countries by a factor of 20 in men and 10 in women.[1] According to the International Agency for Research on Cancer (IARC), in 2002 the overall worldwide, age-standardized incidence and mortality rate for renal tumors was 3.6 and 1.8, respectively (all rates per 100,000 people).[11] The incidences for men and women were 4.7 and 2.5, with mortality rates of 2.3 and 1.2, respectively. The incidence in more developed regions was 7.7 compared with 1.7 in less developed regions, with the highest incidences in the Czech Republic (15.7), Lithuania (11.6), and Hungary (10.7), and the lowest incidences in Cameroon (0.2), Burkinafaso (0.35), and Bangladesh (0.4). In 2002, the regions that had the highest incidences of renal tumors were North America, Australia/New Zealand, and Europe, and the lowest rates were in Asia and Africa (Figure 5.3). Mortality rates were greatest in Central, Eastern and Western Europe, with the highest rates in the Czech Republic, Lithuania, and Hungary (Figure 5.3 and 5.4).

Socioeconomic Factors and Urbanization

The incidence and mortality rates for renal cancer tend to be higher in urbanized centers in countries such as the U.S., England, Wales, Norway, and Denmark.[4] This difference is most pronounced among men in these urban areas and may reflect the higher prevalence of cigarette smoking and the greater availability of medical and

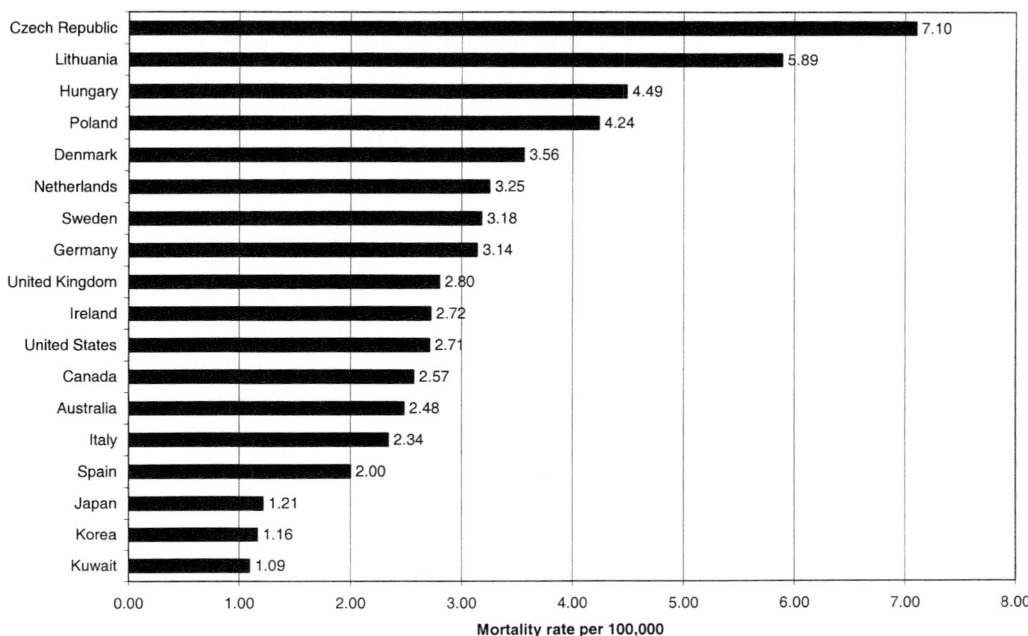

Figure 5.3. Renal cancer world mortality rates for 2000, stratified by selected country. (From International Agency for Research on Cancer 2002 GLOBOCAN database.)

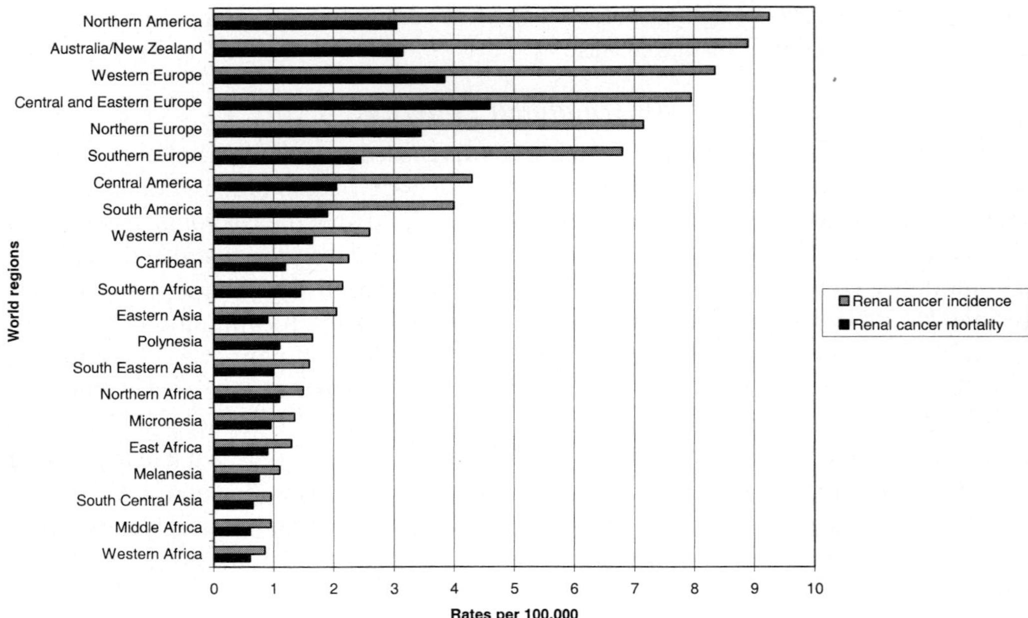

Figure 5.4. Renal cancer world incidence and mortality rates for 2002, stratified by world region. (From International Agency for Research on Cancer 2002 GLOBOCAN database.)

diagnostic services in cities.[4] When comparing the lowest to the highest socioeconomic strata in Denmark, poorer men and women had more than double the probability of developing RCC (for men: odds ratio [OR], 2.2; 95% confidence interval [CI], 1.0–4.6; for women: OR, 2.4; 95% CI, 0.9–5.9). As of now, there are few studies that have shown a link between renal cancer and socioeconomic markers, such as income and education.[12–14]

TUMOR CLASSIFICATION

Renal cell carcinoma was first classified by Grawitz[15] in 1883. He attributed the origin of renal tumors to ectopic adrenal rests, and as a result, called them hypernephromas. Historically, renal parenchymal tumors have been classified on the basis of their cytomorphologic characteristics and presumed cellular origin, comparing the tumor cells with mature counterparts in the renal tubular system.[16] Advances in the understanding of renal tumor genetics have led to the recognition of distinctive tumor types.[16] Kovacs et al.[16] and others[17] have proposed a system of renal tumor histologic classification based on the genetic lesions that underlie the formation of the distinct tumors. Incorporating these concepts, in 1997 the Union Internationale Contre le Cancer (UICC) and the American Joint Committee on Cancer (AJCC) published their recommendations for the classification of renal tumors[18] (Table 5.2).

Benign Renal Parenchymal Neoplasms

PAPILLARY ADENOMA

Papillary adenoma is more common than all other neoplasms of the renal tubular epithelium combined (occurring in as many as 20% of all patients) and is often an

Table 5.2.
Renal tumor frequency and common genetic alterations

	Relative frequency	*Common genetic alterations*
Benign tumors		
Papillary adenoma		Trisomy of chr 7, 17; loss of Y chr
Metanephric adenoma		Unknown
Oncocytoma	3–5%	Loss of chr Y and 1; translocations involving 11q13
Malignant tumors		
Conventional (clear cell) carcinoma	75%	Loss of genetic material at 3p
Papillary carcinoma	10–15%	Trisomy of chr 3q, 7, 12, 16, 17, 20; loss of Y chr
Chromophobe carcinoma	5%	Monosomy of chr 1, 2, 6, 10, 13, 17, 21; hypodiploidy
Collecting duct carcinoma	<1%	No consistent pattern
Unclassified	4–5%	No consistent pattern

chr, chromosome.

incidental finding in adult kidneys at autopsy or accompanying papillary RCC in surgical specimens (Table 5.3).[16–18] The vast majority of these tumors are <3 mm in size, and they microscopically resemble low grade papillary RCC. These tumors often have combinations of genetic alterations, including trisomy of chromosomes 7 and 17 and loss of the Y chromosome.[16] Their benign nature is inferred from their relative high frequency compared with papillary carcinoma.

METANEPHRIC ADENOMA AND ADENOFIBROMA

Metanephric adenoma and metanephric adenofibroma are rare, closely related neoplasms composed of tubular and tubulopapillary structures and glomeruloid bodies of small cuboidal cells with a high degree of maturation and differentiation, reminiscent of Wilms' tumor.[16–18] These tumors are composites of epithelial and stromal elements. Since the number of cases of these tumor types is small, their designation as benign is provisional.

RENAL ONCOCYTOMA

Oncocytomas arise from the distal renal tubule, are made up of cells with abundant eosinophilic cytoplasm and mitochondria, and comprise approximately 3% to 5% of all renal tubular neoplasms.[17,18] They usually exhibit an acinar growth, but solid and trabecular growth can occur, and approximately 5% contain tubules and cysts.[16,18] Two groups can be distinguished genetically: one with a loss of chromosomes Y, 1p, and 14q, and another with translocations between chromosome 11 at 11q13 and other chromosomes.[16,18] Some oncocytomas have a normal karyotype.

Malignant Renal Parenchymal Neoplasms

CONVENTIONAL (CLEAR CELL) CARCINOMA

Conventional (clear cell) renal carcinoma is the most common type of renal tubular carcinoma and accounts for approximately 75% of cases in surgical series.[16] These

Table 5.3.
Adult renal neoplasia syndromes

Syndrome	Renal tumor type	Genetic abnormalities	Result of mutation	Other associated lesions
Von Hippel–Lindau disease	Clear-cell RCC	Mutation of VHL tumor suppressor genes at 3p25–26	Accumulation of HIF-1α with resultant increased transcription of VEGF, GLUT-1, PDGF, TGF-α, and erythropoietin	Pheochromocytoma, pancreatic cysts, islet cell tumors, retinal angiomas, cerebellar or spinal cord hemangioblastomas, epididymal cysts
Familial renal carcinoma	Clear-cell RCC	t(3;8)(p14;q24), t(3;6), t(2;3)	Inconsistent	None known
Hereditary papillary RCC	Papillary type 1 RCC	Mutation of c-*met* proto-oncogene at 7q31.1–34	Constitutive activation of the met tyrosine kinase, promoting angiogenesis, cell motility, and growth	None known
Birt-Hogg-Dubé syndrome	Chromophobe RCC/oncocytoma	Mutation of BHD tumor suppressor gene at 17p11.2	Depletion of folliculin: function unknown	Cutaneous fibrofolliculomas and pulmonary cysts
Tuberous sclerosis complex	Angiomyolipomas and clear-cell RCC	Mutation of TSC1 (chr 9q34) or TSC2 (chr 16p13.3)	Abnormal hamartin (TSC1): involved in cell adhesion; Abnormal tuberin (TSC2): induces cell division	Facial angiofibromas, periungual fibromas, hypopigmented cutaneous macules
Hereditary leiomyomatosis RCC	Papillary type 2 RCC	FH tumor suppressor gene at 1q42–44	Abnormal FH: a Krebs cycle enzyme	Cutaneous and uterine leiomyomas
Hyperparathyroidism–jaw tumor	Renal hamartoma, renal cysts, type 1 papillary RCC	HPT-JT tumor suppressor gene at 1q21–32	Cell cycle abnormalities	Primary hyperparathyroidism and fibroma of the jaw
Familial oncocytoma	Oncocytomas and renal cysts	t(8;9)(q24.1;q34.3)	Unknown	None known

RCC, renal cell carcinoma; VHL, von Hippel–Lindau; HIF-1α, hypoxia induced factor 1α; VEGF, vascular endothelial growth factor; GLUT-1, glucose transporter 1; PDGF, platelet-derived growth factor; TGF-α, transforming growth factor α; BHD, Birt-Hogg-Dubé; TSC, tuberous sclerosis complex; FH, fumarate hydratase; HPT-JT, hyperparathyroidism-jaw tumor.

tumors have been designated as nonpapillary in genetic classification systems and can have solid or cystic patterns.[18] The majority are composed of cells with clear cytoplasm, with occasional foci of cells with eosinophilic cytoplasm.[18] These tumors exhibit loss of genetic material in chromosome 3p, with at least 50% having somatic mutations in the von Hippel–Lindau *(VHL)* gene (3p25), and an additional 10% to 20% showing inactivation of the *VHL* gene by hypermethylation.[18] Duplication of 5q22 and deletion of arms 6q, 8p, 9p, and 14q are also often present.[16] In addition, some studies have shown an association between loss of segments of chromosome 14q and progression of this tumor.[16] Sarcomatoid changes can be found in 5% of these tumors.[18]

PAPILLARY RENAL CARCINOMA

Accounting for 10% to 15% of cases in most surgical series, papillary renal carcinoma is the second most common renal tubular carcinoma.[18] These tumors have been called chromophil renal carcinoma and tubulopapillary carcinomas as well.[18] Papillary architectures dominate the majority of these tumors as do trisomies of chromosomes 3q, 7, 12, 16, 17, and 20, translocations of chromosome 1 and loss of the Y chromosome.[18,19] Papillary renal carcinoma can be further divided into types 1 and 2.[20] Type 1 is a basophilic tumor with papillae and tubular structures covered by cells with scanty cytoplasm, small oval nuclei, foamy macrophages, and frequent psammoma bodies. Type 2 is an eosinophilic tumor consisting of papillae covered by large cells with abundant eosinophilic cytoplasm and large nuclei with prominent nucleoli. Type 2 tends to be the more aggressive form. These tumors are often associated with multiple bilateral microscopic lesions and papillary renal adenomas.[16]

CHROMOPHOBE RENAL CARCINOMA

Chromophobe renal carcinoma is the third most common type of renal tubular carcinoma, accounting for approximately 5% of cases.[18] The cells that comprise this tumor grow in large solid sheets and have pale or eosinophilic cytoplasm containing several microvesicles.[16,18] Solid architecture is most common, and loss of genetic heterozygosity at chromosomes 1, 2, 6, 10, 13, 17, and 21 and hypodiploidy is prevalent.[16]

COLLECTING DUCT CARCINOMA

The histologic appearance of collecting duct carcinoma is quite variable and is most commonly characterized by irregular channels lined by atypical epithelium with a "hobnail" appearance.[18] Since collecting duct carcinoma is rare (accounts for <1% of carcinomas of the renal tubular epithelium) and the morphology is heterogeneous, no consistent pattern of genetic abnormalities has been established.[18]

MEDULLARY RENAL CARCINOMA

Medullary renal carcinoma is a particularly aggressive variant of papillary RCC that arises from the collecting ducts of the renal medulla and occurs most frequently in patients who are sickle cell trait positive.[18,21] It has many histologic characteristics in common with collecting duct carcinoma, and no consistent genetic aberrations has been identified.[22]

RENAL CELL CARCINOMA, UNCLASSIFIED

A renal cell carcinoma is designated as unclassified when it does not readily fit into the above categories, even after genetic analysis. These carcinomas account for up to 4% to 5% of cases.[18]

SARCOMATOID CHANGES

Since there is no evidence that tumors with sarcomatoid changes arise de novo, they are not viewed as a unique renal cancer type, but rather as a manifestation of high-grade carcinoma of the type of its origin.[18] Sarcomatoid changes can occur in all renal tubular carcinomas.

ADULT RENAL NEOPLASIA SYNDROMES AND GENETICS

Although the vast majority of renal parenchymal cancers develop sporadically, there are several inherited forms of the disease that have been characterized over the last three decades. Patients who develop sporadic, noninherited forms of RCC tend to develop a single, unilateral tumor late in life. In contrast, tumors associated with inherited RCC syndromes cluster in families, occur at an earlier age than sporadic tumors, are usually bilateral or multifocal, and are often associated with additional anatomic abnormalities.

Von Hippel–Lindau Disease

Von Hippel–Lindau (VHL) disease has an autosomal dominant inheritance pattern with an estimated incidence of 1 in 36,000 live births and is the best characterized form of familial RCC.[19] Individuals with VHL can develop tumors of the kidney, cerebellum, spinal cord, eyes, inner ear, pancreas, adrenal gland, and epididymis[19]; 40% to 45% of affected individuals develop clear cell renal carcinomas that occur at a mean age of 39 and if untreated account for up to 50% of deaths among VHL patients.[23,24] Approximately 18% of individuals with VHL develop pheochromocytoma, which can be bilateral; VHL patients are also frequently found to have pancreatic cysts and may develop pancreatic islet cell tumors.[19] Nearly 60% of VHL patients develop retinal angiomas, which are benign vascular tumors that can be multiple, bilateral, and can lead to blindness. Benign hemangioblastomas of the cerebellum and spinal cord occur in 60% and can be unifocal or multiple. Seven to 10% of patients develop benign epididymal cystadenomas, which are rarely symptomatic.

Von Hippel–Lindau disease is associated with mutations of the VHL tumor suppressor gene located on chromosome 3p25–26. In VHL-associated renal tumors, the germline copy of VHL is mutated and the second copy of the *VHL* gene is inactivated, most often by deletion of the gene.[19] Inactivation of the *VHL* gene, in the form of mutation, loss of heterozygosity, or hypermethylation, is frequently found in sporadic, noninherited forms of clear cell renal carcinoma as well.[20] The *VHL* gene codes for a protein that binds two additional proteins: elongin C and B.[25] These are part of a family of proteins that regulate gene transcription. This VHL complex targets a protein called hypoxia-inducible factor 1α (HIF-1α) that controls the transcription of vascular endothelial growth factor (VEGF), the glucose transporter (GLUT-1), platelet-derived growth factor (PDGF), transforming growth factor α (TGF-α), and erythropoietin.[22] Inactivation of the VHL gene results in an inability to target HIF-1α for degradation.

Familial Renal Carcinoma

Familial occurrences of clear-cell RCC have also been reported in the absence of manifestation of VHL disease and feature germline alteration involving a balanced translocation affecting chromosome 3p.[26] Approximately 50% of patients with germline translocations of t(3;8)(p14;q24), t(3;6), or t(2;3) have an inherited form of clear-cell RCC called familial renal carcinoma (FRC).[17] Patients with FRC usually develop unilateral clear-cell renal carcinomas between the ages of 50 and 70.[22] Chromosome 3p mutations are observed in 85% of nonpapillary sporadic tumors of the kidneys, suggesting common genetic mechanisms for hereditary and sporadic forms of RCC.[27]

Hereditary Papillary Renal Carcinoma

Hereditary papillary renal carcinoma (HPRC) was first described in 1994 and has an autosomal dominant transmission.[28] Affected individuals are at risk for bilateral, multifocal type 1 papillary renal carcinoma. Hereditary papillary renal carcinoma kidneys can contain over 3000 microscopic tumors per kidney.[22] Tumors in HPRC are often late onset, occurring in the 4th to 6th decades of life. HPRC has been linked to missense mutations in the c-*met* proto-oncogene located at 7q31.1–34, leading to constitutive activation of the Met tyrosine kinase in these papillary cancers.[22] This protein is related to angiogenesis, cellular motility, growth, invasion, and morphogenic differentiation.[20] Mutations of the *met* gene are also found in some sporadic type I papillary renal carcinomas.

Birt-Hogg-Dubé Syndrome

Weirich et al.[29] described a familial form of renal oncocytoma in which tumors were often bilateral and multifocal. Individuals were also found to have cutaneous fibrofolliculomas, trichodiscomas and acrochordons. An inherited autosomal dominant form of fibrofolliculoma was first described by Birt et al.[30] in 1977. Birt-Hogg-Dubé (BHD) exhibits an autosomal dominant pattern of inheritance and is associated with fibrofolliculomas, pulmonary cysts, and renal tumors. Kidney neoplasms develop in 15% to 30% of those affected with BHD at a mean age of 51, with chromophobe RCC, oncocytic-transition neoplasm, and oncocytoma being the most common types.[22,31] One series reported the incidence of chromophobe/oncocytic hybrid, chromophobe RCC, clear-cell RCC, and oncocytoma to be 50%, 34%, 9%, and 5%, respectively, in BHD patients.[32] The fibrofolliculomas tend to appear on the face, neck, and upper trunk. The pulmonary cysts are often asymptomatic, but spontaneous pneumothorax can be seen in up to 25% of affected individuals.[22] The *BHD* gene is located on chromosome 17p11.2, codes for a protein called folliculin, and has characteristics consistent with a tumor suppressor gene.[22]

Tuberous Sclerosis Complex

Tuberous sclerosis complex (TSC) is an autosomal dominant disease with variable or incomplete penetrance and an incidence of 1:9000 to 1:150,000 live births.[33] It involves facial angiofibromas (adenoma sebaceum), periungual fibromas, hypopigmented cutaneous macules, and multiple renal angiomyolipomas.[20] Seizures and learning disabilities are also common. The prevalence of angiomyolipomas in the general population is approximately 12%; in patients with TSC this prevalence is 50% to 80%.[34] Angiomyolipomas associated with TSC tend to be small, multifocal, bilateral, and asymptomatic.[35] Several cases of multifocal clear cell RCC have also been described associated with TSC.[36] Two TSC genes, *TSC1* and *TSC2,* have been mapped to chromosomes 9q34 and 16p13.3, respectively.[20] *TSC1* encodes hamartin, which is involved in cell adhesion, and *TSC2* encodes tuberin, which functions as a guanosine triphosphatase (GTPase) activating protein that induces quiescent cells to enter the S phase of the cell cycle.[20]

Hereditary Leiomyomatosis Renal Cell Carcinoma

Hereditary leiomyomatosis renal cell carcinoma (HLRCC) is a disease characterized by the development of cutaneous and uterine leiomyoma and an aggressive form of unilateral, solitary type 2 papillary renal carcinoma.[28] The gene for HLRCC is the Krebs cycle enzyme fumarate hydratase *(FH),* which acts as a tumor suppressor gene and has been mapped to chromosome 1q42-44.[20,28] The type 2 papillary renal cancers that develop in association with this disease metastasize early and are often fatal.

ilial Renal Hamartomas Associated with Hyperparathyroidism–Jaw Tumor Syndrome

Familial renal hamartomas associated with hyperparathyroidism–jaw tumor (HPT-JT) syndrome is an autosomal dominant disease characterized by primary hyperparathyroidism, ossifying fibroma of the jaw, and renal hamartomas.[20] The *HPT-JT* gene has been mapped to chromosome 1q21-32 and is a tumor suppressor gene that blocks the expression of cyclin D1, a key cell cycle regulator.[37] This syndrome is also associated with renal cysts and type 1 papillary renal cell carcinoma.

Familial Oncocytoma

Familial oncocytoma is a disease unique from Birt-Hogg-Dubé that results in multiple, bilateral renal oncocytomas and cysts associated with the reciprocal translocation (8;9)(q24.1;q34.3).[38]

RISK FACTORS FOR RENAL CANCERS

The most widely accepted risk for the development of RCC is advanced age. The vast majority of sporadic cases of RCC are diagnosed in patients over 50 years old, and for each decade of life beyond age 35, the relative risk (RR) of developing RCC is 2.17 (95% CI, 1.83–2.58) as compared to subjects in the previous decade of life. The majority of the epidemiologic information on other risk factors for RCC has come from case-control studies. These studies have been conducted in several countries around the world and their results often vary. The largest and most comprehensive studies of the epidemiology of renal cancer to date are included in the International Renal-Cell Cancer Study (IRCCS), a multicenter investigation that took place in five countries using a common protocol and included 1732 cases and 2309 controls.[39–45] Despite these studies, the current epidemiologic information regarding a subject's characteristics, comorbidities, habits, and exposures as they relate to the development of RCC is often inconsistent and at times contradictory.

Family History

Only approximately 4% of cases of renal cancer are inherited.[19] In a case-control study, Mellemgaard et al.[13] showed that a family history of RCC was associated with an increased risk of developing RCC in both men (OR, 4.1; 95% CI, 1.1–14.9) and women (OR, 4.8; 95% CI 1.0–23.0). The IRCCS determined that having a first-degree relative with a history of RCC increased a person's odds of developing RCC by 60%.[45]

This is further supported by familial clustering of RCC, likely due to mutations of chromosome 3,[46] and increased risk among individuals with autosomal dominant inherited diseases such as VHL and polycystic kidney disease.[47,48] Family history, though, explains only a small portion of the renal cancers.

Tobacco

Although anti-tobacco campaigns and educational efforts have dramatically reduced the prevalence of tobacco smoking in the U.S., the most recent report from the Centers for Disease Control and Prevention (May 2004) estimated that 22.5% of American adults (46 million people) smoke cigarettes.[49] Smoking is one of the most consistent risk factors for RCC. Out of 17 case-control studies reviewed, representing populations from countries around the world, 15 showed an increased overall probability of developing RCC associated with smoking, with odds ratios ranging from 1.1 to 3.9.[13,14,41,50–63] Of those studies that differentiate between genders, most show that the risk of developing RCC associated with smoking is either more significant in or exclusive to men.[13,51–53,57,59,62] Most studies indicate that a higher number of cigarettes smoked per day and a longer duration of smoking leads to a higher risk of developing RCC, with some studies showing elevated risk only in those subjects who have smoked for more than 40 years or two to three packs per day.[13,41,54,55] Second-hand smoke may also increase the risk for RCC. Hu et al.[52] found that men and women exposed to passive smoke at home or at their place of work for more than 43 years had odds ratios of 3.9 (95% CI, 1.4–10.6) and 1.8 (95% CI, 1.0–3.3), respectively, for developing RCC. Beginning smoking at a younger age may also lead to an increased risk for RCC, with people who start smoking at age 24 or later having two-thirds the risk of those who began smoking at an age 12 or younger.[41] In a case-control study conducted in Los Angeles, California, McLaughlin et al.[57] estimated that 30% of RCC in men and 24% in women are attributable to cigarette smoking. The components of cigarette smoke that promote the development of RCC have not been identified; however, N-nitrosodimethylamine induces kidney tumors in several animal species, and the urine of smokers has known mutagenic potential.[64]

The benefits of smoking cessation with regard to lowering the risk for developing RCC can be seen as soon as 10 years after quitting, and the risk to ex-smokers approximates the risk for those who have never smoked after 30 years of cessation.[63,65] Several studies have found no links between pipe smoking and RCC,[41,63] but one report did find that men who chewed tobacco had a relative risk of 3.2 (95% CI, 1.1–8.7) compared to those who did not chew tobacco[59]; others found no increased risk with chewing tobacco.[41,63]

McLaughlin et al.[66] confirmed the dose-response relationship between cigarette smoking and RCC in a cohort of 250,000 U.S. military veterans studied from 1954 to 1980. The relative risks were 1.31, 1.37, 1.60, and 2.06 for those who smoked 1 to 9, 10 to 20, 21 to 39, and ≥40 cigarettes per day, respectively. Overall, the authors calculated that current smokers had a 47% increased incidence of RCC compared with nonsmokers. Hunt et al.[67] performed a meta-analysis of 19 case-control studies and five cohort studies that examined the relationship between tobacco smoking and RCC risk. This report included 8032 cases, 13,800 controls, and 1,457,754 cohort participants. The authors found that the relative risk for RCC for people who ever smoked as compared to lifetime never-smokers was 1.38 (95% CI, 1.27–1.50); the relative risk for male smokers was 1.54 (95% CI, 1.42–1.68) and 1.22 (95% CI, 1.09–1.36) for female smokers. In a separate study, smokers were also at an increased risk of death from RCC as compared with former smokers and nonsmokers (hazard ratio, 2.5; 95% CI, 1.5–4.3) and were more likely to be diagnosed with metastatic disease (OR, 2.2; 95% CI, 1.4–3.5).[60] In those cases without distant metastases, smokers had a significantly worse overall rate of survival as compared to nonsmokers.[68] In total, the calculated attributable risks indicate that 20% to 30% of RCC among men and 10% to 20% among women are caused by cigarette smoking.[4] Cigarette smoking exerts a significant increase in the risk for developing RCC. There seems to be a dose-dependent relationship and demonstrable benefits to smoking cessation with regard to a person's risk for developing RCC and dying from this disease.

Diet

Thirteen case-control studies and three cohort studies reviewed the influence of diet on the development of RCC. Overall, diet has a role, but many of the associations between RCC and specific food items or nutrients are controversial. Much of the information presented in these studies was collected via patient-administered questionnaires, bringing recall bias into question.

Some case-control studies suggest that high energy or carbohydrate intake leads to an increased incidence of RCC, especially in women.[69,70] Van Dijk et al.[71] performed a prospective cohort study including over 120,000 Danish subjects and found no association between energy intake and RCC. Foods and food groups that have been implicated in RCC include red meat (beef, pork, lamb, sausages, fried meats, processed meats), poultry, dairy products, and oils, along with a high fat intake and a high-protein diet.[55,57,58,61,70,72–74] Beverages that have shown an association with RCC include tea and coffee,[57,62] but some studies have not found this association.[50] Parker et al.[75] found that women who drank at least three alcoholic drinks per week compared to nondrinkers had a 50% lower incidence of RCC, and the effect is most significant in women who drink beer.

The foods that are most commonly found to be protective against RCC include dark-green vegetables, orange vegetables, cruciferous vegetables (i.e., vegetables in the mustard family, including mustard greens, cabbage, broccoli, cauliflower, Brussels sprouts, kohlrabi, radishes, and turnips), and fruits, especially citrus fruits and apples.[58,61,70,72,73,76] These foods affect RCC incidence most significantly in women and at the highest levels of consumption. Supporting this finding, a Swedish cohort study composed of 61,000 women surveyed at baseline and followed for an average 13.4 years claimed a decreased risk of RCC in those women who ate ≥75 servings of fruits and ≥75 servings of vegetables per month as compared to those women who ate ≤11 servings of these per month despite odds ratios that lacked statistical significance (OR, 0.59; 95% CI, 0.26–1.34 and OR, 0.6; 95% CI, 0.31–1.17, respectively).[77] In contrast, van Dijk et al.[78] found no significant protective effect of fruits or vegetables in a cohort of over 120,000 subjects in the Netherlands. As far as specific nutrients are concerned, vitamin E, calcium, iron, α-carotene, β-carotene, β-cryptoxanthin, and lutein have been shown to have a protective effect against RCC, and a low intake of magnesium has been linked to an increased risk of RCC.[70,72,76]

In general, the information regarding diet and its effects on the incidence of RCC is inconsistent and inconclusive. The most convincing data include the negative effects of high protein and carbohydrate diets and the protective effects of diets rich in fruits and vegetables. Nonetheless, these effects are minor and results are only significant for the extreme intake levels of these foods.

Obesity

Several case-control studies have reported that obesity leads to an increased risk of developing RCC, but the findings regarding the prognosis of the disease in obese patients vary. Generally, these studies compare the two extremes in body mass index (BMI) when evaluating for effect.[42,55,57–59,62,79–81] For instance, in comparing the highest to the lowest BMI quartile, Shapiro et al.[80] found that men had an odds ratio of 2.3 (95% CI, 1.2–4.5) and women had an odds ratio of 3.3 (95% CI, 1.2–8.7) for developing RCC.[80] Several authors found obesity results in an increased risk of RCC only in women.[42,57,79] For instance, McLaughlin et al.[57] found that women with a BMI in the highest 5% of their study population were nearly six times as likely to develop RCC as those in the lowest BMI quartile (OR, 5.9; 95% CI, 1.8–20.4); the significance of the risk increased with increasing age. Obesity was not associated with an increased risk in men. Other studies have found that higher BMI brings greater risk, that a higher rate of weight increase is an independent risk factor in women, and that the increased risk associated with BMI is seen only in subjects who also have hypertension.[42,59,79]

A cohort study out of the Netherlands found that for each 1-point increase in BMI, the relative risk of developing RCC increased by 7% (RR, 1.07; 95% CI, 1.02–1.12).[71] Calle et al.[82] conducted a prospective cohort study in 900,000 United States adults and found that death from RCC was 1.7 times more likely in men with a BMI >35 and 4.75 times more likely in women with a BMI >40.[82] Also of note, amphetamines, which are frequently used as components of diet pills, have been found to increase the odds of developing RCC by up to four times, with this effect being most pronounced with regular use and increased dose,[81,83] but the IRCCS study that evaluated amphetamine use found that RCC was unrelated to amphetamines.[42]

Physical Activity

A series of studies have investigated the relationship between a person's level of physical activity and their risk of developing RCC.[42,83–86] Of these five studies, the most extensive was a cohort study conducted by Bergstrom et al.[84] in a group of nearly 11,000 Swedish same-sex twin sets. They found no association between the level of leisure or occupational physical activity and the risk of RCC. Only Lindblad et al.[83] found that high levels of physical activity led to a reduced risk of developing RCC, but this association was only significant in men. As of yet, there is little evidence to support a link between physical activity and RCC.

Urinary Tract Conditions

Urinary tract conditions that have been implicated in the development of RCC include urinary tract infections, kidney stones, and past kidney trauma. The odds ratio of developing RCC in patients who had a history of recurrent urinary tract infection, as established by a set of three case-control studies, ranged from 1.2 to 1.9.[45,53,61] Case-control studies looking at the influence of stone disease on RCC indicate that those patients who have any history of nephrolithiasis have approximately double the risk of developing renal cancers as compared to the general population.[45,55,61] Chow et al.,[87] though, conducted a prospective study of a cohort of over 60,000 Swedes with a history of kidney stones over a 25-year period and determined that these patients had no increased risk RCC. Finally, Schlehofer et al.[45] determined that a history of kidney trauma tripled the risk of developing a subsequent RCC (RR, 3.2; 95% CI, 1.9–5.5).[45] These conditions may be associated with RCC, but the literature to support this as of now is limited.

General Medical Conditions

A number of medical conditions have been linked with RCC, but the evidence is inconsistent. No consistent association between RCC and myocardial infarction, stroke, prostate disease, sexually transmitted diseases, cirrhosis, hepatitis, or cholelithiasis has been shown.[45,64] In one of the more extensive international case-control studies, Schlehofer et al.[45] found a modest increase in risk of developing RCC with diabetes (OR, 1.4; 95% CI, 1.0–1.8) and thyroid disease (OR, 1.6; 95% CI, 1.3–2.2), but these findings have not been supported by others.[64] In addition, one study reported a 40% increased risk of RCC in patients with rheumatoid arthritis and osteoarthritis,[88] but this relationship has not yet been confirmed.

Hypertension (HTN), antihypertensives, and their influences on renal cancer have been widely studied. In general, the results are mixed. In addition, since the use of antihypertensives and HTN is closely linked, it is difficult to use evidence from case-control studies to isolate the pure effects of the individual factors. Shapiro et al.[89] found that being categorized as hypertensive increased the probability of developing RCC in women alone (OR, 2.5; 95% CI, 1.2–5.1), but isolated elevated systolic or diastolic pressures increased the risk in both men and women. Yuan et al.[81] found that HTN was a strong, independent risk factor for RCC in both men and women (OR, 2.2; 95% CI, 1.8–2.6). A cohort study of over 364,000 Swedish adults showed that men with a diastolic blood pressure >90 mm Hg had a twofold increased risk of developing RCC compared with those adults with a diastolic blood pressure <70 mm Hg, and the risk was 60% higher in men with a systolic blood pressure >150 mm Hg compared with men with a systolic blood pressure <120 mm Hg.[90] This effect was most pronounced in those men who were also obese. A final cohort study of nearly 333,000 American adults found that the relative risk of RCC increased 1.12 (95% CI, 1.06–1.18) for each 10 mm Hg of systolic blood pressure greater than the comparison group.[91] This effect was greatest for those subjects with a systolic blood pressure >140 mm Hg and who also smoked more than 26 cigarettes per day.

Several studies have shown that diuretic use in hypertensives is not related to RCC development.[81,89,92] Additionally, the use of diuretics for reasons other than hypertension (i.e., weight control, heart failure) has not been linked to an increased risk of RCC in normotensive subjects (OR, 1.2; 95% CI, 0.7–2.2).[92] Among hypertensive subjects, heavy users of diuretics experienced similar risk as light users (lifetime dose ≥137 g vs. lifetime dose <43 g).[81] In addition, normotensive subjects who took nondiuretic antihypertensives showed no increased risk of RCC.

In contrast, Mellemgaard et al.[93] conducted a prospective cohort study of over 200,000 Danish patients identified as having HTN upon hospital discharge and concluded that the risk of RCC associated with diuretic use was more than doubled. One case-control study found a fourfold increased risk of developing RCC in women who use diuretics,[62] and another found this level of increased risk in women was associated with thiazide diuretics alone.[51] Still others have shown that an increased risk of RCC was only associated with nondiuretic antihypertensives.[94] Grossman et al.[95] reviewed nine case-control studies and three cohort studies that examined the effect that diuretics have on the development of RCC. In the case-control studies, the odds ratio of renal cell carcinoma occurring in patients treated with diuretics averaged 1.55 (95% CI, 1.42–1.71) compared with patients not taking diuretics. In the three cohort studies evaluating over 1,226,000 patients, diuretic therapy was associated with a greater than twofold risk of RCC when compared with patients not on diuretics. One cohort study and the seven case-control studies that stratified the effects by gender reported that women who used diuretics were more likely to develop RCC than men (OR, 2.0; 95% CI, 1.6–2.7; and OR, 1.7; 95% CI, 1.3–2.1, respectively).

In total, it seems that long-standing and significant HTN increases the risk of developing RCC. It is postulated that HTN may induce renal injury or may be associated with metabolic or functional changes within the renal tubules, which in turn may increase renal susceptibility to carcinogens.[43] Although some studies present compelling evidence that diuretics and other antihypertensive medications may bring added risk of developing RCC, especially in women and with long-term use, the number of cases of RCC that can be linked to antihypertensive use alone is likely minimal and would not merit restricting the use of any particular class of medication.

Occupation

Certain occupational exposures are considered risk factors for developing RCC. Industrial exposures, especially organic solvents, are most consistently linked to RCC. The occupation portion of the IRCCS reported that RCC was associated with blast furnace or coke oven exposure, the iron and steel industry, and exposure to asbestos, cadmium, dry cleaning solvents, gasoline, or other petroleum products with odds ratios ranging from 1.4 to 2.0.[39] The risk associated with asbestos, petroleum products, and dry-cleaning solvents was related to the duration of exposure, supporting a hypothesis of a causal role of the exposure to the development of RCC. One study reports that the latency from the time of exposure to the development of RCC for many common occupational exposures is at least 30 years.[96] Table 5.4 lists the industries, occupations, and exposures and the associated odds ratio or range of odds ratios reported.

Analgesics

Several studies have reported that phenacetin use results in an increased risk of developing RCC.[57,58,97,98] In fact, this compound is no longer available in the United States due to its presumed carcinogenic effects on the urinary tract. Other analgesics, though, have also been linked to RCC. For instance, Gago-Dominguez et al.[97] evaluated over 1200 cases of RCC and an equal number of controls matched for age, race, and gender and found that regular use of any analgesics, including phenacetin, acetaminophen, aspirin, and nonaspirin nonsteroidal antiinflammatory medications, was associated with a higher odds of developing RCC (OR, 1.6; 95% CI, 1.4–1.9), and the risk was proportional to the extent of exposure.[97] Importantly, there was no increased risk for those subjects who took a 325-mg aspirin daily for its cardioprotective properties. In contrast, the analgesic portion of the IRCCS reported that, after controlling for age, gender, BMI, tobacco use, and study center, there was no association between phenacetin, pyrazolones, acetaminophen, or aspirin and the development of RCC.[44] These

Table 5.4.
Renal cancer odds ratios or odds ratio ranges for specific industries, occupations, and exposures

Industry	Odds ratio	Occupation	Odds ratio	Occupation	Odds ratio	Exposures	Odds ratio	Exposures	Odds ratio
Construction industry[104,105]	NA–1.4	Aircraft mechanics[106]	2.8	Mechanics[107]	1.9	Jet fuel[106]	3.5	Asbestos[39, 106, 108–110]	NA–1.6
Dry cleaning[14,39,105,106,108]	NA–2.5	Architects[104]	NA	Medical professionals[39,105,106,111]	NA	Lead[110]	2.6	Aromatic amines[110]	NA
Electronic industry[110]	3.2	Auto dealers[107]	3.0	Miners[105]	NA	Nitric acid[106]	NA	Benzene[110]	1.4
Iron and steel industry[39,96,108,111]	NA–1.6	Auto mechanics[107]	4.0	Painters[105,110]	1.8–1.9	Nongasoline petroleum products[39]	1.6	Cadmium[39,110]	1.4–4.3
Leather manufacturing[105,111]	NA	Blast furnace/coke oven workers[39]	1.7	Photographers[105]	NA	Organic solvents[110,112]	1.6–2.3	Carbon tetrachloride[110]	1.2
Metal degreasing[110,113]	NA–5.6	Chemical workers[110]	3.1	Plumbers[105,106]	NA	Ozone[106]	1.8	Chlorinated aliphatic hydrocarbons[109,112]	NA–2.1
Metal working[14,39,106,110]	NA–1.6	Engineers[104]	1.4	Police[105,106]	NA	Pesticides[39]	NA	Chromium[106]	NA
Oil refining[108–111]	NA	Farmers and farm product vendors[105–107]	NA–4.4	Radiation[39,111]	NA	Phosphoric acid[106]	NA	Felt dust[106]	3.6
Printing industry[105,106,110]	NA–3.5	Firefighters[105,106]	NA–4.9	Sales workers[105,114]	NA–2.1	Rubber[105,106,110]	NA–6.0	Gasoline[39]	1.6
Railway industry[110]	6.2	Fishermen[105]	NA	Scientists[105]	NA	Tetrachloroethylene[110]	1.4	Hydrogen sulfide[106]	NA
		Forestry workers[105]	NA	Security guards[106,107]	NA–5.4	Trichloroethylene[110,112,113]	NA–2.0	Inks[106]	NA
		Gardeners[106]	4.1	Textile workers[114]	6.2	Ultraviolet radiation[106]	NA	Inorganic acids[106]	NA
		Glass workers[105]	2.6	University employees[107]	7.6				
		Managers[105,106,110,114]	NA–3.3	Welders[39,106,110]	NA–3.0				
				Wood workers[105]	NA				

NA, no association.

findings are supported by other reports.[92,99] Given this body of evidence, it is likely that analgesics have little to no influence on RCC development.

Reproductive Factors

Hormonal factors are implicated in the development of RCC because normal and malignant renal tissue contains steroid hormone receptors.[100] Exogenous estrogens have been reported to induce renal tumors in animals,[101] and obesity, which is related to elevated estrogen levels, is implicated as a possible risk factor for RCC in women.[86] After adjusting for age, smoking status, BMI, and age at first birth, women with five or more births had an odds ratio of 2.2 (95% CI, 1.2–4.0) of developing RCC.[102] This association was strongest if the women also had hypertension or were obese. There was also an increased chance of developing RCC in those women who had a history of hysterectomy or used postmenopausal hormonal replacements, but long-term oral contraceptive use had a protective effect. A Swedish study of 1465 RCC female cases and 7325 female controls reported odds ratios of 1.4 (95% CI, 1.2–1.7) for ever-parous compared with nulliparous women, 1.9 (95% CI, 1.4–2.6) for women with a history of five or more births compared with nulliparous women, and an odds increase of 15% for each birth.[103] Finally, the reproductive portion of the IRCCS found an odds ratio of 1.8 (95% CI, 1.1–2.9) for women with a history of six or more births compared with women with only one birth.[40] The authors also reported a decreasing risk of RCC with increasing age at first birth. Age at menopause and menarche was unrelated to RCC. Women who had a history of both hysterectomy and oophorectomy were also at increased risk. Women taking oral contraceptives and who were also nonsmokers had decreased odds of developing RCC (OR, 0.5; 95% CI, 0.4–0.8), and this effect increased with increased length of use. Estrogen replacement therapy was not associated with RCC. In general, no consistent association has been shown between RCC and parity, age at first birth, age at menarche or menopause, menopausal status, hysterectomy, or oophorectomy.

CONCLUSION

Renal cell carcinoma accounts for 2%–3% of all malignant cancers and is the third most common urologic neoplasm. The incidence of RCC has increased over the last three decades, especially in black Americans. The 5-year survival rate for this disease has improved by over 20% during the same time period, though. The yearly worldwide incidence of RCC is over 200,000 cases. The world regions that have the highest incidences of renal tumors include North America, Australia/New Zealand, and Europe, with the lowest rates in Asia and Africa. The incidence and mortality rates for renal cancer tend to be higher in urbanized centers in countries such as the United States, England, Wales, Norway, and Denmark. With the increased use of abdominal imaging, small, asymptomatic renal tumors are diagnosed more frequently. Despite this, the rate at which advanced disease is diagnosed and the mortality rate from RCC has also increased, indicating that factors other than greater use of abdominal imaging are contributing to the increasing incidence of this disease.

Family history and the adult renal neoplasia syndromes account for relatively few cases of RCC. The most consistent risk for developing renal parenchymal cancers is advanced age, but other factors, such as smoking, high protein and fat diets, obesity (especially in women), long-standing hypertension, and use of certain categories of antihypertensives, may also increase an individual's risk for this disease. Diets high in certain fruits and vegetables may have a protective effect against developing RCC. The evidence regarding the risk associated with physical activity, urinary tract pathology, occupational exposures, analgesics, and reproductive factors is at this time mixed and inconclusive. Overall, much of the data regarding specific RCC risks are from case-control studies, making it impossible to assert definite causality for these factors.

REFERENCES

1. Motzer RJ, Bander NH, Nanus DM. Renal-cell carcinoma. N Engl J Med 1996;335(12):865–875.
2. Jemal A, Murray T, Ward E, et al. Cancer statistics, 2005. CA Cancer J Clin 2005;55(1):10–30.
3. Ries L, Eisner M, Kosary C, et al. SEER Cancer Statistics Review, 1975–2002. http://seer.cancer.gov/csr/1975_2002/. Bethesda, MD: National Cancer Institute, 2005.
4. McLaughlin JK, Lipworth L. Epidemiologic aspects of renal cell cancer. Semin Oncol 2000;27(2):115–123.
5. Guinan P, Sobin LH, Algaba F, et al. TNM staging of renal cell carcinoma: Workgroup No. 3. Union International Contre le Cancer (UICC) and the American Joint Committee on Cancer (AJCC). Cancer 1997;80(5):992–993.
6. Gettman MT, Blute ML, Spotts B, Bryant SC, Zincke H. Pathologic staging of renal cell carcinoma: significance of tumor classification with the 1997 TNM staging system. Cancer 2001;91(2):354–361.
7. Chow WH, Devesa SS, Warren JL, Fraumeni JF Jr. Rising incidence of renal cell cancer in the United States. JAMA 1999;281(17):1628–1631.
8. Hock LM, Lynch J, Balaji KC. Increasing incidence of all stages of kidney cancer in the last 2 decades in the United States: an analysis of surveillance, epidemiology and end results program data. J Urol 2002;167(1):57–60.
9. Marshall FF, Stewart AK, Menck HR. The National Cancer Data Base: report on kidney cancers. The American College of Surgeons Commission on Cancer and the American Cancer Society. Cancer 1997;80(11):2167–2174.
10. Duchene DA, Lotan Y, Cadeddu JA, Sagalowsky AI, Koeneman KS. Histopathology of surgically managed renal tumors: analysis of a contemporary series. Urology 2003;62(5):827–830.
11. Ferlay J, Bray F, Pisani P, Parkin D. GLOBOCAN 2002: Cancer Incidence, Mortality and Prevalence Worldwide. IARC CancerBase No.5, version 2.0. IARC Press, 2004.
12. McLaughlin J, Blot W, Devesa S, Fraumeni JF Jr. Renal Cancer. In: Schottenfeld D, Fraumeni JF Jr, eds. Cancer Epidemiology and Prevention. New York: Oxford University Press, 1996:1142–1155.
13. Mellemgaard A, Engholm G, McLaughlin JK, Olsen JH. Risk factors for renal cell carcinoma in Denmark. I. Role of socioeconomic status, tobacco use, beverages, and family history. Cancer Causes Control 1994;5(2):105–113.
14. Schlehofer B, Heuer C, Blettner M, Niehoff D, Wahrendorf J. Occupation, smoking and demographic factors, and renal cell carcinoma in Germany. Int J Epidemiol 1995;24(1):51–57.
15. Grawitz P. Die Enstehung von Nierentumoren aus Nebennierengewebe. Arch Klin Chir 1883;30:824.
16. Kovacs G, Akhtar M, Beckwith BJ, et al. The Heidelberg classification of renal cell tumours. J Pathol 1997;183(2):131–133.
17. Zambrano NR, Lubensky IA, Merino MJ, Linehan WM, Walther MM. Histopathology and molecular genetics of renal tumors toward unification of a classification system. J Urol 1999;162(4):1246–1258.
18. Storkel S, Eble JN, Adlakha K, et al. Classification of renal cell carcinoma: Workgroup No. 1. Union Internationale Contre le Cancer (UICC) and the American Joint Committee on Cancer (AJCC). Cancer 1997;80(5):987–989.
19. Linehan WM, Lerman MI, Zbar B. Identification of the von Hippel-Lindau (VHL) gene. Its role in renal cancer. JAMA 1995;273(7):564–570.
20. Takahashi M, Kahnoski R, Gross D, Nicol D, Teh BT. Familial adult renal neoplasia. [Review] [60 refs]. J Med Genet 2002;39(1):1–5.
21. Davis CJ Jr, Mostofi FK, Sesterhenn IA. Renal medullary carcinoma. The seventh sickle cell nephropathy. Am J Surg Pathol 1995;19(1):1–11.

22. Linehan WM, Walther MM, Zbar B. The genetic basis of cancer of the kidney. J Urol 2003;170(6, pt 1):2163–2172.
23. Poston CD, Jaffe GS, Lubensky IA, et al. Characterization of the renal pathology of a familial form of renal cell carcinoma associated with von Hippel-Lindau disease: clinical and molecular genetic implications. J Urol 1995;153(1):22–26.
24. Neumann HP, Zbar B. Renal cysts, renal cancer and von Hippel-Lindau disease. Kidney Int 1997;51(1):16–26.
25. Kibel A, Iliopoulos O, DeCaprio JA, Kaelin WG Jr. Binding of the von Hippel-Lindau tumor suppressor protein to Elongin B and C. Science 1995;269(5229):1444–1446.
26. Cohen AJ, Li FP, Berg S, et al. Hereditary renal-cell carcinoma associated with a chromosomal translocation. N Engl J Med 1979;301(11):592–595.
27. Gnarra JR, Lerman MI, Zbar B, Linehan WM. Genetics of renal-cell carcinoma and evidence for a critical role for von Hippel-Lindau in renal tumorigenesis. Semin Oncol 1995;22(1):3–8.
28. Linehan WM, Vasselli J, Srinivasan R, et al. Genetic basis of cancer of the kidney: disease-specific approaches to therapy. Clin Cancer Res 2004;10(18, pt 2):t-9S.
29. Weirich G, Glenn G, Junker K, et al. Familial renal oncocytoma: clinicopathological study of 5 families. J Urol 1998;160(2):335–340.
30. Birt AR, Hogg GR, Dube WJ. Hereditary multiple fibrofolliculomas with trichodiscomas and acrochordons. Arch Dermatol 1977;113(12):1674–1677.
31. Pavlovich CP, Walther MM, Eyler RA, et al. Renal tumors in the Birt-Hogg-Dube syndrome. Am J Surg Pathol 2002;26(12):1542–1552.
32. Pavlovich CP, Walther MM, Eyler RA, et al. Renal tumors in the Birt-Hogg-Dube syndrome. Am J Surg Pathol 2002;26(12):1542–1552.
33. Tello R, Blickman JG, Buonomo C, Herrin J. Meta analysis of the relationship between tuberous sclerosis complex and renal cell carcinoma. Eur J Radiol 1998;27(2):131–138.
34. Malone MJ, Johnson PR, Jumper BM, Howard PJ, Hopkins TB, Libertino JA. Renal angiomyolipoma: 6 case reports and literature review. [Review] [37 refs]. J Urol 1986;135(2):349–353.
35. Chonko AM, Weiss SM, Stein JH, Ferris TF. Renal involvement in tuberous sclerosis. Am J Med 1974;56(1):124–132.
36. Sampson JR, Patel A, Mee AD. Multifocal renal cell carcinoma in sibs from a chromosome 9 linked (TSC1) tuberous sclerosis family. J Med Genet 1995;32(11):848–850.
37. Woodard GE, Lin L, Zhang JH, Agarwal SK, Marx SJ, Simonds WF. Parafibromin, product of the hyperparathyroidism-jaw tumor syndrome gene HRPT2, regulates cyclin D1/PRAD1 expression. Oncogene 2005;24(7):1272–1276.
38. Teh BT, Blennow E, Giraud S, et al. Bilateral multiple renal oncocytomas and cysts associated with a constitutional translocation (8;9)(q24.1;q34.3) and a rare constitutional VHL missense substitution. Genes Chromosomes Cancer 1998;21(3):260–264.
39. Mandel JS, McLaughlin JK, Schlehofer B, et al. International renal-cell cancer study. IV. Occupation. Int J Cancer 1995;61(5):601–605.
40. Lindblad P, Mellemgaard A, Schlehofer B, et al. International renal-cell cancer study. V. Reproductive factors, gynecologic operations and exogenous hormones. Int J Cancer 1995;61(2):192–198.
41. McLaughlin JK, Lindblad P, Mellemgaard A, et al. International renal-cell cancer study. I. Tobacco use. Int J Cancer 1995;60(2):194–198.
42. Mellemgaard A, Lindblad P, Schlehofer B, et al. International renal-cell cancer study. III. Role of weight, height, physical activity, and use of amphetamines. Int J Cancer 1995;60(3):350–354.
43. McLaughlin JK, Chow WH, Mandel JS, et al. International renal-cell cancer study. VIII. Role of diuretics, other anti-hypertensive medications and hypertension. Int J Cancer 1995;63(2):216–221.
44. McCredie M, Pommer W, McLaughlin JK, et al. International renal-cell cancer study. II. Analgesics. Int J Cancer 1995;60(3):345–349.
45. Schlehofer B, Pommer W, Mellemgaard A, et al. International renal-cell-cancer study. VI. the role of medical and family history. Int J Cancer 1996;66(6):723–726.
46. Cohen AJ, Li FP, Berg S, et al. Hereditary renal-cell carcinoma associated with a chromosomal translocation. N Engl J Med 1979;301(11):592–595.
47. Lynch HT, Walzak MP. Genetics in urogenital cancer. Urol Clin North Am 1980;7(3):815–829.
48. Bernstein J, Evan AP, Gardner KD, Jr. Epithelial hyperplasia in human polycystic kidney diseases. Its role in pathogenesis and risk of neoplasia. [Review] [100 refs]. Am J Pathol 1987;129(1):92–101.

49. Adult Cigarette Smoking in the United States: Current Estimates. http://www.cdc.gov/tobacco/factsheets/AdultCigaretteSmoking_FactSheet.htm. Atlanta: Centers for Disease Control, 2005.

50. Benhamou S, Lenfant MH, Ory-Paoletti C, Flamant R. Risk factors for renal-cell carcinoma in a French case-control study. Int J Cancer 1993;55(1):32–36.

51. Hiatt RA, Tolan K, Quesenberry CP Jr. Renal cell carcinoma and thiazide use: a historical, case-control study. Cancer Causes Control 1994;5(4):319–325.

52. Hu J, Ugnat AM, Canadian Cancer Registries Epidemiology Research Group. Active and passive smoking and risk of renal cell carcinoma in Canada. Eur J Cancer 2005;41(5):770–778.

53. Kreiger N, Marrett LD, Dodds L, Hilditch S, Darlington GA. Risk factors for renal cell carcinoma: results of a population-based case-control study. Cancer Causes Control 1993;4(2):101–110.

54. LaVecchia C, Negri E, D'Avanzo B, Franceschi S. Smoking and renal cell carcinoma. Cancer Res 1990;50(17):5231–5233.

55. Maclure M, Willett W. A case-control study of diet and risk of renal adenocarcinoma. Epidemiology 1990;1(6):430–440.

56. McCredie M, Ford JM, Stewart JH. Risk factors for cancer of the renal parenchyma. Int J Cancer 1988;42(1):13–16.

57. McLaughlin JK, Mandel JS, Blot WJ, Schuman LM, Mehl ES, Fraumeni JF Jr. A population-based case-control study of renal cell carcinoma. J Natl Cancer Inst 1984;72(2):275–284.

58. McLaughlin JK, Gao YT, Gao RN, et al. Risk factors for renal-cell cancer in Shanghai, China. Int J Cancer 1992;52(4):562–565.

59. Muscat JE, Hoffmann D, Wynder EL. The epidemiology of renal cell carcinoma. A second look. Cancer 1995;275(10):2552–2557.

60. Sweeney C, Farrow DC. Differential survival related to smoking among patients with renal cell carcinoma. Epidemiology 2000;11(3):344–346.

61. Talamini R, Baron AE, Barra S, et al. A case-control study of risk factor for renal cell cancer in northern Italy. Cancer Causes Control 1990;1(2):125–131.

62. Yu MC, Mack TM, Hanisch R, Cicioni C, Henderson BE. Cigarette smoking, obesity, diuretic use, and coffee consumption as risk factors for renal cell carcinoma. J Natl Cancer Inst 1986;77(2):351–356.

63. Yuan JM, Castelao JE, Gago-Dominguez M, Yu MC, Ross RK. Tobacco use in relation to renal cell carcinoma. Cancer Epidemiol Biomarkers Prev 1998;7(5):429–433.

64. Tavani A, La VC. Epidemiology of renal-cell carcinoma. J Nephrol 1997;10(2):93–106.

65. Parker AS, Cerhan JR, Janney CA, Lynch CF, Cantor KP. Smoking cessation and renal cell carcinoma. Ann Epidemiol 2003;13(4):245–251.

66. McLaughlin JK, Hrubec Z, Heineman EF, Blot WJ, Fraumeni JF Jr. Renal cancer and cigarette smoking in a 26-year followup of U.S. veterans. Public Health Reports 1990;105(5):535–537.

67. Hunt JD, van der Hel OL, McMillan GP, Boffetta P, Brennan P. Renal cell carcinoma in relation to cigarette smoking: meta-analysis of 24 studies. Int J Cancer 2005;114(1):101–108.

68. Oh WK, Manola J, Renshaw AA, et al. Smoking and alcohol use may be risk factors for poorer outcome in patients with clear cell renal carcinoma. Urology 2000;55(1):31–35.

69. Mellemgaard A, McLaughlin JK, Overvad K, Olsen JH. Dietary risk factors for renal cell carcinoma in Denmark. Eur J Cancer 1996;32A(4):673–682.

70. Wolk A, Gridley G, Niwa S, et al. International renal cell cancer study. VII. Role of diet. Int J Cancer 1996;65(1):67–73.

71. van Dijk BA, Schouten LJ, Kiemeney LA, Goldbohm RA, van den Brandt PA. Relation of height, body mass, energy intake, and physical activity to risk of renal cell carcinoma: results from the Netherlands Cohort Study. Am J Epidemiol 2004;160(12):1159–1167.

72. Hu J, Mao Y, White K, Canadian Cancer Registries Epidemiology Research Group. Diet and vitamin or mineral supplements and risk of renal cell carcinoma in Canada. Cancer Causes Control 2003;14(8):705–714.

73. Lindblad P, Wolk A, Bergstrom R, Adami HO. Diet and risk of renal cell cancer: a population-based case-control study. Cancer Epidemiol Biomarkers Prev 1997;6(4):215–223.

74. Chow WH, Gridley G, McLaughlin JK, et al. Protein intake and risk of renal cell cancer. J Natl Cancer Inst 1994;86(15):1131–1139.

75. Parker AS, Cerhan JR, Lynch CF, Ershow AG, Cantor KP. Gender, alcohol consumption, and renal cell carcinoma. Am J Epidemiol 2002;155(5):455–462.

76. Yuan JM, Gago-Dominguez M, Castelao JE, Hankin JH, Ross RK, Yu MC. Cruciferous vegetables in relation to renal cell carcinoma. Int J Cancer 1998;77(2):211–216.

77. Rashidkhani B, Lindblad P, Wolk A. Fruits, vegetables and risk of renal cell carcinoma: a prospective study of Swedish women. Int J Cancer 2005;113(3):451–455.
78. van Dijk BA, Schouten LJ, Kiemeney LA, Goldbohm RA, van den Brandt PA. Vegetable and fruit consumption and risk of renal cell carcinoma: results from the Netherlands cohort study. Int J Cancer 2005;117(4):648–654.
79. Chow WH, McLaughlin JK, Mandel JS, Wacholder S, Niwa S, Fraumeni JF Jr. Obesity and risk of renal cell cancer. Cancer Epidemiol Biomarkers Prev 1996;5(1):17–21.
80. Shapiro JA, Williams MA, Weiss NS. Body mass index and risk of renal cell carcinoma. Epidemiology 1999;10(2):188–191.
81. Yuan JM, Castelao JE, Gago-Dominguez M, Ross RK, Yu MC. Hypertension, obesity and their medications in relation to renal cell carcinoma. Br J Cancer 1998;77(9):1508–1513.
82. Calle EE, Rodriguez C, Walker-Thurmond K, Thun MJ. Overweight, obesity, and mortality from cancer in a prospectively studied cohort of U.S. adults. N Engl J Med 2003;348(17):1625–1638.
83. Lindblad P, Wolk A, Bergstrom R, Persson I, Adami HO. The role of obesity and weight fluctuations in the etiology of renal cell cancer: a population-based case-control study. Cancer Epidemiol Biomarkers Prev 1994;3(8):631–639.
84. Bergstrom A, Terry P, Lindblad P, et al. Physical activity and risk of renal cell cancer. Int J Cancer 2001;92(1):155–157.
85. Goodman MT, Morgenstern H, Wynder EL. A case-control study of factors affecting the development of renal cell cancer. Am J Epidemiol 1986;124(6):926–941.
86. Mellemgaard A, Engholm G, McLaughlin JK, Olsen JH. Risk factors for renal-cell carcinoma in Denmark. III. Role of weight, physical activity and reproductive factors. Int J Cancer 1994;56(1):66–71.
87. Chow WH, Lindblad P, Gridley G, et al. Risk of urinary tract cancers following kidney or ureter stones. J Natl Cancer Inst 1997;89(19):1453–1457.
88. Mellemgaard A, Moller H, Jensen OM, Halberg P, Olsen JH. Risk of kidney cancer in analgesics users. J Clin Epidemiol 1992;45(9):1021–1024.
89. Shapiro JA, Williams MA, Weiss NS, Stergachis A, LaCroix AZ, Barlow WE. Hypertension, antihypertensive medication use, and risk of renal cell carcinoma. Am J Epidemiol 1999;149(6):521–530.
90. Chow WH, Gridley G, Fraumeni JF Jr, Jarvholm B. Obesity, hypertension, and the risk of kidney cancer in men. N Engl J Med 2000;343(18):1305–1311.
91. Coughlin SS, Neaton JD, Randall B, Sengupta A. Predictors of mortality from kidney cancer in 332,547 men screened for the Multiple Risk Factor Intervention Trial. Cancer 1997;79(11):2171–2177.
92. Mellemgaard A, Niwa S, Mehl ES, Engholm G, McLaughlin JK, Olsen JH. Risk factors for renal cell carcinoma in Denmark: role of medication and medical history. Int J Epidemiol 1994;23(5):923–930.
93. Mellemgaard A, Moller H, Olsen JH. Diuretics may increase risk of renal cell carcinoma. Cancer Causes Control 1992;3(4):309–312.
94. Chow WH, McLaughlin JK, Mandel JS, Wacholder S, Niwa S, Fraumeni JF Jr. Risk of renal cell cancer in relation to diuretics, antihypertensive drugs, and hypertension. Cancer Epidemiol Biomarkers Prev 1995;4(4):327–331.
95. Grossman E, Messerli FH, Goldbourt U. Does diuretic therapy increase the risk of renal cell carcinoma? Am J Cardiol, 1999;83(7):1090–1093.
96. Partanen T, Heikkila P, Hernberg S, Kauppinen T, Moneta G, Ojajarvi A. Renal cell cancer and occupational exposure to chemical agents. Scand J Work Environ Health 1991;17(4):231–239.
97. Gago-Dominguez M, Yuan JM, Castelao JE, Ross RK, Yu MC. Regular use of analgesics is a risk factor for renal cell carcinoma. Br J Cancer 1999;81(3):542–548.
98. McCredie M, Stewart JH, Day NE. Different roles for phenacetin and paracetamol in cancer of the kidney and renal pelvis. Int J Cancer 1993;53(2):245–249.
99. Rosenberg L, Rao RS, Palmer JR, et al. Transitional cell cancer of the urinary tract and renal cell cancer in relation to acetaminophen use. Cancer Causes Control 1998;9(1):83–88.
100. Ronchi E, Pizzocaro G, Miodini P, Piva L, Salvioni R, Di FG. Steroid hormone receptors in normal and malignant human renal tissue: relationship with progestin therapy. J Steroid Biochem 1984;21(3):329–335.
101. Li JJ, Li SA. Estrogen carcinogenesis in hamster tissues: a critical review. Endocr Rev 1990;11(4):524–531.

102. Chow WH, McLaughlin JK, Mandel JS, Blot WJ, Niwa S, Fraumeni JF Jr. Reproductive factors and the risk of renal cell cancer among women. Int J Cancer 1995;60(3):321–324.
103. Lambe M, Lindblad P, Wuu J, Remler R, Hsieh CC. Pregnancy and risk of renal cell cancer: a population-based study in Sweden. Br J Cancer 2002;86(9):1425–1429.
104. McLaughlin JK, Malker HS, Blot WJ, et al. Renal cell cancer among architects and allied professionals in Sweden. Am J Ind Med 1992;21(6):873–876.
105. Delahunt B, Bethwaite PB, Nacey JN. Occupational risk for renal cell carcinoma. A case-control study based on the New Zealand Cancer Registry. Br J Urol 1995;75(5):578–582.
106. Parent ME, Hua Y, Siemiatycki J. Occupational risk factors for renal cell carcinoma in Montreal. Am J Ind Med 2000;38(6):609–618.
107. Zhang Y, Cantor KP, Lynch CF, Zheng T. A population-based case-control study of occupation and renal cell carcinoma risk in Iowa. J Occup Environ Med 2004;46(3):235–240.
108. McCredie M, Stewart JH. Risk factors for kidney cancer in New South Wales. IV. Occupation. Br J Ind Med 1993;50(4):349–354.
109. Poole C, Dreyer NA, Satterfield MH, Levin L, Rothman KJ. Kidney cancer and hydrocarbon exposures among petroleum refinery workers. Environ Health Perspect 1993;101(suppl 6):53–62.
110. Pesch B, Haerting J, Ranft U, Klimpel A, Oelschlagel B, Schill W. Occupational risk factors for urothelial carcinoma: agent-specific results from a case-control study in Germany. MURC Study Group. Multicenter Urothelial and Renal Cancer. Int J Epidemiol 2000;29(2):238–247.
111. Mellemgaard A, Engholm G, McLaughlin JK, Olsen JH. Occupational risk factors for renal-cell carcinoma in Denmark. Scand J Work Environ Health 1994;(3):160–165.
112. Dosemeci M, Cocco P, Chow WH. Gender differences in risk of renal cell carcinoma and occupational exposures to chlorinated aliphatic hydrocarbons. Am J Ind Med 1999;36(1):54–59.
113. Bruning T, Pesch B, Wiesenhutter B, et al. Renal cell cancer risk and occupational exposure to trichloroethylene: results of a consecutive case-control study in Arnsberg, Germany. Am J Ind Med 2003;43(3):274–285.
114. Auperin A, Benhamou S, Ory-Paoletti C, Flamant R. Occupational risk factors for renal cell carcinoma: a case-control study. Occup Environ Med 1994;51(6):426–428.

6

Molecular Genetics in Inherited Renal Cell Carcinoma: Identification of Targets in the Hereditary Syndromes

Nadeem Dhanani, Cathy Vocke, Gennady Bratslavsky, and W. Marston Linehan

KEYWORDS

Molecular genetics
Inherited renal cell carcinoma
Hereditary cancer syndromes
Metastatic kidney cancer
Von Hippel-Lindau
Hereditary papillary renal carcinoma
Heat shock proteins

ABSTRACT

An estimated 12,000 people will die of kidney cancer this year. With the increased use of axial abdominal imaging, kidney tumors are being diagnosed at earlier stages, often incidentally while the patient is still asymptomatic. While extirpative surgery is most often curative in tumors restricted to the kidney, treatment of metastatic disease has proven to be a formidable challenge. As our understanding of the genetic basis of kidney cancer increases, advances in molecular therapies offer new approaches to treatment. Understanding the cellular mechanisms of oncogenesis have the potential to change the face of renal cancer therapy.

An estimated 36,000 people will be diagnosed with kidney cancer this year, and close to 30% of these patients will die of their disease.[1] Based on data from the National Cancer Institute's Surveillance, Epidemiology, and End Results (SEER) Cancer Statistics

From: *Clinical Management of Renal Tumors*
Edited by: R.M. Bukowski and A.C. Novick © Humana Press Inc., Totowa, NJ

Review, 1 out of every 82 men and women will be diagnosed with cancer of the kidney over the course of their lifetime, and the incidence continues to rise. Men are affected almost twice as often as women, and the incidence among blacks is slightly higher than that of whites. With the increased use of axial abdominal imaging, kidney tumors are being diagnosed at earlier stages, oftentimes incidentally while the patient is still asymptomatic. Nonetheless, at the time of presentation, 40% of these tumors will no longer be confined to the kidney, either through local extension or distant metastatic spread.[2] While extirpative surgery is most often curative in tumors restricted to the kidney, treatment of metastatic disease has proven to be a formidable challenge with the traditional therapies currently available. As our understanding of the genetic basis of kidney cancer increases, exciting advances in molecular therapeutics offer novel approaches to treatment for these patients.

IDENTIFICATION OF THE *VHL* GENE

As recently as 30 years ago, very little was known about the contribution of genetic mutations to the development of renal tumors. Like cancer of the colon, breast, and prostate, kidney cancer was known to occur in both sporadic and familial forms. Based on earlier work by Knudson and Strong,[3,4] the concept of tumor suppressor gene inactivation was recognized as an etiologic factor in Wilms' tumor and retinoblastoma. In keeping with this hypothesis, when compared to the sporadic form, familial kidney cancers were more often multifocal, bilateral, and had earlier onset. Still, there was no gene identified that could be implicated in renal cancer.

In 1979, Cohen et al.[5] noted a chromosomal translocation between the short arm of chromosome 3 and the long arm of chromosome 8 in eight of ten affected members of a family known to have heritable kidney cancer. This was followed by several additional reports characterizing chromosomal abnormalities in different families affected with renal cell carcinoma (RCC). In each of these lineages, chromosome 3 was involved, particularly the 3p13–3p14 region. Important insight into the link between the hereditary and sporadic forms of RCC was provided through work by Zbar and colleagues,[6] when they reported loss of alleles at loci on the short arm of chromosome 3 in 11 of 11 evaluable patients with sporadic renal cancers. Shortly thereafter, it was postulated that the genetic mutation responsible for von Hippel–Lindau (VHL) disease was located in a region on chromosome 3p, distinct from the human homologue of RAF1, but apparently linked to it.[7] All evidence was pointing to the existence of a tumor suppressor gene encoded on the short arm of chromosome 3, a mutation of which resulted in renal cell cancer. Unfortunately, gene localization was still not feasible because the region of interest was too large for the cloning techniques available at the time. Research efforts were thus shifted to the heritable form of renal cancer, with VHL being the model for investigation.

VON HIPPEL–LINDAU

Von Hippel–Lindau is transmitted in an autosomal dominant pattern with an estimated incidence of 1 in 36,000 live births.[8,9] With a penetrance of over 95% by the age of 65,[10] affected individuals develop neoplastic tumors in multiple organ systems. Central nervous system lesions include retinal hemangioblastomas, endolymphatic sac tumors of the inner ear, and craniospinal hemangioblastomas in the cerebellum, brainstem, spinal cord, lumbosacral nerve roots, and supratentorial lesions. The pancreas may also be affected in these patients, developing cysts, cystadenomas, and neuroendocrine tumors. Benign epididymal papillary cystadenomas occur with increased frequency than in the general population and can be bilateral. Rarely, women can have analogous lesions with papillary cystadenomas in the broad ligament. Tumors found in the kidney are solid renal cell cancers, simple cysts, and combinations thereof. In the setting of VHL, it has been estimated that a kidney may contain 600 microscopic tumors and over 1000 cysts before the age of 40 years.[11] Although simple cysts in these patients rarely transform to solid masses,[12] complex cysts are known to contain malignant elements and may progress if left untreated. Adrenal lesions found in VHL are pheochromocytomas. Like the kidney tumors, these are frequently multiple and bilateral. Extraadrenal paragangliomas are also known to occur in these patients, arising in peri-aortic tissues, the carotid body, and the glomus jugulare.[13]

In searching for the gene responsible for VHL, researchers explored the applicability of Knudson's two-hit hypothesis to tumor behavior in VHL patients with kidney cancer. Tory et al.[14] evaluated tissue from patients with multiple kidney tumors, and for each patient compared chromosome 3 from one tumor to another. They found that each patient had loss of the same allele of chromosome 3p in all of their tumors. Further analysis of haplotypes revealed that the lost allele was always from the wild-type chromosome, the contribution of the nonaffected parent. This provided strong support for the notion that alteration of a tumor suppressor gene was the causative factor in VHL, and in accordance with Knudson's theory, individuals with a germline mutation were at risk for VHL if they incurred a second hit at the same locus, thus inactivating the wild-type allele.

Expanding upon earlier work by Seizinger et al.,[15] Lerman's group[16] isolated and mapped 2000 single copy DNA fragments of chromosome 3 from humans, thus generating vital tools that would be used for the future cloning of the *VHL* gene. With these reagents newly available, Hosoe and colleagues[17] performed further multipoint linkage analysis to localize the *VHL* gene to an interval between RAF1 and a polymorphic DNA marker, D3S18. Finally, in 1993, researchers at the National Cancer Institute reported identification of the *VHL* gene through cloning studies and described its role in renal cell carcinoma.[18] This small gene, with 854 coding nucleotides on three exons, was found to be located on the short arm of chromosome 3 and responsible for encoding the VHL protein. The gene is evolutionarily conserved, and its product shares homology with only a small region of a surface membrane protein of *Trypanosoma brucei*.

Once the causative gene for VHL had been identified, clinicians were eager to find screening methods to identify patients with genetic mutations. Early laboratory studies generated germline mutation detection rates of 39% to 75%.[19,20] Mutation analyses showed that the type (e.g., insertion, deletion, missense, or nonsense) and location (e.g., codon position) of mutation correlated well with phenotype, thus allowing health care providers to predict the extent of involvement of the various organ systems for any given VHL family. In a study of 469 VHL families from North America, Europe, and Japan, researchers compared the effects of identical *VHL* germline mutations on different families. Based on their findings, VHL was broken down into three distinct phenotypes: pheochromocytoma along with renal cell carcinoma, pheochromocytoma alone, and renal cell carcinoma alone.[21] Later studies correlated the relationship between length and location of germline mutations and the incidence of renal cell carcinomas in VHL patients. A retrospective review of 123 patients from 55 families revealed that individuals harboring a partial deletion suffered a significantly higher rate of renal cell carcinoma when compared to those with complete gene deletions. Moreover, deletion mapping demonstrated the presence of a 30-kilobase (kb) gene on the short arm of chromosome 3, directly adjacent to the *VHL* gene, which, when preserved, may promote the development of RCC.[22]

Further advances were made when Stolle's group[23] developed a new technique that improved germline mutation detection, accurately identifying a mutation in 93 of 93 (100%) VHL families tested. The method involved a combination of tests that each demonstrated high sensitivity for the various types of mutations implicated in VHL. Qualitative Southern blotting to detect gene rearrangements and quantitative Southern blotting for the detection of entire gene deletions were the newly added components responsible for the dramatic increase in sensitivity. In addition, fluorescence in situ hybridization (FISH) and full gene sequencing completed the battery of tests. The 100% sensitivity of the new technique lent support to the notion that VHL is genetically homogeneous, and clinically allowed providers to counsel patients with reasonable certainty that a family member found to lack the gene mutation with the new test combination was unlikely to have VHL.

SPORADIC RENAL CELL CARCINOMA

Discovery of the *VHL* gene in the setting of familial renal cell carcinoma allowed scientists to then investigate its role in sporadic tumors. Gnarra et al.[24] used polymerase chain reaction (PCR) amplification of the three exons of the *VHL* genes of 108 patients with sporadic renal cell carcinoma to analyze the entire coding region in each gene. They identified somatic mutations in the *VHL* gene in 57% of these patients, and nearly all (98%) were found to have loss of heterozygosity. It was clear that the *VHL* gene played a role in the development of sporadic RCC in a majority of patients; however, questions arose as to why gene mutations were not demonstrable in all renal cell cancers. One explanation is offered by an important mechanism for *VHL* gene inactivation as described by Herman and colleagues.[25] They discovered hypermethylation of a CpG island in the 5′ region of the *VHL* gene, a region that is normally unmethylated, in nearly 20% of VHL patients with RCC. No other mutation of the *VHL* gene could be demonstrated in 80% of these patients, and *VHL* gene expression was absent in all. Furthermore, when treated with 5-aza-2′ deoxycytidine, a hypomethylating agent, the *VHL* gene was once again expressed. Additionally, one has to consider the limitations of current investigative techniques. There are still regions of the *VHL* gene that have not yet been thoroughly examined, and this may hinder our ability to fully detect genetic variation. Furthermore, there is always the possibility of normal tissue interspersed with cancerous cells within a given tumor, thus confounding laboratory findings.[26]

CYSTIC LESIONS IN VON HIPPEL–LINDAU

In addition to solid RCCs, patients with VHL are also frequently found to have cystic lesions within their kidneys (Figure 6.1). These lesions range from simple benign cysts, as characterized by radiographic imaging, to complex cystic masses suspicious for malignancy. In this patient population, which can be expected to develop numerous multifocal and bilateral lesions requiring surgical extirpation, maximal nephron preservation relies on the clinician's ability to predict the malignant potential of a cyst or mass, and the likelihood that treatment of that lesion will improve survival. To better characterize the relationship between cysts and solid renal masses, Lubensky et al.[27] analyzed 26 renal lesions from two VHL patients for loss of heterozygosity at the *VHL* region. They found loss of a *VHL* allele in 25 out of the 26 lesions, thereby demonstrating both benign

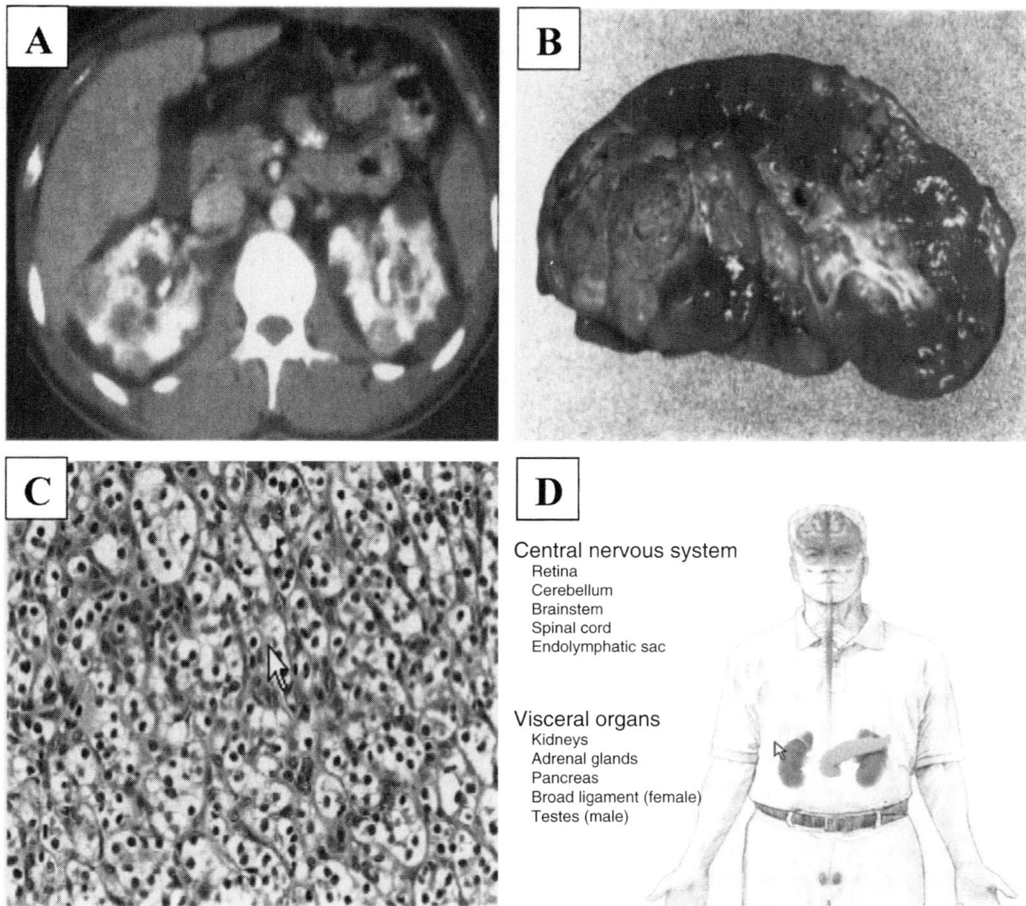

Figure 6.1. Phenotypic manifestations of von Hippel–Lindau (VHL). Renal masses are common in VHL patients. (A) Computed tomography (CT) scan of a VHL patient demonstrating characteristic bilateral multifocal renal lesions consisting of simple and complex cysts as well as enhancing solid masses. (B) Gross specimen removed from a VHL patient showing classic multiple golden-yellow tumors. (C) Hematoxylin and eosin (H&E) stain of a classic clear cell renal carcinoma found in patients with VHL. (D) In addition to renal manifestations, VHL affects organs systems throughout the body. (From Linehan WM, et al. Genetic Basis of Cancer of the Kidney: Disease-Specific Approaches to Therapy. 2004.) (To view this figure in color, see the insert.)

and malignant lesions to share similar genetic aberration. In both sets of lesions, the mutated gene remained while the normal copy was the one that was lost, thus keeping with Knudson's two-hit hypothesis. Further evidence to support the theory that renal cysts potentially represent precursors to malignant renal cell carcinoma in VHL was provided by the work of Lee et al.,[28] when they showed the consistent coexpression of erythropoietin and erythropoietin receptor in RCC as well as many renal cysts.

Knowing that simple cysts harbored the same genetic abnormality as solid malignant lesions, clinicians were then faced with the dilemma of when to act on cysts found in the kidneys of VHL patients. If left untreated, simple cysts may develop malignancy over time, and a plan of observation may prove fatal if progression to metastatic disease ensued. On the other hand, unnecessarily operating on benign lesions could lead to a dramatic increase in morbidity for VHL patients, including the perioperative risks of surgery as well as the subsequent renal insufficiency from loss of parenchyma. Thus, investigators focused on determining the natural history of cystic lesions in the VHL population.[12] Two hundred and twenty eight renal lesions from 28 patients were observed for a mean of 2.4 years with serial computed tomography (CT) scans. Overall, 74% of the cysts remained stable with respect to size, with an additional 9% actually decreasing in size. Only two patients were found to have malignant transformation of their simple cysts based on radiographic criteria. These results supported the practice of conservative management of simple cysts in the VHL population.

FUNCTION OF THE *VHL* GENE

Once the putative gene for RCC was identified, there was an effort to better define the function of the VHL protein, with the hope that this would eventually uncover potential therapeutic targets. One method of determining the function of a protein is to find out what other proteins it complexes with in order to reveal its role in a cellular pathway. In 1995, Duan and colleagues[29] localized the *VHL* gene product to the cytosol and the nucleus, indicating common translocation of the protein. They were also able to identify two additional proteins of 16 kd and 9 kd, which formed a heterotrimeric complex with VHL. When certain missense mutations of the *VHL* gene were investigated, the complex did not form. Subsequent studies offered a more detailed description of the protein complex.[30] They explained the function of a transcription elongation factor, Elongin (SIII), made up of three distinct protein subunits, Elongins A, B, and C, which serves to prevent transient pauses of RNA polymerase II (Pol II) during transcription. Although VHL protein was shown to displace Elongin A and compete for binding with Elongins B and C in vitro, there was no evidence of such function in vivo. Iliopolous et al.[31] demonstrated the effects of VHL protein on certain hypoxia-inducible genes. Under normoxic conditions, intact VHL was shown to downregulate vascular endothelial growth factor (VEGF), platelet-derived growth factor B (PDGF-B), and the glucose transporter GLUT-1 by destabilizing their respective messenger RNAs (mRNAs). Thus, presumably, with a VHL mutation there was unregulated expression of these proteins, a finding that was congruent with the known hypervascular characteristics of VHL-associated RCCs. In a search for proteins that interact with the VHL-B-C complex, Pause and colleagues[32] identified *Hs-CUL-2*, a newly described gene involved in cell cycle regulation of yeast and *Caenorhabditis elegans*. They observed that in the presence of a *VHL* gene mutation, the VHL-B-C–Hs-CUL-2 interaction was markedly diminished, suggesting a tumor suppressor role for this new protein.

It was known that VEGF, GLUT-1, and PDGF are all targets of hypoxia-inducible factor (HIF) and also that the clear cells of renal cell carcinoma express higher levels of these proteins than do nonmalignant cells.[33] The role of VHL was further elucidated when researchers showed that the previously described protein complex of VHL-B-C-CUL functioned as a ubiquitin ligase that targets HIF-1α and HIF-2α for degradation under normoxic conditions.[34] Upon hydroxylation by oxygen-dependent prolyl hydroxylases, HIF-1α binds to VHL and is subsequently degraded.[35] If the hydroxylation does not occur, however, VHL binding is inhibited and ubiquitination of HIF-1α fails.[36] Transcription of HIF-dependent genes ensues, leading to overexpression of VEGF and ultimately increased vascularity. Lending support to this pathway, Maranchie et al.[37]

used a competitive inhibitor of the VHL–HIF-1α binding site to assess functional outcomes. In preventing this interaction, they found accumulation of cellular HIF-1α in normoxia and a conversion to the *VHL*-negative phenotype.

HEREDITARY PAPILLARY RENAL CARCINOMA

While advances were being made in the genetic basis of RCC resulting from *VHL* mutations, in 1994 clinicians were uncovering a distinct familial syndrome that was also manifest by renal tumors. Zbar and colleagues[38] reported on a family in which renal tumors had developed in three generations, and whose tumors were multifocal and bilateral. Pathologically these tumors were papillary variants of RCC, as opposed to the conventional type associated with VHL, and they showed no abnormalities in chromosome 3. This new syndrome, termed hereditary papillary renal cancer (HPRC), appeared to have an autosomal dominant mode of inheritance with incomplete penetrance. Further analysis of 10 families with HPRC suggested renal cancers occur in both sexes, with a male-to-female ratio of 2.2 : 1, have a late age of onset (50 to 70 years), and are bilateral and multifocal in nature.[39] A later study evaluated 88 surgical pathology slides of grossly normal areas of 12 kidneys from patients with HPRC. More than half of these samples were found to contain microscopic papillary renal cancers, thereby predicting the presence of 1100 to 3400 microscopic tumors in a single kidney of a patient with HPRC.[40] Histologically these tumors display a distinct phenotype, with a majority of the architecture in a papillary/tubulopapillary pattern and a chromophil basophilic staining, consistent with a type I papillary renal carcinoma phenotype.[41] Radiographically, in stark contrast to the hypervascular tumors of VHL, tumors of HPRC display poor contrast enhancement and are markedly hypovascular[42] (Figure 6.2).

IDENTIFICATION OF THE GENE FOR HEREDITARY PAPILLARY RENAL CARCINOMA

Three years after describing the disease, researchers reported identification of the gene responsible for HPRC.[43] Findings of chromosomal trisomy in malignant papillary renal carcinomas raised suspicions of proto-oncogene dysfunction, and the defect was mapped to the long arm of chromosome 7. Missense mutations in the tyrosine kinase domain of the *MET* gene ultimately proved responsible for constitutive activation of the MET protein and interference with autoinhibitory mechanisms, resulting in papillary renal cancers. The MET transmembrane protein was found to be a receptor site for hepatocyte growth factor (HGF) also termed Scatter factor (SF).[44] Upon activation by HGF, MET tyrosine phosphorylation induces a host of signaling cascades responsible for embryonic development, cell branching, and invasion.[45]

BIRT-HOGG-DUBÉ SYNDROME

In 1977, three physicians described a familial syndrome in which affected individuals developed multiple small skin-colored papules on the face, neck, and back.[46] Histologically these lesions were found to be fibrofolliculomas, trichodiscomas, and acrochordons, and they were transmitted in an autosomal dominant pattern. Some patients with this constellation of findings, termed Birt-Hogg-Dubé (BHD), were also known to have concurrent visceral tumors, including thyroid carcinoma, colonic polyps, and one case

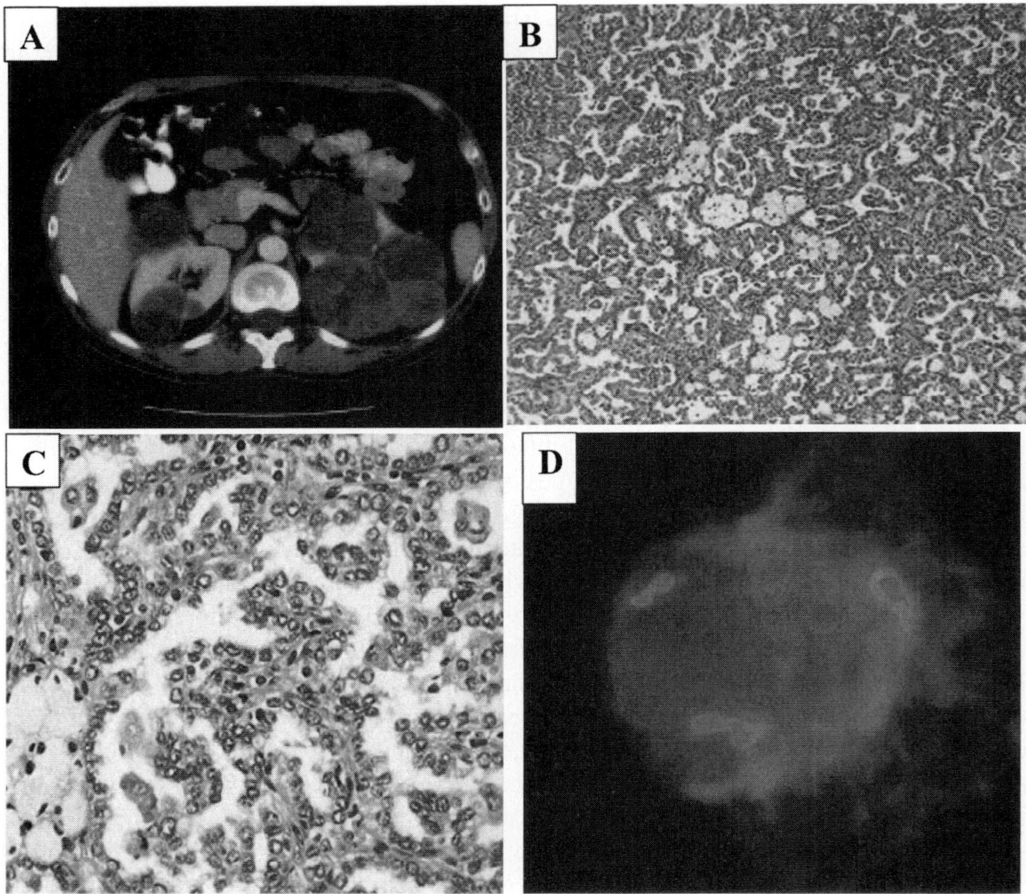

Figure 6.2. Manifestations and genetics of hereditary papillary renal cancer (HPRC). Patients with HPRC primarily develop bilateral multifocal renal masses. (A) Abdominal CT demonstrates HPRC tumors with characteristic poor enhancement on contrasted study that may frequently be mistaken for simple cysts. The tumors are best seen on late phase images of a contrast CT. Low (B) and high (C) power H&E stain of type I papillary renal cell carcinoma (RCC) seen in patients with HPRC. (D) Fluorescence in situ hybridization (FISH) using a MET probe demonstrating trisomy of chromosome 7 (red signal) in papillary type 1 RCC compared with chromosome 11 serving as control (green signal). (From Schmidt et al. Early Onset Hereditary Papillary Renal Carcinoma: Germline Missense Mutations in the Tyrocine Kinase Domain of the MET Proto-Oncogene. 2004.) (To view this figure in color, see the insert.)

of a renal tumor. In 1999, a group of clinicians noted that a significant number of their renal mass patients had these distinctive skin lesions that had previously been described in the dermatologic literature. They therefore set out to evaluate a large cohort of patients with known familial renal tumors and assess the presence of cutaneous findings. As a result, Toro and colleagues[47] found three extended families in which there appeared to be common segregation of renal tumors and the cutaneous lesions of BHD. They concluded that BHD seemed to be associated with renal tumors, both transmitted in an autosomal dominant manner.

As BHD began to attract more attention and closer scrutiny, numerous additional disease processes were identified in BHD patients. Spontaneous pneumothoraces, parotid oncocytomas, multiple lipomas, angiolipomas, parathyroid adenomas, and colonic polyposis were all postulated to have some connection with BHD.[48–51] To better define the

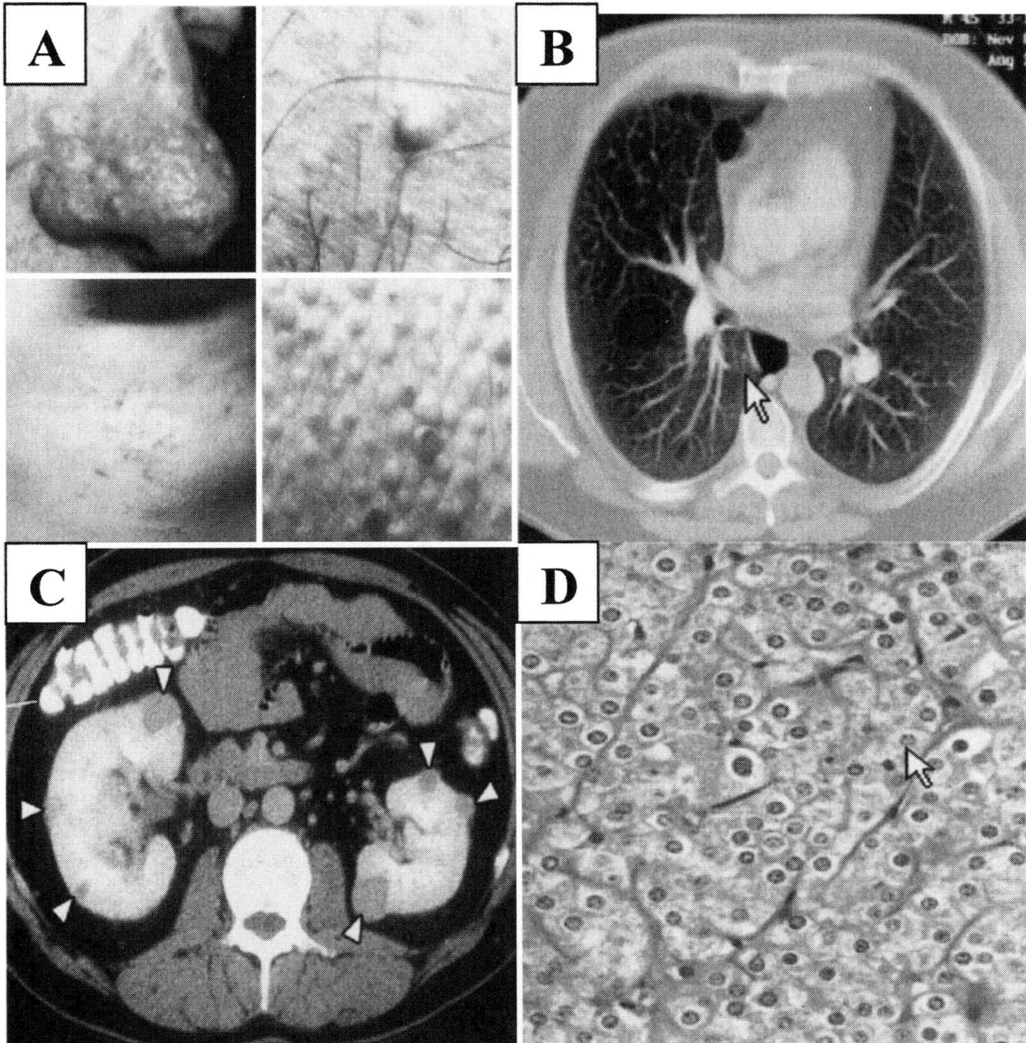

Figure 6.3. Phenotypic manifestations of Birt-Hogg-Dubé (BHD). Classic findings in BHD include (A) characteristic cutaneous fibrofolliculomas, (B) pulmonary cysts that result in a 30–fold increased incidence of spontaneous pneumothoraces, and (C) renal tumors that are usually multifocal and can vary in pathologic subtype, from (D) chromophobe RCC (most common) to oncocytoma, hybrid tumors, or clear cell carcinoma. (From Zbar et al.[52])

spectrum of disease processes associated with BHD, Zbar and colleagues[52] solicited participation from patients who were under the care of dermatologists from across the United States and Canada for classic BHD skin lesions. The patients were evaluated for concomitant health problems, particularly kidney, lung, and colon manifestations. The group eventually found no correlation between BHD and colon cancer or polyps. There was, however, a strong link between BHD and renal tumors, as previously suspected, as well as spontaneous pneumothoraces. On multivariate analysis, patients with BHD had an odds ratio of ~9.0 for developing renal tumors, and a risk of developing spontaneous pneumothoraces 32 times higher than the general population (Figure 6.3).

To better characterize the renal neoplasms associated with BHD, researchers examined the pathologic findings of 130 renal tumors from 30 BHD patients from 19 different

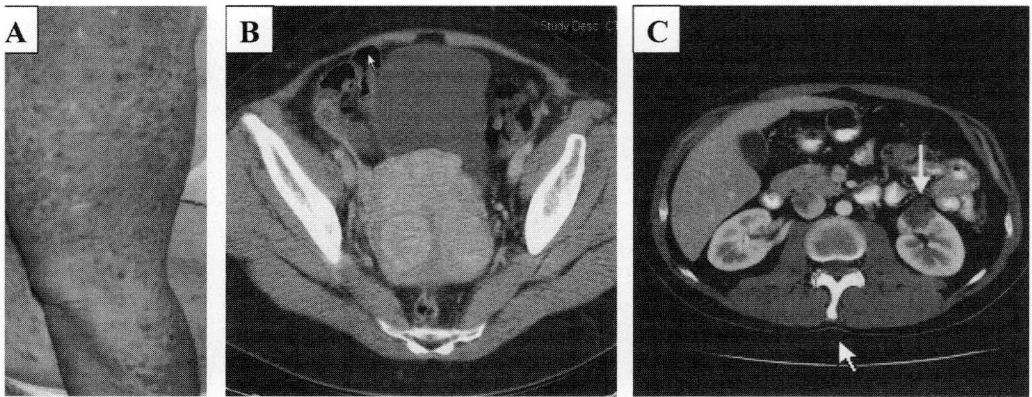

Figure 6.4. Phenotypic manifestations of hereditary leiomyomatosis renal cell carcinoma (HLRCC). (A) Classic cutaneous leiomyomatas presenting as multiple firm and erythematous macules and papules that are frequently painful. (B) Abdominal CT scan showing multiple uterine leiomyomas. This often leads to hysterectomy in HLRCC-affected women in their 20s or 30s. (C) CT abdomen demonstrating anterior upper pole mass in the left kidney. The renal lesions of HLRCC patients may present early and frequently have an aggressive clinical course. (From Toro et al.[61])

families.[53] Close to 35% of the tumors were pure chromophobe variants of renal cell carcinoma, with an additional 50% being a hybrid of chromophobe RCC and oncocytoma. Less than 10% of the entire cohort had elements of clear-cell (conventional) renal cell carcinoma. When present, the clear-cell RCC were larger, with a mean diameter of 4.7 cm, versus the chromophobe tumors, which averaged 3.0 cm, or the hybrid tumors with a mean diameter of 2.2 cm. Furthermore, analysis of grossly normal appearing surrounding renal parenchyma revealed multifocal oncocytosis throughout a majority of the specimens (Figure 6.4).

Identification of the BHD *Gene*

Knowledge of the genetic basis for BHD came largely in part from work by Schmidt and colleagues.[54] Linkage analysis was used to localize the *BHD* gene to a locus on the short arm of chromosome 17 from a screen of the genome of a large BHD kindred. Further work by Nickerson et al. utilized recombination mapping to localize the gene to a region of 17p11.2. A novel gene in this region was determined to exhibit mutations in the germlines of affected patients. The gene product folliculin was truncated as a result of insertions, deletions, or nonsense mutations. The frequency with which *BHD* is inactivated as a result of genetic mutations suggested a tumor suppressor function. Vocke and coworkers[55] found support for this theory when they sequenced the DNA of 77 renal tumors from 12 patients with germline *BHD* mutations. They demonstrated a high frequency of mutations in the wild-type *BHD* allele, thus providing the second "inactivating hit." The 579 amino acid protein, named for the hallmark dermatologic findings of the syndrome, has no known functional domains, but is highly preserved across species. Birt-Hogg-Dubé mRNA expression as measured by fluorescent in situ hybridization has been demonstrated in 17 human tissues, including the kidney, lung, skin, and brain.[56]

HEREDITARY LEIOMYOMATOSIS RENAL CELL CARCINOMA

A fourth familial syndrome of renal cancer was described by Launonen et al.[57] They noted co-segregation of cutaneous leiomyomas and type II papillary renal cell carcinoma in two familial lines (Figure 6.4) This syndrome, termed hereditary leiomyomatosis renal cell carcinoma (HLRCC), was mapped to a 14-cM region on the long arm of chromosome 1.[58] Fumarate hydratase (FH), the product of the putative gene for this syndrome, is a catalyst for the conversion of fumarate to malate in the Krebs cycle, and its activity is diminished in leiomyomatous tumors.[59] The loss of *FH* function and impediment of the Krebs cycle creates reliance upon glycolytic metabolism and upregulation of HIF and HIF-inducible transcripts[60] (Figure 6.5). The resultant environment is ideal for tumor cell survival and proliferation. The largest reported series of HLRCC patients revealed a 93% germline *FH* mutation detection rate in families suspected of

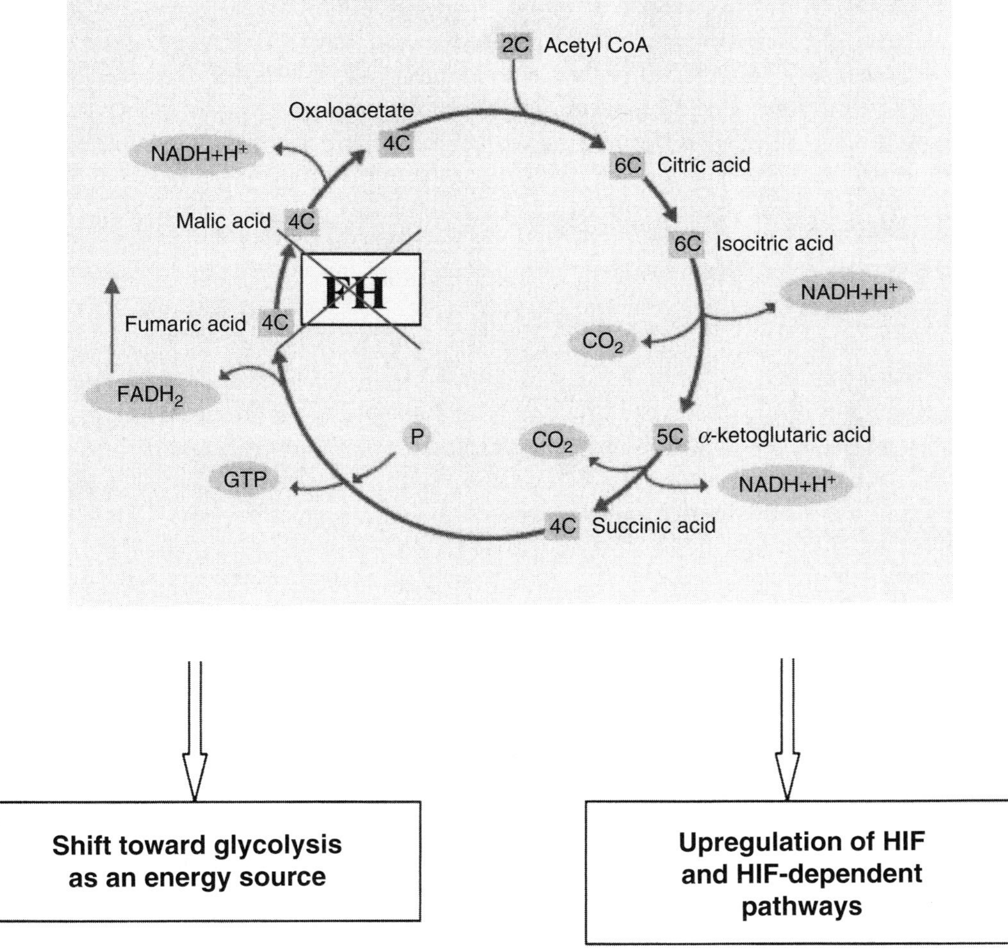

Figure 6.5. In HLRCC, mutation of the *FH* gene leads to dysfunctional fumarate hydratase, one of the key regulatory enzymes in the Krebs cycle, necessary for mitochondrial respiration and oxidative energy production. This in turn leads to accumulation of fumarate but more importantly to preferential energy production from glycolysis, a phenomenon observed in other malignancies as well. It may also lead to upregulation of hypoxia-inducible factor (HIF) and HIF-dependent pathways.

harboring disease with an autosomal dominant inheritance pattern.[61,62] Details of the molecular mechanisms involved in the downstream pathway of this gene are still under investigation, but the renal cancers associated with it appear to be aggressive and lethal if allowed to progress.

TREATMENT

Localized Disease

As our understanding of renal malignancies has evolved, so have our treatment strategies. In 1869 Gustav Simon performed the first planed nephrectomy in the treatment of a ureterovaginal fistula. A century later, Robson and colleagues[63] described refined techniques for radical nephrectomy for renal malignancies. Surgical extirpation remains the gold standard for treatment of localized RCC, although the surgical techniques have become more sophisticated. Since the first laparoscopic radical nephrectomy performed by Clayman et al.,[64] great strides have been made in minimally invasive approaches to removing kidneys. Laparoscopy offers patients decreased morbidity as compared with the historical open surgical procedures, while not appearing to compromise cancer control.

In the setting of localized renal tumors, nephron-sparing surgery is becoming more common. In 1890, Czerny performed the first partial nephrectomy for malignancy. Since that time, the scope has increased with surgeons proposing a wide range of acceptable size limits for nephron-sparing surgery, with the general consensus being about 4 cm in diameter.[65,66] Here, too, minimally invasive approaches are being employed, and laparoscopic partial nephrectomies are now being performed at specialized centers across the country.

Preservation of renal function and maximal sparing of nephrons during therapy is of paramount importance when treating patients with familial syndromes who are at risk of developing multiple, recurrent, bilateral tumors and may require numerous therapeutic interventions over their lifetime. Nonetheless, cancer control cannot be compromised. To minimize the morbidities associated with renal replacement therapy while maintaining vigilance in the containment of cancer, a threshold of 3 cm has been employed whereby tumors are observed until they reach this size criterion.[67] In determining the safety of this guideline, researchers found no patients developed metastatic disease nor did they require dialysis when the 3-cm rule was adhered to.

In addition to surgical extirpation, ablative techniques have also been employed for the treatment of renal tumors. Thermal tissue ablation with radiofrequency energy can be performed either percutaneously or laparoscopically. With higher wattage generators, results of radiofrequency ablation (RFA) appear promising. Hwang et al.[68] reported favorable outcomes for 23 of 24 patients treated with RFA at a mean follow-up of 1 year. Nonetheless, this is still considered an experimental technique, and further studies need to be conducted with longer follow-up and validation of post-RFA imaging criteria.

METASTATIC DISEASE

Despite high success rates with treatment of localized renal cancers, the prognosis for patients with metastatic disease is far grimmer. Although immunotherapy has been used, with interleukin-2 being the standard treatment modality, overall response rates are only in the range of 15% to 22%.[69] It is obvious that new strategies are needed for the successful treatment of these patients, and molecular therapeutics seems to hold the key. The success of the tyrosine kinase inhibitor STI-571 in combating gastrointestinal stromal tumors and chronic myelogenous leukemia has fueled enthusiasm for further investigation into the molecular mechanisms of oncogenesis and potential pharmacologic disruption of these pathways.[70,71]

In the paradigm of renal cancers, molecular therapeutics can be thought of in two broad categories: those that seek to interrupt specific pathways of tumorigenesis and the individual proteins involved, and those that affect the cancer cell's adaptability. Given the variability of each distinct type of renal cancer, it should not be surprising that this heterogeneous group of diseases offers a wide range of unique molecular targets. Our understandings of the mechanisms involved in the familial syndromes greatly impact our ability to direct therapies at their sporadic counterparts.

TARGETING *VHL*

The VHL pathway offers a variety of targets for intervention. In *VHL*-negative cells, the protein complex responsible for promoting HIF degradation is nonfunctional, resulting in the overabundance of HIF in a normoxic state. One therapeutic approach was demonstrated by Rapisarda et al.,[72] when they used a small molecule inhibitor of the HIF-1 pathway, topotecan, to block the transcriptional activity of HIF-1. Although effective in reducing the accumulation of HIF-1α in hypoxic environments, the efficacy of topotecan for VHL remains to be determined since in vitro and in vivo studies in human VHL models suggest HIF-2 to be the major factor in oncogenic pathways.[73,74] Efforts are currently under way to better target HIF-2 function.[75,76]

Several components of the downstream pathways in HIF have also been targeted (Figure 6.6). Failure to adequately inactivate HIF leads to unregulated expression of gene products such as VEGF, PDGF, epidermal growth factor (EGF), transforming growth factor α (TGF-α), and GLUT-1. Pharmacotherapies inhibiting these pathways may offer a systemic modality to combat metastatic disease. Bevacizumab, a monoclonal antibody to VEGF, has been shown to decrease angiogenesis in RCC.[77] Another drug, BAY 43-9006, inhibits signal transduction and subsequent cell proliferation by antagonizing the tyrosine kinase receptors for VEGF and PDGF.[78] The receptor of EGF can be blocked individually through the function of either ZD1839 or erlotinib, or in combination with the VEGF receptor by ZD6474.[79–81]

ALTERING THE C-MET PATHWAY

Type 1 papillary RCC in HPRC has been shown to result from activating mutations in the cell surface tyrosine kinase receptor for HGF, c-MET. Upon activation, the c-MET receptor is autophosphorylated, thus recruiting multiple signaling molecules to its cytoplasmic domain and activating intra- and extracellular cascades, which ultimately contribute to cellular proliferation, scattering, and invasion.[45] Based on this knowledge, several therapeutic strategies have been proposed: inhibition of autophosphorylation by the prevention of adenosine triphosphate (ATP) binding, inhibition of the interaction between HGF and its receptor, and suppression of the downstream signaling cascade of activated c-MET.[75]

HEAT SHOCK PROTEIN 90 INHIBITION

An alternative strategy in the molecular targeting of tumorigenesis is to affect the mechanisms used by the cancer cells to adapt and thrive in surrounding environments. One such group of targets is molecular chaperones, termed heat shock proteins (HSPs),

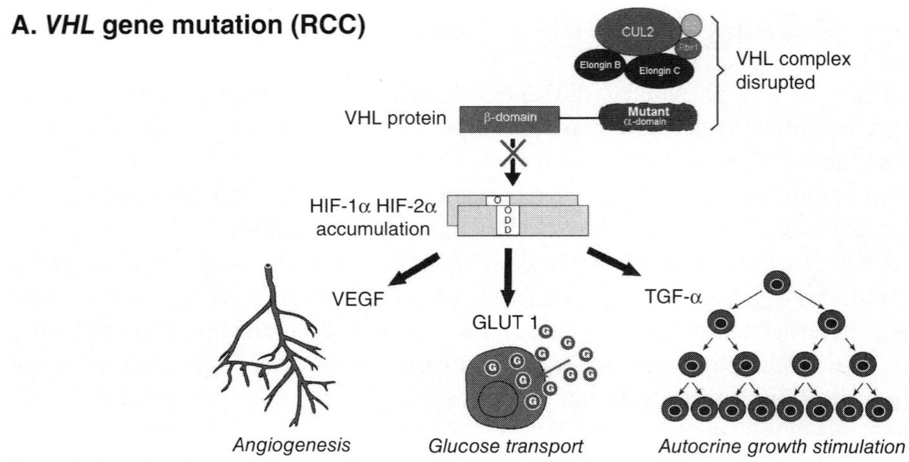

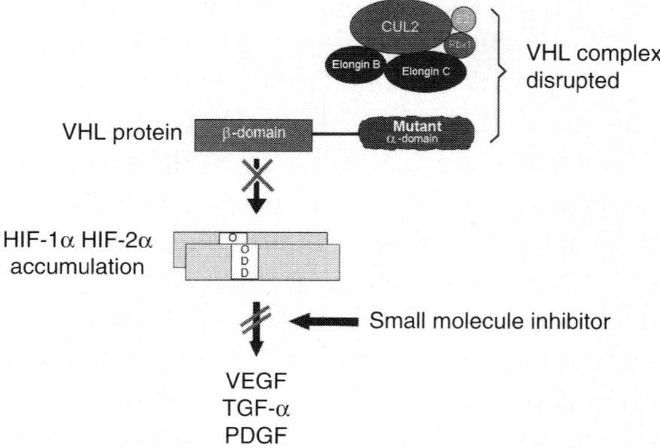

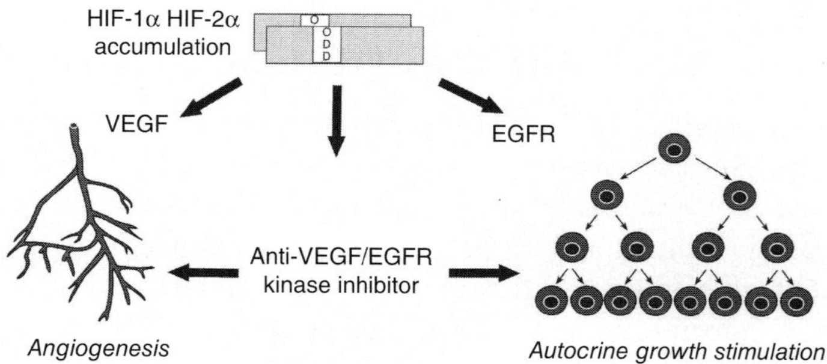

Figure 6.6. *VHL* gene mutation, downstream effects, and molecular targeting of the VHL pathway. (A) With a *VHL* gene mutation, the VHL complex is disrupted and allows for accumulation of HIF with subsequent activation of downstream pathways for angiogenesis, glucose transport, and growth. (B) Inhibition of overaccumulated HIF and prevention of downstream activation with a small molecule is one of the strategies for molecular targeting of the VHL/HIF pathway. (C) New tyrosine kinase inhibitors as well as direct vascular endothelial growth factor (VEGF) and platelet-derived growth factor (PDGF) receptor blockers are examples of downstream targeting. EGFR, epidermal growth factor receptor; TGF, transforming growth factor. (From Linehan WM, et al. Genetic Basis of Cancer of the Kidney: Disease-Specific Approaches to Therapy. 2004.) (To view this figure in color, see the insert.)

which maintain appropriate protein conformation, assist in protein transport, and play a role in antigen presentation. Out of the entire family of molecular chaperones, heat shock protein 90 (HSP-90) has drawn attention for its active role in renal. It is part of a complex that stabilizes and promotes the activity of HIF and the receptor tyrosine kinases MET and KIT.[75] An inhibitor of HSP-90, 17-allylamino-17-desmethoxygeldanamycin (17-AAG), has been shown to disrupt the function of this complex, thus leading to rapid inactivation and degradation of its client proteins.[82] As a result, HIF-dependent transcriptional activity is impaired, thus decreasing the downstream gene products in the HIF pathway.

Heat shock protein 90 has also been shown to play a role in chromophobe and papillary RCC through its effects on KIT and MET and their downstream pathways.[83,84] In addition to direct inhibition of KIT, HSP-90 inhibitors also function on AKT and RAF, transcription promoters that are stimulated by KIT but are also themselves client proteins of HSP-90. Finally, with respect to MET, HSP-90 inhibitors may have a potential role as an adjunct to angiogenesis inhibitors. Hypoxia has been shown to upregulate MET via the HIF pathway, including in vivo after the administration of antiangiogenic agents. Therefore, suppression of MET using HSP-90 inhibitors simultaneously with antagonists of angiogenesis may prove beneficial.[75]

CONCLUSION

Great strides have been made in the understanding of the genetic basis for renal malignancy. Through refined surgical techniques, patients afflicted with localized renal cancer have an excellent chance for survival with continued decrease in treatment-associated morbidities. Unfortunately, the current treatment modalities for those with advanced disease are not nearly as effective. Nonetheless, the future looks promising. Unrelenting research and dedication to understanding the cellular mechanisms of oncogenesis have the potential to change the face of renal cancer therapy and may provide these patients with the hope of a cure.

ACKNOWLEDGMENT

This research was supported by the Intramural Research Program of the National Institutes of Health (NIH), National Cancer Institute, Center for Cancer Research.

REFERENCES

1. Jemal A, Murray T, Ward E, et al. Cancer statistics, 2005. CA Cancer J Clin 2005;55(1):10–30.
2. Surveillance, Epidemiology, and End Results Program, 1992.
3. Knudson AG Jr. Mutation and cancer: statistical study of retinoblastoma. Proc Natl Acad Sci USA 1971;68:820–823.
4. Knudson AG Jr, Strong LC. Mutation and cancer: a model for Wilms' tumor of the kidney. J Natl Cancer Inst 1972;48:313–324.
5. Cohen AJ, Li FP, Berg S, et al. Hereditary renal-cell carcinoma associated with a chromosomal translocation. N Engl J Med 1979;301:592–595.
6. Zbar B, Brauch H, Talmadge C, Linehan WM. Loss of alleles of loci on the short arm of chromosome 3 in renal cell carcinoma. Nature 1987;327:721–724.
7. Seizinger BR, Rouleau GA, Ozelius LJ, et al. Von Hippel-Lindau disease maps to the region of chromosome 3 associated with renal cell carcinoma. Nature 1988;332(6161):268–269.
8. Linehan WM, Walther MM, Zbar B. The genetic basis of cancer of the kidney. J Urol 2003;170: 2163–2172.

9. Lonser R, Glenn G, Walther MM, et al. von Hippel-Lindau disease. Lancet 2003;361(9374): 2059–2067.
10. Maher ER, Yates JRW, Harries R, et al. Clinical features and natural history of von Hippel-Lindau disease. Q J Med, in press.
11. Walther MM, Lubensky IA, Venzon D, Zbar B, Linehan WM. Prevalence of microscopic lesions in grossly normal renal parenchyma from patients with von Hippel-Lindau disease, sporadic renal cell carcinoma and no renal disease: Clinical implications. J Urol 1995;154:2010–2015.
12. Choyke PL, Glenn GM, Walther MM, et al. The natural history of renal lesions in von Hippel-Lindau disease: a serial ct study in 28 patients. Am J Roentgenol 1992;159(6):1229–1234.
13. Lonser R, Glenn G, Walther MM, et al. von Hippel-Lindau disease. Lancet 2003; 361(9374):2059–2067.
14. Tory K, Brauch H, Linehan WM, et al. Specific genetic change in tumors associated with von Hippel-Lindau disease. J Natl Cancer Inst 1989;81:1097–1101.
15. Seizinger BR, Rouleau GA, Ozelius LJ, et al. Von Hippel-Lindau disease maps to the region of chromosome 3 associated with renal cell carcinoma. Nature 1988;332:268–269.
16. Lerman MI, Latif F, Glenn GM, et al. Isolation and regional localization of a large collection (2,000) of single copy DNA fragments on human chromosome 3 for mapping and cloning tumor suppressor genes. Hum Genet 1991;86:567–577.
17. Hosoe S, Brauch H, Latif F, et al. Localization of the von Hippel-Lindau disease gene to a small region of chromosome 3. Genom 1990;8:634–640.
18. Latif F, Tory K, Gnarra JR, et al. Identification of the von Hippel-Lindau disease tumor suppressor gene. Science 1993;260:1317–1320.
19. Whaley JM, Naglich J, Gelbert L, et al. Germ-line mutations in the von Hippel-Lindau tumor-suppressor gene are similar to von Hippel-Lindau aberrations in sporadic renal cell carcinoma. Am J Hum Genet 1994;55:1092–1102.
20. Chen F, Kishida T, Yao M, et al. Germline mutations in the von Hippel-Lindau disease tumor suppressor gene: correlation with phenotype. Hum Mutat 1995;5:66–75.
21. Zbar B, Kishida T, Chen F, et al. Germline mutations in the von Hippel-Lindau disease (VHL) gene in families from North America, Europe and Japan. Hum Mutat 1996;8:348–357.
22. Maranchie JK, Afonso A, Albert P, et al. Solid renal tumor severity in von Hippel Lindau disease is related to germline deletion length and location. Hum Mutat 2004;23(1):40–46.
23. Stolle C, Glenn GM, Zbar B, et al. Improved detection of germline mutations in the von Hippel-Lindau disease tumor suppressor gene. Hum Mutat 1998;12(6):417–423.
24. Gnarra JR, Tory K, Weng Y, et al. Mutation of the VHL tumour suppressor gene in renal carcinoma. Nat Gen 1994;7:85–90.
25. Herman JG, Latif F, Weng Y, et al. Silencing of the VHL tumor suppressor gene by DNA methylation in renal carcinoma. Proc Natl Acad Sci USA 1994;91:9700–9704.
26. Linehan WM, Lerman MI, Zbar B. Identification of the VHL gene: its role in renal carcinoma. JAMA 1995;273(7):564–570.
27. Lubensky IA, Gnarra JR, Bertheau P, Walther MM, Linehan WM, Zhuang Z. Allelic deletions of the VHL gene detected in multiple microscopic clear cell renal lesions in von Hippel-Lindau disease patients. Am J Pathol 1996;149(6):2089–2094.
28. Lee Y-S, Vortmeyer AO, Lubensky IA, et al. Co-expression of erythropoietin and erythropoietin receptor in von Hippel-Lindau disease-associated renal cysts and renal cell carcinoma. Clin Cancer Res 2005;11(3):1059–1064.
29. Duan DR, Humphrey JS, Chen DYT, et al. Characterization of the VHL tumor suppressor gene product: Localization, complex formation, and the effect of natural inactivating mutations. Proc Natl Acad Sci USA 1995;92:6459–6463.
30. Duan DR, Pause A, Burgess WH, et al. Inhibition of transcription elongation by the VHL tumor suppressor protein. Science 1995;269:1402–1406.
31. Iliopoulos O, Jiang C, Levy AP, Kaelin WG, Goldberg MA. Negative regulation of hypoxia-inducible genes by the von Hippel-Lindau protein. Proc Natl Acad Sci USA 1996;93(20):10595–10599.
32. Pause A, Lee S, Worrell RA, et al. The von Hippel-Lindau tumor-suppressor gene product forms a stable complex with human CUL-2, a member of the Cdc53 family of proteins. Proc Natl Acad Sci USA 1997;94(6):2156–2161.
33. Siemeister G, Weindel K, Mohrs K, Barleon B, Martiny-Baron G, Marme D. Reversion of deregulated expression of vascular endothelial growth factor in human renal carcinoma cells by von Hippel-Lindau tumor suppressor protein. Cancer Res 1996;56:2299–2301.

34. Cockman ME, Masson N, Mole DR, et al. Hypoxia inducible factor-alpha binding and ubiquitylation by the von Hippel-Lindau tumor suppressor protein. J Biol Chem 2000;275(33):25733–25741.
35. Epstein AC, Gleadle JM, McNeill LA, et al. C. elegans EGL-9 and mammalian homologs define a family of dioxygenases that regulate HIF by prolyl hydroxylation. Cell 2001;107(1):43–54.
36. Jaakkola P, Mole DR, Tian YM, et al. Targeting of HIF-alpha to the von Hippel-Lindau ubiquitylation complex by O2-regulated prolyl hydroxylation. Science 2001;292:468–472.
37. Maranchie JK, Vasselli JR, Riss J, Bonifacino JS, Linehan WM, Klausner RD. The contribution of VHL substrate binding and HIF1–α to the phenotype of VHL loss in renal cell carcinoma. Cancer Cell 2002;1:247–255.
38. Zbar B, Tory K, Merino M, et al. Hereditary papillary renal cell carcinoma. J Urol 1994;151: 561–566.
39. Zbar B, Glenn GM, Lubensky IA, et al. Hereditary papillary renal cell carcinoma: Clinical studies in 10 families. J Urol 1995;153:907–912.
40. Ornstein DK, Lubensky IA, Venzon D, Zbar B, Linehan WM, Walther MM. Prevalence of microscopic tumors in normal appearing renal parenchyma from patients with hereditary papillary renal cancer. J Urol 2000;163(2):431–433.
41. Lubensky IA, Schmidt L, Zhuang Z, et al. Hereditary and sporadic papillary renal carcinomas with c-met mutations share a distinct morphological phenotype. Am J Pathol 1999;155(2):517–526.
42. Choyke PL, Walther MM, Glenn GM, et al. Imaging features of hereditary papillary renal cancers. J Comput Assist Tomogr 1997;21(1997):737–741.
43. Schmidt L, Duh F-M, Chen F, et al. Germline and somatic mutations in the tyrosine kinase domain of the MET proto-oncogene in papillary renal carcinomas. Nat Gen 1997;16(May):68–73.
44. Bottaro DP, Rubin JS, Faletto DL, et al. Identification of the hepatocyte growth factor receptor as the c-met proto-oncogene product. Science 1991;251(4995):802–804.
45. Zhang YW, Vande Woude GF. HGF/SF-met signaling in the control of branching morphogenesis and invasion. J Cell Biochem 2003;88(2):408–417.
46. Birt AR, Hogg GR, Dube WJ. Hereditary multiple fibrofolliculomas with trichodiscomas and acrochordons. Arch Dermatol 1977;113(12):1674–1677.
47. Toro J, Duray PH, Glenn GM, et al. Birt-Hogg-Dube syndrome: a novel marker of kidney neoplasia. Arch Dermatol 1999;135(10):1195–1202.
48. Binet O, Robin J, Vicart M, Ventura G, Beltzer-Garelly E. Fibromes Perifolliculaires polypose colique familaile pneumothorax spontanes familiaux. Ann Dermotol Venereol 1986;113:928–930.
49. Liu V, Kwan T, Page EH. Parotid oncocytoma in the Birt-Hogg-Dubé syndrome. J Am Acad Dermatol 2000;43:1120–1122.
50. Chung JY, Ramos-Caro FA, Beers B, Ford MJ, Flowers F. Multiple lipomas, angiolipomas, and parathyroid adenomas in a patient with Birt-Hogg-Dube syndrome. Int J Dermatol 1996;35(5):365–367.
51. Hornstein OP. Generalized dermal perifollicular fibromas with polyps of the colon. Hum Genet 1976;33(2):193–197.
52. Zbar B, Alvord G, Glenn G, et al. Risk of renal and colon neoplasms and spontaneous pneumothorax in the Birt Hogg Dube syndrome. Cancer Epidemiol Biomarkers Prev 2002;11(4):393–400.
53. Pavlovich CP, Hewitt S, Walther MM, et al. Renal tumors in the Birt-Hogg-Dube syndrome. Am J Surg Pathol 2002;26(12):1542–1552.
54. Schmidt LS, Warren MB, Nickerson ML, et al. Birt Hogg Dube syndrome, a genodermatosis associated with spontaneous pneumothorax and kidney neoplasia, maps to chromosome 17p11.2. Am J Hum Genet 2001;69:876–882.
55. Vocke CD, Yang Y, Pavlovich CP, et al. High frequency of somatic frameshift BHD gene mutations in Birt-Hogg-Dube-associated renal tumors. J Natl Cancer Inst 2005;97(12):931–935.
56. Warren MB, Torres-Cabala CA, Turner ML, et al. Expression of Birt-Hogg-Dube gene mRNA in normal and neoplastic human tissues. Mod Pathol 2004;17(8):998–1011.
57. Launonen V, Vierimaa O, Kiuru M, et al. Inherited Susceptibility to uterine leiomyomas and renal cell cancer. Proc Natl Acad Sci USA 2001;98(6):3387–3382.
58. Alam NA, Bevan S, Churchman M, et al. Localization of a gene (MCUL1) for multiple cutaneous leiomyomata and uterine fibroids to chromosome 1q42.3–q43. Am J Hum Genet 2001;68(5):1264–1269.
59. Tomlinson IP, Alam NA, Rowan AJ, et al. Germline mutations in FH predispose to dominantly inherited uterine fibroids, skin leiomyomata and papillary renal cell cancer. Nat Gen 2002;30(4):406–410.
60. Isaacs JT, Jung YJ, Mole DR, et al. HIF overexpression correlates with biallilic loss of fumarate hydratase in renal cancer: novel role of fumarate in regulation of HIF stability. Cancer Cell 2005;8(2):143–153.

61. Toro JR, Nickerson ML, Wei MH, et al. Mutations in the fumarate hydratase gene cause hereditary leiomyomatosis and renal cell cancer in families in North America. Am J Hum Genet 2003;73(1):95–106.

62. Wei M-H, Toure O, Glenn GM, et al. Novel mutations in *FH* and expansion of the spectrum of phenotypes expressed in families with hereditary leiomyomatosis and renal cell cancer. J Med Genet 2005.

63. Robson CJ, Churchill BM, Anderson W. The results of radical nephrectomy for renal cell carcinoma. J Urol 1969;101:297–301.

64. Clayman RV, Kavoussi LR, Soper NJ, et al. Laparoscopic nephrectomy: initial case report. J Urol 1991;146:278–282.

65. Butler BP, Novick AC, Miller DP, Campbell SA, Licht MR. Management of small unilateral renal cell carcinomas: radical versus nephron-sparing surgery. Urology 1995;45:34–41.

66. Lerner SE, Hawkins CA, Blute ML, et al. Disease outcome in patients with low stage renal cell carcinoma treated with nephron sparing or radical surgery. J Urol 1996;155:1868–1873.

67. Walther MM, Choyke PL, Glenn GM, et al. Renal cancer in families with hereditary renal cancer: prospective analysis of a tumor size threshold for renal parenchymal sparing surgery. J Urol 1999;161(5):1475–1479.

68. Hwang JJ, Walther MM, Pautler SE, et al. Radio frequency ablation of small renal tumors: intermediate results. J Urol 2004;171(5):1814–1818.

69. Srinivasan R, Linehan WM. Targeted for destruction: the molecular basis for development of novel therapeutic strategies in renal cell cancer. J Clin Oncol 2005;23(3):410–412.

70. Joensuu H, Roberts PJ, Sarlomo-Rikala M, et al. Effect of the tyrosine kinase inhibitor STI571 in a patient with a metastatic gastrointestinal stromal tumor. N Engl J Med 2001;344(14):1052–1056.

71. Druker BJ, Sawyers CL, Kantarjian H, et al. Activity of a specific inhibitor of the BCR-ABL tyrosine kinase in the blast crisis of chronic myeloid leukemia and acute lymphoblastic leukemia with the Philadelphia chromosome. N Engl J Med 2001;344(14):1038–1042.

72. Rapisarda A, Uranchimeg B, Sordet O, Pommier Y, Shoemaker RH, Melillo G. Topoisomerase I-mediated inhibition of hypoxia-inducible factor 1: mechanism and therapeutic implications. Cancer Res 2004;64(4):1475–1482.

73. Kondo K, Kim WY, Lechpammer M, Kaelin WG Jr. Inhibition of HIF2alpha is sufficient to suppress pVHL-defective tumor growth. PLoS Biol 2003;1(3):E83.

74. Seagroves T, Johnson RS. Two HIFs may be better than one. Cancer Cell 2002;1:211–213.

75. Linehan WM, Vasselli J, Srinivasan R, et al. Genetic basis of cancer of the kidney: disease-specific approaches to therapy. Clin Cancer Res 2004;10(18):6282S–6289S.

76. Linehan WM, Zbar B. Focus on kidney cancer. Cancer Cell 2004;6(3):223–228.

77. Yang JC, Haworth L, Sherry RM, et al. A randomized trial of bevacizumab, an anti-vascular endothelial growth factor antibody, for metastatic renal cancer. N Engl J Med 2003;349(5):427–434.

78. Ratain MJ, Flaherty KT, Stadler WM, et al. Preliminary antitumor activity of BAY 43–9006 in metastatic renal cell carcinoma and other advanced refractory solid tumors in a phase II randomized discontinuation trial (RDT). J Clin Oncol (Meeting Abstracts) 2004;22(14_suppl):382.

79. Bennasroune A, Gardin A, Aunis D, Cremel G, Hubert P. Tyrosine kinase receptors as attractive targets of cancer therapy. Crit Rev Oncol/Hematol 2004;50(1):23–38.

80. Ciardiello F, Caputo R, Damiano V, et al. Antitumor effects of ZD6474, a small molecule vascular endothelial growth factor receptor tyrosine kinase inhibitor, with additional activity against epidermal growth factor receptor tyrosine kinase. Clin Cancer Res 2003;9(4):1546–1556.

81. Hainsworth JD, Sosman JA, Spigel DR, et al. Phase II trial of bevacizumab and erlotinib in patients with metastatic renal carcinoma (RCC). J Clin Oncol (Meeting Abstracts) 2004; 22(14_suppl):382–38b.

82. Isaacs JS, Jung YJ, Mimnaugh EG, Martinez A, Cuttitta F, Neckers L. Hsp90 regulates a von Hippel Lindau-independent hypoxia-inducible factor-1 alpha-degradative pathway. J Biol Chem 2002;277(33):29936–29944.

83. Yamazaki K, Sakamoto M, Ohta T, Kanai Y, Ohki M, Hirohashi S. Overexpression of KIT in chromophobe renal cell carcinoma. Oncogene 2003;22(6):847–852.

84. Lin ZH, Han EM, Lee ES, et al. A distinct expression pattern and point mutation of c-kit in papillary renal cell carcinomas. Mod Pathol 2004.

7

T-Cell Unresponsiveness in Renal Cell Carcinoma Patients

James H. Finke and Mahesh Goel

KEYWORDS

T CELLS
APOPTOSIS
DENDRITIC CELLS
T-REGULATORY CELLS
GANGLIOSIDES
CTLA-4

ABSTRACT

There is evidence that immune responses to renal cell carcinoma do occur and in limited cases mediate tumor regression. This notion is supported by the infrequent though detectable occurrences of spontaneous regression in renal cell carcinoma (RCC) patients[1] and by the higher incidence of renal cell tumors in patients that are immuno-suppressed after receiving kidney allografts.[2–4] There is also a significant infiltrate of T lymphocytes in many primary renal tumors,[5] and in some patients tumor-specific T-cell lines and clones have been expanded from their tumors.[6–8] Furthermore, clonal expansion of T-cell receptor (TCR)α/β T cells has been reported in renal cell tumors, most notably in those that are regressing.[9,10] More recently, a number of tumor-associated antigens were found to be expressed on RCC; among these are antigens shared by other tumor types, such as RAGE-1, Mage-3/-6, EphA2, Muc-1, and Her-2/neu, but also several that may be unique to RCC.[11–17] Despite the potential for an effective immune response to RCC, it is not well developed in this patient population even after implement of various forms of immunotherapy designed to stimulate tumor immunity. The presence of an ineffective immune response is likely attributable to suppression induced by the developing tumor.

Recently a paradigm shift has occurred in treatment of metastatic RCC with the demonstration that small molecule inhibitors of receptor tyrosine kinases and antibodies

From: *Clinical Management of Renal Tumors*
Edited by: R.M. Bukowski and A.C. Novick © Humana Press Inc., Totowa, NJ

that antagonize vascular endothelial growth factor (VEGF)/platelet-derived growth factor (PDGF) receptor signaling significantly increased not only the frequency of clinical responses but also their duration.[18] While these targeted therapies are a significant improvement in the treatment of metastatic disease, they are not typically curative. To further improve the outcome for RCC patients' future therapies will likely include combining the VEGF antagonist with strategies that promote antitumor immune responses. Thus, understanding how the tumor microenvironment can hinder the development of effective T-cell response to RCC remains an important issue to address. Here we describe the major suppressive pathways reported in RCC patients and provide some insight into their mechanism of action.

IMMUNE DYSFUNCTION IN RENAL CELL CARCINOMA PATIENTS

Increased Sensitivity of T Cells to Apoptosis

One explanation for the impaired responsiveness of tumor-infiltrating T-cell lymphocytes (TIL) is that these cells are undergoing apoptosis, which is supported by in situ staining of tumor tissue sections from RCC patients demonstrating that a portion of the lymphocytes were indeed showing DNA breaks (Terminal dUTP nick-end labeling [TUNEL] used to detect programed cell death [apoptosis]).[19] To obtain a more precise number of TILs that were apoptotic in RCC tissue, we performed three-color flow cytometry analysis (anti-CD3 antibody, AnnexinV, and the vital dye 7AAD) on digested tissue. Tonsil tissue was used as a control to rule out the possibility that the isolation procedure itself could induce T-cell apoptosis. The examination of 50 clear-cell RCCs revealed that the median number of apoptosis plus late apoptosis/necrosis among the $CD3^+$ TILs was 50%. Most striking was the variability in the level of apoptosis within the TIL population (3% to 70%) that was observed in tumors from different patients. In contrast, very few apoptotic T cells (<10%) were detected in peripheral blood from normal healthy volunteers or tonsil tissue. Our most recent findings with flow analysis of TIL revealed that the level of apoptosis was similar in the two major subsets of T cells ($CD4^+$ and $CD8^+$) ($n = 5$ TIL) (A. Richmond, manuscript in preparation).

Furthermore, peripheral blood T cells from some RCC patients display unique vulnerability to activation-induced cell death (AICD) after either 24 or 48 hours of polyclonal activation.[19] TUNEL assays were available for 51 normal controls, 79 localized RCC, and 93 metastatic RCC patients. T cells from normal individuals displayed little AICD (less that 5%, $n = 51$). Regardless of the duration of activation (24 or 48 hours), the AICD was statistically significantly greater in patients with localized ($n = 79$) or metastatic ($n = 93$) RCC as compared to controls ($p < .001$); there was no significant difference between localized and metastatic patients ($p = .91$). Overall, 59% of RCC patients had elevated activation-induced apoptosis, defined as TUNEL-positive results 2 standard deviations (SD) above the normal control values[19] (J. Finke, unpublished data).

Collectively these findings demonstrate that T cells in RCC patients are more sensitive to apoptosis when compared to T cells from normal healthy controls. These findings are not unique to RCC since others have reported an increase in apoptotic activity in T cells from patients with melanoma as well as squamous cell carcinoma of the head and neck cancer.[20,21] We are currently testing whether the percentage of apoptotic TIL or the sensitivity of peripheral blood T cells correlate with clinical outcome.

T-HELPER-2 CYTOKINE BIAS

Cytokine production is classified as type 1 or type 2, that is, mediated by CD4[+] subsets T-helper-1 (Th1) and Th2 cells, respectively.[22,23] The Th1 cells produce interleukin-2 (IL-2), interferon-γ (IFN-γ), and tumor necrosis factor β (TNF-β),[24] while Th2 cells produce IL-4, -5, -6, −10, and −13.[25] The Th1 cells secrete IFN-γ, and IL-2, which in turn promotes cellular immunity, in part by providing helper signals for cytotoxic CD8[+] T lymphocyte. Type 1 response (Th1) also plays a critical role in the rejection of tumors. The Th2 cells induce an antibody response, whereas Th3/T-regulatory cells produce immunosuppressive cytokines IL-10, and transforming growth factor β (TGF-β), which can dampen both Th1 and Th2 type immune responses.[26] Th1 and Th2 can also exert antagonistic effects. The Th2 cells inhibit Th1 cell functions by secreting IL-10, while IFN-γ secreted by Th1 cells can inhibit the differentiation and proliferation of Th2 cells and also antagonize the effect of IL-4 on its targets. Moreover, animal experiments suggest that antibodies to IL-4, IL-10, and TGF-β1 can block tumor-induced Th2 bias.[27,28]

Several studies have examined the issue of type 1 versus type 2 polarization in RCC patients, and most concluded that within the tumor microenvironment the predominant cytokine profile was type 2. An analysis of freshly isolated tumor infiltrating mononuclear cells[29,30] detected mainly IL-10 and IL-4[31] messenger RNA (mRNA) with minimal levels of either IFN-γ or IL-2. There is also an impaired Th1 response to tumor-associated antigens in peripheral blood T cells from RCC patients with active disease. It was noted that CD4[+] T cells specific for MAGE-6 and EphA2 peptides mediate a Th1 response from patients with no evidence of disease, but in patients with RCC an effective Th1 response is impaired.[31–33] Tatsumi et al.[32] showed that the vast majority of patients with active disease were highly skewed toward a Th2-type response against MAGE-6–derived epitopes regardless of stage, while patients with no evidence of disease had either mixed Th1/Th2 response or the response was strongly polarized toward Th1. In contrast, a disease stage variation in the Th1 response to the receptor tyrosine kinase EphA2 was observed in patients with RCC.[33,34] While the CD4[+] T-cell response to EphA2 epitopes was skewed toward Th2-type reactivity in patients with more advanced disease (stage IV), patients with stage I disease had predominately a Th1-type response, indicating that the response to some tumor antigens can be influenced by tumor stage. The findings that the cytokine response was predominately type 1 (IFN-γ) in patients where the tumor had been resected and that there was no evidence of remaining disease suggest perhaps that the presence of tumor was responsible for the induction of a type 2 response (IL-5) in patients with active disease. Most recently we observed that MAGE-6 and EphA2-specific CD4[+] T cells in the peripheral blood of patients with active disease are clearly more sensitive to apoptosis than influenza-specific T cells from the same individuals.[35] Thus, in some RCC patients the Th2 bias may be related to selective apoptosis of the Th1 population that can recognize tumor antigens.

The diminished type 1 response in the peripheral blood of RCC patients is not limited to MAGE-6 and EphA2-specific CD4[+] T cells. Indeed, following polyclonal activation,

Onishi et al.[36] showed that peripheral blood response changes from predominantly Th1 to Th2 with advancing stage of RCC. They suggested that peripheral blood lymphocytes could be useful for the immunologic assessment of RCC patients. Finally, Zea et al.[37] showed that the suppression in type 1 cytokine response observed in metastatic RCC patients correlated with a loss in the expression of the TCR-ζ (zeta) chain in peripheral blood T cells.

MECHANISMS OF IMMUNE SUPPRESSION IN RENAL CELL CARCINOMA PATIENTS

Dendritic Cell Dysfunction

Dendritic cells (DCs) are antigen-presenting cells derived from bone and are found throughout the body, but are more concentrated in areas of potential antigen entry into the body, especially around the epithelial and mucosal surfaces, where they can capture and process the antigens. Dendritic cells are also found in the thymus (where they have a role in self tolerance) and secondary lymphoid organs, where they present the antigens to specific T cells. Dendritic cells migrate out from blood into the tissue to sample the local environment.[38,39]

There are different subtypes of DC due to different developmental pathways, but this area remains under investigations. Clinically, there are various types of DCs[40]: (1) DCs derived from CD34$^+$ bone marrow precursor cells; (2) DCs derived from CD14$^+$ monocytes; and (3) peripheral blood DC populations either directly isolated or expanded in vivo by growth factors, such as Ftl-3 ligand. Dendritic cells may be immature (predominant phagocytic activity) or mature (less phagocytic and more potent T-cell stimulator activity). Dendritic cells are distinct due to a high concentration of peptides/major histocompatability complexes (MHCs) on their cell surface compared to B cells and other monocytes, and DCs can express both class I and class II molecules. They are capable of stimulating both CD8$^+$ cytotoxic T lymphocytes and CD4$^+$ T-helper cells for (1) enhancing the extent of cytotoxic T lymphocyte (CTL) response during the priming phase, (2) inducing T-cell memory against the presented tumor antigens, and (3) augmenting the primary immune response.[41,42]

Dendritic cell dysfunction is a common feature in a tumor-bearing host, which may partly explain the suppression of T-cell responses in cancer patients. Reduced numbers of DCs may be a bad prognostic sign, as shown in hepatocellular carcinoma, and gastric carcinoma,[43] while others suggest that higher number of DCs in tumors correlates with a better prognosis.[44,45]

One potential mechanism for the reduced number of DCs in tumor-bearing host is their elimination via apoptosis. Indeed, tumors can secrete a number of soluble factors that can induce apoptosis in DCs. Increased apoptosis was observed in DCs incubated with tumor cells and from implanted tumors in murine tumor models.[46,47] Katou et al.[48] studied the mechanism of tumor-induced DC apoptosis using supernatants from melanoma and fibroblastoma cells. It was shown that ceramide mediates tumor-induced apoptosis of DCs by downregulating the P13K pathway. Esche et al.[46] demonstrated that there is an upregulation of Bax (proapoptotic protein) and downregulation of Bcl-2 (antiapoptotic protein) associated with cytochrome-c release from mitochondria of apoptotic DC. Also, it has been suggested that nitrous oxide or S-nitros-*N*-acetylpencillamine (SNAP) may induce apoptosis by downregulating expression of the antiapoptotic protein cIAP.[49] These latter data suggest that tumor-induced nitric oxide (NO) can influence the number of DCs within the tumor microenvironment.

The expression of co-stimulatory molecules on DCs plays an important role in determining T-cell survival, apoptosis, anergy, or productive immunity. It is reported that DCs from tumor-bearing mice have significantly lower expression of important co-stimulatory molecules (CD40, CD80, and CD86) compared to DCs from non–tumor-bearing mice.[50] Moreover, CD40 ligation on DCs from tumor-bearing mice does not lead to expression of IL-12, suggesting impaired CD40 signaling and cytokine production by these DCs.[50] Studies also suggest that upon maturation, DCs from cancer patients have significantly lower expression of human leukocyte antigen (HLA)-DR, CD40, and CD80. It was shown that DCs treated with melanoma supernatant express a marked decrease in adhesion molecules like β_2-integrin and intercellular adhesion molecule (ICAM-1). Troy et al.[51,52] showed that DCs extracted from RCCs are minimally activated and have reduced co-stimulatory activity. These DCs express no or very low levels of co-stimulatory CD80, and CD86 molecules with reduced antigen-presenting function. Thus, abrogation of DC maturation is a common feature of tumor cell–DC interaction both in vivo and in vitro. Hence, decreased expression of co-stimulatory molecules and MHC class II molecules could be partly responsible for decreased induction of T-cell proliferation in cancer patients.

Several studies have demonstrated that different products present in the tumor environment can promote defective differentiation and maturation of DCs as well as suppress their function. This includes VEGF, TGF-β, macrophage colony-stimulating factor (M-CSF), gangliosides, IL-6, IL-10, and prostaglandin E_2 (PGE$_2$).[53–59] Recent studies have shown that the tumor environment via these suppressive products results in impaired differentiation of myeloid cells, which leads to decreased presence of mature and functional DCs and the accumulation of immature myeloid-suppressive cells (IMCs).[59] A number of studies have shown that the accumulation of IMC in tumor-bearing hosts plays an important role in suppressing antigen-specific T-cell responses. Indeed, depletion of the murine IMC (Gr1$^+$ cells) dramatically improved CD8$^+$ T-cell immunity, which coincided with tumor regression.[60,61] These IMCs can suppress immune responses by a variety of mechanisms, including reducing the expression of the T-cell receptor ζ-chain as a consequence of arginine depletion[37] and inhibiting T-cell proliferation by production of reactive nitrogen and oxygen intermediates.[62] In vitro studies by Zea et al.[37] demonstrated that these IMCs are partly responsible for the reduced production of IFN-γ by RCC patients' T cells. Most recently, Mirza et al.[63] demonstrated in metastatic RCC patients that treatment with all-*trans*-retinoic acid improves differentiation of myeloid cells and the ability of patient mononuclear cells to stimulate allogenic T cells. The improved DC function also resulted in greater tetanus toxoid–specific T-cell response, suggesting that all-trans-retinoic acid (ATRA) can improve DC function and T-cell responses in some patients. Whether this translates into improved clinical outcome in RCC patients remains to be determined.

Additional studies suggest that CD40L might increase the resistance of DCs to the tumor-induced inhibition of DC maturation and function.[50] Cytokines may also play a similar role. Menetrier-Caux et al.[64] found that IL-4 and IL-13 can reverse the inhibition of RCC-induced DC differentiation by blocking the expression of IL-6 and M-CSF receptors, and by preventing the loss of granulocyte-macrophage colony-stimulating factor (GM-CSF) receptor expression. Hoffmann et al.[65] found that addition of proinflammatory cytokines or CD40L ± IFN-γ improved DC function, the expression of MHC class I/II, and co-stimulatory molecules on the surface of DCs as well as the induction of IL-12 and IL-15 production. Finally, the administration of DC overexpressing cytokines such as TNF-α or IL-12 at the tumor site induces a strong antitumor response.[66] Increasingly there is evidence that protection of DCs from tumor-induced apoptosis may significantly increase the efficacy of DC-based therapy in cancer.

GANGLIOSIDES

Gangliosides are structurally diverse acidic glycosphingolipids present in the outer leaflet of the plasma membrane of cells.[67] They are composed of ceramide, which is linked to a sialic acid–containing oligosaccharide via a glycosidic bond.[68] It is also known that tumors exhibit augmented synthesis of select gangliosides, which are shed into the tumor microenvironment.[69,70] Malignant melanomas and neuroblastomas overexpress GD3, GD2, and GM2.[68] The elevated GD2 levels in neuroblastoma patients correlated with tumor progression and a lower survival rate for those patients.[71] Increased expression of GD1a, GM1, and GM2 in RCCs, as compared to normal kidney tissue, has been noted,[72] and enhanced RCC expression of several disialogangliosides appears to correlate with increased metastatic potential.[73]

Gangliosides play important roles in cell differentiation, growth, and cell adhesion,[74,75] and can also serve as receptors for microbes and their toxins.[76] Gangliosides associate with lipid rafts in the plasma membrane of cells and can modulate the function of various receptors.[76–78] Gangliosides are also known to inhibit immune responses[79–81] including T-cell proliferation and Th1 cytokine production.[82]

We have recently shown that GM2 is expressed by most clear-cell RCCs and that it is partly responsible for the ability of the RCC tissue–derived gangliosides to induce T-cell death. This conclusion is supported by the observation that all RCC lines tested ($n = 5$) expressed GM2 as did the majority of tumors (15 of 18) derived from patients with clear-cell RCC. Furthermore, the apoptosis induced in peripheral blood T cells from healthy donors by gangliosides isolated from RCC lines and RCC tissue was blocked by over 50% with the addition of a GM2 specific antibody (DMF10.167.4) to the cultures.[83] Additional supporting data demonstrating that GM2 is apoptogenic for T cells is provided by transfecting the tumor lines with siRNA (small interfering RNA) for GM2 synthase. Such treatment causes a specific and significant reduction in the expression of GM2 and GM2 synthase (48 hours), which coincided with a reduction (50%) in the ability of the RCC and GBM lines to induce apoptosis in normal T lymphocytes (G. Sa et al., manuscript in preparation).

The mechanism by which gangliosides induce apoptosis is not well defined except for the bovine brain–derived GD3. GD3 also has a direct effect on mitochondria, resulting in the formation of reactive oxygen species followed by the mitochondrial permeability transition (MPT) and the release of the proapoptotic molecule, cytochrome-c.[84] Once in the cytoplasm, cytochrome-c, and 2′-deoxyadenosine triphosphate (dATP) bind to Apaf-1, which in turn activates the caspase cascade resulting in apoptosis.[85] GD3 is also thought to play a critical role in apoptosis mediated by cross-linking Fas. The ligation of the Fas receptor is known to cause an increase in intracellular ceramide accumulation, which is rapidly converted to GD3 by enhanced GD3 synthase, and apoptosis can be blocked by antisense RNA against GD3 synthase.[86] We recently reported that gangliosides expressed by several RCC and glioblastoma lines also contribute to tumor-induced T-cell apoptosis.[87,88] Like commercial brain gangliosides, tumor-derived gangliosides appear to initiate T-cell apoptosis by a mechanism involving reactive oxygen species (ROS) formation and MPT (P. Rayman et al., manuscript in preparation). The tumor-derived gangliosides also induce caspase-dependent degradation of nuclear factor (NF)-κB (RelA/p50) and a subsequent drop in Bcl-2 and Bcl-XL expression, depriving the mitochondrion of antiapoptotic proteins and rendering the cells even further susceptible to ganglioside-induced death.[89] This scenario was supported by our recent data revealing that, when overexpressed in Jurkat cells, elevated RelA levels abrogate ganglioside-induced caspase activation, NF-κB degradation, the disappearance of Bcl-2 and Bcl-XL, and apoptosis.[89,90]

Findings by Rayman et al.[91] suggest that gangliosides in the tumor microenvironment may partially explain the Th2 bias observed in RCC patients. In vitro studies show that gangliosides present in the supernatants from RCC explants can polarize toward the Th2 response. It was also shown that a mixture of bovine brain–derived gangliosides inhibited IFN-γ production and not IL-4 after T-cell stimulation.[91] Most recently, we have reported that RCC tissue–derived gangliosides could suppress IFN-γ and in some cases IL-4 production by CD4⁺ T cells at concentrations (1 ng/mL to 100 pg/mL) well below those that induced any T-cell death (4 to 20 μg/mL). Additional findings demonstrated that GM2 contributed to the Th1 suppression induced by the RCC tissue–derived gangliosides. This conclusion was supported by the observation that the addition of anti-GM2 antibody to T cells co-incubated with RCC tissue–derived gangliosides partially blocked (50%) the ability of these gangliosides to inhibit IFN-γ production.[83]

Gangliosides like GM2 have been targets for cancer therapy using either monoclonal antibodies or vaccines to promote anti-GM2 antibodies. Indeed, the chimeric anti-GM2 antibody (KM966) reduced the establishment of human tumor xenografts in nude mice.[90] A second antibody specific to GM2 (DMF10.127.4) was also effective at preventing human melanoma and small cell lung carcinomas from establishing in vivo.[92] Livingston et al.[93] have shown that vaccination with GM2/bacille Calmette-Guérin (BCG) did stimulate an antibody response to GM2; however, the clinical benefit was modest and not significantly better than treatment with BCG alone. Our studies suggest that in vitro treatment with anti-GM2 antibody can protect T cells from apoptosis and suppressed Th1 response induced by RCC-derived gangliosides containing GM2. Thus, our interest is in developing strategies that can protect T cells from the suppressive effects of gangliosides. Future preclinical studies will focus on our recent findings that the antioxidants desferoxamine and *N*-acetylcysteine can block ganglioside-induced T-cell apoptosis and Th1 suppression in vitro. We are currently addressing whether these antioxidants, when given to tumor-bearing mice, will promote T-cell survival and improve the efficacy of EphA2 peptide/DC vaccine.

T-REGULATORY CELLS

The depressed type 1 response observed in RCC patients may be mediated by several mechanisms, including the suppressive activity of T-regulatory cells. Typically T-reg cells constitutively bear a CD4⁺CD25⁺ phenotype in situ and appear responsible for protection against autoimmunity in healthy normal donors.[94] It should be noted that only a subset of total CD4$^+$CD25$^+$ T cells in the circulation mediates immune suppression since activated CD4$^+$ effectors also express CD25 (IL-2 receptor IL-2Ra).[94] Another characteristic feature of T-reg cells is the expression of the forkhead box transcription factor FoxP3. It has been shown that expression of FoxP3 is sufficient to confer suppressive activity on naive T cells.[95]

There is growing evidence that CD4$^+$CD25$^+$ T-reg cells may play an important role in suppressing the development of antitumor immunity in cancer patients. The frequency of CD4$^+$CD25$^+$ T-reg cells is elevated in tumor sites or the peripheral blood of patients with advanced tumors.[96–101] It has been shown that T-reg cells can impair induction of both antigen-specific and nonspecific T cells in melanoma patients[102,103] and predict reduced survival in certain types of cancer.[99,104] In these studies T-reg numbers were assessed using multicolor confocal microanalysis (CD3$^+$CD4$^+$CD25$^+$) or by using real-time PCR to detect FoxP3 levels in tumor tissue. In one of these studies the level of Foxp3 correlated with IFN-γ and CD3 expression.[104] Relevant to therapy, experimental models have shown that removal of CD4$^+$CD25$^+$ T cells modifies the immune response to tumors.[105] Depletion of CD4$^+$CD25$^+$ cells in mouse models of RCC has been shown to enhance antitumor activity.[106,107]

Only limited analysis of T-reg has occurred in patients with RCC. The study by Cesana et al.[108] demonstrated that CD4$^+$CD25$^+$ (high expression) T-reg cells were increased in number (7%) compared to the numbers present in the peripheral blood of healthy volunteers (2.2%).[108] These T-reg cells expressed FoxP3 and CTLA-4 and produced the immunosuppressive cytokine IL-10. When isolated, the cells were capable of suppressing the proliferation of CD4$^+$CD25$^-$ autologous lymphocytes.[108] This study also showed that treatment with high-dose IL-2 resulted in a significant decrease of T-reg in those patients who had an objective clinic response to IL-2 therapy.[108] Another study in RCC patients demonstrated that modulating levels of T-regs could enhance vaccine-mediated antitumor immunity.[109] The reduction of CD25$^+$ T-regs by treatment with the recombinant IL-2 diphtheria toxin conjugate DAB$_{389}$IL-2 (ONTAK) did indeed enhance the proliferative and cytotoxic activity of autologous T cells. Furthermore, T-reg elimination with ONTAC followed by vaccination with RNA-transfected DCs did increase the stimulation of tumor-specific T-cell response over that observed with vaccination alone.[109]

One report has examined the role CD4$^+$ T-reg cells play in suppressing the Th1 response of tumor antigen specific CD4$^+$ T cells in the peripheral blood of RCC patients (stage 4).[33] Tatsumi et al.[33] had reported a Th2 bias in CD4$^+$ T cells that recognize the tumor-associated antigen EphA2.[33] In addition to measuring IL-5 and IFN-γ production by enzyme-linked immunosorbent spot (ELISPOT), assays for monitoring immune response (cytokine protection) using patient CD4$^+$ T cells following stimulation with EphA2 peptides/DC, TGF-β, and IL-10 production was also measured. While suppression of a Th1 response (IFN-γ) was noted in all 15 patients, CD4$^+$ T cells from five RCC patients also produced TGF-β after peptide stimulation, with none producing IL-10. Interestingly, in the five patients where the CD4$^+$ T cells produced TGF-β, there was a coordinately weak Th1- and Th2-type (IFN-γ and IL5 ELISPOT) CD4$^+$ T-cell reactivity against EphA2 peptides[33] (Strokus et al., unpublished data). While T-reg cells likely play a role in suppressing Th1/Th2 response to EphA2 peptides in a subset of RCC patients, these findings also suggest that other products may be involved in the development of a Th2 bias in this patient population.[33]

CTLA-4

T cells recognize foreign or self antigens through T-cell receptor interaction with a peptide in the context of "self" MHC. Usually co-stimulation is required for the activation of antigen-specific T cells. Co-stimulation is primarily mediated through CD28 receptor and CD80/CD86 ligand interaction.[110] The interaction between co-stimulatory molecule and its ligand are multifaceted, and the outcome depends on the stage of T-cell maturation.[110] After activation, T cells express a second receptor for B7 (CD80/86) known as CTLA-4, which is an inducible receptor with T-cell inhibitory activity.[111,112] CTL-4 binds CD80/86 molecules with 50-fold greater affinity compared to CD28.[113] Once CTLA-4 molecules become bound to cycling T cells they decrease activation and downregulate effector T-cell function.[112] It was shown that CTLA-4 inhibits T-cell response by blocking IL-2 production, and suppressing cell cycle progression.[113] CTLA-4 appears to be stored in the intracellular vesicles, and activation stimulates its export to the cell surface. Low levels of CTLA-4 expression support high affinity with CD80/86 as compared to CD28.

In the absence of CTLA-4 (knockout mice), T cells may remain chronically activated, supporting the role of CTLA-4 in the regulation of autoimmune disease.[114,115] Indeed, mice with targeted disruption of the CTLA-4 gene develop lymphoproliferation and autoimmune disease. On the other hand, blocking the suppressive activity of CTLA-4 in the setting of cancer can promote T-cell activation and enhance immune-mediated tumor regression. The role of CTLA-4 using surrogate antigens was studied by Shrikant et al.,[116] who found that blockade of CTLA-4 following tumor challenge can prevent tolerance to class I restricted antigen by a CD4 T cell– and IL-2–dependent mechanism. Leach and colleagues[117] reported that the blockade of CTLA-4 accelerates regression of B7$^+$ tumors as well as promotes regression of unmodified tumors (B7$^-$). Tumor immunity was dependent on CD8$^+$ T cells and conferred a long-lasting protection to repeat challenge, but these results were restricted to immunogenic tumors. The role of CTLA-4 blockade has also been studied in the transgenic adenocarcinoma mouse prostate (TRAMP) model. This approach reduced both primary tumor incidence and tumor grade.[118,119] Use of CTLA-4 blockade has also been combined with other immune-mediated and non–immune-mediated cancer therapies. For example, low-dose melphalan administration followed by CTLA-4 blockade shows enhanced tumor regression and improved survival of tumor-bearing mice.[120]

A clinical study in RCC and melanoma patients using an antibody (ipilimumab, MDX-010) specifically against CTLA-4 to block CTLA-4 suppressive activity has demonstrated some antitumor activity.[121] Anti-CTLA-4 antibody treatment did induce durable responses in both melanoma and RCC patients with an overall response rate of 14%. This treatment also induced immune-mediated toxicities including enterocolitis, dermatitis, hypophysitis, uveitis, and nephritis, although the major toxicity was observed in the gastrointestinal tract.[121] Interestingly, the clinical responses were most prevalent in patients with enterocolitis. The response rates in patients with enterocolitis were 36% for melanoma and 35% for RCC, compared to 11% and 2%, respectively, without enterocolitis. The possibility was raised that a plausible mechanism for development of enterocolitis following anti–CTLA-4 antibody treatment could involve T-regs. This idea is supported by the observations that T-reg cells constitutively express high levels of CTLA-4, and blocking CTLA-4 can promote autoimmunity.[122]

The ability of anti–CTLA-4 therapy to promote T-cell reactivity and to possibly reduce T-reg activity is of clinical interest. A number of different approaches that combine suppressing CTLA-4 activity with promoting antitumor immunity are under way and should yield interesting results.

ROLE OF B7-H1

Recent studies demonstrate that B7-H1 is a cell surface glycoprotein that is part of the B7 family of co-stimulatory molecules.[123] It participates in the activation of naive T cells and deletion of activated T cells. Human B7-H1 expression is restricted mainly to monocyte-derived cells, although aberrant expression has also been noted in other cell types. The co-stimulatory function of B7-H1 may be critical for enhancing maturation and differentiation of T cells in lymphoid organs. Conversely, after binding to its receptor, the programmed death-1 (PD-1) receptor on activated T and B cells, B7-H1 may inhibit ongoing T-cell response in peripheral tissues by inducing apoptosis and arresting cell-cycle progression.[124] B7-H1 preferentially co-stimulates IL-10 production in the resting T cells and further induces apoptosis of activated T cells.[125] Expression of B7-H1 is known to enhance apoptosis of activated tumor-specific T cells in vitro. In vivo, it has been shown that monoclonal antibody blockade of B7-H1 increases the antitumoral response in tumor-bearing mice.[126] Although the role of co-stimulatory molecules in the progression of solid tumors is not yet clear, progress is being made in understanding this process. Recent reports suggest that B7-H1 expression by tumor cells themselves stimulates IL-10 production (Th2 bias) in resting T cells and increases the apoptosis of activated T cells in murine models.[127] Hence, tumor-associated expression of B7-H1 may impair the survival of antigen-specific T cells, thus increasing the growth of immunogenic tumors.

Thompson et al.[128] demonstrated that B7-H1 appears to be the first co-stimulatory molecule related to solid tumor aggressiveness and patient survival. Immunostaining of frozen tumor tissue or paraffin-embedded tissue with anti–B7-H1 antibody demonstrated that approximately 60% of clear-cell RCC express B7-H1, although the level of expression does vary among tumors. Moreover, increased levels of B7-H1 expression by RCC does correlate with poor clinical outcome and decreased survival.[128] The same study also demonstrated that B7-H1 was not only expressed on the tumor cells themselves but also the infiltrating mononuclear cells. They demonstrated increased risk of cancer-specific death and tumor progression with high intratumoral B7-H1 expression, suggesting that B7-H1 expression may be used to identify a subset of RCC patients likely to benefit from immunotherapy (anti–B7-H1 antibody) and may also be used to ascertain prognosis. Thompson et al. propose that B7-H1 inhibits T-cell–mediated immunity by inducing apoptosis or inhibiting T-cell clonal expansion or both. Thus, they propose that B7-H1 acts as negative regulator of T-cell–mediated immunity promoting tumor progression.

Recently, a paradoxical relationship has been shown between increased number of infiltrating lymphocytes and poorer prognosis.[129] It was concluded that B7-H1, expressed by RCC tumor cells, may contribute to immunosuppression in RCC patients. It may be that immune suppressed or immunosuppressive lymphocytes accumulate in tumors as a consequence of B7-H1 expression, instead of the accumulation of fully functional T cells capable of mediating antitumor immunity. Although speculative at this time, it is possible that B7-H1 on cells including dendritic cells within the tumor microenvironment may promote the accumulation of immunosuppressive T cells. Indeed, Curiel et al.[130] have shown that VEGF, which is produced by tumors including clear-cell RCC, can induce B7-H1 expression on DC cells, which in turn can promote immune suppression in tumor-bearing mice.

Given the association between B7-H1 expression on RCCs and poor clinical outcome and the ability of B7-H1 to promote T-cell dysfunction, it seems likely that approaches to block or abrogate B7-H1 signaling may be therapeutically beneficial, similar to anti–CTLA-4 monoclonal antibody now in clinical trials for melanoma and RCC patients.[126,131]

REFERENCES

1. Oliver RT, Miller RM, Mehta A, Barnett MJ. A phase 2 study of surveillance in patients with metastatic renal cell carcinoma and assessment of response of such patients to therapy on progression. Mol Biother 1988;1(1):14–20.
2. Edwards MJ, Anderson JA, Angel JR, Harty JI. Spontaneous regression of primary and metastatic renal cell carcinoma. J Urol 1996;155(4):1385.
3. Kliem V, Kolditz M, Behrend M, et al. Risk of renal cell carcinoma after kidney transplantation. Clin Transplant 1997;11(4):255–258.
4. Kunisch-Hoppe M, Hoppe M, Bohle RM, et al. Metastatic RCC arising in a transplant kidney. Eur Radiol 1998;8(8):1441–1443.
5. Finke JH, Rayman P, Hart L, et al. Characterization of tumor-infiltrating lymphocyte subsets from human renal cell carcinoma: specific reactivity defined by cytotoxicity, interferon-gamma secretion, and proliferation. J Immunother Emphasis Tumor Immunol 1994;15(2):91–104.
6. Finke JH, Rayman P, Alexander J, et al. Characterization of the cytolytic activity of CD4+ and CD8+ tumor-infiltrating lymphocytes in human renal cell carcinoma. Cancer Res 1990;50(8):2363–2370.
7. Belldegrun A, Kasid A, Uppenkamp M, Rosenberg SA. Lymphokine mRNA profile and functional analysis of a human CD4+ clone with unique antitumor specificity isolated from renal cell carcinoma ascitic fluid. Cancer Immunol Immunother 1990;31(1):1–10.
8. Schendel DJ, Gansbacher B, Oberneder R, et al. Tumor-specific lysis of human renal cell carcinomas by tumor-infiltrating lymphocytes. I. HLA-A2–restricted recognition of autologous and allogeneic tumor lines. J Immunol 1993;151(8):4209–4220.
9. Angevin E, Kremer F, Gaudin C, Hercend T, Triebel F. Analysis of T-cell immune response in renal cell carcinoma: polarization to type 1–like differentiation pattern, clonal T-cell expansion and tumor-specific cytotoxicity. Int J Cancer 1997;72(3):431–440.
10. Puisieux I, Bain C, Merrouche Y, et al. Restriction of the T-cell repertoire in tumor-infiltrating lymphocytes from nine patients with renal-cell carcinoma. Relevance of the CDR3 length analysis for the identification of in situ clonal T-cell expansions. Int J Cancer 1996;66(2):201–208.
11. Ronsin C, Chung-Scott V, Poullion I, Aknouche N, Gaudin C, Triebel F. A non-AUG-defined alternative open reading frame of the intestinal carboxyl esterase mRNA generates an epitope recognized by renal cell carcinoma-reactive tumor-infiltrating lymphocytes in situ. J Immunol 1999;163(1):483–490.
12. Neumann E, Engelsberg A, Decker J, et al. Heterogeneous expression of the tumor-associated antigens RAGE-1, PRAME, and glycoprotein 75 in human renal cell carcinoma: candidates for T-cell-based immunotherapies? Cancer Res 1998;58(18):4090–4095.
13. Brossart P, Stuhler G, Flad T, et al. Her-2/neu-derived peptides are tumor-associated antigens expressed by human renal cell and colon carcinoma lines and are recognized by in vitro induced specific cytotoxic T lymphocytes. Cancer Res 1998;58(4):732–736.
14. Flad T, Spengler B, Kalbacher H, et al. Direct identification of major histocompatibility complex class I-bound tumor-associated peptide antigens of a renal carcinoma cell line by a novel mass spectrometric method. Cancer Res 1998;58(24):5803–5811.
15. Steffens MG, Oosterwijk-Wakka JC, Zegwaart-Hagemeier NE, et al. Immunohistochemical analysis of tumor antigen saturation following injection of monoclonal antibody G250. Anticancer Res 1999;19(2A):1197–1200.

16. Gaugler B, Brouwenstijn N, Vantomme V, et al. A new gene coding for an antigen recognized by autologous cytolytic T lymphocytes on a human renal carcinoma. Immunogenetics 1996; 44(5):323–330.

17. Hanada K, Perry-Lalley DM, Ohnmacht GA, Bettinotti MP, Yang JC. Identification of fibroblast growth factor-5 as an overexpressed antigen in multiple human adenocarcinomas. Cancer Res 2001;61(14):5511–5516.

18. Motzer RJ, Bacik J, Schwartz LH, et al. Prognostic factors for survival in previously treated patients with metastatic renal cell carcinoma. J Clin Oncol 2004;22(3):454–463.

19. Uzzo RG, Rayman P, Kolenko V, et al. Mechanisms of apoptosis in T cells from patients with renal cell carcinoma. Clin Cancer Res 1999;5(5):1219–1229.

20. Whiteside TL. Immune suppression in cancer: effects on immune cells, mechanisms and future therapeutic intervention. Semin Cancer Biol 2006;16(1):3–15.

21. Saito T, Dworacki G, Gooding W, Lotze MT, Whiteside TL. Spontaneous apoptosis of CD8+ T lymphocytes in peripheral blood of patients with advanced melanoma. Clin Cancer Res 2000; 6(4):1351–1364.

22. Abbas AK, Murphy KM, Sher A. Functional diversity of helper T lymphocytes. Nature 1996;383(6603):787–793.

23. Constant SL, Bottomly K. Induction of Th1 and Th2 CD4+ T cell responses: the alternative approaches. Annu Rev Immunol 1997;15:297–322.

24. Cher DJ, Mosmann TR. Two types of murine helper T cell clone. II. Delayed-type hypersensitivity is mediated by TH1 clones. J Immunol 1987;138(11):3688–3694.

25. Stevens TL, Bossie A, Sanders VM, et al. Regulation of antibody isotype secretion by subsets of antigen-specific helper T cells. Nature 1988;334(6179):255–258.

26. Levings MK, Bacchetta R, Schulz U, Roncarolo MG. The role of IL-10 and TGF-beta in the differentiation and effector function of T regulatory cells. Int Arch Allergy Immunol 2002; 129(4):263–276.

27. Nagai H, Hara I, Horikawa T, Oka M, Kamidono S, Ichihashi M. Elimination of CD4(+) T cells enhances anti-tumor effect of locally secreted interleukin-12 on B16 mouse melanoma and induces vitiligo-like coat color alteration. J Invest Dermatol 2000;115(6):1059–1064.

28. Seo N, Hayakawa S, Takigawa M, Tokura Y. Interleukin-10 expressed at early tumour sites induces subsequent generation of CD4(+) T-regulatory cells and systemic collapse of antitumour immunity. Immunology 2001;103(4):449–457.

29. Wang Q, Redovan C, Tubbs R, et al. Selective cytokine gene expression in renal cell carcinoma tumor cells and tumor-infiltrating lymphocytes. Int J Cancer 1995;61(6):780–785.

30. Elsasser-Beile U, Grussenmeyer T, Gierschner D, et al. Semiquantitative analysis of Th1 and Th2 cytokine expression in CD3+, CD4+, and CD8+ renal-cell-carcinoma-infiltrating lymphocytes. Cancer Immunol Immunother 1999;48(4):204–208.

31. Maeurer MJ, Martin DM, Castelli C, et al. Host immune response in renal cell cancer: interleukin-4 (IL-4) and IL-10 mRNA are frequently detected in freshly collected tumor-infiltrating lymphocytes. Cancer Immunol Immunother 1995;41(2):111–121.

32. Tatsumi T, Kierstead LS, Ranieri E, et al. Disease-associated bias in T helper type 1 (Th1)/Th2 CD4(+) T cell responses against MAGE-6 in HLA-DRB10401(+) patients with renal cell carcinoma or melanoma. J Exp Med 2002;196(5):619–628.

33. Tatsumi T, Herrem CJ, Olson WC, et al. Disease stage variation in CD4+ and CD8+ T-cell reactivity to the receptor tyrosine kinase EphA2 in patients with renal cell carcinoma. Cancer Res 2003;63(15):4481–4489.

34. Tatsumi T, Kierstead LS, Ranieri E, et al. MAGE-6 encodes HLA-DRbeta1–1–presented epitopes recognized by CD4+ T cells from patients with melanoma or renal cell carcinoma. Clin Cancer Res 2003;9(3):947–954.

35. Tatsumi T, Wesa AK, Finke J, Bukowski R, Storkus WJ. CD4 T cell mediated immunity to cancer. In: Finke J, Bukowski R, eds. Cancer Immunotherapy at the Crossroads: How Tumors Evade Immunity and What Can Be Done? Totowa, NJ: Humana Press, 2004:67–86.

36. Onishi T, Ohishi Y, Imagawa K, Ohmoto Y, Murata K. An assessment of the immunological environment based on intratumoral cytokine production in renal cell carcinoma. BJU Int 1999; 83(4):488–492.

37. Zea AH, Rodriguez PC, Atkins MB, et al. Arginase-producing myeloid suppressor cells in renal cell carcinoma patients: a mechanism of tumor evasion. Cancer Res 2005;65(8):3044–3048.

38. Jefford M, Maraskovsky E, Cebon J, Davis ID. The use of dendritic cells in cancer therapy. Lancet Oncol 2001;2(6):343–353.
39. Banchereau J, Steinman RM. Dendritic cells and the control of immunity. Nature 1998; 392(6673):245–252.
40. Siena S, Di Nicola M, Bregni M, et al. Massive ex vivo generation of functional dendritic cells from mobilized CD34+ blood progenitors for anticancer therapy. Exp Hematol 1995;23(14):1463–1471.
41. Volk J, Sel S, Ganser A, Schoffski P. Tumor cell-based vaccination in renal cell carcinoma: rationale, approaches, and recent clinical development. Curr Drug Targets 2002;3(5):401–408.
42. Schwaab T, Schned AR, Heaney JA, et al. In vivo description of dendritic cells in human renal cell carcinoma. J Urol 1999;162(2):567–573.
43. Takahashi A, Kono K, Itakura J, et al. Correlation of vascular endothelial growth factor-C expression with tumor-infiltrating dendritic cells in gastric cancer. Oncology 2002;62(2):121–127.
44. Becker Y. Anticancer role of dendritic cells (DC) in human and experimental cancers–a review. Anticancer Res 1992;12(2):511–520.
45. Shurin GV, Lotze MT, Barksdale EM. Neuroblastoma inhibits dendritic cell differentiation and function. Curr Surg 2000;57(6):637.
46. Esche C, Lokshin A, Shurin GV, et al. Tumor's other immune targets: dendritic cells. J Leukoc Biol 1999;66(2):336–344.
47. Pirtskhalaishvili G, Shurin GV, Esche C, Trump DL, Shurin MR. TNF-alpha protects dendritic cells from prostate cancer-induced apoptosis. Prostate Cancer Prostatic Dis 2001;4(4):221–227.
48. Katou F, Ohtani H, Saaristo A, Nagura H, Motegi K. Immunological activation of dermal Langerhans cells in contact with lymphocytes in a model of human inflamed skin. Am J Pathol 2000; 156(2):519–527.
49. Stanford A, Chen Y, Zhang XR, Hoffman R, Zamora R, Ford HR. Nitric oxide mediates dendritic cell apoptosis by downregulating inhibitors of apoptosis proteins and upregulating effector caspase activity. Surgery 2001;130(2):326–332.
50. Shurin MR, Yurkovetsky ZR, Tourkova IL, Balkir L, Shurin GV. Inhibition of CD40 expression and CD40–mediated dendritic cell function by tumor-derived IL-10. Int J Cancer 2002;101(1):61–68.
51. Troy AJ, Hart DN. Dendritic cells and cancer: progress toward a new cellular therapy. J Hematother 1997;6(6):523–533.
52. Troy AJ, Summers KL, Davidson PJ, Atkinson CH, Hart DN. Minimal recruitment and activation of dendritic cells within renal cell carcinoma. Clin Cancer Res 1998;4(3):585–593.
53. Katsenelson NS, Shurin GV, Bykovskaia SN, Shogan J, Shurin MR. Human small cell lung carcinoma and carcinoid tumor regulate dendritic cell maturation and function. Mod Pathol 2001; 14(1):40–45.
54. Gabrilovich D, Ishida T, Oyama T, et al. Vascular endothelial growth factor inhibits the development of dendritic cells and dramatically affects the differentiation of multiple hematopoietic lineages in vivo. Blood 1998;92(11):4150–4166.
55. Yang L, Carbone DP. Tumor-host immune interactions and dendritic cell dysfunction. Adv Cancer Res 2004;92:13–27.
56. Ohm JE, Gabrilovich DI, Sempowski GD, et al. VEGF inhibits T-cell development and may contribute to tumor-induced immune suppression. Blood 2003;101(12):4878–4886.
57. Caldwell S, Heitger A, Shen W, Liu Y, Taylor B, Ladisch S. Mechanisms of ganglioside inhibition of APC function. J Immunol 2003;171(4):1676–1683.
58. Peguet-Navarro J, Sportouch M, Popa I, Berthier O, Schmitt D, Portoukalian J. Gangliosides from human melanoma tumors impair dendritic cell differentiation from monocytes and induce their apoptosis. J Immunol 2003;170(7):3488–3494.
59. Kusmartsev S, Gabrilovich DI. Role of immature myeloid cells in mechanisms of immune evasion in cancer. Cancer Immunol Immunother 2006;55(3):237–245.
60. Bronte V, Chappell DB, Apolloni E, et al. Unopposed production of granulocyte-macrophage colony-stimulating factor by tumors inhibits CD8+ T cell responses by dysregulating antigen-presenting cell maturation. J Immunol 1999;162(10):5728–5737.
61. Seung LP, Rowley DA, Dubey P, Schreiber H. Synergy between T-cell immunity and inhibition of paracrine stimulation causes tumor rejection. Proc Natl Acad Sci U S A 1995;92(14):6254–6258.
62. Kusmartsev SA, Li Y, Chen SH. Gr-1+ myeloid cells derived from tumor-bearing mice inhibit primary T cell activation induced through CD3/CD28 costimulation. J Immunol 2000;165(2):779–785.

63. Mirza N, Fishman M, Fricke I, et al. All-trans-retinoic acid improves differentiation of myeloid cells and immune response in cancer patients. Cancer Res 2006;66(18):9299–9307.
64. Menetrier-Caux C, Thomachot MC, Alberti L, Montmain G, Blay JY. IL-4 prevents the blockade of dendritic cell differentiation induced by tumor cells. Cancer Res 2001;61(7):3096–3104.
65. Hoffmann TK, Meidenbauer N, Muller-Berghaus J, Storkus WJ, Whiteside TL. Proinflammatory cytokines and CD40 ligand enhance cross-presentation and cross-priming capability of human dendritic cells internalizing apoptotic cancer cells. J Immunother 2001;24(2):162–171.
66. Satoh Y, Esche C, Gambotto A, et al. Local administration of IL-12–transfected dendritic cells induces antitumor immune responses to colon adenocarcinoma in the liver in mice. J Exp Ther Oncol 2002;2(6):337–349.
67. Sorice M, Parolini I, Sansolini T, et al. Evidence for the existence of ganglioside-enriched plasma membrane domains in human peripheral lymphocytes. J Lipid Res 1997;38(5):969–980.
68. Ritter G, Livingston PO. Ganglioside antigens expressed by human cancer cells. Semin Cancer Biol 1991;2(6):401–409.
69. Ladisch S, Gillard B, Wong C, Ulsh L. Shedding and immunoregulatory activity of YAC-1 lymphoma cell gangliosides. Cancer Res 1983;43(8):3808–3813.
70. Black PH. Shedding from the cell surface of normal and cancer cells. Adv Cancer Res 1980;32:75–199.
71. Valentino L, Moss T, Olson E, Wang HJ, Elashoff R, Ladisch S. Shed tumor gangliosides and progression of human neuroblastoma. Blood 1990;75(7):1564–1567.
72. Hoon DS, Okun E, Neuwirth H, Morton DL, Irie RF. Aberrant expression of gangliosides in human renal cell carcinomas. J Urol 1993;150(6):2013–2018.
73. Ito A, Levery SB, Saito S, Satoh M, Hakomori S. A novel ganglioside isolated from renal cell carcinoma. J Biol Chem 2001;276(20):16695–16703.
74. Li R, Manela J, Kong Y, Ladisch S. Cellular gangliosides promote growth factor-induced proliferation of fibroblasts. J Biol Chem 2000;275(44):34213–34223.
75. Sun P, Wang XQ, Lopatka K, Bangash S, Paller AS. Ganglioside loss promotes survival primarily by activating integrin-linked kinase/Akt without phosphoinositide 3–OH kinase signaling. J Invest Dermatol 2002;119(1):107–117.
76. Yates AJ, Rampersaud A. Sphingolipids as receptor modulators. An overview. Ann NY Acad Sci 1998;845:57–71.
77. Rebbaa A, Hurh J, Yamamoto H, Kersey DS, Bremer EG. Ganglioside GM3 inhibition of EGF receptor mediated signal transduction. Glycobiology 1996;6(4):399–406.
78. Yates AJ, VanBrocklyn J, Saqr HE, Guan Z, Stokes BT, O'Dorisio MS. Mechanisms through which gangliosides inhibit PDGF-stimulated mitogenesis in intact Swiss 3T3 cells: receptor tyrosine phosphorylation, intracellular calcium, and receptor binding. Exp Cell Res 1993;204(1):38–45.
79. Kong Y, Li R, Ladisch S. Natural forms of shed tumor gangliosides. Biochim Biophys Acta 1998;1394(1):43–56.
80. Li R, Villacreses N, Ladisch S. Human tumor gangliosides inhibit murine immune responses in vivo. Cancer Res 1995;55(2):211–214.
81. Ladisch S, Li R, Olson E. Ceramide structure predicts tumor ganglioside immunosuppressive activity. Proc Natl Acad Sci U S A 1994;91(5):1974–1978.
82. Irani DN, Lin KI, Griffin DE. Brain-derived gangliosides regulate the cytokine production and proliferation of activated T cells. J Immunol 1996;157(10):4333–4340.
83. Biswas K, Richmond A, Rayman P, et al. GM2 expression in renal cell carcinoma: potential role in tumor-induced T-cell dysfunction. Cancer Res 2006;66(13):6816–6825.
84. Garcia-Ruiz C, Colell A, Paris R, Fernandez-Checa JC. Direct interaction of GD3 ganglioside with mitochondria generates reactive oxygen species followed by mitochondrial permeability transition, cytochrome c release, and caspase activation. FASEB J 2000;14(7):847–858.
85. Hengartner MO. Apoptosis. DNA destroyers. Nature 2001;412(6842):27,29.
86. Birkle S, Zeng G, Gao L, Yu RK, Aubry J. Role of tumor-associated gangliosides in cancer progression. Biochimie 2003;85(3–4):455–463.
87. Kudo D, Rayman P, Horton C, et al. Gangliosides expressed by the renal cell carcinoma cell line SK-RC-45 are involved in tumor-induced apoptosis of T cells. Cancer Res 2003;63(7):1676–1683.
88. Chahlavi A, Rayman P, Richmond AL, et al. Glioblastomas induce T-lymphocyte death by two distinct pathways involving gangliosides and CD70. Cancer Res 2005;65(12):5428–5438.

89. Thornton MV, Kudo D, Rayman P, et al. Degradation of NF-kappa B in T cells by gangliosides expressed on renal cell carcinomas. J Immunol 2004;172(6):3480–3490.
90. Nakamura K, Koike M, Shitara K, et al. Chimeric anti-ganglioside GM2 antibody with antitumor activity. Cancer Res 1994;54(6):1511–1516.
91. Rayman P, Wesa AK, Richmond AL, et al. Effect of renal cell carcinomas on the development of type 1 T-cell responses. Clin Cancer Res 2004;10(18 Pt 2):6360S–6366S.
92. Retter MW, Johnson JC, Peckham DW, et al. Characterization of a proapoptotic antiganglioside GM2 monoclonal antibody and evaluation of its therapeutic effect on melanoma and small cell lung carcinoma xenografts. Cancer Res 2005;65(14):6425–6434.
93. Livingston PO, Wong GY, Adluri S, et al. Improved survival in stage III melanoma patients with GM2 antibodies: a randomized trial of adjuvant vaccination with GM2 ganglioside. J Clin Oncol 1994;12(5):1036–1044.
94. Levings MK, Sangregorio R, Sartirana C, et al. Human CD25+CD4+ T suppressor cell clones produce transforming growth factor beta, but not interleukin 10, and are distinct from type 1 T regulatory cells. J Exp Med 2002;196(10):1335–1346.
95. Hori S, Nomura T, Sakaguchi S. Control of regulatory T cell development by the transcription factor Foxp3. Science 2003;299(5609):1057–1061.
96. Liyanage UK, Moore TT, Joo HG, et al. Prevalence of regulatory T cells is increased in peripheral blood and tumor microenvironment of patients with pancreas or breast adenocarcinoma. J Immunol 2002;169(5):2756–2761.
97. Woo EY, Chu CS, Goletz TJ, et al. Regulatory CD4(+)CD25(+) T cells in tumors from patients with early-stage non-small cell lung cancer and late-stage ovarian cancer. Cancer Res 2001; 61(12):4766–4772.
98. Wolf AM, Wolf D, Steurer M, Gastl G, Gunsilius E, Grubeck-Loebenstein B. Increase of regulatory T cells in the peripheral blood of cancer patients. Clin Cancer Res 2003;9(2):606–612.
99. Curiel TJ, Coukos G, Zou L, et al. Specific recruitment of regulatory T cells in ovarian carcinoma fosters immune privilege and predicts reduced survival. Nature Med 2004;10(9):942–949.
100. Ormandy LA, Hillemann T, Wedemeyer H, Manns MP, Greten TF, Korangy F. Increased populations of regulatory T cells in peripheral blood of patients with hepatocellular carcinoma. Cancer Res 2005;65(6):2457–2464.
101. Alvaro T, Lejeune M, Salvado MT, et al. Outcome in Hodgkin's lymphoma can be predicted from the presence of accompanying cytotoxic and regulatory T cells. Clin Cancer Res 2005; 11(4):1467–1473.
102. Chakraborty NG, Twardzik DR, Sivanandham M, Ergin MT, Hellstrom KE, Mukherji B. Autologous melanoma-induced activation of regulatory T cells that suppress cytotoxic response. J Immunol 1990;145(7):2359–2364.
103. Mukherji B, Guha A, Chakraborty NG, et al. Clonal analysis of cytotoxic and regulatory T cell responses against human melanoma. J Exp Med 1989;169(6):1961–1976.
104. Wolf D, Wolf AM, Rumpold H, et al. The expression of the regulatory T cell-specific forkhead box transcription factor FoxP3 is associated with poor prognosis in ovarian cancer. Clin Cancer Res 2005;11(23):8326–8331.
105. Onizuka S, Tawara I, Shimizu J, Sakaguchi S, Fujita T, Nakayama E. Tumor rejection by in vivo administration of anti-CD25 (interleukin-2 receptor alpha) monoclonal antibody. Cancer Res 1999;59(13):3128–3133.
106. Golgher D, Jones E, Powrie F, Elliott T, Gallimore A. Depletion of CD25+ regulatory cells uncovers immune responses to shared murine tumor rejection antigens. Eur J Immunol 2002;32(11): 3267–3275.
107. Takeuchi T, Konno-Takahashi N, Kasuya Y, Ogushi T, Nishimatsu H, Kitamura T. Interleukin-2 blocks the antitumour activity caused by depletion of CD25 cells in a murine renal adenocarcinoma model. BJU Int 2004;94(1):171–176.
108. Cesana GC, DeRaffele G, Cohen S, et al. Characterization of CD4+CD25+ regulatory T cells in patients treated with high-dose interleukin-2 for metastatic melanoma or renal cell carcinoma. J Clin Oncol 2006;24(7):1169–1177.
109. Dannull J, Su Z, Rizzieri D, et al. Enhancement of vaccine-mediated antitumor immunity in cancer patients after depletion of regulatory T cells. J Clin Invest 2005;115(12):3623–3633.
110. Allison JP. CD28–B7 interactions in T-cell activation. Current opinion in immunology 1994; 6(3):414–419.

111. Walunas TL, Lenschow DJ, Bakker CY, et al. CTLA-4 can function as a negative regulator of T cell activation. Immunity 1994;1(5):405–413.

112. Krummel MF, Allison JP. CTLA-4 engagement inhibits IL-2 accumulation and cell cycle progression upon activation of resting T cells. J Exp Med 1996;183(6):2533–2540.

113. Chambers CA, Kuhns MS, Egen JG, Allison JP. CTLA-4–mediated inhibition in regulation of T cell responses: mechanisms and manipulation in tumor immunotherapy. Annu Rev Immunol 2001; 19:565–594.

114. Waterhouse P, Penninger JM, Timms E, et al. Lymphoproliferative disorders with early lethality in mice deficient in Ctla-4. Science 1995;270(5238):985–988.

115. Chambers CA, Cado D, Truong T, Allison JP. Thymocyte development is normal in CTLA-4–deficient mice. Proc Natl Acad Sci U S A 1997;94(17):9296–9301.

116. Shrikant P, Khoruts A, Mescher MF. CTLA-4 blockade reverses CD8+ T cell tolerance to tumor by a CD4+ T cell- and IL-2–dependent mechanism. Immunity 1999;11(4):483–493.

117. Leach DR, Krummel MF, Allison JP. Enhancement of antitumor immunity by CTLA-4 blockade. Science 1996;271(5256):1734–1736.

118. Hurwitz AA, Foster BA, Kwon ED, et al. Combination immunotherapy of primary prostate cancer in a transgenic mouse model using CTLA-4 blockade. Cancer Res 2000;60(9):2444–2448.

119. Hurwitz AA, Kwon ED, van Elsas A. Costimulatory wars: the tumor menace. Curr Opin Immunol 2000;12(5):589–596.

120. Mokyr MB, Kalinichenko T, Gorelik L, Bluestone JA. Realization of the therapeutic potential of CTLA-4 blockade in low-dose chemotherapy-treated tumor-bearing mice. Cancer Res 1998; 58(23):5301–5304.

121. Beck KE, Blansfield JA, Tran KQ, et al. Enterocolitis in patients with cancer after antibody blockade of cytotoxic T-lymphocyte-associated antigen 4. J Clin Oncol 2006;24(15):2283–2289.

122. Read S, Malmstrom V, Powrie F. Cytotoxic T lymphocyte-associated antigen 4 plays an essential role in the function of CD25(+)CD4(+) regulatory cells that control intestinal inflammation. J Exp Med 2000;192(2):295–302.

123. Dong H, Zhu G, Tamada K, Chen L. B7–H1, a third member of the B7 family, co-stimulates T-cell proliferation and interleukin-10 secretion. Nat Med 1999;5(12):1365–1369.

124. Tamura H, Ogata K, Dong H, Chen L. Immunology of B7–H1 and its roles in human diseases. Int J Hematol 2003;78(4):321–328.

125. Dong H, Chen L. B7–H1 pathway and its role in the evasion of tumor immunity. J Mol Med 2003;81(5):281–287.

126. Hirano F, Kaneko K, Tamura H, et al. Blockade of B7–H1 and PD-1 by monoclonal antibodies potentiates cancer therapeutic immunity. Cancer Res 2005;65(3):1089–1096.

127. Strome SE, Dong H, Tamura H, et al. B7–H1 blockade augments adoptive T-cell immunotherapy for squamous cell carcinoma. Cancer Res 2003;63(19):6501–6505.

128. Thompson RH, Gillett MD, Cheville JC, et al. Costimulatory B7–H1 in renal cell carcinoma patients: Indicator of tumor aggressiveness and potential therapeutic target. Proc Natl Acad Sci U S A 2004;101(49):17174–17179.

129. Bromwich EJ, McArdle PA, Canna K, et al. The relationship between T-lymphocyte infiltration, stage, tumour grade and survival in patients undergoing curative surgery for renal cell cancer. Br J Cancer 2003;89(10):1906–1908.

130. Curiel TJ, Wei S, Dong H, et al. Blockade of B7–H1 improves myeloid dendritic cell-mediated anti-tumor immunity. Nature Med 2003;9(5):562–567.

131. Sanderson K, Scotland R, Lee P, et al. Autoimmunity in a phase I trial of a fully human anti-cytotoxic T-lymphocyte antigen-4 monoclonal antibody with multiple melanoma peptides and Montanide ISA 51 for patients with resected stages III and IV melanoma. J Clin Oncol 2005;23(4):741–750.

8
Renal Cell Carcinoma: *Clinical Presentation and Diagnosis*

Venkatesh Krishnamurthi

KEYWORDS

KIDNEY
KIDNEY NEOPLASMS
RENAL CELL CARCINOMA
DIAGNOSIS
RADIOLOGY

ABSTRACT

Renal cell carcinoma remains the most common malignant kidney tumor. The yearly incidence of renal cancer is rising, which may be related to a number of environmental factors. Due to advances in radiographic imaging modalities and surgical techniques, cure rates for low-stage renal cancer have dramatically improved. Unfortunately, the same cannot be said for advanced kidney cancer, which remains incurable despite medical progress. This chapter reviews the signs, symptoms, common clinical presentations of patients with renal cancer, and discusses the current approaches to establishing a diagnosis of renal cancer.

BACKGROUND

Accounting for 2% to 3% of all new cancer diagnoses in 2004, approximately 36,000 cases of renal cancer will be identified and nearly 13,000 deaths will result from kidney cancer.[1] Renal cell carcinoma (RCC), the most common epithelial neoplasm of the kidney, comprises 80% to 85% of all renal neoplasms. Approximately two thirds of renal cell carcinomas occur in men and most often during the 7th decade of life. Previously thought to be single entity, RCC is now considered a heterogeneous group of kidney tumors based on the cell type and, in many instances, specific genetic mutation. The majority of sporadic RCC cases are of the clear cell type (60% to 70%) and the rest are chromophil (15% to 20%), chromophobe (5% to 7%), oncocytic (5% to 7%), and collecting duct and unclassified types (5%). Within the last decade, four genetic forms of RCC have been discovered and the genetic mutation characterized. Each of

From: *Clinical Management of Renal Tumors*
Edited by: R.M. Bukowski and A.C. Novick © Humana Press Inc., Totowa, NJ

the hereditary forms of renal cell carcinoma, which have been recently reviewed by Linehan et al.,[2] is associated with a specific histologic type.

From an epidemiologic perspective, the incidence of renal cell has increased over the last three decades.[3] Although much of this increase can be attributed to more frequent use of imaging studies, patient-related factors such as obesity, hypertension, and tobacco use may also play a causal role in the increasing incidence of RCC.[3,4]

CLINICAL PRESENTATION

Symptomatic Presentation

Renal cell carcinoma has historically been referred to as the "internist's tumor" due to its predilection to present with unusual clinical manifestations. Notwithstanding this notion, however, a large proportion of patients with RCC present with hematuria. Although it is difficult to elucidate from published series, the occurrence of hematuria generally implies gross hematuria. Communication between the renal cortex and the collecting system, possibly through direct invasion or adjacent contact, are likely explanations for signs of hematuria. Additionally, rapid tumor growth may result in areas of necrosis that slough into the collecting system and manifest as blood in the urine. Tumor-related angiogenesis may also play a role in the development of gross hematuria. Interestingly, despite these potential explanations for the occurrence of hematuria, one study comparing central versus peripheral tumors did not find a higher proportion of symptomatic patients in the central tumor group.[5]

The prevalence of hematuria in patients with RCC varies widely. Prior to the introduction of sensitive abdominal imaging modalities such as ultrasonography (US), and subsequently, computed tomography (CT) and magnetic resonance imaging (MRI), in the majority of patients the diagnosis of RCC was made following the evaluation of signs or symptoms (Table 8.1). In a review of 309 patients treated at the Massachusetts General Hospital from 1935 to 1965, Skinner et al.[6] identified gross hematuria as an isolated finding in 60% of patients. The proportion of patients who may have had hematuria in combination with other signs or symptoms was not clear from this study, but nearly 93% of patients presented with symptoms related to renal cancer. Later series that have reviewed the clinical presentation of renal tumors suggest that the prevalence of hematuria ranges from 24% to 58%.[7–12]

The occurrence of microscopic hematuria must also be considered a distinct possibility with RCC. As mentioned previously, published reports do not distinguish between

Table 8.1.
Percentage of patients with renal cell carcinoma demonstrating common symptoms and signs

	Hematuria	Palpable mass	Pain	Incidentally detected
Skinner, 1971	>60			7
Sweeney, 1996	58	37	46	15
Jayson, 1993	24	8	10	61
Zisman, 2002				
(+) RV/IVC	37			2.3
(−) RV/IVC	21			21
Eggener, 2004	29	30–40	40	35

gross or microscopic hematuria when classifying patients as presenting with "symptomatic" or "incidentally detected" renal tumors; therefore, it is difficult to estimate the exact prevalence of microscopic hematuria in this patient population. It makes intuitive sense, however, that neoplasms involving the tubular architecture of the kidney would have a strong tendency to cause either gross or microscopic hematuria. Accordingly, patients being evaluated for signs of asymptomatic microscopic hematuria should undergo an imaging study of the renal parenchyma such as US, CT, or MRI.

The presence of a palpable abdominal or flank mass and pain in the same region are also common findings in symptomatic patients with RCC. These findings are most likely due to local growth of the tumor and when noted specifically in several studies, ranged in prevalence from 3.4% to 37%.[7–10,12] Likely explanations for such disparity include the difficulty in standardizing symptoms of pain, the varying availability of sensitive imaging modalities, and the referral-based practice pattern of tertiary care centers. Interestingly, the combination of flank or abdominal pain, mass, and hematuria, often referred to as the "classic triad," was seen in less than 10% of patients.[6,7]

Given the propensity to involve the renal vein or inferior vena cava (IVC), RCC can also produce symptoms and signs related to venous obstruction. Patients may notice acute-onset, bilateral lower extremity swelling from IVC obstruction. Acute onset of a varicocele, particularly on the right side, also suggests IVC or renal vein obstruction. Hepatic venous obstruction, or Budd-Chiari phenomenon, can also be seen, and these patients may present with signs and symptoms of liver disease including ascites and variceal bleeding. Not unexpectedly, nearly 90% to 100% of patients with RCC involving the renal vein or IVC present with tumor-related symptoms.[11]

Asymptomatic Presentation (Incidental Detection)

The increased utilization of US, CT, and MRI over the last two decades has brought about a dramatic increase in the proportion of patients with incidentally detected renal tumors. As mentioned previously, nearly four decades ago Skinner et al.[6] identified RCC as an incidental finding in only 7% of patients. In all of these cases, the incidental detection of a renal tumor was made during surgery for an unrelated condition. Several studies have shown a growing trend of an increasing proportion of patients with incidentally detected disease. Thompson and Peek[13] noted that the percentage of asymptomatic patients found to have renal malignancies increased from 6% during the decade from 1946 to 1955 to 25% from 1976 to 1985. In a subsequent review from the same institution, Leslie et al.[14] found that over half of all renal tumors were detected incidentally during the most recent 3-year period (1997 to 1999). Similarly, in the Jayson and Sanders[9] study of 131 patients with RCC, 61% of patients were asymptomatic at the time of diagnosis. Data from these and numerous other studies add to the growing body of literature on increased detection of asymptomatic renal tumors.

The rate at which symptoms develop in patients with incidentally detected renal tumors is unclear. Four studies that have evaluated the growth rates of small (mean tumor size of 1.5 to 3.27 cm), mostly incidentally detected renal tumors, found these tumors to be slow growing (Table 8.2).[15–18] With mean follow-up nearly to 5 years, the average growth rate of the largest diameter in these tumors ranged from 0.216 cm/year to 0.54 cm/year. Of note, only two of the 80 patients (2.5%) were described as having developed worsening symptoms during the period of observation, and these two patients also had "rapidly growing" tumors. From these data, it would appear that, during a

Table 8.2.
Evaluation of the growth rates of small tumors

Study	n	Presenting symptoms	Onset of symptoms	Mean size (diameter)	Growth rate (cm)	Growth rate (cm³)	Pathology	Comment
Bosniak, 1995	40 total (37 pts) 26 surgery 14 observation	Incidental	Not described	1.5 cm (0.2–3.5 cm)	0–1.1 cm/year Mean 0.36 cm/year	0 to 42.05 cm³/year	RCC in 22 (grade 2 in four) Oncocytoma in four	No patient developed metastases Mean F/U 3.25 years (1.8–8.5 years)
Rendon, 2000	13 pts.	7 incidental 4 pain or hematuria 2 w/previous cancer	2/13 developed symptoms	0.9–4.0 cm (2.95 cm)	Only two tumors grew rapidly; symptoms; 0.216 cm/year or 0.144 cm/year (removing two cases)	4.2 cm³/year 1.32 cm³/year	5 pts w/ surgery RCC in all five (no grade)	CT or US q6 months Mean F/U 42 months (5–57 months) Growth rate not different from 0 if 2 rapid tumors are excluded
Oda, 2001	16 primary 16 w/metastases	Incidental Not indicated	Not described	2.0 cm (median) (1.0–4.5 cm) 1.9 cm (median) (1.6–6.0 cm)	0.54 cm/year (0.1–1.35 cm/year) 1.72 cm/year (0.3–5.1 cm/year)			2.1 year mean F/U (1.0–6.0 years) Metastases grow more rapidly than primary Grade 3 metastases more rapid growth No relation of growth rate to initial diameter
Kassouf, 2004	24	2 w/symptoms (8.3%)	Not described	3.27 cm (0.9–10 cm)	0.49 cm/year (only 5 tumors grew)	7.3 cm³/year	RCC in all four who underwent surgery (no grade)	Mean F/U 31.6 months

period of limited follow-up, the onset of symptoms in patients with incidentally detected renal tumors is relatively uncommon, and when symptoms do present, they are more likely to occur in the setting of a rapidly growing neoplasm.

Several additional key points are apparent from studies that have reviewed RCC in asymptomatic patients. These patients tend to have smaller tumors, and as a consequence they tend to have a higher proportion of lower stage (stage I and II) tumors. Additionally, there tends to be a higher proportion of low-grade tumors (grade 1 and 2) in asymptomatic patients. Survival rates tend to be significantly better in asymptomatic versus symptomatic patients, which is almost certainly due to the higher proportion of lower stage and lower grade tumors.[7,10,14,19–21] Interestingly, in a study from the University of California–Los Angeles, asymptomatic patients who were found to have metastatic disease at the time of diagnosis still tended to have lower grade tumors and increased survival in comparison to stage IV patients who were symptomatic at the time of diagnosis.

Presentation with Metastatic Disease

Nearly 25% to 30% of patients with RCC are found to have distant metastases at the time of diagnosis. Presenting signs and symptoms in these patients are, in general, related to the site of metastasis. Lung metastases are the most common site of metastasis, and patients may present with a cough or dyspnea. Bone pain or pathologic fracture may be seen with skeletal metastases. The presence of asymptomatic elevations in alkaline phosphatase and transaminases suggests hepatic metastases.

Renal cell carcinoma also has a propensity to metastasize to a variety of unusual sites and, as such, the clinical presentation is often directly dependent on the site of metastatic spread. Several reports have described metastases to structures of the head and neck, including the orbit and paranasal sinuses.[22,23] Also, when identified clinically, RCC is the most common primary tumor to metastasize to the thyroid gland.[24] Hematogenous dissemination via the paravertebral venous plexus, thereby bypassing the lungs, is the potential explanation by which renal cancers metastasize to craniocervicofacial structures.

Metastatic involvement of numerous other abdominal and pelvic organs has been described. In addition to hepatic metastases, isolated metastases to the gallbladder, pancreas, and intestine have been reported.[25,26] Involvement of gynecologic organs is thought to occur via retrograde spread along the gonadal vein. Interestingly, in two reports of patients presenting with solitary vaginal metastases and a renal tumor, the primary tumor involved the left kidney, supporting the notion of retrograde venous extension from the renal vein to gonadal vein.[27,28]

Paraneoplastic Syndromes

The presence of a paraneoplastic syndrome is a relatively common occurrence with RCC and can be seen in up to 20% of patients. In addition to its excretory function, the kidney provides endocrine function through production of several hormones, which serve to maintain normal homeostasis. The overproduction of these hormones and hormone-like related peptides by renal tumors may produce the clinical effects seen in the endocrine paraneoplastic syndromes. Tumor-related secretion of other proteins, including cytokines, enzymes, and unidentified substances, can lead to the abnormalities seen in the nonendocrine paraneoplastic syndromes. Paraneoplastic syndromes can involve essentially any organ system and often present in a bizarre manner.

Two common hematologic abnormalities include anemia and erythrocytosis. Although blood loss via the urinary tract may be one explanation for anemia, malnutrition leading to iron deficiency, hemolysis secondary to tumor-related products, and cytokine-mediated bone marrow suppression are other potential causes.[29,30] Erythrocytosis can result from increased production of erythropoietin or an erythropoietin-like substance by tumor cells, as well as from adjacent normal renal tissue due to local areas of hypoxia from rapid tumor growth.[30–32] Leukocytosis and thrombocytosis have also been observed in RCC.

Abnormalities in hepatic function, both in coagulation factors and enzyme production, have been seen in patients with RCC. Initially described over four decades ago, Stauffer's syndrome is composed of elevated serum alkaline phosphatase, elevated prothrombin time or hypoalbuminemia, and elevated serum bilirubin and transaminases in the setting of a renal tumor and no evidence of hepatic metastases.[30,33] Increased levels of alkaline phosphatase or an alkaline phosphatase–like precursor isoenzyme are thought to be produced by the renal tumor and, when present, enzyme levels tend to normalize following nephrectomy in the majority of patients.[34] Failure of alkaline phosphatase levels to normalize should prompt further evaluation for metastatic disease and generally portends a poor prognosis even when metastatic disease is not identified.

Hypercalcemia is the most common endocrine paraneoplastic syndrome observed in patients with RCC. As RCC tends to produce osteolytic metastases, hypercalcemia may result from metastatic bone destruction. The paraneoplastic syndrome of hypercalcemia, in contrast, occurs in the absence of skeletal metastases. Several potential mechanisms of hypercalcemia in renal cancer have been proposed by Walther and colleagues.[35] These include tumor-related production of a parathyroid hormone–related protein, local osteolytic hypercalcemia (possibly from tumor-related cytokine production), and prostaglandin-mediated hypercalcemia.[35,36]

New-onset cardiovascular symptoms have also been seen as an uncommon presentation of RCC. Hypertension, a relatively common cardiovascular symptom associated with RCC, may result from renin secretion by the tumor, compression or encasement of the renal artery, effectively creating renal artery stenosis, and arteriovenous fistula within the tumor.[29,31,33] Large arteriovenous fistulas within the tumor can cause significant shunting of oxygenated arterial blood into the venous circulation, which may result in cardiomegaly with congestive heart failure.[36,37]

Renal manifestations of RCC include membranous, minimal change and immune complex glomerulonephritides.[9,36,37] Impaired renal function from tumor-related sarcoid reaction in a contralateral kidney has also been reported.[38]

Neuromuscular syndromes, in particular polyneuromyopathy, polymyositis, and myopathy, are all known to occur with RCC.[36,39,40] These conditions are thought to occur from the presence of an undefined circulating factor since, in the majority of cases, the symptoms resolve after resection of the primary tumor.

Finally, relatively nonspecific abdominal complaints, such as discomfort, bloating, and early satiety, as well as nonspecific systemic complaints, such as fever, night sweats, malaise, and weight loss, can also be observed with renal malignancy, particularly with advanced stages of disease. Tumor-related production of cytokines such as interleukin-6 (IL-6) and tumor necrosis factor α (TNF-α) are thought to mediate symptoms of fever, malaise, and muscle wasting.

Hereditary Renal Cell Carcinoma Syndromes

The discovery of inherited or familial RCC syndromes has established a variety of clinical features that are associated with each of the syndromes.[2] The most common hereditary form of RCC is seen in patients with von Hippel–Lindau (VHL) disease. This condition, which arises from a germline mutation in the *VHL* gene, leads to the development of bilateral, multifocal clear-cell RCC in approximately 35% to 45% of patients with VHL. VHL patients are also at risk of developing multifocal pheochromocytomas, pancreatic tumors and cysts, epididymal cystadenomas, cerebellar and spinal hemangiomas, retinal angiomas, and endolymphatic sac tumors in the inner ear. Hereditary papillary renal carcinoma (HPRC) type I is also an autosomal dominant disorder that is characterized by the development of bilateral, multifocal type I papillary RCCs. These tumors tend to appear later in life, generally during the 4th, 5th, and 6th decades. Furthermore, in contrast to VHL disease, the papillary tumors in HPRC tend to demonstrate an aggressive growth pattern and have been observed to metastasize. Individuals with hereditary chromophobe RCC/oncocytoma, or Birt-Hogg-Dubé (BHD) syndrome, are at risk for the development of cutaneous tumors of the face and neck (fibrofolliculomas), pulmonary cysts, and renal tumors (most commonly chromophobe or hybrid oncocytic neoplasms). Pulmonary cysts are most often asymptomatic but spontaneous pneumothorax can be seen in up to 25% of affected individuals. Lastly, the most recently identified hereditary renal carcinoma is hereditary leiomyomatosis RCC (HLRCC) or multiple cutaneous leiomyoma (MCL). In this disorder, patients may develop multiple cutaneous leiomyomas, uterine leiomyoma, uterine leiomyosarcoma, and kidney cancer (papillary type II).[2] Knowledge of and familiarity with these unusual phenotypic manifestations of the hereditary renal carcinoma syndromes may enable the clinician to diagnose and treat renal tumors in these patients at an earlier stage.

DIAGNOSIS OF RENAL CELL CARCINOMA

Radiologic Diagnosis

As mentioned previously, the widespread availability of cross-sectional imaging modalities, specifically CT and MRI, has permitted rapid and accurate diagnosis of renal malignancy in a high proportion of cases. The overwhelming majority of patients suspected of having a renal tumor ultimately undergo CT or MRI, which, in unequivocal cases, demonstrates a solid mass arising from the renal parenchyma. From a historical perspective, and for the purposes of understanding the evolution of modern renal imaging, it is useful to review the role of intravenous pyelography (IVP) and renal ultrasonography (US) in the evaluation and diagnosis of solid renal masses.

INTRAVENOUS PYELOGRAPHY

Even today, IVP, or excretory urography (EU), remains the initial radiographic study for the evaluation of patients with hematuria. With IVP, a series of plain films inclusive of the kidneys, ureters, and bladder are obtained both prior to and at various intervals following the administration of iodinated intravenous contrast. Additional tomographic images can be obtained to provide greater detail regarding the renal contour. Renal masses may be recognized on IVP by the presence of a mass lesion that distorts the renal contour, displacement of the collecting system (such as splaying of the calyces), or nonvisualization of a reniform structure (due to replacement by tumor or from venous obstruction by tumor). Masses that extend from the anterior or posterior surface of the kidney frequently do not distort the renal contour; consequently, small renal masses that do not produce the above-mentioned radiographic findings may not be detected on IVP. The relative insensitivity of IVP in comparison to CT has been well demonstrated in several studies, including that from Warshauer et al.,[41] which showed a detection rate less than 20% for renal masses under 2cm. Due to this inaccuracy in the detection of renal masses and the inability to illustrate other adjacent structures, IVP has given way to CT and MRI in the diagnosis of renal malignancy.

ULTRASONOGRAPHY

Ultrasonography has also been utilized to diagnose mass lesions of the kidneys. Historically, US was particularly useful in patients who could not undergo IVP, either due to a history of allergic reaction to iodinated contrast agents or renal insufficiency that precluded administration of intravenous contrast. The typical appearance of a renal tumor on US is that of a solid, echogenic mass that distorts the reniform structure of the kidney. Masses may appear homogeneous or heterogeneous depending on the proportion of necrosis within the mass and associated areas of cystic change. The echotexture of the tumor is often different from that of the adjacent normal renal tissue and, as a consequence, the tumor can be identified as a distinct lesion. Larger renal tumors tend to be isoechoic or hypoechoic in comparison to adjacent renal parenchyma, whereas smaller tumors (<3.0cm) are more often hyperechoic.[42]

Ultrasonography offers several advantages in the detection of renal masses. It is easy to perform, widely available, thus low cost, and poses no threat to the patient in terms of radiation exposure or nephrotoxicity. Several studies have attempted to exploit these advantages by using ultrasound to screen large numbers of asymptomatic patients for the presence of renal tumors.[19,43] In nearly 300,000 asymptomatic patients, the prevalence of renal masses ranged from 0.33% to 1.02%. Importantly, many of the masses were small, limited to the kidney, and highly successfully treated with surgical excision, thereby lending support to the use of US as a screening modality. In contrast, however, the ability of US to distinguish malignant versus benign masses was poor, as the false-positive rate ranged between 50% and 62%.

There are several other disadvantages of US that make it impractical for use as a sole modality for RCC detection and diagnosis. The ability to accurately obtain images with US is inherently linked to the experience of the operator. To perform a detailed study that obtains all the available information, a skilled ultrasonographer needs a dedicated and, often variable, amount of time. Additionally, and even in the setting of an experienced ultrasonographer, the patient's anatomy or variations in internal structures, such as overlying bowel gas or abundant retroperitoneal fat, can limit the ability to adequately visualize the kidneys. Although US has enabled the increased detection of small renal masses, the overall sensitivity of US to detect renal masses that were visible on CT was 26% for masses <1.0cm and 60% for masses between 1.0 and 2.0cm.[41] As is the case with IVP, for other than the initial demonstration of a renal mass, in the current era US has very little role in the imaging of renal masses.

COMPUTED TOMOGRAPHY

The mainstay of imaging for RCC remains computed tomography (CT),[44,45] which enables accurate characterization of nearly all renal masses as solid or cystic. The differential diagnosis of a solid renal mass detected on CT includes RCC (all histologic types), renal adenoma, angiomyolipoma, transitional cell carcinoma, and metastatic renal neoplasm. The absence of specific imaging characteristics and pertinent patient history often eliminates the latter three diagnostic possibilities, but, in the setting of small solid tumors limited to the kidney, CT cannot distinguish between malignant renal cell tumors and oncocytoma. Therefore, the identification of a solid renal mass on CT is an RCC until proven otherwise. In addition to the presence of a solid mass, perhaps the most important characteristic of the mass is the demonstration of enhancement following administration of IV contrast. The presence of unequivocal enhancement (>20 Hounsfield units) illustrates lesion vascularity, thereby confirming the diagnosis of a renal neoplasm. In addition to defining the tissue characteristic of the lesion (solid versus cystic, enhancing versus nonenhancing), CT accurately estimates the size of the lesion and allows for precise visualization of adjacent structures such as perinephric fat, lymph nodes, adjacent organs, and vascular structures (renal vein and IVC). These data not only facilitate accurate clinical staging of RCC but also provide a road map for surgical planning.

Several improvements in CT imaging over the last two decades have brought about the current diagnostic accuracy of CT. Helical or spiral CT permits rapid imaging of kidneys during a single breath hold, which effectively eliminates respiratory misregistration.[44–46] Power injection of iodinated contrast agents enables consistent tissue enhancement. Multidetector CT scans enables 1-mm reconstruction, shorter image acquisition times, and improved spatial resolution.[44] The current technique of renal imaging with CT involves three distinct phases. The first phase includes unenhanced scanning from above the diaphragm to below the kidneys. The second, or corticomedullary phase, requires helical scanning with thin sections (≤3–5 mm) beginning approximately 25 seconds following the injection of iodinated contrast. Vascular structures, specifically renal arteries and renal veins/IVC, are best seen during the corticomedullary phase. In the third, or nephrographic phase, thin sections (≤3–5 mm) of the kidneys are again obtained, now approximately 100 seconds following contrast administration. If desired, an additional phase depicting the collecting system structures (excretory phase) can be obtained by scanning 3 to 5 minutes following contrast administration.

With standard three-phase renal imaging, the accuracy of CT in the diagnosis of RCC is nearly 100%. As mentioned previously, lymph node enlargement and venous involvement are also well illustrated with CT. One area in which CT's diagnostic accuracy falls short is in the imaging of cystic renal masses. The Bosniak classification, devised in 1986, is a CT-based classification scheme that places renal cysts into four categories, based on increasing levels of complexity. Category I cysts are simple renal cysts, round, fluid-filled structures with thin imperceptible walls. Following contrast administration, these cysts may enhance only a few Hounsfield units and therefore are not consistent with malignancy. Bosniak category I cysts do not require further follow-up. On the opposite end of the spectrum are Bosniak category IV cysts, which have thick, enhancing irregular walls or septa, small or large amounts of calcification, and associated enhancing soft tissue components. Category IV cysts are RCCs until proven otherwise.

The most frequent diagnostic dilemma occurs with Bosniak category II, IIF, and III cysts. These cysts contain thin septa and fine calcifications (in the case of category II cysts) or thick, irregular walls or septa and variable amounts of calcification (category

III cysts). More complex category II cysts are classified as IIF, meaning further follow-up is required. Not unexpectedly, categorizing lesions based on subjective assessment of the thickness of septa or walls, degree of enhancement, or amount and distribution of calcification is an inexact process and leads to the diagnostic quandary. Accurate distinction between category II and III is important, however, in that the probability of a malignancy among category II lesion is approximately 5%, in contrast to nearly 57% among category III lesions.[47,48] Despite the difficulty in neatly separating lesions as category II or category III, the accuracy of the Bosniak classification scheme has been validated by several studies.[47,48] Given the limitation of CT scanning, Bosniak category III and IV cysts require surgical exploration, whereas category I and II cysts may be followed.

Several other points regarding the imaging of renal masses and cysts are worth mentioning. The degree of enhancement within a mass must be ascertained only during the appropriate postcontrast phase of the CT scan, specifically the nephrographic phase. Attempts to determine enhancement too early following contrast administration, or during the corticomedullary phase, may falsely underestimate the degree of enhancement.[49,50] Additionally, neoplasms that are primarily located in the medullary portion of the kidney may not be visualized very early after contrast administration.[49,50]

The possibility of pseudoenhancement within a mass must also be considered, particularly for small masses. Pseudoenhancement refers to enhancement due to radiographic artifact rather than from tissue characteristics. Pseudoenhancement is particularly problematic during the imaging of small renal cysts. Laboratory-based and clinical studies have demonstrated that pseudoenhancement is more likely to occur with small (<1.0 cm) intrarenal cysts that are evaluated during the peak phase of enhancement or nephrographic phase.[51,52] Pseudoenhancement is even more likely to occur when image thickness is greater than one half of the lesion diameter. Volume averaging and beam hardening are putative mechanisms leading to pseudoenhancement.

Finally, the degree of calcification within a renal mass or cyst was previously thought to be associated with malignancy, but in fact may not offer any additional diagnostic information. The presence of calcification within a solid renal mass is nonspecific and should not change the diagnosis from RCC. Increasing amounts of calcification within complex renal cysts were also thought to be associated with increasing complexity and increasing probability of malignancy. In a recent study, Israel and Bosniak[53] demonstrated that the degree of calcification within renal cysts has no bearing on the diagnosis of RCC and that minimally complex cysts (Bosniak category II) may develop bulky calcification with long-term follow-up.

MAGNETIC RESONANCE IMAGING

In patients who cannot receive iodinated intravenous contrast materials because of allergy or renal insufficiency, the diagnosis of RCC may be obtained through MRI. Renal imaging is best performed by obtaining a combination of T1-weighted images both prior to and following intravenous gadolinium administration and T2-weighted images. As with CT, solid renal masses that show enhancement following administration of gadolinium are highly suggestive of RCC. The diagnostic accuracy of this finding has been shown by Rofsky et al.[54] in a study of patients with moderate to advanced renal dysfunction, which precluded examination with iodinated contrast. Additionally, there was no evidence of renal functional impairment following the administration of gadolinium. Moreover, the overall safety of gadolinium has been well described in a large series of patients.[55] The prevalence of serious and long-lasting side effects following intravenous gadolinium administration is extremely low, even when administered to patients with a history of asthma, allergy, or prior reaction to iodinated or MR contrast agents.[55]

Magnetic resonance imaging has also been utilized to characterize renal masses that are indeterminate on CT. As noted previously, small, intrarenal cysts are more prone to show features of pseudoenhancement, which may result in false diagnosis of renal neoplasia. Evaluation with T1-weighted MRI, before and after gadolinium administration, is unaffected by beam hardening and volume averaging problems that may occur with CT of small, cystic masses. As a result, MRI may be more accurate than CT in the diagnosis of subcentimeter renal masses.

Similarly, MRI has been used to evaluate complex renal cysts. Although a scheme similar to the Bosniak classification scheme has not been established, there are identifiable features on MRI that are highly suggestive of renal malignancy. These include mural irregularity or nodularity and intense mural enhancement.[56] In contrast to CT, the finding of heterogeneous cyst fluid is common on MRI due to the high sensitivity of MRI in depicting the varying signal intensities of the different components in cyst fluid.

Several other features of MRI offered improved imaging prior to the development of multidetector CT. These related primarily to the ability to reconstruct images in multiple planes, which allowed better visualization of vascular structures, such as the IVC, and relationship to adjacent organs. The improvements in CT have resulted in the ability to reconstruct images with equally precise resolution, and currently CT is equivalent to MRI in demonstrating the cephalad extent of tumor thrombi within the IVC. One remaining advantage of MRI is the lack of radiation, which may be relevant in patients who undergo multiple examinations. Despite these issues, at the present time, CT remains the imaging modality of choice in patients who do not have a renal insufficiency or allergic reaction to iodinated intravenous contrast.[45]

Pathologic Diagnosis of Renal Masses

PERCUTANEOUS BIOPSY

The utility of preoperative biopsy of small, radiographically indeterminate renal masses has also been questioned as a potential diagnostic aid. Several studies have attempted to answer this question, and in reviewing these reports, many shortcomings are apparent.[57–60] First, the yield of samples sufficient for pathologic analysis ranges from 40% to 95%.[57,58] In the studies by Campbell et al.[58] and Dechet et al.,[60] in which there was final histopathologic confirmation of all biopsy specimens, the diagnostic accuracy ranged from 40% to 78%. Other studies have suggested a higher accuracy rate but these studies are limited by the lack of histopathologic confirmation on all prospective biopsies.[57,59] Additionally, although the predictive value of a positive biopsy (positive for malignancy) remains high in these studies (93%–100%), the negative predictive value may be prohibitively low, ranging from 0% to 31%. Finally, complications of percutaneous biopsy, including malignant seeding of the biopsy needle tract and subcapsular hematoma formation, have also been reported.[58]

The results of these studies suggest that the diagnosis of a renal mass based on imaging features is more accurate than cytologic analysis of fine-needle aspirates or histopathologic analysis of core biopsies. One potential role for percutaneous biopsy is in cases of a solitary renal mass in patients with known primary malignancies elsewhere. Metastatic renal involvement by hematologic tumors, such as lymphoma and leukemia, and solid tumors of the lung, breast, and gastrointestinal tract is a common finding in patients dying from these cancers.[33] When identified clinically, biopsy of a solitary renal mass, thereby lending histopathologic confirmation of metastatic spread, may impact upon treatment decisions.

REFERENCES

1. Cancer Facts and Figures 2004. American Cancer Society, Atlanta, GA, 2005.
2. Linehan WM, Walther MM, Zbar B. The genetic basis of cancer of the kidney. J Urol 2003;170(6 pt 1):2163–2172.
3. Chow WH, Devesa SS, Warren JL, Fraumeni JF Jr. Rising incidence of renal cell cancer in the United States. JAMA 1999;281(17):1628–1631.
4. Chow WH, Gridley G, Fraumeni JF Jr, Jarvholm B. Obesity, hypertension, and the risk of kidney cancer in men. N Engl J Med 2000;343(18):1305–1311.
5. Hafez KS, Novick AC, Butler BP. Management of small solitary unilateral renal cell carcinomas: impact of central versus peripheral tumor location. J Urol 1998;159(4):1156–1160.
6. Skinner DG, Colvin RB, Vermillion CD, Pfister RC, Leadbetter WF. Diagnosis and management of renal cell carcinoma. A clinical and pathologic study of 309 cases. Cancer 1971;28(5):1165–1177.
7. Sweeney JP, Thornhill JA, Graiger R, McDermott TE, Butler MR. Incidentally detected renal cell carcinoma: pathological features, survival trends and implications for treatment. Br J Urol 1996; 78(3):351–353.
8. Bretheau D, Koutani A, Lechevallier E, Coulange C. A French national epidemiologic survey on renal cell carcinoma. Oncology Committee of the Association Francaise d'Urologie. Cancer 1998;82(3): 538–544.
9. Jayson M, Sanders H. Increased incidence of serendipitously discovered renal cell carcinoma. Urology 1998;51(2):203–205.
10. Tsui KH, Shvarts O, Smith RB, Figlin R, de Kernion JB, Belldegrun A. Renal cell carcinoma: prognostic significance of incidentally detected tumors. [see comment]. J Urol 2000;163(2):426–430.
11. Zisman A, Pantuck AJ, Chao DH, et al. Renal cell carcinoma with tumor thrombus: is cytoreductive nephrectomy for advanced disease associated with an increased complication rate? J Urol 2002;168(3):962–967.
12. Eggener SE, Rubenstein JR, Smith ND, Nadler RL, Kontak J. Renal tumors in young adults. J Urol 2004;171(1):106–110.
13. Thompson IM, Peek M. Improvement in survival of patients with renal cell carcinoma—the role of the serendipitously detected tumor. J Urol 1988;140(3):487–490.
14. Leslie JA, Prihoda T, Thompson IM. Serendipitous renal cell carcinoma in the post-CT era: continued evidence in improved outcomes. Urol Oncol 2003;21(1):39–44.
15. Bosniak MA, Birnbaum BA, Krinsky GA, Waisman J. Small renal parenchymal neoplasms: further observations on growth. [see comment]. Radiology 1995;197(3):589–597.
16. Rendon RA, Stanietzky N, Panzarella T, et al. The natural history of small renal masses. J Urol 2000;164(4):1143–1147.
17. Oda T, Miyao N, Takahashi A, et al. Growth rates of primary and metastatic lesions of renal cell carcinoma. Int J Urol 2001;8(9):473–477.
18. Kassouf WAA. Natural history of renal masses followed expectantly. J Urol 2004;171(1):111–113.
19. Tosaka A, Ohya K, Yamada K, et al. Incidence and properties of renal masses and asymptomatic renal cell carcinoma detected by abdominal ultrasonography. J Urol 1990;144(5):1097–1099.
20. Luciani LG, Cestari R, Tallarigo C. Incidental renal cell carcinoma-age and stage characterization and clinical implications: study of 1092 patients (1982–1997). Urology 2000;56(1):58–62.
21. Licht MR, Novick AC, Goormastic M. Nephron sparing surgery in incidental versus suspected renal cell carcinoma. J Urol 1994;152(1):39–42.
22. Holt BA, Holmes SA, Kirby RS. Renal cell carcinoma presenting with orbital metastases. Br J Urol 1995;75(2):246–247.

23. Sesenna E, Tullio A, Piazza P. Treatment of craniofacial metastasis of a renal adenocarcinoma: report of case and review of literature. J Oral Maxillofac Surg 1995;53(2):187–193.

24. Green LK, Ro JY, Mackay B, Ayala AG, Luna MA. Renal cell carcinoma metastatic to the thyroid. Cancer 1989;63(9):1810–1815.

25. Pagano S, Ruggeri P, Franzoso F, Brusamolino R. Unusual renal cell carcinoma metastasis to the gallbladder. Urology 1995;45(5):867–869.

26. Dousset B, Andant C, Guimbaud R, et al. Late pancreatic metastasis from renal cell carcinoma diagnosed by endoscopic ultrasonography. Surgery 1995;117(5):591–594.

27. Knight EL Jr, Kandzari SJ, Milam DF. Renal cell carcinoma presenting as vaginal bleeding. Urology 1977;10(3):249–250.

28. Torne A, Pahisa J, Castelo-Branco C, Fabregues F, Mallofre C, Iglesias X. Solitary vaginal metastasis as a presenting form of unsuspected renal adenocarcinoma. Gynecol Oncol 1994;52(2):260–263.

29. Cherukuri SV, Johenning PW, Ram MD. Systemic effects of hypernephroma. Urology 1977; 10(2):93–97.

30. Gold PJ, Fefer A, Thompson JA. Paraneoplastic manifestations of renal cell carcinoma. Semin Urol Oncol 1996;14(4):216–222.

31. Sufrin G, Mirand EA, Moore RH, Chu TM, Murphy GP. Hormones in renal cancer. J Urol 1977;117(4):433–438.

32. Da Silva JL, Lacombe C, Bruneval P, et al. Tumor cells are the site of erythropoietin synthesis in human renal cancers associated with polycythemia. Blood 1990;75(3):577–582.

33. Novick AC, Campbell SC. Renal tumors. In: Walsh PC, Retik AB, Vaughn ED, Wein AJ, eds. Campbell's Urology. Philadelphia: Saunders, 2002:2672–2731.

34. Chuang YC, Lin AT, Chen KK, Chang YH, Chen MT, Chang LS. Paraneoplastic elevation of serum alkaline phosphatase in renal cell carcinoma: incidence and implication on prognosis. J Urol 1997;158(5):1684–1687.

35. Walther MM, Patel B, Choyke PL, et al. Hypercalcemia in patients with metastatic renal cell carcinoma: effect of nephrectomy and metabolic evaluation. J Urol 1997;158(3 pt 1):733–739.

36. Papac RJ, Poo-Hwu WJ. Renal cell carcinoma: a paradigm of lanthanic disease. Am J Clin Oncol 1999;22(3):223–231.

37. Cronin RE, Kaehny WD, Miller PD, et al. Renal cell carcinoma: unusual systemic manifestations. Medicine 1976;55(4):291–311.

38. Marinides GN, Hajdu I, Gans RO. A unique association of renal carcinoma with sarcoid reaction in the kidney. Nephron 1994;67(4):477–480.

39. Solon AA, Gilbert CS, Meyer C. Myopathy as a paraneoplastic manifestation of renal cell carcinoma. Am J Med 1994;97(5):491–492.

40. Forman D, Rae-Grant AD, Matchett SC, Cowen JS. A reversible cause of hypercapnic respiratory failure: lower motor neuronopathy associated with renal cell carcinoma. Chest 1999;115(3): 899–901.

41. Warshauer DM, McCarthy SM, Street L, et al. Detection of renal masses: sensitivities and specificities of excretory urography/linear tomography, US, and CT. Radiology 1988;169(2):363–365.

42. Forman HP, Middleton WD, Melson GL, McClennan BL. Hyperechoic renal cell carcinomas: increase in detection at US. Radiology 1993;188(2):431–434.

43. Mihara S, Kuroda K, Yoshioka R, Koyama W. Early detection of renal cell carcinoma by ultrasonographic screening–based on the results of 13 years screening in Japan. Ultrasound Med Biol 1999;25(7):1033–1039.

44. Sheth S, Scatarige JC, Horton KM, Corl FM, Fishman EK. Current concepts in the diagnosis and management of renal cell carcinoma: role of multidetector ct and three-dimensional CT. Radiographics 2001;21(Spec. No.):S237–S254.

45. Zagoria RJ. Imaging of small renal masses: a medical success story. AJR 2000;175(4):945–955.

46. Bosniak MA, Rofsky NM. Problems in the detection and characterization of small renal masses. Radiology 1996;198(3):638–641.

47. Siegel CL, McFarland EG, Brink JA, Fisher AJ, Humphrey P, Heiken JP. CT of cystic renal masses: analysis of diagnostic performance and interobserver variation. AJR 1997;169(3):813–818.

48. Curry NS, Cochran ST, Bissada NK. Cystic renal masses: accurate Bosniak classification requires adequate renal CT. AJR 2000;175(2):339–342.

49. Cohan RH, Sherman LS, Korobkin M, Bass JC, Francis IR. Renal Masses: Assessment of corticomedullary-phase and nephrographic-phase CT scans. Radiology 1995;196:445–451.

50. Birnbaum BA, Jacobs JE, Ramchandani P. Multiphasic renal CT: comparison of renal mass enhancement during the corticomedullary and nephrographic phases. Radiology 1996;200(3):753–758.

51. Bae KT, Heiken JP, Siegel CL, Bennett HF. Renal cysts: is attenuation artifactually increased on contrast-enhanced CT images? Radiology 2000;216(3):792–796.

52. Maki DD, Birnbaum BA, Chakraborty DP, Jacobs JE, Carvalho BM, Herman GT. Renal cyst pseudoenhancement: beam-hardening effects on CT numbers. Radiology 1999;213(2):468–472.

53. Israel GM, Bosniak MA. Calcification in cystic renal masses: is it important in diagnosis? Radiology 2003;226(1):47–52.

54. Rofsky NM, Weinreb JC, Bosniak MA, Libes RB, Birnbaum BA. Renal lesion characterization with gadolinium-enhanced MR imaging: efficacy and safety in patients with renal insufficiency. Radiology 1991;180(1):85–89.

55. Nelson KL, Gifford LM, Lauber-Huber C, Gross CA, Lasser TA. Clinical safety of gadopentetate dimeglumine. Radiology 1995;196(2):439–443.

56. Balci NC, Semelka RC, Patt RH, et al. Complex renal cysts: findings on MR imaging. AJR 1999;172(6):1495–1500.

57. Juul N, Torp-Pedersen S, Gronvall S, Holm HH, Koch F, Larsen S. Ultrasonically guided fine needle aspiration biopsy of renal masses. J Urol 1985;133(4):579–581.

58. Campbell SC, Novick AC, Herts B, et al. Prospective evaluation of fine needle aspiration of small, solid renal masses: accuracy and morbidity. Urology 1997;50(1):25–29.

59. Niceforo J, Coughlin BF. Diagnosis of renal cell carcinoma: value of fine-needle aspiration cytology in patients with metastases or contraindications to nephrectomy. AJR 1993;161(6):1303–1305.

60. Dechet CB, Sebo T, Farrow G, Blute ML, Engen DE, Zincke H. Prospective analysis of intraoperative frozen needle biopsy of solid renal masses in adults. J Urol 1999;162(4):1282–1284.

9

Clinical and Pathologic Staging of Renal Cell Carcinoma

Alison M. Lake, Cara Cimmino, James E. Montie, and Khaled S. Hafez

KEYWORDS

RENAL CELL CARCINOMA
STAGING
PROGNOSTIC FACTORS
KIDNEY NEOPLASMS

ABSTRACT

Renal cell carcinoma (RCC), which accounts for 3% of adult malignancies, is the most lethal of the urologic cancers. It is the third most common urologic malignancy following prostate and bladder cancers; however, approximately 40% of patients eventually die of progression of their RCC, while the mortality rates for prostate and bladder carcinomas are closer to 20%. Traditionally, RCC has been staged according to anatomic staging systems, such as the tumor, node, metastasis (TNM) system. This system takes into account tumor size and extent of local disease, nodal disease, and presence of metastases when grouping patients for both prognosis and treatment. Recent advances in understanding of the pathogenesis, molecular behavior, and progression of RCC, as well as recent investigation of clinical predictive factors, have led to suggestions of new algorithms for staging RCC patients.

This chapter reviews the clinical and pathologic staging of RCC according to current practices, and provides an overview of more recently proposed, comprehensive staging systems.

CLINICAL STAGING

Clinical Factors

SIGNS AND SYMPTOMS

Due to the retroperitoneal location of the kidney, many renal masses remain asymptomatic and nonpalpable until they reach advanced stages. For this reason, the presence of clinical signs and symptoms is often indicative of advanced disease.[1–3] These include

From: *Clinical Management of Renal Tumors*
Edited by: R.M. Bukowski and A.C. Novick © Humana Press Inc., Totowa, NJ

weight loss, decreased performance status, hematuria, flank pain, palpable mass, lower extremity edema, and presence of a varicocele.

The most common presenting symptom in one series of RCC patients was hematuria reported by 35%, followed by flank pain reported in 27%.[4] Suggested etiologies of pain in the RCC patient include compression or infiltration of surrounding tissues, rapid expansion of the renal mass from acute hemorrhage, and compression and obstruction of the renal collecting system. A palpable mass is correlated with tumor size and locally advanced disease. The classic triad of RCC includes hematuria, flank pain, and palpable mass. The combination of these three signs and symptoms is now rarely seen.[5] Renal cell carcinoma has also been associated with paraneoplastic syndromes. Systemic findings such as hypertension, erythrocytosis, and elevated liver function tests can be attributed to this.

Some specific signs on physical exam have been associated with advanced disease. The presence of bilateral lower extremity edema, new nonreducible varicocele, caput medusa, and deep venous thrombosis are indicative of venous involvement.[6,7] It is also widely accepted that palpable lymphadenopathy has a negative impact on RCC stage. Bone metastasis is suggested by pain in the hip, extremity, back, and rib. Similarly, metastasis to the brain is suggested by neurologic symptoms or headache, and lung metastases are a concern in patients with respiratory symptoms. The most common sites of metastases of RCC include lung, liver, bone, and brain.

IMAGING

Computed tomography (CT), or in some cases magnetic resonance imaging (MRI), should be performed to assess local tumor stage. Indications for MRI include suspected venous involvement, intravenous (IV) contrast allergy, obliteration of planes between the tumor and adjacent organs on CT scan, and renal insufficiency. Additionally, a standard posteroanterior and a lateral chest x-ray are mandatory for the initial workup of RCC to rule out pulmonary metastases. Perinephric involvement can be suggested by perinephric stranding or the presence of abnormal soft tissue density within the perinephric fat. Absence of suspicious findings in the perinephric region on CT does not rule out microscopic perinephric fat involvement. Preoperative diagnosis of lymphadenopathy by CT can also alter therapeutic approach significantly. Lymph nodes of size 2 cm or greater are suspicious for malignancy, while those less than 2 cm have a high likelihood of being inflammatory reaction.[8] Computed tomography may also illuminate the presence of venous tumor thrombus by demonstrating venous enlargement, changes in the caliber of the vessel, and intraluminal variations in contrast enhancement. If tumor thrombus is suspected based on CT findings, an MRI is indicated for better venous imaging. In addition to the presence of thrombus, the level of tumor thrombus in relation to the patient's diaphragm will aid in operative planning.

Bone scintigraphy is an additional test that is indicated in the setting of increased alkaline phosphatase, bony pain, or the detection of other metastases in an attempt to rule out bone metastases. Computed tomography of the head is indicated only if the patient reports neurologic symptoms, or if other metastases have been discovered. If lesions are noted on chest x-ray, a CT of the chest is appropriate for further evaluation. Finally, percutaneous biopsy, though not routinely used, can be enlisted to confirm the histology of the primary tumor in patients with evidence of systemic metastases, to assess enlarged lymph nodes, or to sample metastatic lesions.

LABORATORY TESTS

Some other preferred tests for the clinical staging of RCC include the complete blood count, serum creatinine, erythrocyte sedimentation rate, serum calcium, and liver function tests. The complete blood count is helpful for screening for polycythemia or anemia. Serum creatinine is an indication of baseline renal function of the patient, which is important to assess before initiation of therapy. The sedimentation rate, serum calcium, and liver function tests are all important for the screening of paraneoplastic syndromes associated with RCC, as well as possible metastatic disease undetected by radiography.

PATHOLOGIC STAGING

Staging Systems

Tumor staging is recognized as the most important prognostic factor for the clinical behavior and outcome of RCC.[9] The first classification system was the Flocks and Kadesky staging system, which was based on the physical characteristics of the tumor and the location of tumor spread. This system was later modified in 1969, when Robson et al.[10] proposed that criteria for RCC staging should include the impact of vascular involvement on staging. Initially, the Robson staging criteria were widely used, but it was later demonstrated that this system correlated poorly with prognosis.[11] The primary issue with this staging system was that lymphatic metastases, an indicator of very poor prognosis, were grouped together in stage III with those tumors with venous involvement, which can potentially be treated with aggressive surgery. Additionally, the extent of venous involvement was not delineated by this staging system. Ultimately, some studies discovered equivalent survival for patients with stage II and stage III tumors, which substantially decreased the prognostic significance of this staging system.[12]

The TNM system, which is now the predominant staging system, was proposed by the Union Internationale Contre le Cancer (UICC; International Union Against Cancer), and further delineates the difference in prognosis between those tumors with venous involvement and those with lymphatic invasion, quantifies each, and defines the anatomic extent of disease more explicitly.[13] The TNM staging system is particularly notable for its systematic emphasis on local growth, nodal spread, and distant metastases, which more accurately classifies the extent of tumor involvement.[14]

In 2002 the TNM staging system (Table 9.1) was further modified after a collaborative effort by the UICC and the American Joint Committee on Cancer (AJCC), in order to reflect the improved results obtained by the contemporary management of RCC.[15] The previous division of stages T1 and T2 at a tumor size of 2.5 cm was abandoned and changed to 7 cm, because it was noted that the lower cutoff point did not generate statistically significant differences in survival rates.[16,17] Additionally, alterations were proposed in regard to the classification of venous involvement. Tumor thrombus above the diaphragm, previously designated stage T4, was changed to stage T3c, and involvement of the inferior vena cava below the diaphragm was changed to T3b, where it had previously been designated stage T3c. Notably, invasion of the adrenal gland or perinephric tissues within the boundaries of Gerota's fascia continued to be labeled stage T3a.[16]

The TNM staging system was used by Tsui et al.[18] to predict 5-year survival rates depending on patient classification. This study demonstrated survival rates of 91%,

Table 9.1.
American Joint Committee on Cancer (AJCC) staging of renal cell carcinoma (see Chapter 4)

Primary tumor (T)	
TX	Primary tumor cannot be assessed
T0	No evidence of primary tumor
T1	Tumor 7 cm or less in greatest dimension, limited to the kidney
T1a	Tumor 4 cm or less in greatest dimension, limited to the kidney
T1b	Tumor more than 4 cm but not more than 7 cm in greatest dimension, limited to the kidney
T2	Tumor more than 7 cm in greatest dimension, limited to the kidney
T3	Tumor extends into major veins or invades adrenal gland or perinephric tissues but not beyond Gerota's fascia
T3a	Tumor directly invades the adrenal gland or perirenal and/or renal sinus fat but not beyond Gerota's fascia
T3b	Tumor grossly extends into the renal vein or its segmental (muscle-containing) branches, or vena cava below the diaphragm
T3c	Tumor grossly extends into vena cava above diaphragm or invades the wall of the vena cava
T4	Tumor invades beyond Gerota's fascia
Regional lymph nodes (N)	
NX	Regional lymph nodes cannot be assessed
N0	No regional lymph node metastases
N1	Metastases in a single regional lymph node
N2	Metastases in more than one regional lymph node
Distant metastasis (M)	
MX	Distant metastasis cannot be assessed
M0	No distant metastasis
M1	Distant metastasis

74%, 67%, and 32% for stages I through IV, respectively. The Mayo Clinic Kidney Registry was used in a retrospective study to confirm these findings. In that review, Gettman et al.[19] reported 10-year survival rates of 91%, 70%, 53%, 42%, and 43% for stages T1, T2, T3a, T3b, and T3c disease, respectively.

Controversies Regarding Local Tumor Stage

IMPACT OF TUMOR SIZE

Tumor size is one of the criteria outlined by the TNM staging system, and is specifically related to survival differences in patients with organ-confined disease. The 1997 TNM classification system categorized tumors with size less than 7 cm as stage T1. While there was relative agreement that the optimal size for stratifying outcome was somewhere between 4 and 10 cm, there were some studies suggesting that the breakpoint for T1 tumors should be decreased.[20–23] As a result of these studies, the 2002 TNM T1 category was amended to T1a and T1b based on a cutoff of 4 cm.[24] This was an important distinction to make, not only for prognostic accuracy, but also due to the increasing use of nephron-sparing surgery (NSS) and minimally invasive therapies such as cryoablation and radiofrequency ablation for small tumors. Currently there is good evidence to suggest successful NSS for T1a, though emerging data implies that NSS on larger tumors that are anatomically amenable can be performed with good results.[25]

IMPACT OF TUMOR THROMBUS

The TNM staging system currently includes the presence and extent of tumor thrombus as a criterion. Currently stage T3 tumors are divided into those with no vein involvement (T3a), infradiaphragmatic vein involvement (T3b), and those with supra-diaphragmatic vein involvement (T3c). However, the significance of the level of the tumor thrombus, and invasion of the thrombus into the vessel wall remains controversial.

Although the level of tumor thrombus is not the most significant prognostic factor, the presence of venous thrombus does seem to be an ominous predictor. Long-term survival of patients with renal vein involvement is significantly greater than those with involvement of the inferior vena cava.[26] Similar survival has also been shown in patients with renal vein and infradiaphragmatic vein involvement (T3b), while patients with supradiaphragmatic vein involvement (T3c) may have a significantly worse prognosis, even after controlling for grade and Eastern Cooperative Oncology Group (ECOG) performance status.[27]

Direct invasion of the venous wall seems to be a more important prognosticator than the location of the thrombus in relationship to the diaphragm. Decreased survival has been demonstrated in patients with direct invasion of thrombus into the venous wall after complete resection, and survival is profoundly decreased in those patients with direct invasion who undergo incomplete resection.[28]

Although the importance of the level of tumor thrombus is controversial, it is likely that the presence and extent of tumor thrombus are associated with other adverse factors such as lymph node and distant metastases, perinephric fat invasion, and biologic aggressiveness, which do portend a poorer prognosis.

STATUS OF THE ADRENAL GLAND

At this time, the 2002 TNM classification system designates T3a tumors as those with adrenal involvement or invasion into the perinephric fat, but not beyond Gerota's fascia. Of those patients with adrenal involvement, approximately 60% had invasion by direct extension, while in the other 40% it occurred as the result of hematogenous spread.[29]

Reclassification of tumors with adrenal involvement has been suggested. Although there is often a correlation between adrenal invasion and lymph node involvement, metastatic disease, and higher tumor grade, adrenal invasion has been demonstrated as an independent predictor of poor prognosis in multivariate analysis.[30] Adrenal involvement predicts significantly worse survival for tumors with direct extension into the adrenal gland compared to those with perinephric fat invasion alone. This leads to consideration of reclassification of tumors with direct adrenal gland involvement as stage T4 tumors.[30–32]

COLLECTING SYSTEM INVASION

Review of outcomes of RCC patients with collecting system invasion also leads to a consideration of alteration of the current staging system. A lower disease-specific survival rate is observed in patients with collecting system invasion when compared to their counterparts without involvement of the collecting system.[33] The prognosis of high-stage lesions (T3 or greater) with urothelial involvement is poor, but not significantly different from those without urothelial involvement. However, in patients with low-stage tumors (pT2 or less), collecting system invasion was shown to be a significant adverse pathologic finding associated with poor prognosis.[34]

LOCALLY ADVANCED OR NODAL-POSITIVE DISEASE

Approximately 30% of patients with RCC are found to have locally advanced or metastatic disease at presentation, which is generally accepted as portending a significantly poor prognosis.[32] It has been shown that patients with extension of their tumor beyond Gerota's fascia with involvement of contiguous organs rarely survive 5 years, particularly if en bloc resection with negative margins is not possible.[35] Lymph node involvement is also associated with poor prognosis, with 5- and 10-year survival rates of 5% to 30% and 0% to 5%, respectively.[14]

Positive lymph node status is associated with larger, higher grade, more locally advanced tumors that were more likely to demonstrate sarcomatoid features. Patients with lymphadenopathy are also three to four times more likely to have distant metastasis. Additionally, patients with metastatic RCC and positive lymph nodes have a significantly worse 5-year survival rate.[36]

OTHER TUMOR-RELATED FACTORS NOT INCLUDED IN THE TNM STAGING

Tumor Grade

Tumor grade offers valuable information in the prognostication of RCC. However, this is confounded by the existence of multiple systems used by pathologists, which results in unreliable comparison of outcomes between institutions. Although most of these tumor-grading systems have shown prognostic capability, they all suffer to some extent from issues with reproducibility and interobserver variability, as designation of tumor grade is certainly subjective.

The Fuhrman classification system is the most commonly used system in North America, and allocates grades 1 to 4 based on the presence of a nucleolus, size of nucleus, and the magnification at which it can be observed.[37] In Fuhrman's original report, the 5-year survival rates were 64%, 34%, 31%, and 10% for grades 1 through 4, respectively, and nuclear grade proved to be the most significant prognostic factor for stage I tumors in this series.[38] A more recent review of 405 cases suggested 5-year survival rates for grades 1 through 4 of 100%, 94%, 80%, and 35%, respectively.[39] Fuhrman's own analysis failed to distinguish a difference in survival between patients with grade 2 and 3 tumors. This failure has been similarly reproduced in numerous other studies, and these other reports have consistently demonstrated a difference in outcome only when comparing grades 1 and 2 with grades 3 and 4, with the higher grades indicating poorer prognosis.[40–42] Simplifying the grading system for prognostic value was ultimately supported by recommendations of the 1997 UICC/AJCC consensus meeting, where the suggestion was made to convert to a three-tiered system, combining the first two grades of the Fuhrman system and designating them as low grade, designating grade 3 tumors as intermediate, and grade 4 tumors as high grade.[43]

Recently, the Mayo Clinic group retrospectively reviewed the records of 2042 RCC patients, and reported a standardized nuclear grading system. This system designated grade 1 tumors as having small, round nuclei with inconspicuous nucleoli visible at × 400; grade 2 contained round to slightly irregular nuclei with prominent nucleoli visible at ×200; grade 3 had irregular nuclei with prominent nucleoli visible at ×100; and grade 4 contained pleomorphic or giant cells. The investigators proceeded to assess the predictive abilities of this standardized grading system when compared to nonstandardized grading. The reviewed grades were ultimately more predictive of death due to RCC than the original grades for RCC. These differences were apparent even after adjusting for the TNM stage among patients with clear cell and papillary RCC.[32]

Histologic Subtype

The histologic classification of RCC has undergone a major revision since the early 1990s. The Hydelberg classification defines four primary histiotypes, which include conventional (clear cell, granular, or mixed), papillary, chromophobe, and collecting duct. Each subtype has its own characteristics and patterns of disease that may be associated with prognosis.

Conventional RCC accounts for approximately 70% to 80% of all RCCs, and this subtype includes clear cell, granular, and mixed type tumors.[43] These tumors are normally yellow in appearance when bivalved, and are highly vascular, containing a network of vascular sinusoids interspersed between acini of tumor cells. Clear cells are usually round or polygonal with abundant cytoplasm. Conventional RCC histiotype is associated with chromosome 3 alterations, and *VHL* mutations are common in conventional RCC. Mutation or inactivation of this gene has been found in 75% of sporadic cases.[44,45]

Papillary RCC accounts for 10% to 20% of RCCs and is the second most common histiotype after the conventional type. Microscopically, these tumors usually consist of basophilic or eosinophilic cells arranged in papillary or tubular configuration. Recent data from Moch and colleagues[46] on 588 nephrectomy specimens suggests that conventional RCC and papillary RCC carry a similar prognosis when stage and grade are taken into account. Papillary RCC has been separated into two categories, type 1 (basophilic) and 2 (eosinophilic), with type 2 tending to be higher grade, to present at a more advanced stage, and to be more aggressive than type 1.[46–49] The cytogenetic abnormalities associated with papillary histiotype include trisomy of chromosome 7 and 17.[50]

Chromophobe RCC accounts for approximately 5% of RCC, and several large studies have demonstrated that this histiotype portends an excellent prognosis, and overall survival seems to be better than with other types of RCC.[39,46] Most data demonstrate that, while tumors are capable of growing quite large, they tend to be more organ-confined, with relatively low propensity toward metastasis. Case series from both the Mayo Clinic and Memorial Sloan-Kettering Cancer Center demonstrate a low rate of metastasis (10%) in patients with chromophobe histology.[51,52] A recent study compared the 5-year survival rate for conventional, papillary, and chromophobe RCC, and found them to be 69%, 87%, and 87%, respectively.[53] These tumors have a distinctive appearance, and seem to be derived from the cortical collecting duct.[44] The tumor cells exhibit a relatively transparent cytoplasm with a fine reticular pattern and perinuclear halo. This histiotype has been associated with increased incidence of p53 mutations.[54]

The final subtype, collecting duct carcinoma, is the most aggressive, and least common type of RCC, accounting for less than 1% of tumors. Patients with these tumors tend to develop systemic metastasis rapidly, and rarely survive more than 2 years after diagnosis.[46,55] This histologic type includes renal medullary carcinoma, a subtype nearly exclusive to African-American males with sickle cell disease or trait. Collecting duct carcinomas are derived from the medulla, but many are infiltrative, and extension into the cortex is common. Microscopically, these tumors have a mixture of dilated tubules and papillary structures lined by a layer of cuboidal cells, which often creates a cobblestone appearance. Overall, most reported cases demonstrate high grade and advanced stage at diagnosis.[56]

The sarcomatoid variant is no longer considered its own histologic subtype of RCC, as many histologic types have been noted to include sarcomatoid elements. Sarcomatoid features can be found in any of the histologic subtypes of RCC, and has an incidence of 2% to 5% of RCCs. It is typified by a spindle cell growth pattern.[57] Clinically, sarcomatoid RCC is characterized by its locally aggressive nature, metastatic potential, and poor prognosis.[57–59] In a review of 108 patients with the presence of sarcomatoid differentiation, Mian and colleagues[60] noted an overall median survival of 9 months, with metastases present in 77% of these patients at presentation.

A review of 101 cases of RCC with sarcomatoid features reported 5- and 10-year survival rates to be 22% and 15%, respectively. When this group was compared to a similar cohort of patients with RCC, but without sarcomatoid features, those with sarcomatoid features were found to present at a higher stage and had worse survival, even after adjusting for other prognostic factors such as presence of tumor necrosis, stage, and tumor size.[61]

Histologic Tumor Necrosis

The presence of tumor necrosis is another histologic feature that is purported to affect outcome, and is found in approximately one third of RCCs.[46,62] Histologic necrosis is defined as any degree of microscopic tumor necrosis exclusive of degenerative changes, such as hyalinization, hemorrhage, or fibrosis.[62] Several studies have demonstrated the prognostic value of histologic tumor necrosis evidenced by a two- to threefold increased risk of death from RCC if tumor necrosis is present.[39,60,62,63]

SYSTEMIC METASTASIS

As is the case with most malignancies, the presence of systemic metastases conveys a substantially poor prognosis for patients with RCC.[64] Researchers have begun to identify other important factors that impact the prognosis of patients with metastatic RCC such as performance status, the metastasis-free interval, the site and burden of disease, and the presence of significant weight loss and specific laboratory abnormalities.[65] Lung-only metastasis, good performance status, metastasis-free interval of 24 months or greater, less than 10% weight loss, and absence of elevated serum lactate dehydrogenase and calcium levels are predictive of improved survival.[64–67]

THE FUTURE OF STAGING FOR RENAL CELL CARCINOMA

The incorporation of molecular tumor markers into future staging systems has the potential to completely revolutionize the approach to diagnosis, staging, and prognosis of RCC. Methods based on gene arrays, which screen for differential expression of thousands of genes, have identified many new, potentially promising prognostic markers.[68] An extensive variety of markers have been examined, and some have shown enough promise to legitimize further research to prove their value as prognostic tools.

Expanding knowledge of prognostic factors in RCC has fostered the emergence of new comprehensive staging systems. Though the TNM classification system is currently the most widely used system, as new prognostic factors begin to be used clinically, future attempts to form one integrated staging modality will emerge in an attempt to improve prognostication in RCC.

Molecular Markers

Molecular tumor markers are expected to have an enormous impact on future prognostication, diagnosis, and treatment of RCC. In addition to the ability of tumor markers to provide prognostic information, they may also aid in the selection of appropriate therapy and long-term monitoring for tumor recurrence. Currently, a number of tumor markers relating to tumor proliferation, angiogenesis, growth, and loss of cell adhesion are being evaluated, and early studies indicate the emergence of some promising markers. Among those currently being investigated are carbonic anhydrase IX (CA IX), Ki67, argyrophilic nucleolar organizer region (AgNOR), proliferating cell nuclear antigen (PCNA), vascular endothelial growth factor (VEGF), p53, and others.[68] However, more controlled, clinical trials are necessary to thoroughly evaluate their usefulness in everyday clinical practice.

Integrated Staging Systems

As knowledge of prognostic factors in RCC expands, one can expect to see changes made to the current TNM staging system. Though this is currently the most widely used system, several investigators have attempted to combine various prognostic factors in an attempt to develop a new comprehensive staging modality.

UNIVERSITY OF CALIFORNIA–LOS ANGELES INTEGRATED STAGING SYSTEM (UICC)

The University of California–Los Angeles created a system to integrate pathologic staging information with some of the additional prognostic variables that have been discussed in an attempt to improve the prognostic value of the staging system, and to better stratify patients into prognostic categories to accurately define an individual patient's probability of survival.[69] Numerous factors were evaluated in a sample of 661 patients, including age, sex, Fuhrman grade, TNM stage, ECOG performance status, laterality, smoking, number of presenting systems, weight loss histologic type, administration of immunotherapy, inferior vena cava involvement, number of metastatic sites, site of metastasis, and disease-free interval. Ultimately, the most significant factors included TNM stage, grade, and ECOG performance status (Table 9.2). Patients were stratified into five groups depending on survival outcomes. Based on the results of the initial analysis, the system was subsequently revised into a simplified system, separating patients into those with metastatic versus nonmetastatic disease, and assigning them to low-, intermediate-, and high-risk groups.

MAYO CLINIC STAGE, SIZE, GRADE, AND NECROSIS SCORE

The Mayo Clinic group has also created a comprehensive outcome prediction model for patients with conventional (clear-cell) RCC undergoing radical nephrectomy. The

Table 9.2.
UISS categorization

UISS	1997 TNM stage	Fuhrman's grade	ECOG
I	I	1, 2	0
II	I	1, 2	1 or more
	I	3, 4	Any
	II	Any	Any
	III	Any	0
	III	1	1 or more
III	III	2–4	1 or more
	IV	1, 2	0
IV	IV	3, 4	0
		1–3	1 or more
V	IV	4	1 or more

ECOG, Eastern Cooperative Oncology Group; TNM, tumor, node, metastasis; UISS, UCLA Integrated Staging System.

group analyzed the data of 1801 patients and discovered that TNM stage, tumor size 5 cm or greater, nuclear grade, and presence of histologic tumor necrosis were independent predictors of survival. These factors were combined into the stage, size, grade, and necrosis (SSIGN) scoring algorithm. According to this system, decreased survival was shown to correlate with increased SSIGN score. The group demonstrated a 5-year cancer specific survival rate of 99.4% for patients with SSIGN scores of 0 to 1, which decreased to 7.4% for patients with scores of 10 or greater.[63]

THE KATTAN POSTOPERATIVE PROGNOSTIC NORMOGRAM

The Kattan postoperative prognostic normogram is a system that was created to predict the probability of tumor recurrence within 5 years in patients undergoing radical nephrectomy for RCC.[70] This system evaluated several parameters, including presence of symptoms, histology, tumor size, and standard TNM staging criteria, and assigned a numerical score to each of these prognosticators. This nomogram appeared accurate and discriminating in a study of 601 patients with RCC who were treated with nephrectomy.

At this time, none of the integrated models have replaced the current staging systems. However, revisions to the current TNM system can be anticipated in the future given the evolution of prognostication in RCC. In the future, the inclusion of additional clinical, pathologic, and molecular factors can be expected.

REFERENCES

1. Bostwick DG, Murphy GP. Diagnosis and prognosis of renal cell carcinoma: highlights from an international consensus workshop. Semin Urol Oncol 1998;16(1):46–52.
2. Gelb AB. Renal cell carcinoma: current prognostic factors. Union International Contre le Cancer and the American Joint Committee on Cancer. Cancer 1997;80:981–986.
3. Sobin LH, Wittekind CH. International Union Against Cancer (IUCC): TNM Classification of Malignant Tumours, 5th ed. New York: Wiley-Liss, 1997:180–182.
4. Dinney CPN, Awad SA, Gajewski JB, et al. Analysis of imaging modalities, staging systems, and prognostic indicators for RCC. Urology 1992;39:122–129.
5. Jayson M, Saunders H. Increased incidence of serendipitously discovered renal cell carcinoma. Urology 1998;51(2):203–205.

6. Belldegrun A, Dekernion JB. Renal tumors. In: Walsh PC, Retik AB, Vaughan ED Jr, et al., ed. Campbell's Urology, vol 3, 7th ed. Philadelphia: WB Saunders, 1998:2283–2326.

7. Wolf JS Jr. Staging of renal cell carcinoma. In: Belldegrun A, ed. Renal and Adrenal Tumors: Biology and Management. Oxford: Oxford University Press, 2003:61–65.

8. Studer UE, Scherz S, Scheidegger J, et al. Enlargement of regional lymph nodes in renal cell carcinoma is often not due to metastases. J Urol 1990;144:243–245.

9. Thrasher J, Paulson D. Prognostic factors in renal cancer. Urol Clin North Am 1993;20:247–262.

10. Robson CJ, Churchill BM, Anderson W. The results of radical nephrectomy for renal cell carcinoma. J Urol 1969;101:297–301.

11. Pantuck AJ, Zisman A, Belldegrun AS. The changing natural history of renal cell carcinoma. J Urol 2001;166:1611–1623.

12. Skinner DG, Colvin RB, Vermillion CD, et al. Diagnosis and management of renal cell carcinoma: a clinical and pathologic study of 309 cases. Cancer 1971;28:1165–1177.

13. Beahrs OH, Henson DE, Hutter RUP, Myers MH. American Joint Committee on Cancer Manual for Staging of Cancer, 3rd ed. Philadelphia: JB Lippincott, 1988.

14. Bassil BA, Dosoretz DE, Prout GR. Validation of the tumor, nodes, and metastasis classification of renal cell carcinoma. J Urol 1985;134:450–454.

15. Greene FL, Page DL, Fleming ID, et al (eds). AJCC (American Joint Committee on Cancer) Cancer Staging Manual, 6th ed. Springer-Verlag, New York 2002. p. 323.

16. Guinan P, Frank W, Saffrin R, et al. Staging and survival of patients with renal cell carcinoma. Semin Surg Oncol 1994;10:47–50.

17. Hermaneck P, Schrott KM. Evaluation of the new tumor, nodes, and metastases classification of renal cell carcinoma. J Urol 1990;144:238–241.

18. Tsui KH, Shvarts O, Smith RB, Figlin RA, DeKernion JB, Belldegrun AS. Prognostic indicators for renal cell carcinoma: a multivariate analysis of 643 patients using the revised 1997 TNM criteria. J Urol 2000;163:1090–1095.

19. Gettman MT, Blute ML, Spotts B, Bryant SC, Zincke H. Pathologic staging of renal cell carcinoma: significance of tumor classification with the 1997 TNM staging system. Cancer 2001;91(2): 354–361.

20. Frank I, Blute ML, Leibovich BC, et al. pT2 classification for renal cell carcinoma. Can its accuracy be improved. J Urol 2005;173:380–384.

21. Lau WK, Cheville JC, Blute ML, et al. Prognostic features of pathologic stage T1 renal cell carcinoma after radical nephrectomy. Urology 2002;59:532–537.

22. Zisman A, Pantuck AJ, Chao D, et al. Reevaluation of the 1997 TNM classification for renal cell carcinoma: T1 and T2 cutoff point at 4.5 rather than 7 cm better correlates with clinical outcome. J Urol 2001;166:54–58.

23. Hafez KS, Fergany AF, Novick AC. Nephron sparing surgery for localized renal cell carcinoma: impact of tumor size on patient survival, tumor recurrence, and TNM staging. J Urol 1999;162: 1930–1933.

24. Sobin, LH, Wittekind. TNM Classification of Malignant Tumours, 6th ed. UICC International Union Against Cancer. New York: Wiley-Liss, 2003:193.

25. Patard JJ, Shvarts O, Lam JS, et al. Safety and efficacy of partial nephrectomy for all T1 tumors based on an international multicenter experience. J Urol 2004;171:2181–2185.

26. Moinzadeh A, Libertino JA. Prognostic significance of tumor thrombus level in patients with renal cell carcinoma and venous tumor thrombus extension. Is all T3b the same? J Urol 2004; 171:598–601.

27. Kim HL, Zisman A, Wieder JA, Han KR, Figlin RA, Belldegrun AS. Prognostic significance of venous thrombus in renal cell carcinoma. Are renal vein and inferior vena cava involvement different? J Urol 2004;171:588–591.

28. Hatcher PA, Anderson EE, Paulson DF, Carson CC, and Robertson JE. Surgical management of and prognosis of renal cell carcinoma invading the vena cava. J Urol 1995;154:1681–1684.

29. Tsui KH, Schvarts O, Barbarie Z, et al. Is adrenalectomy a necessary component of radical nephrectomy? UCLA experience with 511 radical nephrectomies. J Urol 2000;163:437–441.

30. Han KR, Bui MH, Pantuck AJ, et al. TNM T3a renal cell carcinoma: adrenal gland involvement is not the same as renal fat invasion. J Urol 2003;169:899–903.

31. Siemer S, Lehmann J, Loch A, et al. Current TNM classification for renal cell carcinoma evaluated: revising stage T3a. J Urol 2005;173:33–37.

32. Lohse CM, Blute ML, Zincke H, et al. Comparison of standardized and nonstandardized nuclear grade of renal cell carcinoma to predict outcome among 2042 patients. Am J Clin Pathol 2002; 118:877–886.
33. Palapattu GS, Pantuck AJ, Dorey F, Said JW, Figlin RA, Belldeggrun AS. Collecting system invasion in renal cell carcinoma: impact on prognosis and future staging strategies. J Urol 2003; 170:768–772.
34. Uzzo RG, Cherullo EE, Myles J, Novick AC. Renal cell carcinoma invading the urinary collecting system: implications for staging. J Urol 2002;167:2392–2396.
35. Thrasher JB, Paulson DF. Prognostic factors in renal cancer. Urol Clin North Am 1993;20:247–262.
36. Pantuck AJ, Zisman A, Dorey F, et al. Renal cell carcinoma with retroperitoneal lymph nodes: role of lymph node dissection. J Urol 2003;169:2076–2083.
37. Gominbu M, Tessler A, Al-Askari S, Joshi P, Sperber A, Morales P. Renal cell carcinoma: survival and prognostic factors. Urology 1986;27:291–301.
38. Fuhrman SA, Lasky LC, Limas C. Prognostic significance of morphologic parameters in renal cell carcinoma. Am J Surg Pathol 1982;6:655–663.
39. Amin MB, Tamboli P, Javidan J, et al. Prognostic impact of histologic subtyping of adult renal epithelial neoplasms: an experience of 405 cases. Am J Surg Pathol 2002;26:281–291.
40. Selli C, Hinshaw WM, Woodard BH, and Paulson DF. Stratification of risk factors in renal cell carcinoma. Cancer 1983;52:899–903.
41. Bibbo M, Galera-Davidson H, Dytch HE, et al. Karyometry and isometry of renal-cell carcinoma. Anal Quant Cytol Histol 1987;9:182–187.
42. Bretheau D, Lechevallier E, de Fromont M, Sault MC, Rampal M, Coulange C. Prognostic value of nuclear grade of renal cell carcinoma. Cancer 1995;76:2543–2549.
43. Medeiros L, Gelb A, Weiss L. Renal cell carcinoma: prognostic significance of morphologic parameters in 121 cases. Cancer 1988;61:1639–1651.
44. Storkel S, Eble JN, Adlakha K, et al. Classification of renal cell carcinoma: Workgroup No 1. Union Internationale Contre le Cancer (UICC) and the American Joint Committee on Cancer (AJCC). Cancer 1997;80:987–989.
45. Clifford SC, Prowse AH, Affara NA, Buys CH, Maher ER. Inactivation of the von Hippel-Lindau (VHL) tumour suppressor gene and allelic losses at chromosome arm 3p in primary renal cell carcinoma: evidence for a VHL-independent pathway in clear cell renal tumourigenesis. Genes Chromosomes Cancer 1998;22:200–209.
46. Moch H, Grasser T, Amin MB, Torhorst J, Sauter G, Mihatsch MJ. Prognostic utility of the recently recommended histologic classification and revised TNM staging system of renal cell carcinoma: a Swiss experience with 588 tumors. Cancer 2000;89:604–614.
47. Amin M, Corless C, Renshaw A, Icko S, Kubus J, Schuktz D. Papillary (chromophil) renal cell carcinoma: histomorphologic characteristics and evaluation of conventional pathologic prognostic parameters in 62 cases. Am J Surg Pathol 1997;21:621–635.
48. Delahunt B, Nacey JN. Renal cell carcinoma: histological indicators of prognosis. Pathology 1987; 19:258–263.
49. Delahunt B. Histopathologic prognostic indicators for renal cell carcinoma. J Urol 2001;166:63–67.
50. Oyasu R. Renal cancer: histologic classification update. Int J Clin Oncol 1998;3:125–133.
51. Crotty TB, Faroon GM, Lieber MM. Chromophobe cell renal carcinoma: clinicopathological features of 50 cases. J Urol 1995;154:964–967.
52. Campbell SC, Russo P, Hamed G, et al. Chromophobe cell carcinoma of the kidney: a clinicopathologic study. J Urol 1996;155:385A.
53. Cheville JC, Lohse CM, Zincke H, et al. Comparisons of outcome and prognostic features among histologic subtypes of renal cell carcinoma. Am Surg Pathol 2003;27:612–624.
54. Contractor H, Zariwala M, Bugert P, Zeisler J, Kovacs G. Mutation of the p53 suppressor gene occurs preferentially in the chromophobe type of renal cell tumour. J Pathol 1997;181:136–139.
55. Kennedy SM, Merino MJ, Linehan WM, et al. Collecting duct carcinoma of the kidney. Hum Pathol 1990;21:449–456.
56. Carter MD, Tha S, McLoughlin MG, Owen DA. Collecting duct carcinoma of the kidney: a case report and review of the literature. J Urol 1992;147:1096–1098.
57. Tomera KM, Farrow GM, Leiber MM. Sarcomatoid renal carcinoma. J Urol 1983;130:657–659.
58. Oda H, Machinami R. Sarcomatoid renal cell carcinoma: a study of its proliferative activity. Cancer 1993;71:2292–2298.

59. Sella A, Logothetis CJ, Ro JY, et al. Sarcomatoid renal cell carcinoma: a treatable entity. Cancer 1987;60:1313–1318.
60. Mian BM, Bhadakankar N, Slaton JW, et al. Prognostic factors and survival of patients with sarcomatoid renal cell carcinoma. J Urol 2002;167:65–70.
61. de Peralta-Venturina M, Moch H, Amin M, et al. Sarcomatoid differentiation in renal cell carcinoma: a study of 101 cases. Am J Surg Pathol 2001;25:275–284.
62. Cheville JC, Blute ML, Zincke H, et al. Stage pT1 conventional (clear cell) renal cell carcinoma: pathological features associated with cancer specific survival. J Urol 2001;166:453–456.
63. Frank I, Blute ML, Cheville JC, Lohse CM, Weaver AL, Zincke H. An outcome prediction model for patients with clear cell renal cell carcinoma treated with radical nephrectomy based on tumor stage, size, grade and necrosis: the SSIGN score. J Urol 2002;168:2395–2400.
64. Motzer RJ, Mazumdar M, Bacik J, et al. Survival and prognostic stratification of 670 patients with renal cell carcinoma. J Clin Oncol 1999;17:2530–2540.
65. Elson PJ. Prognostic factors of metastatic renal cell carcinoma. In: Budowski RM, Novick AC, eds. Renal Cell Carcinoma: Molecular Biology, Immunology, and Clinical Management. Totowa, NJ: Humana Press, 2000:147–160.
66. Maldazys JD, deKernion JB. Prognostic factors in metastatic renal cell carcinoma. J Urol 1986;136:376–379.
67. Kavolius JP, Mastorakos DP, Pavolvich C, et al. Resection of metastatic renal cell carcinoma. J Clin Oncol 1998;16:2261–2266.
68. Kononen J, Bubendorf L, Kallioniemi A, et al. Tissue microarrays for high-throughput molecular profiling of tumor specimens. Nat Med 1998;4:844–887.
69. Zisman A, Pantuck AJ, Wieder J, et al. Risk group assessment and clinical outcome algorithm to predict the natural history of patients with surgically resected renal cell carcinoma. J Clin Oncol 2002;20:4559–4566.
70. Kattan MW, Reuter V, Motzer RJ, Katz J, Russo P. A postoperative prognostic normogram for renal cell carcinoma. J Urol 2001;166:63–67.

10   Active Surveillance of Localized Renal Tumors

Paul L. Crispen, Sameer N. Chawla, and Robert G. Uzzo

KEYWORDS

OBSERVATION
RENAL CANCER
SURVEILLANCE
GROWTH KINETICS

ABSTRACT

The incidental detection of small enhancing renal masses presumed to be renal cell carcinoma has increased due to the widespread use of cross-sectional body imaging. Active surveillance of these lesions has been pursued in elderly or infirm patients. Here we review the current data regarding the growth kinetics, pathology, stage progression, and clinical management of renal masses under active surveillance. The limitations of these data are discussed.

Incidental detection of renal cell carcinoma (RCC) has increased over the past two decades.[1–3] This is a direct effect of renal lesions identified on radiographic images performed to evaluate unrelated abdominal symptomatology. Although this increase has been noted across all clinical stages of RCC, the greatest increase is in low-stage, localized tumors.[4] The current standard of care for all suspected renal malignancies is prompt surgical resection, while the long-term efficacy of minimally invasive ablative therapies is yet to be determined.[5,6] Five-year survival for patients with T1 disease following surgical resection with negative margins is excellent, approaching 97%.[7] As a result of earlier detection, excellent surgical outcomes, and the failure of systemic therapies for advanced disease, the natural history of untreated incidental localized renal cancers is poorly established.

Patients who are either medically unfit or unwilling to undergo surgical intervention present a unique opportunity to study the natural history of RCC through serial radiographic evaluations. During the last decade, several single institutional series have been published characterizing the radiographic appearance and clinical behavior of unresected small enhancing renal masses over time. This chapter reviews the biologic

From: *Clinical Management of Renal Tumors*
Edited by: R.M. Bukowski and A.C. Novick © Humana Press Inc., Totowa, NJ

behavior of untreated incidental enhancing renal masses in regard to indications for observation, determination of lesion size, growth rate, clinical and pathologic predictors of lesion growth, indications for surgical intervention, pathology of lesions undergoing observation, and rate of progression to metastatic disease.

INDICATIONS AND GOALS OF ACTIVE SURVEILLANCE

Given the excellent outcomes associated with surgical extirpation of localized RCC, the patient population meeting indications for active surveillance, observation, or non-treatment of a suspected renal malignancy is highly select. Most series reporting growth kinetics of observed renal masses are small, retrospective, and fail to identify the initial indications for surveillance. Therefore, the true impact that an untreated asymptomatic localized kidney mass has on a patient's life expectancy and quality of life (QOL) is yet to be fully quantitated.

For purposes of clarity, it is best to classify the indications for observation of a presumed renal malignancy as absolute, relative, or elective. Absolute indications include patients in whom surgery is contraindicated due to severe medical comorbidities. Excessive health risks making surgery unsafe or associated with a high mortality may force both patients and physicians to accept the uncertainty of active surveillance. Relative indications for observation include other concomitant disease states that must be addressed prior to planned treatment or alternatively observation. Medical comorbidities, competing longevity risks, and implications of nontreatment are the major considerations when evaluating a patient for surgery of any type. These factors provide both subjective and less often objective data with which to perform a trade-off evaluation regarding the necessity and ultimately the ability of an individual to undergo surgical intervention. In cases where loss of a vital organ would require replacement therapy, the treatment trade-off requires an even more compelling surgical benefit. In the case of incidental, asymptomatic kidney cancer, this is particularly true in patients with preexisting medical renal disease, a solitary kidney, or bilateral disease, whereby extirpation or any surgical manipulation may contribute to immediate or delayed permanent renal dysfunction or failure. Lastly, some patients may simply wish to undergo a period of observation despite being low-risk surgical candidates. This constitutes an elective indication for active surveillance and requires the treating physician to inform the patient of the available data on renal tumor growth kinetics and risk for progression in an unbiased fashion. No matter what the indication for surveillance of a presumed renal cancer, it must be understood that the patient and physician are taking a calculated risk due to the heterogeneous and occasional unpredictable behavior of RCC.

Once a patient and physician have mutually decided to observe a presumed renal malignancy, a follow-up schedule must be established to meet defined goals of observation. The primary goal of surveillance is obvious—to avoid death from disease. Currently, the development of systemic disease is a surrogate end point for cancer specific mortality in RCC, whereas the median time to death in these patients is between 4 and 28 months depending on performance status, disease burden, and response to systemic therapies.[8] A second goal of observation is to avoid the development of symptoms that can impair QOL. In this regard, the clinician must recognize not only the limitations of existing QOL data as they pertain to surveillance of renal masses, but also that the perceived risk of a patient developing symptoms is likely overemphasized.[9] A final goal to be considered is the need to detect local tumor growth and understand the implications of local growth kinetics as they relate to the tumor's biology and overall risks to the patient. For example, although a patient may elect an initial period of observation, radiographic tumor growth or the development of symptoms associated with the mass must be considered in the appropriate clinical context before deciding on maintaining a course of further observation versus initiating surgical intervention.

To meet these goals, the treating physician must formally quantitate medical comorbidities and performance status, perform a thorough initial clinical and radiographic assessment, carefully plan appropriate radiographic follow-up at regular time intervals to detect disease progression, and be aware of the current data regarding the natural history of untreated RCC.

CORRELATION BETWEEN CLINICAL AND PATHOLOGIC PARAMETERS IN RENAL CELL CARCINOMA

The most well-established prognostic variables in patients with RCC are pathologic and include histologic type, nuclear grade, and pathologic stage. Of these, stage has been identified consistently as the single most important variable.[8] Currently, the most widely used clinical and pathologic staging system is that published by the American Joint Commission on Cancer and is represented by the tumor, node, metastases (TNM) system.[10] Although clinical staging is a useful initial measure of tumor extent, the pathologic stage provides much more detailed prognostic information as it relates to the tumor's biology. Thus, during the initial clinical evaluation of an enhancing renal mass, little useful information is available to accurately predict tumor grade, histology, or pathologic stage, and therefore its biologic potential. Of the information available on initial imaging, tumor size and nodal or metastatic involvement are most easily quantitated, while the local pathologic extent of the tumor measured by cross-sectional imaging is unreliable, especially in small lesions. For example, upstaging of clinical T1a lesions to pathologic T3a (perirenal fat) occurs in as many as 31% to 38% of cases.[11,12] Furthermore, although a relationship between tumor grade and lesion size has been postulated in RCC, up to 28% of tumors less than 4 cm are of high nuclear grade.[11] This paucity of pathologic information at initial assessment has led some to recommend percutaneous biopsy of renal lesions, particularly prior to initiating a course of active surveillance; however, the practice of routine percutaneous biopsy of enhancing renal masses is not widely accepted secondary to poor histologic and pathologic correlation between biopsy and surgical specimens.[13–15]

Several investigators have suggested that renal tumor size at initial presentation is an important predictor of future growth and prognosis in both sporadic[10] and hereditary RCC.[16] We have recently identified that renal tumor size on presentation is a significant predictor of the presence of synchronous metastatic disease.[17] In our series, the incidence of pathologically confirmed synchronous metastatic disease in tumors 3 cm or less was only 6.1% (5/82) and rose significantly with increasing tumor size (Table 10.1).

Table 10.1.
Correlation between renal lesion size and presence of synchronous metastatic disease

Tumor size (cm)	Total	Metastatic	Nonmetastatic	Percent metastatic
0–1.0	6	0	6	0
1.1–2.0	27	0	27	0
2.1–3.0	49	5	44	10.2
3.1–4.0	53	7	46	13.2
4.1–5.0	32	7	25	21.9
5.1–6.0	37	9	28	24.3
6.1–7.0	27	10	17	37
7.1–8.0	26	17	9	65.4
8.1–9.0	21	12	9	57.1
9.1–10.0	26	15	11	61.1
10.1–11.0	18	11	7	50
11.1–12.0	10	5	5	20
12.1–13.0	10	2	8	16.7
13.1–14.0.	6	1	5	42.9
14.1–15.0	7	3	4	75
15.1–16.0	4	3	1	33.3
16.1–17.0	3	1	2	0
17.1–18.0	1	0	1	0
18.1–19.0	0	0	0	0
19.1–20.0	1	0	1	0

DETERMINATION OF RADIOGRAPHIC TUMOR SIZE

To characterize and follow the growth kinetics of a renal mass accurately, tumor size must be measured in a reliable and consistent manner. Computed tomography (CT) scan is the most common imaging modality used for the diagnosis and follow-up of RCC with thin (5-mm) cuts through the kidneys recommended. For patients with poor renal function, contrast-based magnetic resonance imaging (MRI) may be utilized. Measurement of tumor size can be accomplished in several ways. The maximal cross-sectional diameter of the tumor is determined first. Currently available software on most modern imaging display systems provides a simple and reproducible means of measuring cross-sectional diameter by CT or MRI. When digital images are not available, hand calipers can be used to obtain the maximal axial diameter of the lesion. The estimated standard deviation of error while using calipers is ±2 mm. Whether computer software or hand calipers are used to determine maximal tumor diameter, potential misregistration may result based on slice thickness and artifact. When using axial diameter for tumor size, it is assumed that the tumor is spherical and grows in a uniform fashion in all directions, an assumption that is not always correct. Nonetheless, measuring the maximal cross-sectional diameter of a single lesion over time is a simple and relatively reproducible means of assessing growth.

A drawback of expressing tumor growth by following changes in maximal diameter is that it is not reflective of overall change in tumor volume. This is because calculating the volume of a sphere requires cubing the radius. For example, a change in maximal axial diameter of a renal mass from 1 cm to 2 cm is not just double the volume as would be implied, but rather represents a change in volume from 0.52 cm^3 to 4.19 cm^3, or over

Table 10.2.
Renal lesion volume determination based on number of
available cross-sectional dimensions

Available dimensions	Equation
1	$0.5326x^3$
2	$0.532xy\ (x + y/2)$
3	$0.5326xyz$

eightfold. Tumor volume can be calculated in several ways, depending on how many dimensions are available. Table 10.2 lists useful equations to calculate tumor volume based on the number of measured dimensions available. Another argument for using tumor volume instead of axial diameter is that volume provides a better representation of changes in total tumor cell number.

The relationship between radiographic size and pathologic size has been questioned. Although CT and MRI produce reliable and consistent measurements of renal lesions, discordance of radiographic tumor size and pathologic tumor size is often encountered. Herr[18] examined the relationship between radiographic and pathologic tumor size and noted a greater decrease in tumor size with RCC compared to benign lesions. This size discrepancy is largely thought to be a function of the hypervascular nature of renal malignancies and the effect of tumor engorgement when in situ. Irani et al.[19] also evaluated concordance rates between radiographic and pathologic tumor size. In this series, a greater size discrepancy was noted among smaller lesions than larger ones, possibly reflecting a decreased ability to accurately size smaller lesions radiographically. In contrast to the above findings, Yaycioglu et al.[20] failed to demonstrate a significant discordance between radiographic and pathologic tumor size.

AVAILABLE DATA REGARDING ACTIVE SURVEILLANCE OF RENAL MASSES

The practice of observing a known renal malignancy is almost certainly underreported. There have been several small retrospective series published addressing the natural history of small renal tumors under active surveillance and a single meta-analysis aggregating all available data (Table 10.3).

To date the only published prospective study on the natural history of observed small renal masses was performed by Volpe et al.[21] In an update of a prior report on 13 patients,[22] they analyzed 29 patients with 32 localized renal masses. All masses were less than 4 cm in greatest dimension with a mean initial size of 2.48 cm (median 2.40, range 0.9–3.9). Imaging characteristics of all masses were consistent with solid (88%) or cystic (22%) enhancing renal masses. Lesions grew on average 0.1 cm/year over a mean follow-up interval of 35 months (median 28, range 5.3–143). The overall average growth rate in this series was not found to be statistically greater than zero. Nine masses were removed in eight patients revealing eight clear-cell RCCs and one oncocytoma. No patient experienced stage progression or metastatic disease. The authors found that only 25% (8/32) of the masses they observed demonstrated significant interval growth. From these data they concluded that it may be appropriate to recommend a period of initial observation of small masses, especially in the elderly or infirm, with surgical

Table 10.3.
Growth rate of clinically localized and metastatic lesions

Author	Year	n	Clinical extent of disease	Average size on presentation (cm)	Size range (cm)	Duration of follow up (average months)	Growth rate average	Growth rate range (cm/year)
Oda	2003	16	Localized	2.0*	1.0–4.5	25*	0.54* cm/year	0.1–1.35
		16	Metastatic	1.9*	1.0–3.0	12*	1.72* cm/year	0.08–7.87
Ozono	2004	56	Localized and metastatic	2.7	0.5–11.0	NA	0.96 cm/year	NA
Kato	2004	18	Localized	1.98	0.8–3.4	27	0.42 cm/year	0.08–1.60
Volpe	2004	32	Localized	2.48	0.9–3.9	35	0.1 cm/year	NA
Kassouf	2004	26	Localized	2.37	1.0–7.0	32	0.09 cm/year	0–1.2
Bosniak	1995	40	Localized	1.73	0.2–3.5	39	0.47 cm/year	0–1.1
Wehe	2004	29	Localized	1.83	0.4–3.5	32	0.12 cm/year	NA
Lamb	2004	36	Localized	7.2	3.5–20.0	28	0.39** cm/year	0–1.76
Sowery	2004	22	Localized	4.08	2.0–8.8	26	0.86 cm/year	NA
Fujimoto	1995	6	Localized	2.47	1.8–3.4	29	0.47 cm/year	0.05–0.73
		12	Metastatic	0.84	0.4–1.6	7	1.78 cm/year	0.42–4.47
Takebayashi	2000	17	Localized and metastatic	1.9	0.8–3.4	25	1.61 cm/year	0.41–2.56
Chawla	2006	61	Localized	2.97	1.0–12.0	36	0.20 cm/year	−1.64–1.80
Meta-analysis	2006	234	Localized	2.60	0.2–20.0	34	0.28 cm/year	0–1.76

n, number of lesions observed in each series; NA, not available.
*Median values.
**Does not represent all lesions presented in the series.

treatment reserved for patients who have tumors that grow rapidly or reach a size that is deemed unsafe.

The remaining published reports on the topic have all been retrospective. In data from New York University presented by Bosniak et al.,[23,24] the authors followed 40 localized tumors over a mean interval of 3.25 years (range 1.75–8.5) and demonstrated an average growth rate of 0.36 cm/year (range 0–1.10). No patient developed metastatic disease in this series. The majority of tumors showed little to no growth, and a small proportion of tumors accounted for the overall average growth. The authors concluded that most small, incidentally discovered parenchymal neoplasms grow slowly, and may be safely watched in those who are elderly or are not suitable surgical candidates.

Fujimoto et al.[25] examined renal tumor volume doubling time in a series from Japan. The authors compared tumor growth rates between six localized lesions and 12 metastatic lesions. Although smaller in size at presentation, metastatic lesions demonstrated accelerated growth rates compared to localized lesions. Pathology was available on all lesions that were confirmed RCC. The authors found that nonmetastatic RCC lesions grow relatively slowly, especially when compared to metastatic lesions. These findings are consistent with prior reports comparing the growth rates of primary and metastatic lesions of rectal and colon cancers.[26]

A report by Kassouf et al.[27] from McGill University examined 24 patients with renal masses who were followed expectantly because of age, poor medical condition, or the presence of a mass in a solitary kidney. Interestingly, of the 24 patients, only five (21%) had tumors that demonstrated growth over a mean follow-up interval of 32 months (median 24, range 8–86). Those that grew did so at a mean rate of 0.49 cm/year (median 0.43, range 0.13–1.2), with a combined growth rate of 0.09 cm/year when including all 24 patients. Four of the patients underwent surgery either due to patient choice or tumor growth and all resected lesions proved to be RCC. The authors concluded that most small renal masses undergo limited growth when followed expectantly and that without tumor growth, the risk of metastases seems low.

Oda et al.[28] reported their experience in Sapporo, Japan, with 16 patients who did not receive immediate surgical treatment for solid renal masses (median size 2.0 cm, range 1–4.5) that were detected incidentally and 16 patients with metastatic RCC (median size 1.9 cm, range 1.0–3.0). All of these lesions were later proven to be RCC. Of the patients with metastatic disease, all had previously failed interferon therapy and 56% (9/16) had the primary lesion removed. Median follow-up time was 2.1 years for localized lesions and 1 year for metastatic lesions. The median growth rate of localized lesions was 0.54 cm/year (range 0.10–1.35) and 1.72 cm/year (range 0.08–7.87) for metastatic lesions. The difference in growth rates between localized and metastatic lesions was statistically significant despite the lesions having a similar size at presentation. The authors concluded that although some patients with localized lesions may be candidates for "watchful waiting," they should be selected with great caution.

In a retrospective review, Wehle et al.[29] analyzed their experience with 29 lesions in 29 patients who were followed with serial imaging. All masses were enhancing on CT and had an average size of 1.83 cm (range 0.4–3.5). Tumors were followed an average of 32 months (range 10–89) with a mean growth rate of 0.12 cm/year. No growth was observed in 52% (15/29) of the lesions followed. Of the 29 patients, five had known pathology via either biopsy or nephrectomy. Of these four were RCCs. No patient developed metastatic disease during follow-up. The authors concluded that when surgical therapy is contraindicated or undesirable, it is safe to manage small renal masses expectantly.

In another study from Japan, Kato et al.[30] examined the growth rate of initially observed lesions and correlated this with tumor histopathology. This group looked at a total of 18 tumors in 18 patients that had been followed for at least 12 months and were subsequently removed. All lesions were pathologically confirmed RCCs, with 15 clear cell and three papillary histologic subtypes. The overall mean growth rate was 0.42 cm/year over a median 22.5 months (mean 26.9, range 12–63) follow-up. Individual lesion growth rate ranged from 0.08 to 1.60 cm/year. The authors concluded that for elderly or high-risk surgical patients, watchful waiting is acceptable if the lesion has a slow growth rate. They did caution that the range of tumor growth rates is wide and may change depending on tumor histology.

Lamb et al.[31] reported their experience with 36 solid renal masses in 36 patients who were either medically unfit or unwilling to undergo surgical treatment. Twelve (33%) patients were symptomatic on presentation, tumor size at diagnosis was 7.2 cm (range 3.5–20.0 cm) and the mean growth rate in 20 of 36 patients evaluated was 0.39 cm/year (median 0, range 0–1.76). No patient in this series underwent nephrectomy. Biopsy was performed in 24/36 (66.7%) patients and 96% (23/24) were RCC. Metastatic disease developed in one patient at 132 months despite an initial negative renal biopsy. Additionally, 5.6% (2/36) of patients required tumor embolization for persistent hematuria. This series is especially notable since the average lesion size on presentation was large (7.2 cm) yet the mean growth rate (0.39 cm/year) was not appreciably different from other series with smaller initial tumor sizes. The authors concluded that in selected elderly and medically unfit patients, observation of renal masses is a safe and reasonable approach, with little impact on life expectancy.

Sowery and Siemens[32] published their series of 22 patients undergoing surveillance of enhancing renal tumors. Reasons for observation were medical comorbidities in 15 patients and patient preference in seven patients. Seven (32%) patients had enhancing cystic lesions. Duration of follow-up was an average of 26 months. Mean tumor size on presentation was 4.08 cm in greatest diameter and average growth was 0.86 cm/year. Tumors presenting with a diameter of greater than 4 cm did not have a faster growth rate than tumors less than 4 cm. Two patients underwent nephrectomy and both specimens contained RCC. One patient developed metastatic disease during follow-up. This patient presented with an 8.8-cm renal mass that grew at 0.2 cm/year over a 111-month period. The authors concluded that metastases are unlikely in tumors that do not exhibit interval growth.

The Japanese Society of Renal Cancer presented its collective experience with observation of RCC in 56 patients.[33] Mean lesions size on presentation was 2.7 cm (range 0.5–11.0 cm). Tumor doubling time was 603.1 days with a mean growth rate of 0.96 cm/year. Thirty-eight patients eventually underwent surgical intervention. The authors attempted to correlate doubling time and growth rate with age of onset, TNM classification, lesion size, grade, and RCC histologic subtype. Of the variables examined, only growth rate correlated with lesion size in tumors ≥ 4 cm. The authors suggested that further elucidation of the natural history of enhancing renal lesions will help optimize treatment strategies.

Takebayashi et al.[34] examined the growth rate and doubling time of RCCs in patients with acquired cystic disease of the kidney. Seventeen patients were included in the review, all of whom were on chronic hemodialysis. Mean tumor size on presentation was 1.9 cm (range 0.8–3.4 cm). The combined growth rate of localized and metastatic tumors was 1.61 cm/year, with a mean doubling time of 5.09 years. All tumors were surgically removed and were confirmed RCC with 15 tumors confined to the renal capsule, one tumor extending into the perirenal fat, and one tumor with an associated liver metastasis. The authors suggest that observation may be safe in slow-growing tumors and recommend immediate surgical removal of tumors exhibiting short doubling times.

A recent review of the tumor database at the Fox Chase Cancer Center revealed 61 enhancing renal lesions in 42 patients with at least 12 months follow-up.[35] To our knowledge, this is the largest single institutional experience to date. The mean lesion growth rate in this population was 0.20 cm/year (median 0.12, range −1.64–1.80 cm/year); 34% (21/61) of lesions underwent pathologic assessment, the majority of which were malignant (81%; 17/21). Figure 10.1 presents a case report from the series in

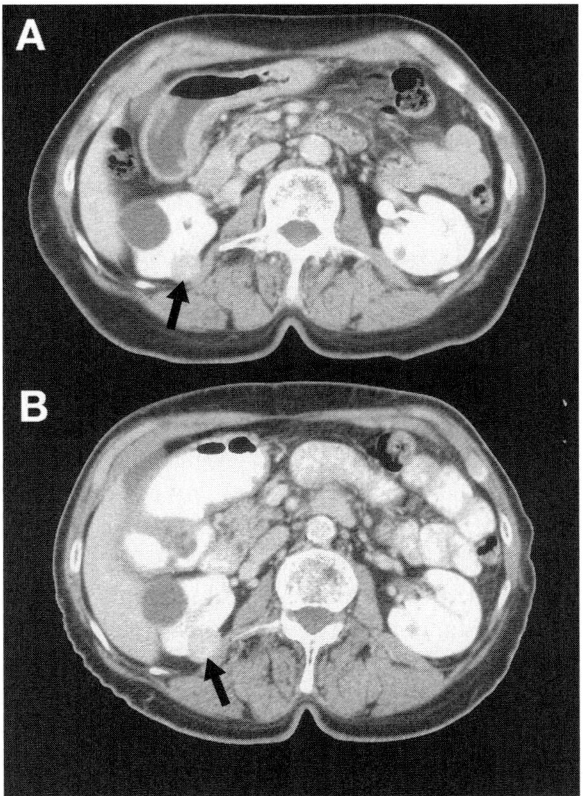

Figure 10.1. An 81-year-old woman presenting with an incidental 1.9-cm enhancing right renal mass in March 1999. Past medical history was significant for coronary artery disease, peripheral vascular disease, hypothyroidism, and hypercholesterolemia. The patient initially elected active surveillance and then requested surgical intervention due to a small interval increase in renal mass size from 1.9 cm to 2.3 cm over 63 months of follow-up (growth rate = 0.08 cm/year). Laparoscopic cryoablation was performed, with pre-cryoablation biopsy revealing a grade 2 clear cell RCC in June 2004. Computed tomography scan images of the renal mass from September 2001 (A) and December 2003 (B) are shown, demonstrating small interval renal mass growth. Black arrows point to the enhancing renal mass.

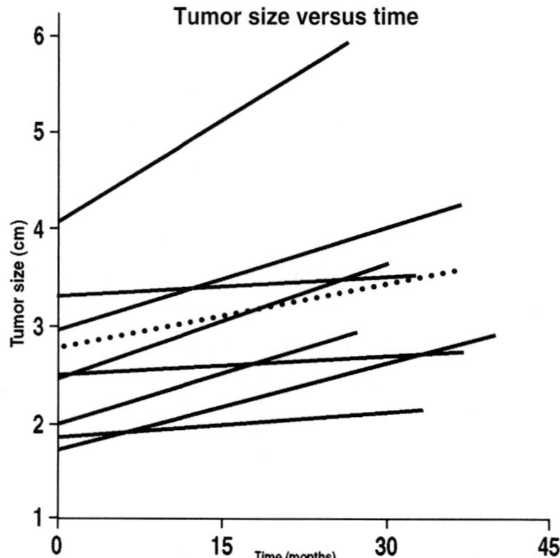

Figure 10.2. Graph comparing the growth rates (slope of line) of published reports evaluating solid renal masses under active surveillance. Solid lines represent individual series. Dotted line represents combined data.

which a lesion was followed over a period of 63 months and demonstrated a growth rate of 0.08 cm/year. One patient in our series developed metastatic disease during observation—an 84-year-old patient who presented with a 2.0-cm incidental mass that grew to 8.0 cm during 54 months of follow-up. These observations are in agreement with the previously published series, demonstrating that enhancing renal lesions have a slow growth rate and rarely metastasize.[35]

A meta-analysis on the growth rate of 234 localized renal tumors undergoing observation, including the above listed series, revealed an overall mean growth rate of 0.28 cm/year (median 2.48, range 0.09–0.86).[35] Figure 10.2 demonstrates the growth rate and duration of follow-up in the series included in the meta-analysis; 92% of the lesions followed with evaluable pathologic data were confirmed RCC variants. Progression to metastatic disease was noted in 1% (3/286) of the lesions followed.

Taken together these studies demonstrate that the growth rate of enhancing renal lesions, although potentially variable, is most often slow and averages 0.28 cm/year (range 0.09–0.86 cm/year).[35] However, there are several limitations to the presented data that must be recognized. Only one of the studies presented above was prospective; the rest were retrospective. This is a potential source of selection bias since some patients were successfully followed at an outside institution prior to referral to a tertiary care center. Furthermore, the indication for initial observation was not stated in many of the series discussed. This information is potentially helpful in establishing guidelines for observation. Finally, the imaging modalities utilized in each series were not uniform, and significant observer variability may have been introduced when evaluating follow-up studies.

ENHANCING LESIONS THAT DO NOT DEMONSTRATE GROWTH OVER TIME

A substantial number of enhancing renal lesions under observation do not demonstrate any radiographic tumor growth. The number of lesions that do not increase in size varies between series and ranges from 0% to 73% of all lesions followed. Table 10.4 summarizes the available data on zero-growth renal masses under observations and notes that approximately 26% of lesions show no radiographic growth during a period of active surveillance. Although some observed lesions that remain static do not represent RCC, many are pathologically confirmed renal cancer. To date, no study has investigated the clinical, radiographic, or clinical characteristics that may distinguish these lesions from those that do demonstrate radiographic growth. Bosniak et al.[23,24] confirmed a grade 1 RCC in a 2.30-cm lesion that was followed for 2 years without demonstrating radiographic growth. Wehle et al.[29] observed no increase in tumor size in 52% (15/29) of the lesions followed in their series. Three of the lesions in this series that did not demonstrate any interval growth underwent nephrectomy and two were RCCs with a single case of oncocytoma. Pathology was available in an additional six lesions from the Fox Chase Cancer Center series, of which five were RCCs and one was an oncocytoma. These findings suggest that the lack of interval radiographic growth does not correlate with malignant potential or pathological findings.

Table 10.4.
Zero net growth rates during active surveillance

Author	Total No. of lesions	No. exhibiting no growth	Percentage	No. with available pathology	Pathology
Bosniak	40	2	5%	1	RCC = 1
Chawla	61	21	34%	6	RCC = 5 Oncocytoma = 1
Fujimoto	6	0	0		
Kassouf	26	19	73%	NA	NA
Kato	18	0	0		
Oda	16	0	0		
Sowery	22	3	14%	NA	NA
Volpe	32	4	12%	NA	NA
Whele	29	15	52%	3	RCC = 2 Oncocytoma = 1
Total	250	64	26%	10	RCC = 8 Oncoyctoma = 2

Note: Enhancing renal lesions that did not demonstrate interval growth radiographically during active surveillance. Pathology is representative of lesions that did not demonstrate growth in the individual series.

PATHOLOGY OF OBSERVED LESIONS

Before drawing conclusions regarding the natural history of observed enhancing renal masses based on this literature, it is important to confirm that the lesions studied are in fact renal carcinomas. Table 10.5 reviews the pathology available in each of the aforementioned series. There was some pathologic data available in all series ranging from 9% to 100% of individual lesions reported. The majority of lesions undergoing pathologic assessment were surgically removed. However, this is not the case in the series by Lamb et al.[31] in which all presented pathology was obtained from percutaneous biopsies. The authors of this series report that the diagnosis of RCC was confirmed in 23 of 24 tumors sampled and that a histologic subtype of RCC could be assigned in 19 of 23 cases. Paradoxically, the one case in the series that was not confirmed to be RCC via percutaneous biopsy later developed metastatic renal carcinoma after 10 years of observation.

Table 10.5.
Available pathology on renal lesions undergoing a period of observation

Author	No. of lesions	Pathology available (%)	Benign (%)	Positive for RCC (%)	Grade*	Histology
Fujimoto	6	6 (100)	0	6 (100)	G2 = 5	Clear cell = 5
Bosniak	40	26 (65)	4 (15)	22 (85)	G1 = 18 G2 = 4	NA
Oda	16	16 (100)	0	16 (100)	G1 = 6 G2 = 9 G3 = 1	NA
Kassouf	26	4 (15)	0	4 (100)	NA	Clear cell = 3 Papillary = 1
Volpe	32	9 (28)	1 (11)	8 (89)	G2 = 4 G3 = 2 G4 = 2	Clear cell = 8
Wehle	29	5 (17)	1 (20)	4 (80)	NA	NA
Kato	18	18 (100)	0	18 (100)	G1 = 7 G2 = 8 G3 = 3	Clear cell = 15 Papillary = 3
Lamb*	36	24 (67)	1 (4)	23 (96)	G1 = 3 G3 = 1	Clear cell = 18 Papillary = 1
Sowery	22	2 (9)	0	2 (100)	NA	NA
Takebayashi	17	17 (100)	0	17 (100)	G1 = 9 G2 = 5 G3 = 3	Papillary = 8 Tubular = 4 Alveolar = 4 Solid = 1
Ozono	56	38 (68)	0	38 (100)	G1 = 12 G2 = 23 G3 = 3	Clear cell = 25 Granular = 5 Mixed = 7 Spindle = 1
Meta-analysis	286	131 (46)	11 (8)	120 (92)	NA	NA

*Pathology presented in the Lamb et al. series represents pathologic assessment of percutaneous biopsies.

Overall, the majority of observed renal lesions with available pathology represented kidney cancer including 80% to 100% of sampled lesions in each series. Clear-cell RCC was the most common histologic subtype identified, consistent with contemporary series reviewing pathologic findings in RCC. While nuclear grade assessment was inconsistently applied throughout the individual series, it should be noted that where information was available regarding nuclear grade, most lesions were grade 1 or 2.

All benign lesions in these series were oncocytomas, which accounted for 0% to 20% of tumors in any individual series (Table 10.5). The incidence of benign lesions observed is in agreement with other large contemporary series that report benign lesions in 10% to 30% of all enhancing renal masses.[36,37] Although the percentage of benign versus malignant lesions in observation series is consistent with other published pathology data regarding enhancing renal masses, these results must be viewed with caution because of several potential sources of bias. First, not all lesions undergoing observation have pathology available for review. Second, the decision to remove a lesion after surveillance may have been influenced by clinical findings suggestive of a more aggressive phenotype, such as rapid radiographic growth or the onset of symptoms. Lastly, in series reporting a 100% incidence of RCC in observed lesions, the authors do not state if benign lesions were excluded from their analyses.

MORBIDITY OF OBSERVATION

Most of the lesions reported were incidentally discovered during the evaluation of other medical conditions. Although the lesions were asymptomatic on presentation, the potential exists for symptoms to develop, especially in those that demonstrate growth. Two series commented on the development of tumor-related symptoms in patients undergoing observation. Lamb et al.[31] noted the development of hematuria in 11% (4/36) of patients undergoing observation. In two patients this resolved without intervention, while the remaining two patients required tumor embolization. One patient in the Sowery and Siemens[32] series developed hematuria during follow-up and required embolization. Importantly, there were no reports of flank or abdominal pain directly attributed to an observed renal mass, although it is possible that the development of symptoms in patients undergoing observation is under reported.

PROGRESSION TO METASTATIC DISEASE

The greatest risk of active surveillance of RCC is the potential for progression to metastatic disease. This is especially relevant given the current lack of effective systemic therapies for the treatment of metastatic disease.[8] In the series reported to date, only three cases of enhancing renal lesions undergoing observation have progressed to metastatic disease, representing 1% (3/286) of all published cases.[35] The first was from Lamb et al.,[31] in which a patient developed metastatic disease 132 months after the initial diagnosis of an enhancing renal lesion. The patient underwent a percutaneous biopsy on initial presentation, which was negative for malignancy, and was then lost to follow-up. The initial lesion size and growth rate for this patient was not presented. The second case was reported by Sowery and Siemens[32] in which an 8.8-cm lesion was observed for 111 months, and grew at 0.2 cm/year before metastasizing. Both of these patients were symptomatic with hematuria, with one patient requiring embolization. The third patient developing metastatic disease was from our own institution as reported in our meta-analysis. The patient presented with a 2.0-cm mass that grew at a rate of 1.2 cm/year during 54 months of observation to a final diameter of 8.0 cm. Multiple pulmonary nodules were noted on repeat imaging.[35]

PREDICTORS OF GROWTH

The current series examining the growth rate of enhancing renal lesions demonstrate that most lesions grow at a slow rate and have a low likelihood of metastasis. However, some lesions grow rapidly and may have a greater propensity to become symptomatic or metastasize. With this in mind it would be helpful to identify lesions with the potential for rapid growth in order to follow these lesions more closely or institute early intervention. Several authors have attempted to correlate clinical, radiographic, and pathologic characteristics of renal lesions with their observed growth rate. Only one series attempted to correlate patient symptoms to observed renal lesion growth rate. Sowery and Siemens[32] compared renal lesion growth rates in patients who were symptomatic ($n = 6$) on presentation to those who were asymptomatic ($n = 16$). Lesions that were symptomatic on presentation grew at a higher rate than asymptomatic lesions (45.03 cc/year vs. 16.12 cc/year); however, the authors did not compare lesion size on presentation between symptomatic and asymptomatic patients.

Potential radiographic predictors of renal lesion growth include lesion size on presentation and presence of cystic components. Lesion size on presentation was not found to correlate with observed growth rates in multiple series. Bosniak et al.[23,24] compared growth rates of tumors ≤2 cm to tumors >2 cm and did not find a difference. Similarly, Sowery and Siemens[32] did not notice a significant difference in growth rates comparing lesions >4 cm to those <4 cm in diameter. Furthermore, Volpe et al.[21] could not associate growth rate with lesion size ($p = .23$). In the case of hereditary renal carcinoma associated with von Hippel–Lindau (VHL), Duffey et al.[16] report a correlation of tumor size with metastatic potential. In their series of 108 patients with VHL and renal tumors <3 cm, none developed metastases over a mean follow-up of 58 months compared with 20/73 (27%) patients with tumors ≥3 cm. Based on these findings, it was the authors' recommendation and has become their practice to observe RCC in cases of VHL until the size of the lesion exceeds 3 cm. This recommendation was based not only on the metastatic potential of the lesion, but also on the inevitability of RCC in patients with VHL; therefore, the applicability of this rule to patients with sporadic RCC remains to be demonstrated.

Recent reports have suggested that cystic RCC presents with a smaller mean tumor size and may have a better prognosis compared to conventional clear cell RCC.[38–41] Although the diagnosis of cystic RCC can only be made after pathologic examination, renal lesions with substantial enhancing cystic components likely represent cystic RCC.[42] Theoretically, the growth rate of cystic lesions may differ from solid lesions due to the relative differences between tumor cell volume and total mass volume of cystic and solid lesions. However, in at least two of the aforementioned series, the growth rates of cystic lesions did not differ significantly from that of solid masses.[21,32]

Studies investigating the relationship among renal tumor size, histologic subtype, and nuclear grade have been performed. Frank et al.,[36] in their review of a large series of renal tumors, demonstrated that for each centimeter increase in tumor size there was a 17% increase in the odds of the lesion being malignant. The authors also correlated tumor size to histologic subtype, with larger lesions having a greater likelihood of clear cell or chromophobe carcinoma compared to papillary RCC. In their data, nuclear grade also increased as the size of both papillary and clear cell lesions grew. To date there have been no series comparing growth rates of benign and malignant lesions or growth rates of different histologic subtypes of RCC in sporadic cases. Takebayashi et al.[34] attempted to correlate growth rate and histologic subtype in patients with acquired cystic kidney disease who developed RCC. Papillary tumors in this select population appeared to have a slower growth rate and a longer doubling time compared to other tumors, but the difference did not reach statistical significance.

Several authors attempted to correlate nuclear grade to growth rates in renal lesions undergoing active surveillance prior to operative intervention. Oda et al.[28] failed to demonstrate an association between nuclear grade and growth rate in localized RCC, but did note a significant relationship between nuclear grade and growth rate in metastatic RCC. Kato et al.[30] compared growth rates of grade 1, 2, and 3 renal cancers. Grade 1 and 2 tumors demonstrated similar growth rates, while grade 3 tumors grew at a significantly faster rate when compared to grade 2 tumors. Importantly this series only reported on a total of 18 lesions, limiting the applicability of their conclusions. Takebayashi et al.[34] noted significantly increased growth rates in grade 3 compared to grade 1 and 2 carcinomas in 17 patients with acquired cystic kidney disease.

Other potential pathologic predictors of lesions growth rate include markers of cellular proliferation and apoptosis. Three series have evaluated the relationship of molecular markers to the growth rates of RCCs undergoing surveillance prior to removal. Fujimoto et al.[25] analyzed argyrophilic nucleolar organizer regions (AgNORs) and proliferating cell nuclear antigen (PCNA) activity in localized and metastatic lesions. Tumor doubling time was inversely and significantly correlated with AgNORs and PCNA activity in localized tumors. A similar relationship was found between metastatic lesions and AgNORs but not PCNA. Kato et al.[30] examined the relationship of another marker of cellular proliferation, Ki-67, and the apoptotic index to growth rates in localized RCC, and found that while Ki-67 immunostaining did not correlate with RCC growth ($p = .36$), the degree of apoptosis did ($p = .0013$). Oda et al.[28] investigated the relationship of Ki-67 and measures of apoptosis and angiogenesis to RCC growth rates. In 16 patients who underwent a period of observation prior to surgical excision, the Ki-67 labeling index, apoptosis index, and microvessel density did not correlate with RCC growth, although the balance between cell proliferation and apoptosis, as determined by the ratio of Ki-67 labeling index/apoptotic index, did.

Unfortunately, there are no current markers to predict which renal lesions will grow rapidly or metastasize. For this reason the development of both urine and serum biomarkers are needed for molecular diagnosis and prognosis.[43–46] Such diagnostic and prognostic tools would be invaluable in deciding which patients are appropriate candidates for observation and which should undergo surgical intervention, even in the face of significant competing health risks.

GUIDELINES FOR RADIOGRAPHIC FOLLOW-UP

Once the patient and physician have agreed on instituting a course of observation for presumed RCC, several important guidelines should be followed. The radiologist must be informed of the purpose of the follow-up imaging and should be provided with all available prior studies. The treating physician should also personally review follow-up studies to ensure that the renal lesion of interest is being compared appropriately to previous exams. This is particularly important in patients with multiple renal cysts, enhancing cystic lesions, and multiple solid enhancing lesions. Care must also be taken to measure the lesion at equivalent levels in the kidney when comparing lesion size to prior studies. Patients should be evaluated with periodic assessments for metastatic disease and the development of symptoms related to the observed renal tumor.

The frequency of radiographic follow-up should be every 3 to 6 months during the first 2 years of evaluation. This is done initially to assess the growth kinetics of the lesion. If the tumor being observed demonstrates zero net growth or radiographic stability, the follow-up interval can be increased. The type of imaging modality employed during follow-up is also important. Contrast imaging with CT or MRI is preferable to ultrasound (US), as these modalities will introduce less technician-dependent variability. Once an imaging modality has been selected, it should be used consistently throughout follow-up.

CONCLUSION

The majority of enhancing lesions under active surveillance demonstrate slow growth rates and a low rate of progression to metastatic disease. On pathologic assessment, most of these lesions represent renal carcinoma. While the gold standard in the management of enhancing renal lesions remains surgical extirpation, an initial period of active surveillance is likely safe but remains a calculated risk until prospective data are available. The only true indications for conservative therapy at the present time are absolute or relative competing health risks, which remain difficult to quantitate as they relate to treatment trade-offs. When undertaking observation of an enhancing renal mass, both the patient and physician assume inherent risks of nontreatment, which must be weighed against the risk of surgical intervention. Finally, the data summarized here regarding active surveillance of renal carcinomas must be remembered when evaluating the short to intermediate cancer specific results of new technologies in the treatment of localized cancer of the kidney.

REFERENCES

1. Jayson M, Sanders H. Increased incidence of serendipitously discovered renal cell carcinoma. Urology 1998;51(2):203–205.
2. Chow WH, et al. Rising incidence of renal cell cancer in the United States. JAMA 1999; 281(17):1628–1631.
3. Smith SJ, et al. Renal cell carcinoma: earlier discovery and increased detection. Radiology 1989;170(3pt 1):699–703.
4. Hock LM, Lynch J, Balaji KC. Increasing incidence of all stages of kidney cancer in the last 2 decades in the United States: an analysis of surveillance, epidemiology and end results program data. J Urol 2002;167(1):57–60.
5. Derweesh IH, Novick AC. Small renal tumors: natural history, observation strategies and emerging modalities of energy based tumor ablation. Can J Urol 2003;10(3):1871–1879.
6. Parsons JK, Schoenberg MS, Carter HB. Incidental renal tumors: casting doubt on the efficacy of early intervention. Urology 2001;57(6):1013–1015.
7. Edwards BK, et al. Annual report to the nation on the status of cancer 1975–2002, featuring population-based trends in cancer treatment. J Natl Cancer Inst 2005;97(19):1407–1427.

8. Mekhail TM, et al. Validation and extension of the Memorial Sloan-Kettering prognostic factors model for survival in patients with previously untreated metastatic renal cell carcinoma. J Clin Oncol 2005;23(4):832–841.
9. Montie JE. Prognostic factors for renal cell carcinoma. J Urol 1994;152(5pt 1):1397–1398.
10. Greene F, Page DL, Fleming ID, et al. AJCC Cancer Staging Handbook, 6th ed. Chicago: Springer, 2002.
11. Hsu RM, Chan DY, Siegelman SS. Small renal cell carcinomas: correlation of size with tumor stage, nuclear grade, and histologic subtype. AJR Am J Roentgenol 2004;182(3):551–557.
12. Roberts WW, et al. Pathological stage does not alter the prognosis for renal lesions determined to be stage T1 by computerized tomography. J Urol 2005;173(3):713–715.
13. Dechet CB, et al. Prospective analysis of computerized tomography and needle biopsy with permanent sectioning to determine the nature of solid renal masses in adults. J Urol 2003;169(1):71–74.
14. Campbell SC, et al. Prospective evaluation of fine needle aspiration of small, solid renal masses: accuracy and morbidity. Urology 1997;50(1):25–29.
15. Rybicki FJ, et al. Percutaneous biopsy of renal masses: sensitivity and negative predictive value stratified by clinical setting and size of masses. AJR Am J Roentgenol 2003;180(5):1281–1287.
16. Duffey BG, et al. The relationship between renal tumor size and metastases in patients with von Hippel-Lindau disease. J Urol 2004;172(1):63–65.
17. Kunkle DA, et al. Enhancing renal masses with zero net growth during active surveillance. J Urol 2007;177(3):848–854.
18. Herr HW. Radiographic vs surgical size of renal tumours after partial nephrectomy. BJU Int 2000;85(1):19–21.
19. Irani J, et al. Renal tumor size: comparison between computed tomography and surgical measurements. Eur Urol 2001;39(3):300–303.
20. Yaycioglu O, et al. Clinical and pathologic tumor size in renal cell carcinoma; difference, correlation, and analysis of the influencing factors. Urology 2002;60(1):33–38.
21. Volpe A, et al. The natural history of incidentally detected small renal masses. Cancer 2004;100(4):738–745.
22. Rendon RA, et al. The natural history of small renal masses. J Urol 2000;164(4):1143–1147.
23. Bosniak MA. Observation of small incidentally detected renal masses. Semin Urol Oncol 1995;13(4):267–272.
24. Bosniak MA, et al. Small renal parenchymal neoplasms: further observations on growth. Radiology 1995;197(3):589–597.
25. Fujimoto N, et al. Observations on the growth rate of renal cell carcinoma. Int J Urol 1995;2(2):71–76.
26. Spratt JS Jr, Spratt TL. Rates of growth of pulmonary metastases and host survival. Ann Surg 1964;159:161–171.
27. Kassouf W, et al. Natural history of renal masses followed expectantly. J Urol 2004;171(1):111–113; discussion 113.
28. Oda T, et al. Growth rates of primary and metastatic lesions of renal cell carcinoma. Int J Urol 2001;8(9):473–477.
29. Wehle MJ, et al. Conservative management of incidental contrast-enhancing renal masses as safe alternative to invasive therapy. Urology 2004;64(1):49–52.
30. Kato M, et al. Natural history of small renal cell carcinoma: evaluation of growth rate, histological grade, cell proliferation and apoptosis. J Urol 2004;172(3):863–866.
31. Lamb GW, et al. Management of renal masses in patients medically unsuitable for nephrectomy—natural history, complications, and outcome. Urology 2004;64(5):909–913.
32. Sowery RD, Siemens DR. Growth characteristics of renal cortical tumors in patients managed by watchful waiting. Can J Urol 2004;11(5):2407–2410.
33. Ozono S, et al. Tumor doubling time of renal cell carcinoma measured by CT: collaboration of Japanese Society of Renal Cancer. Jpn J Clin Oncol 2004;34(2):82–85.
34. Takebayashi S, et al. Renal cell carcinoma in acquired cystic kidney disease: volume growth rate determined by helical computed tomography. Am J Kidney Dis 2000;36(4):759–766.
35. Chawla SN, et al. The natural history of observed enhancing renal masses: meta-analysis and review of the world literature. J Urol 2006;175(2):425–431.
36. Frank I, et al. Solid renal tumors: an analysis of pathological features related to tumor size. J Urol 2003;170(6pt 1):2217–2220.

37. Gill IS, et al. Comparative analysis of laparoscopic versus open partial nephrectomy for renal tumors in 200 patients. J Urol 2003;170(1):64–68.
38. Nassir A, et al. Multilocular cystic renal cell carcinoma: a series of 12 cases and review of the literature. Urology 2002;60(3):421–427.
39. Koga S, et al. Outcome of surgery in cystic renal cell carcinoma. Urology 2000;56(1):67–70.
40. Han KR, et al. Cystic renal cell carcinoma: biology and clinical behavior. Urol Oncol 2004; 22(5):410–414.
41. Corica FA, et al. Cystic renal cell carcinoma is cured by resection: a study of 24 cases with long-term followup. J Urol 1999;161(2):408–411.
42. Aubert S, et al. Cystic renal cell carcinomas in adults. Is preoperative recognition of multilocular cystic renal cell carcinoma possible? J Urol 2005;174(6):2115–2119.
43. Dulaimi E, et al. Promoter hypermethylation profile of kidney cancer. Clin Cancer Res 2004;10(12pt 1):3972–3979.
44. Mizutani Y, et al. Downregulation of Smac/DIABLO expression in renal cell carcinoma and its prognostic significance. J Clin Oncol 2005;23(3):448–454.
45. Shvarts O, et al. p53 is an independent predictor of tumor recurrence and progression after nephrectomy in patients with localized renal cell carcinoma. J Urol 2005;173(3):725–728.
46. Skates S, Iliopoulos O. Molecular markers for early detection of renal carcinoma: investigative approach. Clin Cancer Res 2004;10(18pt 2):6296S–6301S.

11 Radical Nephrectomy

Benjamin I. Chung and John A. Libertino

KEYWORDS

RADICAL NEPHRECTOMY
RENAL CELL CARCINOMA

ABSTRACT

Renal cell carcinoma as we know today is primarily a surgical disease. The modern era of radical nephrectomy for the treatment of renal cell carcinoma was described by Robson et al.[1] The technique of radical nephrectomy can be performed in a variety of ways, but the firm principles outlined by Robson remain relevant today. Robson and associates described removing the kidney with early ligation of the renal artery and vein to minimize tumor emboli, and a lymph node dissection, removing the paraaortic and paracaval nodal packets from the crus of the diaphragm superiorly to the aortic bifurcation inferiorly. Since that time, the technique of radical nephrectomy has undergone some modification, but the general principles outlined remain germane to today's contemporary practice.

TECHNIQUE

At our institution, we typically employ a supra–11th rib incision for radical nephrectomy, as per Turner-Warwick.[2] The rib is not removed during the procedure. The patient is placed in the full 90-degree flank position (Figure 11.1). The intercostal muscles are divided and the lumbodorsal fascia is exposed (Figures 11.2 and 11.3). The pleura is avoided during the dissection and the lumbodorsal fascia is divided off of the tip of the 11th rib, thus entering the retroperitoneal space. The incision is carried medially to the lateral border of the rectus muscle. The muscles are divided off the superior edge of the rib. The fascia of the latissimus dorsi and external oblique muscles are encountered and divided. The internal oblique and serratus posterior inferior muscle layers are divided next. The neurovascular bundle running between the transversalis muscle and internal oblique muscle is avoided and spared if possible. Dividing the intercostal

From: *Clinical Management of Renal Tumors*
Edited by: R.M. Bukowski and A.C. Novick © Humana Press Inc., Totowa, NJ

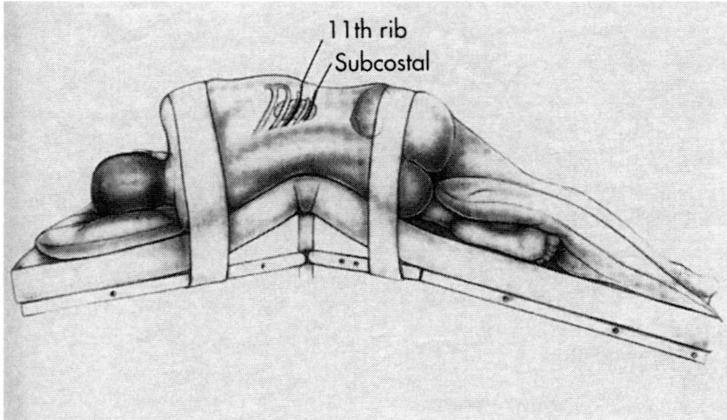

Figure 11.1. Full flank positioning for open radical nephrectomy with locations of incisions relative to ribs and kidney.

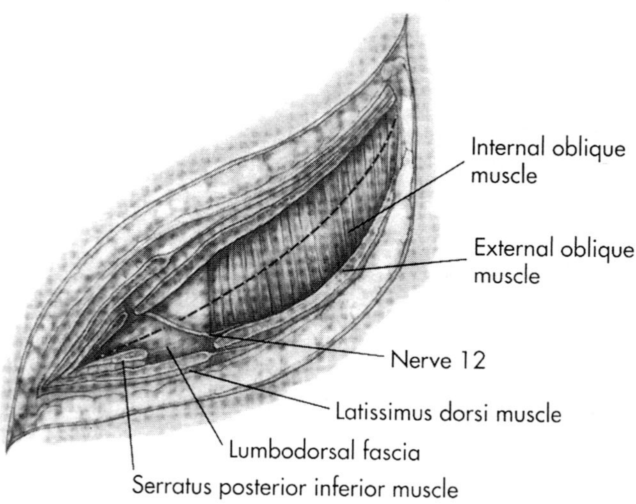

Figure 11.2. Muscle layers and anatomic location of lumbodorsal fascia during flank incision.

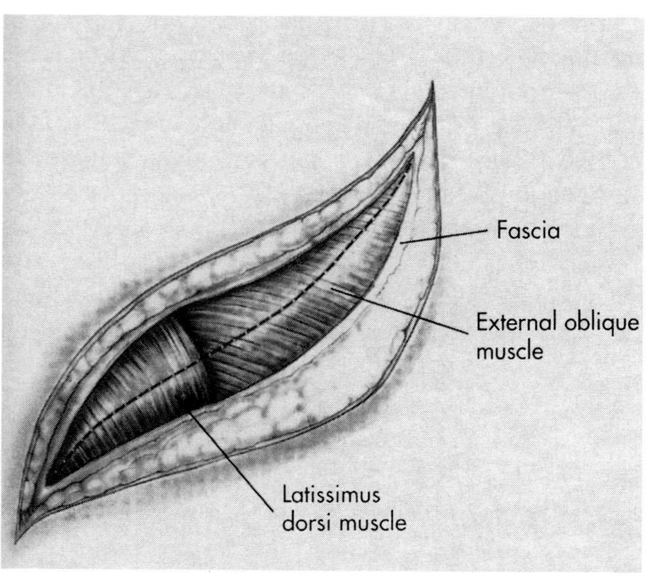

Figure 11.3. Superficial muscle layers encountered during flank incision.

ligament provides for greatly improved exposure. At this point, the intercostal muscle attachments to the upper surface of the rib are carefully divided centimeter by centimeter. Eventually, the intercostal nerve is visualized running on the undersurface of the rib. This nerve can then be used as a landmark to avoid entering the pleural cavity. By entering the investing fascia that lies around the neurovascular bundle, one can stay extrapleural by remaining in this plane. The diaphragmatic attachments to the undersurface of the rib can then be divided.

Gerota's fascia is kept intact and mobilized free away from the psoas and quadratus lumborum muscles, keeping the psoas fascia intact posteriorly. The peritoneum and the diaphragm are freed from Gerota's fascia anteriorly and superiorly. The approach to the hilum is both anterior and posterior, with the renal artery initially digitally identified via its pulsations in the posterior aspect of Gerota's fascia. The artery is ligated followed by vein ligation. The ureter is then ligated and the specimen removed.

With larger tumors or tumors with a large upper pole component, a thoracoabdominal approach may be needed for added exposure. The patient is placed in a modified flank position and the incision is begun over the 10th or 11th rib in the midaxillary line and continued obliquely across the rectus and caudally toward the umbilicus (Figure 11.4). The rectus abdominis muscle is divided along with the external oblique, internal oblique, latissimus dorsi, and transversus abdominis muscles. The exposure to the kidney is the same as the supracostal exposure, except that the pleural cavity is entered underneath the intercostal muscles, taking care not to injure the underlying lung. The diaphragm too is visualized and divided, taking care not to injure the phrenic nerve as it courses along the diaphragm. On the right side, the surface of the liver lies just beneath the

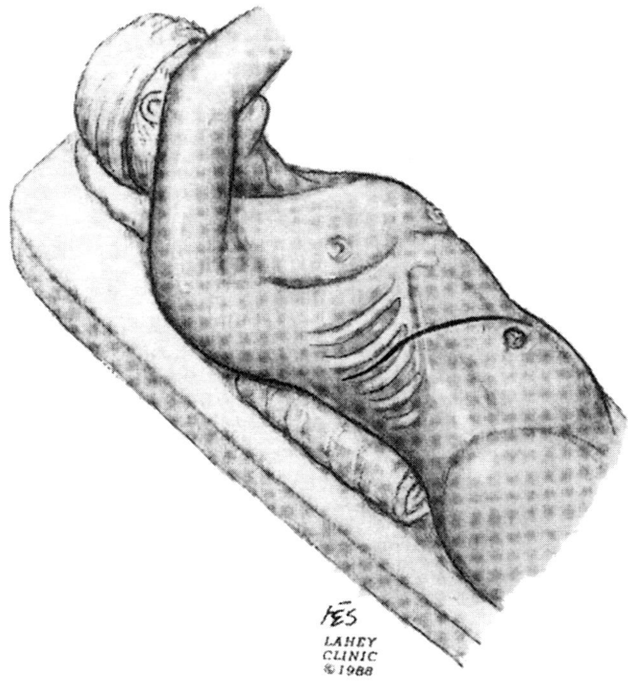

Figure 11.4. Line of incision for thoracoabdominal approach.

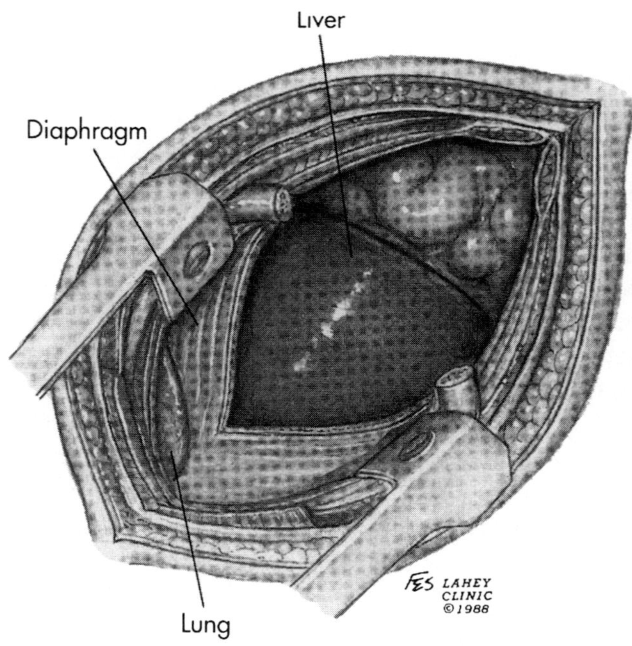

Figure 11.5. Location of liver directly below diaphragm during thoracoabdominal approach.

diaphragm, and on the left side it is the spleen, both of which can be inadvertently injured in the course of division of the diaphragm (Figure 11.5).

CANCER CONTROL WITH RADICAL NEPHRECTOMY

To date, open radical nephrectomy remains the gold standard to which all other extirpative therapies for renal cell carcinoma (RCC) are compared. Robson et al.'s[1] original article details the cancer outcome of 88 cases of RCC treated with radical nephrectomy. In this series, the authors demonstrated an overall 52% five-year survival and a 66% five-year survival for patients with localized disease. Other contemporary series illustrate similar or improved survival to Robson et al.'s series when stratified by stage. Skinner and associates[3] found a very similar 65% five-year survival for Robson stage 1 RCC (organ confined). In the literature, large reported series of radical nephrectomy show between a 65% and 93% five-year survival rates for Robson stage 1 organ confined disease.[4–6] Predictably, overall survival is linked closely with pathologic staging.

CONTROVERSIES IN RADICAL NEPHRECTOMY

Radical Nephrectomy and the Removal of the Ipsilateral Adrenal Gland

Radical nephrectomy, as defined by Robson et al.,[1] required removal of the ipsilateral adrenal gland, as it lies within the "perinephric fat envelope" that they recommend be removed. However, as time has passed, the necessity of this practice has been thrown into question. Currently, it remains a controversial issue. With advancements in cross-sectional imaging, namely computed tomography (CT) and magnetic resonance imaging (MRI), the presence of ipsilateral adrenal extension of tumor can often be delineated.

For this and other reasons, some authors have advocated adrenal sparing radical nephrectomy, in selected cases. Sagalowsky and coworkers,[7] in their review of 695 cases of radical nephrectomy at their institution, noted an overall incidence of ipsilateral adrenal metastasis of 4.3%. They also found that ipsilateral adrenal metastasis was correlated with upper pole tumors, left-sided tumors, advanced pathologic stage, and large tumors replacing the entire kidney. They also found that of the 30 patients with adrenal metastasis, nine (30%) had evidence of widespread metastatic disease. The long-term survival of these patients was uniformly poor; of the 21 patients who underwent surgical resection with adrenal metastasis, 17 died, with 14 of these 17 succumbing of metastatic disease at a mean of 26 months. The authors contention is that the benefit of removing the ipsilateral adrenal during radical nephrectomy is extremely limited. They note that the morbidity associated with adrenal gland removal is not trivial and, in their estimation, the risks probably outweigh the benefits.

In another study, Robey and Schellhammer[8] explored this same issue. They came to a similar conclusion: ipsilateral adrenalectomy does not need to be a routine part of every radical nephrectomy. They found that 5- and 9-year survival was equivalent between those patients who had their adrenal gland removed and those who did not (79% and 65% vs. 78%). Also, if the ipsilateral adrenal is removed, the finding of a contralateral adrenal lesion would leave the patient with lifelong adrenal insufficiency. The authors state that the adrenal gland lies within a separate fascial envelope within Gerota's fascia and that a normal preoperative CT scan should allow selection of those patients in whom adrenal sparing is appropriate. They recommend that patients with a contralateral adrenal lesion found preoperatively should be spared ipsilateral adrenalectomy if that gland is normal on the CT scan. Also, they suggest that those patients with lower pole lesions do not routinely need ipsilateral adrenalectomy. Another factor that leads the authors to advocate this approach is the minimal rates of recurrence RCC in the partial nephrectomy literature.

Winter and coworkers[9] examine this issue and reach a different conclusion. Of 138 patients who underwent radical nephrectomy with concomitant adrenalectomy at their institution, eight were found to have ipsilateral adrenal metastasis. Of those eight, three had solitary adrenal metastases and five had concomitant lymph node metastasis. Those five patients eventually died within 35 months, but the three with solitary adrenal metastasis all survived with a follow-up interval of 4 years. The authors point out that all of these patients had micrometastases to the adrenal gland and were not detectable on preoperative CT imaging. The authors' contention is that with routine ipsilateral adrenalectomy, the three patients with adrenal involvement without lymph node involvement were cured. The authors state that the performance of the concomitant adrenalectomy, in their opinion, adds minimal morbidity. Their recommendation is that routine adrenalectomy should be an integral part of the performance of radical nephrectomy.

Tsui and colleagues[10] come to the conclusion that patients with early-stage RCC typically do not have adrenal involvement, and therefore do not require concomitant adrenalectomy. However, those with higher stage RCC have a much higher incidence of adrenal involvement, with a quoted 8.1% incidence. The authors stress the need for good, cross-sectional imaging studies performed preoperatively to evaluate the adrenal gland. However, given the potential shortcomings of imaging, the authors feel that in high-stage, upper-pole, multifocal RCC tumors, adrenalectomy can potentially eradicate micrometastatic disease.

With the evolution of radical nephrectomy, most authors would agree that adrenalectomy is not a necessary component of the procedure in every single case. Currently, most would agree that it can be safely omitted in those cases with mid- to lower-pole, low clinical stage tumors. However, the data from Winter et al.[9] does give one pause with their findings of micrometastatic disease invisible on cross-sectional imaging, even in cases of mid- to lower-pole, apparently organ-confined disease. One must balance routine removal of the adrenal gland with the possibility that, should the other adrenal gland need to be removed for whatever reason, the patient will need lifelong steroid replacement therapy, which is not a trivial issue. Because of these conflicting findings and opinions, the routine removal of the adrenal gland remains a controversial issue.

Extended Lymphadenectomy During Radical Nephrectomy and Survival Benefit

In the past, various authors have voiced their opinion regarding the benefit of extended lymphadenectomy. Peters and Brown[11] report on their series of patients undergoing radical nephrectomy for RCC, who underwent an extended lymphadenectomy. They specifically looked at those patients with stage C tumors, which include those with tumors extending beyond Gerota's fascia or from the main renal vein into the vena cava, or those having regional lymph node involvement from the diaphragm superiorly to the bifurcation of the common iliac artery inferiorly. When Peters and Brown compared the survival of their patient cohort pathologically staged to stage C, they found that those who had undergone lymphadenectomy had an 87.5% one-year survival and a 43.75% five-year survival. Those who did not undergo lymphadenectomy had a 56.5% one-year survival and 25.69% five-year survival. Therefore, the authors concluded that although their sample size is small ($n = 31$ patients in stage C), there is a suggestion of a survival benefit in those patients undergoing a lymphadenectomy as part of their procedure.

Giuliani and associates[12] presented their data regarding 200 consecutive patients who underwent radical nephrectomy and extended lymphadenectomy for renal cell carcinoma. Their extended lymphadenectomy comprised the paracaval, retrocaval, precaval, interaortocaval, and preaortic lymph node packets for right-sided tumors from the diaphragm to the aortic bifurcation. For left-sided tumors, they removed the paraaortic, preaortic, retroaortic, interaortocaval, and precaval lymph node packets from the diaphragm to the aortic bifurcation. They found that on average, 30 to 40 nodes were removed during their dissection. In their cohort of 20 patients with node-positive disease, without distant metastases, their 5- and 10-year survival was 52% and 26%. On the flip side, once patients were found to have distant metastases, their 5- and 10-year survival was a dismal 7% and 0%, respectively. The authors concluded that given the excellent survival results in the N+ cohort, extended lymphadenectomy had a positive impact upon survival.

In a different light, De Kernion[13] addresses this question as well. He states that the drainage pattern of lymphatic metastases from RCC is neither orderly nor predictable. Part of the problem is that the neovascularity of RCC leads to lymphatic drainage to any point in the retroperitoneum from the diaphragm to the pelvis. This uncertainty makes it difficult to be sure that the lymphadenectomy that is being performed is truly excising the true drainage from the kidney and the tumor. Also, De Kernion points out that the potential morbidity of the lymphadenectomy may not be justified, especially if there is no survival benefit or a very small benefit. Another point is that many patients with node-negative disease die from metastatic disease, suggesting that hematogenous spread of tumor may be the culprit in these cases. If hematogenous spread is indeed contributing to the spread of metastatic RCC, then the benefit of lymphadenectomy is indeed dubious. The author does admit that there are studies in the literature that seem to suggest a survival benefit; however, he states that selection bias may play a role. He points out that in the series by Robson et al.,[1] 5- and 10-year survival rates were approximately 35% for patients with node-positive disease. However, in this series, patients with mediastinal metastases were excluded from the analysis.

In another study, Siminovitch and associates[14] examined 102 patients who underwent variable lymphadenectomy during radical nephrectomy. The extent of lymphadenectomy was dictated by the surgeon during the procedure and was dependent on gross operative findings or personal preference. Nineteen patients had extended lymphadenectomy from the crus of the diaphragm to the aortic bifurcation; 70 received a regional lymphadenectomy defined as the removal of the packet between the hilar vessels to the inferior mesenteric artery; and the remaining 13 patients had either a node biopsy or incidental removal of nodes with the specimen. The authors discovered that of these 102 patients, nine had positive nodes. Of these nine patients, only one was a long-term survivor and that particular individual had minimal involvement, with only one hilar lymph node involved with metastatic disease. The authors conclude that the survival benefit incurred by lymphadenectomy is minimal given the findings of their study.

The overall issue in the above studies is whether lymphadenectomy is therapeutic or primarily beneficial for staging purposes. Marshall[15] believes that given the high rate of incidentally diagnosed tumors and the resultant smaller size of these tumors, lymphadenectomy is less important than it had been in the past, due to less chance of nodal metastases. However, his points echo the above issues. Like De Kernion,[13] he feels that the pattern of nodal drainage from the kidney is variable and not constant and the performance of a lymphadenectomy is somewhat inexact. Also, since RCC metastasizes by both hematogenous and lymphatic routes, if nodal involvement is limited to the regional nodes, then there may be some benefit in removing these nodes, especially in those with limited microscopic disease. However, in those with more extensive nodal metastases, the chance of hematogenously spread distant metastases is high, in which case almost uniformly dismal prognosis awaits. The morbidity in performing an extended lymph node dissection in these cases, Marshall feels, outweighs the benefit.

Pantuck et al.,[16] on a slightly different note, feels that clinically negative nodes do not require resection. However, their viewpoint is that in carefully selected patients with clinically positive nodal disease, a thorough lymphadenectomy followed by cytoreductive nephrectomy and postoperative immunotherapy, may yield a survival benefit.

Thus, although many different viewpoints exist regarding the subject, there is no clear consensus about the necessity or utility of a lymphadenectomy during radical nephrectomy. Given the above data, I believe that most would agree that routine lymphadenectomy during the performance of a radical nephrectomy with clinically negative nodes is not necessary. However, I also believe that given clinical lymphadenopathy in the face of renal cell carcinoma, for staging purposes, those lymph nodes should be removed. Whether or not the removal of such lymph nodes can be curative is debatable.

RENAL CELL CARCINOMA WITH CAVAL THROMBUS

As RCC becomes more advanced in its presentation, it can present many obstacles to its surgical extirpation. One of the characteristics of RCC is the ability of tumor to extend into the venous outflow of the kidney via the renal vein and inferior vena cava. In most published studies, the incidence of this occurrence is approximately 4% to 10% of cases.[17]

The description of surgical extirpation of RCC with caval extension dates back to the early part of the 20th century when Berg[18] described the removal of an RCC with caval extension. When RCC presents in this fashion, the management becomes tailored to the level of caval extension. The level of tumor thrombus can greatly affect whether or not the procedure involved is a relatively minor or, on the contrary, a major undertaking.

Diagnosis and Workup

Assessment of the tumor extent is made upon initial diagnosis of the renal mass, whether that be for incidental reasons or because of signs and symptoms, such as hematuria. Other physical signs that may lead one to suspect caval involvement include a right-sided varicocele, a varicocele that does not regress when the patient lies down, lower extremity edema, or pulmonary embolism. The removal of secondary caval tumor thrombi can be among the most challenging procedures in urologic surgery; therefore, extensive preprocedure planning should be undertaken. Usually a contrast CT scan is obtained for initial cross-sectional imaging. Three-dimensional reconstructions can be helpful to further delineate anatomy. If the CT scan is inconclusive as to caval thrombus extent, an MRI scan can help to better define the superior extent of the tumor. The advantage inherent in CT and MRI is the minimally invasive nature of these radiologic studies.

At our institution, we routinely obtain an MRI to elucidate the extent of tumor thrombus. We have found that a good-quality MRI is invaluable for surgical planning. If the information gleaned from CT and MRI is not conclusive, then a more invasive test such as vena cavography may be necessary. Ultimately, the surgeon must know the superior extent of the thrombus to plan the correct procedure and to decide if the patient needs to be placed on bypass to remove the tumor. Without confident knowledge as to the exact level of tumor thrombus extension, one should not proceed with the surgery. In situations where tumor thrombus appears to be extending into the atrium, transesophageal echocardiography can provide accurate real-time information. If tumor is found to extend above the hepatic veins or into the atrium on preoperative imaging, cardiology and cardiac surgery services are consulted. We generally recommend having a full cardiologic workup done, including a transesophageal echocardiogram (TEE) and a cardiac catheterization in cases of thrombi above the hepatic veins. Clearly, if caval thrombi that are entering the atrium are missed preoperatively, the consequences are not trivial. Namely, if one is not prepared to put a patient on cardiopulmonary bypass (CPB) for a thrombus extending into the atrium, it makes for a complicated intraoperative situation. Therefore, we cannot stress enough the importance of a complete and thorough preoperative investigation.

Preoperatively, our protocol at the Lahey Clinic has been to routinely angioinfarct any patient with caval extension. In doing so, we feel that the advantages are several.

First, during the initial dissection, attention need not be directed solely at ligating the renal artery. Instead, because the renal artery has been thrombosed by the infarction procedure, dissection can proceed at the renal vein. Second, overall blood loss is minimized by devascularizing both the kidney and the tumor. Also, there is a possibility that the angioinfarction can decrease the size of the tumor thrombus, although this possibility is small. A vena cavagram can be performed concurrently with the angioinfarction to confirm the superior extent of tumor. Typically, the angioinfarction is performed by our interventional radiologists, who instill pure ethanol into the renal artery. The patients are then admitted for observation. Usually, the patients experience fevers and flank discomfort postprocedure. On a nephrologic level, we have found also that they also become hyponatremic, due to mechanisms not well understood.[19] The postinfarction syndrome is one that is well described in the literature and consists of fever, pain, and nausea for approximately 36 hours.[20] Also, the use of ethanol instead of Gelfoam as an embolic agent seems to be associated with less complications and postinfarction symptoms.[20]

The patient also undergoes a metastatic workup with a bone scan and CT of the chest, abdomen, and pelvis. The presence of metastatic disease on imaging studies rules out surgical management due to the poor survival observed at our institution.[21]

Technical Aspects

Because of the complexity of the procedure, knowledge of vascular surgical principles is mandatory. Based on general principles, the following general surgical guidelines are recommended. With minimal renal vein thrombus, often the tumor thrombus can be "milked" back into the proximal renal vein and a vascular clamp applied above the level of tumor thrombus. With extensive caval thrombus extending into the right atrium, however, cardiovascular attending support is necessary, with the capability of performing CPB and deep hypothermic circulatory arrest. If the extent of the tumor lies somewhere in between these two extremes, extensive caval surgery will still be required to remove the tumor with adequate vascular control to render the procedure safe.

The surgical approach of the procedure is dictated by the anatomy of the involved structures. Because of the involvement of the vena cava, the procedure should be considered primarily a right-sided one. We have found that the optimal approach, therefore, is one that keeps this principle in mind, even in the case of a left-sided renal tumor. A subcostal chevron incision or a supra-eighth or -ninth rib thoracoabdominal approach offers excellent exposure of the retrohepatic cava and the chest. For left-sided tumors, the incision is carried across the midline to the lateral border of the left rectus abdominis muscle. The second important principle is that the kidney should not be mobilized in its entirety before attempting removal of the caval thrombus. The third important principle is that manipulation of the vena cava and renal vein should be kept to a minimum until a DeWeese clip or substitute can be placed above the tumor thrombus to prevent dislodgment of the thrombus and consequent pulmonary embolism (Figure 11.6). If a DeWeese clip cannot be obtained, a substitute or caval interruption created by using interrupted silk sutures to approximate the front and back walls of the cava together is effective. Initially, the abdominal portion of the incision should be opened and the abdomen and its contents should be carefully palpated and examined to rule out the presence of metastatic disease. If there is gross metastatic disease, the procedure is

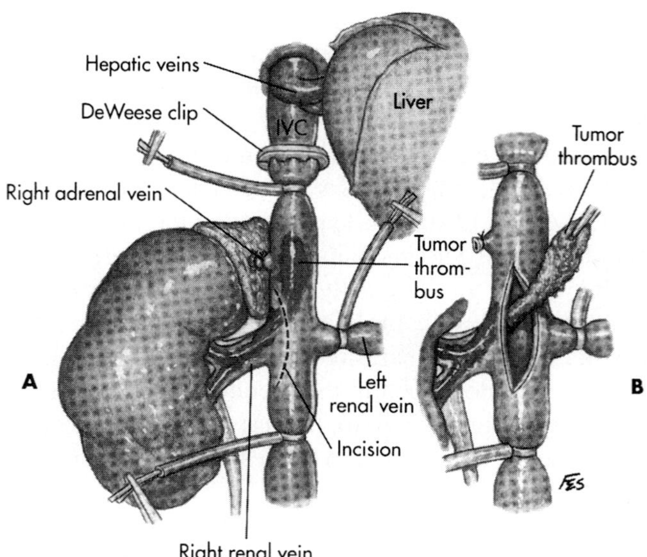

Figure 11.6. (A) Langenbuch maneuver with placement of DeWeese clip, Rummel tourniquets, and subsequent removal of tumor thrombus. (B) Creation of cavotomy with subsequent thrombus removal.

aborted due to a uniformly poor prognosis. If no metastatic disease is palpable, the thoracic portion of the incision is then opened.

For a right-sided tumor, the right colon is mobilized from the cecum to the hepatic flexure. The small bowel is then mobilized superiorly to the ligament of Treitz to effect maximal exposure. The duodenum and pancreas are kocherized medially, exposing the vena cava. The colon and small bowel are then placed into a Lahey bag and placed on the chest wall. In doing this, the superior mesenteric artery (SMA) is elevated and exposes the left renal vein as it crosses over the aorta. One must be careful not to exert too much tension on the SMA to avoid bowel ischemia.

If the tumor involves only the renal vein or a small portion of the vena cava, then usually the tumor thrombus can be milked back into the renal vein or proximal cava and encircled with a Satinsky or C-shaped DeBakey clamp. This allows for removal of the kidney and tumor with a cuff of cava without needing to clamp the vena cava.

If the tumor thrombus extends into the vena cava to a level where it cannot be milked back into this level, then the cava needs to be mobilized to a level above the tip of the tumor thrombus. Depending on the level, the liver may need to be mobilized medially by dividing the right triangular and coronary ligaments and rotating the right lobe of the liver medially as in the Langenbuch maneuver (Figures 11.6 and 11.7). This exposes the retrohepatic cava up to the level of the diaphragm. In exposing this section of cava, one must be cognizant of minor and major hepatic veins, and the minor hepatic veins should be divided to prevent disruption and consequent bleeding.

In performing the procedure, the surgeon must be cognizant of the collateral venous drainage of the kidneys and adrenal glands. The right kidney has little collateral venous drainage, whereas the left kidney has abundant collaterals through the gonadal, adrenal, and lumbar veins. The surgical implications of this pattern of collateral drainage is that the left renal vein can be clamped or divided at the level of the cava with relative impunity if the need arises to resect the vena cava. We ascertain the integrity of venous collaterals by cross-clamping the left renal vein and occluding the right ureter. Failure to observe bluish discoloration of the urine 10 to 12 minutes after the intravenous injection of methylene blue indicates a lack of collateral venous flow. However, in the case of a left nephrectomy with caval tumor extraction, should the need arise for complete resection of the vena cava, the surgeon must create a venous outflow for the right kidney by means of a saphenous vein graft from the right renal vein to either the portal system or the cava above the point of resection.

Because, at our institution, these kidneys are routinely angioinfarcted, early ligation of the renal arterial blood supply is not necessary. The DeWeese clip is placed prior to dissection. The lumbar veins are divided and ligated. Failure to perform this step leads to hemorrhage after cavotomy. In patients with a right renal tumor, depending on the collateral venous outflow, the left renal artery may need to be occluded with a vascular bulldog clamp prior to occluding the left renal vein and vena cava. Dissection is then carried out to mobilize the right kidney in its entirety from its adjacent structures. The infarcted artery is divided and the adrenal vein ligated and divided. After complete mobilization has been achieved, the only structure holding the kidney in place should be the renal vein (Figure 11.6). The renal vein should not be divided or ligated at this point. Umbilical tapes are passed around the cava both above and below the tumor thrombus and cinched down creating Rummel tourniquets. A longitudinal cavotomy is created and the clot removed with blunt dissection or, if needed, a Penfield elevator. The cavotomy is extended down toward the ostium of the right renal vein so that a cuff of vena cava is excised in continuity with the right renal vein. Therefore, the kidney and tumor thrombus are removed en bloc (Figure 11.8). After complete removal of tumor thrombus, the cavotomy is closed with a running 5-0 polypropylene (Prolene) suture. Before the cavotomy is completely closed, the distal caval tourniquet is released to allow for debris and air to be vented from the cavotomy and prevent a pulmonary

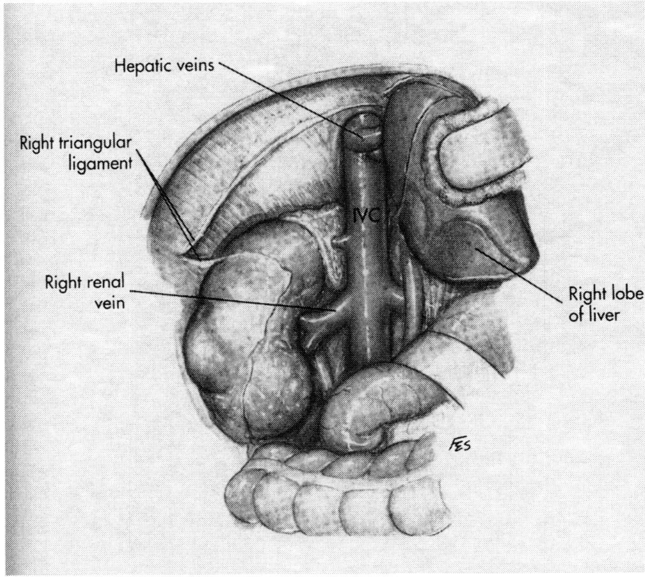

Figure 11.7. Langenbuch maneuver exposing retrohepatic vena cava and hepatic veins.

embolus. The cavotomy is closed and the tourniquets are removed in the following order: proximal cava, left renal vein, left renal artery, and distal cava. If the tumor extends above the hepatic veins, it may be necessary to place a Fogarty vascular clamp on the porta hepatis (Pringle maneuver) to control the arterial and venous inflow into the liver and also across the major hepatic veins to prevent back-bleeding when the cavotomy is created.

When the presence of right atrial tumor thrombus exists, then CPB/deep hypothermia and circulatory arrest (DHCA) must be performed to safely remove the thrombus (Figure 11.9). In the past, this has been performed with median sternotomy and placement of the bypass circuit with arterial return via the ascending aorta and the venous drainage via the superior vena cava and right common femoral vein. The patient is placed on CPB and DHCA with cooling to below 20°C. Circulatory arrest is achieved and the right atrium is opened and explored. The tumor can then be manually pushed caudally into the inferior vena cava. After this maneuver, the complete removal of tumor thrombus is completed by the "shoeshine" maneuver. A sponge is passed through the atriotomy and down into the inferior vena cava and passed to and fro to dislodge any remaining pieces of thrombus. After this is completed, the cavotomy and atriotomy are closed and circulating blood flow restored to the patient. At our institution, we have also utilized venacavoscopy to confirm complete removal of intracaval tumor thrombus. Also, should the need exist, and the tumor is densely adherent to the caval wall, vena caval replacement with Gore-Tex or pericardial patch repair can be instituted.

With the presence of a left-sided tumor, the surgical principles are identical. The difference lies in the exposure of the left kidney, which is still accessed through either a chevron incision or a right thoracoabdominal incision, which is extended across the midline. The collateral network of veins to the left renal vein should be divided, including the left gonadal vein, the left adrenal vein, and any lumbar veins draining into the left renal vein. The tourniquets are placed in the same fashion on the cava, and the right renal artery and vein will also need to be occluded. The removal of tourniquets after cavotomy closure is done in the same order as in the right-sided tumor: venting proximal cava, contralateral vein, contralateral artery, and finally distal cava.

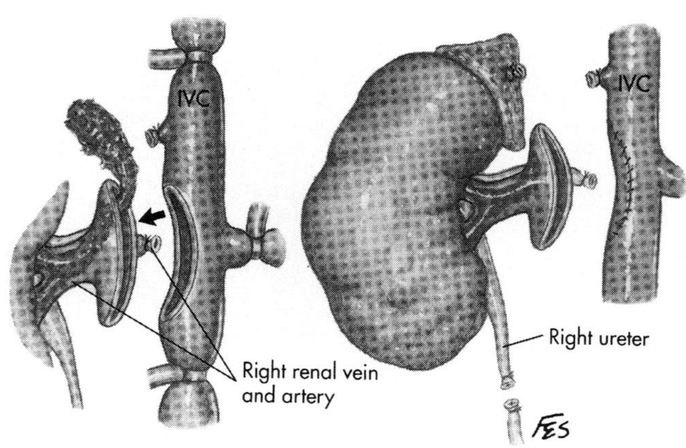

Figure 11.8. Removal of the kidney and tumor thrombus en bloc. IVC, inferior vena cava.

Figure 11.9. Cardiopulmonary bypass (CPB) diagram for tumor thrombus extending into right atrium.

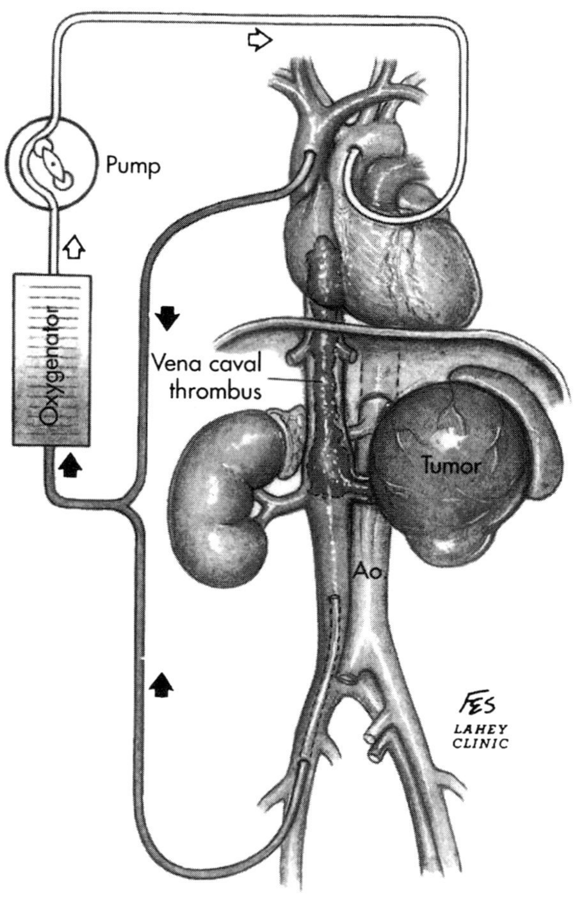

Minimal Access Technique

As mentioned above, since 1997 at our institution,[22] we have developed and described a minimally invasive CPB technique, obviating the need for traditional median sternotomy (Figure 11.10). The kidney is not mobilized but the vena cava is exposed with minimal mobilization. A small 2- to 3-cm incision is made over or under the right clavicle, exposing the right subclavian artery for arterial inflow. A second 2- to 3-cm right parasternal incision exposes the heads of the third and fourth ribs and the pericardium underneath. The pericardium is opened and the right atrium, aorta, and right superior pulmonary vein are exposed. The right subclavian artery is cannulated, and a two-stage venous cannula is inserted into the right atrium with its tip swung up into the superior vena cava via a purse-string suture. Then CPB/DHCA is instituted in the standard fashion.

When the traditional technique of CPB was compared with the minimal access technique in 52 patients, we found with the latter technique that there was a statistically significant decrease in morbidity indices, such as operative time, hospital stay, and transfusion requirements. There was no difference in perioperative mortality. Although there were no statistical differences in survival between the two cohorts, the median

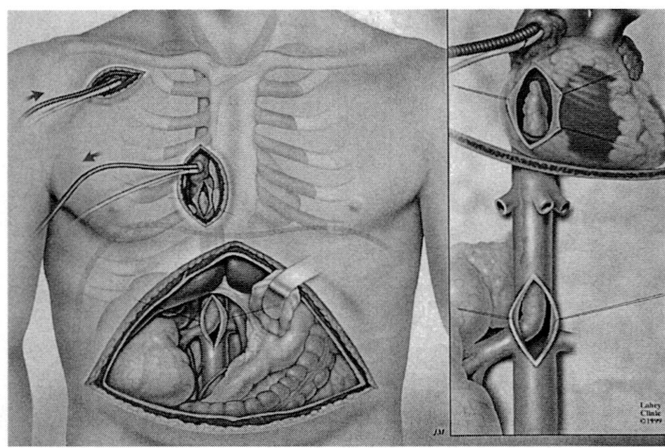

Figure 11.10. The Lahey Clinic's minimally invasive CPB technique, which obviates the need for traditional median sternotomy.

survival of the traditional sternotomy access was 0.62 years and the minimal access group, 2.84 years, which approached statistical significance ($p = .06$).[23]

Survival with Caval Thrombus

Most authors report that between 4% and 10% of patients presenting with RCC have tumor extension into the inferior vena cava. Sogani et al.[24] found in their series of 16 patients a predominance of right-sided tumors, with 12 on the right and four on the left. Kearney et al.[17] also found that most of their patients had right-sided tumors, with 88% of their patients having tumors arising from the right kidney. Historically, the enthusiasm of the surgical management of RCC with caval tumor thrombus has waxed and waned due to variable published survival results. Kearney and associates reported a mean survival of only 21 months and, in their reported series of 24 patients, only four were still alive at last follow-up. On the other hand, if the tumor is surgically resectable and there are no lymph node metastases, survival at 5 years has been reported to be as high as 68%.[25] Sogani and associates reported a 50% survival in those patients with no evidence of metastasis at surgery over a mean duration of 93 months.

At the Lahey Clinic, we have reported survival in these patients in two separate series, the first study showing a survival of 68.8% at 5 years and 60.2% at 10 years in a patient cohort of 32 patients stratified into the ideal and favorable categories.[21] The definition of ideal or favorable was if the disease was not metastatic or had, at most, extension into the perinephric fat, respectively.[21] The more recent study reported an overall survival of 54% at 5 years and 46% at 10 years in a cohort of 100 patients, with an overall median survival of 5.1 years.[26] In 72 of the 100 patients, there was no evidence of nodal or metastatic disease, and the median survival was 21.1 years, with a 5-year survival of 64% and a 10-year survival of 57%. On the other hand, the 28 patients found to have metastatic or nodal disease had a median survival of 2.5 years and a 5-year survival of 20%.

A study by Skinner and associates[27] underscores some important points about RCC with caval thrombus. In their series, if the tumor was confined to Gerota's fascia without regional lymph node involvement, 5- and 10-year survival was 55% and 43%, respectively. But if regional lymph nodes were involved in tumor, there was a dramatic decrease in survival, with 5- and 10-year survival of 16% and 8%, respectively. Also, if there was direct extension to contiguous visceral structures, the 5- and 10-year survivals were dismal, each at 0%.

If the tumor thrombus is not completely removed, there is a poor 5-year survival (17.5%) compared to the 5-year survival with complete removal (68%).[25] However, most large studies have demonstrated acceptable 5- and 10-year survival in such patients in the absence of metastatic disease. Despite a few studies in the literature that report modest survival with adjuvant immunotherapy for metastatic disease in such cases,[28] most other authors report uniformly dismal survival with metastatic disease.[21,29]

The Consequence of Incomplete Tumor Removal

Hatcher et al.[30] performed a retrospective study that underscores the need for complete removal of tumor thrombus, including that thrombus that invades the caval wall. In their series, they found that in those patients with free-floating tumor thrombus that was completely removed with a primary tumor confined to Gerota's fascia, the survival was 69% at 5 years, compared to those patients with tumor invading the caval wall, whose survival was 26% at 5 years. In those patients with caval wall extension of tumor, which was completely resected, the 5-year survival was 57%. The authors' surgical technique included utilizing frozen-section analysis of the cava until a negative margin was obtained. This study underscores other authors' findings that residual tumor thrombus will lead to greatly diminished survival. Neves and Zincke[25] found that in patients with incomplete thrombus removal, 5-year survival was 17.5% as opposed to 68% when thrombus was completely removed. The authors also found that the grade of tumor significantly affected survival, as patients with grade 1 and 2 tumors did significantly better than those with grades 3 and 4 tumors (approximately 70% vs. 40% five-year survival). Skinner and colleagues[31] also found that if a complete tumor resection was not possible, the patients uniformly did poorly, with only 8% survival at 1 year postoperatively.

Does Level of Tumor Thrombus Make a Difference in Survival?

Sosa and colleagues[32] explored the significance of the level of vena caval involvement in overall survival. In their series of 24 patients, the 10 patients who had infrahepatic involvement had a 2-year survival of 80% and a mean survival of 61.4 months, whereas the 14 patients with thrombus to the level of the hepatic veins or above had a 2-year survival of 21% and a mean survival of 22.9 months, suggesting a survival advantage for the lower level of thrombus involvement.

Other authors have not found a difference in survival based on the level of tumor thrombus.[33] At our institution, we examined the prognostic significance of tumor thrombus level in our cohort of 153 patients.[34] We found no statistically significant survival differences based on tumor thrombus level. The 10-year overall cancer-specific survival was 30%, 19%, and 29% for level I, II, and III, respectively ($p = .48$).[34] However, others have found a survival difference based on the level of tumor thrombus. Kim et al.[35] found that patients with T3c disease, meaning tumor extending above the diaphragm, had significantly worse survival than those with tumor involvement below the diaphragm. The authors also found no difference in survival between patients with renal vein involvement of tumor and those with tumor extending below the diaphragm. The question regarding a difference in survival based on tumor thrombus therefore remains unanswered and controversial.

Lymph Node–Positive Disease and Metastatic Tumor in Caval Thrombus

In a study in our institution, we found that patients with caval tumor thrombus and concomitant lymph node involvement or metastatic disease had a median survival of only 1.2 years, with no patient surviving beyond 4.8 years.[21] Skinner et al.[27] showed that if the tumor was confined to Gerota's fascia without regional lymph node involvement, the 5- and 10-year survivals were 55% and 43%, respectively. In their series, however, if regional lymph nodes were involved in tumor, there was a dramatic decrease in survival, with 5- and 10-year survivals at 16% and 8%. Also, if there was direct extension to contiguous visceral structures, 5- and 10-year survivals were dismal, each at 0%. However, most large studies have demonstrated acceptable 5- and 10-year survival rates in such patients in the absence of metastatic disease. Despite a few studies in the literature that reported modest survival with adjuvant immunotherapy for metastatic disease in such cases,[28] most other authors reported uniformly dismal survival with metastatic disease.[21,29]

PULMONARY EMBOLI FORMATION WITH CAVAL THROMBUS

A devastating complication of caval thrombi is pulmonary embolization of tumor. Often, patients presenting with the diagnosis are found to have pulmonary emboli (PEs) during metastatic workup with CT images of the chest. Sometimes these emboli do not produce symptoms and the question arises as to whether or not preoperative anticoagulation will be of any benefit. At our institution, we have come to the conclusion that patients should be routinely anticoagulated before the procedure to decrease the risk of PE. In situations where patients present with large PEs preoperatively, a therapeutic dilemma ensues. In such cases, especially when patients need CPB, the presence of large PEs can provide a hazardous situation due to the increased difficulty in discontinuing CPB in such cases. In the past, we have utilized interventional radiologic vascular dissolution and removal of clot with excellent operative and postoperative results. Such a minimally invasive approach can obviate the need for open clot removal, in and of itself a risky venture, with high morbidity and mortality rates.[36] These procedures have literally saved the lives of patients who presented with this difficult clinical scenario. The possibility of accidental tumor thrombus dislodgment during the procedure also underscores the need of ensuring proximal caval interruption via DeWeese clip or sutures.

Laparoscopic Radical Nephrectomy with Caval Thrombectomy

To date, the open surgical removal of caval thrombi is the gold standard. However, with the recent advances in laparoscopic urologic technique, a laparoscopic approach has been described. Desai and associates[37] report 16 patients who underwent laparoscopic radical nephrectomy in cases with level I renal vein involvement. The technique involves first ligating the renal artery and then using a laparoscopic vascular stapler to ligate the renal vein distal to the visualized bulging tumor thrombus. In certain cases, milking of the tumor thrombus proximal to a more favorable location was required to safely apply the stapler. In all cases, the vascular margin of the renal vein was negative.

In an animal study, a laparoscopic approach to a level III or IV tumor thrombus was simulated and a combined laparoscopic nephrectomy, tumor thrombectomy, CPB with DHCA was accomplished in six male calves.[38] Further future studies are necessary to validate the feasibility of this technique and possible applicability in the clinical realm.

A laparoscopic assisted approach to caval tumor thrombectomy has been reported.[39] The advantage to performing the procedure in this manner is a smaller incision, with potential improved convalescence, although this particular study showed equivalent results to an open series in operative time, blood loss, and hospital stay.[39] Sundaram et al.[40] reported a purely hand-assisted approach performing radical nephrectomy and caval thrombectomy with endoscopic vascular control. The procedure was successfully completed without conversion and with 500 cc of blood loss.

CONCLUSION

The surgical management of RCC is constantly evolving. Optimization of our existing surgical procedures continues, and newer, minimally invasive techniques are being developed. As advancing technology is incorporated, safer techniques are utilized to address more complex clinical cases. Renal cell carcinoma still remains a primarily surgical disease, and at present our techniques that are involved in even difficult cases give patients an ever-improving survival rate.

REFERENCES

1. Robson CJ, Churchill BM, Anderson W. The results of radical nephrectomy for renal cell carcinoma. J Urol 1969;101:297.
2. Turner-Warwick RT. The supracostal approach to the renal area. Br J Urol 1965;37:671–672.
3. Skinner DG, Vermilion CD, Colvin RB. The surgical management of renal cell carcinoma. J Urol 1972;107:705.
4. Selli C, Hinshaw WM, Woodard BH, et al. Stratification of risk factors in renal cell carcinoma. Cancer 1983;52:899.
5. Golimbu M, Joshi P, Sperber A, Tessler A, Al-Askari S, Morales P. Renal cell carcinoma: survival and prognostic factors. Urology 1986;27(4):291–301.
6. McNichols DW, Segura JW, DeWeerd JH. Renal cell carcinoma: long term survival and late recurrences. J Urol 1981;126:17.
7. Sagalowsky AI, Kadesky KT, Ewalt DM, Kennedy TJ. Factors influencing adrenal metastasis in renal cell carcinoma. J Urol 1994;151:1181–1184.
8. Robey EL, Schellhammer PF. The adrenal gland and renal cell carcinoma: is ipsilateral adrenalectomy a necessary component of radical nephrectomy? J Urol 1986;135:453–455.
9. Winter P, Miersch WD, Vogel J, Jaeger N. On the necessity of adrenal extirpation combined with radical nephrectomy. J Urol 1990;144:842–844.
10. Tsui KH, Shvarts O, Barbaric Z, Figlin R, deKernion JB, Belldegrun A. Is adrenalectomy a necessary component of radical nephrectomy? UCLA experience with 511 radical nephrectomies. J Urol 2000; 163:437–441.
11. Peters PC, Brown GL. The role of lymphadenectomy in the management of renal cell carcinoma. Urol Clin North Am 1980;7(3):705–709.
12. Giuliani L, Giberti C, Martorana G, Rovida S. Radical extensive surgery for renal cell carcinoma: long-term results and prognostic factors. J Urol 1990;143:468–474.
13. De Kernion JB. Lymphadenectomy for renal cell carcinoma. Urol Clin North Am 1980; 7(3):697–703.
14. Siminovitch JP, Montie JE, Straffon RA. Lymphadenectomy in renal adenocarcinoma. J Urol 1982;127:1090–1091.
15. Marshall FF. Lymphadenectomy for renal cell carcinoma. BJU Int 2005;95(suppl 2):34.

16. Pantuck AJ, Zisman A, Dorey F, et al. Renal cell carcinoma with retroperitoneal lymph nodes. Impact on survival and benefits of immunotherapy. Cancer 2003;97(12):2995–3002.
17. Kearney GP, Waters WB, Klein LA, Richie JP, Gittes RF. Results of inferior vena cava resection for renal cell carcinoma. J Urol 1981;125:769.
18. Berg AA. Malignant hypernephroma of the kidney. Its clinical course and diagnosis with a description of the author's method of radical operative cure. Surg Gynecol Obstet 1913;17:463.
19. Huang WC, Rhee HK, Mourtzinos AP, et al. Hyponatremia is a potentially serious complication following renal angioinfarction. J Urol 2003;169(4, suppl):abstr 115.
20. Munro NP, Woodhams S, Nawrocki JD, Fletcher MS, Thomas PJ. The role of transarterial embolization in the treatment of renal cell carcinoma. BJU Int 2003;92:240–244.
21. Libertino JA, Zinman L, Watkins E. Long term results of resection of renal cell cancer with extension into inferior vena cava. J Urol 1987;137:21–24.
22. Fitzgerald JM, Tripathy U, Svensson LG, Libertino JA. Radical nephrectomy with vena caval thrombectomy using a minimal access approach for cardiopulmonary bypass. J Urol 1998;159(4):1 292–1293.
23. Wotkowicz C, Libertino JA, Sorcini A, Mourtzinos AP. Management of renal cell carcinoma with vena cava and atrial thrombus: minimal access versus median sternotomy with circulatory arrest. BJU Int 2006;98(2):289–297.
24. Sogani PC, Herr HW, Rains MS, Whitmore WF. Renal cell carcinoma extending into inferior vena cava. J Urol 1983;130:660–663.
25. Neves RJ, Zincke H. Surgical treatment of renal cancer with vena cava extension. Br J Urol 1987;59:390–395.
26. Swierzewski DJ, Swierzewski MJ, Libertino JA. Radical nephrectomy in patients with renal cell carcinoma with venous, vena caval, and atrial extension. Am J Surg 1994;168(2):205–209.
27. Skinner DG, Pfister RF, Colvin R. Extension of renal cell carcinoma into the vena cava: the rationale for aggressive surgical management. J Urol 1972;107:711.
28. Naitoh J, Kaplan A, Dorey F, Figlin R, Belldegrun A. Metastatic renal cell carcinoma with concurrent inferior vena caval invasion: long-term survival after combination therapy with radical nephrectomy, vena caval thrombectomy, and postoperative immunotherapy. J Urol 1999;162:46–50.
29. Suggs WD, Smith RB, Dodson TF, Salam AA, Graham SD. Renal cell carcinoma with inferior vena caval involvement. J Vasc Surg 1991;14:413–418.
30. Hatcher PA, Anderson EE, Paulson DF, Carson CC, Robertson JE. Surgical management and prognosis of renal cell carcinoma invading the vena cava. J Urol 1991;145:20–24.
31. Skinner DG, Pritchett TR, Lieskovsky G, Boyd SD, Stiles QR. Vena caval involvement by renal cell carcinoma. Ann Surg 1989;210(3):387–394.
32. Sosa RE, Muecke EC, Vaughan ED, McCarron JP. Renal cell carcinoma extending into the inferior vena cava: the prognostic significance of the level of vena caval involvement. J Urol 1984;132:1097–1100.
33. Nesbitt JC, Soltero ER, Cinney CPN, et al. Surgical management of renal cell carcinoma with inferior vena cava tumor thrombus. Ann Thorac Surg 1997;63:1592–1600.
34. Moinzadeh A, Libertino JA. Prognostic significance of tumor thrombus level in patients with renal cell carcinoma and venous tumor thrombus extension. Is all T3b the same? J Urol 2004;171: 598–601.
35. Kim HL, Zisman A, Han KR, Figlin RA, Belldegrun A. Prognostic significance of venous thrombus in renal cell carcinoma. Are renal vein and inferior vena cava involvement different? J Urol 2004;171:588–591.
36. Mattox KL, Feldtman RW, Beall AC, DeBakey ME. Pulmonary embolectomy for massive pulmonary embolism. Ann Surg 1982;195(6):726–731.
37. Desai MM, Gill IS, Ramani AP, Matin SF, Kaouk JH, Campero JM. Laparoscopic radical nephrectomy for cancer with level I renal vein involvement. J Urol 2003;169:487–491.
38. Meraney AP, Gill IS, Desai MM, et al. Laparoscopic inferior vena cava and right atrial thrombectomy utilizing deep hypothermic circulatory arrest. J Endourol 2003;17(5):275–282.
39. Varkarakis IM, Bhayani SB, Allaf ME, Inagaki T, Gonzalgo ML, Jarrett TW. Laparoscopic-assisted nephrectomy with inferior vena cava tumor thrombectomy: preliminary results. Urology 2004;64: 925–929.
40. Sundaram CP, Rehman J, Landman J, Oh J. Hand assisted laparoscopic radical nephrectomy for renal cell carcinoma with inferior vena caval thrombus. J Urol 2002;168:176–179.

12 Laparoscopic Radical Nephrectomy

Benjamin I. Chung, Jose R. Colombo, Jr., and Inderbir S. Gill

KEYWORDS

LAPAROSCOPY
RADICAL NEPHRECTOMY
RETROPERITONEOSCOPY
RENAL CELL CARCINOMA

ABSTRACT

Laparoscopic radical nephrectomy (LRN) was first reported by Clayman and associates[1] in 1991. The authors described removing the right kidney of an 85-year-old woman with a 3-cm renal mass. Since then, the procedure has evolved from one that was performed at relatively few centers of excellence to one that has become standard urologic practice in both community and academic centers, and is now considered a standard-of-care procedure for most patients with renal malignancy who are not eligible for a nephron-sparing procedure.

TECHNIQUE

Three methods of LRN are in wide use in clinical practice: transperitoneal approach, retroperitoneal approach, and hand-assisted approach.

The *transperitoneal approach* employs a three- or four-port configuration. The patient is positioned in the flank position, at a 45-degree angle. Access is obtained to the peritoneal cavity with a Veress needle, typically at the most inferior port, at the junction of the lateral border of the rectus abdominal muscle and the line connecting the umbilicus and the anterior-superior iliac spine. The most superior port is typically at the junction between the subcostal margin and the lateral border of the rectus abdominal muscle. The middle port is placed in between these two other ports, preferably at the level of

From: *Clinical Management of Renal Tumors*
Edited by: R.M. Bukowski and A.C. Novick © Humana Press Inc., Totowa, NJ

the renal hilum. If a right-sided nephrectomy is planned, a fourth port is placed at the midline near the xiphoid process to allow for a liver retractor. On the right side, the ascending colon is reflected medially along the avascular line of Toldt. The duodenum is then kocherized medially, exposing the vena cava. More inferiorly, the gonadal vein and ureter are identified running along the psoas muscle. The plane between the ureter and psoas muscle is developed and traced to the level of the renal hilum. The renal artery or arteries are clipped with Hem-o-Lock clips (Weck Closure System, Research Triangle Park, NC) and the vein typically divided with an endoscopic stapler. The specimen is entrapped in a laparoscopic removal sack, and either a Gibson incision or the port site is extended to accommodate removal of the specimen. On the left side, the procedure is the same, except that the duodenum is not encountered and the tail of the pancreas and spleen are mobilized away from Gerota's fascia. The hilar vessels are controlled in the same fashion.

The *retroperitoneal approach* is the one favored at our institution. The patient is placed into the full 90-degree flank position and the table is flexed. A round distention balloon (U.S. Surgical Corp., Norwalk, CT) expands the potential space in the retroperitoneum, and the balloon is inflated between the fascia atop the psoas muscle and the posterior reflection of Gerota's fascia. Approximately 800cc of air is used to distend the balloon. Then the laparoscope is placed into the balloon to ensure that it has been placed into the correct location. Dissection is then carried out in this plane between the psoas muscle and Gerota's fascia, maintaining the psoas fascial layer on top of the psoas muscle during dissection. Because of the possibility of confusion due to the lack of anatomic landmarks, the psoas muscle must be oriented horizontally. Depending on the side of the kidney, either the horizontally placed vena caval or aortic pulsations are used for identification, and then a vertical pulsation is identified, signifying the renal artery. Once the artery is identified and dissected free from surrounding attachments, the vein is usually found anterior and caudal to the artery. In a right-sided procedure, care is taken to identify the renal vein and also the cava, to avoid mistaking the renal vein with the cava.

After the hilum is dissected, the artery can be clamped with Hem-o-Lock clips and the vein divided with an endoscopic vascular stapler. The remainder of the procedure consists of mobilizing Gerota's fascia away from the peritoneal reflection anteriorly and dividing the ureter distally. The adrenal gland may or may not be taken along with the kidney, depending on the size and location of the tumor and the extent of disease. The advantage of this approach is the quick access to the hilum, especially the posteriorly located renal artery and the avoidance of entering the peritoneal cavity, which is especially useful in those patients who have had multiple previous abdominal procedures. In obese patients, the retroperitoneal approach may provide better exposure than the transperitoneal approach. However, we have found that in very obese patients, the retroperitoneal approach can be difficult due to severe limitations in the expansibility of the retroperitoneum. The main disadvantages of the retroperitoneal approach are the limited working space and the lack of landmarks to guide the dissection, which for the novice retroperitoneoscopist can lead to confusion.

The *hand-assisted approach* is one that has been utilized and described by many as a "bridge" to a purely laparoscopic approach. A hand port for the surgeon's nondominant hand is placed usually in the midline either above or below the umbilicus. A transperitoneal approach is usually used because of the larger working space. The steps thereafter are the same as for transperitoneal LRN. The advantages of this approach include direct tactile feedback for the surgeon and the capability of digital dissection and compression. The disadvantages include further decrease in working space for the hand, ergonomic discomfort, and hand discomfort due to the pneumoperitoneum.[2]

SURGICAL APPROACH

The relative advantages and disadvantages of any approach for LRN have been minimally examined. Nambirajan et al.[3] performed a prospective, randomized trial comparing transperitoneal LRN and retroperitoneal LRN; 20 patients were randomized to each group. Demographically and in terms of tumor characteristics, the two groups were equivalent. All procedures were successfully completed laparoscopically, without open conversion. On perioperative and postoperative indices, the authors found that, somewhat surprisingly, all transperitoneal LRN patients tolerated postoperative intake on day 1, compared with only 75% of patients in the retroperitoneal group. Also, this group attempted to use the AESOP (Computer Motion, Inc., Goleta, CA) robotic assist device with both cases and found that although it is easily used with the transperitoneal approach, it could not be used with the retroperitoneal approach. Also, the retroperitoneal approach did take longer, but this was not found to be statistically significant.

The initial feasibility of retroperitoneal LRN was explored by Gaur,[4] who described an insufflated dissecting balloon created from a red rubber catheter and a latex surgeon's glove. Further horizons were explored when Rassweiler et al.[5] described a hydraulic retroperitoneal balloon dissector to expand the potential space. Nadu et al.[6] correlated the retroperitoneal approach with less interference in the ventilatory and hemodynamic functions when comparing to the transperitoneal approach.

At our institution, the retroperitoneal approach is preferred. In a study by Gill et al.,[7] the mean surgical time for retroperitoneoscopic LRN was 2.9 hours, mean tumor size was 4.6 cm, and a mean blood loss was 128 cc. Patients undergoing the procedure had a mean inpatient stay of 1.6 days and a mean analgesic requirement of 31 mg of morphine sulfate equivalent. More recently, Desai et al.[8] also found no statistical differences between the two approaches regarding blood loss, hospital stay, intraoperative and postoperative complications, and analgesic requirements.

When comparing LRN to open radical nephrectomy (ORN), the former entailed significantly less blood loss, shorter hospital stay, fewer analgesic requirements, and shorter convalescence. The complication rate was 17% in the LRN group and 24% in the ORN group.[9] Lee et al.[10] compared hand-assisted LRN to ORN in 54 and 50 patients, respectively. The operative time was statistically equivalent, but the amount of blood loss, the mean days to oral intake, and the mean hospital stay statistically favored the hand-assisted LRN group. No open conversions or major complications occurred in the hand-assist group.

Baldwin et al.[11] also compared the hand-assisted LRN and ORN in patients at high anesthetic risk. The authors concluded that LRN and hand-assisted LRN result in the administration of fewer analgesics and in a faster oral intake when compared to the ORN. In this series, LRN also had a lower cost comparing with the other two techniques.

CONTRAINDICATIONS

General contraindications to the laparoscopic approach include uncorrected coagulopathy and intraabdominal sepsis. In morbidly obese patients, the full flank position required for retroperitoneoscopic LRN allows the pannus to fall away from the flank, thus allowing for less subcutaneous fat to interfere with port placement. Also, with added insufflation to the retroperitoneal balloon dissector, the hilum can be quickly identified and controlled with the retroperitoneal approach. Fugita et al.[12] reported a series of 32 transperitoneal LRN in obese patients, with no significant difference in the outcomes comparing to a group of nonobese patients. Greater insufflation pressure and a lateral shift in trocar site position were recommended in this study.

In our experience, large tumors, even up to 20 cm in size, can be addressed with laparoscopic techniques. Often, these tumors are too large to be entrapped with standard sacks and therefore must be removed without them. An effective incision for removal is a midline, muscle-splitting incision into the linea alba below the umbilicus. After the rectus abdominis muscles are spread, ample space exists for specimen removal and, in general, we find that postoperative discomfort is minimal with the muscle-splitting approach.

Caval thrombi, bulky lymphadenopathy, and locally extensive disease are better addressed with an open approach.

ONCOLOGIC EFFICACY AND OPERATIVE INDICES

Dunn et al.[13] reported 44 LRNs with one open conversion, mean operative time of 5.5 hours, mean blood loss of 172 mL, and an overall transfusion rate of 12%. At a mean follow-up of 25 months, the cancer-specific survival in this series was 91%. Chan et al.[14] presented 66 LRNs, with one conversion, mean blood loss of 289 mL, mean operative time of 4.2 hours, and mean hospital stay of 3.8 days. At a mean follow-up of 35 months, the overall survival and cancer-specific survival were 85% and 95%, respectively.

Ono et al.[15] published a series of 102 LRNs, with four open conversions, mean operative time of 4.7 hours, blood loss of 254 mL, and a transfusion rate of 5%. With a follow-up of 29 months, the estimated 5-year overall and cancer-specific survival was 95%. Portis et al.[16] reported a multiinstitutional analysis of 64 patients undergoing LRN, with a mean operative time of 4.7 hours, blood loss of 219 mL, and hospital stay of 4.8 days. At a mean follow-up of 54 months, the estimated 5-year overall and cancer-specific survival were 81% and 98%, respectively.

In the report of Saika et al.[17] including 195 LRNs, with seven open conversions, mean operative time was 4.6 hours, and mean blood loss was 248 mL. Over a median follow-up of 40 months, both estimated 5-year overall and cancer-specific survival were 94% in this study.

More recently, Permpongkosol et al.[18] analyzed 67 LRNs, with median follow-up of 73 months, with two of major complications (37%), including one case of open conversion, mean blood loss of 280 mL, operative time of 4.2 hours, and hospital stay of 3.8 days. The projected 10-year overall and cancer-specific survival were 97% and 76%, respectively, in this study (Table 12.1).

At our institution, a series with 63 LRNs with a median follow-up of 65 months showed 5-year overall, cancer-specific, and recurrence-free survivals of 78%, 91%, and

Table 12.1.
Laparoscopic radical nephrectomy oncological outcomes

Author	n	Follow-up (years)	Conversion	Minor/major complication	Recurrence-free survival	Projected 5-year cancer-specific survival	5-year overall survival	CRI
Dunn 2000[13]	44	2.1	1	34%/3%	N/A	91%	N/A	N/A
Chan 2001[14]	66	2.9	1	12%/3%	N/A	95%	85%	N/A
Ono 2001[15]	102	2.4	4	N/A/10%	N/A	95%	95%	N/A
Portis 2002[16]	64	4.5	N/A	N/A /N/A	92%	98%	81%	N/A
Saika 2003[17]	195	3.3	7	9%/5%	N/A	94%	94%	N/A
Permpongkosol 2005[18]	67	6	1	12%/3%	N/A	97%*	85%	N/A
Colombo Jr (submitted)[19]	48	5.4	0	20%/3%	91%	91%*	78%	8%

*Actual 5-year survival.
CRI, chronic renal insufficiency.
Source: Adapted from Colombo et al.[19]

91%, respectively, while the 7-year overall, cancer-specific, and recurrence-free survivals were 72%, 91%, and 91%, respectively. Local renal fossa recurrence developed in one patient (2%) in the LRN group with a pT4N0 sarcomatoid tumor invading the psoas muscle and negative surgical margins; this patient died at 17 months from metastatic disease. The mean interval to development of metastatic disease was 19 months (8 to 32) (Table 12.1).[19]

Steinberg et al.[20] examined the relation of increasing size on the performance of LRN. They compared LRN groups stratified by tumors 7 cm or less (LAPT1), greater than 7 cm in size (LAPT2), and an ORN group with tumors greater than 7 cm in size (OpenT2). The authors discovered that the LAPT1 and LAPT2 groups were equivalent in operative time, analgesic requirements, hospital stay, convalescence, and complications. The blood loss was found to be significantly higher in the LAPT2 group than in LAPT1. When LAPT2 and OpenT2 were compared, blood loss, operative time, and hospital stay were shorter and convalescence was more rapid in LAPT2.

Dunn et al.'s[13] study also stratified the LRN cohort by size, comparing those with tumors less than 4 cm to those with tumors 4 to 10 cm in size. The two groups were compared over demographic, operative, and convalescent data. The authors found that there were no statistically significant differences found in every variable, including blood loss, operative time, hospital stay, analgesic use, and weeks to full recovery.

FUNCTIONAL OUTCOMES

The renal functional results comparing LRN and ORN were performed at the authors' institution. After a median follow-up of 51 months, compared to preoperative serum creatinine and estimated creatinine clearance, postoperative values deteriorated significantly and comparably within the LRN and ORN groups (p <.005 for each). (Table 12.2) At last follow-up, a serum creatinine level >1.5 mg/dL was noted in 21% and 33% patients in the LRN and ORN groups, respectively. Over the long-term, renal functional outcomes were similar in the LRN and ORN groups, with serum creatinine increasing by 33% and 25%, and estimated creatinine clearance decreasing by 31% and 23% from baseline, respectively. Chronic renal insufficiency developed in 4% of patients in each group.[19]

Table 12.2.
Renal function outcome at median follow-up of 51 months (18–80 months)

| | *Preoperative* | | *Postoperative* | | p-*value* | |
	LRN	*ORN*	*LRN*	*ORN*	*Between groups*	*Within groups*
Serum creatinine (mg/dL)	1.0 ± 0.3	1.0 ± 0.3	1.4 ± 0.4	1.3 ± 0.3	0.89	<0.05*
Estimated creatinine clearance (mL/min)**	91 ± 32	99 ± 40	58 ± 17	75 ± 32	0.80	<0.05*

*For both groups.
**Lean body mass [140—age (yrs)]/(stable serum creatinine)^2 (multiply by 0.85 for women).
LRN, laparoscopic radical nephrectomy; ORN, open radical nephrectomy.
Source: Adapted from Colombo et al.[19]

SPECIMEN EXTRACTION

Another issue of contention that is unique to LRN is the removal of the specimen. The specimen can be removed intact either by extending the port-site incision, creating a new incision, or, in the case of hand-assisted LRN, by removing the kidney from the hand port. Another method of removal is morcellating the kidney within a specialized morcellation sack, thus obviating the need for lengthening the port incisions. This appears to be an obvious advantage of morcellation. However, the disadvantages of morcellation are obvious as well, including the inability to obtain accurate pathologic staging, the potential for injury to intraabdominal organs during the morcellation process, and spillage of tumor into the peritoneal or retroperitoneal space.[21]

A recent prospective study performed by Varkarakis et al.[22] showed that there was no significant advantage in pain, operating time, or duration of hospital stay when specimens were morcellated versus removed intact. Cohen et al.,[23] in a retrospective study, found that 21.9% of their patients with clinical stage T1 or T2 disease were understaged when the final pathologic stage was ascertained. Given these results, despite the cosmetic benefit, there seems to be little data to recommend morcellation over intact extraction, given the potential risk for major complications.

Vaginal extraction of specimen has been reported.[24] In 10 select female patients, LRN specimen was extracted vaginally in patients. Of note, in five patients, previous uterine surgery had been performed, including hysterectomy in three patients and cesarean section in two. Each specimen was successfully removed transvaginally by locating the posterior fornix laparoscopically via a vaginal sponge stick. A colpotomy was created laparoscopically and, after specimen extraction, the colpotomy was closed transvaginally. No intraoperative or postoperative complications occurred and postoperative questionnaires indicated excellent satisfaction.

Typically, the specimen is removed by a Gibson incision in both transperitoneal and retroperitoneal approaches. In cases where a large specimen must be removed from the retroperitoneal space, we perform an intentional peritoneotomy and then use the larger working space to entrap and remove the specimen. Matin and Gill[25] described a novel way of removing the kidney after retroperitoneal LRN. Using a Pfannenstiel incision, the pelvic extraperitoneal space is manually developed up to the upper retroperitoneum, and after specimen entrapment the kidney is removed from the Pfannenstiel incision, affording improved cosmesis.

COMPLICATIONS

In large LRN series, various complication rates have been reported. Dunn et al.[13] reported a minor complication rate of 34% and a major complication rate of 3% in a series of 44 LRNs. Chan et al.,[14] in their series of 66 LRNs, had a 15% rate of overall complications, with a blood transfusion rate of 8%. Saika et al.[17] reported that intraoperative complications occurred in 10%, and postoperative complications occurred in 5% of patients, in a series of 195 LRNs.

Siqueira et al.[26] published a study addressing complications with 213 laparoscopic nephrectomies, with 61 LRNs. The open conversion rate was 6.1%, transfusion rate was 1.9%, and mortality rate was 0.5%. Shuford et al.[27] reported a complication rate in an LRN series of 12%, compared to 10% and 17% of open and hand-assisted laparoscopic nephrectomies, respectively.

A series with 628 LRNs at our institution showed a perioperative complication rate of 14% (95% confidence interval [CI], 11.5–16.9). Intraoperative complications occurred in 5.8% of the cases (95% CI, 4.3–8), with 3.3% of hemorrhage and 1.9% of visceral injury. Four cases were converted to open surgery. Postoperative complications occurred in 8.2% (95% CI, 7–10.7). Ileus, hemorrhage, and acute renal failure were the more frequent postoperative complications in this series.[28]

SPECIAL SITUATIONS

To date, the open surgical removal of renal vein/caval thrombi is the gold standard. However, with the recent advances in laparoscopic urologic technique, a laparoscopic approach has been described. The technique involves first ligating the renal artery. The renal vein is then dissected as completely as possible toward the vena cava to ensure that an adequate length of tumor free renal vein will be ligated. Usually, the tumor thrombus is clearly visible bulging the renal vein, as the vein is usually relatively flat during pneumoperitoneum. Then, using a laparoscopic vascular stapler, the renal vein is ligated proximal to the visualized, bulging tumor thrombus. In certain cases, "milking" of the tumor thrombus distally to a more favorable location may be required to safely apply the stapler. Desai et al.[29] report 16 patients who underwent laparoscopic radical nephrectomy in cases with level I renal vein involvement. In all cases, the vascular margin of the renal vein was negative. In an animal study, a laparoscopic approach to a level III or IV tumor thrombus was simulated and a combined laparoscopic nephrectomy, tumor thrombectomy, and cardiopulmonary bypass with deep hypothermic circulatory arrest was accomplished in six male calves.[30] Further future studies are necessary to validate the feasibility of this technique and possible applicability in the clinical realm.

Hsu et al.[31] report utilizing a similar technique as described above to remove a level I right renal vein thrombus, but with the addition of a laparoscopic ultrasound probe to confirm the proximal extent of tumor thrombus. The procedure was completed successfully by using the endoscopic stapler to divide the right renal vein proximal to the thrombus. Margins were negative and no intraoperative or postoperative complications occurred.

A pilot study examining this issue reviewed 11 patients who underwent LRN, comparing to 19 patients who underwent ORN for *cytoreductive nephrectomy*. The authors found that the procedure was feasible and that there was no difference between the groups with regard to surgical complications and renal tumor size.[32] Also, the patients who underwent tumor morcellation had the shortest interval postoperatively to undergoing immunotherapy, the shortest time to discharge, and the lowest postoperative narcotic requirements. Rabets et al.[33] examined a series with 22 patients who had undergone LRN for cytoreductive purposes prior to immunotherapy for metastatic disease. This group was compared to a contemporary group of 42 patients with equivalent disease characteristics, who had undergone an ORN. The two groups were equivalent in regard to operative time and complications, but the laparoscopic group had significantly less blood loss and shorter hospital stay, and the patients received their systemic therapy on average almost a month sooner than their ORN counterparts. The mean tumor size was larger in the ORN group overall (9.5 cm vs. 7.9 cm). Although the performance of this surgery can present technical challenges, including perihilar adenopathy, local invasion of tumor, and parasitic vasculature, both studies support the feasibility and applicability of the laparoscopic approach in this population of patients.

CONCLUSION

Laparoscopic radical nephrectomy is a technique that, despite its relatively recent inception, has gained wide acceptance worldwide for the treatment of renal cell carcinoma. It is practiced both in academic and community settings and provides the benefits of similar oncologic outcomes combined with greatly decreased hospital length of stay and convalescence. It can be performed via a variety of surgical approaches and probably represents the most widely disseminated minimally invasive urologic procedure practiced today. With increasing experience and technologic advances, the performance of this procedure will continue to become more refined and widen the already broad indications for removing renal masses from a minimally invasive, laparoscopic approach.

REFERENCES

1. Clayman RV, Kavoussi LR, Soper NJ, et al. Laparoscopic nephrectomy: initial case report. J Urol 1991;146:278.
2. Saranchuk JW, Savage SJ. Laparoscopic radical nephrectomy: current status. BJU Int 2005;95(suppl 2):21.
3. Nambirajan T, Jeschke S, Al-Zahrani H, et al. Prospective, randomized controlled study: transperitoneal laparoscopic versus retroperitoneoscopic radical nephrectomy. Urology 2004;64:919.
4. Gaur DD. Laparoscopic operative retroperitoneoscopy: use of a new device. J Urol 1992;148: 1137–1139.
5. Rassweiler JJ, Henkel TO, Stoch C, et al. Retroperitoneal laparoscopic nephrectomy and other procedures in the upper parietoperitoneum using a balloon dissection technique. Eur Urol 1994;25:229–236.
6. Nadu A, Ekstein P, Szold A, et al. Ventilatory and hemodynamic changes during retroperitoneal and transperitoneal laparoscopic nephrectomy: a prospective real-time comparison. J Urol 2005;174(3):1013–1017.
7. Gill IS, Schweizer D, Hobart MG, Sung GT, Klein EA, Novick AC. Retroperitoneal laparoscopic radical nephrectomy: the Cleveland Clinic experience. J Urol 2000;165:1665–1670.
8. Desai MM, Strzempkowski B, Matin SF, et al. Prospective randomized comparison of transperitoneal versus retroperitoneal laparoscopic radical nephrectomy. J Urol 2005;173:38–41.
9. Gill IS, Meraney AP, Schweizer DK, et al. Laparoscopic radical nephrectomy in 100 patients. A single center experience from the United States. Cancer 2001;92(7):1843–1855.
10. Lee SE, Ku JH, Kwak C, Kim HH, Paick SH. Hand assisted laparoscopic radical nephrectomy: comparison with open radical nephrectomy. J Urol 2003;170:756–758.
11. Baldwin DD, Dunbar JA, Parekh DJ, et al. Single-center comparison of purely laparoscopic, hand-assisted laparoscopic, and open radical nephrectomy in patients at high anesthetic risk. J Endourol 2003;17(3):161–167.
12. Fugita OE, Chan DY, Roberts WW, Kavoussi LR, Jarrett TW. Laparoscopic radical nephrectomy in obese patients: outcomes and technical considerations. Urology 2004;63(2):247–252.
13. Dunn MD, Portis AJ, Shalhav AL, et al. Laparoscopic versus open radical nephrectomy: a 9 year experience. J Urol 2000;164:1153–1159.
14. Chan DY, Cadeddu JA, Jarrett TW, Marshall FF, Kavoussi LR. Laparoscopic radical nephrectomy: cancer control for renal cell carcinoma. J Urol 2001;166:2095–2100.
15. Ono Y, Kinukawa T, Hattori R, Gotoh M, Kamihira O, Ohshima S. The long term outcome of laparoscopic radical nephrectomy for small renal cell carcinoma. J Urol 2001;165:1867–1870.
16. Portis AJ, Yan Y, Landman J, et al. Long-term followup after laparoscopic radical nephrectomy. J Urol 2002;167:1257.

17. Saika T, Ono Y, Hattori R, et al. Long-term outcome of laparoscopic radical nephrectomy for pathologic T1 renal cell carcinoma. Urology 2003;62:1018.
18. Permpongkosol S, Chan DY, Link RE, et al. Long-term survival analysis after laparoscopic radical nephrectomy. J Urol 2005;174:1222.
19. Colombo JR Jr, Haber GP, Lane B, Jelovsek JE, Novick A, Gill IS. Seven years after laparoscopic radical nephrectomy: oncologic and renal functional outcomes. J Urol (submitted).
20. Steinberg AP, Finelli A, Desai MM, et al. Laparoscopic radical nephrectomy for large (greater than 7 cm, T2) renal tumors. J Urol 2004;172:2172–2176.
21. Novick AC. Laparoscopic radical nephrectomy: specimen extraction. BJU Int 2005;95(suppl 2):32.
22. Varkarakis I, Rha K, Hernandez F, Kavoussi LR, Jarrett TW. Laparoscopic specimen extraction: morcellation. BJU Int 2005;95(suppl 2):27–31.
23. Cohen DD, Matin SF, Steinberg JR, Zagone R, Wood CG. Evaluation of the intact specimen after laparoscopic radical nephrectomy for clinically localized renal cell carcinoma identifies a subset of patients at increased risk for recurrence. J Urol 2005;173:1487–1491.
24. Gill IS, Cherullo EE, Meraney AM, Borsuk F, Murphy DP, Falcone T. Vaginal extraction of the intact specimen following laparoscopic radical nephrectomy. J Urol 2002;167:238–241.
25. Matin SF, Gill IS. Modified Pfannenstiel incision for intact specimen extraction after retroperitoneoscopic renal surgery. Urology 2003;61:830–832.
26. Siqueira TM Jr, Kuo RL, Gardner TA, et al. Major complications in 213 laparoscopic nephrectomy cases: the Indianapolis experience. J Urol 2002;168(4 pt 1):1361–1365.
27. Shuford MD, McDougall EM, Chang SS, LaFleur BJ, Smith JA Jr, Cookson MS. Complications of contemporary radical nephrectomy: comparison of open vs. laparoscopic approach. Urol Oncol 2004;22(2):121–126.
28. Colombo JR Jr, Haber GP, Jelovsek JE, Gill IS. Complications in laparoscopic surgery for urologic cancer. J Urol (submitted).
29. Desai MM, Gill IS, Ramani AP, Matin SF, Kaouk JH, Campero JM. Laparoscopic radical nephrectomy for cancer with level I renal vein involvement. J Urol 2003;169(2):487–491.
30. Meraney AM, Gill IS, Desai MM, et al. Laparoscopic inferior vena cava and right atrial thrombectomy utilizing deep hypothermic circulatory arrest. J Endourol 2003;17(5):275–282.
31. Hsu THS, Jeffrey RB, Chon C, Presti JC. Laparoscopic radical nephrectomy incorporating intraoperative ultrasound for renal cell carcinoma with renal vein tumor thrombus. Urology 2003;61:1246–1248.
32. Walther MM, Lyne JC, Libutti SK, Linehan WM. Laparoscopic cytoreductive nephrectomy as preparation for administration of systemic interleukin-2 in the treatment of metastatic renal cell carcinoma: a pilot study. Urology 1999;53:496–501.
33. Rabets JC, Kaouk J, Fergany A, Finelli A, Gill IS, Novick AC. Laparoscopic verus open cytoreductive nephrectomy for metastatic renal cell carcinoma. Urology 2004;64:930–934.

13 Open Nephron-Sparing Surgery for Renal Cell Carcinoma

Andrew C. Novick

KEYWORDS

KIDNEY CANCER
RENAL CELL CARCINOMA
TUMOR
NEPHRON-SPARING SURGERY
PARTIAL NEPHRECTOMY
OPEN SURGERY

ABSTRACT

Partial nephrectomy or nephron-sparing surgery (NSS) provides effective curative therapy for patients with localized renal cell carcinoma. In patients with imperative indications, it represents an alternative to renal replacement therapy. For selected patients with systemic comorbidities that threaten global renal function, NSS preserves unaffected nephrons with excellent cancer-specific survival. Elective partial nephrectomy for patients with a small (≤4 cm), unifocal tumor, and a normal contralateral kidney is associated with a low risk (0% to 3%) of local recurrence and cancer-specific survival rates of 90% to 100%. Comparisons between radical and partial nephrectomy demonstrates equivalent cancer control over 5 years.

Surgical resection remains the standard treatment for renal cell carcinoma (RCC). The concept of wide excision of the affected kidney outside its investing (Gerota's) fascia to include the perirenal fat and ipsilateral adrenal gland has dictated surgical thinking and management of this tumor for over a half a century. Compared to simple nephrectomy, this approach was favored due to the recognition that extrarenal involvement of the adjacent perirenal fat and adrenal gland may contribute to surgical failure, thus necessitating the maintenance of anatomic planes of resection in order to obtain the widest surgical margin possible. Today, a better understanding of the biology of RCC, standardized staging, and changing patterns of presentation for patients with this tumor permit a refined surgical approach, limiting potential long-term morbidity by maximizing preservation of functional renal parenchyma.

From: *Clinical Management of Renal Tumors*
Edited by: R.M. Bukowski and A.C. Novick © Humana Press Inc., Totowa, NJ

Nephron-sparing treatment of renal tumors dates to the 1800s, when Wells[1] described the technique for removal of a perirenal fibrolipoma. In 1887, Czerny was the first to use partial nephrectomy for therapy of a renal malignancy.[2] The initial enthusiasm for this approach abated after significant problems were encountered with renal bleeding, urinary fistulas, and postoperative death. Such postoperative morbidity limited utilization of nephron-sparing techniques until 1950, when Vermooten[3] suggested that peripheral encapsulated renal neoplasms could be locally excised, leaving a margin of normal parenchyma around the tumor. Following the observations by Robson et al.[4] of better survival rates after extrafascial nephrectomy, the use of partial nephrectomy in patients with RCC fell into disfavor. Since that time, radical nephrectomy has remained the standard against which all other forms of surgical treatment for RCC must be measured.

Interest in nephron-sparing surgery (NSS) has been stimulated by several developments, including advances in renal imaging, improved surgical techniques and methods to prevent ischemic renal injury, better postoperative management including renal replacement therapy, and long-term prospective cancer-free survival data. Extended experience has now established that NSS can be performed safely, with low morbidity and low local recurrence rates, high patient satisfaction,[5,6] and equal cost-effectiveness to radical nephrectomy.[7]

INDICATIONS FOR NEPHRON-SPARING SURGERY

Standard indications for NSS fall into three categories: absolute, relative, and elective. Absolute indications for NSS include circumstances where radical nephrectomy would render the patient anephric, with the subsequent immediate need for dialysis. This encompasses patients with bilateral RCC or RCC involving a solitary functioning kidney, whether resulting from unilateral renal agenesis, prior removal of the contralateral kidney, or irreversible impairment of contralateral renal function. Patients with bilateral synchronous renal tumors also have an absolute indication for NSS, and an attempt should be made to preserve as much functioning parenchyma as possible. Preservation involves performing bilateral partial nephrectomy when feasible, usually as a staged procedure with the less involved side done first. When partial nephrectomy is not indicated on one side due to tumor size or anatomy, initial partial nephrectomy is performed as a separate procedure on the less involved side, followed by contralateral radical nephrectomy. Such an ordering precludes the need for temporary dialysis in the immediate postoperative period should acute tubular necrosis arise following partial nephrectomy, and it also affords flexibility when preparing the contralateral operation.[8]

Relative indications for NSS include patients with unilateral RCC and a functioning opposite kidney, and when the opposite kidney is affected by a condition that might threaten its future function, such as calculus disease, chronic pyelonephritis, renal artery stenosis, and ureteral reflux, or systemic diseases such as diabetes and nephrosclerosis. In such patients, the risks and benefits of NSS must be considered in the context of the general clinical status including age, comorbidities, risk of disease progression, and the possibility that these conditions will negatively affect remaining renal function.[8]

Relative indications for NSS also include patients with hereditary forms of RCC such as von Hippel–Lindau (VHL) disease, where there is a high likelihood of subsequent lesions developing in the remaining renal parenchyma. The natural history of RCC in patients with VHL differs from sporadic RCC in that the diagnosis is made at a younger age, and there usually are multiple bilateral renal tumors.[9] In patients with VHL or other hereditary renal malignancies, NSS is offered based on the genetic predisposition to recurrence. Furthermore, preservation of renal function in young patients often poses an important clinical concern.

Elective indications for NSS include patients with localized unilateral RCC and a normal contralateral kidney. Studies have clarified the role of NSS in such patients.[10–14] With evolving longer-term data, a size criterion has gained gradual acceptance for elective NSS. Data from our institution[15] as well as from the Mayo Clinic[16] and Memorial Sloan-Kettering Cancer Center[17] indicate that radical nephrectomy and NSS provide equally effective curative treatment for such patients who present with a single, small (<4 cm), and clearly localized RCC. The results of NSS are less satisfactory in patients with larger (≥4 cm) or multiple localized RCCs, and radical nephrectomy should remain the treatment of choice in such cases when the opposite kidney is normal.

Except in exceptional circumstances, NSS is contraindicated in the presence of lymph node metastasis because the prognosis for these patients is poor. Enlarged or suspicious looking lymph nodes should be biopsied before initiating the renal resection.

PREOPERATIVE EVALUATION

Evaluation of patients with RCC prior to NSS must include a detailed history and physical examination, a laboratory evaluation including serum creatinine, liver function tests, and urinalysis or urine dipstick check to screen for preoperative proteinuria. Radiographic testing is used to rule out locally extensive or metastatic disease, including chest x-ray and abdominal computed tomography (CT) as well as possible bone scan and chest or head CT depending on the clinical circumstances.

However, NSS is technically challenging and requires a more detailed understanding of renal anatomy than en bloc removal of the kidney by radical nephrectomy.[18] Knowledge of the relationship of the tumor to the collecting system and adjacent normal parenchyma, and of the renal and tumor vascular supply is essential for preoperative planning. Therefore, more extensive and invasive preoperative imaging studies are often necessary before NSS. These include renal CT, arteriography, and occasionally venography. Arteriography has been used to delineate the intrarenal vasculature and may aid in excision of the tumor while minimizing blood loss and injury to normal adjacent parenchyma. It is most useful for nonperipheral tumors encompassing two or more renal arterial segments. Selective renal venography is performed in patients with large or centrally located tumors to evaluate the presence of intrarenal venous thrombosis and assess adequacy of venous drainage of the planned renal remnant. These studies provide a two-dimensional map to aid complete excision of tumors, assess arterial and venous involvement, and plan complex reconstruction of the renal remnant. However, these studies yield only limited information on the anatomic spatial relationships among the tumor, normal renal parenchyma, collecting system, and vascular supply. Furthermore, the risks and costs of conventional arteriography or venography are not insignificant.

Computed tomography is widely accepted as the preferred imaging technique for detecting and staging RCC because of its low cost, high accuracy, and ready accessibility.[19] Advances in helical CT image acquisition and computer technology allow production of high-quality three-dimensional (3D) images of the renal vasculature and soft tissue anatomy.[20,21] The latest development in 3D imaging is volume rendering, which allows real-time interactive stereoscopic viewing and presents complex anatomy not possible with conventional axial CT. By combining helical CT and 3D volume rendering, a single noninvasive preoperative test has the potential to provide all of the critical information needed for planning and intraoperative management of renal mass lesions. New volume-rendering software allows real-time interactive stereoscopic viewing of these images and provides a topographical map of the renal surface and multiplanar views of the intrarenal anatomy. This permits evaluation of the complex renal anatomy using a single, unified study in a format that is familiar to the surgeon and consistent with intraoperative findings, thereby obviating the need for mental reconstruction of several 2D imaging studies. A detailed prospective study at the Cleveland Clinic demonstrated the utility of 3D volume-rendering CT in accurately depicting the renal parenchyma and vascular anatomy necessary for the performance of NSS.[22] The data from 3D CT integrate essential information from angiography, venography, excretory urography, and conventional 2D CT into a single preoperative staging test that diminishes the need for more invasive imaging. The use of a 3- to 5-minute videotape in the operating room provides concise, accurate, and immediate 3D information to the surgeons during the dissection, allowing them to anticipate the subtleties of the anatomy. The 3D volume-rendered CT has become the imaging modality of choice prior to NSS, allowing hilar dissection, tumor removal, and reconstruction to proceed quickly and confidently.

OPERATIVE TECHNIQUE

It is usually possible to perform open partial nephrectomy for malignancy in situ by using an operative approach that optimizes exposure of the kidney and by combining meticulous surgical technique with an understanding of the renal vascular anatomy in relation to the tumor.[18] Generally an extraperitoneal flank incision through the 11th and 12th ribs is preferred. Occasionally a thoracoabdominal incision is utilized for very large tumors involving the upper portion of the kidney. These incisions allow the surgeon to operate on the mobilized kidney almost at skin level and provide excellent exposure of the peripheral renal vessels. With an anterior subcostal transperitoneal incision, the kidney is invariably located in the depth of the wound, and the surgical exposure is not as good.

The kidney is mobilized within Gerota's fascia, leaving the perirenal fat around the tumor undisturbed. The surface of the kidney is then evaluated for small abnormalities that may occasionally be missed by noninvasive imaging. In most cases, and in particular with large or intrarenal tumors, temporary occlusion of the renal artery is useful for decreasing bleeding and renal tissue turgor. For central tumors the renal vein is also temporarily occluded. To prevent renal ischemic injury, the patient is briskly hydrated and mannitol is given intravenously 5 to 10 minutes before arterial occlusion to decrease intracellular swelling. It is readministered after the vascular clamp is removed to promote a brisk diuresis. If the anticipated time of arterial occlusion is greater than 30 minutes, in situ renal hypothermia is used to minimize ischemic injury to the kidney. Surgical hypothermia is established immediately after renal artery clamping and maintained for 10 minutes to decrease core temperature to 15° to 20°C prior to initiating tumor resection. Surface cooling of the kidney allows as much as 3 hours of safe ischemia without permanent injury.[23]

An assortment of surgical techniques is available for performing partial nephrectomy in patients with renal tumors. These include polar (apical and basilar) segmental nephrectomy, wedge resection, and transverse resection. Extracorporeal NSS with autotransplantation is required only in rare cases with exceptionally large and anatomically challenging tumors.[24] Hemostasis is accomplished by ligation of arterial and venous bleeders during and after tumor excision with fine absorbable suture and coagulation with electrocautery, laser, or argon beam devices. Closure of the renal defect with adjacent fat, fascia, peritoneum, or Oxycel, and watertight closure of the collecting system with fine absorbable suture are critical in prevention of urinary fistula development.[24]

Whichever technique is used, the tumor is removed with a thin margin of adjacent normal-appearing renal parenchyma. Although some renal tumors are surrounded by a distinct pseudocapsule of fibrous tissue, and simple enucleation has been used in such cases to achieve tumor removal, most recent studies have linked enucleation with a higher risk of leaving residual malignancy in the kidney.[25,26] Histopathologic studies have demonstrated frequent microscopic tumor penetration of the pseudocapsule that surrounds the neoplasm,[27,28] and thus it is not always possible to be assured of complete tumor encapsulation. Every attempt should be made to prevent local tumor recurrence, and therefore a surrounding margin of normal parenchyma should be removed with the tumor whenever possible. Enucleation is currently used only in patients with VHL disease who have multiple low-stage encapsulated tumors involving both kidneys.[9]

With respect to the precise amount of normal renal parenchyma that must be removed to ensure a safe surgical margin after NSS, Sutherland et al.[29] investigated the effect of surgical margin size on local tumor recurrence after partial nephrectomy for RCC. They found that no patient with negative parenchymal margins after NSS for stages of T1-2 renal cell carcinoma had local recurrence at the resection site at a mean follow-up of 49 months. Based on these data, they concluded that a margin of normal renal parenchyma of less than 5 mm must be removed during partial nephrectomy for localized RCC. Though the sample size was 44 patients, the authors confirmed outcome data from other institutions by explicitly addressing the important question of margin thickness.

Although intraoperative ultrasonography is not superior to CT in identifying multifocal tumors, it can determine tumor extent and achieve accurate tumor localization, particularly for intrarenal lesions that are not visible or palpable from the external surface of the kidney.[30] Furthermore, determination of venous extension and associated cysts may also be aided by intraoperative sonography. Intraoperative ultrasound is therefore a particularly useful tool in renal exploration in patients with hereditary forms of RCC or those undergoing reoperation, who are at a high risk for having multiple intrarenal lesions that may otherwise go unrecognized.

When NSS is performed, after excision of all gross tumor, absence of malignancy in the remaining portion of the kidney should be verified intraoperatively by frozen-section examinations of biopsy specimens obtained at random from the renal margin of excision. It is unusual for such biopsies to demonstrate residual tumor, but if they do, additional renal tissue must be excised.

The frequency of postoperative complications after NSS continues to decline as patient selection, operative techniques, perioperative care, and cumulative surgical experience improve. In the last decade, most large series have shown a dramatic decrease in the complication rate following NSS. Operative mortality is rare and reported to be 1% to 2% in most studies. A number of technical complications specific to NSS have been described (Table 13.1). Of these, urinary fistula is the most common,

Table 13.1.
Reported major perioperative surgical complications after in situ nephron-sparing surgery for solid renal lesions

Reference	No. of Pts.	No. of deaths (%)	No. of urinary fistula (%)	No. of prolonged ATN/chronic renal insufficiency (%)	No. on dialysis (%)	No. of infections/ abscesses (%)	No. of spleen injuries (%)	No. with bleeding (%)	No. needing reoperation (%)	Total No. (%)
Lerner et al.[31]	169	1 (0.6)	3 (1.8)	—	0	1 (0.6)	—	—	3 (1.8)	7 (4.1)
Belldegrun et al.[32]	146	3 (2.1)	2 (1.4)	—	—	—	—	3 (2.1)	3 (2.1)	8 (5.5)
Thrasher et al.[35]	42	2 (4.8)	2 (4.8)	2 (4.8)	1 (2.4)	1 (2.4)	—	1 (2.4)	1 (2.4)	8 (19)
VanPoppel et al.[33]	76	1 (1.3)	—	—	—	—	1 (1.4)	6 (7.9)	2 (2.6)	8 (11)
Duque et al.[36]	66	—	6 (9.1)	10 (15)	3 (4.5)	2 (3.0)	—	3 (4.5)	2 (3.0)	18 (27)
Campbell et al.[34]	259	4 (1.5)	45 (17.4)	19 (7.3)	14 (5.4)	11 (4.2)	1 (0.4)	6 (2.3)	8 (3.1)	78 (30)
Steinbach et al.[11]	140	2 (1.4)	3 (2.1)	1 (0.7)	—	—	1 (0.7)	2 (1.4)	2 (1.4)	12 (8.6)
Moll et al.[14]	164	—	11 (6.7)	—	—	—	—	6 (3.7)	1 (0.6)	16 (9.8)

*Majority of patients had a solitary kidney.

with a reported incidence of 1.4% to 17.4%. Diagnosis is made when persistent drainage demonstrates elevated creatinine (drainage fluid-to-serum ration greater than 2). Almost all fistulas may be managed conservatively by observation, Foley catheter placement, or insertion of a ureteral stent. If a urinoma develops, percutaneous drainage may be necessary. Prolonged acute tubular necrosis (ATN) with or without acute renal failure is the second most common complication after NSS, with a frequency of occurrence between 0.7% and 7.3%. The primary etiology of ATN is ischemic renal injury and a decreased renal mass, although other causes of ATN/acute renal failure must be considered, including prerenal and postrenal causes. Operative maneuvers to prevent ATN include vigorous hydration and administration of mannitol to promote a brisk intraoperative diuresis.[18] The need for temporary or permanent dialysis occurs in 2.4% to 5.4%, and patients should be advised of this risk preoperatively. Other reported complications are postoperative hemorrhage in 2.4% of cases, infection with or without retroperitoneal abscess formation in 0.6% to 6.0%, injury to adjacent viscera such as the spleen in 0.4% to 1.3%, and perioperative medical complications. Bleeding (1.4% to 7.9%) after NSS may be acute or delayed and occasionally requires reexploration. Careful intraoperative attention to hemostasis and precise reconstruction of the remnant kidney is mandatory to avoid this and other complications.[18] The overall reoperative rate after NSS remains low in most series (0% to 3.1%). Particular tumor characteristics are strongly associated. Patients with an increased risk of technical complications after NSS include those with imperative indications (functionally solitary kidney or bilateral lesions) and large or centrally located tumors.[34]

Postoperative follow-up after NSS involves serum creatinine measurement and excretory urography at 4 to 6 weeks to document renal function and anatomy. Subsequent surveillance strategies (Table 13.2) follow stage-specific guidelines[37] and are no more extensive or expensive than surveillance after radical nephrectomy for low-stage pT1 or pT2 disease. Locally recurrent disease may be treated with repeat partial or

Table 13.2.

Recommended postoperative surveillance after nephron-sparing surgery (NSS) for sporadic localized renal cell carcinoma (RCC)

Pathologic tumor stage	History, exam, blood test*	Chest x-ray	Abdominal CT scan
T1	Yearly	—	—
T2	Yearly	Yearly	Every 2 years
T3	Yearly	Yearly	Every 6 months for 2 years, then every 2 years

*Medical history, physical examination, and measurement of serum calcium, alkaline phosphatase, liver function, and renal function.

Note: The need for postoperative radiographic surveillance studies varies according to the initial pathologic tumor (pT) stage. Patients who undergo NSS for pT1 RCC do not require radiographic imaging postoperatively in view of the very low risk of recurrent malignancy. A yearly chest radiograph is recommended after NSS for pT2 or pT3 RCC because the lung is the most common site of postoperative metastasis in both groups. Abdominal or retroperitoneal tumor recurrence is uncommon in pT2 patients, particularly early after NSS, and these patients require only occasional follow-up abdominal CT scanning. Patients with pT3 RCC have a higher risk of developing local tumor recurrence, particularly during the first 2 years after NSS, and they may benefit from more frequent follow-up abdominal CT scanning initially.

complete nephrectomy depending on the clinical circumstances and the anatomy of the remnant kidney.[38]

CLINICAL RESULTS OF NEPHRON-SPARING SURGERY FOR RENAL CELL CARCINOMA

The technical success rate with NSS for RCC is excellent, and long-term patient survival free of cancer is comparable to that obtained after radical nephrectomy. Table 13.3 lists results of NSS for RCC in 1262 patients reported in the literature since 1990. The reported mean cancer specific survival for all patients undergoing NSS for localized RCC is 88% to 97.5%. Mean follow-up for these studies ranged between 3 and 6 years.

Fergany et al.[41] reviewed the results of NSS in 107 patients with localized sporadic RCC treated prior to 1988 and who were followed a minimum of 10 years at the Cleveland Clinic. Tumors were symptomatic in 73 patients (68%) and indications for surgery were imperative in 96 (90%). All patients were followed for at least 10 years or until death. Cancer-specific survival was 88.2% at 5 years and 73% at 10 years, and 26% of the patients died of metastatic disease. Long-term preservation of renal function was achieved in 93% of patients. Cancer-specific survival for tumors 4 cm or less was 98% at 5 years and 92% at 10 years regardless of the indication for partial nephrectomy. Important negative predictors of survival included high tumor grade, high tumor stage, bilateral disease, and tumors greater than 4 cm. These data are consistent with other shorter term previously published series that confirm that tumor stage, grade, and size remain the most important prognostic indicators determining outcome after NSS.[42] On the other hand, there are no significant biologic differences between centrally versus peripherally located small, solitary, unilateral RCCs, and treatment with NSS or radical nephrectomy is equally effective regardless of tumor location in these patients.[43]

In another recent study from the Cleveland Clinic, we reviewed the long-term results of open NSS in 400 patients with RCC in a solitary kidney. Postoperatively, 97% of patients maintained satisfactory renal function without the need for dialysis. Cancer-specific survival was 89% at 5 years and 82% at 10 years.

Table 13.3.
Outcome in patients undergoing nephron-sparing surgery for localized renal cell carcinoma

References	*No. of Pts.*	*Disease-specific survival (%)*	*No. of local recurrences*	*Mean follow-up (months)*
Moll et al.[14]	142	98	1.4	34.8
Provert et al.[12]	44	88	2	36
Lee et al.[17]	79	96	0	40
Lerner et al.[31]	185	89	5.9	44
Steinbach et al.[11]	121	90	4.1	47
Hafez et al.[15]	485	92	3.2	47
Barbalias et al.[39]	41	97.5	7.3	59
Armiento et al.[40]	19	95	0	70
Belldegrun et al.[32]	146	93	2.7	74

NEPHRON-SPARING SURGERY WITH A NORMAL CONTRALATERAL KIDNEY

Although radical nephrectomy remains the standard treatment for localized RCC in patients with an anatomically and functionally normal opposite kidney, a growing number of authors are reporting excellent results with NSS in this setting. Disease-specific survival in this setting is 90% to 100% with extended follow-up in several series. In a recent study from Memorial Sloan-Kettering Cancer Center, Herr[44] reported the 10-year results of elective NSS in the setting of a normal contralateral kidney. With an average tumor size of 3 cm with predominantly low-grade, low-stage tumors, of the 70 patients, 69 (98.6%) had no local recurrence, and 68 (97%) survived free of metastasis.

Although the long-term functional advantage of NSS when there is a normal opposite kidney remains to be definitely demonstrated, the benefit of maximal nephron preservation may include a decreased risk of progression to chronic renal insufficiency and end-stage renal disease. In studies by McKiernan et al.[45] from Memorial Sloan-Kettering Cancer Center and Lau et al.[46] from the Mayo Clinic, patients who underwent radical nephrectomy were compared with patients who underwent elective NSS. Each institution's groups were well matched for age, grade, stage, tumor size, preoperative creatinine, and year of surgery. Although they identified no significant difference in cancer-free survival, Lau et al. demonstrated that at 10 years, renal insufficiency (defined as an increase in serum creatinine to greater than 2 mg/dL) was significantly different between the groups, occurring in 12.4% of radical nephrectomy cases compared with only 2.3% of NSS cases. Similarly, McKiernan et al. found that the chance of progression to renal insufficiency was significantly higher in the radical nephrectomy group. In both groups, differences in functional renal reserve were thought to be responsible for these findings. Therefore, given the excellent short-term and long-term results of elective NSS for cancer control and the increasingly recognized functional benefits of this approach, patients with a single, small, unilateral, localized RCC may now be considered suitable candidates for NSS even when the opposite kidney is completely normal.

INDICATIONS AND OUTCOMES FOR NEPHRON-SPARING SURGERY IN SPECIAL CIRCUMSTANCES

Hereditary Renal Tumors and Nephron-Sparing Surgery

Hereditary conditions that predispose patients to renal tumors include VHL disease associated with clear-cell renal cell carcinoma, hereditary papillary renal cell carcinoma, hereditary oncocytoma, and the Birt-Hogg-Dubé syndrome. Considerations regarding the treatment of solid renal malignancies in these patients differ significantly from treatment of those with sporadic renal neoplasms, primarily due to the propensity for hereditary lesions to be bilateral, multifocal, and often microscopic. Treatment of RCC in patients with VHL disease differs significantly from that of patients with sporadic renal neoplasms primarily due to the tendency of lesions in VHL to be bilateral, multifocal, and often microscopic. This reflects the changes in the germline of the *VHL* gene located on the short arm of chromosome 3 (3p25-26). For this reason, RCC occurs at a much younger age in patients with hereditary renal tumors such as VHL, and the entire renal parenchyma has a higher lifetime risk of developing subsequent tumors.

Additionally, the malignant potential of cysts is often underappreciated on ultrasound or CT in such patients, and histologically these cysts frequently contain either frank carcinoma or a hyperplastic clear cell lining that may represent incipient tumor.[47] For instance, adequate surgical treatment of localized RCC in VHL therefore requires complete excision of all solid and cystic renal lesions. Available options include observation of lesions less than 3 cm, NSS with close surveillance, and subsequent resection of recurrent disease or bilateral radical nephrectomy, thereby rendering the patient anephric with the potential for subsequent transplantation.[48,49] Walther et al.[50] evaluated a 3-cm surgical threshold for performing NSS in 52 patients with VHL and hereditary papillary renal carcinoma. No patient was noted to have metastatic disease during observation with a dominant tumor of less than 3 cm during a median follow-up of 60 months. Regardless of the treatment course elected, the patient must be advised of the need for strict lifelong follow-up, the possible need for resection of recurrent disease in the setting of NSS, and the risks of immune suppression in the setting of previous RCC if transplantation is elected.

The role of NSS in preserving renal function and avoiding or postponing dialysis in patients with VHL disease was examined in a multicenter study of 49 patients who underwent NSS for RCC.[49] The 5- and 10-year cancer-specific survival rates were 100% and 81%, respectively. At a mean follow-up of 68 months, 51% of the patients treated with NSS had local recurrence, of whom most underwent salvage by repeat NSS or removal of the renal remnant. Whether these recurrences represent de novo tumors or microscopic, clinically undetected foci present at the time of the original surgery is not known. Survival free of local recurrence was 71% at 5 years but only 15% at 10 years. These data underscore the need for diligent surveillance in these patients. Therefore, NSS is feasible in well-selected patients with VHL and can preserve renal function without compromising cancer-free survival in most patients.

Nephron-Sparing Surgery with Coexistent Renal Artery Disease

Occasionally, preoperative history and radiographic imaging reveal both RCC and renal artery stenosis (RAS) in the same patient. This can complicate the clinical picture. When RCC and RAS are found in the same kidney and a normal contralateral kidney is present, the treatment of choice is radical nephrectomy. Involvement of all functional renal parenchyma by either or both of these processes poses a more difficult therapeutic dilemma. Management of such cases must be individualized to achieve maximal cancer control while balancing the need to preserve overall renal function.

Campbell et al.[51] reviewed their experience in the management of 34 patients with concurrent RCC and RAS affecting all of the functioning renal parenchyma. The mean patient age was 67, and 88% of cases of RAS were due to atherosclerotic disease. Patients were divided into four groups: patients with a solitary kidney with RCC and RAS; patients with bilateral RCC and bilateral RAS; patients with unilateral RCC and contralateral RAS; and patients with unilateral RCC and bilateral RAS. All patients underwent complete surgical excision of their tumor and a nephron-sparing approach was utilized in 88%. Eight patients underwent simultaneous partial or radical nephrectomy and surgical renal revascularization with excellent cancer-free survival and maintenance of renal function in all but one patient, who ultimately required dialysis. In recent years, improved endovascular management of RAS has increased the number of therapeutic options available for the management of patients with RCC and coexisting renal artery disease.[52]

Nephron-Sparing Surgery for Advanced Renal Cell Carcinoma

Nephron-sparing surgery in patients with locally advanced or metastatic disease is primarily indicated to avoid rendering the patient anephric and in need of renal replacement therapy, and to obtain tissue for adoptive immunotherapy protocols. Under these circumstances, it is possible to provide symptomatic relief for locally advanced disease and in some cases to aggressively resect all clinically evident tumor while maintaining acceptable renal function. Few studies have examined the role of partial nephrectomy in these selected circumstances. Angermeier et al.[53] reviewed nine patients who underwent partial nephrectomy for tumor with venous involvement in a solitary kidney. Although all cases were technically successful and renal function was preserved, many patients developed local or distant metastasis. Krishnamurthi et al.[54] reviewed the clinical outcome of 15 patients with metastatic RCC who underwent NSS and surgical or systemic treatment of metastases. All cases were technically successful and the need for renal replacement therapy was obviated in all but one patient. In patients with metachronous metastases in a solitary kidney, death from disease occurred later than in patients with synchronous lesions resected from the kidney and other soft tissues. Although these preliminary data are from highly selected patient populations, they suggest that partial nephrectomy can occasionally provide effective treatment for patients with locally advanced or completely resected metastatic RCC.

REFERENCES

1. Wells S. Successful removal of two solid circumrenal tumours. Br Med J 1884;1:758–774.
2. Hercel E. Ueber Nierenexitirpation Bietr. Klinich Khirurg 1890;6:485.
3. Vermooten V. Indications for conservative surgery in certain renal tumors: a study based on the growth patterns of clear cell carcinoma. J Urol 1950;64:200–207.
4. Robson CJ, Churchill BM, Anderson W. The results of radical nephrectomy for renal cell carcinoma. J Urol 1969;101:297.
5. Clark PE, Shover LR, Uzzo RG, Hafez KS, Rybicki LA, Novick AC. Quality of life and psychological adaptation after surgical treatment for localized renal cell carcinoma: impact of the amount of remaining renal tissue. Urology 2001;57:252–256.
6. Shinohara N, Harabayashi T, Sato S, Hioka T, Tsuchiya K, Koyangi T. Impact of nephron-sparing surgery on quality of life in patients with localized renal cell carcinoma. Eur Urol 2001;39:114–119.
7. Uzzo RG, Wei JT, Hafez K, et al. Comparison of direct hospital costs and length of stay for radical nephrectomy versus nephron-sparing surgery in the management of localized renal cell carcinoma. Urology 1999;54:994–998.
8. Licht MR, Novick AC. Nephron-sparing surgery for renal cell carcinoma. J Urol 1993;149:1–7.
9. Spencer WF, Novick AC, Montie JE, Streem SB, Levin HS. Surgical treatment of localized renal cell carcinoma in von Hippel-Lindau's disease. J Urol 1988;139:507–509.
10. Pertritsch PH, Rauchenwald M, Zechner O, et al. Results after organ-preserving surgery for renal cell carcinoma. An Austrian multicenter study. Eur Urol 1990;18:84–87.
11. Steinbach F, Stockle M, Hohenfellner R. Clinical experience with nephron-sparing surgery in the presence of a normal contralateral kidney. Semin Urol Oncol 1995;13:288–291.
12. Provert J, Tessler A, Brown J, Golimbu M, Bosniak M, Morales P. Partial nephrectomy for renal cell carcinoma indications, results and implications. J Urol 1991;145:472–476.
13. Butler BP, Novick AC, Miller DP, Campbell SA, Licht MR. Management of small unilateral renal cell carcinoma: radical versus nephron-sparing surgery. Urology 1995;45:34–40.
14. Moll V, Becht E, Ziegler M. Kidney preserving surgery in renal cell tumors: indications, techniques and results in 152 patients. J Urol 1993;150:319–323.

15. Hafez KS, Fergany AF, Novick AC. Nephron sparing surgery for localized renal cell carcinoma: impact of tumor size on patient survival, tumor recurrence and TNM staging. J Urol 1999;162:1930–1933.
16. Lerner SE, Hawkins CA, Blute ML, et al. Disease outcome in patients with low stage renal cell carcinoma treated with nephron sparing or radical surgery. J Urol 2002;167:884–889.
17. Lee CT, Katz J, Shi W, Thaler HT, Reuter VE, Russo P. Surgical management of renal tumors 4cm or less in a contemporary cohort. J Urol 2000;163:730–736.
18. Campbell SA, Novick AC. Surgical technique and morbidity of elective partial nephrectomy. Semin Urol Oncol 1995;13:281–287.
19. McClennan BL, Deyoe LA. The imaging evaluation of renal cell carcinoma: diagnosis and staging. Radio Clin North Am 1994;32:55–69.
20. Wyatt SH, Urban BA, Fishman EK. Spiral CT of the kidneys: role in characterization of renal disease. Part II: neoplastic disease. Crit Rev Diag Imag 1995;36:39–72.
21. Smith PA, Marshall FF, Fishman EK. Spiral computed tomography evaluation of the kidneys: state of the art. Urology 1998;51:3–11.
22. Coll DM, Uzzo RG, Herts BB, Davros WJ, Wirth SL, Novick AC. 3–dimensional volume rendered computerized tomography for preoperative evaluation and intraoperative treatment of patients undergoing nephron sparing surgery. J Urol 1999;161:1097–1102.
23. Novick AC. Renal hypothermia: in vivo and ex vivo. Urol Clin North Am 1983;10:637–644.
24. Novick AC. Partial nephrectomy for renal cell carcinoma. Urol Clin North Am 1987;14:419–433.
25. Marshall FF, Taxy JB, Fishman ED, Chang R. The feasibility of surgical enucleation for renal cell carcinoma. J Urol 1986;135:231–234.
26. Novick AC, Zincke H, Neves RJ, Topley HM. Surgical enucleation for renal cell carcinoma. J Urol 1986;135:235–238.
27. Kurozumi T, Yagi H, Omoto T, Iwata Y. Extracapsular tumor invasion in renal cell carcinoma: with special reference to limitation of surgical enucleation. Nippon Hinyokika Gakkai Zasshi 1993;84:1943–1947.
28. Constantini E, Mearini E, Ficola F, et al. Renal cell carcinoma: histological findings in peritumoral tissue after organ-preserving surgery. Eur Urol 1996;29:279–283.
29. Sutherland SE, Resnick MI, Maclennan GT, Goldman HB. Does the size of the surgical margin in partial nephrectomy for renal cell cancer really matter? J Urol 2002;167:61–64.
30. Campbell SC, Fichtner J, Novick AC, et al. Intraoperative evaluation of renal cell carcinoma: a prospective study of the role of ultrasonography and histopathological frozen sections. J Urol 1996;155:1191–1195.
31. Lerner SE, Hawkins CA, Blute ML, et al. Disease outcome in patients with low stage renal cell carcinoma treated with nephron sparing or radical surgery. J Urol 1996;155:1868–1873.
32. Belldegrun A, Tsui KH, deKernion JB, Smith RB. Efficacy of nephron-sparing surgery for renal cell carcinoma: analysis based on the new 1997 tumor-node-metastasis staging system. J Clin Oncol 1999;17:2868–2875.
33. Van Poppel H, Barnelis B, Oyen R, Baert L. Partial nephrectomy for renal cell carcinoma can achieve long-term tumor control. J Urol 1998;160:674–678.
34. Campbell SC, Novick AC, Streem SB, Klein E, Licht M. Complications of nephron-sparing surgery for renal tumors. J Urol 1994;151:1177–1180.
35. Thrasher JB, Robertson JE, Paulson DF. Expanding indications for conservation renal surgery in renal cell carcinoma. Urology 1994;43:160–168.
36. Duque JL, Loughlin KR, O'Leary MP, Kumar S, Richie JP. Partial nephrectomy: alternative treatment for selected patients with renal cell carcinoma. Urology 1998;52:584–590.
37. Hafez KS, Novick AC, Campbell SC. Patterns of tumor recurrence and guidelines for follow-up after nephron-sparing surgery for sporadic renal cell carcinoma. J Urol 1997;157:2067–2070.
38. Campbell SC, Novick AC. Management of local recurrence following radical nephrectomy or partial nephrectomy. Urol Clin North Am 1994;21:593–599.
39. Barbalias GA, Liatsikos EN, Tsintayis A, Nikiforidis G. Adenocarcinoma of the kidney: nephron-sparing surgical approach vs. radical nephrectomy. J Surg Oncol 1999;72:156–161.
40. D'Armiento M, Damiano R, Felepa B, Perdona S, Oriana G, DeSio M. Elective conservative surgery for renal carcinoma versus radical nephrectomy: a prospective study. Br J Urol 1997;79:15–19.
41. Fergany AF, Hafez KS, Novick AC. Long-term results of nephron-sparing surgery for localized renal cell carcinoma: 10-year follow-up. J Urol 2000;163:442–445.
42. Bostwick DG, Murphy GP. Diagnosis and prognosis of renal cell carcinoma: highlights from an international consensus workshop. Semin Urol Oncol 1998;16:46–52.

43. Hafez KS, Novick AC, Butler BP. Management of small solitary unilateral renal cell carcinomas: impact of central versus peripheral tumor location. J Urol 1998;159:1156–1160.
44. Herr HW. Partial nephrectomy for unilateral renal carcinoma and a normal contralateral kidney: 10-year follow-up. J Urol 1999;161:33–34.
45. McKiernan J, Simmons R, Katz J, Russo P. Natural history of chronic renal insufficiency after partial and radical nephrectomy. Urology 2002;59:816–820.
46. Lau WK, Blute ML, Weaver AL, Torres VE, Zincke H. Matched comparison of radical nephrectomy vs. nephron-sparing surgery in patients with unilateral renal cell carcinoma and a normal contralateral kidney. Mayo Clin Proc 2000;75:1236–1242.
47. Christenson PJ, Craig JP, Bibro MC, O'Connell KJ. Cysts containing renal cell carcinoma in von Hippel-Lindau disease. J Urol 1982;128:798–800.
48. Goldfarb DA, Neumann HP, Penn I, Novick AC. Results of renal transplantation in patients with renal cell carcinoma and von Hippel-Lindau disease. Transplant 1997;64:1726–1729.
49. Steinbach F, Novick AC, Zincke H, et al. Treatment of renal cell carcinoma in von Hippel-Lindau disease. A multicenter study. J Urol 1995;153:1812–1816.
50. Walther MM, Choyke PL, Glenn G, et al. Renal cancer in families with hereditary renal cancer: prospective analysis of a tumor size threshold for renal parenchymal sparing surgery. J Urol 1999;161:1475–1479.
51. Campbell SC, Novick AC, Streem SB, Klein EA. Management of renal cell carcinoma with coexistent renal artery disease. J Urol 1993;150:808–813.
52. Hafez KS, Krishnamurthi V, Campbell SC, Novick AC. Contemporary management of renal cell carcinoma with coexistent renal artery disease: update of the Cleveland Clinic experience. Urology 2000;56:382–386.
53. Angermeier KW, Novick AC, Streem SB, Montie JE. Nephron-sparing surgery for renal cell carcinoma with venous involvement. J Urol 1990;144:1352–1355.
54. Krishnamurthi V, Novick AC, Bukowski R. Nephron-sparing surgery in patients with metastatic renal cell carcinoma. J Urol 1996;156:36–39.

14   Minimally Invasive Nephron-Sparing Surgery for Renal Tumors:
Laparoscopic Partial Nephrectomy and Probe Ablative Treatments

Monish Aron, Georges-Pascal Haber, and Inderbir S. Gill

KEYWORDS

KIDNEY
RENAL
TUMOR
NEPHRON-SPARING SURGERY
LAPAROSCOPIC PARTIAL NEPHRECTOMY
CRYOABLATION
RADIOFREQUENCY ABLATION
RADIOSURGERY
HIGH-INTENSITY FOCUSED ULTRASOUND
CHEMOABLATION
MICROWAVE THERMOTHERAPY
LASER INTERSTITIAL THERMOTHERAPY

ABSTRACT

Objectives: To review the evolution and current status of extirpative and probe-ablative methods of minimally invasive nephron sparing surgery (MINSS) for renal tumors. **Methods:** The English language literature of past 10 years was reviewed using the National Library of Medicine database and the following key words: kidney, renal, tumor, nephron sparing surgery, laparoscopic partial nephrectomy, cryoablation, radiofrequency ablation, radiosurgery, high-intensity focused ultrasound, chemoablation, microwave thermotherapy, and laser interstitial thermotherapy. Over 500 articles were identified. A total of 100 articles were selected for this review based on their contribution to knowledge pertaining to: a) evolution of concepts, b) development and refinement of techniques, and c) intermediate and long-term clinical outcomes with minimally invasive nephron sparing surgery. **Results:** Open partial nephrectomy (OPN) is the

From: *Clinical Management of Renal Tumors*
Edited by: R.M. Bukowski and A.C. Novick © Humana Press Inc., Totowa, NJ

reference standard for nephron sparing surgery agianst which all minimally invasive techniques should be measured. Given the requisite skills for time-sensitive intracorporeal suturing, laparoscopic partial nephrectomy (LPN) can provide long-term cancer cure comparable to the reference standard. The initial 5-year data of 50 patients have just become available and have shown overall and cancer-specific survival of 84% and 100%, respectively. Although the initial outcomes of cryoablation and radiofrequency ablation (RFA) are encouraging, long-term studies are necessary to confirm lasting efficacy. The optimal modality for tumor targeting, monitoring therapy, and follow-up remains to be determined. These ablative techniques should be reserved for carefully selected patients, data should be prospectively accrued, and the long-term cancer cure rates should be compared to the reference standard. **Conclusions:** As of this writing, the technique and global acceptance of LPN is evolving, although it remains restricted by the complexity of laparoscopic renal reconstruction. In expert hands cancer cure and renal functional outcomes are similar to OPN. Of the probeablative techniques, promising long-term data are available for cryoablation. RFA is still developmental and instances of incomplete cell-kill, despite negative enhancement are concerning. Other modalities are still experimental.

Since the 1970s, the routine evaluation of abdominal symptoms by ultrasonography (US) and computed tomography (CT) scan has led to a 2.3% to 4.3% increase in detection of renal cell carcinoma (RCC) annually. Consequently, the rate of incidental detection of small (≤4 cm) renal tumors of low stage and low metastatic potential has increased by 60%.[1] These tumors usually occur in patients older than 70 years of age who may have significant comorbidity. Radical nephrectomy appears to be unnecessary in many of these patients. Several minimally invasive nephron-sparing surgery (NSS) options are advocated for select patients with small renal tumors (SRTs), with the aim of providing comparable oncologic control with reduced morbidity. These include excisional (laparoscopic partial nephrectomy) as well as probe ablative procedures. Laparoscopic partial nephrectomy (LPN) is technically challenging and requires advanced laparoscopic dexterity and time-sensitive intracorporeal suturing.[2] Ablative techniques destroy tissue in situ rather than by excision. Potential benefits of ablative versus excisional procedures are decreased morbidity, shorter hospitalization, earlier return to normal activities, preservation of renal function, and the ability to treat patients who are poor surgical risks. Techniques that are used either clinically or experimentally for renal tumor ablation are cryoablation, radiofrequency ablation (RFA), high-intensity focused ultrasound (HIFU), microwave thermotherapy (MT), laser interstitial thermotherapy (LITT), chemoablation with or without radiofrequency, and radiosurgery.

Epithelial tumors of the kidney account for 3% of all adult malignancies. Multifocality is seen in 7% to 25% of RCCs overall, and in 0% to 5% when the primary tumor is ≤4 cm. Risk of local recurrence after NSS is <10% and is a manifestation of undetected microscopic RCCs in the renal remnant. No predictable relationship between multifocality and local recurrence has been reported.[3] To minimize local recurrence, tumor excision with an adequate margin of normal parenchyma is essential. A negative margin is the primary criterion, with margin width having no practical consequence.[4] During LPN a margin of about 0.5 cm is aimed for to prevent a tumor breach. Most incidental small renal tumors have a slow growth rate and hence may take several years to become a clinically significant threat to the patient. This should be kept in mind when considering treatment options, especially in elderly patients with major comorbidity. In such instances, a "wait and watch" policy may be a prudent alternative.

THE REFERENCE STANDARD

For patients in whom therapy is indicated, open partial nephrectomy (OPN) is considered the reference standard for treatment of renal tumors ≤4 cm. For such tumors, the cancer cure rate is comparable to that of radical nephrectomy.[5] Minimally invasive nephron-sparing surgery (MINSS) options strive to achieve similar cancer control with reduced morbidity. Although reducing morbidity is a laudable goal, it is essential not to lose sight of the primary goal—cancer cure. Hence, 5-year oncologic data are of critical importance.

The goal of NSS is twofold: (1) complete tumor excision, and (2) preservation of a well-functioning renal remnant. Cancer-specific survival after NSS for small (≤4 cm) RCC is comparable to that after radical nephrectomy. For RCC ≤4 cm, Lee et al.[6] reported a 5-year disease-free survival of 96% after NSS and 96% after radical nephrectomy, with no local recurrence in each group. Reporting a 10-year follow-up of NSS, Fergany et al.[5] documented cancer-specific survival of 88% at 5, and 73% at 10 years. Recurrences occurred locally in 4%, at metastatic sites in 21%, or at both sites in 6.5%. Cancer-specific survival in patients with a renal mass ≤4 cm was 100% at 10 years with no local recurrence.

LAPAROSCOPIC PARTIAL NEPHRECTOMY

Laparoscopic partial nephrectomy (LPN) is a minimally invasive alternative to the reference standard. It is imperative that oncologic principles not be compromised, and hence laparoscopic surgeons must endeavor to duplicate techniques of open NSS during LPN.

Indications and Contraindications—2006

Indications and contraindications of LPN are essentially the same as OPN, with the caveat that this procedure should be performed only by surgeons who possess advanced laparoscopic skills.

Absolute indications include synchronous bilateral RCC, tumor in solitary kidney, or unilateral tumor with poorly/nonfunctioning contralateral kidney, wherein radical nephrectomy would render the patient anephric. Ghavamian et al.[7] showed that open NSS in a solitary kidney can be performed safely; 5- and 10-year cancer-specific survival was 81% and 64%, respectively, and local recurrence-free survival was 89% and 80%, respectively.

Relative indications include circumstances wherein the contralateral kidney is at risk for future compromise: hereditary RCC syndromes, genetic diseases with risk of metachronous kidney cancer, diabetes, hypertension, stone disease, and renovascular disease. Elective indications for partial nephrectomy are a renal mass ≤4 cm in size, and suspicious cysts with malignant potential in the presence of a normal contralateral kidney.

Elective NSS is beginning to gain acceptance within the urologic community. Novick[8] reported NSS for localized RCC in 315 patients with a normal opposite kidney. Accurate patient selection with tumor size <3.5 cm resulted in a cancer-specific survival of 95%

with local tumor recurrence in only two patients at approximately 3-year follow-up. Herr[9] reported a 97% ten-year cancer-free survival after elective NSS for small (mean size 3 cm), unifocal, low-grade and low-stage tumors and a normal contralateral kidney.

Current contraindications for LPN include a central intrarenal tumor, and prior open kidney surgery. Morbid obesity and more than two tumors increase the technical difficulty of LPN. Patients with impaired coagulation and platelet dysfunction must be approached cautiously. Patients with atherosclerotic renovascular disease or those who have undergone renal artery stenting are at risk of intimal injury during clamping.

Foundations

Before LPN can be widely recommended, reproducible technical, perioperative, pathologic, functional, and oncologic outcomes comparable to OPN must be confirmed.[2,10] Advances in laparoscopic techniques and technology have allowed effective renal hilar control, renal hypothermia (if required), tumor excision, caliceal suture repair, and hemostatic parenchymal renorrhaphy.[2,10]

Clinical LPN was first performed transperitoneally by Winfield et al.[11] and retroperitoneally by Gill et al.[12] It was initially limited to the treatment of select small, solitary, peripheral, exophytic tumors.[13,14] With increasing experience, these indications have been carefully extended to include tumors infiltrating into the renal sinus or up to the collecting system, completely intrarenal tumors, tumors abutting the hilum, tumors in a solitary kidney, large tumors requiring heminephrectomy, and tumors in the presence of concomitant renovascular disease.[15–19]

Technical Considerations

The specific technical challenge of LPN lies in achieving a bloodless field for tumor excision, pelvicaliceal repair, and renal hemostasis in a time-sensitive manner, with minimal compromise of renal function.

HEMOSTASIS

Various methods have been used to achieve hemostasis. Gettman et al.[20] performed LPN with the assistance of radiofrequency (RF) coagulation in 10 patients. A spherical area of coagulation, including the lesion and a 1-cm margin, was created with a percutaneous RF probe, followed by laparoscopic excision with cold scissors or ultrasound shears. Median estimated blood loss (EBL) was 125 mL. In six patients, Bak et al.[21] used thrombin gel slurry application to the cut surface after tumor excision, followed by a 1- to 2-minute compression with a sponge stick with a clamped hilum. Median warm ischemia (WI) time was 13 minutes, and median EBL was 200 mL.

The hemostatic sealant Floseal® (Baxter Healthcare, Deerfield, IL) was evaluated at our institute where patients undergoing LPN with adjunctive use of Floseal were compared with patients who underwent LPN without Floseal.[22] The Floseal group had significantly decreased overall complications (37% vs. 16%), and a lower rate of hemorrhagic complications (12% vs. 3%).

A monopolar RF device that achieves simultaneous dissection, hemostasis, and coagulation has been reported for LPN without clamping on 10 patients with a mean tumor size of 3.9 cm.[23] Mean EBL was 352 mL (range, 20–1000 mL) with open conversion in one patient.

HILAR CONTROL AND WARM ISCHEMIA

Modalities of hilar control during LPN include clamping the renal artery alone, both renal artery and vein, and intermittent occlusion. Advantages and disadvantages of these modalities remain under debate. Critical renal warm ischemia time has generally been considered to be a 30-minute cutoff. Laparoscopic partial nephrectomy may require longer warm ischemia times compared to OPN.[24] Complete recovery of renal function after 60 minutes of warm ischemia has been reported.[25]

Shekarriz et al.[26] evaluated the impact of warm ischemia on renal function in 17 patients undergoing LPN. Mean warm ischemia time was 22.5 minutes (10–44 minutes). Warm ischemia time did not correlate with change in renal function, or change in glomerular filtration rate. Desai et al.[27] evaluated the impact of warm ischemia on renal function in 179 patients, with special emphasis on 15 patients with a solitary kidney and 12 patients with both kidneys who had radionuclide differential renal function data. In patients with a solitary kidney the mean warm ischemia time was 29 minutes, mean percent renal parenchyma excised was 29%, and serum creatinine at baseline and last follow-up (mean 4.8 months) was 1.3 and 1.8 mg/dL, respectively. In the second group, assessed by renal scintigraphy, the function of the operated kidney was reduced by a mean of 29%, commensurate with the amount of parenchyma excised.

RENAL HYPOTHERMIA

The initial description of renal hypothermia by minimally invasive techniques was reported by Gill et al.[28] Twelve patients underwent intracorporeal surface hypothermia during LPN. The kidney was entrapped in an Endocatch-II bag (U.S. Surgical, Norwalk, CT). The hilum was occluded with a Satinsky clamp, the bottom of the bag retrieved through a 12-mm port site, and 600 to 750 mL of ice slush delivered into the bag over 4 to 7 minutes to achieve core renal temperatures of 5° to 19°C. Subsequently, Janetschek et al.[29] achieved hypothermia by continuous perfusion of lactated Ringer's at 4°C through an angiocatheter in the clamped renal artery in 15 patients. At a steady-state perfusion of 25 to 33 mL/min, a parenchymal temperature of 25°C was maintained. Since optimal temperature for renal protection is <15°C, this technique needs further refinement. Hypothermia with cortical and medullary temperatures of 24°C and 21°C, respectively, has also been achieved by retrograde pelvicaliceal cold saline perfusion via a ureteral access sheath in one patient.[30] Ames et al.[31] reported a technique to cool the kidneys to 15° to 25°C during LPN in a porcine model using fine ice slush delivered through a 10-mm laparoscopic end-effector.

PELVICALICEAL REPAIR

Desai et al.[10] compared the perioperative data of 27 LPNs with pelvicaliceal entry with 37 LPNs with no pelvicaliceal entry. Pelvicaliceal suture repair was associated with longer hospital stay and longer warm ischemia time. No patient undergoing pelvicaliceal repair developed urinary leak. Bove et al.[32] evaluated the necessity of ureteral stenting during LPN for single ≤4.5 cm renal tumors. Patients undergoing 5 French (F) ureteral catheter placement prior to LPN ($n = 54$) were compared to those without ureteral catheter ($n = 49$). Postoperative urinary leak occurred in one patient in each group.

At the Cleveland Clinic, we routinely employ a ureteral catheter for the following reasons: (1) it allows precise identification of the site of pelvicaliceal entry; (2)

pelvicaliceal entry can occur at more than one location, which may be difficult to locate without retrograde injection; and (3) retrograde injection allows testing the water-tightness of the pelvicaliceal system repair.

Our current technique of laparoscopic partial nephrectomy[33] is described in Table 14.1.

Worldwide Data

Gill et al.[24] compared patients undergoing LPN ($n = 100$) with OPN ($n = 100$) for a solitary ≤7-cm tumor. The median tumor size was 2.8 cm vs. 3.3 cm. Median operating room (OR) time and EBL were lesser in the LPN group, while warm ischemia time was longer during LPN (28 vs. 18 minutes). The LPN patients required less analgesia and shorter hospitalization, and had a quicker convalescence. Positive surgical margins occurred in 3% and 0%, respectively. Intraoperative and urologic complications were 5% and 11%, respectively, in the LPN group vs. 0% and 2%, respectively, in the OPN group. The senior author's experience now exceeds 550 LPN cases. In the initial 100 patients, each with ≥3 years of follow-up, no recurrence or metastases were noted. At a mean follow-up of 42.6 months (24.3–62.5), overall survival was 86% and cancer specific survival was 100%.[34] Five-year data are now available in 50 patients treated at our center, with a mean tumor size of 3 cm (1.4–7 cm). Renal cell carcinoma was confirmed in 64% with tumor stage pT1a in 91%. Surgical margin was positive in one patient. At median follow-up of 5.2 years, overall and cancer-specific survival was 84% and 100%, respectively.[35]

In a multicenter European experience of 53 patients,[36] the mean tumor size was 2.3 cm (1–5 cm). Transperitoneal approach was used in 28%. Mean OR time was 191 minutes (90–320), and EBL 725 mL (20–1500). Intraoperative complications included pneumothorax in one patient, and bleeding in four patients, of whom two were converted to an open procedure. Postoperative complications included bleeding in one, and urine leak in five. Two patients required subsequent nephrectomy. Histology showed 69% pT1 RCC and 100% cancer specific survival at 3 years.

Jeschke et al.[37] reported LPN without hilar clamping in 51 patients with renal tumors <2 cm, using ultrasonic shears and bipolar coagulation with fibrin glue-coated cellulose. The OR time was 132 minutes (70–300 minutes), EBL was 282 mL (20–800 mL), and no open conversion was necessary. Complications occurred in 10%. At a mean follow-up of 34 months (3–78 months), neither local recurrence nor distant metastases occurred.

Weld et al.[38] reported 60 LPNs without any conversion. Renal cell carcinoma was documented in 60%, with no positive margins or recurrence at 25 months. Overall complication rate was 30% (13% urologic and 17% nonurologic). The authors' technique includes hilar control, cold excision of tumor, and sutured renal reconstruction.

Wille et al.[39] reported 44 LPNs for exophytic tumors with a median diameter of 3 cm (1–5 cm), performed by three surgeons. The hilum was clamped in 56%. Mean surgical time was 210 minutes (115–355 minutes); warm ischemia time was 21 minutes (7–41 minutes). Positive margins on frozen section were seen in 16%, and these were addressed at the time of surgery. At a mean follow-up of 15 months (6–37 months), no recurrence was observed.

(text continues on p. 228)

Table 14.1.
Our current technique of laparoscopic partial nephrectomy

Technical nuances	*Caveat/comment*
Retrograde 5-French (F) ureteral catheter placement in the renal pelvis for intraoperative injection of dilute methylene blue	Use a guide wire to prevent ureteral trauma
Patient is placed in a 45-degree flank position for the transperitoneal approach, and 90-degree lateral position for the retroperitoneal approach	All pressure points must be padded and the patient secured to the table
Renal hilum is identified initially; for the retroperitoneal procedure we circumferentially mobilize the artery and the vein separately for subsequent application of bulldog clamps; for the transperitoneal approach, space is created all around the hilum for application of the Satinsky clamp, but the vessels are not individually mobilized	En bloc clamping is safer than individual vessel dissection; in case of multiple arteries, ensure all are clamped
Strategic defatting of the kidney, maintaining perirenal fat over the tumor; additional "handles" of perirenal fat and areolar tissue may be left in place for manipulation of the kidney during tumor excision	The kidney should be well mobilized; do not compromise the capsule, which is essential for the renorrhaphy sutures to hold
Perform intraoperative ultrasound to map the tumor limits and score an adequate margin of surrounding normal parenchyma with cautery J-hook	Expert ultrasound significantly reduces chances of a positive margin
Intravenous mannitol 12.5 g, 15 to 30 minutes prior to hilar clamping	Good renal perfusion and diuresis is critical for optimal functional outcomes
Clamp hilum en bloc with Satinsky clamp (Figure 14.1) for transperitoneal approach, and with bulldog clamps for the retroperitoneal approach	The Satinsky clamp is inherently more reliable than bulldog clamps
Excise the tumor and overlying fat with cold Endoshears (Figure 14.2) in a near-bloodless field; the point of entry into the collecting system is confirmed by retrograde injection of dilute methylene blue (Figure 14.3)	The curve of the Endoshears should face away from the tumor to minimize chances of entry into tumor base
Occasionally, obtain targeted biopsies from the tumor bed for frozen section	Only if there is doubt
Collecting system is suture repaired with a running 200 Vicryl on CT-1 needle (Figure 14.4); water tightness of the caliceal repair is confirmed by repeat retrograde injection of methylene blue	For hilar tumors, take care not to include the main renal vessels in the running suture

(Continued)

Table 14.1. Continued

Technical nuances	Caveat/comment
Renal parenchymal repair is performed with 1–0 Polyglactin on a CTX needle; 3 to 5 interrupted sutures (Figure 14.5) are placed over a pre-prepared Surgicel bolster (Johnson & Johnson, New Brunswick, NJ) that has been positioned over the cut surface of the kidney (Figure 14.6); a Hem-o-Lok clip (Weck Closure System, Research Triangle Park, NC) is secured on the suture to prevent it from pulling through; biologic hemostatic gelatin-matrix-thrombin tissue sealant FloSeal (Baxter Healthcare, Deerfield, IL) is applied to the cut renal parenchymal surface underneath the bolster; another Hem-o-Lok clip is applied to the suture flush with the opposite renal surface, compressing the kidney; the suture is then tightly tied across the bolster, maintaining adequate parenchymal compression	We have tried various techniques, such as running stitch, Lapra-Ty, and no cross-tying over the bolster; with our experience in over 550 cases, we believe that the technique described here is the most reliable
Mannitol 12.5 g and furosemide 10–20 mg are given intravenously and the hilum is unclamped	Administer 2 to 3 minutes prior to unclamping
The abdomen is reinspected after 5 to 10 minutes of zero pneumoperitoneum to ensure good hemostasis	This is important to confirm absolute hemostasis in each and every case
The specimen is removed in an endocatch bag and a Jackson-Pratt (JP) drain is placed prior to exiting the abdomen	We prefer a Penrose drain for retroperitoneal cases

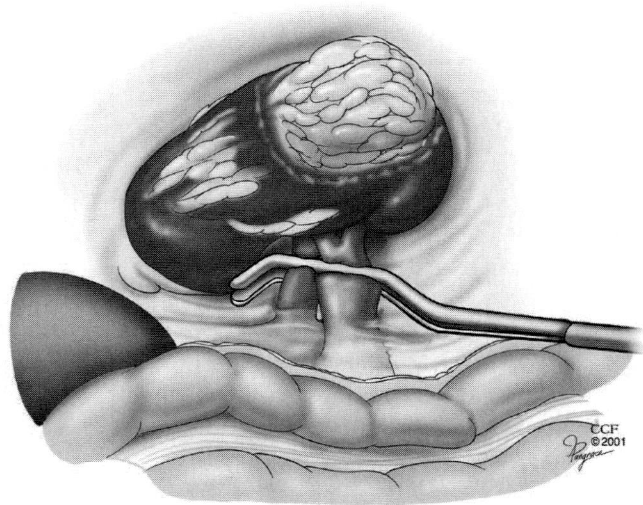

Figure 14.1. During a transperitoneal procedure, the hilum is clamped en bloc with a Satinsky clamp.

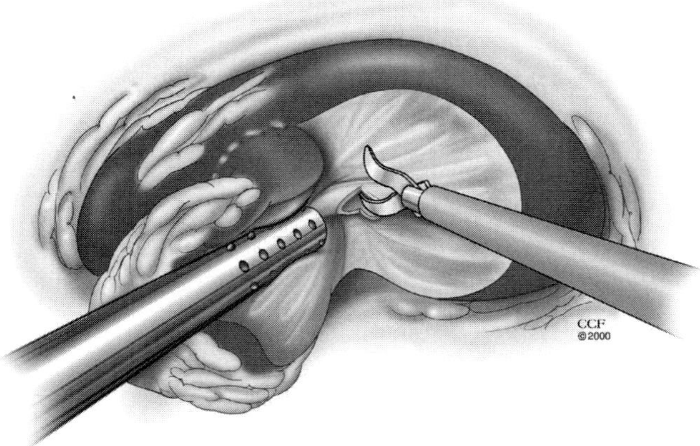

Figure 14.2. The tumor is excised using cold Endoshears in a near bloodless field while the hilum is clamped.

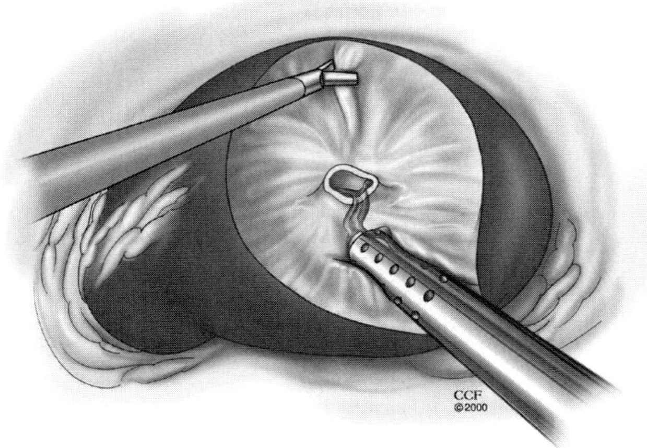

Figure 14.3. The point of entry into the collecting system is confirmed with retrograde injection of dilute methylene blue.

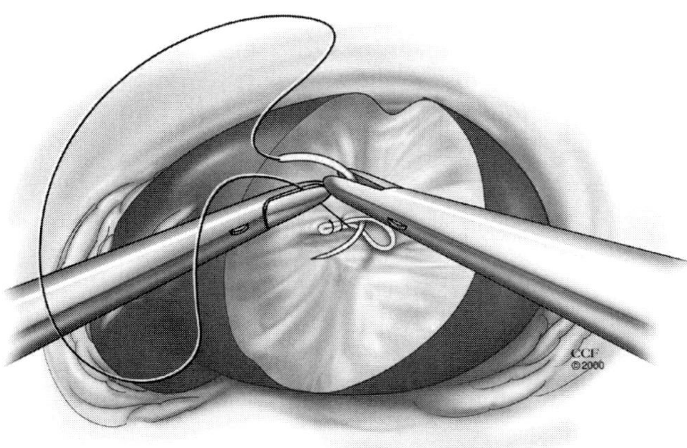

Figure 14.4. The collecting system is suture repaired using a running 2-0 Vicryl suture on a CT-1 needle.

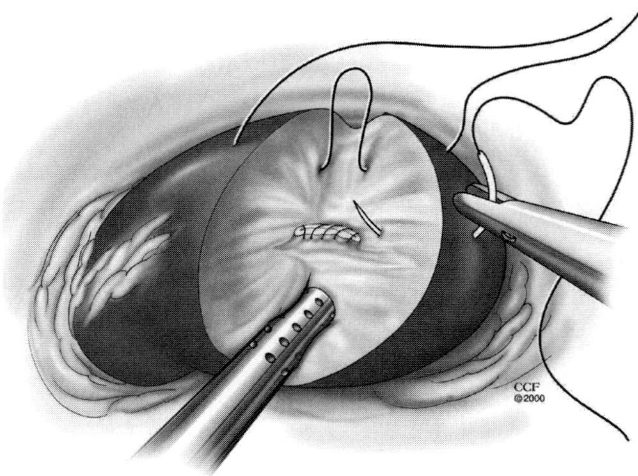

Figure 14.5. Interrupted renorrhaphy sutures are placed through the parenchymal edges ensuring that the renal capsule is included.

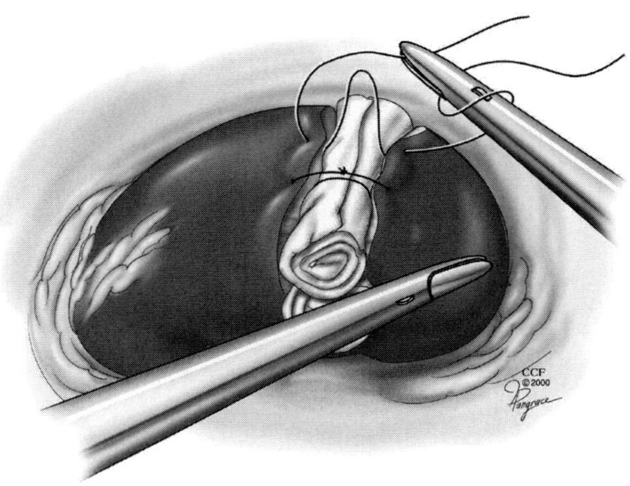

Figure 14.6. The renorrhaphy sutures are tied over a Surgicel bolster placed in the partial nephrectomy bed.

Rais-Bahrami et al.[40] reported a conversion rate of 13.6% to laparoscopic radical nephrectomy and 1.6% to open surgery among 257 operations that started as LPN. They found age >70 years and tumor size >4 cm to significantly increase (fourfold) the risk of conversion.

MULTIPLE TUMORS

Steinberg et al.[41] from the Cleveland Clinic reported treatment of 27 tumors in 13 patients (with an imperative indication in 92%) using a combination of MINSS techniques. Treatments included en bloc excision of adjacent tumors during LPN (in three patients); individual LPN of discrete masses (in two patients); LPN of one mass and laparoscopic cryoablation of the other (in two patients); and cryoablation of all masses (in six patients). Mean tumor size treated by LPN was 2.5 cm (1–4.1 cm), mean size treated by cryoablation was 1.8 cm (0.9–3.2 cm), mean OR time was 4.3 hours, and mean EBL was 169 mL. Mean warm ischemia time was 40 minutes in patients treated with LPN for adjacent masses, and 30 minutes in patients undergoing LPN and cryo-ablation. After a mean follow-up of 16.4 months (range, 1–54 months), there were no recurrences.

ADRENAL INVOLVEMENT

Ramani et al.[42] reported adrenalectomy during LPN in four patients with an upper pole tumor and suspected adrenal involvement. Using a transperitoneal approach, adre-nalectomy was performed first, followed by LPN. The adrenal gland was maintained en bloc with the partial nephrectomy specimen. Warm ischemia was limited to LPN only. No intraoperative complication occurred, and open conversion was not necessary.

TUMOR SEEDING

In a recent survey, 18,750 urologic laparoscopic procedures performed between 1990 and 2003 were assessed, of which 10,912 were for tumor, and 555 were LPN.[43] The overall incidence of tumor seeding was 0.1% (13 of 10,912); however, no cases of tumor seeding after LPN were noted.

HEMINEPHRECTOMY

Finelli et al.[17] evaluated laparoscopic heminephrectomy in 41 patients requiring a resection ≥30% of renal parenchyma, compared to a contemporary group of 41 consecu-tive patients who underwent LPN with <30% resection. The laparoscopic heminephrec-tomy group had larger tumors (3.7 vs. 2.3 cm), which were more commonly central (41% vs. 9.8%). Warm ischemia time was longer for laparoscopic heminephrectomy (39 vs. 33 minutes); however EBL (150 vs. 100 mL) and OR time (220 vs. 190 minutes) were comparable.

CENTRAL TUMORS

Frank et al.[15] compared LPN for central tumors ($n = 154$) with LPN for peripheral tumors ($n = 209$). Central tumors were defined as those abutting or invading the col-lecting system on preoperative CT. Central tumors were larger (3.0 vs. 2.4 cm) than peripheral tumors. Although EBL was similar (150 cc), central tumors required longer OR time (210 vs. 180 minutes), warm ischemia time (33.5 vs. 30.0 minutes), and hos-pital stay (67 vs. 60 hours). The incidence of margin positivity was 0.8% vs. 1.7%. There were more early postoperative complications in the central group (6% vs. 2%).

HILAR TUMORS

Gill et al.[16] reported the outcomes of LPN for hilar tumors. In 362 patients under-going LPN, 25 (6.9%) had a hilar tumor. Hilar tumor was defined as one located in the renal hilum and in contact with the renal vessels. No open conversion or operative reintervention was necessary. Mean tumor size was 3.7 cm (1–10.3 cm), and four patients (16%) had a solitary kidney. Pelvicaliceal repair was performed in 22 patients (88%). Warm ischemia time was 36.4 minutes (27–48 minutes), EBL was 231 cc (50–900 xx), and OR time was 3.6 hours (2–5 hours). Hemorrhagic complications occurred in three patients (12%).

SOLITARY KIDNEYS

Gill et al.[18] reported 22 patients (5%) with a tumor in a solitary kidney out of 430 LPNs. Mean tumor size was 3.6 cm (1.4 to 8.3 cm), median EBL was 200 cc (50 to 500 cc), warm ischemia time was 29 minutes (14 to 55 minutes), OR time was 3.3 hours (2.2 to 4.5 hours) and hospital stay was 2.8 days (1.3 to 12 hours). Two cases (9%) were electively converted to open surgery. Median preoperative and postoperative serum creatinine (1.2 and 1.5 mg/dL) and estimated glomerular filtration rate (67.5 and 50 mL/min/1.73 m^2) reflected a change of 33% and 27%, respectively, commensurate with the 23% parenchyma excised.

UNCLAMPED LAPAROSCOPIC PARTIAL NEPHRECTOMY

Guillonneau et al.[44] compared 12 patients undergoing LPN with hilar clamping vs. 16 patients without clamping. The nonclamped group had greater EBL (708 vs. 270 mL) and longer OR time (179 vs. 121 minutes) compared to LPN with clamping. Postoperative serum creatinine was not significantly different (1.3 vs. 1.45 mg/dL).

TRANSPERITONEAL VERSUS RETROPERITONEAL LAPAROSCOPIC PARTIAL NEPHRECTOMY

Ng et al.[45] retrospectively compared 100 transperitoneal and 63 retroperitoneal LPN. Transperitoneal access was elected for anterior or lateral lesions, and retroperitoneal access for posterior or posterolateral lesions. En bloc hilar control was achieved with a Satinsky clamp during transperitoneal LPN, while during retroperitoneal LPN individual control of the renal artery and vein was obtained with bulldog clamps. Transperitoneal LPN was associated with significantly larger tumors (3.2 vs. 2.5 cm), more pelvicaliceal repairs (79% vs. 57%), longer warm ischemia time (31 vs. 28 minutes), longer OR time (3.5 vs. 2.9 hours), and longer hospital stay (2.9 vs. 2.2 days) compared to retroperitoneal LPN. Blood loss, perioperative complications, postoperative serum creatinine, analgesic requirements, and histologic outcomes were comparable.

Complications

Urinary fistula is the most frequent complication following OPN. Other complications include hemorrhage, ureteral obstruction, and acute or chronic renal insufficiency. In a report on 259 patients undergoing OPN, Campbell et al.[46] reported urinary fistula in 17%, bleeding in 2.3%, reoperation in 3%, acute hemodialysis in 5%, and perioperative mortality in 1.5%. Corman et al.[47] compared complications after open radical nephrectomy ($n = 1373$) and OPN ($n = 512$) and did not find any significant difference in specific complication rates.

The most common complications of LPN include intraoperative or delayed hemorrhage, urine leak, and open conversion. In the first 200 LPN at the authors' institute, perioperative complications occurred in 66 patients (33%).[48] Open conversion was required in two patients (1%). Reoperative laparotomy was necessary in four patients (2%). Overall, hemorrhagic complications occurred in 19 patients (9.5%). Urine leak occurred in nine patients (4.5%). Other urologic complications occurred in 4.5%. Nonurologic complications occurred in 15% of patients. Since we began using Floseal as an adjunct, our complication rates have decreased significantly. When comparing LPN without Floseal to LPN with Floseal,[22] the Floseal group had decreased overall complications (37% vs. 16%), a lower rate of hemorrhagic complications (12% vs. 3%), and lesser urine leak (6% vs. 1.5%).

Our Current Concerns

Laparoscopic partial nephrectomy has come a long way in a short span of 5 years. The technique is becoming standardized and the procedure more prevalent at centers of excellence around the world. Nevertheless, it continues to be a technically challenging procedure that requires advanced laparoscopic skills allowing tumor excision and sutured renal reconstruction within a reasonable time period. In the hands of experienced surgeons, the rate of hemorrhagic complications, positive margins, and urinary leakage is now comparable to contemporary OPN series. However, such results are not yet reproducible at all centers. In addition, 5-year oncologic data are currently available in only 50 patients worldwide. Laparoscopic renal hypothermia is still evolving. A user-friendly method that reproducibly reduces renal temperature to 15°C may extend the indications of LPN to more complex renal tumors.

Our Future Expectations

Future directions could include potentially bloodless renal parenchymal incision without hilar clamping with the use of hydro-jet technology[49] or lasers.[50] Hydro-jet technology employs a high-pressure water jet to perform selective tissue dissection in a relatively bloodless manner.[49] Spared intrarenal vessels may then be controlled with clips or bipolar coagulation, and the renal collecting system suture repaired. Moinzadeh et al.[50] investigated the technical feasibility and short-term outcomes of the 80-watt potassium-titanyl-phosphate (KTP) laser LPN without hilar clamping in the survival calf model. Two techniques, ablative vaporization ($n = 5$) and wedge resection ($n = 7$), were evaluated. Renal parenchymal resection and hemostasis were achieved solely with the laser, without any adjunctive hemostatic sutures or bioadhesives. All 12 procedures were successful without open conversion, 11 (92%) without hilar clamping. Blood loss was 119 cc (25–300 cc). Shortcomings of such technique included considerable smoke generation during laser LPN leading to increased operative time, and higher CO_2 inflow-rate requirement.

Nearly 25% of all renal tumors treated with LPN are benign on final histopathology. At this time no consistently reliable method exists to make this determination preoperatively. Advances in imaging with adjunctive needle biopsies could make this a possibility in the future.

CRYOABLATION

Cryoablation causes tumor destruction by rapid freeze and thaw cycles, at a temperature below minus 20°C. Liquid argon and liquid nitrogen are the two most commonly used cryogens.

Indications and Contraindications—2006

Currently, renal cryoablation should be restricted to a small (<3 cm) solid enhancing renal tumor in older patients with high operative risk. Relative contraindications are young age, tumors >4 cm, hilar tumors, intrarenal tumors, and cystic tumors. Irreversible coagulopathy is an absolute contraindication.

Foundations

TISSUE–ICE INTERACTIONS

Acute tissue injury results from ice formation in tissues. Initial ice formation occurs in the extracellular space and leads to movement of water from inside the cells to the extracellular compartment. This eventually leads to changes in intracellular solute composition, pH, and protein denaturation. Extracellular ice formation also leads to mechanical disruption of the cell membranes and hence intracellular ice formation. Delayed tissue injury occurs in the hours and days following cryoablation and is an indirect damage due to injury to the microvasculature of the target tissue leading to diminished tissue perfusion and delayed cell death.[51,52]

Freeze–Thaw Cycles

Double freezing has been shown to produce a larger area of necrosis in an animal model, when compared to a single freeze. Whether slow thawing confers any advantage over rapid active thawing in the clinical context is not entirely clear.[53] Our personal preference is for a double-freeze thaw cycle.

Temperature and Ice-Ball Monitoring

Chosy et al.[54] found renal tissue needed exposure to or below −19.4°C. This was substantiated by Campbell et al.,[55] who observed complete necrosis 3.1 mm inside the edge of the ice ball. This physical location correlated with a temperature of −19.4°C. Clinical protocols err on the side of caution and freeze to −40°C. Such an end point can be determined by thermocouples at the tumor margin, or ultrasound[56] can be used to verify extension of the ice ball 1 cm beyond the tumor margin.[57]

Effects on the Collecting System

In an experimental study Sung et al.[58] found that in the absence of direct puncture into the collecting system with the cryoprobe, the cryoinjured collecting system heals in a watertight manner and does not lead to urinary fistulas. Other authors have reported similar experiences with cryoablation but found that RFA was associated with a greater risk of urinary leakage.[59,60]

Effects on Renal Function

In a canine solitary kidney model, Campbell et al.[55] found that renal function remained stable after cryoablation. Gill et al.[61] found no significant deleterious effect of cryoablation on renal function. In a cohort of 56 patients with 3-year follow-up, preoperative and postoperative serum creatinine was 1.2 mg/dL vs. 1.4 mg/dL. Ten patients had a solitary kidney. In this subgroup mean preoperative and postoperative serum creatinine was 2.2 and 2.6 mg/dL, respectively. In 13 patients with baseline renal insufficiency, mean preoperative and postoperative serum creatinine were 3.0 and 2.7 mg/dL, respectively.

Technical Considerations

The main features of renal cryotherapy are real-time imaging of the tumor, planning the depth and angle of entry of the cryoprobe, needle biopsies of the tumor, cryoprobe insertion through the center of the tumor up to or just beyond the deep margin, creating a cryolesion about 1 cm larger than the tumor under real-time US control, and securing hemostasis after removal of the probe and thawing of the ablated tissue.

Currently renal cryoablation is performed laparoscopically or percutaneously. Laparoscopic renal cryoablation (LRC) offers the advantage of precise cryoprobe positioning and monitoring of the evolving ice ball under real-time ultrasonic and visual control. Ultrasound shows the ice ball as a hyperechoic advancing crescent with a posterior acoustic shadow. In addition, adjacent structures can be mobilized away from the

Table 14.2.
Our current technique of laparoscopic renal cryoablation

Technical nuances	*Caveat/comment*
Access	
Retroperitoneal for posterior or posterolateral tumors	
Transperitoneal for anterior or anteromedial tumors	
Mobilization of kidney to expose tumor	The surface of the kidney opposite to the tumor must also be mobilized for placement of the ultrasound probe
Perform intraoperative ultrasound to map the tumor limits	Expert ultrasonography is needed
Resect overlying fat for histopathology	
Obtain needle biopsy under visual and ultrasonic control	
Insert cryoprobes into center of tumor up to the deep margin of the tumor (Figure 14.7)	The probe must enter at right angles to the tumor surface
Real-time ultrasound monitoring of the evolving ice ball (Figure 14.8) during a double freeze thaw cycle	
Extend ice ball 1 cm beyond tumor margin	
Remove cryoprobes and obtain hemostasis with surgical, argon beam, and FloSeal (Baxter)	The cryoprobe is removed once it is mobile within the thawing ice ball; perform hemostatic maneuvers at this stage
MR imaging on postoperative day 1, and at 3, 6, 12, 18, 24, 36, 48, and 60 months	
CT-guided needle biopsy at 6 months, repeated if MRI findings are abnormal	

planned ablation site. A transperitoneal approach is used for anterior and anteromedial tumors, while a retroperitoneal approach is used for posterior and posterolateral tumors.[62,63] Anterior or medial tumors, which would be difficult to target percutaneously, can be safely approached laparoscopically. Our preference is for the argon-based cryomachine, and we now use the 3.8 mm cryoprobes. Our current technique of LRC is outlined in Table 14.2.

Percutaneous renal cryoablation (PRC) is currently performed using open gantry magnetic resonance imaging (MRI)[64] or CT scan guidance. Recently percutaneous cryoablation under general anesthesia with ultrasound guidance alone has been reported in a pilot study of four patients.[65] Percutaneous ablation is usually reserved for posterior tumors. Patients with von Hippel–Lindau disease are particularly suited for the percutaneous technique.

Worldwide Data

Khorsandi et al.[66] reported open renal cryoablation on 17 patients with lesions smaller than 4 cm in diameter. The median length of follow-up was 30 months (range, 10–60 months), with eight patients followed up for more than 20 months. The procedure was

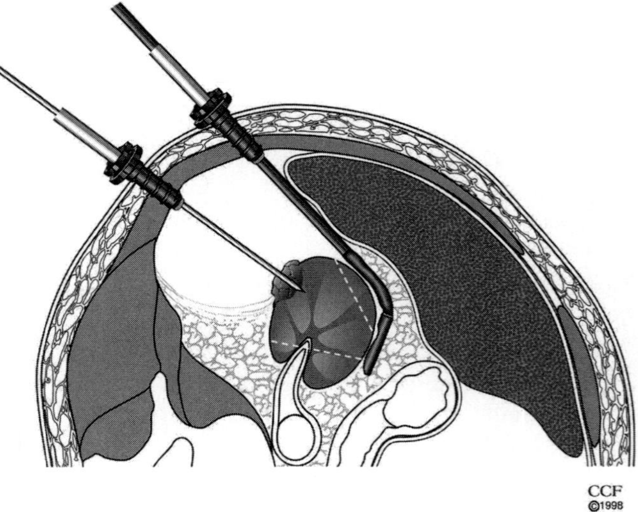

Figure 14.7. The cryoprobe enters the tumor in its center and at right angles under direct laparoscopic and ultrasound guidance.

accomplished in 3 hours through a 5- to 7-cm subcostal incision. The median blood loss was 100 mL, and the median hospital stay was 2 days (range, 2–8 days). Postoperative serum creatinine levels were unchanged. Follow-up MRI scans demonstrated infarction and a reduction of lesion size in 15 of 16 cases.

Shingleton and Sewell reported MRI-guided PRC[64] in 20 patients with mean tumor diameter of 3 cm (1.8–7.0 cm). Average treatment time was 97 minutes (56–172 minutes). One patient had evidence of persistent tumor on follow-up imaging and required retreatment. Mean follow-up was 9 months (3–14 months) with no radiographic evidence of recurrence or new tumor development.

Gupta et al.[67] reported CT-guided PRC on 27 tumors ≤5 cm. Blood transfusion was required in one patient. Sixteen tumors in 12 patients have follow-up ≥1 month (mean 5.9 months). Five of these were centrally located and 11 were peripheral; 15 showed no enhancement on follow-up.

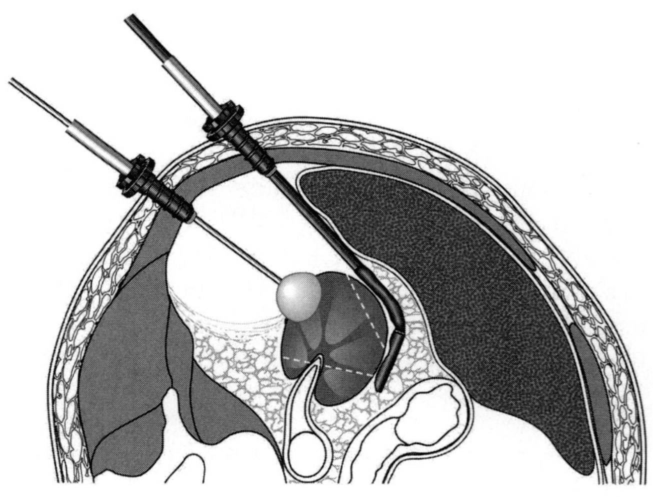

Figure 14.8. The evolving ice ball is monitored in real time with laparoscopic ultrasound. The ultrasound probe is placed on the surface of the kidney opposite the tumor.

Three-year follow-up data on 56 patients (including 10 with solitary kidneys) treated with LRC was reported by Gill et al.[61] CT-guided biopsy of the cryolesion was performed 6 months postoperatively and repeated if MRI findings were abnormal. A 75% reduction in size of cryolesion was seen at 3 years. Needle biopsy identified locally persistent/recurrent tumor in two patients. In the 51 patients undergoing LRC for a unilateral, sporadic tumor 3-year cancer-specific survival was 98%. There was no open conversion, kidney loss, urinary fistula, dialysis requirement, or perirenal or port site recurrence in any patient.

Lawatsch et al.[68] reported LRC of 81 tumors (median size 2.5 cm) in 59 patients. Open surgery was required in two patients including nephrectomy in one. Two recurrences were noted at a median follow-up of 27 months.

Cestari et al.[69] reported LRC on 37 patients with a mean tumor size of 26 mm (10–60 mm). There were no conversions to open procedures. Mean operating time was 194 minutes, and mean blood loss was 165 mL. Of the 35 patients with at least 6 months follow-up, CT-guided biopsy was performed in 25, who were negative for neoplasm.

Moon et al.[70] reported LRC in 16 patients with one conversion. The mean blood loss was 40 mL. The mean hospital stay was 1.9 days. With a mean follow-up of 9.6 months, all tumors remained nonenhancing.

Desai et al.[71] compared laparoscopic partial nephrectomy (group 1, $n = 153$) with LRC (group 2, $n = 78$) for the small (≤3 cm) renal tumor. Laparoscopic partial nephrectomy was associated with greater blood loss and more delayed complications. Both groups were comparable as regards operating time, intraoperative and postoperative complications, hospital stay, convalescence, and postoperative serum creatinine. Local recurrence was detected over a mean follow-up of 5.8 months in group 1 (0.6%) and 24.6 months in group 2 (3%).

Hruby et al.[72] reported a comparison of 12 LPNs and 11 LRCs on patients with hilar tumors. There were no conversions. The mean operating time for LPN and LRC was 2.8 hours and 2.3 hours, respectively. The mean blood loss was 197 mL for LPN and 70 mL for LRC. The hospital stay for patients in the LPN and LRC groups was 3.9 days vs. 3.2 days, respectively. No intraoperative complications occurred in either group. Nine complications were seen in the LPN group, including four urine leaks versus none in the LRC group. No disease recurrence was seen in the LRC or the LPN group at about 1-year follow-up.

Shingleton and Sewell[73] reported MRI-guided PRC on solitary kidneys in 14 patients. Fifteen tumors (mean 3.1 cm) were treated; the mean treatment time was 96.7 minutes (30–143 minutes). There were no complications during treatment. Two patients had gross hematuria afterward that resolved within 24 hours. The mean follow-up was 17 months (2–30 months), with three patients requiring retreatment for incomplete ablation. There was no evidence of local recurrence as of the last follow-up. In two patients the tumor was not completely ablated.

Complications

The most common complications are pain and paresthesias at the operative site. Complications such as renal fracture, perirenal hematoma, liver injury, pancreatic injury, ureteropelvic junction obstruction, and paralytic ileus occur rarely. Renal fracture can occur as a result of poorly planned cryoprobe entry and can be prevented by perpendicular insertion of the probe and maintaining it in a fixed position throughout the procedure. A multiinstitutional review revealed a total of 20 complications following 139 cryoablation, procedures of which 1.4% were major and 12.2% were minor[74]; 16 of these 20 complications were observed in the percutaneous group.

Our Current Concerns

The major limitation to the use of ablative techniques is the lack of histologic confirmation of complete tumor ablation, hence the need for rigorous radiologic follow-up. Absence of contrast enhancement on follow-up CT or MRI is considered oncologic success. To date only 6-month follow-up biopsy data are available, although the optimum biopsy schedule is yet to be determined. Reliable 5-year survival data are needed.

Our Future Expectations

A proportion of renal masses treated with ablative techniques could be benign, which may tend to overestimate the efficacy of these procedures. The amount of energy used, mode of energy delivery, and duration of treatment, which have a major influence on the results, differ between various studies, which make comparisons between studies unreliable. These parameters need to be standardized and techniques need to be refined to improve outcome. Intralesional use of apoptosis promoters may enhance the cytocidal efficacy of cryotherapy. Although the short and intermediate-term results are encouraging, long-term 5-year follow-up data remain critically important.

RADIOFREQUENCY ABLATION

Radiofrequency ablation involves coagulating tumors by directly applying temperatures above 50°C via needle electrodes.

Indications and Contraindications—2006

Radiofrequency ablation may be indicated in patients with advanced age and comorbidity, multiple bilateral RCC (von Hippel–Lindau disease), and RCC in a solitary kidney. Tumors >5 cm, hilar tumors, and central tumors are not suitable. The only absolute contraindication is an irreversible coagulopathy. Radiofrequency ablation has also been used in patients with intractable hematuria due to RCC[75] and tumor recurrence in the nephrectomy bed.[76]

Foundations

Radiofrequency ablation acts by converting RF waves to heat, resulting in thermal damage. High-frequency current flows from needle electrode to target tissue result in ionic agitation and heat-producing molecular friction, denaturation of proteins, and cell membrane disintegration. These changes take 4 to 6 minutes at temperatures >50°C and almost immediately above 60°C. Temperatures >105°C result in vaporization of tissue, resulting in gas formation and inefficient creation of an RF lesion. The goal of RFA is to induce temperatures of 50° to 100°C throughout the tumor.[77] In dry RFA, the increase in temperature around the probe increases tissue impedance, preventing expansion of the lesion. In wet RFA, saline irrigated through tissue increases conductivity and helps in dissipation of the energy, preventing an increase in impedance.[78] This results in larger RF lesions. Bipolar RFA decreases the risk of accidental burns associated with monopolar RFA.[79] Exophytic tumors that are draped by avascular perirenal fat are better ablated than central tumors surrounded by vascular parenchyma that acts as a heat sink.[80] In contrast to cryotherapy, temporary renal artery occlusion may enhance the efficacy of RFA.[81]

Technical Considerations

Open, laparoscopic, and percutaneous techniques have been employed for renal RFA. Laparoscopic RFA has the advantage of mobilizing the tumor and avoiding adjacent organ damage and placement of the probe under direct vision, while percutaneous RFA (pRFA; currently the most prevalent) is well tolerated and can be performed under sedation on an outpatient basis. The size of the ablated tissue depends on tissue impedance, ablation time, amount of energy delivered, and surface area of the electrodes. The RFA probes can be inserted under ultrasound, CT, and MRI guidance. The formation of microbubbles and the hyperechoic rim limits the use of ultrasound for real-time imaging of RFA. As coagulated tissue is not perfused, administration of intravenous contrast prior to retracting the probe helps estimate the result of RFA during CT or MRI guidance. Imaging immediately after the procedure can be difficult to interpret because of peripheral inflammation. The success of RFA is usually assessed typically by CT scan 1 month after treatment by demonstrating absence of enhancement in the ablated tissue.

Worldwide Data

Zagoria et al.[80] reported 27 CT-guided pRFA in 22 patients. No serious complications were noted. No residual tumor was detected on follow-up contrast-enhanced CT or MRI, 1 to 35 months (mean, 7 months) after final tumor ablation in 20 (91%) of 22 patients. Complete ablation was achieved after a single session in 83% of patients, and in 8% after subsequent sessions. Size was the major determinant for success with a single session, with all 11 tumors ≤3 cm being completely ablated after one session.

Gervais et al.[82] report RFA of 100 renal tumors in 85 patients. All 52 small (≤3 cm) and all 68 exophytic tumors underwent complete necrosis regardless of size, although many large tumors (>3 cm) required a second ablation session. The authors found that both small size and noncentral location were independent predictors of complete necrosis after a single session. Complications were self-limited or readily treated and included hemorrhage (major in two patients and minor in three), inflammatory track mass in one patient, transient lumbar plexus pain in two patients, ureteral injury in two patients, and skin burns in one patient.

Matsumoto et al.[83] reported 109 small renal tumors (91 patients) treated with CT-guided pRFA ($n = 63$) or laparoscopic RFA ($n = 46$). The mean tumor size was 2.4 cm (0.8–4.7 cm). The initial ablation was successful in 107 (98%) tumors. Of the 60 patients with at least 1 year of follow-up, 60% had biopsy proven RCC. One local recurrence (1.7%) was detected during a mean follow-up of 19.4 months (12–33 months), and in those with known RCC, none had evidence of distant progression (0%).

Weizer et al.[84] reported complications in 24 patients with 32 renal tumors treated with pRFA. Average tumor size was 2.4 cm (0.5–8.6 cm). Five patients experienced complications: perinephric hematoma in two patients, persistent urinoma and proximal ureteral stricture in one patient, and colonic injury in two patients. Three of these five patients had undergone prior partial nephrectomy on the pRFA-treated kidney. Two of four patients treated for multiple tumors and 57% of patients with anteriorly located tumors experienced complications.

Merkle et al.[85] reported 18 patients treated with MRI-guided pRFA. The mean follow-up time was 16.1 months (6–41 months). Thermal ablation zones were uniformly hypointense and had a surrounding bright rim on T2–weighted images, and were predominantly hyperintense on T1–weighted images. Thin rim enhancement with central hypointensity was noted on the gadolinium-enhanced images. Residual tumor was detected after RFA in two cases, best seen on unenhanced T2–weighted and gadolinium-enhanced T1–weighted MR images.

Mahnken et al.[86] reported CT-guided pRFA in 14 patients. Tumors >3 cm ($n = 6$) were embolized within 24 hours prior to RFA. Average tumor size was 3 ± 1 cm. With the exception of one renocutaneous fistula, which was treated conservatively, no major complications were observed. No local recurrence was observed (follow-up: 14 ± 12 months), while extrarenal tumor progression occurred in four patients.

Ahrar et al.[87] reported 29 patients with 30 renal tumors (mean diameter, 3.5 ± 0.24 cm) who underwent CT-guided pRFA. Overall, 88 overlapping ablations were performed (mean 2.6 ablations per tumor per session) in 34 sessions. There were four major complications (12%), including three with gross hematuria. There were no significant changes in renal function after RFA. Technical success was achieved in all cases. Follow-up images were available for 26 patients. The primary tumor was completely ablated in 23 of 24 patients (96%) in whom eradication of the primary tumor was attempted (mean follow-up of 10 months).

Su et al.[88] reported CT-guided pRFA in 29 patients with 35 small (≤4 cm) renal lesions using a dry RFA technique. Of 37 RFA treatments, 35 (95%) were successfully performed under intravenous sedation and 32 (86%) treatments were performed on an outpatient basis. Over a mean radiographic follow-up period of 9 months, 33 of 35 (94%) renal lesions have required only a single RFA treatment, and two patients required a second, successful retreatment for residual enhancement. Of 13 renal lesions with a ≥12-month radiographic follow-up interval, 11 (85%) have demonstrated no residual enhancement.

Clark et al.[89] reported their experience with pRFA using multi-tined expandable electrodes along with an aggressive treatment strategy to displace adjacent viscera away from probe tines. Over a 36-month period, 22 patients with 26 sporadic RCC underwent 43 ablations during 27 pRFA sessions under CT guidance. The mean age was 71 years and mean tumor diameter was 2.2 cm (1–4 cm). Technical success in targeting and ablation was 100%. Mean follow-up was 11 months (1–31 months). One patient had local recurrence and underwent repeat pRFA. Adjunctive techniques included water injection for displacement of the tail of the pancreas ($n = 1$) or the descending colon ($n = 3$). Penetration of tines beyond the margins of the kidney was performed in 41% of cases; no hemorrhage occurred in these cases. No major complications occurred. Minor complications occurred in 17% of patients, including asymptomatic pneumothorax, perirenal hematomas, subcutaneous hematoma, and subcutaneous abscess. After 6 months, mean involution of the ablation zone was 15% from baseline volume per year.

Complications

The most common complication is pain and paresthesias at the percutaneous probe insertion site. Other complications, such as perinephric hematoma, transient hematuria, ureteropelvic junction obstruction, and liver burns, have been described. The ability to avoid tract bleeding and tumor seeding by coagulating the puncture channel during probe withdrawal results in decreased bleeding complications associated with this procedure. A multiinstitutional review showed major and minor complications associated with RFA to be 2.2% and 6%, respectively.[74]

Our Current Concerns

Viable residual tumor has been found in radical and partial nephrectomy specimens of patients treated with previous RFA,[90,91] which raises concerns about the oncologic efficacy of this technique, and makes a cogent argument for the need for further refinements and close follow-up.

Our Future Expectations

Radiofrequency ablation lacks reliable real-time monitoring of the evolving lesion. Recently, contrast-enhanced ultrasonography (CEUS) has been reported to be accurate in predicting the progression of the thermolesion during RFA in a porcine model.[92] Five pigs underwent laparoscopic RFA twice, separated by a 1-week interval. Post-RFA ultrasound imaging was performed immediately after ablation. The kidneys were assessed for a contrast void corresponding to the ablated tissue. The kidneys were then harvested and the gross RFA lesions measured to compare lesion size with that measured using CEUS.

OTHER TECHNIQUES

Experience with the following techniques is limited, and considerable research is required to define their role in the current context.

High-Intensity Focused Ultrasound

A high-intensity ultrasonic beam is focused onto a small volume of target lesion, which causes a rise in the tissue temperature leading to protein denaturation and cell death. The transducer is used to both deliver and monitor therapy. High-intensity focused ultrasound (HIFU) causes tissue insult by two mechanisms: a thermal and a cavitational effect. Thermal effects are due to the absorption of sound energy by the tissue as the ultrasonic waves pass through the tissue, leading to heat formation and protein denaturation. It is obtained by using low-intensity energy over long periods. With high-intensity energy over shorter periods, cavitational effects are achieved by bubble implosion leading to mechanical disruption. Experimental studies in animals have shown that HIFU lesions are consistent with coagulative necrosis.[93] The main limitation of this technique is the difficulty in lesion localization and targeting. Respiratory movements and overlying ribs are a limiting factor with the use of HIFU for renal tumors.[94]

To date, the role of HIFU remains unproven in clinical studies. Hacker et al.[95] applied HIFU to the healthy tissue of 24 kidneys, monitored by ultrasound, with a maximum power of 400 W and a spatially averaged intensity in the focus of $1192\,W/cm^2$. For an in vivo study, 14 kidneys were removed immediately after ablation, and 10 kidneys were removed after 1, 7, and 10 days. The clinical study consisted of 19 patients requiring radical nephrectomy for a renal tumor. High-intensity focused ultrasound was applied to the healthy tissue of 19 kidneys (up to 1600 W, averaged intensity = 4768 W/cm^2) before proceeding with the radical nephrectomy. Side effects included grade 3 skin burns in two patients. During the follow-up there were no further HIFU-specific side effects. In one case (in vivo study) there was a thermal lesion of the small intestine, which the authors attributed to poor focusing. The HIFU effects in the focal zone immediately after application were interstitial hemorrhages, fiber rupture, shrinking of the collagen fibers, and coagulation necrosis. These effects occurred sporadically, and their number and size did not correspond to the number of HIFU pulses applied. After 7 and 10 days, there was a well-demarcated coagulation necrosis in vivo. The authors concluded that refinements in technology are essential to establish HIFU as a noninvasive treatment option.

Microwave Thermotherapy

Microwave thermotherapy (MT) involves the passage of microwave energy (300–3000 MHz) from flexible antennae into the tissue, which causes the setting up of a rapidly alternating electromagnetic field leading to oscillation of ions, and this increase in kinetic energy is converted to heat resulting in coagulative necrosis.[96] In comparison to other ablative modalities microwave thermotherapy causes a smaller zone of ablation. Experimental data in the VX-2 rabbit model suggests equivalent survival in rabbits treated with MT and nephrectomy.[97] Currently, MT is being used for achieving hemostasis during partial nephrectomy. No clinical experience has been reported to date regarding the use of MT in renal tumor ablation.

Laser Interstitial Thermal Therapy

Laser interstitial thermal therapy (LITT), also known as laser thermal ablation (LTA), involves the placement of laser fibers into the tumor and applying laser energy to ablate the tumor. Laser energy raises the tissue temperature and causes coagulative necrosis. Diode and neodymium:yttrium-aluminum-garnet (Nd:YAG) lasers have been used. Laser energy at 20 to 25 W for 20 minutes raises the tissue temperature to 55°C. Application of 480 J laser energy causes coagulative necrosis, while 720 J causes vaporization with a peripheral zone of coagulative necrosis. Laser interstitial thermal therapy has been tried in a laparoscopic environment experimentally and with MR guidance in inoperable tumors clinically.[98,99] Studies regarding the use of LTA are sparse, and it should be considered purely experimental at the current stage.

Chemoablation

Injecting several chemical agents into the tumor causes cellular destruction by a direct cytotoxic effect. Hypertonic saline (23.4%), absolute ethanol (95%), and acetic acid (50%) have been tried either alone or in combination with monopolar or bipolar radiofrequency in experimental studies in pigs.[79] These agents when used alone failed to produce consistent cellular necrosis and contained skip areas, while, when used in combination with RF, produced larger areas of more complete necrosis.

Radiosurgery

Radiosurgery for renal tumors is analogous to the use of gamma knife radiosurgery for intracranial lesions. Ponsky et al.[100] reported experience with Cyberknife® technology in 10 swine. The Cyberknife® is a frameless image-guided radiosurgery device that uses a linear accelerator mounted on a robotic arm, and divides the high-dose radiation into up to 1200 beams. Thus the individual dose of each beam is relatively benign to adjacent tissue, although, at the focal point of these beams, the dose is additive, and the desired ablative dose is attained. Ponsky et al. also treated 16 kidneys with single doses of 24 to 40 Gy. Eight weeks after treatment, the lesions showed complete fibrosis. The first human trials of this promising technology are currently underway at the authors' institution.

CLEVELAND CLINIC EXPERIENCE

We have analyzed our experience over the last 9 years with MINSS. In the initial 5 years (1997–2001), we performed 91 LPNs for patients with a mean age of 64 years and mean body mass index (BMI) of 30; 61% of patients had American Society of Anesthesiologists (ASA) score ≥3. Mean tumor size was 2.9 cm, with 35% of patients having tumors ≥3 cm. An imperative indication for LPN existed in 30%, and 13% of patients had renal insufficiency (serum creatinine >1.4 mg/dL). In the ensuing 4 years (2002–2005) our experience with LPN increased fivefold, and we performed 408 such procedures with mean age of 58 years, mean BMI of 29, and mean tumor size of 2.8 cm; 31% of patients had tumor size >3 cm. Renal insufficiency existed in 9% of patients, and an imperative indication was found in 27% (including solitary kidneys in 6%). Five LPNs were performed on renal remnants after previous partial nephrectomy. Overall, of the 499 tumors, 55% were peripheral, 39% were central, and 6% were hilar. Tumor location was anterior in 350 patients and posterior in 149. Final pathology revealed RCC in 75%.

Perioperative parameters in the latter 408 patients revealed a mean OR time of 204 minutes, mean EBL of 265 mL, mean warm ischemia time of 31.7 minutes, and hospital stay of 3.2 days. Intraoperative complications occurred in 7.8%, and postoperative complications in 15%. Blood transfusion was required in 3%. Open conversion was seen in five patients (1.2%), including two (0.4%) for nephrectomy.

For the initial 91 patients, the mean follow-up duration is 42 months. There have been no local recurrences, although one patient developed distant metastases. There have been seven deaths, all due to unrelated causes.

In the initial 5 years (1997–2001), we performed 74 LRCs for patients with a mean age of 66 years and mean BMI of 28; 60% of patients had ASA score ≥3. Mean tumor size was 2.3 cm, with 16% of patients having tumors ≥3 cm. An imperative indication for LRC existed in 47%, and 19% of patients had renal insufficiency (serum creatinine >1.4 mg/dL). Fifteen patients (20%) had a solitary kidney. No RFA were performed in these 5 years. In the ensuing 4 years (2002–2005) we performed another 72 LRCs with mean age of 67 years, mean BMI of 29, and mean tumor size of 2.6 cm; 23% of patients had tumor size >3 cm. Renal insufficiency existed in 35% of patients, and an imperative indication was found in 37% (including solitary kidneys in 16%). Overall, 17 of the 146 LRC (12%) were performed on renal remnants after previous partial nephrectomy. Multiple tumors were treated in 12 patients (8%). Pre-procedure needle biopsy revealed RCC in 23%. Overall mean operating time, blood loss, and hospital stay were 174 minutes, 115 mL, and 2.4 days, respectively. Intraoperative complications occurred in 3% and postoperative complications in 2%. Blood transfusion was required in 2%. Open conversion and nephrectomy were not required in any patient. Mean follow-up duration is 40 months. There have been no local recurrences, although five patients (3%) developed distant metastases and subsequently died.

In the last 4 years (2002–2005) we have performed 68 pRFAs for SRT. Mean age was 66 years and 66% patients had ASA ≥3. Mean tumor size was 2.5 cm with 20% >3 cm. Renal insufficiency was seen in 26%. An imperative indication existed in 66%, including 35 patients (51%) with a solitary kidney. Twenty-three pRFAs (33%) were performed on renal remnants and 10 (14%) for multiple tumors. Preprocedure needle biopsy confirmed RCC in 66%. No patient required blood transfusion, open conversion, or nephrectomy. Current mean follow-up is 12 months. There have been seven local recurrences (10%) and three distant metastases (4%).

CONCLUSION

We have reviewed the evolution and current status of extirpative and probe-ablative methods of MINSS for renal tumors. Open partial nephrectomy is the reference standard for nephron-sparing surgery against which all minimally invasive techniques should be measured. Given the requisite skills for time-sensitive intracorporeal suturing, LPN can provide long-term cancer cure comparable to the reference standard. The initial 5-year data of 50 patients have just become available and have shown overall and cancer-specific survival of 84% and 100%, respectively. Preliminary 3-year data for renal cryoablation indicate that this modality could be at the forefront of probe-ablative therapies for small renal tumors, where a partial nephrectomy is not considered suitable. Long-term data for RFA are still awaited. Concerns about residual tumor after RFA, despite negative enhancement, need to be addressed. The optimal modality for tumor targeting, monitoring therapy, and follow-up remains to be determined. These ablative techniques should be reserved for carefully selected patients, the data should be prospectively accrued, and the long-term cancer cure rates should be compared to the reference standard.

REFERENCES

1. Luciani LG, Cestari R, Tallarigo C. Incidental renal cell carcinoma-age and stage characterization and clinical implications: study of 1092 patients. Urology 2000;56:58–62.
2. Gill IS, Desai MM, Kaouk JH, et al. Laparoscopic partial nephrectomy for renal tumor: duplicating open surgical techniques. J Urol 2002;167:469–476.
3. Uzzo RG, Novick AC. Nephron sparing surgery for renal tumors: indications, techniques and outcomes. J Urol 2001;166:6–18.
4. Castilla EA, Liou LS, Abrahams NA, et al. Prognostic importance of resection margin width after nephron-sparing surgery for renal cell carcinoma. Urology 2002;60:993–997.
5. Fergany AF, Hafez KS, Novick AC. Long term results of nephron sparing surgery for localized renal cell carcinoma: 10-year follow-up. J Urol 2000;163:442–445.
6. Lee CT, Katz J, Shi W, Thaler HT, Reuter VE, Russo P. Surgical management of renal tumors 4 cm or less in a contemporary cohort. J Urol 2000;163:730–736.
7. Ghavamian R, Cheville JC, Lohse CM, Weaver AL, Zincke H, Blute ML. Renal cell carcinoma in the solitary kidney: an analysis of complications and outcome after nephron sparing surgery. J Urol 2002;168:454–459.
8. Novick AC. Partial nephrectomy for renal cell carcinoma. Urology 1995;46:149–152.
9. Herr HW. Partial nephrectomy for unilateral renal carcinoma and a normal contralateral kidney: 10-year followup. J Urol 1999;161:33–34.
10. Desai MM, Gill IS, Kaouk JH, Matin SF, Novick AC. Laparoscopic partial nephrectomy with suture repair of the pelvicaliceal system. Urology 2003;61:99–104.

11. Winfield HN, Donovan JF, Godet AS, Clayman RV. Laparoscopic partial nephrectomy: initial case report for benign disease. J Endourol 1993;7:521–526.

12. Gill IS, Delworth MG, Munch LC. Laparoscopic retroperitoneal partial nephrectomy. J Urol 1994;152:1539–1542.

13. McDougall EM, Elbahnasy AM, Clayman RV. Laparoscopic wedge resection and partial nephrectomy—the Washington University experience and review of the literature. JSLS 1998;2:15–23.

14. Janetschek, G, Jeschke K, Peschel R, Strohmeyer D, Henning K, Bartsch G. Laparoscopic surgery for stage T1 renal cell carcinoma: radical nephrectomy and wedge resection. Eur Urol 2000;38: 131–138.

15. Frank I, Colombo JR Jr, Rubinstein M, Desai M, Kaouk J, Gill IS. Laparoscopic partial nephrectomy for centrally located renal tumors. J Urol 2006;175:849–852.

16. Gill IS, Colombo JR Jr, Frank I, Moinzadeh A, Kaouk J, Desai M. Laparoscopic partial nephrectomy for hilar tumors. J Urol 2005;174:850–853.

17. Finelli A, Gill IS, Desai MM, et al. Laparoscopic heminephrectomy for tumor. Urology 2005;65:473–478.

18. Gill IS, Colombo JR Jr, Moinzadeh A, et al. Laparoscopic partial nephrectomy in solitary kidney. J Urol 2006;175:454–458.

19. Steinberg AP, Abreu SC, et al. Laparoscopic nephron-sparing surgery in the presence of renal artery disease. Urology 2003;62:935–939.

20. Gettman MT, Bishoff JT, Su LM, et al. Hemostatic laparoscopic partial nephrectomy: initial experience with the radiofrequency coagulation-assisted technique. Urology 2001;58:8–11.

21. Bak JB, Singh A, Shekarriz B. Use of gelatin matrix thrombin tissue sealant as an effective hemostatic agent during laparoscopic partial nephrectomy. J Urol 2004;171:780–782.

22. Gill IS, Ramani AP, Spaliviero M, et al. Improved hemostasis during laparoscopic partial nephrectomy using gelatin matrix thrombin sealant. Urology 2005;65:463–466.

23. Urena R, Mendez F, Woods M, Thomas R, Davis R. Laparoscopic partial nephrectomy of solid renal masses without hilar clamping using a monopolar radio frequency device. J Urol 2004;171: 1054–1056.

24. Gill IS, Matin SF, Desai MM, et al. Comparative analysis of laparoscopic versus open partial nephrectomy for renal tumors in 200 patients. J Urol 2003;170:64–68.

25. Novick AC. Renal hypothermia: in vivo and ex vivo. Urol Clin North Am 1983;10:637–644.

26. Shekarriz B, Shah G, Upadhyaya J. Impact of temporary hilar clamping during laparoscopic partial nephrectomy on postoperative renal function: a prospective study. J Urol 2004;172:54–57.

27. Desai MM, Gill IS, Ramani AP, Spaliviero M, Rybicki L, Kaouk JH. The impact of warm ischaemia on renal function after laparoscopic partial nephrectomy. BJU Int 2005;95:377–383.

28. Gill IS, Abreu SC, Desai MM, et al. Laparoscopic ice slush renal hypothermia for partial nephrectomy: the initial experience. J Urol 2003;170:52–56.

29. Janetschek G, Abdelmaksoud A, Bagheri F, Al-Zahrani H, Leeb K, Gschwendtner M. Laparoscopic partial nephrectomy in cold ischemia: renal artery perfusion. J Urol 2004;171:68–71.

30. Landman J, Venkatesh R, Lee D, et al. Renal hypothermia achieved by retrograde endoscopic cold saline perfusion: technique and initial clinical application. Urology 2003;61:1023–1025.

31. Ames CD, Venkatesh R, Weld KJ, et al. Laparoscopic renal parenchymal hypothermia with novel ice-slush deployment mechanism. Urology 2005;66:33–37.

32. Bove P, Bhayani SB, Rha KH, Allaf ME, Jarrett TW, Kavoussi LR. Necessity of ureteral catheter during laparoscopic partial nephrectomy. J Urol 2004;172:458–460.

33. Haber GP, Gill IS. Laparoscopic partial nephrectomy: contemporary technique and outcomes. Eur Urol 2006;49:660–665.

34. Moinzadeh A, Gill IS, Finelli A, Kaouk J, Desai M. Laparoscopic partial nephrectomy: 3-year followup. J Urol 2006;175:459–462.

35. Lane BR, Gill IS. Five-year outcomes of laparoscopic partial nephrectomy. J Urol 2007; 177:70–74.

36. Rassweiler JJ, Abbou C, Janetschek G, Jeschke K. Laparoscopic partial nephrectomy. The European experience. Urol Clin North Am 2000;27:721–736.

37. Jeschke K, Peschel R, Wakonig J, Schellander L, Bartsch G, Henning K. Laparoscopic nephron-sparing surgery for renal tumors. Urology 2001;58(5):688–692.

38. Weld KJ, Venkatesh R, Huang J, Landman J. Evolution of surgical technique and patient outcomes for laparoscopic partial nephrectomy. Urology 2006;67(3):502–506; discussion 506–507.

39. Wille AH, Tullmann M, Roigas J, Loening SA, Deger S. Laparoscopic partial nephrectomy in renal cell cancer—results and reproducibility by different surgeons in a high volume laparoscopic center. Eur Urol 2006;49(2):337–342; discussion 342–343. Epub 2005 Dec 27.

40. Rais-Bahrami S, Lima GC, Varkarakis IM, et al. Intraoperative conversion of laparoscopic partial nephrectomy. J Endourol 2006;20(3):205–208.

41. Steinberg AP, Kilciler M, Abreu SC, et al. Laparoscopic nephron-sparing surgery for two or more ipsilateral renal tumors. Urology 2004;64:255–825.

42. Ramani AP, Abreu SC, Desai MM, et al. Laparoscopic upper pole partial nephrectomy with concomitant en bloc adrenalectomy. Urology 2003;62:223–226.

43. Micali S, Celia A, Bove P, et al. Tumor seeding in urological laparoscopy: an international survey. J Urol 2004;171:2151–2154.

44. Guillonneau B, Bermudez H, Gholami S, et al. Laparoscopic partial nephrectomy for renal tumor: single center experience comparing clamping and no clamping techniques of the renal vasculature. J Urol 2003;169:483–486.

45. Ng CS, Gill IS, Ramani AP, et al. Transperitoneal versus retroperitoneal laparoscopic partial nephrectomy: patient selection and perioperative outcomes. J Urol 2005;174:846–849.

46. Campbell SC, Novick AC, Streem SB, Klein E, Licht M. Complications of nephron sparing surgery for renal tumors. J Urol 1994;151:1177–1180.

47. Corman JM, Penson DF, Hur K, et al. Comparison of complications after radical and partial nephrectomy: results from the National Veterans Administration Surgical Quality Improvement Program. BJU Int 2000;86:782–789.

48. Ramani AP, Desai MM, Steinberg AP, et al. Complications of laparoscopic partial nephrectomy in 200 cases. J Urol 2005;173:42–47.

49. Moinzadeh A, Hasan W, Spaliviero M, et al. Water jet assisted laparoscopic partial nephrectomy without hilar clamping in the calf model. J Urol 2005;174:317–321.

50. Moinzadeh A, Gill IS, Rubenstein M, et al. Potassium-titanyl-phosphate laser laparoscopic partial nephrectomy without hilar clamping in the survival calf model. J Urol 2005;174:1110–1114.

51. Hoffmann, NE, Bischof JC. The cryobiology of cryosurgical injury. Urology 2002;60:40–49.

52. Gill IS, Novick AC. Renal cryosurgery. Urology 1999;54:215–219.

53. Woolley ML, Schulsinger DA, Durand DB, Zeltser IS, Waltzer WC. Effect of freezing parameters (freeze cycle and thaw process) on tissue destruction following renal cryoablation. J Endourol 2002;16:519–522.

54. Chosy SG, Nakada SY, Lee FT, Warner TF. Monitoring renal cryosurgery: predictors of tissue necrosis in swine. J Urol 1998;159:1370–1374.

55. Campbell SC, Krishnamurthi V, Chow G, Hale J, Myles J, Novick AC. Renal cryosurgery: experimental evaluation of treatment parameters. Urology 1998;52:29–33.

56. Onik GM, Reyes G, Cohen JK, Porterfield B. Ultrasound characteristics of renal cryosurgery. Urology 1993;42:212–215.

57. Rukstalis DB, Khorsandi M, Garcia FU, Hoenig DM, Cohen JK. Clinical experience with open renal cryoablation. Urology 2001;57:34–39.

58. Sung GT, Gill IS, Hsu TH, et al. Effect of intentional cryo-injury to the renal collecting system. J Urol 2003;170:619–622.

59. Janzen NK, Perry KT, Han KR, et al. The effects of intentional cryoablation and radio frequency ablation of renal tissue involving the collecting system in a porcine model. J Urol 2005;173:1368–1374.

60. Brashears JH III, Raj GV, Crisci A, et al. Renal cryoablation and radio frequency ablation: an evaluation of worst case scenarios in a porcine model. J Urol 2005;173:2160–2165.

61. Gill IS, Remer EM, Hasan WA, et al. Renal cryoablation: outcome at 3 years. J Urol 2005;173:1903–1907.

62. Moinzadeh A, Spaliviero M, Gill IS. Cryotherapy of renal masses: intermediate-term follow-up. J Endourol 2005;19(6):654–657.

63. Bachmann A, Sulser T, Jayet C, et al. Retroperitoneoscopy-assisted cryoablation of renal tumors using multiple 1.5 mm ultrathin cryoprobes: a preliminary report. Eur Urol 2005;47:474–479.

64. Shingleton WB, Sewell PE. Percutaneous renal tumor cryoablation with MRI guidance. J Urol 2001;165:773–776.

65. Bassignani MJ, Moore Y, Watson L, Theodorescu D. Pilot experience with real time ultrasound guided percutaneous renal mass cryoablation. J Urol 2004;171:1620–1623.

66. Khorsandi M, Foy RC, Chong W, Hoenig DM, Cohen JK, Rukstalis DB. Preliminary experience with cryoablation of renal lesions smaller than 4 centimeters. J Am Osteopath Assoc. 2002;102:277–281.

67. Gupta A, Allaf ME, Kavoussi LR, et al. Computerized tomography guided percutaneous renal cryoablation with the patient under conscious sedation: initial clinical experience. J Urol 2006;175: 447–452.

68. Lawatsch EJ, Langenstroer P, Byrd GF, See WA, Quiroz FA, Begun FP. Intermediate results of laparoscopic cryoablation in 59 patients at the Medical College of Wisconsin. J Urol 2006;175:1225–1229.

69. Cestari A, Guazzoni G, dell'Acqua V, et al. Laparoscopic cryoablation of solid renal masses: intermediate term followup. J Urol 2004;172:1267–1270.

70. Moon TD, Lee FT Jr, Hedican SP, Lowry P, Nakada SY. Laparoscopic cryoablation under sonographic guidance for the treatment of small renal tumors. J Endourol 2004;18:436–440.

71. Desai MM, Aron M, Gill IS. Laparoscopic partial nephrectomy versus laparoscopic cryoablation for the small renal tumor. Urology 2005;66:23–28.

72. Hruby G, Reisiger K, Venkatesh R, Yan Y, Landman J. Comparison of laparoscopic partial nephrectomy and laparoscopic cryoablation for renal hilar tumors. Urology 2006;67:50–54.

73. Shingleton WB, Sewell PE Jr. Cryoablation of renal tumours in patients with solitary kidneys. BJU Int 2003;92:237–239.

74. Johnson DB, Solomon SB, Su LM, et al. Defining the complications of cryoablation and radiofrequency ablation of small renal tumors: a multi-institutional study. J Urol 2004;172:874–877.

75. Neeman Z, Sarin S, Coleman J, Fojo T, Wood BJ. Radiofrequency ablation for tumor related massive hematuria. J Vasc Intervent Radiol 2005;16:417–421.

76. McLaughlin CA, Chen MY, Torti FM, Hall MC, Zagoria RJ. Radiofrequency ablation of isolated local recurrence of renal cell carcinoma after radical nephrectomy. Am J Roentgenol 2003;181: 93–94.

77. Goldberg SN, Gazelle GS, Mueller PR. Thermal ablation therapy for focal malignancy: a unified approach to underlying principles, techniques and diagnostic imaging guidance. Am J Roentgenol 2000;174:323–331.

78. Hoey MF, Mulier PM, Leveillee RJ, Hulbert JC. Transurethral prostate ablation with saline electrode allows controlled production of larger lesions than conventional methods. J Endourol 1997;11:279.

79. Rehman J, Landman J, Lee D, et al. Needle based ablation of renal parenchyma using microwave, cryoablation, impedance and temperature based monopolar and bipolar radiofrequency, and liquid gel chemoablation: laboratory studies and review of the literature. J Endourol 2004;18:83–104.

80. Zagoria RJ, Hawkins AD, Clark PE, et al. Percutaneous CT guided radiofrequency ablation of renal neoplasms: factors influencing success. AJR 2004;183:201–207.

81. Corwin TS, Lindberg G, Traxer O, et al. Laparoscopic radiofrequency thermal ablation of renal tissue with and without hilar occlusion. J Urol 2001;166:281–284.

82. Gervais DA, McGovern FJ, Arellano RS, McDougal WS, Mueller PR. Radiofrequency ablation of renal cell carcinoma: part 1, Indications, results, and role in patient management over a 6-year period and ablation of 100 tumors. AJR Am J Roentgenol 2005;185:64–71.

83. Matsumoto ED, Johnson DB, Ogan K, et al. Short-term efficacy of temperature-based radiofrequency ablation of small renal tumors. Urology 2005;65:877–881.

84. Weizer AZ, Raj GV, O'Connell M, Robertson CN, Nelson RC, Polascik TJ. Complications after percutaneous radiofrequency ablation of renal tumors. Urology 2005;66:1176–1180.

85. Merkle EM, Nour SG, Lewin JS. MR imaging follow-up after percutaneous radiofrequency ablation of renal cell carcinoma: findings in 18 patients during first 6 months. Radiology 2005;235: 1065–1071.

86. Mahnken AH, Rohde D, Brkovic D, Gunther RW, Tacke JA. Percutaneous radiofrequency ablation of renal cell carcinoma: preliminary results. Acta Radiol 2005;46:208–214.

87. Ahrar K, Matin S, Wood CG, et al. Percutaneous radiofrequency ablation of renal tumors: technique, complications, and outcomes. J Vasc Interv Radiol 2005;16:679–688.

88. Su LM, Jarrett TW, Chan DY, Kavoussi LR, Solomon SB. Percutaneous computed tomography-guided radiofrequency ablation of renal masses in high surgical risk patients: preliminary results. Urology 2003;61:26–33.

89. Clark TW, Malkowicz B, Stavropoulos SW, et al. Radiofrequency ablation of small renal cell carcinomas using multitined expandable electrodes: preliminary experience. J Vasc Intervent Radiol 2006;17:513–519.

90. Michaels MJ, Rhee HK, Mourtzinos AP, Summerhayes IC, Silverman ML, Libertino JA. Incomplete renal tumor destruction using radiofrequency interstitial ablation. J Urol 2002;168:2406–2409.
91. Rendon RA, Kachura JR, Sweet JM, et al. The uncertainty of radiofrequency treatment of renal cell carcinoma: findings at immediate and delayed nephrectomy. J Urol 2002;167:1587–1592.
92. Johnson DB, Duchene DA, Taylor GD, Pearle MS, Cadeddu JA. Contrast enhanced ultrasound evaluation of radiofrequency ablation of the kidney: reliable imaging of the thermolesion. J Endourol 2005;19:248–252.
93. Chapelon JY, Margonari J, Theillere Y, et al. Effects of high energy focused ultrasound on kidney tissue in the rat and the dog. Eur Urol 1992;22:147–152.
94. Marberger M, Schatzl G, Kranston D, Kennedy JE. Extracorporeal ablation of renal tumors with high intensity focused ultrasound. BJU Int 2005;95(suppl 2):52–55.
95. Hacker A, Michel MS, Marlinghaus E, Kohrmann KU, Alken P. Extracorporeally induced ablation of renal tissue by high-intensity focused ultrasound. BJU Int 2006;97:779–785.
96. Ankem MK, Nakada SY. Needle ablative nephron sparing surgery. BJU Int 2005;95(suppl 2):46–51.
97. Kigure T, Harada T, Yuri Y, Satoh Y, Yoshida K. Laparoscopic microwave thermotherapy on small renal tumors: experimental studies using implanted VX-2 tumors in rabbits. Eur Urol 1996;30: 377–382.
98. Lofti MA, Mccue P, Gomella LG. Laparoscopic interstitial contact laser ablation of renal lesions: an experimental model. J Endourol 1994;8:153–156.
99. de Jode MG, Vale JA, Gedroyc WM. MR guided laser thermoablation of inoperable renal tumors in an open configuration interventional MR scanner: preliminary clinical experience in 3 cases. J Magn Reson Imaging 1999;10:545–549.
100. Ponsky LE, Crownover RL, Rosen MJ, et al. Initial evaluation of cyberknife technology for extracorporeal renal tissue ablation. Urology 2003;61:498–501.

15 The Role of Angioinfarction in the Management of Renal Tumors

Bryan T. Kansas, Paul L. Crispen, and Robert G. Uzzo

KEYWORDS

KIDNEY CANCER
ANGIOINFARCTION
RENAL CELL CARCINOMA
EMBOLIZATION
ANGIOMYOLIPOMA

ABSTRACT

Hypervascularity is a radiographic and pathologic hallmark of most solid tumors of the kidney. Angioinfarction targets the end product of altered angiogenesis pathways by eliminating the tumor's blood supply. Angioinfarction of renal tumors may be used to both the surgeon's and patient's advantage. Here we review the history, indications, techniques, and complications of angioinfarction in the management of primary renal tumors and their metastases.

Hypervascularity is a radiographic and pathologic hallmark of renal cell carcinoma (RCC) and is directly attributable to alteration of specific genes involved in the regulation of angiogenesis. Increased neovascularization in RCC has been linked to mutations in the von Hippel–Lindau tumor suppressor gene, via effects on the hypoxia-induced pathway. Angioinfarction targets the end product of altered angiogenesis pathways by eliminating the tumor's blood supply.

There are many techniques and tools employed in the treatment of renal tumors. Surgical approaches include open and laparoscopic procedures. Secondary approaches include cryotherapy or radiofrequency ablation, which are most often reserved for smaller lesions. Angioinfarction of renal tumors may be used to the advantage of both the surgeon and the patient. This chapter reviews the indications and techniques of angioinfarction for solid enhancing renal masses.

From: *Clinical Management of Renal Tumors*
Edited by: R.M. Bukowski and A.C. Novick © Humana Press Inc., Totowa, NJ

HISTORY

Angiography and its techniques date back to the 1940s. It was a German urologist, Werner Forssmann, who first developed a technique for catheterization of the living heart. He accomplished this by inserting a cannula into his own antecubital vein through which he passed a catheter for 65 cm and then walked to the x-ray department, where a radiograph was taken of the catheter positioned in his right atrium. His experience, for the first time, demonstrated the ability to catheterize a functioning organ for both diagnostic and potentially therapeutic purposes. Subsequent extensions of these experiments have given rise to the field of modern angiography, invasive cardiology, as well as diagnostic and therapeutic interventional radiology. For his efforts he and his colleagues André Frédéric Cournand and Dickinson W. Richards, Jr. were awarded the Nobel Prize in Medicine in 1956.[1]

Currently, angioinfarction is a technique most often performed by interventional radiologists and vascular surgeons. The principal advantage of embolization is immediate control of ongoing or impending hemorrhage. It is used therapeutically in situations involving trauma, gastrointestinal bleeding, arterial aneurysms and pseudoaneurysms, neoplasms, vascular malformations, varicoceles, and pulmonary or obstetrical hemorrhage.

The goals and limitations of embolization must be considered before performing the procedure. The vessels must be readily accessible for selective catheterization to prevent inadvertent blockage of a nontargeted vessel. Embolization can be classified as proximal and distal. Proximal embolization refers to the occlusion of a vessel near its origin (e.g., segmental renal artery), whereas distal embolization refers to the occlusion of a smaller branch (e.g., interlobular artery). Therapeutically, proximal and distal occlusions achieve different goals. Proximal occlusion aims to reduce end organ perfusion in order to obtain hemostasis without regard to possible tissue necrosis, while the primary goal of a distal occlusion is to achieve selective vascular occlusion with the preservation of surrounding parenchyma.[2]

Proponents of transcatheter embolization of RCC have advocated its use for varied indications, including control of persistent hematuria due to neovascularization in an unresectable tumor or severely debilitated patient, treatment of symptomatic primary or metastatic lesions, facilitation of subsequent surgical dissection, and possible stimulation of an antitumor immune response.[3] Embolizing agents used for these purposes are best delivered through an end-hole catheter. A selective angiogram is necessary to delineate vascular anatomy and provides a vascular roadmap for subsequent manipulations. Once the therapeutic purpose and plan are carefully established, the catheter must be placed selectively so as to avoid reflux of embolic agents into nontargeted vessels. For this reason, embolization of large tumors or vascular malformations is often performed in stages.[2]

EMBOLIZATION MATERIALS

Embolization materials are classified as either temporary or permanent (Table 15.1). The size of the material primarily determines its use as a proximal or distal occlusion agent. Short-term embolizing agents are sometimes used when permanent occlusion is not desired, such as in cases of trauma and gastrointestinal bleeding.[4] The classic example of a short-term embolization material is autologous clot. The drawbacks of an

Table 15.1.
Embolization materials utilized in angioinfarction of renal tumors

Embolization techniques (temporary)	Situation employed	Advantages	Disadvantages
Autologous clot	Traumatic or gastrointestinal bleeding	Ease of use, low cost	Easily fragmented and readily lysed
Gelfoam	Traumatic or gastrointestinal bleeding	Contact hemostasis, ease of use, recanalization in 3 weeks	Cost
Polyvinyl alcohol (PVA) particles	Arterial bed of a tumor, small vessel bleeding of a bronchial artery, nidus of a vascular malformation	Suspended in contrast material for ease of use with fluoroscopy	Distal migration or reflux of particles
Alcohol	Tissue sclerosing agent of choice for peripheral congenital AVMs	Ease of use, permanent sclerosis, and protein precipitation causing thrombosis	Intoxication, transient pulmonary hypotension
Boiling contrast agents	Varicocele	Visualization of the delivery agent	Only useful in low-flow situations as high flow dissipates heat rapidly
Gianturco coils (steel coil with attached Dacron strands)	AV fistulas, small pulmonary AVMs, situations when ligation of an artery is desired	Equivalent of ligating vessel	Choice of size of coil important to avoid migration and to ensure coiling in vessel
Platinum microcoils	Embolize the lumen of aneurysms	Precise delivery via microcatheters into small peripheral aneurysms or arterial lesions	Small size requires multiple coils to fill lumen
Silk thread	Embolize the lumen of aneurysms	Precise delivery via microcatheters into small peripheral aneurysms or arterial lesions	Small size may require multiple passes to fill lumen
Detachable balloons	Pulmonary AVMs and occlude aneurysms	Embolic effect of the balloon could be tested before detachment	Balloon deflation and subsequent migration or recurrence

AV, ateriovenous; AVM, ateriovenous malformation.

autologous clot are that it is easily fragmented and readily lysed by the patient's own natural thrombolytic system. For these reasons Gelfoam (Upjohn, Kalamazoo, MI) is the temporary embolic agent of choice. Gelfoam is a surgical packing agent that provides contact hemostasis. Because it is absorbable, the occlusion process may result in recannulation within 3 weeks. Therefore, Gelfoam is often used in situations of traumatic or gastrointestinal bleeding.[5]

Permanent embolic agents include particles, liquids, and blocking agents. Polyvinyl alcohol (PVA) particles are used to embolize the arterial bed of a tumor, small vessel bleeding from a bronchial artery, or the nidus of a vascular malformation. The PVA particles range in size from 150 to 1000 μm. The particles are suspended in contrast and selectively injected under fluoroscopy. They cause permanent occlusion by mechanical impaction within the vascular bed.[5]

Alcohol, Sotradecol (Elkins-Sinn, Saint Davids, PA), 50% glucose, and boiling contrast solutions are examples of liquid embolic agents. Liquid sclerosants are useful in venous embolization since the slower flow rates allow better control while delivering the agent. Alcohol is a tissue sclerosing agent that produces occlusion at all levels from the capillary bed to the main artery. Alcohol causes protein precipitation within the vascular bed with clot formation and subsequent infarction. Absolute alcohol is the agent of choice for embolizing peripheral congenital arteriovenous malformations. Although alcohol embolization is a relatively safe procedure, it may be complicated by intoxication.[5]

Boiling contrast agents offer the advantage of visualization of the delivery agent during the procedure. Occlusion occurs by heat-induced thrombosis. The poor thermal conductivity of catheter materials prevents heat loss and protects transited vessels from undesired thrombosis. It has been used successfully in varicocele embolization but is less useful in vascular malformations, whereas the high flow rate dissipates the heat before thrombosis can occur.[2]

Mechanical blocking agents include steel coils, platinum microcoils, balloons, and silk thread. Gianturco coils (Cook, Bloomington, IN) are steel coils with attached Dacron strands that cause permanent thrombosis. Gianturco coil embolization is the angiographic equivalent of ligating an artery. The coils come in several sizes ranging from 3 to 15 mm in diameter. The coil is advanced through a catheter over a guidewire under fluoroscopic guidance. Properly sizing the coil is important, as too large a coil will stay in an unraveled position, occluding more proximal vessels, while too small a coil will embolize distal to the targeted vessel. Neoplasms and arteriovenous malformation (AVMs) are inadequately embolized with Gianturco coils, as there is often significant collateralization that remains. Gianturco coils are used to embolize arteriovenous fistulas, small pulmonary AVMs, and other situations where complete occlusion or angiographic ligation of an artery is desired and there is little concern of significant collateralization.[6]

Platinum microcoils were developed to embolize the lumen of aneurysms. These are 0.010 to 0.018 inch in diameter and come in a variety of shapes from straight to complex helical coils. Their advantage is precise delivery via microcatheters into small peripheral aneurysms or arterial lesions. The Guglielmi detachable coil (GDC) (Target Therapeutics, Fremont, CA) is a soft platinum helical microcoil that is packed inside the lumen of an aneurysm and detached from the delivery wire by an electrical current. The GDC system is used in the setting of inoperable intracranial aneurysms. Typically five to six coils are used to fill the lumen of the aneurysm.[6]

Silk thread can be used in a similar manner as platinum microcoils to fill the lumen of aneurysms. Detachable balloons are not commercially available in the United States. Balloons have been used to treat pulmonary AVMs and occlude aneurysms. The advantage of microballoons is that the embolic effect of the balloon could be tested before detachment. A disadvantage is that balloon deflation may result in recurrence or uncontrolled migration.[2]

THERAPEUTIC ANGIOINFARCTION FOR RENAL CELL CARCINOMA

Primary Therapy

Angioinfarction can be utilized as a primary treatment of RCC in highly selected situations. If a patient has a small to moderate-sized tumor and multiple comorbidities that preclude other extirpative or curative invasive procedures, angioinfarction has been used with modest, albeit anecdotal success. Figure 15.1 presents a patient who

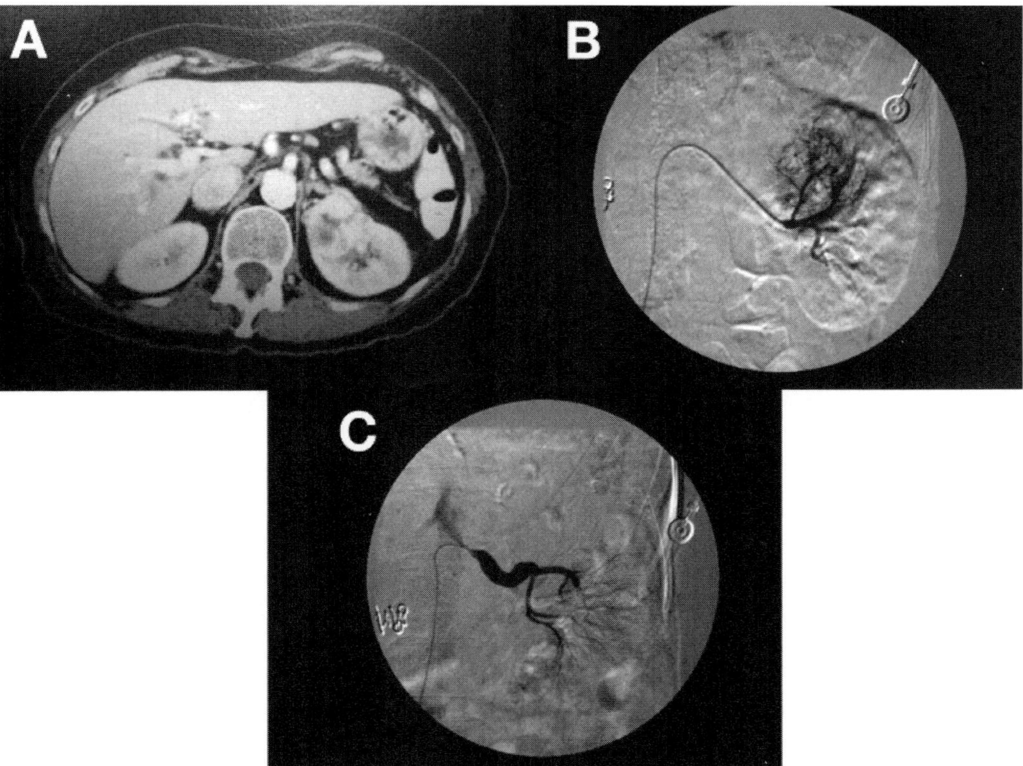

Figure 15.1. Angioinfarction as primary therapy in RCC. An 87-year-old woman with hypertension, emphysema, diabetes, chronic renal insufficiency, and cardiovascular disease presented with painless hematuria. Workup revealed a 3.6-cm left enhancing renal mass (A). Given her performance status (Eastern Cooperative Oncology Group [ECOG] 2), active surveillance was elected. Interval growth and persistent hematuria mandated treatment. Selective renal angioinfarction to the upper pole lesion was performed. Selective injection demonstrated neovascularity of the superior-anterior branch of the left renal artery (B). This division of the renal artery was selectively ablated with a total of 8 cc of ethanol. Follow-up injection of the main renal artery demonstrates selective occlusion of the upper pole vessels (C).

underwent angioinfarction as the primary treatment of a left-sided renal tumor due to her advanced age, poor performance status, and persistent bleeding.

Jafri et al.[7] compared computed tomography (CT) findings in nine patients after renal tumor embolization. All tumors were ablated using absolute alcohol, Gelfoam particles, or occlusion coils. A rim of peripheral enhancement surrounding a central low-density area, presumed to represent the necrotic infarcted tumor, was a typical postinfarction CT appearance of these lesions. Intratumoral gas was seen in three patients and persisted in some for up to 6 months before resolution. A mild postinfarction syndrome was experienced in nearly all cases. These authors concluded that although the role of renal embolization as primary therapy is limited, if the procedure is used, the natural course of the neoplasm can be best evaluated and followed by serial CT scans.

Munro et al.[8] reviewed 25 patients undergoing transarterial embolization who were unable or unwilling to undergo surgical extirpation for treatment of their disease. More than half of the patients (56%) presented with localized or locally advanced disease, and the rest presented with distant metastases. The median age of patients with localized and regional disease was 80 years. Symptoms from the primary tumor were well controlled in patients with symptomatic disease on presentation. Ten of the 14 patients with localized and regional disease underwent follow-up radiographic restaging of their disease. Tumor size was noted to increase in two patients, remain unchanged in four patients, and decrease in four patients. Progression to distant metastases was not identified in any patients presenting with localized disease over a median follow-up of 39 months. The authors concluded that transarterial embolization is associated with minimal morbidity and relatively few complications, and can accomplish adequate control of tumor related symptoms.

Demirci et al.[9] retrospectively investigated the value of embolization alone compared to radical nephrectomy and immunochemotherapy in 20 patients with metastatic RCC. Patients receiving embolization alone had a lower median survival time (1 month) compared to combined therapy (11 months), but the difference did not reach statistical significance due to a small sample size and existing selection bias.

Preoperative Angioinfarction for Surgical Assistance

There are several surgical situations in which preoperative selective or complete angioinfarction may be of benefit. When properly performed, blood loss during a technically difficult nephrectomy may be decreased, and the procedure itself may be facilitated. These situations include those in which access to the renal artery may be hindered by bulky hilar nodal disease or venous clot. Under these circumstances, embolization of the main renal artery can allow the surgeon to ligate the renal vein first with less concern of complications associated with continued arterial inflow to the kidney. Also it has been suggested that the size and extent of an inferior vena caval thrombus may be reduced by preoperative renal artery embolization, particularly if the vena caval clot demonstrates arterialization. Proponents of preoperative embolization also hypothesize that angioinfarction may create edema along surgical tissue planes, thereby facilitating operative dissection.[10] Figure 15.2 illustrates a case in which preoperative angioinfarction was performed prior to radical nephrectomy and thrombectomy.

Swanson et al.[11] treated 100 patients with metastatic RCC by angioinfarction of the primary tumor followed by radical nephrectomy. Their findings included an overall response rate of 28% including complete regression of all metastatic lesions in seven

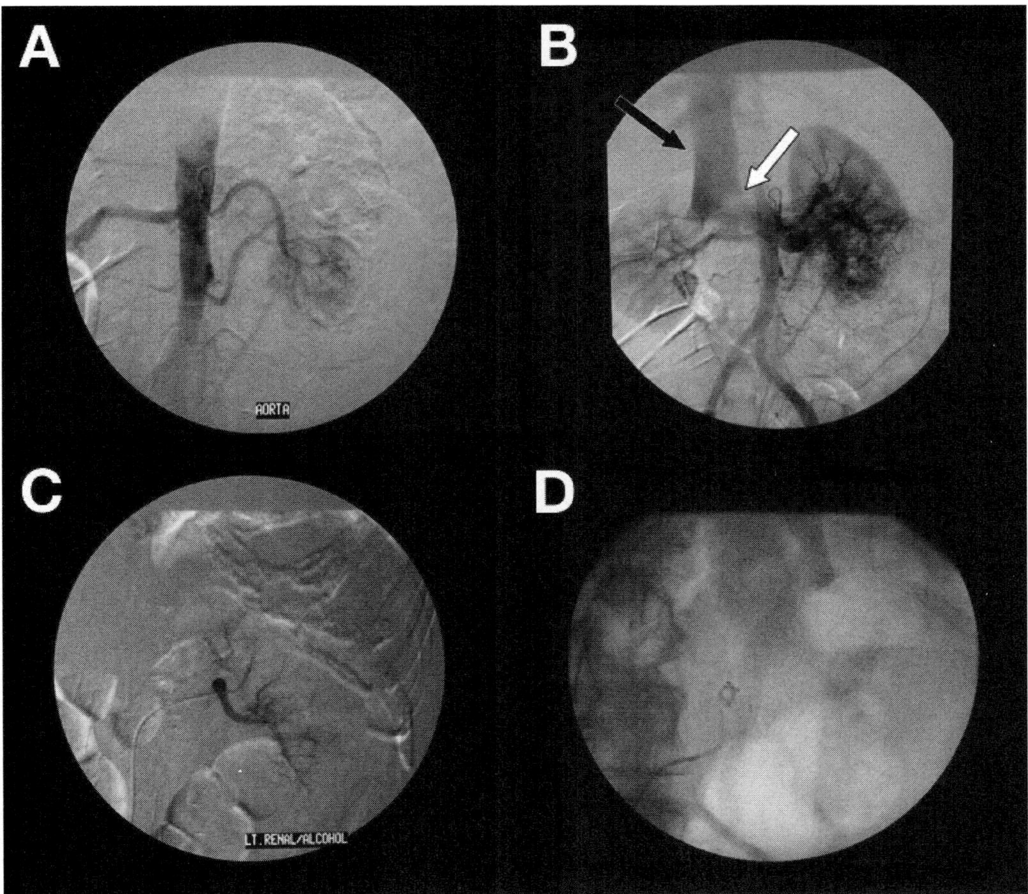

Figure 15.2. Preoperative angioinfarction preceding radical nephrectomy. A 69-year-old woman with hypertension, hepatitis, and peptic ulcer disease presented with painless hematuria. Radiographic evaluation noted a large centrally located enhancing renal mass clinical stage T3bN2M1. Given her extensive hilar adenopathy and bleeding, preoperative embolization was performed the morning of surgery. Early postinjection aortogram noted three renal arteries to the left kidney (A). Rapid arteriovenous shunting (black arrow) and a level 2 inferior vena cava (IVC) thrombus (white arrow) were noted during subsequent aortic films (B). A total of 20 cc of denatured ethanol were injected, resulting in incomplete angioinfarction (C). Two steel coils were then deployed in the inferior segmental branch resulting in complete infarction (D). The patient subsequently underwent uncomplicated radical nephrectomy and thrombectomy.

patients, regression greater than 50% in eight, and stabilization for at least 1 year in 13. Unfortunately, they could not demonstrate any survival benefit as a result of preoperative angioinfarction.

Several series have evaluated the advantages and disadvantages of preoperative angioinfarction. Klimberg et al.[3] reported on a total of 25 patients with RCC who underwent preoperative angioinfarction using absolute ethanol. Complete cessation of renal arterial flow was demonstrated in all cases. The postembolization syndrome of pain, nausea, vomiting, hypertension, and fever was minimal. Of the patients in this series, 62% (21/34) underwent postinfarction transabdominal radical nephrectomy without intraoperative or postoperative complications directly attributable to the injection of absolute ethanol. No damage to extrarenal tissue was noted at the time of surgery. These authors subjectively report that subsequent surgical dissection was facilitated, particularly in cases of large tumors where control of the renal pedicle was difficult. Median blood loss in their series was 725 mL (range, 75–2500 cc). This series was among the first to demonstrate the safety of preoperative angioinfarction with absolute ethanol.

Mebust et al.[12] found that the early mortality rate in 46 patients who underwent preoperative angioinfarction for RCC was 4%. The postembolization syndrome was noted in 86% to 90% of patients. In their series, however, the use of absolute ethanol as a medium for renal infarction was associated with a significant incidence of damage to other organs, a finding markedly different than reported by Klimberg et al.[3] As much as a 30% decrease in tumor volume following angioinfarction was noted in 75% of patients in the series. There was no evidence of metastatic tumor reduction after angioinfarction of the primary lesion, and these investigators could not document any significant decrease in operative time or blood loss. In fact, their study found that blood loss was substantially greater in the postinfarction population. Using a thoracoabdominal incision, they report a median blood loss of 1014 cc without infarction (mean tumor size 332 cm^3) versus 1976 cc with angioinfarction (mean tumor size 591 cm^3). In cases where a chevron incision was used, average blood loss was 959 cc without infarction (mean tumor size 184.3 cm^3) and 1718 cc after angioinfarction (mean tumor size 364 cm^3). Although angioinfarction in this series was associated with a higher blood loss, the difference was most likely attributable to selection bias with larger masses more often treated with preoperative angioinfarction.

Sweeney et al.[10] reviewed their experience with angioinfarction in 96 patients with vena caval thrombus. The thrombus levels were classified according to the classification system of Neves and Zincke[13] as modified by Nesbitt et al.,[14] and were infrahepatic (level I) in 39 cases, intrahepatic (level II) in 28 cases, suprahepatic (level III) in seven cases, into the atrium (level IV) in 14 cases, and undefined in eight cases.[10] Preoperative angioinfarction was performed in 44% (42/96) of the cases including all 14 level IV thrombi. Median blood loss was 1400 cc in level I, 3500 cc in level II, 4400 cc in level II, and 5000 cc in level IV. In their series, cardiopulmonary bypass was avoided in five of the 14 patients with level IV thrombi. Blood loss was found to be similar in all groups regardless of whether bypass was employed. These authors also report facilitation with dissection when employing preoperative angioinfarction, a finding they did not objectify.

Selective Embolization Following Nephron-Sparing Surgery

The role of nephron-sparing surgery (NSS) in the management of RCC continues to expand. With detailed preoperative imaging and improved surgical techniques, postoperative complications following NSS remain low. Postoperative hemorrhage from the tumor resection bed has been reported in 0% to 5% of cases. Typically, the bleeding is self-limited and does not require additional intervention. However, severe retroperitoneal or intraabdominal hemorrhage or hematuria may require immediate or delayed intervention. Heye et al.[15] described their experience with the use of angiographic diagnosis and selective embolization of postoperative bleeding following NSS. The authors report a 2.8% (7/251) rate of postoperative hemorrhage following NSS requiring transcatheter embolization. Presenting symptoms included macroscopic hematuria (five patients), flank pain (one patient), and anemia (one patient). Angiographic findings include extravasation of contrast in three patients, and pseudoaneurysm or arteriovenous fistula in four. All patients were successfully managed with superselective embolization, and only one patient had a transient increase in serum creatinine. No patient required further intervention for bleeding.

Albani and Novick[16] described their experience in the treatment of three cases of pseudoaneurysm formation following NSS. These cases represent 0.43% (3/698) of patients undergoing NSS during a 3-year period. Two of the cases were managed successfully with selective embolization, while the third pseudoaneurysm persisted despite multiple attempts at embolization. In this case the pseudoaneurysm eventually resolved spontaneously.

Vascular Conditions Associated with Tumors

Renal arteriovenous malformations (AVMs) are abnormal communications between the intrarenal arterial and venous systems and may be congenital or acquired. Renal AVMs are uncommon, but have been discovered with increasing frequency since first described by Varela in 1928.[17] They are most often identified incidentally or during the evaluation of gross hematuria. The estimated rate in large autopsy series is less than 1 case per 30,000 patients.[18] Treatment must be tailored to the individual patient since options for therapy range from observation to embolization to nephrectomy.[18]

Two types of renal AVMs have been described: congenital and acquired.[19] The term *arteriovenous malformation* usually refers to a congenital lesion since acquired arteriovenous anomalies of the kidney are often termed renal arteriovenous fistula. The incidence of arteriovenous fistula has increased significantly secondary to a higher incidence of both blunt and penetrating renal trauma; more complex open, endoscopic, and laparoscopic renal surgery; and the use of percutaneous needle biopsies, particularly in renal allografts.[17] Idiopathic renal arteriovenous fistulas have the radiographic characteristics of acquired fistulas but without any identifiable cause. They are often associated with renal artery aneurysms.[18]

Congenital AVMs account for approximately 25% of all renal vascular malformations. Most of these are the classic cirsoid type. Congenital cirsoid AVMs have a dilated, corkscrew appearance with multiple communications between the main or segmental renal arteries.[20,21] Cavernous AVMs, with single dilated vessels, account for the remainder of congenital malformations. Although they are considered congenital, they rarely present before the third or fourth decade of life. Women are affected three times as often as men, with the right kidney involved slightly more often than the left.[21]

Acquired arteriovenous fistulas are more common and represent as many as 75% to 80% of renal vascular malformations. An estimated 15% to 50% of renal biopsies result in some degree of fistula formation. In one study in which arteriograms were performed after every renal biopsy, radiographic evidence of fistula was identified in 15% of patients. Trauma is another important cause of acquired renal fistulas. In patients with penetrating trauma, arteriovenous fistulas may affect as many as 80% of patients presenting with hypertension following the initial injury. Idiopathic renal arteriovenous fistulas represent less than 3% of renal vascular malformations. Idiopathic arteriovenous fistulas are thought to arise from the spontaneous erosion or controlled rupture of a segmental renal artery into a nearby vein.[18] These lesions are usually located in the upper pole of the kidney (45%), but can be found in the midportion (30%) or lower pole (25%) as well.[22]

The precise cause of congenital AVMs is unclear. Theories exist that they may be present at birth or that a congenital aneurysm erodes into an adjacent vein and then slowly enlarges.[23] The pathophysiology and the symptoms caused by the fistula are variable and based on their size, location, and rate of development and progression.[24] Hemodynamic derangements often produce a loud bruit, and renin-mediated hypertension occurs secondary to relative renal ischemia distal to the fistula.[25] An increased venous return and high cardiac output may result in left ventricular hypertrophy and high output cardiac failure.[19]

Gross hematuria is the initial sign or symptom in as many as 75% of patients with renal AVMs. Renal colic may result from obstructing vermiform blood clots. Rarely, during the evaluation of asymptomatic microscopic hematuria, an AVM is found and presumed to be the cause of trace blood. A significant percentage of patients with renal AVMs are hypertensive, with as many as 50% of patients with acquired and 25% of patients with congenital renal AVMs developing hypertension. Furthermore, preexisting hypertension is thought to be a risk factor for developing a fistula following a renal biopsy.[26]

While small and asymptomatic renal AVMs are often managed conservatively, the initial means of treating symptomatic lesions is by angiographic embolization.[27,28] Signs and symptoms due to a renal AVM may be elusive and can include pain, bleeding, and hypertension. Pain from renal AVMs results from either obstruction of the collecting system by clots or expansion of the renal capsule due to hemorrhage. Persistent gross hematuria, especially in patients with anemia, may also prompt treatment.[29] Hypertension is another important indication for treatment. Attempts have been made preoperatively to determine whether the malformation is responsible for the hypertension. However, selective renal vein renin levels have not been helpful in discriminating which patients' hypertension will respond to therapy. Congestive heart failure from severe shunting is an unusual yet compelling indication for treatment.[30]

Indications for surgical therapy have become more limited as the ability to treat renal AVMs with angiographic embolization has improved. Nephrectomy and partial nephrectomy are more extensive treatment options reserved for very large lesions or those refractory to minimally invasive techniques.[18] The AVMs due to malignancy also require surgical extirpation. Renal cell carcinoma has a predilection toward neovascularization, with renal vein extension and parasitic tumor vessels both being relatively common. Angiogenic tumor factors, such as overproduction of vascular endothelial growth factor (VEGF), have been implicated in tumor hypervascularity and may explain the development of AVMs within renal carcinomas.[18] Significant metastatic disease and poor performance status may limit the use of nephrectomy and in these cases embolization may be palliative. Figure 15.3 presents the treatment of a symptomatic AVM associated with an RCC in a solitary kidney. Symptomatic hematuria and intratumoral hemorrhage is definitively treated by nephrectomy. In most cases hypertension and pain refractory to less invasive attempts may also respond to radical nephrectomy.[31]

Role of Embolization of Renal Cell Carcinoma Metastatic Lesions

Metastatic lesions associated with RCC can be profoundly symptomatic and debilitating. This is especially true of bony metastases, which can lead to mechanical instabil-

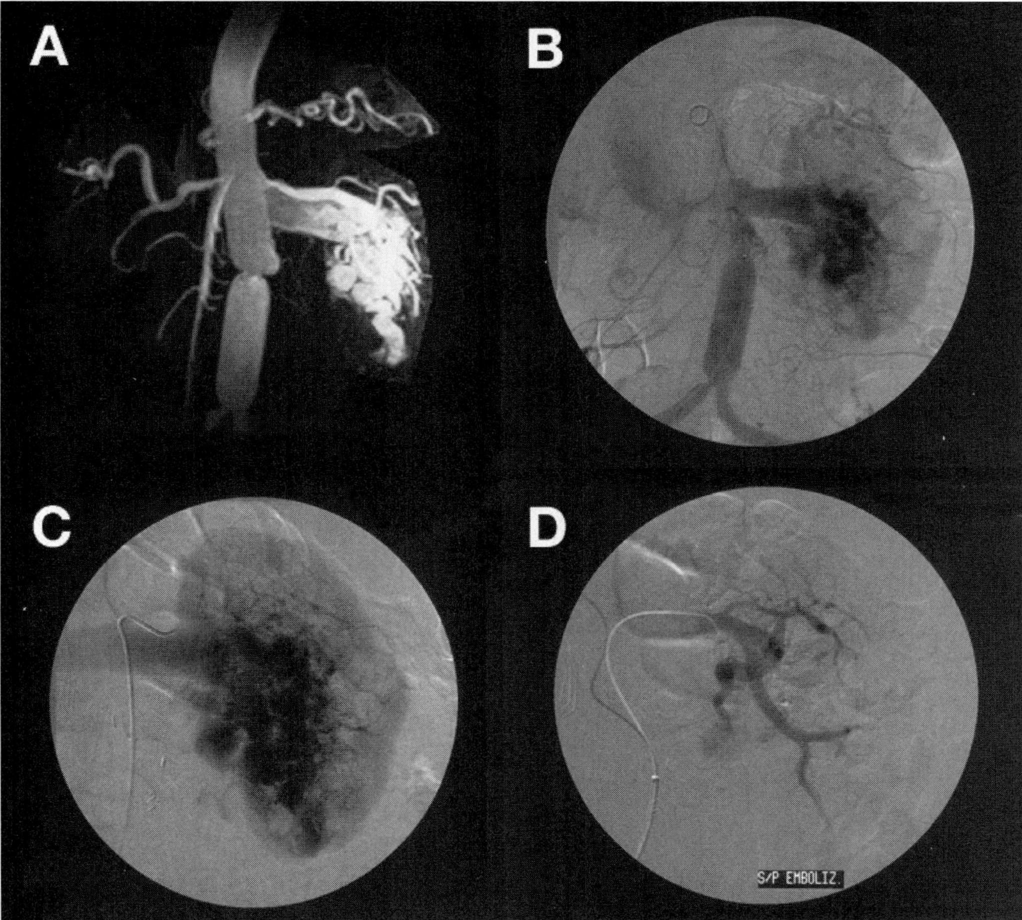

Figure 15.3. Embolization of arterial venous fistula associated with renal carcinoma. A 78-year-old man with coronary artery disease, peripheral vascular disease, a large abdominal aneurysm, and a solitary kidney presented with recurrent hematuria. He became extremely debilitated after aneurysmal tube grafting and several prolonged hospitalizations (ECOG performance status 2–3). Magnetic resonance angiography (MRA) revealed a single renal artery with rapid venous filling consistent with an AVM (A). Cross-sectional magnetic resonance imaging confirmed the AVM and noted a renal vein thrombus extending to the vena cava (data not shown). After considering removal of a solitary kidney, it was decided to proceed with placement of an inferior vena caval filter and embolization of the large associated AV fistula. Flush aortogram noted rapid arteriovenous filling secondary to a lower pole AVM (B and C). Selective embolization utilizing 900- to 1200-μm-diameter embospheres (Guerbet Biomedical, Louvres, France) resulted in a significantly decreased AV shunting while maintaining overall renal function (postprocedure serum creatinine 2.4 mg/dL) (D).

ity, intractable pain, and symptoms of cord compression in the case of spinal metastases. Symptomatic bony metastases are primarily treated with radiation, with surgical intervention reserved for younger patients with long disease-free intervals and a good performance status or for radiation-resistant unstable lesions. Often bony metastases cannot be fully resected but rather simply stabilized. A common complication of the surgical treatment of these lesions is the potential for massive intraoperative blood loss secondary to the increased vascularity of these lesions.[32] Manke et al.[33] evaluated the efficacy of preoperative embolization of spinal metastases secondary to RCC in 29 patients. Ten patients had complete embolization, nine patients had partial embolization, and 10 had no embolization prior to surgical intervention. Intraoperative blood loss was significantly lower in patients with complete or partial embolization compared to control subjects without preoperative embolization. No significant difference in intraoperative blood loss was noted between patients with complete embolization and those with partial embolization. Additionally, there were no differences in long-term neurologic complications related to preoperative embolization. Given these findings, the authors concluded that preoperative embolization, complete or partial, prior to surgical resection of spinal metastases secondary to RCC was effective in reducing operative blood loss and was associated with few side effects.

Chatziioannou et al.[34] also compared intraoperative blood loss in patients with complete or partial embolization prior to surgical resection of bone metastases secondary to RCC. In contrast to the findings by Manke et al.,[33] the authors noted a significant decrease in blood loss in patients with complete embolization compared to partial embolization. Furthermore, patients with complete embolization had a significantly decreased transfusion requirement compared to patients with partial embolizations. Based on their findings, the authors advocate complete angiographic devascularization prior to surgical resection of bony metastases in RCC.

Palliative Angioinfarction

As many as 25% to 30% of patients with RCC present with locally advanced or metastatic disease. Although some patients are candidates for cytoreduction, others with multiple comorbidities or a poor performance status may progress and develop significant symptoms from the primary tumor or its metastases. These symptoms include, but are not limited to, severe bleeding and pain. Often these symptoms can be controlled with conservative and supportive measures, but occasionally they may not respond or may even progress further. Angioinfarction has been used in these situations for palliation. The success rate of these procedures varies given the heterogeneity of the population in published reports; however, angioinfarction can be a very useful tool in the clinician's armamentarium. These procedures can reduce the number of days in the hospital, analgesic use, transfusion risk and cost, and most importantly improve the patient's quality of life. Nurmi et al.[35] reviewed their experience with palliative embolization of 20 renal tumors, and reported that as many as 50% of embolizations utilized to reduce tumor-related pain were beneficial, while 79% of embolizations for persistent gross hematuria were successful. The mortality rate as a consequence of embolization in this series was 5%.

EMBOLIZATION FOR ANGIOMYOLIPOMA

The angiographic appearance of angiomyolipomas (AMLs) is characterized by aneurysmal dilation within the tumor, a whorled vessel pattern, and the absence of arteriovenous shunting; however, these findings are not specific to AMLs, and similar findings can be found in RCC. For this reason, angiography is used primarily in the treatment of AMLs rather than in its diagnosis. Nelson and Sanda[36] reviewed the published experience of selective angioembolization of AMLs. Their review evaluated 76 reported cases. The most common indications for selective embolization included acute hemorrhage, patient comorbidities limiting surgical options, and renal insufficiency. Ten percent of patients experienced postoperative complications, with 85% of patients developing postembolization syndrome. Additionally, 14% of patients required repeat embolization for recurrent symptoms and 16% of patients went on to require operative intervention. Kothary et al.[37] reviewed their long-term results of 19 patients undergoing embolization of AMLs with a mean follow-up time of 52 months. Of these patients, 32% were noted to have a recurrence defined as a 2-cm increase in tumor size at any time following embolization. The median time to recurrence was 79 months. Although the overall need for future intervention appears high following selective embolization for AML, the technique presents a useful alternative to surgical intervention in patients who are poor surgical candidates or as a treatment for acute hemorrhage from an AML, as may happen during pregnancy.[38]

POSTEMBOLIZATION IMMUNE FUNCTION

In addition to eliminating or reducing the blood supply of renal malignancies, angioinfarction has been theorized to stimulate the antitumor response of the host immune system. Tumor antigen release following tumor embolization is thought to be a potential catalyst for an increased host immune response. Several investigators have evaluated this concept by measuring the immune response in patients following embolization. Nakada et al.[39] measured the proliferative response of lymphocytes in patients before and after renal tumor embolization. Patients with RCC were noted to have significantly lower lymphocyte response to phytohemagglutinin before treatment compared to control subjects. Following embolization lymphocyte response was increased, but was not significantly different from preembolization levels. Another report by Bakke et al.[40] investigated natural killer (NK) cell activity following embolization of RCCs. The NK cell activity was noted to be significantly elevated 48 hours following embolization. The observed increase in NK cell activity was postulated to be the result of increased interferon production by macrophages. Although these studies suggest an increased host immune response following tumor embolization, there are no direct data to support defined changes in the immune response affecting tumor biology or overall patient survival following angioinfarction.[40,41]

COMPLICATIONS OF ANGIOINFARCTION

Angioinfarction offers a less invasive treatment option for patients with medical risk factors that preclude standard surgical intervention for renal tumors and may be used as part of a multimodal approach in the management of this disease. Overall, complications following embolization of renal tumors have been reported in 5% to 14% of cases.[42] Associated mortality, although low, still remains a potential risk, occurring in 0% to 5% of cases.[43,44] Risk factors have been identified that predispose patients to an increased occurrence of postembolization complications and include tumor size, indications for embolization, embolization material, and preexisting comorbidities.[42] Patients undergoing embolization for palliation were noted to have a 20% complication rate and a 7.3% mortality rate compared to patients undergoing preoperative embolization who have a reported complication rate of 4.9% and a 1.2% mortality rate.[42] While the overall incidence of postembolization syndrome (PES) following renal tumor embolization is as high as 30% to 60%,[45,46] a lower incidence of PES was noted when ethanol is used as an embolizing agent compared to Gelfoam.[47,48]

Postembolization complications can be categorized as non-target organ and target organ specific. Non-target organ complications include the unintentional embolization of adjacent organs and complications related to technical failures. Unintentional embolization of non-target organs can result from misplaced catheters, reflux of embolization particles, and vascular anomalies within the tumor. The manifestations of non-target organ embolization depend on the organ inadvertently embolized. Non-target organ embolization can occur even with proper placement of the embolization material secondary to reflux or the subsequent migration of the embolization material to other sites.[42,49] Vascular injuries occur infrequently but may require surgical intervention to either remove a misplaced coil or repair an injured vessel.[49] Target organ complications refer to those that directly result from tumor embolization. Postprocedure renal insufficiency is largely dependent on the patient's preexisting renal function. Renal failure following embolization occurs in 3.3% to 8.8% of patients and is typically transitory.[42] Limiting the amount of contrast agent utilized and assuring adequate hydration can help reduce the risk of renal failure in patients with preexisting renal insufficiency. The role of acetylcysteine in preventing contrast-induced nephropathy is still being established.[50,51]

Infectious complications include sepsis and abscess formation. The rate of sepsis ranges from 0.8% to 1.9% in published series.[42,49] Although rare, death secondary to postembolization sepsis has been reported.[49] Renal abscess formation has also been described following embolization. Figure 15.4 demonstrates a patient who developed emphysematous pyelonephritis following palliative embolization of a symptomatic large left renal tumor. Although abscess formation was documented in this particular case, the presence of air within the renal parenchyma following embolization does not always indicate infection.[49,52] The greatest risk factor for complex infectious complications following embolization is a preexisting urinary tract infection. A preembolization urinalysis and culture provides a simple and effective means of screening for potential preexisting urinary tract infections, with delay of embolization or prophylactic antibiotics in patients with bacteriuria or pyuria.

Postembolization syndrome is the most common complication following renal tumor embolization and is characterized by fever, pain, nausea, transient hypertension, malaise, leukocytosis, and an elevated lactate dehydrogenase. This syndrome is not specific to renal tumor embolization and has been associated with embolization for acute gastrointestinal bleeding, primary tumors in other organs, and AVMs.[52,53] It is often difficult to distinguish PES from infection following embolization. Patients with persistent fevers and leukocytosis following embolization should be evaluated for potential infections. Preembolization administration of IV steroids followed by an oral steroid taper may help reduce the incidence of PES as demonstrated by Bissler et al.,[54] who reported a lower rate of PES with the prophylactic use of steroids in patients undergoing embolization of AMLs.

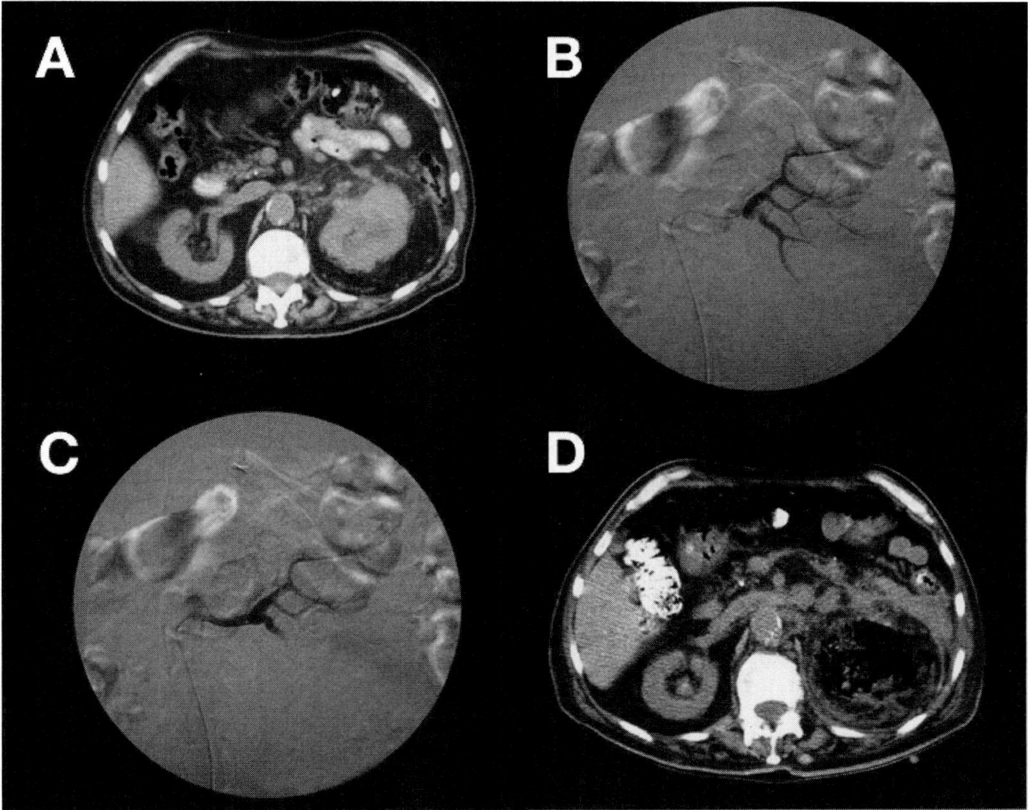

Figure 15.4. Emphysematous pyelonephritis following palliative angioinfarction. An 81-year-old man with renal insufficiency, coronary artery disease, and macular degeneration presented with hematuria. A large left renal mass was noted on CT examination, with associated adenopathy and liver nodules (A). The patient refused cytoreductive nephrectomy and adjuvant therapy after consultation with a medical oncologist. Following repeated episodes of gross hematuria, requiring blood transfusions, the patient underwent palliative angioinfarction. Selective catheterization of left renal artery was performed and demonstrated hypervascularity consistent with the known renal neoplasm (B). Ethanol ablation was performed using 20 cc of absolute ethanol, with resultant decreased blood flow to the left kidney (C). Four weeks following the palliative angioinfarction, the patient presented with left flank pain and fever. (D) CT examination revealed a large abscess in the area of the left renal fossa consistent with emphysematous pyelonephritis.

CONCLUSION

This chapter has been a review of the diagnostic and therapeutic indications for renal embolization. The technique is best performed by a skilled interventional radiologist at the direction and discretion of the treating urologist. Indications include preoperative infarction to facilitate surgery, postoperative infarction in the setting of hemorrhage, primary therapy for arteriovenous malformations, and highly selected AMLs or RCC, or for symptomatic control of metastatic RCC. Many studies, mostly subjective and retrospective, have evaluated the techniques, efficacy, and consequences of embolizing renal lesions. Currently, its use is fairly limited in the daily management of patients with RCC and should be undertaken in highly selected and well-defined circumstances.

Nonetheless, the ability to selectively employ angioinfarction must remain within the purview of practicing urologists. As angioinfarction techniques and materials continue to improve and new effective targeted therapies for RCC are developed, the role of angioinfarction in the diagnosis and management of this disease will continue to evolve.

REFERENCES

1. Truss MC, Stief CG, Jonas U. Werner Forssmann: surgeon, urologist, and Nobel Prize winner. World J Urol 1999;17(3):184–186.
2. Braun MN, AA, Vogelzang RL. Embolization. In: Interventional Radiology Procedure Manual, 1st ed. New York: Churchill Livingstone, 1997:272.
3. Klimberg I, Hunter P, Hawkins IF, Drylie DM, Wajsman Z. Preoperative angioinfarction of localized renal cell carcinoma using absolute ethanol. J Urol 1985;133(1):21–24.
4. Ward JFaV, Thomas E. Transcatheter therapeutic embolization of genitourinary pathology. Rev Urol 2000;2:236–245.
5. Coldwell DM, Stokes KR, Yakes WF. Embolotherapy: agents, clinical applications, and techniques. Radiographics 1994;14(3):623–643; quiz 645–646.
6. Uflacker R. Embolization Procedures: Techniques and Materials. New York: McGraw-Hill, 1991.
7. Jafri SZ, Ellwood RA, Amendola MA, Farah J. Therapeutic angioinfarction of renal carcinoma: CT follow-up. J Comput Assist Tomogr 1989;13(3):443–447.
8. Munro NP, Woodhams S, Nawrocki JD, Fletcher MS, Thomas PJ. The role of transarterial embolization in the treatment of renal cell carcinoma. BJU Int 2003;92(3):240–244.
9. Demirci D, Tatlisen A, Ekmekcioglu O, Ozcan N, Kaya R. Does radical nephrectomy with immuno-chemotherapy have any superiority over embolization alone in metastatic renal cell carcinoma? A preliminary report. Urol Int 2004;73(1):54–58.
10. Sweeney P, Wood CG, Pisters LL, et al. Surgical management of renal cell carcinoma associated with complex inferior vena caval thrombi. Urol Oncol 2003;21(5):327–333.
11. Swanson DA, Johnson DE, von Eschenbach AC, Chuang VP, Wallace S. Angioinfarction plus nephrectomy for metastatic renal cell carcinoma—an update. J Urol 1983;130(3):449–452.
12. Mebust WK, Weigel JW, Lee KR, Cox GG, Jewell WR, Krishnan EC. Renal cell carcinoma—angio-infarction. J Urol 1984;131(2):231–235.
13. Neves RJ, Zincke H. Surgical treatment of renal cancer with vena cava extension. Br J Urol 1987;59(5):390–395.
14. Nesbitt JC, Soltero ER, Dinney CP, et al. Surgical management of renal cell carcinoma with inferior vena cava tumor thrombus. Ann Thorac Surg 1997;63(6):1592–1600.
15. Heye S, Maleux G, Van Poppel H, Oyen R, Wilms G. Hemorrhagic complications after nephron-sparing surgery: angiographic diagnosis and management by transcatheter embolization. AJR Am J Roentgenol 2005;184(5):1661–1664.
16. Albani JM, Novick AC. Renal artery pseudoaneurysm after partial nephrectomy: three case reports and a literature review. Urology 2003;62(2):227–231.
17. Bauer SB. Anomalies of the upper urinary tract. In: Walsh P, ed. Campbell's Urology, 8th ed., vol 3. Philadelphia: Saunders, 2002:1885–1925.
18. Wakefield M. Renal arteriovenous malformation. E-Medicine, 2004. www.emedicine.com/med/topic2861.htm.
19. Maldonado JE, Sheps SG, Bernatz PE, Deweerd JH, Harrison EG Jr. Renal arteriovenous fistula. A reversible cause of hypertension and heart failure. Am J Med 1964;37:499–513.
20. Crummy AB Jr, Atkinson RJ, Caruthers SB Jr. Congenital renal arteriovenous fistulas. J Urol 1965;93:24–26.
21. Cho KJ, Stanley JC. Non-neoplastic congenital and acquired renal arteriovenous malformations and fistulas. Radiology 1978;129(2):333–343.
22. Yazaki T, Tomita M, Akimoto M, Konjiki T, Kawai H, Kumazaki T. Congenital renal arteriovenous fistula: case report, review of Japanese literature and description of non-radical treatment. J Urol 1976;116(4):415–418.
23. Thomason WB, Gross M, Radwin HM, Hulse CM, Dobbs RM Jr. Intrarenal arteriovenous fistulas. J Urol 1972;108(4):526–529.

24. Messing E, Kessler R, Kavaney PB. Renal arteriovenous fistulas. Urology 1976;8(2):101–107.
25. McAlhany JC Jr, Black HC Jr, Hanback LD Jr, Yarbrough DR 3rd. Renal arteriovenous fistula as a cause of hypertension. Am J Surg 1971;122(1):117–120.
26. Honda H, Onitsuka H, Naitou S, et al. Renal arteriovenous malformations: CT features. J Comput Assist Tomogr 1991;15(2):261–264.
27. Yakes WF, Luethke JM, Merland JJ, et al. Ethanol embolization of arteriovenous fistulas: a primary mode of therapy. J Vasc Intervent Radiol 1990;1(1):89–96.
28. Clouse ME, Adams DF. Congenital renal arteriovenous malformation: angiography in its diagnosis. Urology 1975;5(2):282–285.
29. Yakes WF, Haas DK, Parker SH, et al. Symptomatic vascular malformations: ethanol embolotherapy. Radiology 1989;170(3 pt 2):1059–1066.
30. Takebayashi S, Hosaka M, Kubota Y, Ishizuka E, Iwasaki A, Matsubara S. Transarterial embolization and ablation of renal arteriovenous malformations: efficacy and damages in 30 patients with long-term followup. J Urol 1998;159(3):696–701.
31. Crotty KL, Orihuela E, Warren MM. Recent advances in the diagnosis and treatment of renal arteriovenous malformations and fistulas. J Urol 1993;150(5 pt 1):1355–1359.
32. Olerud C, Jonsson B. Surgical palliation of symptomatic spinal metastases. Acta Orthop Scand 1996;67(5):513–522.
33. Manke C, Bretschneider T, Lenhart M, et al. Spinal metastases from renal cell carcinoma: effect of preoperative particle embolization on intraoperative blood loss. AJNR Am J Neuroradiol 2001;22(5):997–1003.
34. Chatziioannou AN, Johnson ME, Pneumaticos SG, Lawrence DD, Carrasco CH. Preoperative embolization of bone metastases from renal cell carcinoma. Eur Radiol 2000;10(4):593–596.
35. Nurmi M, Satokari K, Puntala P. Renal artery embolization in the palliative treatment of renal adenocarcinoma. Scand J Urol Nephrol 1987;21(2):93–96.
36. Nelson CP, Sanda MG. Contemporary diagnosis and management of renal angiomyolipoma. J Urol 2002;168(4 pt 1):1315–1325.
37. Kothary N, Soulen MC, Clark TW, et al. Renal angiomyolipoma: long-term results after arterial embolization. J Vasc Intervent Radiol 2005;16(1):45–50.
38. Morales JP, Georganas M, Khan MS, Dasgupta P, Reidy JF. Embolization of a bleeding renal angiomyolipoma in pregnancy: case report and review. Cardiovasc Intervent Radiol 2005; 28(2):265–268.
39. Nakada T, Koike H, Katayama T. Changes of vasoactive substances following embolization for renal cell carcinoma. Int Urol Nephrol 1988;20(6):569–576.
40. Bakke A, Gothlin JH, Haukaas SA, Kalland T. Augmentation of natural killer cell activity after arterial embolization of renal carcinomas. Cancer Res 1982;42(9):3880–3883.
41. Nakano H, Nihira H, Toge T. Treatment of renal cancer patients by transcatheter embolization and its effects on lymphocyte proliferative responses. J Urol 1983;130(1):24–27.
42. Lammer J, Justich E, Schreyer H, Pettek R. Complications of renal tumor embolization. Cardiovasc Intervent Radiol 1985;8(1):31–35.
43. Goldstein HM, Medellin H, Beydoun MT, et al. Transcatheter embolization of renal cell carcinoma. Am J Roentgenol Radium Ther Nucl Med 1975;123(3):557–562.
44. Rabe FE, Yune HY, Richmond BD, Klatte EC. Renal tumor infarction with absolute ethanol. AJR Am J Roentgenol 1982;139(6):1139–1144.
45. Zielinski H, Szmigielski S, Petrovich Z. Comparison of preoperative embolization followed by radical nephrectomy with radical nephrectomy alone for renal cell carcinoma. Am J Clin Oncol 2000; 23(1):6–12.
46. Klimberg IW, Locke DR, Hawkins IF Jr, Drylie DM. Absolute ethanol renal angioinfarction for control of hypertension. Urology 1989;33(2):153–158.
47. Wells IP, Hammonds JC, Franklin K. Embolisation of hypernephromas: a simple technique using ethanol. Clin Radiol 1983;34(6):689–692.
48. Lanigan D, Jurriaans E, Hammonds JC, Wells IP, Choa RG. The current status of embolization in renal cell carcinoma—a survey of local and national practice. Clin Radiol 1992;46(3):176–178.
49. Chuang VP, Wallace S, Swanson DA. Technique and complications of renal carcinoma infarction. Urol Radiol 1981;2(3):223–228.
50. Zagler A, Azadpour M, Mercado C, Hennekens CH. N-acetylcysteine and contrast-induced nephropathy: a meta-analysis of 13 randomized trials. Am Heart J 2006;151(1):140–145.

51. Morcos SK. Prevention of contrast media-induced nephrotoxicity after angiographic procedures. J Vasc Intervent Radiol 2005;16(1):13–23.
52. Hemingway AP, Allison DJ. Complications of embolization: analysis of 410 procedures. Radiology 1988;166(3):669–672.
53. Jacobson AI, Amukele SA, Marcovich R, et al. Efficacy and morbidity of therapeutic renal embolization in the spectrum of urologic disease. J Endourol 2003;17(6):385–391.
54. Bissler JJ, Racadio J, Donnelly LF, Johnson ND. Reduction of postembolization syndrome after ablation of renal angiomyolipoma. Am J Kidney Dis 2002;39(5):966–971.

16 Surveillance Strategies Following Curative Therapy for Localized Renal Cell Carcinoma

Vitaly Margulis, Surena F. Matin, and Christopher G. Wood

KEYWORDS

RENAL CELL CARCINOMA
SURVEILLANCE
STAGING
PROGNOSTIC MODELS
BIOMARKERS

ABSTRACT

Advances in the diagnosis, staging, and treatment of patients with renal cell carcinoma (RCC) have resulted in improved survival pf patients with locally recurrent and metastatic disease. Assuming that success of clinical intervention at the time of relapse is inversely proportional to the disease burden at the time of salvage treatment, ideal surveillance protocol should allow the earliest identification of potentially treatable recurrences while minimizing unnecessary examinations and patient anxiety. In addition, optimal surveillance regimen would take into account primary tumor characteristics; initial treatment modality; incidence, timing, and pattern of recurrence; and effectiveness of available salvage treatments. Anatomic tumor stage remains the most important prognosticator of outcome in RCC and a cornerstone of several currently proposed surveillance strategies. Nonetheless, recent identification of novel clinical and pathologic prognostic factors in RCC have resulted in gradual transition from the use of solitary clinical factors, such as tumor, node, metastasis staging system, to the introduction of systems that integrate multiple validated prognostic factors. Finally, development of new and meaningful biomarkers and their incorporation into integrated staging algorithms will likely revolutionize the staging and surveillance of RCC patients.

Historically, 25% to 50% of patients who present with and are treated for localized renal cell carcinoma (RCC) will develop local or systemic recurrence, which can be

From: *Clinical Management of Renal Tumors*
Edited by: R.M. Bukowski and A.C. Novick © Humana Press Inc., Totowa, NJ

associated with a dismal prognosis.[1] Without effective therapeutic modalities available for treatment of disease relapse, development of effective surveillance strategies was deemed a measure in futility as nothing meaningful could be done at the time of disease relapse. Significant recent advances in the diagnosis, staging, and treatment of patients with RCC have resulted in improved survival of patients with locally recurrent and metastatic disease. In recent reports, 30% to 50% of patients with isolated local recurrence are found to be free of disease progression following aggressive extirpative treatment with or without adjuvant therapy.[2,3] Response rates of 10% to 30% have been reported following systemic immunotherapy for patients with metastatic RCC.[4] Recently, small molecule kinase inhibitors have demonstrated impressive activity as single agents in the second-line setting in advanced RCC, and phase 3 trials comparing these drugs with interferon as first-line therapy are encouraging.[5,6] Mounting evidence indicates that the success of clinical intervention for locally recurrent or metastatic RCC is inversely proportional to the disease volume at the time of salvage treatment. Consequently, an ideal surveillance protocol would allow the earliest identification of potentially treatable recurrences while minimizing unnecessary examinations and patient anxiety.

Although no universally accepted follow-up schema exist, the ideal surveillance regimen would take into account primary tumor characteristics; initial treatment modality; incidence, timing, and pattern of recurrence; and effectiveness of available salvage treatments. As documented by several large clinical series, tumor stage remains the most important prognosticator of outcome in RCC and a cornerstone of several currently proposed surveillance strategies (Table 16.1).[7–11] Recent identification of novel clinicopathologic prognosticators in RCC have resulted in gradual transition from the use of solitary clinical factors, such as tumor, node, metastasis (TNM) staging system, to the introduction of systems that integrate multiple validated prognostic factors.[12–15] Development of new and meaningful biomarkers and their incorporation into integrated staging algorithms will likely revolutionize the staging and surveillance of RCC patients.[16]

In this context, follow-up of patients with RCC after curative treatment should allow detection of local recurrence and distant metastases as early as possible, facilitating delivery of salvage therapies when disease burden is minimal.

SURVEILLANCE FOR RENAL CELL CARCINOMA AFTER DEFINITIVE THERAPY

pT1 Renal Cell Carcinoma

Five-year cancer specific survival rates of 85% to 100% have been reported after radical or partial nephrectomy for pT1 RCC.[8,9,11] The vast majority of relapses after radical nephrectomy are systemic and rarely occur within the first year after treatment. Stephenson et al.[11] reported a median time to relapse of 35 months (range 2 to 93 months) in 16 of 310 pT1 RCC patients. Only one isolated local recurrence was detected after radical nephrectomy. All thoracic or bone metastases were detected on routine chest x-ray (CXR) surveillance or clinical examination. Similarly, Levy et al.[8] reported only systemic relapse in eight of the 113 patients with pT1 primary tumor at a median follow-up of 39 months (range 6 to 126 months). None of the four patients with a pulmonary metastasis were symptomatic but had detectable lesions on CXR, while all of the remaining metastases (bone, brain, etc.) were symptomatic at presentation.

Table 16.1.
Surveillance guidelines after therapy for clinically localized renal cell carcinoma

	Stage[a]	H&P lab[b]	Chest imaging[c]	Abdominal imaging[d]
		Radical nephrectomy		
M.D. Anderson Cancer Center	T1	Q 1 y	Q 1 y	None
	T2	Q 6 mo × 3 y, then q 1 y	Q 6 mo × 3 y, then q 1 y	At 24 mo, at 60 mo
	T3	At 3 mo, Q 6 mo × 3 y, then q 1 y	At 3 mo, Q 6 mo × 3 y, then q 1 y	At 24 mo, at 60 mo
Cleveland Clinic	T1	Q 1 y	None	None
	T2	Q 1 y	Q 1 y	At 24 mo, then q 2 y
	T3	Q 6 mo	Q 6 mo	At 12 mo, then q 2 y
Umea University	T1[e]	At 3 mo, Q 6 mo × 3 y, then q 1 y	At 3 mo, Q 6 mo × 3 y, then q 1 y	None
	T2[e]	At 3 mo, Q 6 mo × 3 y, then q 1 y	At 3 mo, Q 6 mo × 3 y, then q 1 y	At 6 mo, at 12 mo
	T3	At 3 mo, Q 6 mo × 3 y, then q 1 y	At 3 mo, Q 6 mo × 3 y, then q 1 y	At 6 mo, at 12 mo
UCLA	LR	Q 1 y × 5 y	Q 1 y × 5 y	At 2 y, at 4 y
	IR	Q 6 mo × 5 y, then q 2 y	Q 6 mo × 5 y, then q 2 y	At 1 y, then q 2 y
	HR	Q 6 mo × 5 y, then q 2 y	Q 6 mo × 5 y, then q 2 y	Q 6 mo × 2 y, then q y
	LN+	At 3 mo, q 6 mo × 2 y, then q 1 y	At 3 mo, q 6 mo × 2 y, then q 1 y	At 3 mo, q 6 mo × 2 y, then q 1 y
		Partial nephrectomy		
	T1	Q 1 y	None	None
	T2	Q 1 y	Q 1 y	At 24 mo, then q 2 y
	T3	Q 6 mo	Q 6 mo	Q 6 mo × 3 y, then q 1 y
		Energy ablation		
	T1	Q 1 y	Q 1 y	At 1, 3, 6, 12 mo, then q 1 y

[a]2002 American Joint Committee on Cancer TNM staging of renal cell carcinoma.
[b]Complete blood count, serum chemistries and liver function tests.
[c]CXR; UCLA protocol: chest CT alternating with CXR.
[d]Abdominal MRI if abdominal CT clinically contraindicated.
[e]No follow-up recommended if tumor <5 cm or diploid.

Rates of tumor recurrence after partial nephrectomy for pT1 RCC have been shown to parallel those after radical nephrectomy. A study from Cleveland Clinic, reviewing data on 327 patients treated with partial nephrectomy for sporadic RCC documented 0% local and systemic relapse rate for pT1 group at 62 month follow-up.[17]

Given the low overall risk of relapse in patients with sporadic pT1 RCC, few recurrences within 12 months of partial or radical nephrectomy, and rare abdominal relapse, this patient group can be surveyed with annual clinical examination, laboratory evaluation, and CXR (Table 16.1). Routine abdominal computed tomography (CT) can safely be avoided in this patient population.

pT2 Renal Cell Carcinoma

Several large series report 81% to 90% five-year relapse-free survival after radical or partial nephrectomy for sporadic pT2 RCC. In a series reported by Levy et al.,[8] 17 (27%) of 64 patients with pT2 disease developed metastasis within 32 months after radical nephrectomy. At time of relapse, the majority of patients had single site metachronous lesions involving lungs in eight of 17 patients, and bone, pancreas, and contralateral adrenal in one each. The vast majority of asymptomatic pulmonary lesions were detected with routine CXR, while liver and bone metastasis were detected secondary to symptoms or abnormal laboratory evaluation. Likewise, a median time to relapse in 14 of 84 patients with pT2 RCC treated with radical nephrectomy reported by Stephenson et al.[11] was 25 months (range 3 to 95 months). All patients with recurrence had symptoms, abnormal laboratory evaluation, or asymptomatic lung metastases detected on routine CXR. Isolated abdominal failure after radical nephrectomy for pT2 RCC is a rare event, and routine abdominal CT can likely be omitted, while instituting an annual clinical examination, laboratory evaluation, and CXR (Table 16.1).

Hafez et al.[17] followed patients after nephron-sparing surgery for stage pT2 RCC according to a uniform schedule of semiannual CXR, laboratory evaluation, and abdominal CT for 4 years and annually thereafter. Only three of 151 patients (2.0%) had local recurrence, which was detected more than 4 years postoperatively. Eight patients (5.3%) had systemic metastases, with six being isolated pulmonary relapse detected on routine CXR.[17] Investigators from Cleveland Clinic advocate abdominal CT at 2 years and every 2 years thereafter, in addition to annual clinical examination, laboratory evaluation, and CXR for patients after partial nephrectomy for sporadic pT2 RCC (Table 16.1).

pT3 Renal Cell Carcinoma

The current primary tumor classification for pT3 RCC incorporates the features of tumor thrombus, fat invasion, and direct ipsilateral adrenal extension. The relative impact of tumor thrombus level and direct adrenal involvement has recently been debated. According to investigators from University of California–Los Angeles, disease specific survival for patients with renal vein involvement (T3b) and inferior vena cava (IVC) involvement below the diaphragm (T3b) was identical after controlling for Fuhrman grade and Eastern Cooperative Oncology Group (ECOG) performance status in a multivariate analysis.[18] Moinzadeh and Libertino,[19] however, challenged this notion, reporting that patients with tumor thrombus involving the renal vein only were less likely to die of RCC compared to patients with larger tumor thrombus burden. Currently patients with perinephric fat extension and renal vein/IVC involvement are assigned a T stage based on the level of the thrombus, yet Gettman et al.[20] demonstrated that perinephric fat invasion portends a worse prognosis among patients with venous tumor thrombus. Furthermore, patients with direct extension of the tumor into the ipsilateral adrenal gland are currently staged as pT3a, despite several large series clearly documenting decreased median survival for patients with direct ipsilateral adrenal involvement compared to patients with fat invasion only.[21–23] Lastly, Thompson et al.[24] and others have shown that patients with renal sinus fat invasion (pT3a) were more likely to die of RCC then patients with perinephric fat invasion (pT3a).

Clearly, patients with pT3 RCC represent a heterogeneous group in terms of relapse risk; nonetheless, relapse after radical or partial nephrectomy for pT3 RCC generally is more frequent, more likely to be systemic, and occurs at significantly shorter interval than for the other stages. Ljungberg et al.[9] reported that of 48 patients with pT3a/b node negative disease, 26 (54%) recurred following a mean interval of 17 months after radical nephrectomy. Similarly, in a series reported by Stephenson et al.,[11] 37 (34%) of 108 pT3a/b patients treated with radical nephrectomy relapsed at a median time of 12 months after treatment. Investigators from M.D. Anderson Cancer Center detailed similar relapse rates for pT3 disease, stressing that 26% of relapses were detected within 6 months of treatment.[8]

Uniformly, with the exception of bone and brain metastases, the majority of relapses detected after radical nephrectomy for pT3 lesions were asymptomatic. Moreover, large series report the abdominal cavity being one of the relapse sites in 9% to 22% of patients and as the sole sight of relapse in 5% to 20% of patients with metastases.[8,9,11]

In a partial nephrectomy series from Cleveland Clinic, local and metastatic recurrence was observed in pT3 RCC patients in 9.3% and 13.0%, respectively. Initial site of metastasis was solitary intraabdominal/retroperitoneal in 20% of patients who relapsed.[17]

To summarize, patients with pT3 disease recur often and early (shorter time from nephrectomy to relapse), and an increased number of them present with asymptomatic pulmonary or abdominal metastases. With this background in mind, routine surveillance with abdominal CT should be instituted. Proposed schema range from abdominal CTs every 6 months for 3 years and yearly thereafter, to abdominal imaging at 12 and 60 months after treatment (Table 16.1). Clinical and laboratory evaluation, as well as chest imaging should be performed at 6-month intervals for the first 3 years posttreatment and annually thereafter.

pT4/N+ Renal Cell Carcinoma

Tumor invasion beyond Gerota's fascia (pT4), without concomitant nodal or metastatic disease, is relatively unusual. Large retrospective series report a 5% to 15% incidence of pT4 RCC, the majority of which were associated with synchronous metastases.[1,23] Not surprisingly, 5-year disease-specific survival after nephrectomy with en-bloc resection of involved organs for pT4N0M0 RCC is reported to be in the range of 5% to 30%.[3] While follow-up data are limited, local and distant relapse is expected and occurs frequently within 6 month of therapy.

Regional lymphadenopathy, while present in about 25% of patients with metastatic RCC, is uncommon in patients with clinically localized renal lesions.[25] Because of the rarity of nodal disease in the absence of systemic metastatic disease, the natural history of this patient group is poorly understood. Canfield et al.,[26] among others, evaluated a group of patients with nonmetastatic node-positive disease treated with radical nephrectomy and complete retroperitoneal lymph node dissection. With a median follow-up of 17 months, 30% of patients had no evidence of disease, while the rest of the patients recurred at a median of 5 months. A 5-year recurrence-free rate of 36% following nephrectomy and limited lymphadenectomy in the N+M0 RCC patient population was reported by the UCLA group.[27] The chest was the site of recurrence in 58.8% and the abdomen in 76.5% of patients who recurred. Of the chest recurrences, 25% recurred within the first 3 months, and 63% within the first year of treatment. Of those with abdominal recurrences, 29% recurred within the first 3 months, and 72% within the first year of follow-up.[27] Given the high risk of early local and distal relapse in the pT4 or N+ group of patients, intensive follow-up with history and physical examination, laboratory studies, chest imaging, and abdominal CT at 3, 6, 12, 18, and 24 months and yearly thereafter is advised (Table 16.1).[28]

Energy-Based Tissue Ablation of RCC

Over the past decade, cryoablation and radiofrequency ablation (RFA) have emerged as treatment alternatives for a select group of patients with localized renal tumors. Although long-term follow-up has not been achieved, intermediate oncologic effectiveness is comparable to the current "gold standard" treatment modalities.[29,30] Because tissue is left in place following thermoablative therapy, cross-sectional imaging with CT or magnetic resonance (MR) is utilized to document the lack of enhancement in the ablated tumor.[31,32] Whether this actually correlates with the lack of viable cancer remains a subject of much debate.

Currently, there are no evidence-based follow-up guidelines that exist for patients after renal energy-ablative therapy. A combined multiinstitutional analysis by Matin et al.[33] of 616 patients treated with cryoablation or RFA revealed residual or recurrent disease after primary treatment in 63 (10.2%) patients. Virtually all failures were in the category of incomplete ablation or local recurrence detected within 6 months, and in 70% of cases detected within 3 months after treatment. Salvage thermal ablation was feasible and effective in the majority of local failures. The authors advocate a minimum of three or four abdominal imaging studies in the first year after treatment, at months 1, 3, 6, and 12 in addition to routine clinical, laboratory, and chest surveillance (Table 16.1).

Integrated Staging Algorithms

While the TNM staging system is the most extensively used staging and prognostic tool for RCC, new clinical, pathologic, and molecular markers have recently been shown to correlate with clinical tumor behavior and patient survival (Table 16.2).[34–36] In an attempt to improve risk assessment in RCC, combinations of the TNM staging system with various other prognostic factors has allowed for the emergence of new comprehensive staging or risk assessment paradigms that may influence how patients are followed postoperatively in the future. Investigators at UCLA have developed the UCLA Integrated Staging System (UISS), a novel staging system based on TNM stage, grade, and ECOG performance status (PS).[37] Patients are stratified into three risk groups according to the probability of tumor recurrence and survival, and risk group–specific surveillance guidelines are offered. The UISS has been internally and externally validated and has been demonstrated to be superior to TNM staging.[38] While effectively risk-stratifying the patients, UISS does not predict a probability of failure.

Based on a large sample of patients, investigators from the Mayo Clinic devised the stage, size, grade, and necrosis (SSIGN) score, in which patients with clear-cell RCC were assigned a score based on tumor stage, tumor size, nuclear grade, and the presence of necrosis.[13] Using a SSIGN score, cancer-specific survival at 1 to 10 years posttreat-

Table 16.2.
Prognostic factors in renal cell carcinoma

Clinical	Pathohistologic	Molecular
Symptoms at presentation	TNM stage	Ki-67
↓ Performance status	Grade	VEGF
↑ Acute-phase reactants	Size	VEGF-R
↑ Corrected calcium	Histologic type	CA IX
↑ Alkaline phosphatase	Architecture	CA XII
↑ Lactate dehydrogenase	Lymphovascular invasion	EpCAM
	Coagulative necrosis	PTEN
	DNA ploidy	
↓Albumin		p53
↓ Hemoglobin		p21
↑ Neutrophil count		Vimentin
		Gelsolin
		Clusterin
		Osteopontin

CA IX, carbonic anhydrase IX; CA XII, carbonic anhydrase XII; EpCAM, epithelial cell adhesion molecule; PTEN, phosphatase and tensin homologue; VEGF, vascular endothelial growth factor; VEGF-R, VEGF receptor.

ment can be estimated for an individual patient. Predictive ability of the SSIGN score was recently validated externally and has been shown to be superior to TNM staging alone.[39]

Investigators from Memorial Sloan-Kettering Cancer Center combined tumor stage, tumor size, histologic subtype, and symptoms at presentation into a nomogram that predicts the probability of freedom from recurrence at 5 years after treatment.[14] This nomogram has recently been updated for the clear cell variant of RCC and includes tumor stage, tumor size, nuclear grade, necrosis, vascular invasion, and symptoms at presentation as prognostic factors.[15]

It is certain that the future of RCC staging will rely on a combined and structured analysis of clinical information, anatomic extent of the disease, histopathologic criteria, and molecular markers. A glimpse into the future of RCC staging has recently been offered by the UCLA group, which demonstrated that addition of expression data from five markers, including carbonic anhydrase IX (CA IX), Ki-67, gelsolin, vimentin, and p53, significantly improved the discriminating ability of the UISS.[16]

CONCLUSION

The surveillance guidelines delineated in this chapter enable cost-effective detection of potentially curable or treatable relapse at a time when tumor burden is minimal and salvage treatment most effective. To date, pathologic tumor stage remains the strongest single determinant of risk and pattern of relapse after curative therapy for localized renal cell carcinoma. Yet, emerging comprehensive staging algorithms are likely to further enhance our ability to predict tumor behavior by integrating clinical information, pathologic tumor characteristics, and molecular markers of disease.

REFERENCES

1. Pantuck AJ, Zisman A, Belldegrun AS. The changing natural history of renal cell carcinoma. J Urol 2001;166:1611–1623.
2. Kavolius JP, Mastorakos DP, Pavlovich C, et al. Resection of metastatic renal cell carcinoma. J Clin Oncol 1998;16:2261–2266.
3. Figlin RA. Renal cell carcinoma: management of advanced disease. J Urol 1999;161:381–386; discussion 386–387.
4. Lam JS, Belldegrun AS, Figlin RA. Advances in immune-based therapies of renal cell carcinoma. Expert Rev Anticancer Ther 2004;4:1081–1096.
5. Motzer RJ, Rini BI, Bukowski RM, et al. Sunitinib in patients with metastatic renal cell carcinoma. JAMA 2006;295:2516–2524.
6. Reddy GK, Bukowski RM. Sorafenib: recent update on activity as a single agent and in combination with interferon-alpha2 in patients with advanced-stage renal cell carcinoma. Clin Genitourin Cancer 2006;4:246–248.
7. Janzen NK, Kim HL, Figlin RA, et al. Surveillance after radical or partial nephrectomy for localized renal cell carcinoma and management of recurrent disease. Urol Clin North Am 2003;30:843–852.
8. Levy DA, Slaton JW, Swanson DA, et al. Stage specific guidelines for surveillance after radical nephrectomy for local renal cell carcinoma. J Urol 1998;159:1163–1167.
9. Ljungberg B, Alamdari FI, Rasmuson T, et al. Follow-up guidelines for nonmetastatic renal cell carcinoma based on the occurrence of metastases after radical nephrectomy. BJU Int 1999;84:405–411.
10. Mickisch G, Carballido J, Hellsten S, et al. Guidelines on renal cell cancer. Eur Urol 2001;40:252–255.
11. Stephenson AJ, Chetner MP, Rourke K, et al. Guidelines for the surveillance of localized renal cell carcinoma based on the patterns of relapse after nephrectomy. J Urol 2004;172:58–62.
12. Zisman A, Pantuck AJ, Figlin RA, et al. Validation of the UCLA Integrated Staging System for patients with renal cell carcinoma. J Clin Oncol 2001;19:3792–3793.
13. Frank I, Blute ML, Cheville JC, et al. An outcome prediction model for patients with clear cell renal cell carcinoma treated with radical nephrectomy based on tumor stage, size, grade and necrosis: the SSIGN score. J Urol 2002;168:2395–2400.
14. Kattan MW, Reuter V, Motzer RJ, et al. A postoperative prognostic nomogram for renal cell carcinoma. J Urol 2001;166:63–67.
15. Sorbellini M, Kattan MW, Snyder ME, et al. A postoperative prognostic nomogram predicting recurrence for patients with conventional clear cell renal cell carcinoma. J Urol 2005;173:48–51.
16. Lam JS, Leppert JT, Figlin RA, et al. Role of molecular markers in the diagnosis and therapy of renal cell carcinoma. Urology 2005;66:1–9.
17. Hafez KS, Novick AC, Campbell SC. Patterns of tumor recurrence and guidelines for followup after nephron sparing surgery for sporadic renal cell carcinoma. J Urol 1997;157:2067–2070.
18. Kim HL, Zisman A, Han KR, et al. Prognostic significance of venous thrombus in renal cell carcinoma. Are renal vein and inferior vena cava involvement different? J Urol 2004;171:588–591.
19. Moinzadeh A, Libertino JA. Prognostic significance of tumor thrombus level in patients with renal cell carcinoma and venous tumor thrombus extension. Is all T3b the same? J Urol 2004;171:598–601.
20. Gettman MT, Boelter CW, Cheville JC, et al. Charlson co-morbidity index as a predictor of outcome after surgery for renal cell carcinoma with renal vein, vena cava or right atrium extension. J Urol 2003;169:1282–1286.
21. Han KR, Bui MH, Pantuck AJ, et al. TNM T3a renal cell carcinoma: adrenal gland involvement is not the same as renal fat invasion. J Urol 2003;169:899–903; discussion 903–904.
22. Leibovich BC, Cheville JC, Lohse CM, et al. Cancer specific survival for patients with pT3 renal cell carcinoma-can the 2002 primary tumor classification be improved? J Urol 2005;173:716–719.
23. Thompson RH, Cheville JC, Lohse CM, et al. Reclassification of patients with pT3 and pT4 renal cell carcinoma improves prognostic accuracy. Cancer 2005;104:53–60.
24. Thompson RH, Leibovich BC, Cheville JC, et al. Is renal sinus fat invasion the same as perinephric fat invasion for pT3a renal cell carcinoma? J Urol 2005;174:1218–1221.
25. Motzer RJ, Mazumdar M, Bacik J, et al. Survival and prognostic stratification of 670 patients with advanced renal cell carcinoma. J Clin Oncol 1999;17:2530–2540.

26. Canfield SE, Kamat AM, Sanchez-Ortiz RF, et al. Renal cell carcinoma with nodal metastases in the absence of distant metastatic disease (clinical stage TxN1–2M0): the impact of aggressive surgical resection on patient outcome. J Urol 2006;175:864–869.
27. Pantuck AJ, Zisman A, Dorey F, et al. Renal cell carcinoma with retroperitoneal lymph nodes: role of lymph node dissection. J Urol 2003;169:2076–2083.
28. Lam JS, Shvarts O, Leppert JT, et al. Postoperative surveillance protocol for patients with localized and locally advanced renal cell carcinoma based on a validated prognostic nomogram and risk group stratification system. J Urol 2005;174:466–472; discussion 472; quiz 801.
29. Gill IS, Remer EM, Hasan WA, et al. Renal cryoablation: outcome at 3 years. J Urol 2005; 173:1903–1907.
30. Anderson JK, Matsumoto E, Cadeddu JA. Renal radiofrequency ablation: technique and results. Urol Oncol 2005;23:355–360.
31. Wagner AA, Solomon SB, Kavoussi LR. Imaging following cryoablation of a renal lesion. Nat Clin Pract Urol 2005;2:52–57; quiz 58.
32. Matsumoto ED, Johnson DB, Ogan K, et al. Short-term efficacy of temperature-based radiofrequency ablation of small renal tumors. Urology 2005;65:877–881.
33. Matin SF CJ, Gervais DA, et al. Residual and recurrent disease following renal energy ablative therapy: implications for management—a multi-institutional study. Am Urol Assoc 2006;abstr 709.
34. Lam JS, Shvarts O, Leppert JT, et al. Renal cell carcinoma 2005: new frontiers in staging, prognostication and targeted molecular therapy. J Urol 2005;173:1853–1862.
35. Lehmann J, Retz M, Nurnberg N, et al. The superior prognostic value of humoral factors compared with molecular proliferation markers in renal cell carcinoma. Cancer 2004;101:1552–1562.
36. Motzer RJ, Bacik J, Schwartz LH, et al. Prognostic factors for survival in previously treated patients with metastatic renal cell carcinoma. J Clin Oncol 2004;22:454–463.
37. Zisman A, Pantuck AJ, Wieder J, et al. Risk group assessment and clinical outcome algorithm to predict the natural history of patients with surgically resected renal cell carcinoma. J Clin Oncol 2002;20:4559–4566.
38. Patard JJ, Kim HL, Lam JS, et al. Use of the University of California Los Angeles integrated staging system to predict survival in renal cell carcinoma: an international multicenter study. J Clin Oncol 2004;22:3316–3322.
39. Ficarra V, Martignoni G, Lohse C, et al. External validation of the Mayo Clinic Stage, Size, Grade and Necrosis (SSIGN) score to predict cancer specific survival using a European series of conventional renal cell carcinoma. J Urol 2006;175:1235–1239.

17 Local Recurrence of Renal Cell Carcinoma: *Management*

Brian K. McNeil and Steven C. Campbell

KEYWORDS

RENAL CELL CARCINOMA
LOCAL RECURRENCE
SALVAGE NEPHRECTOMY
EN BLOC EXCISION

ABSTRACT

Local recurrence (LR) after surgery for renal cell carcinoma is relatively uncommon, which is likely due to the tendency of RCC to be unifocal and well encapsulated. Local recurrence presents unique challenges. This chapter reviews the incidence, risk factors, and management of local recurrence for patients with RCC. Local recurrence occurs primarily as ipsilateral recurrence in the renal fossa after radical nephrectomy and within the residual parenchyma after partial nephrectomy or thermal ablative procedures. In each of these settings, a fundamental issue must be resolved: is this an isolated LR or does it occur in the setting of disseminated disease? Due to the trend toward thermal ablative therapies, for which long-term efficacy has not yet been established, LR for RCC has become a particularly relevant topic.

Local recurrence (LR) after surgery for renal cell carcinoma (RCC) is a relatively uncommon event, with an incidence much lower than for prostate or bladder cancer after definitive radical surgery. This is likely due to the tendency of RCC to be unifocal and well encapsulated in the majority of cases, while the other common urologic malignancies are more likely to be multifocal and infiltrative. Nevertheless, LR does occur after definitive local therapy for RCC, and presents a number of unique challenges. This chapter reviews the incidence, risk factors, and management of LR for patients with RCC.

Local recurrence for RCC occurs primarily in two settings: ipsilateral recurrence in the renal fossa after radical nephrectomy (RNx), and within the residual parenchyma after partial nephrectomy (PNx) or thermal ablative procedures. From a management standpoint, each of these scenarios presents distinct challenges that must be accounted for during counseling and decision making. However, in each of these scenarios a

From: *Clinical Management of Renal Tumors*
Edited by: R.M. Bukowski and A.C. Novick © Humana Press Inc., Totowa, NJ

fundamental issue must be resolved: is this an isolated LR or does it occur in the setting of disseminated disease? Local recurrence for patients with RCC has become a particularly relevant topic due to the trend toward thermal ablative therapies, which are relatively novel and for which long-term efficacy has not yet been established.

INCIDENCE AND PREDISPOSING FACTORS FOR LOCAL RECURRENCE

Local recurrence has been reported after all forms of definitive local therapy, with incidence rates that correlate with treatment modality, stage of RCC, and presence of genetic syndromes. Local recurrence is much more common in patients with von Hippel–Lindau (VHL) syndrome and other familial forms of RCC, since these tend to be multifocal, and nephron-sparing approaches are preferred, leaving behind parenchyma that is clearly at risk. Walther and Linehan have shown that kidneys from patients with VHL or hereditary papillary RCC typically harbor several hundred microscopic malignant or premalignant lesions.[1] Local recurrence rates for patients with VHL approach 80% a decade after PNx, reflecting this striking tumor diathesis.[2]

INCIDENCE AFTER OPEN RADICAL NEPHRECTOMY

In the modern era, LR after open RNx occurs in approximately 2% to 4% of cases. Uson[3] reported a 3.3% rate of LR after 518 open RNx, but 60% of these patients were found to have concomitant disseminated disease. The incidence of isolated LR in this series was thus 1.4%. These recurrences were diagnosed between 3 and 60 months after surgery, although the majority were found within 2 years. All patients with LR in this series originally had Robson stage II or III disease, highlighting the importance of tumor stage as a predisposing factor for LR. A more recent series from the Mayo Clinic looked at 1925 patients treated with RNx between 1970 and 2000, and found 73 total LR (3.8%), while an earlier report from this same database quoted a 1.7% incidence of isolated LR.[4,5] Fifty-seven percent of these patients originally had primary T stage of T3 or greater, and the mean time to LR was 33.6 months. Table 17.1 reviews the published literature on LR after open RNx.

Table 17.1.
Local recurrence after open radical nephrectomy for renal cell carcinoma

Reference	Year	n	LR	Isolated LR	Mean time to LR
DiMarco[4]	2004	1925	73 (3.8%)	NA*	39.6 months
Stephenson[6]	2004	495	12 (2.4%)	NA	NA
Schrodter[7]	2002	1031	NA	8 (0.8%)	NA
Itano[5]	2000	1737	NA	30 (1.7%)	33.6 months
Ljungberg[8]	1999	187	7 (3.7%)	NA	NA
Levy[9]	1998	286	9 (3.1%)	NA	NA
Sandock[10]	1995	137	5 (3.6%)	3 (2.2%)	8.4 months
Uson[3]	1982	518	17 (3.3%)	7 (1.4%)	NA

NA, data not available.

INCIDENCE AFTER OPEN PARTIAL NEPHRECTOMY

Local recurrence was previously thought to be more likely after PNx than after RNx, since the remaining parenchyma remains at risk on a long-term basis, and LR rates after PNx traditionally were reported to be in the 4% to 10% range.[11-15] More recent data demonstrates LR rates for PNx ranging from 1.4% to 6%, similar to RNx.[16-24] This incidence is even lower (1% to 2%) in highly select patients with small (<3 cm), incidentally discovered, unifocal renal tumors undergoing PNx on an elective basis (Table 17.2). The largest review of PNx in the modern era involving 485 patients managed at

Table 17.2.
Local recurrence after open partial nephrectomy for renal cell carcinoma

All indications					
Reference	*Year*	n	*LR*	*Isolated LR*	*Mean time to LR (mo)*
Krejci[16]	2003	344	6 (1.7%)	NA*	34.8
Lee[17]	2000	79	0 (0%)	0%	NA
Belldegrun[18]	1999	146	4 (2.7%)	NA	NA
Hafez[19]	1999	485	16 (3.3%)	7 (1.4%)	42.6
van Poppel[20]	1998	76	0 (0%)	0 (0%)	NA
Lerner[21]	1996	185	11 (5.9%)	NA	NA
Moll[22]	1993	142	2 (1.4%)	2 (1.4%)	NA
Steinbach[23]	1992	121	5 (4.1%)	5 (4.1%)	32
Provet[24]	1991	44	1 (2%)	NA	NA
Selli[11]	1991	56	2 (4%)	NA	NA
Morgan[12]	1990	104	6 (5.8%)	5 (4.8%)	57
Bazeed[13]	1986	51	2 (4%)	NA	NA
Marberger[14]	1981	72	6 (8.3%)	NA	NA
Jacobs[15]	1980	51	5 (9.8%)	NA	NA
Total		1956	66 (3.4%)		
Elective indications					
Reference	*Year*	n	*LR*	*Isolated LR*	*Mean tumor size (cm)*
Leibovich[28]	2004	91	5 (5.6%)	NA*	4–7
Barbalias[29]	1999	41	3 (7.3%)	NA	3–5
Belldegrun[18]	1999	63	2 (3.2%)	NA	2.6–4.3
Hafez[19]	1999	45	0 (0%)	0 (0%)	<4.0
Herr[30]	1999	70	1 (1.4%)	1 (1.4%)	3.0
van Poppel[20]	1998	51	0 (0%)	0 (0%)	3.0
Belussi[31]	1997	320	5 (1.6%)	NA	NA
D'Armiento[32]	1997	19	0 (0%)	0 (0%)	3.3
Moll[22]	1993	105	1 (1%)	1 (1%)	4.0
Steinbach[23]	1992	72	2 (2.8%)	NA	3.3
Provet[24]	1991	19	0 (0%)	0 (0%)	2.6
Selli[11]	1991	20	0 (0%)	0 (0%)	<3.5
Morgan[12]	1990	20	0 (0%)	0 (0%)	NA
Carini[33]	1988	10	0 (0%)	0 (0%)	3.5
Bazeed[13]	1986	23	0 (0%)	0 (0%)	3.3
Total		969	19 (2.0%)		

NA, data not available.

the Cleveland Clinic reported 16 LR (3.3%), with seven of these patients having isolated LR (1.4%) and nine with LR in the presence of metastatic disease.[19] The incidence of isolated LR in this series is thus very similar to those reported after RNx, likely reflecting careful patient selection and improved surgical techniques. Previous studies have shown that the incidence of clinically and radiographically occult microscopic satellite lesions at the time of RNx for RCC is 4% to 6%, and these lesions likely account for most LR after PNx.[25–27] In support of this is the observation that most LRs after PNx occur at sites distant from the tumor bed, suggesting a secondary tumor development rather than an incomplete resection of the primary lesion.

INCIDENCE AFTER LAPAROSCOPIC SURGERY

Laparoscopic RNx is now a well-accepted procedure for the management of select patients with renal masses, with the major advantages being reduced convalescence and lower analgesic requirements. Initial concerns regarding the perceived difficulty in replicating open techniques now appear to be unfounded, although long-term efficacy data are still awaited. One early concern was LR, possibly related to morcellation, tumor spillage, or port-site implantation. However, recently published data suggest LR rates comparable to those of open RNx. A multicenter series reported by Cadeddu and colleagues[34] documented only one LR among 157 patients undergoing laparoscopic RNx, and there were no port-site recurrences. A more recent series reported no LR or port-site recurrences after 402 laparoscopic RNx, and a review of the published literature (Table 17.3) suggests that these may be relatively uncommon events.[35] Follow-up in some of these series is relatively limited and may thus underestimate the true incidence of LR after laparoscopic RNx.

Table 17.3.
Local recurrence after laparoscopic surgery for renal cell carcinoma

Author	Year	n	LR	Mean tumor size (cm)	Mean follow-up (mo)
Laparoscopic radical nephrectomy					
Peschel[35]	2004	402	0 (0%)	5.2	38
Wille[36]	2004	125	0 (0%)	5.1	24
Rassweiler[37]	2003	45	1 (2.2%)	NA*	NA
Portis[38]	2002	64	1 (1.6%)	4.3	54
Chan[39]	2001	67	0 (0%)	NA	21
Ono[40]	2001	103	1 (1.0%)	<5	29
Dunn[41]	2000	38	1 (2.6%)	NA	25
Fentie[42]	2000	57	2 (3.5%)	NA	33
Cadeddu[34]	1998	157	1 (0.6%)	NA	19
Total		1058	7 (0.7%)		
Laparoscopic partial nephrectomy					
Kaouk[43]	2004	275	1 (0.4%)	2.9	1–48
Allaf[44]	2004	48	2 (4.2%)	2.4	37.7
Rassweiler[37]	2003	12	0 (0%)	NA*	NA
Harmon[45]	2000	15	0 (0%)	2.3	8
Janetschek[46]	2000	25	0 (0%)	1.9	22
Total		375	3 (0.8%)		

NA, data not available.

The experience with laparoscopic PNx is limited and long-term data are not yet available (Table 17.3). Adequate hemostasis and tumor margins remain the greatest challenges associated with this procedure, and most centers initially selected patients with relatively small (<3 cm) exophytic tumors. In this setting, LR after laparoscopic PNx has been an uncommon event. However, the indications for this procedure are rapidly evolving, with some centers reporting laparoscopic PNx for larger tumors and for tumors abutting the collecting system or renal hilum. Two LRs were reported by Allaf and colleagues[44] after 48 laparoscopic PNx, with one occurring in a patient with VHL syndrome. The largest experience to date is from Kaouk and colleagues,[43] who have now performed over 275 laparoscopic PNx and have observed only one LR, despite increasing tumor size and less favorable tumor location. This suggests that surgeon expertise combined with sensible patient selection may allow this procedure to replicate the results of open PNx.

INCIDENCE AFTER THERMAL ABLATION

Laparoscopic renal cryoablation and radiofrequency ablation (RFA) have recently been investigated as minimally invasive options for the management of small renal tumors. In both cases the ablated tissue remains in place, theoretically leaving the patient at risk for LR if tumor kill is incomplete. Diagnosis of LR is also challenging, since differentiation between fibrosis within the tumor bed and emerging LR can be difficult. Of these two modalities, experience with cryoablation is more extensive with several series now reported in the literature (Table 17.4). Most series have included

Table 17.4.
Local recurrence after thermal ablative therapies for renal cell carcinoma

Author	Year	n	Exposure	LR*	Mean tumor size (cm)	Mean follow-up (mo)
Cryoablation						
Cestari[47]	2004	37	Laparoscopic	1 (3.4%)	2.6	NA
Hasan[48]	2004	40	Laparoscopic	2 (5%)	2.4	48+
Shingleton[49]	2004	90	Image guided	7 (7.8%)	3.0	30
Lee[50]	2003	20	Laparoscopic	0 (0%)	2.6	14
Nadler[51]	2003	15**	Laparoscopic	1 (10%)	2.2	15

*LR = treatment failure.
**10/15 had RCC on intraoperative biopsy prior to treatment.

Author	Year	n	Exposure	LR*	Mean tumor size (cm)	Mean follow-up (mo)
Radiofrequency ablation						
Hwang[53]	2004	24	Image guided	1 (4.2%)	2.2	13
Matsumoto[54]	2004	28	Laparoscopic	1 (3.6%)	3.6	13
Zagoria[55]	2004	24	Image guided	0 (0%)	3.5	7
Farrell[56]	2003	35	Image guided	0 (0%)	1.7	9
Gervais[57]	2003	34	Image guided	6 (17.6%)	3.2	13
Mayo-Smith[58]	2003	32	Image guided	0 (0%)	2.6	9
Su[59]	2003	29	Image guided	0 (0%)	2.2	9

n = number of tumors.
* LR = treatment failure.

primarily patients for whom laparoscopic exposure has been obtained, but percutaneous treatment has also been advocated. Local recurrence, which in most cases represents inadequate tumor kill, has been a relatively uncommon event, with reported incidence ranging from 0% to 10%. Reported incidences of LR in these series may be underestimates since 10% to 20% of patients with small renal masses may have benign disease rather than RCC. For example, in the series from Nadler and colleagues,[51] five of 15 patients had benign pathology, so the true incidence of LR was 10%, not 6.7%. Patients may also recur at other sites in the kidney, and this should also be considered LR, although the mechanism (novel tumor occurrence rather than treatment failure) is different. Hasan and colleagues[48] reported two (5%) such occurrences when their patients were followed for longer than 48 months, so the total incidence of LR after cryoablation may be higher than previously appreciated. Enhancement in the tumor bed has been considered diagnostic for LR in this setting, and the clinical experience has supported this thus far. Twenty-three patients in Gill's series also underwent image-guided biopsy of the tumor bed, and none were positive.[52] Most other series have not included routine posttherapy biopsies, and many include only limited follow-up, so the true incidence of LR after cryoablation is still not well defined.

From a technical standpoint, most authors advocate a double freeze/thaw protocol, and animal studies suggest that this protocol may optimize tumor cell kill. Ideally, the ice ball should extend at least 1 cm beyond the edge of the lesion, which may be facilitated by the emerging ultrasound technology that provides improved visualization. Finer probes are also now available that minimize the risk of tumor fragmentation and allow for more accurate placement. These recent developments along with increasing surgeon experience may reduce the risk of LR with this modality in the future.

Radiofrequency ablation has emerged as an alternative ablative modality for renal tumors in select patients, with most series reporting image-guided percutaneous access. Again, most patients selected for this modality have had small tumors, and CT guidance is most commonly used in these protocols. Failure rates ranging from 0% to 21% have been reported (Table 17.4), but follow-up is very limited in most series, and routine posttherapy biopsies have not been reported. Patients with large tumors (>3 cm) and those abutting the collecting system are at highest risk for failure, and in the series by Gervais and colleagues[57] all treatment failures fell into these groups. As with cryoablation, the diagnosis of LR after RFA is challenging, and exact criteria have not been well defined, although enhancement within the tumor bed appears to be the diagnostic finding.[60]

RISK FACTORS FOR LOCAL RECURRENCE

Tumor stage is the most important factor that influences the risk of LR of RCC after RNx or PNx, but histology, multifocality, and margin status may also play a role. After RNx tumor stage has directly correlated with risk of LR, with several recent series documenting this correlation. Sandock and colleagues[10] reported incidences of LR of 0%, 2.4%, and 8.4% after RNx for stages pT1, pT2, and pT3, respectively. The mean time to recurrence was 6.7 months in patients with pT3 RCC compared to 11 months for patients with pT2 RCC, further highlighting the influence of stage on the development of LR in this population. In the M.D. Anderson Cancer Center series, there were no LRs in 177 patients with pT1 or pT2 disease after RNx, and all nine patients (9/43,

21%) with LR in renal fossa or adjacent retroperitoneal LNs had pT3 disease.[9] As expected, the risk of LR is even higher for patients with N+ disease. Saidi and colleagues[61] reported 17 patients with LR out of 45 (37.8%) patients with $pT_{any}N+M0$ RCC enrolled in an adjuvant therapy protocol after RNx. As expected, many of these patients also failed systemically. It is interesting to note that 13/30 (43%) patients with isolated LR in the series from Itano and colleagues had pT3b or pT3c disease, and 5/13 (38.5%) patients with isolated LR in the series from Esrig and colleagues[62] had Robson stage III disease. Venous involvement and locally advanced disease thus represent strong risk factors for LR after RNx.

Stage is also a strong predictor of LR after PNx, but tumor size, grade, location, and factors that are associated with multifocality may also be important. In the series from the Cleveland Clinic, the incidences of LR after PNx were 0%, 2%, 8.2%, and 10.6% for patients with stages pT1, pT2, pT3a, and pT3b, respectively.[63] Again, the mean time to LR was also shorter in patients with higher stage disease (62.0, 36.4, and 30.4 months for stages pT2, pT3a, and pT3b, respectively). Tumor size is also prognostic for LR as suggested by the series from Leibovich and colleagues,[28] who reported the outcomes of 91 patients treated with PNx for stage pT1b (4 to 7 cm) RCC in an elective setting.[28] The incidence of LR in this series was 5.5% (5/91), substantially higher than the observed rate of LR in our meta-analysis of elective PNx, which is summarized in Table 17.2. Excluding the Liebovich data, and thereby focusing on patients with smaller tumor size, the incidence of LR was 1.6%. Nuclear grade may also correspond with an increased risk of LR after PNx, and Krejci and colleagues[16] from the Mayo Clinic have presented data in support of this finding. One could also hypothesize that central tumor location would predispose to LR since these tumors may be more challenging to excise, increasing the likelihood of positive surgical margins. However, surgical expertise and experience can overcome this to some extent, and the incidence of LR for centrally located tumors has been relatively low (5.3% and 6.1%) in two series that focused on this patient population.[64,65]

Factors that are associated with tumor multifocality could further increase the risk of LR after PNx, and this is definitely true for patients with familial RCC, as discussed earlier. Papillary histology is known to be associated with an increased risk of multifocality, but a clinical correlation with increased incidence of LR after PNx has not been reported.[4] Finally, surgical margin status has also been investigated, and previous recommendations were to try to obtain a 1.0 cm or greater margin to reduce the risk of LR after PNx. However, several reports have shown that margin width does not correlate with LR or other oncologic outcomes, as long as the final margin is negative.[66,67] In other words, a negative margin is a negative margin for RCC, a fact that can be of considerable practical importance when performing difficult or challenging procedures, or when preservation of functioning parenchyma is of paramount importance.

SYMPTOMS OF LOCAL RECURRENCE

Historically, patients with LR of RCC presented with constitutional symptoms or localized signs due to the compression or involvement of adjacent organs. Local recurrence after RNx faces no natural barriers and can invade adjacent organs, compress nerves within the retroperitoneum, or lead to bowel obstruction. Hence, malaise, weight loss, poor appetite, nausea, gastrointestinal bleed, and back pain were common presentations in the past.[5,10,62,68] Invasion of the duodenum and pancreas can be particularly problematic, and is well described in this setting.[68] Even in the modern era many patients with LR after RNx present symptomatically. Eighty percent of the patients in Parienty, et al.'s[69] series complained of back pain prior to computed tomography (CT) confirmation of LR of RCC. Similarly, 82% of Esrig, et al.'s[62] and 60% of Itano, et al.'s[5] patients with LR were symptomatic. Two of nine LRs in the series from Levy and colleagues[9] were symptomatic, but five others were detected on physical exam. Routine CT surveillance for high-risk patients after RNx is no doubt now diagnosing more LR in an asymptomatic state, but substantial series to confirm this have not yet been published.

Partial nephrectomy was not popularized until CT scan was in routine use, and this patient population has traditionally been followed more intensively, particularly with serial cross-sectional imaging. Most LRs after PNx are thus diagnosed in an asymptomatic state, although some patients still present with hematuria or flank pain due to obstruction of the collecting system.

EVALUATION OF PATIENTS WITH LOCAL RECURRENCE OF RENAL CELL CARCINOMA

The evaluation of individuals suspected of having recurrent disease should include a full history and physical examination and thorough assessment for metastatic disease. Constitutional symptoms or palpable abdominal mass or lymphadenopathy suggest advanced disease, and lower extremity edema suggests recurrence with venous obstruction. Localizing symptoms and neurologic examination may indicate invasion of adjacent organs or compression of nerves in the vicinity of the tumor. A combination of symptoms and elevated liver function tests were identified in 92% of patients with abdominal recurrences after RNx in Sandock, et al.'s[10] series.

Computed tomography continues to play the primary role in the diagnosis and evaluation of LR of RCC. After RNx, soft tissue density within the renal fossa or adjacent retroperitoneum that is invading adjacent organs or increasing in size on serial imaging indicates LR (Figure 17.1). After PNx or ablative therapies, enhancement within a renal mass is indicative of LR, particularly if serial studies suggest increasing size (Figure 17.2). Enhancing pseudotumors can be seen early after PNx but almost always resolve

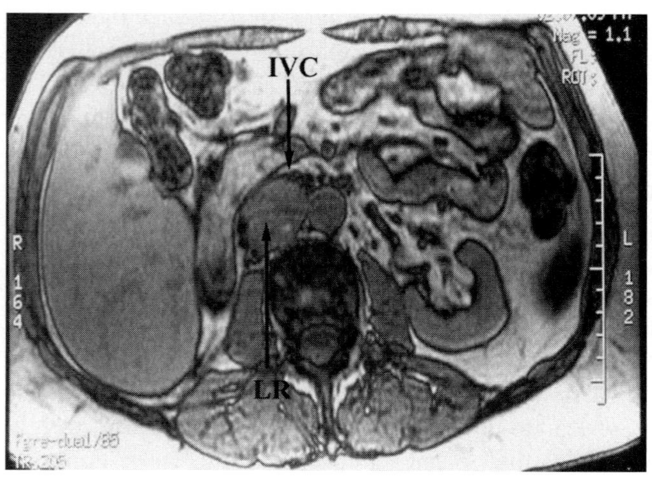

Figure 17.1. A 67-year-old man with local recurrence (LR) 1 year after right radical nephrectomy (RNx). The inferior vena cava (IVC) is compressed and draped over this mass, which lies posteriorly. The patient underwent successful excision of LR with negative margins. The IVC was mobilized away and preserved in continuity.

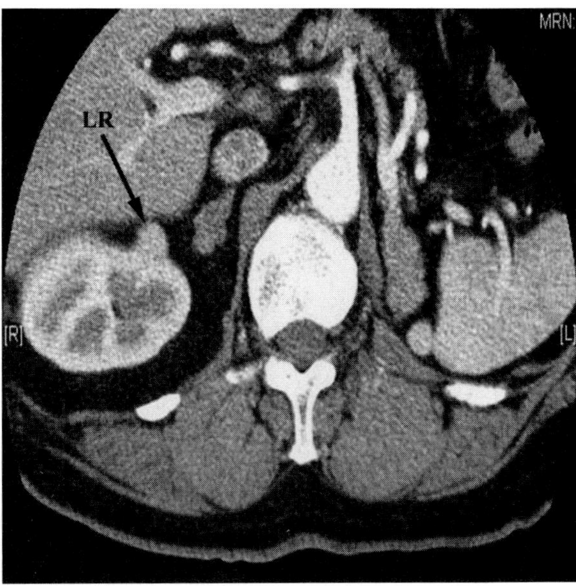

Figure 17.2. A 69-year-old man with LR in a solitary kidney after left RNx and right partial nephrectomy (PNx). This lesion enhances with contrast and was successfully treated with cryoablation.

on subsequent imaging, eventually leaving a fibrotic scar. This entity is well described by Kshirsagar and colleagues,[70] who reported resolution in all 13 such lesions in their series with a mean time of 13 months after PNx. The authors hypothesized that initial enhancement of these lesions was secondary to granulation tissue involving the lattice of absorbable gelatin sponge used during surgery. An initial increase in lesion size and enhancement is also often seen after cryoablation, but most successfully treated lesions will then regress. Progressive or subsequent increase in size when combined with peripheral or nodular enhancement is particularly suspicious for LR after cryoablation or radiofrequency ablation.

The CT should also be carefully reviewed for evidence of locally invasive behavior, particularly if the patient has undergone RNx. Other abdominal sites that commonly harbor metastases of RCC, such as the liver, should also be assessed. Further evaluation with magnetic resonance imaging (MRI) may be indicated since it may provide information about tissue planes around the cancer and the status of adjacent organs and the venous system (Figure 17.3). Magnetic resonance imaging may be particularly useful in patients with LR after RNx to facilitate preoperative planning and counseling, since these tumors often require en-bloc resection of adjacent organs, and proximity to or involvement of vital structures can also present unique surgical challenges that are best recognized prospectively.

Metastatic evaluation should include at least a chest radiograph and comprehensive metabolic panel, but in high-risk patients or those suspected of having advanced disease, strong consideration should be given to chest CT and bone scan. Additional imaging should be based on clinical presentation and exam findings. A major goal in the evaluation of patients with LR of RCC is to determine whether the lesion is isolated and potentially resectable or associated with disseminated disease, in which case systemic treatments will predominate.

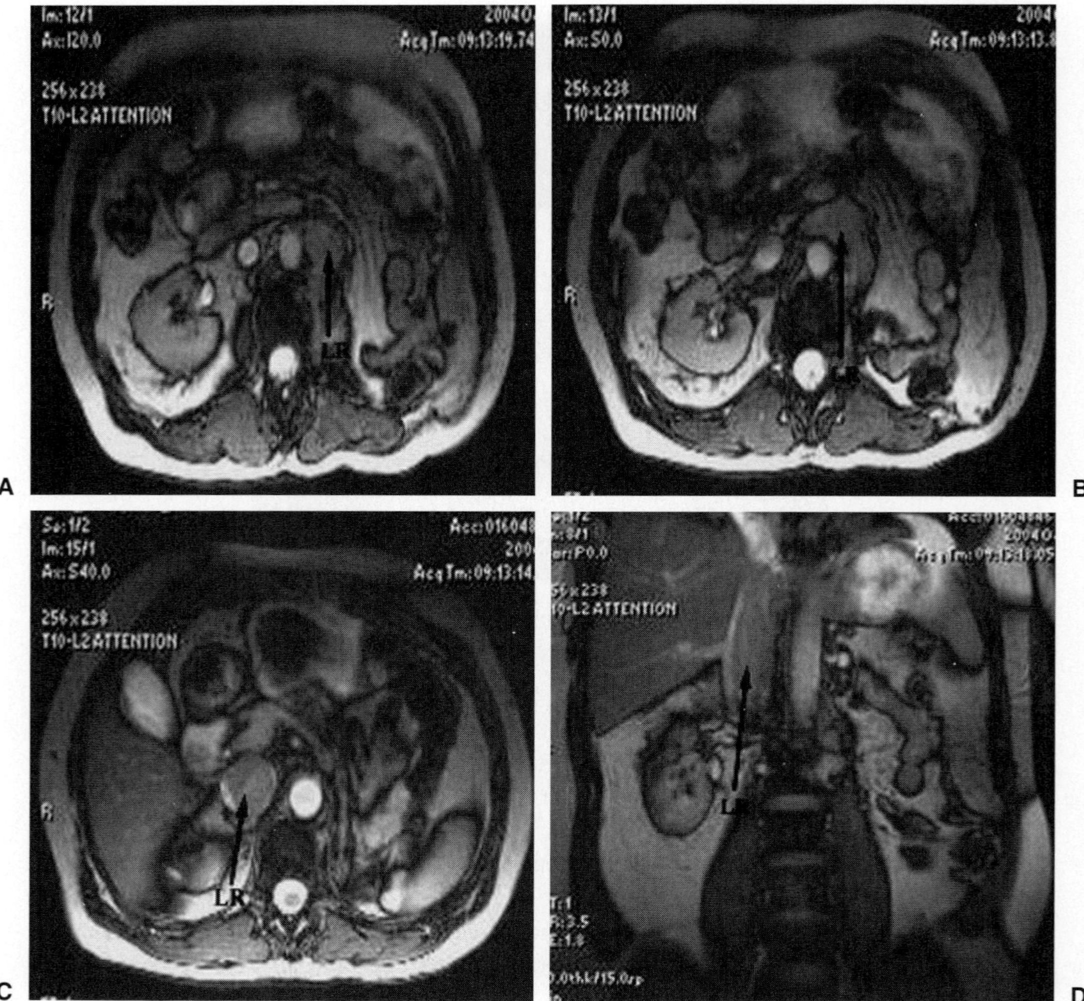

Figure 17.3. A 57-year-old man with LR involving the IVC and retroperitoneal lymph nodes 1 year after left RNx for T3bNxMx RCC. MRI demonstrates (A) tumor in left retroperitoneum invading the psoas muscle; (B) tumor invading into or arising from the left renal vein stump; (C) tumor extending up IVC; and (D) coronal section showing cephalad extension to top of liver near diaphragm. This tumor was invading the nerve roots along the spine posteriorly on the left and was not resectable.

MANAGEMENT OF LOCAL RECURRENCE

Surgery has always played a central role in the management of patients with isolated LR of RCC, and at times surgical efforts have bordered on the heroic.[71] One early report of LR after RNx from Bloom and colleagues[72] detailed the course of a 53-year-old man who was 19 years out from RNx and cobalt treatment to the tumor bed. He was then hospitalized for malaise, weight loss, and an enlarging right flank mass. Metastatic evaluation was negative, and a thoracoabdominal approach was taken to excise this mass, which filled the entire right side of the abdomen, extending down into the inguinal canal. The tumor weighed 14 pounds, and a total of 40 units of blood, along with plate-lets and fresh frozen plasma, were required during the perioperative period. One year later this patient was without evidence of recurrent disease. Surgery continues to play a primary role in the management of isolated LR of RCC, as it represents the only realistic curative option for most patients in this unfortunate circumstance.

LOCAL RECURRENCE AFTER RADICAL NEPHRECTOMY

As highlighted by the above case and the series detailed in Table 17.5, surgical resection of LR after RNx can be a formidable challenge. Local invasion of adjacent organs is common since these tumors are no longer constrained by natural barriers and en-bloc resection with splenectomy, hemicolectomy, distal pancreatectomy, or partial hepatectomy is often required. The Whipple procedure has also been reported for excision of LR of RCC involving the head of the pancreas.[68] In addition, venous thrombectomy or partial resection of the IVC wall are occasionally required, and venovenous bypass may facilitate this procedure. Partial resection of the adjacent psoas muscle or diaphragm is occasionally needed, and care should be taken to avoid the femoral nerve or other retroperitoneal nerves if at all possible. Local recurrence after RNx is often sizable; even the most recent series from Schrodter et al.[7] in 2002 and Gogus et al.[73] in 2003 reported mean tumor sizes of 5.92 and 8.45 cm, respectively.

Given all of these considerations, open surgical approaches have been preferred, and exposure can be at a premium in these cases. Esrig and colleagues[62] favored a thoracoabdominal incision, but most agree that the surgical approach can be tailored to the location of the recurrence, size of the lesion, and proximity to or involvement of adjacent organs. Laparoscopic approaches may also be appropriate in highly select cases, with one report describing the use of a hand-assisted procedure to excise a small LR.[76] Another case report described the use of RFA for the management of LR after RNx, but this approach could be associated with substantial morbidity if the bowel or pancreas were adherent to the mass.[77] Wide excision to achieve negative margins is essential given the natural history and tumor biology of RCC, and this must be the goal. An extensive retroperitoneal lymph node dissection has also been advocated by Esrig and colleagues, and should be considered based on interoperative findings and patient comorbidities. Preoperative planning should include adequate bowel preparation, coordination with appropriate surgical colleagues as necessary, and judicious counseling of the patient about realistic expectations.

Even a cursory review of the literature about these procedures (Table 17.5) reveals that they can be associated with substantial morbidity, and as expected, this is particularly true if the pancreas or duodenum are involved. Blood transfusions are often required, and mean blood loss in the Itano, et al.[5] series was 2800 cc. Hospital stay averaged 12 days (range 5–19 days) in this series. Four postoperative deaths were reported in the six series listed in Table 17.5, representing 5.8% of patients undergoing excision of LR in these studies.

These sobering statistics are counterbalanced by data showing long-term survival in about 30% to 40% of cases, and direct comparison of patients managed with surgery vs. medical approaches or observation shows a distinct advantage to surgery. Patient selection no doubt contributes to these results, but based on what we know about RCC's status as primarily a surgical disease, these observations are not surprising. One could argue that isolated LR of RCC after RNx is similar to a solitary metastasis of RCC, and should be managed in a similar manner, although surgical excision of LR may be

Table 17.5.
Management of local recurrence after radical nephrectomy

Author	Year	n	Isolated LR	Mean time to LR (mo)	Symptomatic	Management	Outcome	Major complications of surgery
Gogus (73)	2003	10	10	33.6	3 (30%)	Surgery, 10 Complete excision, 9 Splenectomy, 3 Hemicolectomy, 2 Distal pancreatectomy, 1	7 NED at 16.6 mo mean f/u 2 dead of mets after 8.5 mo	Death from anastomotic fistula and sepsis, 1
Schrodter (7)	2002	16	16	45.5	2 (12.5%)	Surgery, 16, confirmed LR in 13 Adjuvant immunotherapy, 4 Splenectomy, 1 Hemicolectomy, 1	5 NED at 52.4 mo mean f/u 7 died of mets after mean of 23.1 1 alive with mets	Subcutaneous seroma, 1
Wiesner (74)	2002	15	8	23.0	NA	Surgery, 9 Surgery alone, 4 Surgery + XRT, 3 Surgery + immunotherapy, 1 Surgery + XRT + immunotherapy, 1 Immunotherapy, 5 Observation, 1	Tumor specific survival (mean) Surgery alone = 62.2 mo Surgery + adjuvant Rx = 26 mo Immunotherapy = 9.2 mo	Death from cardiopulmonary failure, 1
Itano (5)	2000	30	30	34	18 (60%)	Surgery ± adjuvant Rx, 10 Partial hepatectomy, 1 Splenectomy, 1 Bowel resection, 1 Psoas resection, 1 Diaphragm resection, 1 Medical Rx, 11 Observation, 9	5 year survival Surgery = 51% Medical Rx = 18% Observation = 13% Overall = 28%	Prolonged ileus, 1 Pneumonia, 1 Hydropneumothorax, 1

| Tanguay (75) | 1996 | 16 | 15 | 16.5 median | 6 (38%) | Surgery alone, 8
Surgery + immunotherapy, 8
Splenectomy, 2
Hemicolectomy, 1
Distal pancreatectomy, 2
Partial hepatectomy, 2
Partial psoas resection, 2
Partial resection diaphragm, 4 | 7 NED at mean of 43 mo
5 alive with disease at mean of 26 mo
4 dead from disease at mean of 16 mo
Surgery + immunotherapy: 50% NED
Surgery alone: 25% NED | Subphrenic abscess and emphysema, 1
Pneumonia, 1
Supraventricular tachycardia, 1
Pulmonary edema, 1
Pyelonephritis, 1 |
| Esrig (62) | 1992 | 11 | 10 | 31 | 9 (82%) | Surgery, 11
RPLND in all
Most required partial psoas resection
Partial hepatectomy, 1
Distal pancreatectomy
Splenectomy, 1
IVC thrombectomy, occasional
Bowel resection, occasional | 4 NED at mean of 85 mo
2 died of mets at 8 and 22 mo
3 died of unrelated causes at 4, 6, and 120 mo | Death from jejunal necrosis and sepsis, 1
Death from ARDS, coagulopathy, hemorrhage, 1
Retroperitoneal abscess, 1
Duodenal obstruction, 1 |

NED, no evidence of disease; f/u, follow-up; mets, metastatic disease; XRT, radiotherapy.

associated with an increased risk of morbidity and this should be taken into account. The Tanguay et al.[75] series is notable in that it demonstrated a potential advantage to adjuvant immunotherapy therapy after surgical excision, and this should be considered in highly motivated patients with good performance status.

LOCAL RECURRENCE AFTER PARTIAL NEPHRECTOMY

Isolated LR after PNx can be addressed with radical surgery to remove the remnant, with repeat PNx, or with thermal ablative therapies. Repeat PNx should be considered if preservation of renal function is important, but tumor location and multifocality should also be taken into account. The first report of successful repeat PNx was from Gittes and Blute,[78] who performed repeat bench surgery on a solitary kidney in an effort to obviate the need for dialysis. This patient then developed a second LR 2 years later and a third PNx was performed using an in situ approach. This patient then remained cancer-free for 5 years and maintained adequate renal function. Moll and colleagues[22] also reported success with this approach; their patient developed three LRs in the same kidney and required three repeat PNx. This patient also maintained cancer-free status and adequate renal function (serum creatinine = 2.1 mg/dL) for prolonged periods of time (13 years).

These experiences highlight the potential for preservation of renal function and long-term cancer-free survival that can be achieved with repeat PNx, and several other groups have reported success with this approach. However, these procedures can be challenging to perform due to fibrosis within the renal fossa, and in the modern era another option is thermal ablative therapy. The LR shown in Figure 17.2 was treated with cryoablation, and short-term follow-up is favorable, but further experience will be required to define the role of these approaches in this challenging situation. Finally, for many patients with LR after PNx, strong consideration should be given to radical excision of the remaining remnant. This is the preferred approach in the presence of a normal contralateral kidney, and is often required if hilar location or other factors preclude nephron-sparing approaches. Prognosis for patients with isolated LR after PNx is better than patients with LR after RNx, and the current literature suggests that about 60% to 70% can be salvaged with repeat surgery.

Local recurrence after PNx for patients with familial RCC is a special case and should be managed accordingly. As discussed above, most patients with familial RCC will recur after PNx if they are followed long-term, and injudicious management would lead to multiple procedures with substantial risk for morbidity and loss of functioning renal parenchyma. Data from the National Cancer Institute (NCI) demonstrates that a threshold of 3.0 cm can be used as a trigger point for repeat intervention.[79] In the NCI's extensive experience with this patient population, metastasis is extremely rare until this threshold has been eclipsed. More recently, thermal ablative approaches have been investigated in this population, and if validated for efficacy, would offer a number of distinct advantages for this patient population.

LOCAL RECURRENCE AFTER THERMAL ABLATIVE THERAPIES

Thermal ablative therapies are relatively novel, and data about the management of LR, which in this case most often represents inadequate tumor kill, is quite limited.

Both LR in the series by Hasan and colleagues[48] were managed with laparoscopic RNx, but repeat thermal ablation has also been described, and in some cases this may be part of the original treatment plan. One important consideration in this patient population is that many are elderly and have substantial comorbidities and may not be reasonable candidates for traditional surgical approaches.

REFERENCES

1. Herring JC, Enquist EG, Chernoff A, et al. Parenchymal sparing surgery in patients with hereditary renal cell carcinoma: 10–year experience. J Urol 2001;165(3):777–781.
2. Steinbach F, Novick AC, Zincke H, et al. Treatment of renal cell carcinoma in Von Hippel-Lindau disease: a multicenter study. J Urol 1995:153(6):1812–1816.
3. Uson AC. Tumor recurrence in the renal fossa and/or the abdominal wall after radical nephrectomy for renal cell cancer. In: Renal Tumors: Proceedings of the First International Symposium on Kidney Tumors. New York: Alan R. Liss, 1982:549–560.
4. DiMarco DS, Lohse CM, Zincke H, et al. Long-term survival of patients with unilateral sporadic multifocal renal cell carcinoma according to histologic subtype compared with patients with solitary tumors after radical nephrectomy. Urology 2004;64(3):462–467.
5. Itano NB, Blute ML, Spotts B, Zincke H. Outcome of isolated renal cell carcinoma fossa recurrence after nephrectomy. J Urol 2000;164:322–325.
6. Stephenson AJ, Chetner MP, Rourke K, et al. Guidelines for the surveillance of localized renal cell carcinoma based on the patterns of relapse after nephrectomy. J Urol 2004;172:58–62.
7. Schrodter S, Hakenberg OW, Manseck A, et al. Outcome of surgical treatment of isolated local recurrence after radical nephrectomy for renal cell carcinoma. J Urol 2002;167:1630–1633.
8. Ljungberg B, Alamdari FI, Rasmuson T, Roos G. Follow-up guidelines for nonmetastatic renal cell carcinoma based on the occurrence of metastases after radical nephrectomy. BJU Int 1999;84: 405–411.
9. Levy DA, Slaton JW, Swanson DA, Dinney CPN. Stage specific guidelines for surveillance after radical nephrectomy for local renal cell carcinoma. J Urol 1998;159:1163–1167.
10. Sandock DS, Seftel AD, Resnick MI. A new protocol for the followup of renal cell carcinoma based on pathological stage. J Urol 1995;154:28–31.
11. Selli C, Lapini A, Carini M. Conservative surgery of kidney tumors. Prog Clin Biol Res 1991; 370:9.
12. Morgan WR, Zincke H. Progression and survival after renal-conserving surgery for renal cell carcinoma: Experience in 104 patients and extended follow-up. J Urol 1990;144:852.
13. Bazeed MA, Scharfe T, Becht E, et al. Conservative surgery for renal cell carcinoma. Eur Urol 1986;12:238.
14. Marberger M, Pugh RCG, Auvert J, et al. Conservative surgery for renal cell carcinoma: the EIRSS experience. Br J Urol 1981;53:528.
15. Jacobs SC, Berg SI, Lawson RK. Synchronous bilateral renal cell carcinoma: total surgical excision. Cancer 1980;46:2341.
16. Krejci KG, Blute ML, Cheville JC, et al. Nephron-sparing surgery for renal cell carcinoma: clinico-pathologic features predictive of patient outcome. Urology 2003;62(4):641–646.
17. Lee CT, Katz J, Shi W, et al. Surgical management of renal tumors 4 cm or less in a contemporary cohort. J Urol 2000;163:730.
18. Belldegrun A, Tsui KH, deKernion JB, Smith RB. Efficacy of nephron-sparing surgery for renal cell carcinoma: Analysis based on the new 1997 tumor-node-metastasis staging system. J Clin Oncol 1999;17:28–68.
19. Hafez KS, Fergany AF, Novick AC. Nephron sparing surgery for localized renal cell carcinoma: Impact of tumor size on patient survival, tumor recurrence and TNM staging. J Urol 1999;162:1930.
20. van Poppel H, Bamelis B, Oyen R, Baert L. Partial nephrectomy for renal cell carcinoma can achieve long term tumor control. J Urol 1998;160:674.
21. Lerner SE, Hawkins CA, Blute ML, et al. Disease outcome in patients with low stage renal cell carcinoma treated with nephron sparing or radical surgery. J Urol 1996;155:1868–1873.

22. Moll V, Becht E, Ziegler M. Kidney preserving surgery in renal cell tumors: Indications, techniques and results in 162 patients. J Urol 1993;150:319.

23. Steinbach F, Stockle M, Muller SC, et al. Conservative surgery of renal cell tumors in 140 patients: 21 years of experience. J Urol 1992;148:24.

24. Provet J, Tessler A, Brown J, et al. Partial nephrectomy for renal cell carcinoma: indications, results and implications. J Urol 1991;145:472.

25. Kletscher BA, Qian J, Bostwick DG, et al. Prospective analysis of multifocality in renal cell carcinoma: influence of histological pattern, grade, number, size, volume and deoxyribonucleic acid ploidy. J Urol 1995:153:904–906.

26. Campbell SC, Fichtner J, Novick AC, et al. Intraoperative evaluation of renal cell carcinoma: a prospective study of the role of ultrasonography and histopathological frozen sections. J Urol 1996;155: 1191–1195.

27. Uzzo RG, Novick AC. Nephron sparing surgery for renal tumors: indications, techniques and outcomes. J Urol 2001;166:6–18.

28. Leibovich BC, Blute ML, Cheville JC, et al. Nephron sparing surgery for appropriately selected renal cell carcinoma between 4 and 7 cm results in outcome similar to radical nephrectomy. J Urol 2004; 171:1066–1070.

29. Barbalias GA, Liatsikos EN, Tsintavis A, Nikiforidis G. Adenocarcinoma of the kidney: Nephron sparing surgical approach versus radical nephrectomy. J Surg Oncol 1999;72:156.

30. Herr HW. Partial nephrectomy for unilateral renal carcinoma and a normal contralateral kidney: 10-year follow-up. J Urol 1999;161:33.

31. Belussi D, Chinaglia D, Micheli E, Lembo A. Conservative surgery of parenchymal renal carcinoma: urologic data from Lombardy. Arch Ital Urol Androl 1997;69(2):87–91.

32. D'Armiento M, Damiano R, Feleppa B, et al. Elective conservative surgery for renal carcinoma versus radical nephrectomy: a prospective study. Br J Urol 1997;79:15.

33. Carini M, Selli C, Barbanti G, et al. Conservative surgical treatment of renal cell carcinoma: clinical experience and reappraisal of indications. J Urol 1988;140:725.

34. Cadeddu JA, Ono Y, Clayman RV, et al. Laparoscopic nephrectomy for renal cell cancer: evaluation of efficacy and safety: a multicenter experience. Urology 1998;52(5):773–777.

35. Peschel R, Neururer R, Bartsch G, et al. Long term outcome of laparoscopic radical nephrectomy for renal cell cancer. J Urol 2004;171(4, suppl):470.

36. Wille AH, Roigas J, Deger S, et al. Laparoscopic radical nephrectomy: techniques, results and oncological outcome in 125 consecutive cases. Eur Urol 2004;45:483–489.

37. Rassweiler J, Tsivian A, Ravi Kumar AV, et al. Oncological safety of laparoscopic surgery for urological malignancy: experience with more than 1,000 operations. J Urol 2003;169:2072–2075.

38. Portis AJ, Yan Y, Landman J, et al. Long term follow up after laparoscopic radical nephrectomy. J Urol 2002;167:1257–1262.

39. Chan DY, Cadeddu JA, Jarrett TW, et al. Laparoscopic radical nephrectomy: Cancer control in renal carcinoma. J Urol 2001;166:2095.

40. Ono Y, Kinukawa T, Hattori R, et al. The long-term outcome of laparoscopic radical nephrectomy for small renal cell carcinoma. J Urol 2001;165:1867–1870.

41. Dunn MD, Portis AJ, Shalhav AL, et al. Laparoscopic versus open radical nephrectomy: a 9-year experience. J Urol 2000;164:1153–1159.

42. Fentie DD, Barrett PH, Taranger LA. Metastatic renal cell cancer after laparoscopic radical nephrectomy: long-term follow-up. J Endourol 2000;14(5):407–411.

43. Kaouk J, Desai MM, Spaliviero M, et al. Laparoscopic partial nephrectomy: single institution experience with 275 patients. J Urol 2004;171(4, suppl):129.

44. Allaf ME, Bhayani SB, Rogers C, et al. Laparoscopic partial nephrectomy: evaluation of long-term oncological outcome. J Urol 2004;172:871–873.

45. Harmon WJ, Kavoussi LR, Bishoff JT. Laparoscopic nephron-sparing surgery for solid renal masses using the ultrasonic shears. Urology 2000;56:274.

46. Janetschek G, Jeschke K, Peschel R, et al. Laparoscopic surgery for stage T1 renal cell carcinoma: radical nephrectomy and wedge resection. Eur Urol 2000;38(2):131–138.

47. Cestari A, Guazzoni G, Dell'Acqua V, et al. Laparoscopic cryoablation of solid renal masses: intermediate term follow up. J Urol 2004;172:1267–1270.

48. Hasan W, Gill IS, Spaliviero M, et al. Renal cryoablation: 4-year follow up. J Urol 2004;171(4, suppl):438.

49. Shingleton WB, Sewell PE. Percutaneous renal tumor cryoablation: results in the first 90 patients. J Urol 2004;171(4, suppl):463.

50. Lee DI, McGinnis DE, Feld R, Strup SE. Retroperitoneal laparoscopic cryoablation of small renal tumors: intermediate results. Urology 2003;61(1):83–88.

51. Nadler RB, Kim SC, Rubenstein JN, et al. Laparoscopic renal cryosurgery: the Northwestern experience. J Urol 2003;170:1121–1125.

52. Gill IS, Novick AC, Meraney AM, et al. Laparoscopic renal cryoablation in 32 patients. Urology 2000;56(5):748–753.

53. Hwang JJ, Walther MM, Pautler SE, et al. Radio frequency ablation of small renal tumors: intermediate results. J Urol 2004;171:1814–1818.

54. Matsumoto ED, Johnson DB, Ogan K, Cadeddu JA. Laparoscopic radiofrequency ablation of small renal tumors. J Urol 2004;171(4, suppl):127.

55. Zagoria RJ, Hawkins AD, Clark PE, et al. Percutaneous CT-guided radiofrequency ablation of renal neoplasms: factors influencing success. AJR 2004;183:201–207.

56. Farrell MA, Charboneau WJ, DiMarco DS, et al. Imaging-guided radiofrequency ablation of solid renal tumors. AJR 2003;180:1509–1513.

57. Gervais DA, McGovern FJ, Arellano RS, et al. Renal cell carcinoma: clinical experience and technical success with radio-frequency ablation of 42 tumors. Radiology 2003;226(2):417–424.

58. Mayo-Smith WW, Dupuy DE, Parikh PM, et al. Imaging-guided percutaneous radiofrequency ablation of solid renal masses: techniques and outcomes of 38 treatment sessions in 32 consecutive patients. AJR 2003;180:1503–1508.

59. Su L, Jarrett TW, Chan DY, et al. Percutaneous computed tomography-guided radiofrequency ablation of renal masses in high surgical risk patients: preliminary results. Urology 2003;61(suppl 4A):26–33.

60. Hines-Peralta A, Goldberg S. Review of radiofrequency ablation for renal cell carcinoma. Clin Cancer Res 2004;10:6328–6334.

61. Saidi JA, Newhouse JH, Sawczuk IS. Radiologic follow-up of patients with T1–3a,b,c or T4N+M0 renal cell carcinoma after radical nephrectomy. Urology 1998;52:1000–1003.

62. Esrig D, Ahlering TE, Lieskovsky G, Skinner DG. Experience with fossa recurrence of renal cell carcinoma. J Urol 1992;147:1491–1494.

63. Hafez KS, Novick AC, Campbell SC. Patterns of tumor recurrence and guidelines for follow up after nephron sparing surgery for sporadic renal cell carcinoma. J Urology 1997;157:2067–2070.

64. Hafez KS, Novick AC, Butler BP. Management of small solitary unilateral renal cell carcinomas: impact of central versus peripheral tumor location. J Urol 1998;159(4):1156–1159.

65. Black P, Filipas D, Fichtner J, et al. Nephron sparing surgery for central renal tumors: experience with 33 cases. J Urol 2000;163:737–743.

66. Castilla EA, Liou LS, Abrahams NA, et al. Prognostic importance of resection margin width after nephron-sparing surgery for renal cell carcinoma. Urology 2002;60(6):993–997.

67. Sutherland SE, Resnick MI, Maclennan GT, Goldman HB. Does the size of the surgical margin in partial nephrectomy for renal cell cancer really matter? J Urology 2002;167:61–64.

68. Benjamin DS, Ruckle HC, Hadley HR. Local recurrence of renal cell carcinoma causing duodenal-inferior vena caval fistula: case report and review of the literature. Urology 1996;48(4):636–638.

69. Parienty RA, Richard F, Pradel J, Vallancien G. Local recurrence after nephrectomy for primary renal cancer: computerized tomography recognition. J Urology 1984;132:246–249.

70. Kshirsagar AV, Choyke PL, Linehan WM, Walther MM. Pseudotumors after renal parenchymal sparing surgery. J Urology 1998;159:1148–1151.

71. Campbell SC and Novick SC. Management of local recurrence following radical nephrectomy or partial nephrectomy. Urol Clin North Am 1994;21(4):593–599.

72. Bloom DA, Kaufman JJ, Smith RB. Late recurrence of Renal Tubular Carcinoma. J Urol 1981;126:546–548.

73. Gogus C, Baltaci S, Beduk Y, et al. Isolated local recurrence of renal cell carcinoma after radical nephrectomy: experience with 10 cases. Urology 2003;61:926–929.

74. Wiesner C, Jakse G, Rohde D. Therapy of local recurrence of renal cell carcinoma. Oncol Rep 2002;9:189–192.

75. Tanguay S, Pisters L, Lawrence DD, Dinney CPN. Therapy of locally recurrent renal cell carcinoma after nephrectomy. J Urology 1996;155:26–29.

76. Nakada SY, Brooke Johnson D, Hahnfield L, Jarrard DF. Resection of isolated fossa recurrence of renal-cell carcinoma after nephrectomy using hand assisted laparoscopy. J Endourol 2002;16(9): 687–868.
77. McLaughlin CA, Chen MY, Torti FM, et al. Radiofrequency ablation of isolated local recurrence of renal cell carcinoma after radical nephrectomy. AJR 2003;181:93–94.
78. Gittes RF, Blute RD. Repeat bench surgery on a solitary kidney. J Urology 1982;127:530–532.
79. Linehan WM, Walther MM, Zbar B. The genetic basis of cancer of the kidney. J Urol 2003; 170:2163–2172.

18   Adjuvant Therapy of Renal Cell Carcinoma

Ronald M. Bukowski

KEYWORDS

ADJUVANT THERAPY
RENAL CELL CARCINOMA

ABSTRACT

A series of adjuvant studies are reviewed that have been conducted in patients with localized renal cell carcinoma following nephrectomy. The randomized studies available do not demonstrate an advantage for pre- or postoperative therapy. Patient selection criteria have varied, but generally high risk groups with T_{2-4} tumors and lymph node metastases (N_+) disease have been included. In the future, adjuvant trials conducted in this group of patients must take into account histology, as well as selection of patients by pathologic stage. Trail design is of importance and randomized studies in which a control population is included are required. The issue of placebo controls will depend upon the agent utilized and its toxicity. External review of radiologic data will be of importance to validate results if a surrogate endpoint such as disease free survival is utilized. In view of our current knowledge of the biology of clear cell carcinoma, studies utilizing medications such as sunitinib, sorafenib, or bevacizumab are considerations.

RATIONALE

Renal cell carcinoma (RCC) can be cured by surgical excision; however, this approach fails to prevent recurrence or death in a significant proportion of patients. In 1973, Bloom[1] noted that 50% of patients undergoing nephrectomy ultimately developed recurrent disease. In the ensuing 30 years, changes in staging systems and clarification of prognostic factors have occurred; however, patients with early-stage RCC continue to relapse. Cumulative 5-year survival rates following nephrectomy and lymphadenectomy range from 47% to 100% in stage T2N0M0 to 34% to 51% in patients with stage T3N0M0.[2] When regional lymph nodes are involved, 5-year survival rates are even lower, and range from 6% to 43%.[2] Nodal status at surgery is often difficult to define, for reasons such as matted lymph nodes or use of lymph node sampling rather than lymphadenectomy.

From: *Clinical Management of Renal Tumors*
Edited by: R.M. Bukowski and A.C. Novick © Humana Press Inc., Totowa, NJ

Patterns of recurrence in patients following resection of RCC have been reviewed[3]; 172 patients undergoing nephrectomy were identified, and the majority (N = 162) had N_0 disease. Distant metastases developed in 26% and local recurrence in 5%. In this latter group, four of six patients also had distant metastases. Positive lymph-node status and renal-vein extension were independent prognostic factors associated with recurrence.

Recently, a series of investigators have utilized clinical databases to assess risk of relapse and death in patients with resected renal cell carcinoma. Studies such as these have identified patients with resected renal tumors who are appropriate candidates for adjuvant therapy trials. Zisman et al.[4] investigated 661 patients who underwent nephrectomy from 1989 to 1999. They developed a novel approach utilizing the American Joint Committee on Cancer (AJCC) tumor, node, metastasis (TMN) stage, tumor grade, and Eastern Cooperative Oncology Group (ECOG) performance status, referred to as the UISS (UCLA Integrated Staging System). Five patient groups were identified (I to V) with 5-year survival rates of 94% (I), 67% (II), 39% (III), 23% (IV), and 0% (V). This system was validated utilizing an international cohort of 4202 patients[5] with localized renal cell carcinoma. Recently, this group has utilized molecular markers such as carbonic anhydrase IX, Ki–67, and epithelial cell adhesion molecule (EpCAM),[6,7] which may also be useful biomarkers to predict outcomes.

Kattan et al.[8] utilized the data from Memorial Hospital (New York, NY) to develop a postoperative prognostic nomogram for localized RCC. Similarly, Zisman et al.[9] have developed a mathematical model to estimate survival after nephrectomy. Application of these methods and approaches to assist in selecting patients with a significant risk of relapse and limited survivals should be considered.

Previous adjuvant trials utilized staging systems such as these developed by Robson[10] and the tumor, node, metastasis (TNM) system[11] to define high-risk populations. In these trials, the issue of histology was not considered, and pathology review not included. This resulted in heterogeneous populations, with 10 to 20% of patients having non–clear-cell histology. Additionally, selected trials have included patients with more advanced disease, such as those with multiple lymph nodes involved (N2), and in some instances resected metastatic disease (M1). In view of these issues, a review of previously conducted trials is relevant, not only as a survey of previous results, but also to examine and contrast the patient population included.

End points in adjuvant trials have included progression-free survival (PFS), time to progression (TTP), and survival. These latter two surrogates of clinical benefit are difficult to assess in trials in which investigators are not blinded, and the control treatment defined as surgery alone. The surrogates of TTP or PFS require either a placebo-controlled and blinded trial, or an independent review of radiographic and clinical data. To date, the majority of adjuvant trials in renal cancer have been underpowered to assess differences in survival, and the progression end points are difficult to assess in view of the study designs.

The modalities and therapeutic agents investigated previously are summarized in Table 18.1. The trials reviewed were randomized and generally contained a control arm defined as standard of care. This has generally been defined as observation, with no study utilizing a placebo control. The patterns of recurrence in patients with RCC suggest that systemic therapeutic approaches are most appropriate, and in the majority of trials, except for those involving radiotherapy, this type of therapy has been employed.

Table 18.1.
Adjuvant therapy employed in patients following resection of
renal cell carcinoma

Progestational agents
Radiotherapy
Cytokines
Vaccines

MEDROXYPROGESTERONE ACETATE

In 1971, Bloom[12] reviewed his experience with hormonal therapy of metastatic RCC in 80 patients (79 received medroxyprogesterone acetate [MPA], and one received Delalutin). Eleven patients demonstrated improvement in radiologic or clinical signs associated with their tumors. Subsequent reports suggested that hormonal therapy for metastatic RCC produces responses in 15% to 20% of cases. Recent data from randomized trials in which tamoxifen[13] or medroxyprogesterone[14] have been used as reference arms have not confirmed this level of activity. Uncontrolled trials suggested that adjuvant MPA could decrease relapse rates compared to historical controls.[15] In view of this finding, prospective studies were undertaken.

Pizzocaro et al.[16] conducted a randomized controlled trial comparing 500 mg of MPA t.i.w. for 1 year following surgery with observation in patients undergoing radical nephrectomy. Individuals with Robson stages I, II, and III were eligible; 136 patients were entered, and 120 were evaluable. Results are summarized in Table 18.2, and demonstrated no differences in relapse rates, time to recurrence, or survival. The authors concluded that the toxicity of MPA and similar 5-year disease-free survivals for MPA-treated and control patients indicate it should not be utilized in the adjuvant setting.

RADIATION THERAPY

Radiotherapy has been used as an adjuvant following nephrectomy since the 1940s.[17] A series of historically controlled studies were published in the 1950s and 1960s, which

Table 18.2.
Adjuvant trial of medroxyprogesterone acetate (MPA) following
radical nephrectomy in patients with renal cell carcinoma

	Treatment group	
	Observation	MPA
No. of patients		
Entered	70	66
Evaluable	62	58
Stages		
I	29	29
II and III	33	29
Relapses (%)	33.9	32.7
Median time to recurrence (months)	11.0	20.0
5-year disease-free survival (%)	67.3	67.1

Source: Pizzocaro et al.[16]

Table 18.3.
Clinical results of adjuvant radiotherapy trials in renal cell carcinoma patients

Reference	Therapy arms	No. patients	Stage distribution			5-year survival (percent)	Comments
			P1	P2	P3		
I. Preoperative trials							
van der Werf-Messing[21]	30 Gy in 3 wk	64	22	12	30	59%[a]	No differences in recurrence rates or survival
	Surgery	62	21	19	22	64%[a]	
Juusela et al.[22]	30–36 Gy in 3 wk	38	8	12	18	47 + 9%	No differences in 5-yr survival rates
II. Postoperative trials			I	II	III		
Kjaer et al.[23]	50 Gy in 20 fractions	32	—	17	15	50%[b]	No differences in survival/ unacceptable toxicity
	Surgery	33	—	17	16	62%[b]	
Finney[24]	55 Gy in 27 fractions in 52 wk	52	23	9	19	36%	No influence on local recurrence or distant mets
	Surgery	49	20	11	18	47%	

[a]Overall survival %.
[b]2-yr survival rates.
P1, P2, P3, pathologic stages.
I, II, III, Robson stages.

suggested this modality improved survival in RCC patients.[18,19] In the 1970s, a series of randomized and controlled trials were initiated to evaluate the effects of adjuvant radiation. Recent reviews[3,20] of failure sites in patients undergoing nephrectomy suggests that local failure is uncommon, and therefore modalities like radiation therapy for control of local disease are unlikely to be of value. The results outlined in Table 18.3 are consistent with this conclusion.

Retrospective reviews in which patients undergoing nephrectomy were treated with postoperative irradiation suggested 5- and 10-year survival rates could be improved at least 10%.[25,26] The prospective trials reported by Kjaer et al.[23] and Finney[24] could not confirm these reports. In the latter study, significant postradiation complications developed in 44% of patients. The size of these trials (69 and 101 patients) probably precludes detection of the anticipated differences. Additionally, in the trial reported by Finney, 40% of patients had clinical stage I tumors, a group in which recurrence rates are expected to be low.

Preoperative radiation therapy for RCC was reported to produce a decrease in tumor size and vascularization, increase fibrosis, and induce loss of proliferative capacity.[26,27] The two clinical trials[21,22] utilizing preoperative radiation therapy are also summarized in Table 18.3. No differences in recurrence rates or survival were found, and in both studies, significant numbers of patients with T1 tumors were included. The authors also analyzed their findings by tumor stage, and found no effect in any category. As in the postoperative trials, the number of patients included was limited. The studies available, therefore, do not demonstrate an effect of pre- or postoperative adjuvant radiation therapy in RCC patients undergoing nephrectomy.

AUTOLOGOUS TUMOR VACCINES

A series of clinical and laboratory observations in patients with RCC suggest the presence of an antitumor immune response.[28,29] Among the most compelling findings are those of spontaneous regression of metastatic tumor sites,[30] and tumor responses in patients receiving T-cell adoptive immunotherapy.[31] A series of tumor-associated antigens has now been defined for RCC,[32] with demonstration of T-cell responses to selected antigens.[33] In patients with advanced RCC, it has been recognized that the immune response is impaired (immune dysfunction), and a series of tumor-related mechanisms have been proposed.[34] In patients with localized RCC, similar findings have been noted,[35] but following nephrectomy, the majority of patients demonstrate normal T-cell function. This series of observations and the reversal of immune dysfunction postnephrectomy suggest that immunologic approaches to adjuvant therapy, such as active specific immunotherapy with tumor cell vaccines, are reasonable.

Active specific immunotherapy (ASI) employing autologous tumor preparations with or without various adjuvants has been utilized to immunize RCC patients in the postoperative setting. In patients with metastatic disease, this approach has been associated with clinical tumor regression in selected patients.[36] Three adjuvant studies have been reported,[37–40] with one trial being historically controlled,[37,38] and the remaining two designed as prospective randomized studies.[39,40] Repmann et al.[37,38] treated 162 patients (116 evaluable) with various stages (T2–4N0M0, T1–4N1–3M0, T1–4N0–3M1). Results were compared to a matched historical group of 106 patients. The vaccine utilized employed autologous tumor cells incubated with interferon-γ and tocopherol acetate for 3 hours. Following this, cells were washed and devitalized with rapid freezing and thawing at −82°C (Lipo Nova, Hannover, Germany). Vaccine aliquots were then stored at −82°C until use. When compared to the matched control group of 106 patients, a significant improvement in survival ($p = .0007$) was found. Two-year survival probability was 92.2% in the vaccine group compared to 75% in the control group. Analysis of various stages demonstrated no differences for Robson stages I and IV, whereas in patients with stages II and III, survival probability remained significantly improved in the treatment group. Toxicity of the vaccine preparation was reported as minimal.

Randomized trials utilizing various autologous tumor cell vaccines are summarized in Table 18.4. The first prospective randomized controlled trial utilizing ASI was reported by Galligioni et al.[39] This was a randomized controlled trial in which patients were allocated to observation or three intradermal injections of 10^7 autologous irradiated tumor cells with 10^7 bacillus Calmette-Guérin (first two injections). Patients with resected RCC TNM stages 1, 2, or 3 were eligible; 184 patients were evaluated, and 120 were entered. Sixty-four patients were not randomized for reasons including insufficient cells for vaccination (24 patients) locally advanced or distant metastases (32 patients), and incomplete resection (three patients). At a median followup of 61 months, the 5-year disease-free survival rates were 63% in vaccine patients and 72% in controls. The overall 5-year survival rates were 69% and 78%, respectively. The differences were not statistically significant. The sample size employed was capable of detecting a 20% to 25% difference in disease-free survival.

Jocham et al.[40] recently reported the results with an autologous tumor cell vaccine in patients with T2–3bN0–3M0 renal cell carcinoma. This was a prospective trial in which 553 patients were randomly allocated to vaccine therapy or observation. The autologous vaccine employed was similar to that utilized by Repmann et al.[37,38] and was prepared by Lipo Nova (Hannover, Germany). The vaccine was administered intradermally in the upper extremities every 4 weeks for a total of six doses. Fifty-five centers participated in this study. In the group of 553 patients randomized, 177 received vaccine and 202 were followed in the control arm (total 379 patients). Reasons for excluding 174 patients included the following: no primary RCC, 46 patients; incorrect stage, 43; metastatic disease, 10; postoperative mortality, three; vaccine preparation not possible, nine; lost to follow-up in ≤6 months, 32; and miscellaneous, 31. Seventy-two percent of the patients included in the analysis had clear cell carcinoma. Other patient characteristics including tumor stages, prognostic score,[42] and performance status appeared evenly distributed. The 379 patients analyzed are referred to as the intent-to-treat group, but exclusion of patients after randomization can introduce potential bias, and an actual intent-to-treat analysis was not conducted by the investigators.

The results of this trial are summarized in Table 18.4. The primary end point was improvement in PFS as defined by local recurrence or development of metastases. Imaging studies obtained every 6 months included ultrasound, chest x-rays, and abdominal computed tomography (CT) or magnetic resonance imaging (MRI). At 5 years, the PFS rates were significantly improved for the vaccine-treated group ($p = .0204$). This trial was not blinded and did not involve a placebo control or external review of radiographic data. Additionally, over 30% of randomized patients were excluded, and it is unclear if an interim analysis was performed. In view of these issues, the results of this trial should be questioned, and a confirmatory study required.

Table 18.4.
Randomized trials with autologous tumor cell preparations: renal cell carcinoma

Reference	Patient seligible	Treatment groups	No. of patients	5-year PFS	5-year OS
Galligioni et al.[39]	T1–3, N0–1, M0	Evaluated	184	—	
		Control	60	72%	78%
		Vaccine + BCG	60	63%	69%
Jocham et al.[40]	T2–3b, N0–3, M0	Evaluated	553	NS	NS
		Control	202	67.8%	NS
		Vaccine	177	77.4%	NS
Wood et al.[41]	T2N0M0 (Gr 3/4) T3a–c, N0–1, M0 T4, N1–2, M0	Evaluated	2024	—	
		Control	409	TE	TE
		HSPPC-96	409	TE	TE

NS, not stated; TE, too early; PFS, progression-free survival; OS, overall survival.

Finally, the largest clinical trial utilizing an autologous tumor vaccine preparation has been conducted by Antigenics (Lexington, MA).[41] A series of studies reported by Srivastava and colleagues[43,44] have demonstrated that heat shock proteins can act as chaperones for various antigenic peptides, and facilitate antigen presentation by dendritic cells. A therapeutic effect utilizing heat shock proteins from tumors has been found,[45] and this approach is now being tested in a variety of solid tumors including RCC. The vaccine contains HSPPC-96, and is prepared by extraction from tumor cells. Preliminary data utilizing HSPPC-96 (Oncophage®) in patients with metastatic RCC demonstrated an excellent safety profile and evidence of antitumor effects in selected patients.[46,47] An adjuvant trial has been conducted in patients with clear cell carcinoma (Table 18.4). The trial design involved identifying patients with tumors ≥5 cm, and preparation of HSPPC-96 by Antigenics. Over 1400 patients were evaluated, and 644 were eligible and randomized to vaccine treatment (25 mg weekly ×4, then every 4 weeks until the vaccine supply is used up) or observation. As in other vaccine trials, a placebo was not utilized for patients in the control arm, but an independent review of all radiologic studies is planned, with independent determination of progression by the review committee. Accrual to this trial is completed, and the primary end point is time to progression. Additional follow up is now required before a planned analysis of PFS is performed.

The series of vaccine trials conducted have utilized different autologous preparations. The report by Jocham et al.[40] suggests improvement in PFS, but methodologic problems with study design and the analysis exist. The largest adjuvant trial to date utilizing HSPPC-96 has completed accrual, but results are pending. It remains unclear if a tumor vaccine administered postoperatively to RCC patients can influence the natural history of this neoplasm. Clearly, the nature of the preparation utilized, the population included, and trial design are the major issues to consider.

CYTOKINE ADJUVANT TRIALS

A variety of cytokines have been utilized to treat metastatic RCC. Interferon-α (IFN-α) and interleukin-2 (IL-2) have modest effects in this patient population. Reviews suggest that IFN-α produces a response rate of 10% to 15%[48,50] and a 2.5-month improvement in overall survival compared to a control population[14] in patients with metastatic disease. Interleukin-2 has a similar response rate, but in selected patients produces complete durable responses.[48] Investigation of both cytokines in the adjuvant setting is therefore reasonable.

Cockerell et al.[49] administered IFN-α at a dose of 3 million units (MU) subcutaneously 3 days prior to surgery and for 14 days postsurgery to a group of 13 RCC patients with minimal metastatic disease. No major toxicity was encountered, and the authors concluded that IFN-α was safe enough to be tested in larger studies. Takahashi et al.[51] treated 20 patients with stages I to III with IFN-α_{2b} following nephrectomy. Interferon-α was administered at a dose of 3.0 MU daily intramuscularly for 28 days followed by 6.0 MU weekly for 12 months. Three patients developed recurrent disease, and significant increases in natural killer (NK) activity were noted in the treated patients. The authors suggest the IFN-α should be administered for a minimum of 5 to 7 months when used as an adjuvant following nephrectomy in view of the delayed antitumor effects previously reported.[37] These trials demonstrated the feasibility of postoperative IFN-α administration.

Three randomized studies were then performed to further evaluate the effects of this cytokine (Table 18.5). No improvements in disease-free or overall survival for interferon-treated patients have been found. The studies differ in the types of interferons utilized (lymphoblastoid IFN [L-IFN], IFN-α_{2a}, IFN-α_{2b}), doses utilized, and duration of therapy (6 to 12 months). Messing et al.[54] utilized L-IFN in escalating doses (3 to 20 MU/m^2). A total of 283 eligible patients were randomized, with 130 receiving L-IFN. At a median follow-up of 10.4 years, median survivals for the control and IFN cohorts were 7.4 and 5.1 years respectively ($p = .09$). Median PFS was 3.0 years for the control patients and 2.2 years for IFN-treated individuals ($p = .33$). Three- and five-year progression free survivals are outlined in Table 18.5 and show no significant differences, but a trend in favor of the observation arm is evident. The study was designed to detect a 15% increase in 5-year survival rates (50% to 65%) with the addition of L-IFN. All histologic subtypes were eligible, with clear cell tumors representing 69% of patients. Of interest were the 83 patients with lymph nodes involved (N1–2). In the N1 group, median survival was 7.7 years (33 patients), compared to 2.1 years for the N2 patients ($n = 50$). Follow-up radiographic examinations (chest x-rays, bone scans, CT chest/abdomen/pelvis) were obtained every 3 months in the first year and then semiannually.

The two other trials investigating the adjuvant effects of IFN utilized recombinant preparations. Pizzocaro et al.[53] reported a study in which patients were randomized to IFN-α_{2b} (6 MU IM t.i.w. for 6 months) or observation. Patients in the control group were to receive IFN-α_{2b} (10 MU IM t.i.w.) or best available therapy at relapse. Two hundred sixty-four patients with Robson stages II/III (T3bN0M0, T2–3N1–3M0) were randomized (Table 18.5). The 5-year overall survival probabilities in both arms were 66%, and relapse-free survivals were 67% and 57% for observation patients and IFN-treated patients, respectively ($p = .107$). This study was designed to detect a 20% improvement in event-free survival (50% to 70%). All histologic subtypes of RCC were eligible and no information was collected on tumor types for individual patients. Follow-up in this trial was every 6 months, with physical examinations, chest x-rays, and abdominal ultrasound. Bone scans, CTs, and MRIs were not required.

The last randomized trial utilizing IFN compared 12 months of IFN-α_{2a} (9 MU SC t.i.w.) to observation. This trial has been reported only in a preliminary fashion,[52] but

Table 18.5.
Randomized trials with interferon: renal cell carcinoma

Reference	Patients eligible	Treatment groups	No. of patients	3-year RFS	5-year OS	5-year PF	5 years SOS
Porzolt et al.[52]	T3–4, N0/+, MO	IFN-α_{2a} 9 MIU TIW (12 mos)	133	60%[1]	80%	—	—
		Control	137	60%[1]	80%	—	—
Pizzocaro et al.[53]	T3aN0M0 T3bN0M0	IFN-α_{2b} 6 MU TIW (6 mos)	123	64%	83%	67%	66%
	T2/3N1–3M0	Control	124	75%	80%	57%	66%
Messing et al.[54]	T1–2N1–3M0	IFN-α NL 3 MU/m²d 1 5 MU/m²d 2	140	44%	62%	37%	51%
	T3a-c N0–3M0	20 MU/m²d 3–5 (12 cycles q 3 wks)					
	T4aN0–3M0	Control	143	48%	70%	41%	62%

[1]Time to treatment failure at 30 months.

MO, MIU, million International Units; MU, million units; NL, normal limits; TIW, three times a week.

is still of interest since 270 patients with T3–4N0–2MOR were registered. No differences at 3 years were noted (Table 18.5), and data for 5-year and median survival in the two groups is not available. The authors do note that relapses and death were most frequent in patients with lymph node involvement and poorly differentiated tumor (grades 3/4). No information on histology is available. Finally, follow-up (examinations not specified) was required every 3 months for 2 years and then every 6 months.

The results of these theer trials demonstrate no benefit from postoperative adjuvant IFN, but only one trial[54] utilized survival as the primary end point. Additionally, the inclusion of all histologic subtypes may not be optimal, in view of the limited effects of systemic IFN-α in non–clear-cell histologies.[55] Finally, absence of external review of radiographic studies and/or a blinded design do not permit conclusions regarding time to progression. Given the modest survival benefit reported with IFN-α administration in metastatic RCC patients, further adjuvant trials with IFN-α may be warranted in selected populations, such as those with clear cell tumors.

A second cytokine utilized for treatment of patients with metastatic RCC is recombinant IL-2 (rIL-2). Reviews have indicated that objective responses are seen in 15% of patients receiving IL-2, with a subset of patients having durable remissions.[56] Recently, randomized trials have investigated the importance of IL-2 dose in patients with metastatic RCC.[57,58] Both trials found approximately 5% of highly selected patients have durable complete responses with high-dose IL-2 (600,000 U/kg q8h), but did not demonstrate improvement in survival when compared to low-dose outpatient regimens. Studies utilizing IL-2 in the postoperative adjuvant setting are limited. Table 18.6 outlines two trials, one in which patients were randomized to high-dose IL-2 or observation,[59] and the second utilizing randomization to different IL-2 doses and schedules.[60]

Table 18.6.
Randomized trials with interleukin-2: renal cell carcinoma

Reference	Patients eligible	Treatment groups	No. of patients	Median (mos)		3-year (%)	
				PFS	OS	PFS	OS
Clark et al.[59]	T3a-cN1–3M0 T4N1–3M0 $T_{any}N_{any}$MIR	IL-2 600,000 U/kg q 8 hrs d 1–5 & 15–19	33	19.5	NA	32%	80%
		Control	36	36.0	NA	45%	86%
Olencki et al.[60]	T3–4N1–2M0 $T_{any}N_{any}$MIR	IL-2 (SC) 4–8 MIU/m²/d (4 different schedules) D1–5, 8–10, etc.	39	21.6	NA	36%	70%

NA, not available.

Clark et al.[59] randomized patients to high-dose IL-2 (600,000 U/kg q8h on days 1 to 5 and 15 to 19) or observation. Sixty-nine patients were registered, 25 of whom had resected M1 disease. All histologies were eligible, with 32/69 (46%) patients reported as having clear-cell RCC. The study design was powered to detect an increase from 40% to 70% in the disease-free survival, and required 68 patients with resected RCC. An interim analysis was conducted after 38 patients with locally advanced, resected RCC had been accrued, and the data safety monitoring board recommended closure, since there was no evidence IL-2 would have the desired effect. The results of this trial are outlined in Table 18.6. The authors concluded that high-dose IL-2 could be safely administered in this patient population. Clinically meaningful benefit of high-dose IL-2 was not seen. In the group of patients with resected metastatic disease (12 received IL-2, and 11 observation), the 3-year disease-free survivals were 40% (IL-2 group) and 56% (observation), and 3 year overall survivals were similar.

A second trial utilized subcutaneous IL-2 in varying doses and schedules.[60] In this trial, 39 patients were allocated to four different IL-2 regimens administered for 6 months to determine tolerance to the various regimens. No differences in toxicity were seen, and overall at 3 years, 70% of patients remain alive and 36% disease free.

These results demonstrate that IL-2 can be administered in the postoperative setting, but conclusions regarding the efficacy are not possible. Additional studies utilizing IL-2 in patients with resected clear cell neoplasms are required with adequately powered trial designs. Given the toxicity and limited applicability of high-dose IL-2 schedules, the use of outpatient regimens should be considered.

COMBINATION REGIMENS

The use of combination regimens such as rIL-2 and IFN-α or chemoimmunotherapy employing this combination and 5-fluorouracil (5-FU) is of interest in view of the increased response rates reported with these approaches.[61,62] Toxicity is also increased, and therefore may limit their utility in the adjuvant setting.

                                303

Migliari et al.[63] have conducted a pilot study utilizing IFN-α and vinblastine in patients following nephrectomy and lymphadenectomy. Thirty patients with T2-3N0M0 RCC were treated. rIFN-α_{2a} was administered intramuscularly three times weekly in gradually increasing doses (from 3.0 to 18.0 MU over 4 weeks) and vinblastine (IV bolus 0.1 mg/kg) every 3 weeks for a total of four cycles. Moderate toxicity was reported, and 4/30 patients discontinued therapy. The results were contrasted with a historical cohort of 32 patients. Five-year survival rates in the two groups were 83% and 50%, respectively ($p = .003$). The investigators suggest that additional trials with this approach should be considered. Recent reports utilizing IFN-α and vinblastine in patients with metastatic disease, however, do not suggest that this combination is superior to IFN-α alone.[64] Therefore, the rationale for further trials with this combination is unclear.

VASCULAR ENDOTHELIAL GROWTH FACTOR TYROSINE KINASE INHIBITORS AND BEVACIZUMAB

Recent reports in patients with metastatic clear cell carcinoma have suggested that three agents may have activity in cytokine refractory patients. SU011248,[65] BAY 43-9006,[66] and Bevacizumab[67] appear to have clinical and biologic effects. The two tyrosine kinase inhibitors (SU011248, BAY 43-9006) are oral agents with acceptable toxicity profiles that are multifunctional and appear to inhibit vascular endothelial growth factor receptor 2 (VEGFR2) and platelet-derived growth factor receptor (PDGFR) as well as other receptors. The high response rates ($\geq$40%) with SU01124[65] and improvement in time to progression with BAY 43-9006[66] suggest that use in the postoperative setting should be explored. Bevacizumab may increase TTP in cytokines refractory patients, and likewise may be a reasonable agent to explore in adjuvant trials in view of its acceptable toxicity profile.[67] These studies should be adequately powered and can be randomized and blinded, permitting use of PFS as a primary endpoint.

CONCLUSION

A series of adjuvant studies have been conducted in patients with localized RCC following nephrectomy. Currently, randomized studies have not demonstrated an advantage for pre- or postoperative therapy. Patient selection criteria have varied, but generally high-risk group with T2–4 tumors and N1–3 disease have been included. In the future, adjuvant trials conducted in this group of patients must take into account histology as well as selection of patients by pathologic stage. Trial design is of importance, and randomized studies in which a control population is included are required. The issue of placebo controls will depend on the agent utilized and its toxicity. External review of radiologic data will be of importance to validate results if PFS/TTP is utilized as a clinical benefit surrogate. In view of our current knowledge of the biology of clear cell carcinoma, use of novel medications such as SU011248, BAY 43-9006 or Bevacizumab should be considered.

REFERENCES

1. Bloom HJG. Adjuvant therapy for adenocarcinoma of the kidney: present position and prospects. Br J Urol 1973;45:237–257.

2. Linehan WM, Shipley WV, Parkinson D. Cancer of the kidney and ureter. In: DeVita VT, Hellman S, Rosenberg SA, eds. Cancer Principles and Practice of Oncology. Philadelphia: Lippincott-Raven, 1997:1271–1299.

3. Rabinovitch RA, Zelefsky MJ, Fuks Z. Patterns of failure following surgical resection of renal cell carcinoma: implications for adjuvant local and systemic therapy. J Clin Oncol 1994;11:206–212.

4. Zisman A, Pantuck AJ, Dorey F, et al. Improved prognostication of renal cell carcinoma using an integrated staging system. J Clin Oncol 2001;19:1649–1957.

5. Patard J, Kim HL, Lam JS, et al. Use of the University of California Los Angeles Integrated Staging System to predict survival in renal cell carcinoma: an international multicenter study. J Clin Oncol 2004;22:3316–3322.

6. Bui MHT, Visapaa H, Seligson D, et al. Prognostic value of carbonic anhydrase IX and Ki67 as predictors of survival for renal clear cell carcinoma. J Urol 2004;171:2461–2455.

7. Seligson DB, Pantuck A, Liu X, et al. Epithelial cell adhesions molecule (KSA) expression: pathobiology and its role as an independent predictor of survival in renal cell carcinoma. Clin Can Res 2004;10:2659–2669.

8. Kattan MW, Reuter V, Motzer RJ, Katz J, Russo P. A postoperative prognostic monogram for renal cell carcinoma. J Urol 2001;166:63–67.

9. Zisman A, Pantuck AJ, Dorey F, et al. Mathematical model to predict individual survival for patients with renal cell carcinoma. J Clin Oncol 2002;20:1368–1374.

10. Robson CJ, Churchill BM, Anderson W. The results of radical nephrectomy for renal cell carcinoma. J Urol 1969;101(3):297–301.

11. Gunan P, Sobon LH, Algaba F, et al. TNM staging of renal cell carcinoma: wordgroup No. 3—Union International Contre le Cancer (UICC) and the American Joint Committee on Cancer (AJCC). Cancer 1997;80:992–993.

12. Bloom HJG. Medroxyprogesterone acetate (Provera) in the treatment of metastatic renal cancer. Br J Cancer 1971;25:250–256.

13. Henriksson R, Nilsson S, Colleen S, et al. Survival in renal cell carcinoma—a randomized evaluation of tamoxifen vs interleukin 2, α-interferon (leukocyte) and tamoxifen. Br J Cancer 1998;77: 1311–1317.

14. Medical Research Council Renal Cancer Collaborators. Interferon-α and survival in metastatic renal cell carcinoma: early results of a randomized control trial. Lancet 1999;353:14–17.

15. Satomi Y, Takai S, Kondo I, Fukushima S, Furuhata A. Postoperative prophylactic use of progesterone in renal cell carcinoma. J Urol 1982;128:919–922.

16. Pizzocaro G, Piva L, DiFonzo G, et al. Adjuvant medroxyprogesterone acetate to radical nephrectomy in renal cancer: 5-year results of a prospective randomized study. J Urol 138 1987;138:1379–1381.

17. Peeling WB, Mantell BS, Shepheard BCF. Postoperative irradiation in the treatment of renal cell carcinoma. Br J Urol 1969;41:23–31.

18. Cox CE, Lacy SS, Montgomery WG, Boyce WH. Renal adenocarcinoma: 28-year review, with emphasis on rationale and feasibility of preoperative radiotherapy. J Urol 1970;104:53–61.

19. Rafla S. Renal cell carcinoma. Natural history and results of treatment. Cancer 1970;25:26–40.

20. Aref I, Bociek RG, Salhani D. Is postoperative radiation for renal cell carcinoma justified: Radiother Oncol 1997;43:155–157.

21. van der Werf-Messing B. Carcinoma of the kidney. Cancer 1973;32:1056–1061.

22. Juusela H, Malmio K, Afthan O, Oravisto J. Preoperative irradiation in the treatment of renal adenocarcinoma. Scand J Urol Nephrol 1977;11:277–281.

23. Kjaer M, Frederiksen PL, Emgelholm SA. Postoperative radiotherapy in stage II and III renal adenocarcinoma. A randomized trial by the Copenhagen renal cancer study group. Int J Radiat Oncol Biol Phys 1987;13:665–672.

24. Finney R. An evaluation of postoperative radiotherapy in hypernephroma treatment—a clinical trial. Cancer 1973;32:1332–1340.

25. Flocks RH, Kadesky MC. Malignant neoplasms of the kidney—an analysis of 353 patients followed for five years or more. J Urol 1958;79:196–201.

26. Waters CA. Preoperative irradiation of cortical renal tumors. AJR 1935;33(1):149–158.

27. Riches E. The place of radiotherapy in the management of parenchymal carcinoma of the kidney. J Urol 1966;93:313–320.

28. Finke JH, Kierstead LS, Ranieri E, Storkus WJ. Immunologic response to renal cell carcinoma. In: Bukowski RM, Novick AC, eds. Renal Cell Caracinoma: Molecular Biology, Immunology and Clinical Management. Totowa, NJ: Humana Press, 2000:39–62.

29. Rayman P, Wesa AK, Richmond AL, et al. Effect of renal cell carcinomas on the development of type 1 T-cell responses. Clin Cancer Res 2005;10:6360S–6366S.
30. Gleave M, Slilali M, Fradet Y, et al. Interferon gamma-1b compared with placebo in metastatic renal cell carcinoma. N Engl J Med 1998;228:1265–1271.
31. Figlin R, Gitlitz B, Franklin J, et al. Interleukin-2 based immunotherapy for the treatment of metastatic renal cell carcinoma: an analysis of 203 consecutively treated patients. Cancer J Sci Am Suppl 1997;1:592–597.
32. Tatsumi T, Kierstead LS, Ranieri E, et al. MAGE-6 encodes DR B1–1–presented epitopes recognized by CD4+ T cells derived from patients with melanoma or renal cell carcinoma. Clin Cancer Res 2003;9:947–954.
33. Tatsumi T, Herrem CJ, Olson WC, et al. Disease stage variance in CD4+ and CD8+ T cell reactivity against the receptor tyrosine kinase EphA2 in patients with renal cell carcinoma. Cancer Res 2003;63:4481–4489.
34. Rayman P, Uzzo RG, Kolenko V, et al. Tumor-induced dysfunction in interleukin-2 production and interleukin-2 receptor signaling: a mechanism of immune escape. Cancer J Sci Am 2000;6:581–587.
35. Uzzo RG, Clark PE, Rayman P, et al. Alterations in NP kappa B activation in T lymphocytes of patients with renal cell carcinoma. J Natl Cancer Inst 1999;91:718–721.
36. Tallberg T, Tykka H. Specific active immunotherapy in advanced renal cell carcinoma: a clinical long term follow up study. World J Urol 1986;3:234–244.
37. Repmann R, Wagner S, Richter A. Adjuvant therapy of renal cell carcinoma with active-specific immunotherapy (ASI) using autologous tumor vaccine. Anticancer Res 1997;17:2879–2882.
38. Repmann R, Goldschmidt AJ, Richter A. Adjuvant therapy of renal cell carcinoma patients with an autologous tumor cell lysate vaccine: a 5-year follow up analysis. Anticancer Res 2003;23:969–974.
39. Galligioni E, Quaia M, Merlo A, et al. Adjuvant immunotherapy treatment of renal carcinoma patients with autologous tumor cells and bacillus Calmette-Guerin. Five-year results of a prospective randomized study. Cancer 1996;77:2560–2566.
40. Jocham D, Richter A, Hoffmann L, et al. Adjuvant autologous renal tumor cell vaccine and risk of tumor progression in patients with renal cell carcinoma after radical nephrectomy: phase III randomized controlled trial. Lancet 2004;363:594–599.
41. Wood CG, Escudier B, Gorelov S, et al. A multicenter randomized study of adjuvant heat-shock protein peptide-complex 96 (HSPCC-96) vaccine in patients with high-risk of recurrence after nephrectomy for renal cell carcinoma (RCC). Proc ASCO 2004;23:192.
42. Störkel S, Thomas W, Jacobs GH, Lippold R. Prognostic parameters in renal cell carcinoma: a new approach. Eur Urol 1989;16:416–422.
43. Udono H, Srivastava PK. Comparison of tumor-specific immunogenicities of stress-induced proteins gp96, hsp90 and hsp70. J Immunol 1994;152:5395–5403.
44. Li Z, Srivastava PK. A critical contemplation on the role of heat shock proteins in transfer of antigenic peptides during antigen presentation. Boering Inst Mitteilungen 1994;94:37–47.
45. Janetzki S, Blachere NE, Daou M, et al. Generation of tumor specific cytotoxic T lymphocytes and memory T cells by immunization with tumor derived heat shock protein gp96. J Immunother 1998;21:269–276.
46. Amato RJ, Wood LS, Savary C, et al. Patients with renal cell carcinoma (RCC) using autologous tumor-derived heat shock protein peptide complex (HSPPC-96) with or without interleukin-2 (IL-2). Proc ASCO 2000;abstr 1782.
47. Amato RJ, Murray L, Wood L, et al. Active specific immunotherapy in patients with renal cell carcinoma (RCC) using autologous tumor derived heat shock protein-peptide complex 96 (HSPPC-96) vaccine. Proc ASCO 1999;abstr 1278.
48. Bukowski RM, Novick AC. Clinical practice guidelines: renal cell carcinoma. Cleve Clin J Med 1997;64:S1–S48.
49. Cockerell OC, Oliver RTD, Nethersall A. Nephrectomy combined with perioperative alpha-interferon in the treatment of advanced local and minimally metastatic renal cell cancer. Urol Int 1991;46:46–49.
50. Quesada JR, Rios A, Swanson D, et al. Antitumor activity of recombinant-cloned interferon alpha in metastatic renal cell carcinoma. J Clin Oncol 1985;3:1522–1528.
51. Takahashi S, Tanigawa T, Imagawa M, Mimata H, Nomura Y, Ogata J. Interferon as adjunctive treatment for non-metastatic renal cell carcinoma. Br J Urol 1994;74:11–14.

52. Porzsolt F, on behalf of the Delta-P Study Group. Adjuvant therapy of renal cell cancer (RCC) with interferon alfa-s. Proc Am Soc Clin Oncol 1992;22:202(abstr).
53. Pizzocaro G, Diva L, Colavita M, et al. Interferon adjuvant to radical nephrectomy in Robson stages II and III renal cell carcinoma: a multicenter randomized study. J Clin Oncol 2001;19:425–431.
54. Messing EM, Manola J, Wilding G, et al. Phase III study of interferon alfa-NL as adjuvant treatment for resectable renal cell carcinoma: an Eastern Cooperative Oncology/Intergroup trial. J Clin Oncol 2003;21:1214–1222.
55. Motzer RJ, Bacik J, Mariani T, Russo P, Mazumdar M, Reuter V. Treatment outcome and survival associated with metastatic renal cell carcinoma of non-clear cell histology. J Clin Oncol 2002;20:2376–2381.
56. Bukowski RM. Natural history and therapy of metastatic renal cell carcinoma: role of interleukin 2. Cancer 1997;80:1198–1220.
57. Yang JC, Skorry RM, Steinberg SM, et al. Randomized study of high-dose and low-dose interleukin-2 in patients with metastatic renal cancer. J Clin Oncol 2003;21:3127–3132.
58. McDermott DF, Regan MM, Clark JI, et al. Randomized phase III trial of high-dose interleukin-2 versus subcutaneous interleukin-2 and interferon in patients with metastatic renal cell carcinoma. J Clin Oncol 2005;23:133–141.
59. Clark J, Atkins M, Urba W, et al. Adjuvant high dose bolus interleukin-2 for patients with high risk renal cell carcinoma: a cytokine working group randomized trial. J Clin Oncol 2003;21:3133–3140.
60. Olencki T, Bukowski RM, Zuccaro K, et al. Adjuvant administration of subcutaneous (SC) interleukin-2 (rIL-2) in patients following resection of renal cell carcinoma: preliminary results of a pilot study. Proc Am Soc Clin Oncol 1998;17:339a (abstract).
61. Atzpodien J, Kirchner H, Jonas U, et al. Interleukin-2- and interferon alfa-2a-based immunochemotherapy in advanced renal cell carcinoma: a prospectively randomized trial of the German Cooperative Renal Carcinoma Chemoimmunotherapy Group (DGCIN). J Clin Oncol 2004;1;22(7):1188–1194.
62. Negrier S, Escudier B, Lasset C, et al. Recombinant human interleukin-2, recombinant interferon alfa-2a or both in metastatic renal cell carcinoma. N Engl J Med 1996;338:1272–1279.
63. Migliari R, Muscas G, Solinas A, et al. Is there a role for adjuvant immunochemotherapy after radical nephrectomy in $pT_{2-3}N_0M_0$ renal cell carcinoma J Chemother 1995;7:240–245.
64. Fossa SD, Martinelli G, Otto U, et al. Recombinant interferon alfa-2a with or without vinblastine in metastatic renal cell carcinoma: results of a European multi-center phase III study. Ann Oncol 1992;3:301–305.
65. Motzer RJ, Rini BJ, Michaelson MD, et al. Phase II trials of SU11248 show antitumor activity in second-line therapy for patients with metastatic renal cell carcinoma. Proc ASCO J Clin Oncol 2005;23:Abstr.4508.
66. Escudier B, Szczylik T, Eisen T, et al. Randomized phase III trial of the RaF-kinase and VEGFR inhibitor sorafenib (BAY 43–9006) in patients with advanced renal cell carcinoma (RCC). Proc ASCO J Clin Oncol 2005;23:Abstr.4510.
67. Yang JC, Haworth L, Skerry M, et al. A randomized trial of bevacizumab, an anti-vascular endothelial growth factor antibody, for metastatic renal cancer. N Engl J Med 2003;349:427–434.

19 Prognostic Factors for Survival in Metastatic Renal Cell Carcinoma

Paul J. Elson

KEYWORDS

METASTATIC RENAL CELL CARCINOMA
PROGNOSTIC FACTORS
SURVIVAL

ABSTRACT

Despite recent advances in treatment, metastatic renal cell carcinoma remains incurable. The poor outlook for these patients coupled with the disease's variable natural history makes the identification and understanding of the factors that impact outcome an important consideration for patient care, the development of new therapies, and study planning and interpretation, Numerous well designed retrospective studies examining clinical factors have been conducted over the past two decades. Although there is no consensus on which set of factors is best, performance status is perhaps the most important clinical factor identified to date. It is a subjective measure of overall health, yet it has consistently, albeit not universally, been shown to have excellent prognostic value in numerous studies. With the exception of performance status most studies have examined different combination of factors, used varying definitions, and/or treated different patient populations, and therefore, it is difficult to fully assess their value as independent prognostic indicators.

In addition to these "classical" predictors, new molecular based technologies are helping to better define the biology of renal cell carcinoma and identify new prognostic factors. Their value as independent prognostic indicators however needs to be confirmed by evaluating them in homogeneous patient groups and in conjunction with the more classical predictors.

The incidence of renal cell carcinoma (RCC) is increasing worldwide,[1] and currently, in 2006, it is expected that over 220,000 new cases will be reported with approximately 39,000 patients being diagnosed in the United States.[2] If detected early, RCC can be treated surgically, and 5-year survival rates approaching 85% can be achieved for patients with organ confined disease (stage $T_1T_2N_0$).[3] Unfortunately, 40% to 50% of patients can be expected to either present with metastatic disease (30%) or relapse distantly following curatively intended nephrectomy for localized disease (20–30%).[3]

From: *Clinical Management of Renal Tumors*
Edited by: R.M. Bukowski and A.C. Novick © Humana Press Inc., Totowa, NJ

Treatment options for these patients are limited, and expected 5-year survival is on the order of 10%.[3]

Metastatic RCC (mRCC) is generally resistant to chemotherapy and hormonal therapy, and marginally responsive to immunotherapy. Recently, however, the importance of mutations in the *VHL* gene and the resulting overexpression of the proangiogenic protein vascular endothelial growth factor (VEGF) in RCC have been recognized, and much attention has been focused on developing agents that target the VEGF-VEGFR signaling pathway. Two new drugs, sorafenib and sunitinib malate, inhibit multiple tyrosine kinases in this pathway and have been shown to cause objective tumor response or significantly delay time to progression in patients with mRCC.[4,5] Both have recently received U.S. Food and Drug Administration approval.

Despite this advance in treatment, mRCC remains incurable. The poor outlook for these patients combined with a variable natural history makes understanding and identifying factors that impact outcome an important consideration for patient care, and the development and evaluation of new treatments for this disease. Knowledge of prognostic factors can be used clinically, for example, to help counsel patients and optimize care by directing specific therapies to the patient groups most likely to benefit from them. Known prognostic factors can also be used to help design and interpret clinical studies. At the design stage of comparative studies, they can be used to stratify patients in order to ensure balance between the treatment arms, improve treatment comparisons, and fine-tune sample size calculations. During analysis, adjustment for known prognostic factors can be used to help clarify differences between the treatments and help determine the extent to which they are altering the natural history of the disease. In drug development knowledge of molecular predictors can aid in the design of new, targeted therapies.

Research on prognostic factors of outcome in mRCC has mainly focused on predictors of survival; however, a number of reports have considered objective response or time to progression. The focus of this chapter likewise is on survival because it is well defined and objective, and ultimately it is the end point that we want to impact.

DEMOGRAPHIC AND CLINICAL FACTORS

A number of retrospective studies of demographic and clinical predictors of survival in mRCC have been conducted over the approximately past two decades.[6–24] These studies have generally included fairly large numbers of patients treated primarily on clinical trials, and have been analyzed using statistically sound methods, including multivariable analysis and in some cases internal and/or external validation. Table 19.1 summarizes these studies. However, for completeness, studies that employed only univariable analyses, examined only a limited number of predictors, or included both metastatic and nonmetastatic patients are also discussed.

Demographics

None of the studies summarized in Table 19.1 have reported an association between survival and age,[6–9,11–19,21–23] sex,[6–9,11–14,16–19,21,22] or race.[7,12] Exceptions to these results are an early study of 101 stage IV patients by Klugo et al.,[25] which suggested that males have a better prognosis than females, and a study by Vaglio et al.[26] of 51 patients treated with interleukin-2 (IL-2) and interferon-α (IFN-α), in which younger patients (≤60 years of age) had a better prognosis than older patients (>60 years).

Constitutional and Presenting Symptoms

Performance status (PS) is a subjective measure of overall well-being that is commonly used in oncology. One of the most frequently used PS scales is the Eastern Cooperative Oncology Group (ECOG) score,[27] which measures PS on a scale from 0 to 5, with 0 indicating asymptomatic patients with no restrictions on their activities, and 5 indicating death. Although it is subjective, it is perhaps the one factor that has most consistently been identified as an independent prognostic factor in mRCC. With the exception of the reports by Mekhail et al.[14] and Leibovich et al.,[19] all of the studies summarized in Table 19.1 that assessed PS found it to be a strong independent predictor of survival.[7–13,15–17,20–24]

Patients with mRCC often present with constitutional symptoms such as weight loss, fatigue, decreased appetite, musculoskeletal pain, and respiratory symptoms. Taken individually or together these paraneoplastic symptoms can also be considered measures of general health. Constitutional symptoms, particularly weight loss, are highly correlated with PS; however, several studies have identified them as independent prognostic factors. Elson et al.[7] and Fossa et al.,[8] for example, found weight loss to be an independent predictor of outcome even after adjusting for PS. Neves et al.[6] did not assess PS, but found recent weight loss in excess of 10% to impact negatively on survival. Leibovich et al.[19] found a constellation of symptoms to be prognostic, which included weight loss, decreased appetite, musculoskeletal pain, respiratory symptoms, gastrointestinal disturbances, sweats, and rashes, but not PS. Other studies, however, such as those by Mani et al.,[12] Palmer et al.,[13] and Negrier et al.[22] found no association between constitutional symptoms (weight loss) and survival, possibly because these studies included relatively few patients with weight loss (11–15%) and were restricted to good PS patients (ECOG scores 0 and 1) or included few poor PS patients.

Other paraneoplastic symptoms, such as anemia, fever, hypercalcemia, liver dysfunction, neutrophilia, and thrombocytosis, can also be present at presentation, and a number of investigators have assessed the impact of related hematologic and laboratory parameters.

The most consistent finding with respect to these symptoms is an association between elevated serum markers of inflammation and poor survival.[8,11,18,22,28,29] Ljungberg et al.,[28] for example, evaluated six acute phase reactants—erythrocyte sedimentation rate (ESR), C-reactive protein (CRP), ferritin, haptoglobin, orosomucoid, and α_1-antitrypsin—in an unselected series of 170 metastatic and nonmetastatic RCC patients. All six markers were highly correlated with each other ($p < .001$ in all cases) and with grade. In univariable analysis all six markers were negatively associated with survival; however, in multivariable analysis only ESR was seen to be an independent predictor once adjustments were made for stage and nuclear grade. Hoffmann et al.,[29] on the other hand, found CRP as well as ESR to be independent predictors in a study of 99 mRCC patients treated with IFN-α and IL-2 with or without 5-fluorouracil. Similarly, Negrier et al.[22] found a composite factor consisting of elevated CRP ($\geq$50 mg/L) and/or ESR ($\geq$100 mm/h) to be an independent predictor of poor outcome in a database study of 782 mRCC patients. Other investigators assessing only ESR have also found it to be an independent predictor of survival.[8,11,30] In contrast to these studies, Atzpodien et al.[18] found CRP but not ESR to be of prognostic value in a database study of 425 mRCC patients who received immunotherapy-based treatments. Negrier et al.[30] also assessed

Table 19.1.
Multivariable analyses of clinical and tumor-related prognostic factors

Reference	n	Treatment period	Treatment[1]	Prior systemic therapy allowed?	PS	Factors associated with poor survival in multivariable analysis	Factors evaluated but not found to influence survival	Validated?
Neves[6]	158	1970–1980	N/A	No	N/A	Recent weight loss ≥10% >1 metastatic site; Nuclear grade >2	Sex and age; Size of the primary; Tumor side	No
Elson[7]	610	1975–1984	Chemotherapy Hormones	Yes	0–3	Increased PS[2]; Recent weight loss MFI ≤12 months; >1 metastatic site[3]; Prior chemotherapy	Sex, age, and race; Prior Nx and RT	Yes, training and validation data sets
Fossa[8]	295	1975–1990	Chemotherapy Immuno-based	N/A	0–3	PS >1; Recent weight loss >10%; MFI ≤12 months; Elevated ESR[4]	Sex and age; Prior Nx; Metastatic sites	No
Landonio[9]	156	1978–1993	Chemotherapy Hormones Immuno	Yes	0–4	PS >2; MFI <24 months; >2 metastatic sites; No prior Nx	Sex and age	No
Motzer[10]	463	1982–1996	Immuno-based	No	0–2	PS >1; MFI <12 months; Hemoglobin <LLN; LDH >1.5 × ULN; Corrected calcium[5] >10mg/dL	Prior Nx and RT; Location and no. of metastatic sites; Serum alkaline phosphatase and albumin	Yes, bootstrap validation, also refs. 14 and 24
Ljungberg[11]	106	1982–1999	Chemotherapy Hormones Radiotherapy Supportive care	No	0–4	PS >1; >1 metastatic site; Elevated ESR[4]; Serum calcium >ULN; Renal vein invasion	Sex and age; Tumor size; Nuclear grade; DNA ploidy; Serum albumin	No
Mani[12]	84	1983–1991	Immuno	Yes	0–1	PS 1; Bone metastasis; Sarcomatoid histology	Sex, age, and race; MFI; Recent weight loss; Prior Nx, RT, and chemotherapy; Lung, liver, lymph node metastasis; Local recurrence	No

Study	N	Years	Treatment		PS range	Poor prognostic factors	Other variables	Validation
Palmer[13]	327	1986–1990	Immuno	Yes	0–1	PS 1; MFI ≤24 months; >1 metastatic site[6]	Sex and age; Recent weight loss; Prior Nx, RT, and chemotherapy	Yes, training and validation data sets
Mekhail[14]	353	1987–2002	Chemotherapy Immuno-based	No	0–1	MSKCC score[7]; Prior RT; >1 metastatic site[8]; Histology[9]	Sex and age; Tumor side; Nuclear grade; Prior Nx; Neutrophil count; Serum albumin, creatinine, and alkaline phosphatase	No
Fyfe[15]	255	N/A	Immuno	Yes	0–4	PS >0; No prior Nx; Short MFI[4]	Age; Prior chemotherapy; Number of metastatic sites; Lung only disease	No
Citterio[16]	109	1988–not specified	Chemotherapy Radiotherapy Immuno Supportive care	No	0–3	PS >1; Hemoglobin ≤10 g/dL	Sex and age; MFI Stage; Nuclear grade; Metastatic sites; Serum creatinine, ferritin, albumin, calcium, LDH, alkaline phosphatase, and triglycerides	No
Canobbio[17]	73	1988–1992	Immuno	Yes	0–2	PS >0; >1 metastatic site	Sex and age; Prior Nx and chemotherapy; MFI	No
Atzpodien[18]	425	1988–1998	Immuno-based	Yes	0–1	MFI <3 years; Bone metastasis; >2 metastatic sites; LDH ≥220 U/L; CRP ≥11 mg/L; Neutrophils ≥6500/μL	Sex and age; ESR; Hemoglobin	No

(Continued)

Table 19.1. *Continued*

Multivariable analyses of clinical and tumor-related prognostic factors

Reference	n	Treatment period	Treatment[1]	Prior systemic therapy allowed?	PS	Factors associated with poor survival in multivariable analysis	Factors evaluated but not found to influence survival	Validated?
Leibovich[19]	173	1989–2000	Immuno-based	No	0–2	Constitutional symptoms[10]; Regional lymph nodes Location of metastases[11]; Sarcomatoid component; TSH>2 mIU/L	Sex and age; PS; T stage; Tumor size; Nuclear grade; Paraneoplastic syndrome[12]	No
Motzer[20]	137	1990–2002	Chemotherapy Immuno	Yes[13]	0–2	PS >1; Hemoglobin <LLN; Corrected calcium[5] ≥10 mg/dL	Metastatic sites; Prior RT and Nx; Time from diagnosis to salvage therapy	Yes, bootstrap validation
Fumagalli[21]	266	1991–1996	Immuno	No	0–2	PS ≥1; MFI <2 years; >1 metastatic site; Lack of partial or complete response; Low pretreatment lymphocyte count; Low maximum lymphocyte count during first treatment cycle	Sex and age	Yes, bootstrap validation
Negrier[22]	782	1992–1998	Immuno-based	N/A	0–2	PS ≥1; MFI ≤12 months >1 metastatic site; Liver, bone, mediastinal metastases; Hemoglobin <LLN; ESR ≥100 mm/h or CRP ≥50 mg/L; Neutrophils ≥7500/µL; Alkaline phosphatase >100 U/L	Sex and age; Recent weight loss; Stage; Prior Nx; Lymphocyte count; Platelet count	No

| Stadler[23] | 153 | 1997–2001 | Chemotherapy | Yes | 0–2 | PS >1; No prior Nx; >2 metastatic sites; Corrected calcium; >10 mg/dL; Alkaline phosphatase >ULN; Albumin <4.0 g/dL | Age; Prior immunotherapy; Histology; Nuclear grade; Hemoglobin; LDH | No |
| Donskov[24] | 85–120[14] | 1999–2002 | Immuno | No | 0–1 | PS 1 Bone and/or lymph node metastases; Hemoglobin <LLN; LDH >1.5 times ULN; Neutrophils >6000/µL; Presence of intratumoral neutrophils; <50 intratumoral $CD57^+$ natural killer cells/m^2 of tumor tissue | MFI; Lung and liver metastases; Number of metastatic sites; Lymphocyte and monocyte counts; Intratumoral lymphocyte subsets, macrophages, and $CD56^+$ natural killer cells | No |

N/A, not applicable; PS, Eastern Cooperative Oncology Group (ECOG) performance status; RT, radiotherapy; Nx, nephrectomy; ULN (LLN), upper (lower) limit of the laboratory's reference range; MFI, metastasis-free interval; ESR, erythrocyte sedimentation rate; LDH, lactate dehydrogenase; CRP, C-reactive protein.

[1]Immuno: Immunotherapy only, generally IFN-α and/or IL-2; Immuno-based: immunotherapy ± chemotherapy, generally vinblastine or 5-fluorouracil.

[2]Analyzed as an ordinal variable, 0 vs. 1 vs. 2 vs. 3.

[3]Based on lung, hepatic, brain, and "other."

[4]Analyzed as a continuous measure.

[5]Total calcium, 0.707 × (albumin − 3.4).

[6]Based on lung, bone, and "other."

[7]Memorial Sloan-Kettering Cancer Center score based on PS, MFI, hemoglobin, LDH, and corrected calcium[10] (see Motzer table entry).

[8]Based on lung, liver, and retroperitoneal nodes.

[9]In a subset of patients after adjustment for other identified prognostic factors.

[10]Rash, sweats, weight loss, early satiety or decreased appetite, other gastrointestinal disturbances, musculoskeletal pain, respiratory symptoms.

[11]Multiple sites and single sites other than lung or bone.

[12]Hypercalcemia (>10 mg/dL), polycythemia (hematocrit >54%), anemia (hematocrit <40%), abnormal liver function test (AST or ALT >50 U/L, alkaline phosphatase >105 U/L).

[13]Restricted to previously treated patients.

[14]120 patients included in assessment of clinical factors; 85 analyzed with respect to immunologic parameters.

serum levels of IL-6, a proinflammatory cytokine, in a subset of 138 patients treated on the Cancer Renal Cytokine (CRECY) trial of IFN-α vs. IL-2 vs. the combination[31] and found elevated levels to be an independent prognostic factor of poor survival. Stadler et al.,[32] on the other hand, did not find serum IL-6 levels to be an independent predictor of outcome in a small phase I trial of the anti-CD3 monoclonal antibody OKT-3.

Anemia, generally defined simply as hemoglobin values below the lower limit of the laboratory's reference range, and hypercalcemia, generally defined as corrected (free) serum calcium above 10 mg/dL, are additional paraneoplastic symptoms that have frequently, though not universally, been identified as independent predictors of poor survival. The studies by Motzer et al.[10,20] and Mekhail et al.[14] that are summarized in Table 19.1, for example, identified both anemia and hypercalcemia as independent prognostic factors. Similarly, studies by Citterio et al.,[16] Negrier et al.,[22] Donskov et al.,[24] and Wittke et al.[33] identified anemia as prognostic; and Ljungberg et al.[11] and Stadler et al.[23] identified hypercalcemia as important. Citterio et al., however found no association between serum calcium levels and survival, and Stadler et al. found no association with hemoglobin. Atzpodien et al.[18] and Hoffmann et al.[29] likewise found no association between survival and hemoglobin levels.

The prognostic value of lactate dehydrogenase (LDH) and serum alkaline phosphatase has been evaluated by several investigators, but with mixed results. Motzer et al.,[10] Mekhail et al.,[14] and Donskov et al.,[24] using a cutoff of 1.5 times the upper limit of the laboratory's reference range, and Atzpodien et al.[18] and Wittke et al.[33] using cutoffs of 220 to 240 U/L all found elevated LDH to be independently associated with poor survival, whereas Citterio et al.,[16] Stadler et al.,[23] and Hoffmann et al.[29] found no such association. Stadler et al., however, did identify elevated alkaline phosphatase as an independent predictor of poor survival, as did Negrier et al.[22] Motzer et al.,[10] Mekhail et al.,[14] and Citterio et al.,[16] however, found no association between levels of serum alkaline phosphatase and outcome.

Hematologic parameters, such as neutrophil, lymphocyte, and platelet counts, have also been assessed in a limited number of studies, but again with mixed results. Using predetermined cutoffs of 6000 to 7500 cells/μL, Atzpodien et al.,[18] Negrier et al.,[22] and Donskov et al.[24] all found elevated pretreatment neutrophil count to be an independent predictor of poor survival, whereas Mekhail et al.[14] and Hoffmann et al.[29] found neutrophil count to be unrelated to outcome in multivariable analysis, although it was in univariable analysis. Similarly, Suppiah et al.[34] identified a pretreatment platelet count >400,000 cells/μL as prognostic for poor survival in a database study of 700 previously untreated patients, while Negrier et al.[22] found no such association in multivariable analysis, although thrombocytosis was prognostic in univariable analysis. Fumagalli et al.[21] found a low lymphocyte count at baseline or during the first cycle of treatment to be associated with a poor outcome in 266 patients treated with IL-2 with or without IFN-α. Negrier et al.[22] and Donskov et al.,[24] in contrast found no association between lymphocyte count and survival.

In addition to these presenting symptoms, a number of other biochemical markers have been assessed to a very limited extent and found to be associated (thyroid-stimulating hormone[19] and urinary albumin[26]) or not associated (serum creatinine,[14,16] triglyceride levels,[16] β₂-microglobulin,[35] and β-human chorionic gonadotropin [β-HGC][36]) with survival.

Disease-Related Factors

Common sites of metastatic spread in RCC are the lungs, liver, bone, and brain.[3] The impact on survival of specific sites of metastatic disease as well as tumor burden, as measured by the number of involved sites, and tumor aggressiveness, as measured by the interval between diagnosis and the development or treatment of metastatic disease (the metastasis-free interval [MFI]), have been extensively studied. As noted in Table 19.1, most investigators who assessed these features have found them to be independent predictors of survival.

A number of studies have identified individual sites of metastatic disease as being of prognostic significance; however, most have found the number of involved sites to be a good surrogate for those individual sites, and in multivariable analysis to be a strong independent prognostic factor.[6,7,9,11,13,14,17,18,21–23] How and what to count, however, has varied. Most investigators have simply counted all involved sites[6,9,11,17,18,21–23]; however, some have restricted the count to specific organs. Elson et al.,[7] for example, restricted the count to the presence or absence of lung, liver, brain, and "other" metastases, where "other" represented all other metastatic sites regardless of the number. Palmer et al.[13] similarly based their count on lung, bone, and "other" metastases. In contrast, Mekhail et al.[14] counted only lung, liver, and retroperitoneal nodal metastases. In addition, investigators have used both one[6,7,11,13,14,17,21,22] or two[9,18,23] metastatic sites as a cutoff for determining prognosis. Although these investigators have all identified the number of metastatic sites as an independent predictor of survival, the estimated increased risk of death due to more extensive disease ranged from 24% to 286%. This wide range in effect is partly due to the variable definitions used, but it is also likely due at least in part to the fact that imaging technologies have advanced considerably during the 30-year time period during which these patients were treated, making it easier to detect metastatic deposits. It should be noted that several investigators have found no prognostic value to the location or number of metastatic sites.[8,10,15,16,20,24]

Similar to tumor burden, MFI has been assessed in a variety of ways. Most studies that investigated its prognostic value used a similar definition of MFI; however, some investigators have defined prognosis in terms of the MFI being less than or greater than 1 year,[7,8,10,14,22] 2 years,[9,13,21] 3 years,[18] or measured on a continuum.[15] Despite these variations, these studies have consistently demonstrated a 43% to 95% increased risk of death for patients with a short MFI. The value of MFI as an independent predictor, however, is not a universal finding, and the studies by Mani et al.,[12] Citterio et al.,[16] Canobbio et al.,[17] and Danskov et al.[24] did not find it to be of prognostic value after adjusting for other factors. A study by Motzer et al.[20] also found no association between MFI and outcome, but this was a study of prognostic factors for survival in the second-line setting, and it is not clear that MFI in the salvage and front-line settings can be interpreted similarly.

In addition to disease extent and MFI, several investigators have examined tumor size,[6,11,19] stage,[16,19,22] and location of the primary (right versus left kidney)[6,14]; however, none of these factors appear to impact survival once other factors are accounted for.

Prior Treatment

Prior treatment does not appear to impact survival in patients with mRCC. The few studies that have assessed the effect of radiotherapy have generally found no association between treatment and outcome.[7,10,12,13,20] Similarly, most studies examining prior systemic therapy have found it not to be of prognostic value.[12,13,15,17,23] Exceptions to these results are studies by Mekhail et al.[14] and Elson et al.,[7] which respectively found prior radiotherapy and prior systemic therapy to impact negatively on survival even after adjusting for other predictors.

Adjunctive cytoreductive nephrectomy appears to improve outcome in prospective randomized trials[37]; retrospective studies by Landonio et al.,[9] Fyfe et al.,[15] and Stadler et al.[23] also found a history of nephrectomy to be associated with improved survival. Most of the studies summarized in Table 19.1, however, found no association between survival and prior nephrectomy in multivariable analysis.[7,8,10,12–14,17,20,22] It should be noted that in these studies prior nephrectomy was frequently associated with improved survival in univariable analysis. Prior nephrectomy and MFI are highly correlated, however, and once MFI was accounted for in multivariable analysis, nephrectomy tended to lose its prognostic value. In addition, these studies did not assess the timing of the nephrectomy, only whether or not it was performed at some point in time during the patient's treatment.

PATHOLOGY

A number of investigators have assessed pathologic features such as nuclear grade and morphometry, DNA ploidy, and histology as potential prognostic factors.

In unselected series of patients with RCC, nuclear grade is frequently identified as a strong independent predictor of survival (see, for example, Zisman et al.,[38] Frank et al.,[39] and Patard et al.[40]). Once RCC metastasizes, however, there is little evidence that grade impacts survival after other important factors are taken into account.[11,14,16,19,23] An exception to this is the study by Neves et al.,[6] in which patients with grade 3 and 4 tumors had significantly worse outcomes than patients with well or moderately well differentiated tumors, even after adjusting for weight loss and number of involved metastatic sites.

Tumor grade as a potential prognostic factor has been criticized because of the subjectivity associated with its evaluation and the various systems used to assess it.[41] This has led a number of investigators to suggest assessing nuclear morphology using more quantitative measures that describe the size of the nuclei and/or their shape. The proposed size parameters include nuclear perimeter or area, length of the major and minor axes, and a measure of mean nuclear volume (MNV). The shape parameters that have been studied are primarily measures of the extent to which the contour of the nuclei deviate from a perfect circle. Many of these parameters are correlated with histopathologic factors such as stage and grade, and in univariable analyses, with survival.[42–46] Most studies, however, have not evaluated the same set of parameters, and the results of multivariable analyses have been mixed. Ruiz et al.,[42] for example, evaluated nuclear area, perimeter, length of the major and minor axes, and a shape factor, and found that none was prognostic in patients with advanced disease. Similarly, van der Poel et al.[43] found a measure of chromatin texture, but no size or shape parameters to be prognostic. Delahunt et al.,[44] on the other hand, found departures from nuclear roundness to be the only independent predictor of survival after adjusting for other important factors such as disease stage, and Artacho-Perula et al.[45] found only MNV to be important. Soda et al.,[46] evaluating only MNV, also found it to be of prognostic value after adjusting for disease stage and grade.

Results from studies of DNA ploidy have been similarly mixed. Several studies have reported that patients with aneuploid tumors have a poor prognosis compared to patients with diploid tumors,[47,48] whereas others have found no association between ploidy and outcome,[11,49–51] or that aneuploidy is positively associated with survival.[52] A possible explanation for these contradictory findings is that RCC tumors are heterogeneous, and therefore the likelihood of defining a tumor as diploid or aneuploid is highly dependent on the number of samples assessed.[47,48]

A retrospective analysis by Patard et al.[40] of over 4000 RCC patients seen at multiple institutions demonstrated a clear trend in outcome based on histologic subtype in univariable analysis. Considering all patients, those with clear cell tumors had an estimated 5-year survival of 64% compared to 70% for patients with papillary tumors and 84% for patients with chromophobe tumors ($p < .001$). The prognostic significance of histology was lost, however, in multivariable analysis once adjustments were made for the effects of tumor, node, metastasis (TNM) stage, nuclear grade, and ECOG PS. Stadler et al.[23] likewise found no association between survival and histology. In contrast, Mani et al.[12] and Leibovich et al.[19] both identified the presence of sarcomatoid features as an independent predictor of poor outcome, and Mekhail et al.[14] identified any non–clear-cell histology (mostly papillary) as being a poor prognostic factor. These latter studies should be viewed cautiously, however, because they included relatively small numbers of patients with sarcomatoid features (6% and 12%, respectively) or non–clear-cell histologies (13%).

IMMUNOLOGIC FACTORS

Interleukin-6 and IL-10 have a number of immunologic functions that can positively or negatively impact the immune response to RCC, and several investigators have assessed their prognostic value. The impact of serum levels of IL-6 on survival is described above in the discussion of inflammatory markers, and therefore only IL-10 is discussed here. Interleukin-10 is an immunosuppressive cytokine that inhibits the growth of T lymphocytes,[53] and has been shown to downregulate major histocompatibility complex (MHC) class I and II molecules on antigen presenting cells, thereby leading to impaired antigen presentation.[33] Wittke et al.[33] found serum IL-10 levels greater than 1 pg/mL to be an independent predictor of poor survival after correcting for the effects of elevated ESR, LDH, and anemia. In contrast, Negrier et al.[30] did not find an association between detectable IL-10 levels and outcome in their study of a subset of patients treated on the CRECY trial.

Several investigators have studied the impact on survival of the absolute or relative numbers of various lymphocyte subsets and other immune cells. Hernberg et al.,[54] for example, found an increasing CD4[+]/CD8[+] T-cell ratio during treatment with vinblastine plus IFN-α to be correlated with improved survival. Donskov et al.,[24] on the other hand, found a significant association between low numbers of intratumoral CD57[+] natural killer (NK) cells and poor survival, but no association with intratumoral T-cell subsets (CD4[+], CD8[+], CD20[+]), macrophages, or CD56[+] NK cells in a retrospective study of 120 patients treated with IL-2 alone or in combination with IFN-α and/or histamine dihydrochloride.

GENETIC FACTORS

Cytogenetics

Although not extensively studied, several investigators have examined the relationship between chromosomal abnormalities and survival in RCC. In small series of unselected patients Wu et al.,[55] Moch et al.,[56] and Elfving et al.[57] suggest that indicators of genetic instability may be of prognostic value. Wu et al., for example, found that loss of the long arm of chromosome 14 was associated with poor survival in a study of 30 patients with nonpapillary RCC. Moch et al., on the other hand, found loss of chromosome 9p, but not 14q, to be associated with poor outcome in a study of 41 non-mRCC patients. Moch et al. also found that patients with a total of three or more chromosomal deletions had a poorer prognosis than patients with fewer than three deletions. Similarly Elfving et al. reported that among 50 consecutive RCC patients, those with fewer than six chromosomal alterations (additions plus deletions) had significantly better prognosis than patients with six or more aberrations.

Gene Expression

The advent of gene expression and tissue microarray technologies has enabled rapid molecular and protein expression profiling of tissue samples, thereby allowing investigators to screen large numbers of potential genetic prognostic factors. Increasing attention is being paid to these methodologies, and markers associated with cell cycle regulation, tumor proliferation and growth, cellular adhesion, and angiogenesis are being assessed. To date, however, relatively few studies have focused specifically on mRCC.

One example of an investigation that has specifically targeted mRCC is a recent study by Vasselli et al.[58] of 58 patients that used a general complementary DNA (cDNA) microarray and both unsupervised and supervised analysis methods to identify prognostic subgroups of patients based on global expression patterns in the primary tumors. Using this approach two groups of patients that differed significantly with respect to survival (18.2 months versus 5.9 months, $p < .05$) could be identified based on the expression patterns of 45 genes. In addition, vascular cell adhesion molecule 1 (VCAM-1) was identified as the most highly predictive marker in the set, with patients expressing high levels having significantly better survival than patients with low expression levels. This result is somewhat different from an earlier study by Hoffmann et al.[29] that selectively looked at serum levels of soluble forms of VCAM-1, intercellular adhesion molecule 1 (ICAM-1), and E-selectin. In that study the soluble form of ICAM-1 but not VCAM-1 was identified as an independent predictor of survival.

In another recent study, Kim et al.[59] used a tissue array composed of samples from 150 mRCC patients with clear cell tumors who underwent nephrectomy prior to treatment with immunotherapy, to focus attention on eight genes that have previously been reported in the literature as being associated with the development and progression of cancer, and in some cases have also been reported to be of prognostic significance in RCC. The set included Ki67 and p53, which are associated with cellular proliferation; gelsolin, vimentin, and epithelial cell adhesion molecule (EpCAM), which are involved in cell motility and cancer progression; and carbonic anhydrase IX (CA IX), CA XII, and phosphatase and tensin homologue (PTEN), which are critical components of the hypoxia pathway that allow growing tumors to adapt to an oxygen-poor microenvironment. Adjusting for the effects of T stage, nuclear grade, and ECOG PS, CA IX, p53, PTEN, and vimentin were all seen to be independent prognostic factors for survival, with high expression levels of CA IX and PTEN, and low levels of p53 and vimentin being associated with improved outcome. Atkins et al.[60] likewise found CA IX expression to be an independent predictor of survival in a study of 66 mRCC patients treated on IL-2–based trials conducted by the Cytokine Working Group.

CONCLUSION

Clinical factors have been studied extensively as potential prognostic factors in mRCC. However, from the studies summarized in Table 19.1, it is clear that they cannot be fully assessed with respect to their value as independent predictors. This is because different studies have examined different sets of factors, definitions and codings have varied, and different patient populations have been studied. To address this issue, a comprehensive database of approximately 4000 previously untreated patients who were entered into controlled clinical trials has been developed by an international consortium of researchers. The goal of this effort is to define a single, validated prognostic model for survival in mRCC that is based on clinical factors.[61,62]

In addition to "classical" prognostic factors, new molecular-based technologies are leading to a better understanding of the underlying biology of RCC, and are helping to identify new prognostic factors. As discussed above, a number of immunologic and genetic factors appear to be correlated with outcome. Their value as independent prognostic factors needs to be confirmed, however, by examining them uniformly in relatively homogeneous groups of patients and in conjunction with the classical predictors.

REFERENCES

1. Matthew A, Devesa SS, Fraument JF, Chow WH. Global increases in kidney cancer incidence, 1973–1992. Eur J Cancer Prev 2002;11:171–178.
2. Jemal A, Siegel R, Ward E, Murray T, Xu J, Smigal C, Thun MJ. Cancer statistics, 2006. CA Cancer J Clin 2006;56:106–130.
3. Motzer RJ, Bander NH, Nanus DM. Renal cell carcinoma. N Engl J Med 1996;335:865–875.
4. Escudier B, Szczylik C, Eisen T, et al. Randomized phase III trial of the raf kinase and VEGFR inhibitor sorafenib (BAY 43–9006) in patients with advanced renal cell carcinoma. J Clin Oncol 2005;23:380s.
5. Motzer RJ, Michaelson MD, Redman BG, et al. Activity of SU11248, a multitargeted inhibitor of vascular endothelial growth factor receptor and platelet-derived growth factor receptor, in patients with metastatic renal cell carcinoma. J Clin Oncol 2006;24:16–24.
6. Neves RJ, Zincke H, Taylor WF. Metastatic renal cell cancer and radical nephrectomy: identification of prognostic factors and patient survival. J Urol 1988;139:1173–1176.
7. Elson PJ, Witte RS, Trump DL. Prognostic factors for survival in patients with recurrent or metastatic renal cell carcinoma. Cancer Res 1988;48:7310–7313.
8. Fossa SD, Kramar A, Droz JP. Prognostic factors and survival in patients with metastatic renal cell carcinoma treated with chemotherapy or interferon-alpha. Eur J Cancer 1994;30:1310–1314.
9. Landonio G, Baiocchi C, Cattaneo D, et al. Retrospective analysis of 156 cases of metastatic renal cell carcinoma: evaluation of prognostic factors and response to different treatments. Tumori 1994;80:468–472.
10. Motzer RJ, Bacik J, Murphy BA, Russo P, Mazumdar M. Interferon-alfa as a comparative treatment for clinical trials of new therapies against advanced renal cell carcinoma. J Clin Oncol 2002;20:289–296.

11. Ljungberg B, Landberg G, Alamdari FI. Factors of importance for prediction of survival in patients with metastatic renal cell carcinoma, treated with or without nephrectomy. Scand J Urol Nephrol 2000;34:246–251.
12. Mani S, Todd MB, Katz K, Poo W-J. Prognostic factors for survival in patients with metastatic renal cancer treated with biological response modifiers. J Urol 1995;154:35–40.
13. Palmer PA, Vinke J, Philip T, et al. Prognostic factors for survival in patients with advanced renal cell carcinoma treated with recombinant interleukin-2. Ann Oncol 1992;3:475–480.
14. Mekhail TM, Abou-Jawde RM, BouMerhi G, et al. Validation and extension of the Memorial Sloan-Kettering prognostic factors model for survival in patients with previously untreated metastatic renal cell carcinoma. J Clin Oncol 2005;23:832–840.
15. Fyfe G, Fisher RI, Rosenberg SA, Sznol M, Parkinson DR, Louis AC. Results of treatment of 255 patients with metastatic renal cell carcinoma who received high-dose recombinant interleukin-2 therapy. J Clin Oncol 1995;13:688–696.
16. Citterio G, Bertuzzi A, Tresoldi M, et al. Prognostic factors for survival in metastatic renal cell carcinoma: retrospective analysis from 109 consecutive patients. Eur Urol 1997;31:286–291.
17. Canobbio L, Rubagotti A, Miglietta L, et al. Prognostic factors for survival in patients with advanced renal cell carcinoma treated with interleukin-2 and interferon-α. J Cancer Res Clin Oncol 1995;121:753–756.
18. Atzpodien J, Royston, P, Wandert T, Reitz M, and CGCIN—German Cooperative Renal Carcinoma Chemo-Immunotherapy Trials Group. Metastatic renal carcinoma comprehensive prognostic system. Br J Cancer 2003;88:348–353.
19. Leibovich BC, Han K, Bui MHT, et al. Scoring algorithm to predict survival after nephrectomy and immunotherapy in patients with metastatic renal cell carcinoma: a stratification tool for prospective clinical trials. Cancer 2003;98:2566–2575.
20. Motzer RJ, Bacik J, Schwartz LH, et al. Prognostic factors for survival in previously treated patients with metastatic disease. J Clin Oncol 2004;22:454–463.
21. Fumagalli LA, Vinke J, Hoff W, Ympa E, Brivio F, Nespoli A. Lymphocyte counts independently predict overall survival in advanced cancer patients: a biomarker for IL-2 immunotherapy. J Immunol 2003;26:394–402.
22. Negrier S, Escudier B, Gomez F, et al. Prognostic factors of survival and rapid progression in 782 patients with metastatic renal carcinomas treated by cytokines: a report from the Groupe Francais d'Immunotherapie. Ann Oncol 2002;13:1460–1468.
23. Stadler WM, Huo D, George C, et al. Prognostic factors for survival with gemcitabine plus 5-fluorouracil based regimens for metastatic renal cancer. J Urol 2003;170:1141–1145.
24. Donskov F, von der Maase H. Impact of immune parameters on long-term survival in metastatic renal cell carcinoma. J Clin Oncol 2006;24:1997–2004.
25. Klugo R, Detmers M, Stiles R, Talley R, Cerny J. Aggressive versus conservative management of stage IV renal cell carcinoma. J Urol 1977;118:244–246.
26. Vaglio A, Buzio L, Cravedi P, Pavone L, Garini G, Buzio C. Prognostic significance of albuminuria in patients with renal cell cancer. J Urol 2003;170:1135–1137.
27. Oken MM, Creech RH, Tormey DC, et al. Toxicity and response criteria of the Eastern Cooperative Oncology Group. Am J Clin Oncol 1982;5:649–655.
28. Ljungberg B, Grankvist K, Rasmuson T. Serum acute phase reactants and prognosis in renal cell carcinoma. Cancer 1995;76:1435–1439.
29. Hoffmann R, Franzke A, Buer J, et al. Prognostic impact of in vivo soluble cell adhesion molecules in metastatic renal cell carcinoma. Br J Cancer 1999;79:1742–1745.
30. Negrier S, Perol D, Menetrier-Caux C, et al. Interleukin-6, interleukin-10, and vascular endothelial growth factor in metastatic renal cell carcinoma: prognostic value of interleukin-6. J Clin Oncol 2004;22:2371–2378.
31. Negrier S, Escudier B, Lasset C, et al. Recombinant human interleukin-2, recombinant human interferon alfa-2a, or both in metastatic renal-cell carcinoma. N Engl J Med 1998;338:1272–1278.
32. Stadler WM, Richards JM, Vogelzang NJ. Serum interleukin-6 levels in metastatic renal cell cancer: correlation with survival but not an independent prognostic indicator. J Natl Cancer Inst 1992;84:1835–1836.
33. Wittke F, Hoffmann R, Buer J, et al. Interleukin 10 (IL-10): an immunosuppressive factor and independent predictor in patients with metastatic renal cell carcinoma. Br J Cancer 1999;79:1182–1184.

34. Suppiah R, Shaheen PE, Elson P, et al. Thrombocytosis as a prognostic factor for survival in patients with metastatic renal cell carcinoma. Cancer 2006;107:1793–1800.
35. Rasmuson T, Grankvist K, Ljungberg B. Serum β_2-microglobulin and prognosis of patients with renal cell carcinoma. Acta Oncol 1996;35:479–482.
36. Hotakainen K, Ljungberg B, Haglund C, Nordling S, Paju A, Stenman UH. Expression of the free β-subunit of human chorionic gonadotropin in renal cell carcinoma: prognostic study on tissue and serum. Int J Cancer 2003;104:631–635.
37. Flanigan RC, Mickisch G, Sylvester R, Tangen C, Van Poppel H, Crawford DE. Cytoreductive nephrectomy in patients with metastatic renal cell cancer: a combined analysis. J Urol 2004;171: 1071–1076.
38. Zisman A, Pantuck AJ, Dorey F, et al. Improved prognostication of renal cell carcinoma using an integrated staging system. J Clin Oncol 2001;19:1649–1657.
39. Frank I, Blute ML, Cheville JC, Lohse CM, Weaver AL, Zincke H. An outcome prediction model for patients with clear cell renal cell carcinoma treated with radical nephrectomy based on tumor stage, size, grade, and necrosis: the SSIGN score. J Urol 2002;168:2395–2400.
40. Patard JJ, Leray E, Rioux-Leclercq N, et al. Prognostic value of histologic subtypes in renal cell carcinoma: a multicenter experience. J Clin Oncol 2005;23:2763–2771.
41. Lanigan D, Conroy R, Barry-Walsh C, Loftus B, Royston D, Leader MA. Comparative analysis of grading systems in renal adenocarcinoma. Histopathology 1994;24:473–476.
42. Ruiz JL, Hernandez M, Martinez J, Vera C, Jimenez-Cruz JF. Value of morphometry as an independent prognostic factor in renal cell carcinoma. Eur Urol 1995;27:54–57.
43. van der Poel HG, Mulders PFA, Oosterhof GON, et al. Prognostic value of karyometric and clinical characteristics in renal cell carcinoma. Cancer 1993;72:2667–2674.
44. Delahunt B, Becker RL, Bethwaite PB, Ribas JL. Computerized nuclear morphometry and survival in renal cell carcinoma: comparison with other prognostic indicators. Pathology 1994;26:353–358.
45. Artacho-Perula E, Roldan-Villalobos R, Martinez-Cuevas JF, Lopez-Rubio F. Nuclear quantitative grading by discriminant analysis of renal cell carcinoma samples. A patient survival evaluation. J Pathol 1994;173:105–114.
46. Soda T, Fujikawa K, Ito T, Sasaki, Nishio Y, Miyakawa M. Volume-weighted mean nuclear volume as a prognostic factor in renal cell carcinoma. Lab Invest 1999;79:859–867.
47. Ljungberg B, Mehle C, Stenling R, Roos G. Heterogeneity in renal cell carcinoma and its impact on prognosis—a flow cytometric study. Br J Cancer 1996;74:123–127.
48. Ruiz-Cerda JL, Hernandez M, Sempere A, O'Connor JE, Kimler B, Jimenez-Cruz F. Intratumoral heterogeneity of DNA content in renal cell carcinoma and its prognostic significance. Cancer 1999;86:664–671.
49. Nakano E, Kondoh M, Okatani K, Seguchi T, Sugao H. Flow cytometric analysis of nuclear DNA content in renal cell carcinoma correlated with histologic and clinical features. Cancer 1993;72:1319–1323.
50. Lanigan D, McLean PA, Murphy DM, Donovan MG, Curran B, Leader M. Ploidy and prognosis in renal carcinoma. Br J Urol 1993;71:21–24.
51. van Bezooijen RL, Goey H, Stoter G, Hermans J, Fleuren GJ. Prognostic markers for survival in patients with metastatic renal cell carcinoma treated with interleukin-2. Cancer Immunol Immuother 1996;43:293–298.
52. Eskelinen M, Lipponen P, Nordling S. Prognostic evaluation of DNA flow cytometry and histomorphological criteria in renal cell carcinoma. Anticancer Res 1995;15:2279–2284.
53. Taga KH, Mostowski H, Tosato G. Human interleukin-10 can directly inhibit T-cell growth. Blood 1993;81:2964–2971.
54. Hernberg M, Muhonen T, Pyrhonen S. Can the CD4+/CD8+ ratio predict the outcome of interferon-α therapy for renal cell carcinoma? Ann Oncol 1997;8:71–77.
55. Wu SQ, Hafez GR, Xing W, Newton M, Chen SR, Messing E. The correlation between the loss of chromosome 14q with histologic tumor grade, pathologic stage, and outcome of patients with nonpapillary renal cell carcinoma. Cancer 1996;77:1154–1160.
56. Moch H, Presti JC, Sauter G, et al. Genetic aberrations detected by comparative genomic hybridization are associated with clinical outcome in renal cell carcinoma. Cancer Res 1996;56: 27–30.
57. Elfving P, Mandahl N, Lundgren R, et al. Prognostic implications of cytogenetic findings in kidney cancer. Br J Urol 1997;80:698–706.

58. Vasselli JR, Shih JH, Iyengar SR, et al. Predicting survival in patients with metastatic kidney cancer by gene-expression profiling in the primary tumor. Proc Natl Acad Sci 2003;100:6958–6963.

59. Kim HL, Seligson D, Liu X, et al. Using tumor markers to predict the survival of patients with metastatic renal cell carcinoma. J Urol 2005;173:1496–1501.

60. Atkins M, Regan M, McDermott D, et al. Carbonic anhydrase IX expression predicts outcome of interleukin 2 therapy for renal cancer. Clin Cancer Res 2005;11:2721–3714.

61. Bukowski RM, Negrier S, Elson P. Prognostic factors in patients with advanced renal cell carcinoma: development of an international kidney cancer working group. Clin Cancer Res 2004;10: 6310s–6314s.

62. Elson PJ, Manola JB, Mazumdar M, Bacik JM, Supers SJ. Prognostic factors for survival in patients with renal cell carcinoma: a study from the Kidney Cancer Association's International Kidney Cancer Working Group (IKCWG). J Clin Oncol 2005;23:386s.

20 Functional Imaging of Renal Cell Carcinoma

Navneet S. Majhail and
Ronald M. Bukowski

KEYWORDS

POSITRON EMISSION TOMOGRAPHY
RENAL CELL CARCINOMA

ABSTRACT

F-18 fluorodeoxyglucose (FDG) positron emission tomography (PET) has been increasingly used in oncology and has been applied for the diagnosis, staging, and followup of several cancers. The role of FDG PET in renal cell carcinoma is currently evolving. Current evidence suggests that this imaging modality has limited sensitivity, but in selected situations PET might complement conventional imaging techniques in further delineating suspicious lesions. Improvements in image acquisition and processing techniques, use of radioisotopes other than FDG and increasing experience with combined PET and computed tomography scanners will increase the applicability of functional imaging in renal cell carcinoma.

Functional imaging represents a variety of imaging techniques where the emphasis is on the extraction of quantitative information about physiologic function from the image-based data instead of simple visual interpretation. Positron emission tomography (PET) is the most widely used tool for functional imaging, with its main clinical application being oncologic imaging. The ability to noninvasively characterize in vivo metabolic reactions makes PET particularly attractive in oncology. Current applications for PET in oncology include initial diagnosis and staging of various malignancies, monitoring response to therapy, and follow-up posttreatment.

Positron emission tomography has been extensively studied and established as a useful modality in the management of a variety of malignancies such as the malignant lymphomas and cancers of the head and neck, lung, gastrointestinal tract, and breast. Feasibility of PET in renal cell carcinoma (RCC) was initially reported by Wahl et al.[1] in 1991; however, its role in RCC is still evolving and is yet to be clearly defined.

"

BASIC PRINCIPLES OF POSITRON EMISSION TOMOGRAPHY

F-18 Fluorodeoxyglucose

F-18 fluorodeoxyglucose (FDG) is the most common radioisotope used for PET imaging in oncology. The accelerated glucose utilization characteristic of malignant cells compared to surrounding normal cells forms the basis of FDG-PET imaging of cancer.[2–4] The enhanced rate of glucose metabolism in cancer cells has been attributed to impaired aerobic glycolysis with a resultant increase in the need for glucose for adenosine triphosphate (ATP) production. A membrane glucose-transporter system mediates the enhanced uptake of FDG, which is subsequently phosphorylated to the intermediate metabolite FDG-6-phosphate. Unlike glucose-6-phosphate, FDG-6-phosphate cannot be metabolized further and remains trapped in the cell. The decay of trapped radioisotope leads to the release of positrons (antimatter counterparts of electrons with the same mass but a positive charge). The positron eventually collides with and annihilates a nearby electron, resulting in the production of two 511-KeV photons (positron decay). Coincident detection of the two photons characterizes the distribution of FDG in the body, which is subsequently reconstructed into cross-sectional images.

The accumulation of FDG within a cell depends on the rate of transport through the cell membrane and has been shown to be mediated by a family of facilitative glucose transporters (GLUTs). Among them, GLUT-1 in particular is a high-affinity glucose transporter with a wide distribution and no tissue specificity; it is overexpressed in a variety of malignancies, is recognized as an early marker of cellular malignant transformation, and has been shown to correlate with cellular proliferation, tumor invasiveness, and poor survival.[5,6] GLUT-1 facilitates the uptake of FDG in malignant tumors, and decreased expression of GLUT-1 has been observed to correlate with low FDG uptake in certain tumor types.[7–12] Expression of hexokinase and glucose-6-phosphatase, two enzymes of the glycolytic pathway, also regulate FDG uptake into the cell.[13–15]

The expression of GLUT-1 in RCC and its impact on prognosis and outcome is as yet unclear. Miyakita et al.[16] observed variable expression of GLUT-1 in RCC and found no correlation with GLUT-1 immunoreactivity and tumor grade, clinical stage, or PET positivity. Nineteen patients with RCC were examined preoperatively with PET; 11 (58%) tumors expressed GLUT-1 but only six (31.6%) had significant uptake of FDG on PET. The authors suggested that although RCC consists of glycogen rich cells, it has a low propensity for metabolizing glucose. Larger tumors, however, had a higher likelihood of being GLUT-1 and PET positive; of the eight tumors larger than 5 cm, five (62.5%) were PET positive and seven (87.5%) were GLUT-1 positive. This observation was corroborated by another study by Nagase et al.,[17] who found heterogeneous expression of GLUT-1 in 75 patients with RCC. GLUT-1 expression was increased in 55 (73%) tumors; GLUT-1 staining was positive in 84.6% tumors with clear cell histology, whereas none with spindle cell type was positive. Positive staining was recognized only in areas of clear cell carcinomas in the mixed cell subtype. The authors did not observe any significant correlation of GLUT-1 positivity with tumor grade or stage.

EVALUATION AND STAGING OF PRIMARY RENAL CELL CARCINOMA WITH POSITRON EMISSION TOMOGRAPHY

The initial step in the management of any malignancy is effective and accurate tumor staging. This is true for RCC as well, where stage has been demonstrated to be an independent predictor of survival.[18,19] Though PET has been found to be a reliable technique for staging many cancer types, its role in the initial staging of RCC remains unclear.

Ramdave et al.[20] found FDG-PET to have an overall accuracy of 94% in the assessment of suspected primary renal tumors. Of the 17 patients evaluated, PET was true positive in 15 patients, true negative in one patient, and false negative in one patient; no patient had a false-positive PET. Computed tomography (CT) had comparable accuracy (94%). Retroperitoneal lymph node spread in one patient was detected by PET but not CT, and neither PET nor CT could detect renal vein extension in one patient. Furthermore, PET influenced treatment decisions in six (35%) patients. These included three patients who did not undergo their planned radical nephrectomy; two patients were found to have unsuspected metastatic disease not detected by CT, and one patient with an equivocal renal lesion on CT was diagnosed with a benign tumor. Three patients ended up having nephron-sparing surgery or partial nephrectomy instead of radical nephrectomy based on PET findings.

Aide et al.,[21] however, did not observe the same encouraging results. Among 35 patients undergoing partial or radical nephrectomy for suspicious renal masses, preoperative FDG-PET was true positive in 14 and false negative in 16 patients. The overall sensitivity, specificity, and accuracy of PET in characterizing renal masses was 47%, 80%, and 51%, respectively. Comparative CT had a sensitivity of 97%, specificity of 0%, and an accuracy of 83%. The median size of tumors positive on PET was significantly larger than that of negative lesions (7.75 cm vs. 4.25 cm). Of the two patients with regional lymph node involvement, PET was positive in only one patient, whereas the CT correctly identified both cases.

The relatively low sensitivity of PET in detecting RCC was confirmed by Kang et al.[22] In their cohort of 17 patients with renal masses undergoing nephrectomy, preoperative FDG-PET exhibited a sensitivity of 60%. Computed tomography, on the other hand, was 92% sensitive. Both PET and CT had specificities of 100%. Similar results were reported by Bachor et al.,[23] who reported a sensitivity of 77% in 29 patients evaluated by FDG-PET prior to nephrectomy.

Though varying sensitivities of PET for the detection of primary RCC has been reported in the literature, it does not seem to offer any advantage over CT in the staging of primary tumor or locoregional lymph node disease (Table 20.1). Lack of contrast between RCC and normal kidney, variable GLUT-1 expression, and subsequent FDG uptake by RCC are the purported reasons for the low diagnostic yield of PET in this setting.

Table 20.1.
Positron emission tomography in the evaluation of primary
renal cell carcinoma

Study	Sensitivity	Specificity
Bachor et al. (1996)[23]	77%	—
Ramdave et al. (2001)[20]	94%	100%
Aide et al. (2003)[21]	47%	80%
Kang et al. (2004)[22]	60%	100%

RESTAGING OF RENAL CELL CARCINOMA WITH POSITRON EMISSION TOMOGRAPHY

Few studies have evaluated the role of PET in restaging RCC. Conventional imaging techniques like CT have limitations in detecting local recurrences in the nephrectomy bed and differentiating them from scarring, inflammation, or edema associated with surgery, radiation, or chemotherapy, or from benign disease. Early and accurate detection of locally recurrent disease while simultaneously ruling out distant metastases would have obvious therapeutic implications.

Safaei et al.[24] evaluated FDG-PET for restaging 36 patients with advanced RCC and demonstrated that PET provided staging information comparable to that obtained from CT, bone scans, and ultrasound. Overall, PET correctly classified the clinical stage in 89% patients with a sensitivity of 87% and a specificity of 100%. Twenty-five suspicious lesions in 20 patients were biopsied; PET accurately identified 84% of these lesions, yielding a sensitivity and specificity of 88% and 75%, respectively. In a retrospective study conducted by Ramdave et al.,[20] FDG-PET effectively confirmed the presence of renal bed recurrence in only two of eight patients in whom the CT was inconclusive. Positron emission tomography was able to differentiate local recurrence from post–radiation therapy changes in one patient. Kang et al.[22] reported a sensitivity of 75% and a specificity of 100% with FDG-PET for detecting renal bed recurrence or retroperitoneal lymph node metastases. The sensitivity and specificity of CT for the same lesions was 93% and 98%, respectively.

The reported results of PET for restaging of RCC are mixed. Overall, PET has modest accuracy and sensitivity in detecting local recurrences. In this scenario, the role of PET will largely be limited to the detection of distant metastases since the presence of metastatic disease would obviate surgical resection of any local recurrence. It is hoped that the improvement in PET technology and the advent of PET-CT will increase the diagnostic yield of PET in this setting.

EVALUATION OF DISTANT METASTASES WITH POSITRON EMISSION TOMOGRAPHY

Distant metastases are independent predictors of poor outcome in RCC.[18,19] One of the goals of using imaging studies in cancer staging is to improve diagnostic yield with a high degree of accuracy noninvasively, especially in the setting of advanced disease, while precluding the need for a tissue diagnosis. Presently available anatomic imaging techniques have limited accuracy for the detection of distant metastases. Positron emission tomography has been shown to be a sensitive imaging modality for the diagnosis of distant metastases from certain tumor sites, especially breast and lung cancers.[25,26] Until recently, the role of PET in the detection of distant metastases from RCC was not well established.

In a study conducted at the Cleveland Clinic, we investigated the role of FDG-PET in 24 patients with clear-cell RCC who underwent surgical resection of distant metastases.[27] Of the 36 sites resected, distant metastases from RCC were confirmed on histology in 33 sites (21 patients). Overall sensitivity of PET for detecting these lesions was 63.6% (21 of 33) while the specificity and positive predictive value was 100% (3 of 3) and 100% (21 of 21), respectively. The mean size of distant metastases in patients with true positive PET was 2.2 cm compared with 1.0 cm in patients with false-negative PET.

Sensitivity increased as a function of lesion size; it was 25% for lesions less than 1 cm versus 93% for lesions more than 2 cm (Figure 20.1).

Jadvar et al.[28] used FDG-PET to restage 25 patients with known or suspected metastatic RCC. They demonstrated modest diagnostic accuracy of PET in this setting and reported a sensitivity of 71%, specificity of 75%, accuracy of 72%, negative predictive value of 33%, and a positive predictive value of 94%.

In another study, Ramdave et al.[20] observed FDG-PET to accurately identify distant metastases from RCC in six of six patients; however, the presence of metastatic RCC was confirmed histologically in only one of these six patients. Positron emission tomography also picked up unsuspected metastatic disease not seen on CT in two of 17 patients undergoing staging workup for primary RCC.

Brouwers et al.[29] studied the role of FDG-PET scintigraphy in 20 patients with 112 sites of distant metastases followed clinically; PET detected 69% (77 of 112) of the metastatic lesions. Of these, 32 lesions had not been detected by CT. The overall sensitivity of PET and CT, however, was comparable (69% vs. 70%, respectively).

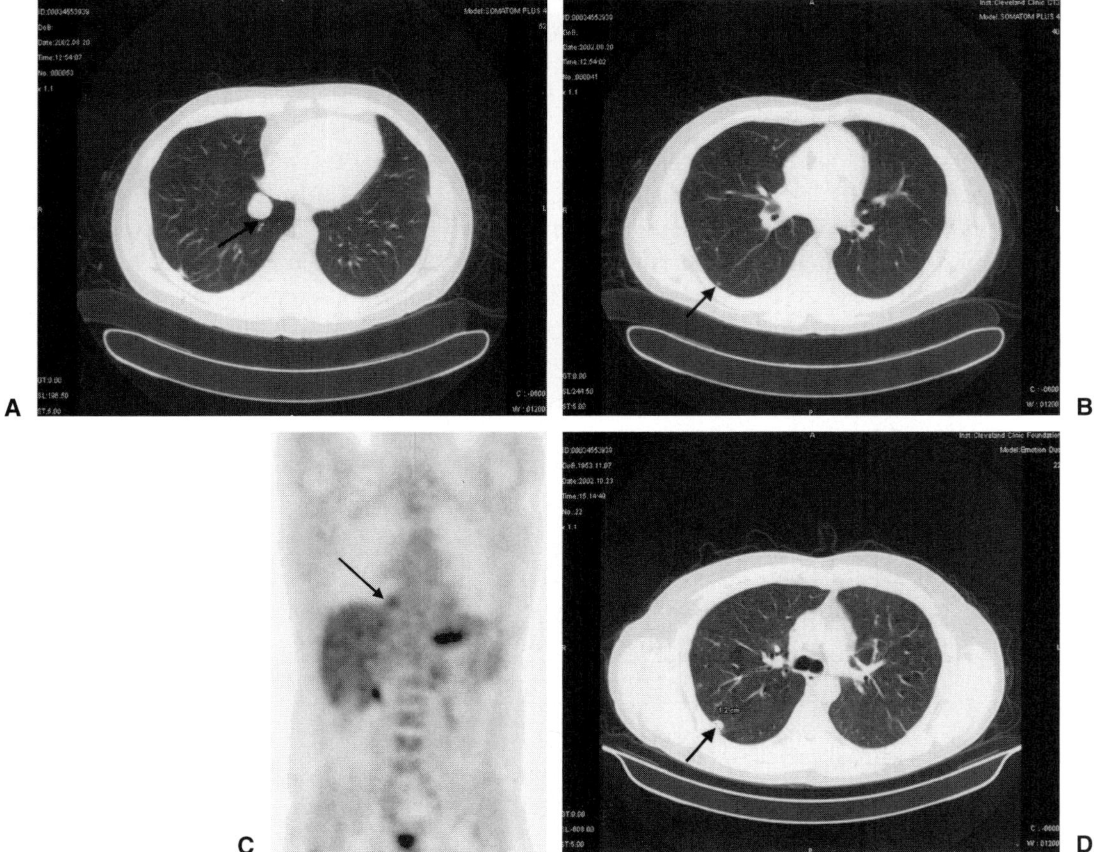

Figure 20.1. Computed tomography (CT) of the chest showing 2.5-cm (A) and 0.5-cm (B) lung nodules (arrow); only the right lower lobe nodule (arrow) was hypermetabolic on positron emission tomography (PET) (C). The subpleural nodule (arrow) had increased in size on repeat CT 2 months later (D). Pathologic evaluation of both nodules revealed metastatic renal cell carcinoma (RCC). (From Majhail et al.,[27] with permission.)

In one of the largest series reported to date, Kang et al.[22] assessed the diagnostic yield of FDG-PET imaging in RCC. Positron emission tomography detected 115 of 172 (66.9%) metastatic lesions. In almost 45% cases, PET failed to identify lesions detected by conventional imaging modalities. For pulmonary metastases, the sensitivity and specificity of PET was 75% and 97% compared to 91% and 73% for chest CT. Positron emission tomography had a sensitivity of 77% and specificity of 100% for detecting bone metastases compared to 94% and 87% for combined CT and bone scan.

In a prospective study of 53 patients conducted by Aide et al.,[21] the sensitivity and specificity of FDG-PET for detecting distant metastases was 100% and 93%, respectively, compared to a sensitivity of 80% and specificity of 91% with CT. Positron emission tomography detected all sites of distant metastases revealed by CT, and in addition picked up eight additional metastatic sites, leading to an accuracy of 94% versus 89% for CT. However, PET results altered the treatment plan in a relatively small proportion (9%) of patients.

Chang et al.[30] reported FDG-PET to be an accurate modality for characterizing indeterminate solitary lesions in 15 patients with RCC. Positron emission tomography correctly identified nine true-positive and four true-negative lesions; however, it failed to interpret one false-positive and one false-negative lesion. Using a standard uptake value (SUV) of more than 2.5 as the cutoff to diagnose malignancy, the sensitivity, specificity, and accuracy of PET in characterizing these lesions were 90%, 80%, and 87%, respectively.

To summarize, currently reported experience with FDG-PET suggests a limited role for this modality in detecting distant metastases from RCC (Table 20.2). In most cases, PET does not provide any additional information beyond that obtained by conventional anatomic imaging modalities. Although PET is not very sensitive for picking up metastatic disease, it can be used as an adjunct to conventional imaging in selected circumstances. Its relatively high specificity and positive predictive value in this setting suggest that it might be suitable for the evaluation of distant metastases not accurately characterized by anatomic radiologic imaging techniques, especially for lesions larger than 1.5 cm.

Table 20.2.
Positron emission tomography in the evaluation of metastatic renal cell carcinoma

Study	Sensitivity	Specificity
Ramdave et al. (2001)[20]	100%	100%
Brouwers et al. (2002)[29]	69%	—
Aide et al. (2003)[21]	100%	93%
Chang et al. (2003)[30]	90%	80%
Jadvar et al. (2003)[28]	71%	75%
Majhail et al. (2003)[27]	64%	100%
Kang et al.* (2004)[22]	75%	97%
Kang et al.# (2004)[22]	77%	100%

*Pulmonary metastases.
#Bone metastases.

POSITRON EMISSION TOMOGRAPHY–COMPUTED TOMOGRAPHY

One of the limitations of currently available PET technology is the difficulty in accurate anatomic localization of visualized functional abnormality. Moreover, nonspecific uptake of the radioisotope in organs such as the brain, heart, liver, and muscles and its excretion through the kidneys and urinary bladder make interpretation of abnormalities in these areas challenging. Complementing the detailed and high-resolution images obtained by conventional anatomic imaging modalities such as CT with physiologic information acquired by PET would have obvious advantages. Two approaches have been used for the fusion of anatomic and functional images: the software approach and the hardware approach. The former employs sophisticated software algorithms and uses specified anatomic landmarks to visually align images obtained from separate CT/magnetic resonance imaging (MRI) and PET scanners. Such an approach has the inherent limitations of temporal and spatial differences between the two sets of images because of patient positioning and internal organ movement.

The hardware approach to image fusion involves the use of a combined PET-CT and has rapidly evolved since the introduction of its first prototype in 1998.[31–33] Positron emission tomography–CT comprises a CT scanner placed in tandem with a PET scanner with a common table for patient positioning; image acquisition is performed within a short time span in a single imaging session, thereby minimizing motion artifacts with resultant accurately aligned anatomic and functional images. Besides dramatically decreasing scanning time and acquiring high-quality images, there is increasing evidence to suggest that PET-CT has greater diagnostic accuracy and provides additional staging information compared to PET alone and to visually correlated PET and CT.[34–37]

The experience with PET-CT in RCC is very limited, and further studies are needed to further define its role in the imaging of RCC. The fusion capability of PET-CT has the potential for improving localization of abnormalities in the urinary tract region that are currently difficult to evaluate by stand alone PET scanners.

OTHER FUNCTIONAL IMAGING TECHNIQUES

Besides PET, the repertoire of functional imaging modalities for oncology includes dynamic contrast-enhanced MRI (DCE-MRI), contrast-enhanced and Doppler ultrasound, x-ray contrast-enhanced dynamic CT, and optical imaging.[38–41] Dynamic contrast-enhanced MRI enables the noninvasive characterization of angiogenic and microcirculatory properties of lesions. Rapid diffusion property of a small contrasting molecule such as gadolinium–diethylenetriamine pentaacetic acid (Gd-DTPA) is used to visualize neo-angiogenesis, and this technique is being studied for assessment of response to therapy and in the development of newer antiangiogenic agents. The majority of these modalities are still investigational, and currently there is essentially no experience with their applicability in RCC.

FUTURE DIRECTIONS

The role of PET imaging in oncology is constantly evolving. Emerging indications include measurement of tumor grade and aggressiveness, assessment of response to therapy, in vivo imaging of drug action and pharmacokinetics, and molecular and functional evaluation of individual tumors. Positron emission tomography is also being studied as a technique to augment conventional anatomic imaging techniques in delineating treatment volumes for radiation therapy. All these are potential areas for investigation in RCC.

Though FDG is the most commonly used radioisotope for PET imaging, it is not specific for malignancy. Certain nonmalignant processes, such as granulomatous diseases, also take up glucose and FDG, albeit to a lesser extent; this can often confound image interpretation. Cancer-specific positron emitting radioisotopes other than FDG are being explored for functional imaging in oncology. F-18– and C-11–labeled thymidine and tyrosine analogue ligands are currently being investigated for tumor characterization at the molecular level for a variety of cancers.[42] Positron emission tomography using these novel radioisotopes would provide information regarding cellular proliferation and growth. F-18– and I-124–labeled nitroimidazole compounds, Cu-64–labeled selenosemicarbazones, and a variety of other F-18–, C-11–, C-15–, and O-15–labeled ligands are being studied for detecting and quantifying tumor hypoxia and angiogenesis.[43–45] Carbon-11 acetate has been reported to have promising activity in RCC.[46] The relatively short half-life of most radioisotopes other than those incorporating F-18 has been a major disadvantage; for example, the half-life of C-11 is 20 minutes compared to 110 minutes for F-18.

Molecular and functional imaging is also playing an integral role in the investigation of newer agents in cancer therapy. Increasing availability of techniques for imaging hypoxia and angiogenesis has provided the impetus for development of novel drugs. Positron emission tomography using F-18–, O-15–, and C-15–labeled analogues have been used in clinical trials of novel antiangiogenic agents in RCC to perform in vivo measurements of tumor and normal tissue perfusion.[47,48] Radioimmunoscintigraphy using PET (immuno-PET) is another exciting area of research; it combines the specific localization properties of a monoclonal antibody with the high resolution of PET. I-131–labeled monoclonal antibody G250, which recognizes a cell surface antigen expressed by human RCC, is currently under clinical development.[29,49,50]

Rapid advances are also being made in improving currently available PET technology. Positron emission tomography systems with shorter image acquisition times and better image resolution are under development, as are software for better image fusion between PET and CT images. Many centers have already adopted integrated PET-CT, which, as described earlier, has certain inherent advantages compared to stand-alone PET. New generation high-performance three-dimensional PET scanners are being developed to achieve high sensitivity and reduce patient imaging times.[51]

Currently available evidence largely suggests that PET has relatively low sensitivity in RCC, especially for small lesions. Positron emission tomography might have a role in further delineating suspicious lesions, particularly when results of other imaging studies are equivocal. The technique should be considered complementary to conventional anatomic imaging techniques and in selected situations may alleviate the need for biopsy; a negative result, however, does not rule out active malignancy. The advent of PET-CT will possibly increase the applicability and accuracy of PET in RCC, but more experience is needed, and its role currently remains under investigation.

REFERENCES

1. Wahl RL, Harney J, Hutchins G, Grossman HB. Imaging of renal cancer using positron emission tomography with 2-deoxy-2-(18F)-fluoro-D-glucose: pilot animal and human studies. J Urol 1991;146(6):1470–1474.

2. Kubota K. From tumor biology to clinical PET: a review of positron emission tomography (PET) in oncology. Ann Nucl Med 2001;15(6):471–486.

3. Bomanji JB, Costa DC, Ell PJ. Clinical role of positron emission tomography in oncology. Lancet Oncol 2001;2(3):157–164.

4. Rohren EM, Turkington TG, Coleman RE. Clinical applications of PET in oncology. Radiology 2004;231(2):305–332.

5. Younes M, Lechago LV, Somoano JR, Mosharaf M, Lechago J. Wide expression of the human erythrocyte glucose transporter Glut1 in human cancers. Cancer Res 1996;56(5):1164–1167.

6. Smith TA. Facilitative glucose transporter expression in human cancer tissue. Br J Biomed Sci 1999; 56(4):285–292.

7. Kurokawa T, Yoshida Y, Kawahara K, et al. Expression of GLUT-1 glucose transfer, cellular proliferation activity and grade of tumor correlate with [F-18]-fluorodeoxyglucose uptake by positron emission tomography in epithelial tumors of the ovary. Int J Cancer 2004;109(6):926–932.

8. Kato H, Takita J, Miyazaki T, et al. Correlation of 18–F-fluorodeoxyglucose (FDG) accumulation with glucose transporter (Glut-1) expression in esophageal squamous cell carcinoma. Anticancer Res 2003;23(4):3263–3272.

9. Yen TC, See LC, Lai CH, et al. 18F-FDG uptake in squamous cell carcinoma of the cervix is correlated with glucose transporter 1 expression. J Nucl Med 2004;45(1):22–29.

10. Higashi K, Ueda Y, Sakurai A, et al. Correlation of Glut-1 glucose transporter expression with. Eur J Nucl Med 2000;27(12):1778–1785.

11. Higashi T, Tamaki N, Torizuka T, et al. FDG uptake, GLUT-1 glucose transporter and cellularity in human pancreatic tumors. J Nucl Med 1998;39(10):1727–1735.

12. Chung JK, Lee YJ, Kim SK, Jeong JM, Lee DS, Lee MC. Comparison of [18F]fluorodeoxyglucose uptake with glucose transporter-1 expression and proliferation rate in human glioma and non-small-cell lung cancer. Nucl Med Commun 2004;25(1):11–17.

13. Hooft L, van der Veldt AA, van Diest PJ, et al. [18F]fluorodeoxyglucose uptake in recurrent thyroid cancer is related to hexokinase I expression in the primary tumor. J Clin Endocrinol Metab 2005;90(1): 328–334.

14. Bos R, van Der Hoeven JJ, van Der Wall E, et al. Biologic correlates of (18)fluorodeoxyglucose uptake in human breast cancer measured by positron emission tomography. J Clin Oncol 2002;20(2): 379–387.

15. Smith TA. FDG uptake, tumour characteristics and response to therapy: a review. Nucl Med Commun 1998;19(2):97–105.

16. Miyakita H, Tokunaga M, Onda H, et al. Significance of 18F-fluorodeoxyglucose positron emission tomography (FDG-PET) for detection of renal cell carcinoma and immunohistochemical glucose transporter 1 (GLUT-1) expression in the cancer. Int J Urol 2002;9(1):15–18.

17. Nagase Y, Takata K, Moriyama N, Aso Y, Murakami T, Hirano H. Immunohistochemical localization of glucose transporters in human renal cell carcinoma. J Urol 1995;153(3 pt 1):798–801.

18. Ficarra V, Righetti R, Pilloni S, et al. Prognostic factors in patients with renal cell carcinoma: retrospective analysis of 675 cases. Eur Urol 2002;41(2):190–198.

19. Tsui KH, Shvarts O, Smith RB, Figlin RA, deKernion JB, Belldegrun A. Prognostic indicators for renal cell carcinoma: a multivariate analysis of 643 patients using the revised 1997 TNM staging criteria. J Urol 2000;163(4):1090–1095; quiz 1295.

20. Ramdave S, Thomas GW, Berlangieri SU, et al. Clinical role of F-18 fluorodeoxyglucose positron emission tomography for detection and management of renal cell carcinoma. J Urol 2001;166(3): 825–830.

21. Aide N, Cappele O, Bottet P, et al. Efficiency of [(18)F]FDG PET in characterising renal cancer and detecting distant metastases: a comparison with CT. Eur J Nucl Med Mol Imaging 2003;30(9): 1236–1245.

22. Kang DE, White RL Jr, Zuger JH, Sasser HC, Teigland CM. Clinical use of fluorodeoxyglucose F 18 positron emission tomography for detection of renal cell carcinoma. J Urol 2004;171(5): 1806–1809.

23. Bachor R, Kotzerke J, Gottfried HW, Brandle E, Reske SN, Hautmann R. [Positron emission tomography in diagnosis of renal cell carcinoma]. Urologe A 1996;35(2):146–150.

24. Safaei A, Figlin R, Hoh CK, et al. The usefulness of F-18 deoxyglucose whole-body positron emission tomography (PET) for re-staging of renal cell cancer. Clin Nephrol 2002;57(1):56–62.

25. Byrne AM, Hill AD, Skehan SJ, McDermott EW, O'Higgins NJ. Positron emission tomography in the staging and management of breast cancer. Br J Surg 2004;91(11):1398–1409.

26. Birim O, Kappetein AP, Stijnen T, Bogers AJ. Meta-analysis of positron emission tomographic and computed tomographic imaging in detecting mediastinal lymph node metastases in nonsmall cell lung cancer. Ann Thorac Surg 2005;79(1):375–382.
27. Majhail NS, Urbain JL, Albani JM, et al. F-18 fluorodeoxyglucose positron emission tomography in the evaluation of distant metastases from renal cell carcinoma. J Clin Oncol 2003;21(21): 3995–4000.
28. Jadvar H, Kherbache HM, Pinski JK, Conti PS. Diagnostic role of [F-18]-FDG positron emission tomography in restaging renal cell carcinoma. Clin Nephrol 2003;60(6):395–400.
29. Brouwers AH, Dorr U, Lang O, et al. 131 I-cG250 monoclonal antibody immunoscintigraphy versus [18 F]FDG-PET imaging in patients with metastatic renal cell carcinoma: a comparative study. Nucl Med Commun 2002;23(3):229–236.
30. Chang CH, Shiau YC, Shen YY, Kao A, Lin CC, Lee CC. Differentiating solitary pulmonary metastases in patients with renal cell carcinomas by 18F-fluoro-2–deoxyglucose positron emission tomography—a preliminary report. Urol Int 2003;71(3):306–309.
31. Townsend DW, Carney JP, Yap JT, Hall NC. PET/CT today and tomorrow. J Nucl Med 2004;45(suppl 1):4S–14S.
32. Beyer T, Townsend DW, Brun T, et al. A combined PET/CT scanner for clinical oncology. J Nucl Med 2000;41(8):1369–1379.
33. Martinelli M, Townsend D, Meltzer C, Villemagne VV. 7. Survey of results of whole body imaging using the PET/CT at the University of Pittsburgh Medical Center PET facility. Clin Positron Imaging 2000;3(4):161.
34. Bar-Shalom R, Yefremov N, Guralnik L, et al. Clinical performance of PET/CT in evaluation of cancer: additional value for diagnostic imaging and patient management. J Nucl Med 2003;44(8): 1200–1209.
35. Lardinois D, Weder W, Hany TF, et al. Staging of non-small-cell lung cancer with integrated positron-emission tomography and computed tomography. N Engl J Med 2003;348(25):2500–2507.
36. Schoder H, Yeung HW, Gonen M, Kraus D, Larson SM. Head and neck cancer: clinical usefulness and accuracy of PET/CT image fusion. Radiology 2004;231(1):65–72.
37. Keidar Z, Haim N, Guralnik L, et al. PET/CT using 18F-FDG in suspected lung cancer recurrence: diagnostic value and impact on patient management. J Nucl Med 2004;45(10):1640–1646.
38. Knopp MV, von Tengg-Kobligk H, Choyke PL. Functional magnetic resonance imaging in oncology for diagnosis and therapy monitoring. Mol Cancer Ther 2003;2(4):419–426.
39. Sahani DV, Kalva SP, Hamberg LM, et al. Assessing Tumor Perfusion and Treatment Response in Rectal Cancer with Multisection CT: Initial Observations. Radiology 2005;234(3):785–792.
40. Montemurro F, Martincich L, De Rosa G, et al. Dynamic contrast-enhanced MRI and sonography in patients receiving primary chemotherapy for breast cancer. Eur Radiol 2005;15:1224–1233.
41. Martincich L, Montemurro F, De Rosa G, et al. Monitoring response to primary chemotherapy in breast cancer using dynamic contrast-enhanced magnetic resonance imaging. Breast Cancer Res Treat 2004;83(1):67–76.
42. Mankoff DA, Shields AF, Krohn KA. PET imaging of cellular proliferation. Radiol Clin North Am 2005;43(1):153–167.
43. Piert M, Machulla HJ, Picchio M, et al. Hypoxia-specific tumor imaging with 18F-fluoroazomycin arabinoside. J Nucl Med 2005;46(1):106–113.
44. McQuade P, Martin KE, Castle TC, et al. Investigation into (64)Cu-labeled Bis(selenosemicarbazone) and Bis(thiosemicarbazone) complexes as hypoxia imaging agents. Nucl Med Biol 2005; 32(2):147–156.
45. Rajendran JG, Krohn KA. Imaging hypoxia and angiogenesis in tumors. Radiol Clin North Am 2005;43(1):169–187.
46. Shreve P, Chiao PC, Humes HD, Schwaiger M, Gross MD. Carbon-11–acetate PET imaging in renal disease. J Nucl Med 1995;36(9):1595–1601.
47. Anderson H, Yap JT, Wells P, et al. Measurement of renal tumour and normal tissue perfusion using positron emission tomography in a phase II clinical trial of razoxane. Br J Cancer 2003; 89(2):262–267.
48. Lara PN, Jr, Quinn DI, Margolin K, et al. SU5416 plus interferon alpha in advanced renal cell carcinoma: a phase II California Cancer Consortium Study with biological and imaging correlates of angiogenesis inhibition. Clin Cancer Res 2003;9(13):4772–4781.

49. Divgi CR, O'Donoghue JA, Welt S, et al. Phase I clinical trial with fractionated radioimmunotherapy using 131I-labeled chimeric G250 in metastatic renal cancer. J Nucl Med 2004;45(8):1412–1421.
50. Divgi CR, Bander NH, Scott AM, et al. Phase I/II radioimmunotherapy trial with iodine-131–labeled monoclonal antibody G250 in metastatic renal cell carcinoma. Clin Cancer Res 1998;4(11): 2729–2739.
51. Lartizien C, Kinahan PE, Comtat C. A lesion detection observer study comparing 2–dimensional versus fully 3–dimensional whole-body PET imaging protocols. J Nucl Med 2004;45(4):714–723.

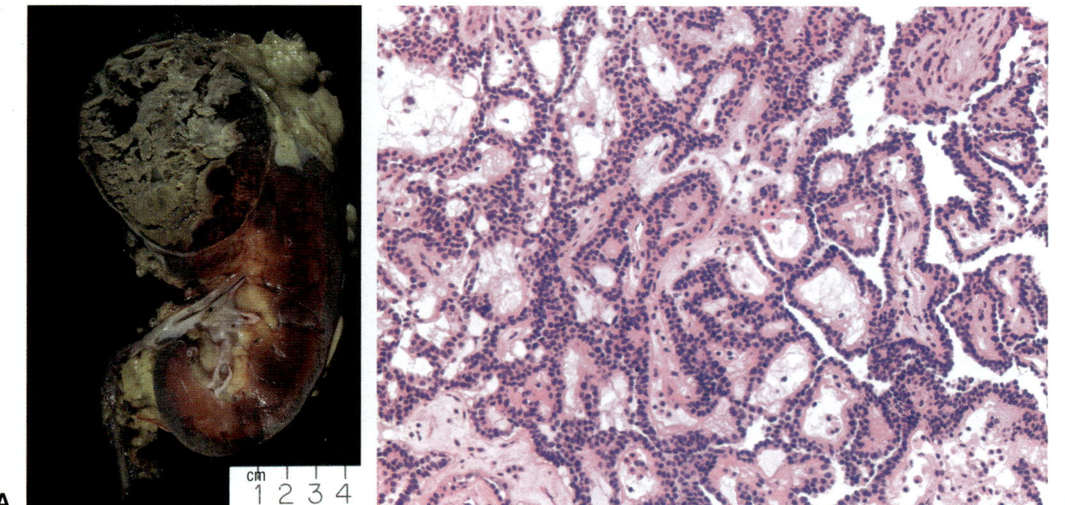

Figure 4.2. (A) Papillary renal cell carcinoma (PRCC) has a pseudocapsule and extensive hemorrhage and necrosis. (B) It is composed of papillae covered by a single layer of tumor cells with scant cytoplasm. The fibrovascular cores are expanded with foamy histiocytes.

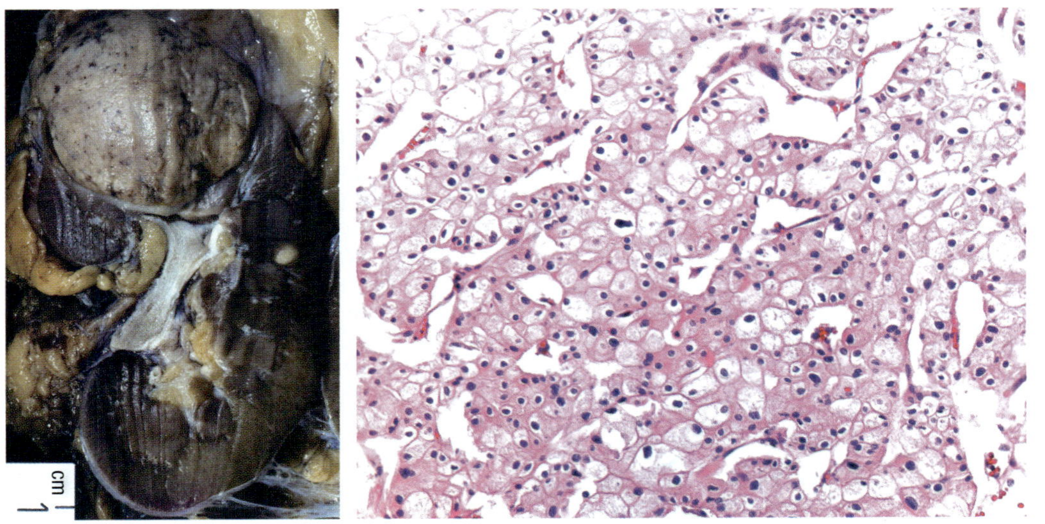

Figure 4.3. (A) Renal cell carcinoma, chromophobe type (ChRCC) forms a circumscribed, nonencapsulated mass with a homogeneous light brown cut surface. (B) The large and polygonal tumor cells have finely reticulated cytoplasm, prominent cell border, and irregular nuclei with perinuclear clearing.

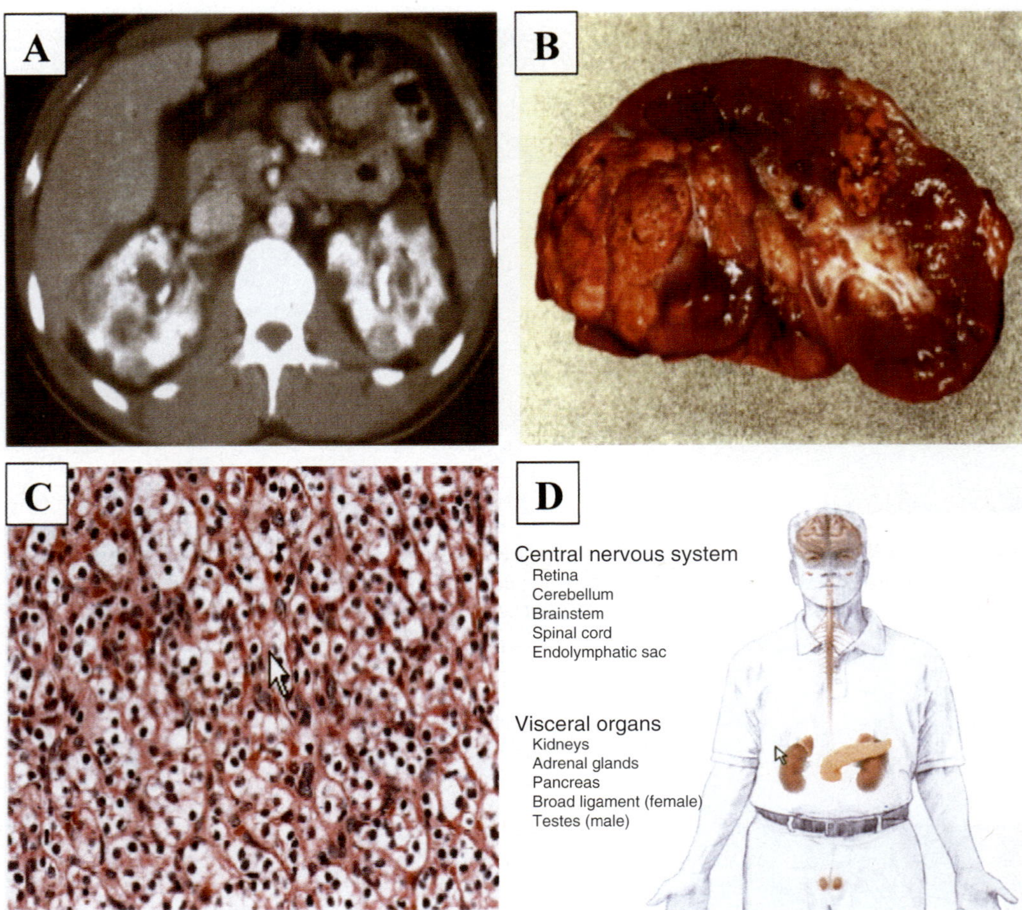

Figure 6.1. Phenotypic manifestations of von Hippel–Lindau (VHL). Renal masses are common in VHL patients. (A) Computed tomography (CT) scan of a VHL patient demonstrating characteristic bilateral multifocal renal lesions consisting of simple and complex cysts as well as enhancing solid masses. (B) Gross specimen removed from a VHL patient showing classic multiple golden-yellow tumors. (C) Hematoxylin and eosin (H&E) stain of a classic clear cell renal carcinoma found in patients with VHL. (D) In addition to renal manifestations, VHL affects organs systems throughout the body. (From Linehan WM, et al. Genetic Basis of Cancer of the Kidney: Disease-Specific Approaches to Therapy. 2004.)

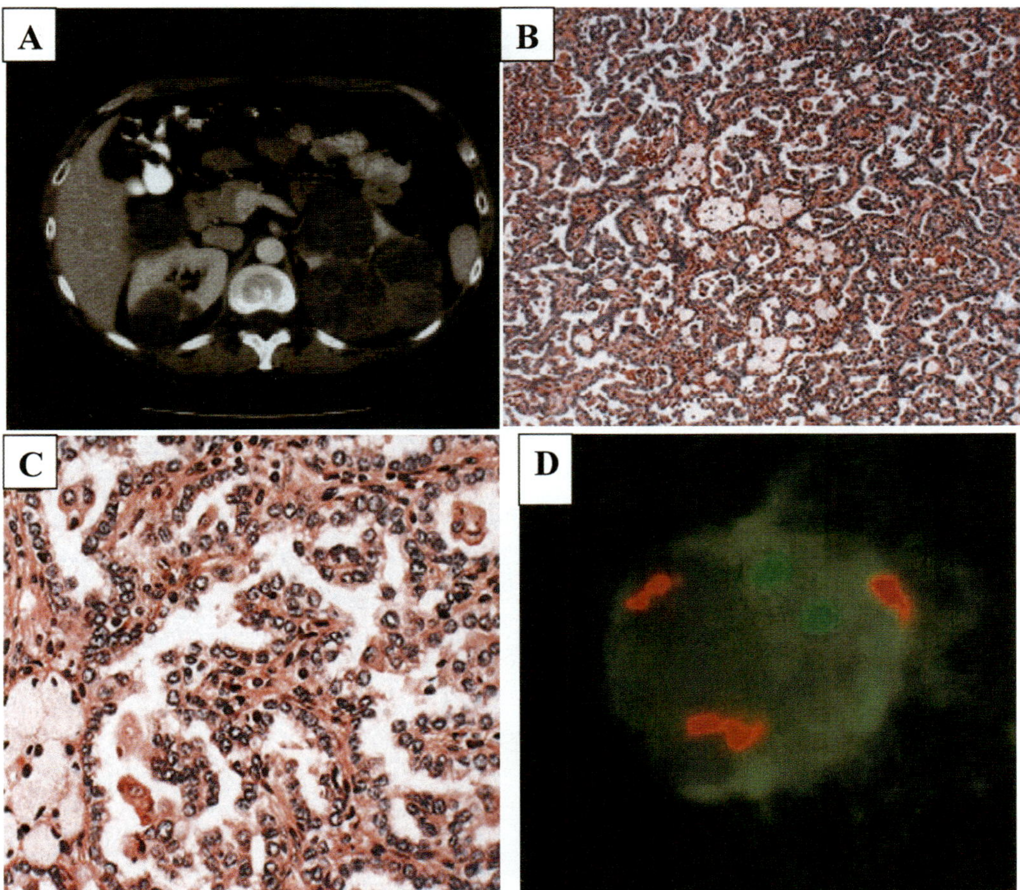

Figure 6.2. Manifestations and genetics of hereditary papillary renal cancer (HPRC). Patients with HPRC primarily develop bilateral multifocal renal masses. (A) Abdominal CT demonstrates HPRC tumors with characteristic poor enhancement on contrasted study that may frequently be mistaken for simple cysts. The tumors are best seen on late phase images of a contrast CT. Low (B) and high (C) power H&E stain of type I papillary renal cell carcinoma (RCC) seen in patients with HPRC. (D) Fluorescence in situ hybridization (FISH) using a MET probe demonstrating trisomy of chromosome 7 (red signal) in papillary type 1 RCC compared with chromosome 11 serving as control (green signal). (From Schmidt et al. Early Onset Hereditary Papillary Renal Carcinoma: Germline Missense Mutations in the Tyrocine Kinase Domain of the MET Proto-Oncogene. 2004.)

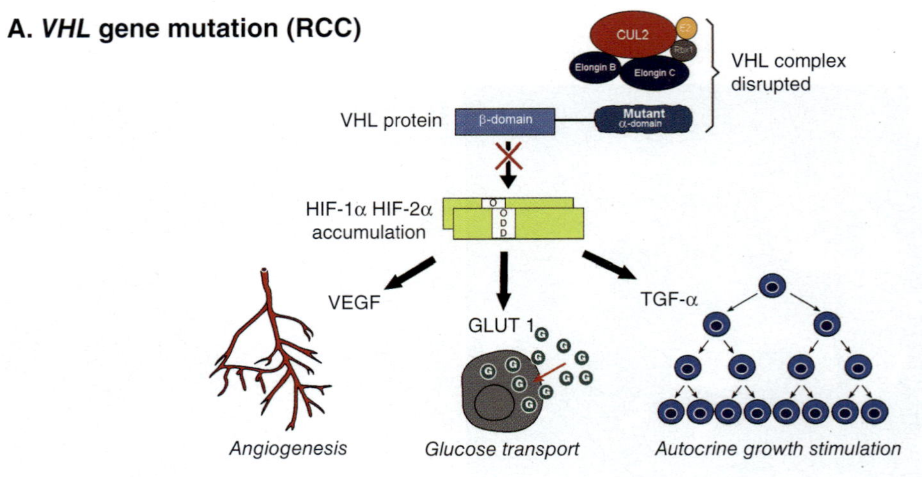

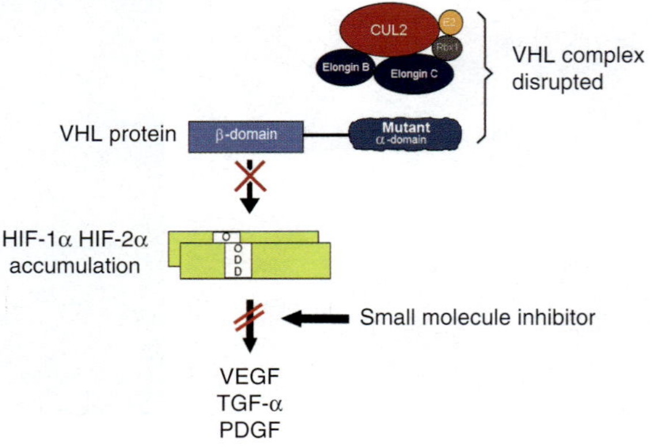

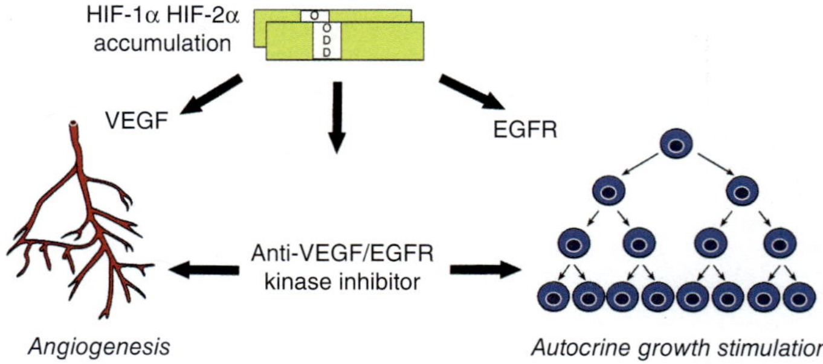

Figure 6.6. *VHL* gene mutation, downstream effects, and molecular targeting of the VHL pathway. (A) With a *VHL* gene mutation, the VHL complex is disrupted and allows for accumulation of HIF with subsequent activation of downstream pathways for angiogenesis, glucose transport, and growth. (B) Inhibition of overaccumulated HIF and prevention of downstream activation with a small molecule is one of the strategies for molecular targeting of the VHL/HIF pathway. (C) New tyrosine kinase inhibitors as well as direct vascular endothelial growth factor (VEGF) and platelet-derived growth factor (PDGF) receptor blockers are examples of downstream targeting. EGFR, epidermal growth factor receptor; TGF, transforming growth factor. (From Linehan WM, et al. Genetic Basis of Cancer of the Kidney: Disease-Specific Approaches to Therapy. 2004.)

21 Nephrectomy in Patients with Metastatic Renal Cell Carcinoma: *Clinical and Biologic Effects*

Bradley G. Orris and Robert C. Flanigan

KEYWORDS

NEPHRECTOMY
RENAL CELL CARCINOMA
METASTATIC RENAL CANCER
IMMUNOSUPPRESSION
SPONTANEOUS REGRESSION
IMMUNOTHERAPY

ABSTRACT

Up to one third of patients with renal cell carcinoma present with metastatic disease, and 20% to 40% of those with clinically localized disease eventually are found to have metastatic involvement. Prognosis continues to be poor for this population with a 2-year survival of only 10% to 30%; however, progress is being made. The role of surgery in those patients with advanced disease is currently being defined. There is a growing body of literature documenting the clinical effects of cytoreductive nephrectomy on patient outcomes. In addition, recent phase III trials have shown that nephrectomy prior to initiation of immunotherapy significantly improves survival in certain well-selected patients with metastatic renal call carcinoma (MRCC). Advances in our understanding of tumor-induced immune dysfunction have allowed greater insight into the biologic effects of nephrectomy on these patients, as well. Fortunately, there are new treatments for MRCC on the horizon, and nephrectomy will likely continue to play a role in these therapies as well.

BIOLOGIC EFFECTS OF NEPHRECTOMY FOR METASTATIC RENAL CELL CARCINOMA

It has been reported for over 30 years that RCC and other cancers cause immune dysfunction in the host.[1] Many different abnormalities have been described, including

From: *Clinical Management of Renal Tumors*
Edited by: R.M. Bukowski and A.C. Novick © Humana Press Inc., Totowa, NJ

dysfunction of various cellular elements of the immune system, as well as alterations in production of cytokines. The ability of removal of the primary tumor to reverse this immune dysfunction when metastatic disease is present is debatable; however, several studies have reported improved immune function with removal of the primary tumor. An extreme example of this is the phenomenon of spontaneous regression of metastatic deposits of RCC after removal or infarction of the primary tumor, which is likely a reflection of an increased immune reaction against the metastatic sites once the primary tumor is removed.

Immunosuppression from Renal Cell Carcinoma

Renal cell carcinoma continues to progress despite the fact that there are often significant numbers of tumor infiltrating lymphocytes (TILs) within the tumor. This phenomenon suggests that there is a local host immune response to the tumor, but that impairment of immune function prevents effective killing of tumor cells. The exact mechanism of immune system evasion by tumor cells is unknown at this time, and is a matter of much speculation and research. One possibility is that the host immune system becomes tolerant of the tumor antigens, likely via a tumor-induced activation of systems that diminish proinflammatory danger-signal production and sensing.[2] Another possibility is T-cell dysfunction rendering them unable to properly respond to malignant cells. Lymphocytes from patients with MRCC have been shown to have defective T-cell receptors,[3] increased apoptosis,[4,5] and defective signal transduction,[6,7] with TILs often showing greater dysfunction than peripheral blood lymphocytes.[8] Renal cell carcinoma has been shown to produce T-cell–inhibitory soluble products such as interleukin-8 (IL-8), IL-6, granulocyte-macrophage colony-stimulating factor (GM-CSF), tumor necrosis factor-α (TNF-α), IL-10, and transforming growth factor-β_1 (TGF-β_1), which interfere with the immunologic response.[9,10] Data have also shown increased numbers of immature myeloid cells that are able to suppress T-cell immune responses.[11,12]

Reversal of Immunosuppression by Surgery

The ability of surgical removal of the primary tumor to reverse immune system dysfunction has been studied in animal models. Danna et al.[13] investigated 4T1 mammary carcinoma, an established model for metastatic carcinoma in mice. They demonstrated suppression of antigen-specific antibody responses in tumor-bearing mice. These responses then returned to normal after resection of the primary tumor, despite the continued presence of metastatic disease. In addition, T-cell responses to inoculation with antigen were impaired in these tumor-bearing mice, but again returned to baseline after primary tumor resection. 4T1 tumors have been shown to secrete TGF-β, vascular endothelial growth factor (VEGF), and IL-10. The authors surmise that resection of the primary tumor shifts the cytokine balance, at least temporarily, away from immunosuppression, allowing the immune system to recover. Salvadori et al.[14] studied a fibrosarcoma tumor in a mouse model. After resection of the tumor, the abnormal phenotype of immune cells found in the spleen returned to normal, and there was normalization of some signal transduction pathways. Reinoculation of the mouse with the same tumor cells that were resected resulted in no new tumors developing due to a specific T-cell response. This was not a model of metastatic disease, but does show that tumor resection can promote a significant return of cellular immunity.

Several studies evaluating the beneficial effects of surgery on the immune system have been conducted in humans. Dadian et al.[15] evaluated various parameters of immune function in patients before and after undergoing nephrectomy. They noted increased immune responses and reversal of defects in natural killer (NK) cell activity and lymphokine-activated killer (LAK) activation after nephrectomy. Almand et al.[16] showed that removal of the tumor in patients with advanced but nonmetastatic head and neck, breast, or lung cancer considerably decreased the numbers of immunosuppressive immature myeloid cells in the blood within 3 to 4 weeks after surgery. They postulated that the abnormal numbers of these immature cells is caused by increased production of some soluble factor produced by the tumor such as GM-CSF, macrophage colony-stimulating factor (M-CSF), IL-6, or VEGF, and that removal of the primary tumor favorably decreases the number of these immunosuppressive cells. Uzzo et al.[17] evaluated defects in the intracellular transcription factor NF-κB that is important for development of T-cell immunity. Of 17 patients with RCC who had defective NF-κB binding activity preoperatively, six (35%) had reversal of this defect within 8 weeks of complete tumor removal. The authors also showed that soluble products derived from renal tumor explants could suppress NF-κB activation in T-cells from healthy volunteers in 23 of 34 cases.

Immunosuppression Caused by Surgery

While it is important to evaluate the beneficial effects that nephrectomy can have on reducing immunosuppression caused by the primary tumor, it is also important to review the deleterious effects that surgery can have on the immune system. Since various aspects of surgery temporarily decrease immunity, there could be rapid progression of metastatic disease in the period after surgery, or decreased response to adjuvant immunotherapy. Rapid tumor progression at metastatic sites after removal of the primary tumor, which has been reported in up to 33% of patients with MRCC, is a common cause of the inability to proceed to immunotherapy after nephrectomy.[18,19] Aspects of surgery that have been shown to decrease immunity include anesthesia and analgesic drugs, hypothermia, tissue damage, blood loss and transfusion, nociception, pain, and perioperative stress or anxiety.[20]

Many animal and human studies have been done to evaluate the effects of surgery on the immune system and metastatic disease. Eggermont et al.[21] demonstrated in a mouse model using melanoma and sarcoma cells that intraperitoneal surgical trauma could temporarily augment tumor growth and inhibit the effects of IL-2 and LAK cells on the tumor cells. It was theorized that this phenomenon was caused by peptide growth factors such as platelet-derived growth factor (PDGF), TGF-α, and TGF-β that are increased in the perioperative period. Ben-Eliyahu et al.[22] studied NK cell activity after surgical stress using a rat model with a variety of tumors. They demonstrated a decrease in resistance to tumors in the period immediately after intraperitoneal surgery that was mediated via decreased NK cell activity, as well as through other unknown mechanisms. Ogawa et al.[23] studied 20 patients undergoing surgery for stage I gastrointestinal cancers and showed decreased peripheral blood lymphocytes that started during surgery and lasted for at least 2 weeks after surgery. In addition, the T-helper-1 (Th1)/Th2 cell balance was changed with an increase in suppressor T cells, and a net suppression of host immunity. Increased levels of cortisol, adrenal corticosteroids, cytokines such as IL-6, and acute phase reactants such as immunosuppressive acidic protein (IAP) and

C-reactive protein (CRP) were theorized to be responsible for these changes in T-cell subsets and the resulting immunosuppression. Studies evaluating nephrectomy for RCC have shown an increase in the level of immunosuppressive cytokines IL-6 and IL-10 for several days after surgery when compared to patients undergoing extracorporeal shock-wave lithotripsy (ESWL) or nephrectomy for reasons other than cancer.[24]

Although the specific effects of nephrectomy on the immune system remain to be elucidated, there is strong evidence of a decrease in immunity at least in the immediate postoperative period. Techniques that may minimize these effects include evaluation and treatment for depression, maximizing pain control in the perioperative period, maintaining core body temperature during surgery, minimizing blood transfusions, and maximizing nutritional status.[25]

Surgery for eradication of a primary tumor is believed to promote progression of metastatic deposits for reasons other than a decrease in cell-mediated immunity.[20] Surgery can lead to a disruption of the tumor or its vascularity, causing release of tumor cells into the circulation.[26,27] Second, the primary tumor is believed to induce the release of angiogenesis inhibitors, which prevent small metastases from growing beyond a certain size. With resection of the primary tumor this inhibition of angiogenesis is removed, theoretically leading to increased growth of metastases.[28,29] This, however, has not been shown to date in humans with RCC.[30] It is also theorized that the release of growth factors due to surgery may promote the development of metastases elsewhere in the body.[31,32]

CLINICAL EFFECTS OF NEPHRECTOMY FOR METASTATIC RENAL CELL CARCINOMA

There are essentially five clinical scenarios in which to consider performing a nephrectomy in the presence of metastatic disease. The first situation is for possible palliation of symptoms that are related to the primary tumor. The second is in the hopes of provoking a spontaneous regression of the metastatic lesions. The third scenario is in the hopes of rendering the patient disease free by combining nephrectomy with complete metastectomy. The fourth reason for nephrectomy is for cytoreduction in combination with adjuvant immunotherapy in hopes of improving response to treatment and, therefore, survival. The final reason is to supply tumor cells and antigens for immunotherapy protocols.

Palliative Nephrectomy

Patients with metastatic RCC may be debilitated with symptoms directly related to their primary tumor.[33] Flank pain, persistent hemorrhage, and large arteriovenous malformations leading to high-output heart failure and hypertension have all been reported, but fortunately are uncommon manifestations of advanced local disease. Although nephrectomy has been advocated as a treatment for all of these conditions, it is rarely necessary considering the effectiveness of less invasive treatments. Most patients with hematuria can be managed by angioembolization, and intractable flank pain can often be managed by more intensive efforts in pain management in coordination with pain specialists. It is important to remember the poor overall survival of patients in this group when considering the morbidity of a surgical procedure simply for palliation.

Renal cell carcinoma is also known to cause a number of debilitating paraneoplastic syndromes such as hypercalcemia, fever, hepatic dysfunction (Stauffer syndrome), and erythrocytosis. While nephrectomy may sporadically be necessary for treatment of these conditions, paraneoplastic symptoms are also often produced by metastatic disease.[34] Walther and associates[35] reported that nephrectomy for hypercalcemia in advanced RCC caused reduction of calcium levels in only seven of 12 patients, with median survival remaining short in either group, and limited to only 6 months.

In general, palliative nephrectomy alone for MRCC without subsequent systemic therapy does not improve survival, and has a significant chance of causing morbidity or death.[36] Nephrectomy should only be undertaken in the rare patient where more conservative measures have been unable to adequately control symptoms from the primary tumor, and when the surgeon feels that surgery has a good chance of alleviating those symptoms.

Spontaneous Regression

One of the more fascinating aspects of RCC is the occasional occurrence of spontaneous regression or stabilization of metastatic lesions. This is typically thought to be due to immunologic host-mediated cytotoxicity against the lesions, although this remains unproven. Spontaneous regression of distant metastases in RCC has been estimated to occur in 0.4% to 0.8% of patients.[37] Spontaneous regression nearly always follows nephrectomy or some other treatment of the primary tumor such as radiofrequency ablation,[38] angioembolization, or radiation. Of 51 cases of spontaneous regression reviewed by Freed and associates,[39] 45 involved pulmonary lesions. The duration of regression was not given, but it was indicated that some cases had greater than 20 years of follow-up without evidence of recurrence. The National Cancer Institute (NCI) reported a much higher rate of spontaneous regression than previous series. They reported that four of 91 total patients experienced complete regression of metastatic disease after cytoreductive nephrectomy, prior to immunotherapy. The mean time of regression was 24.3 months and pulmonary-only metastases were present in all four patients.[40] They noted that their group of patients was younger, and had a better performance status than most patients with MRCC. It is important to note that regression of RCC metastases is a real phenomenon, but that many reported cases have not involved biopsy proven lesions, which may instead have been old granulomas, fungal lesions, or pulmonary infarcts. Since spontaneous regression of metastases is such a rare and unpredictable event, it alone is not considered a valid indication for nephrectomy.

Metastectomy at the Time of Nephrectomy

Several reports have described the potential benefit of nephrectomy with simultaneous or subsequent resection of all identifiable metastatic disease when solitary or low-volume metastatic disease is present. Unfortunately, these potentially curable patients only represent an estimated 1.6% to 3.6% of patients diagnosed with metastatic RCC.[41,42] Patients with synchronous metastases removed at the time of nephrectomy are less likely to do well than those with recurrence after nephrectomy. O'Dea et al.[43] reported on 44 patients undergoing surgery for solitary metastases. Of 18 patients with synchronous metastases, there was only one survivor at 5 years compared to 26 patients with metachronous metastases who had a 50% 5-year survival rate. Tolia and Whitmore[44] reported on 15 patients undergoing complete metastectomy at the time of nephrectomy, with a 5-year overall survival of 20%.

Patient selection is paramount in achieving long-term cures in patients undergoing nephrectomy with metastectomy. Patients most likely to benefit are those with solitary or pulmonary-only metastatic foci and good performance status. Most studies indicate that a disease-free interval after nephrectomy greater than 1 year is also associated with a better outcome.[41,44,45] Recurrences after initial metastectomy should not preclude further attempts at curative resection if the surgeon feels that complete resection is possible and performance status remains good.[45]

Cytoreductive Nephrectomy

Previously, the most effective systemic treatment for metastatic renal cell carcinoma was cytokine-based immunotherapy, but it has now been replaced by agents such as sunitinib and sorafenib. The role of nephrectomy in this treatment paradigm, either before or after system therapy, remains a controversial topic. Two randomized prospective trials suggest an advantage to preimmunotherapy cytoreductive nephrectomy in appropriately selected patients.[46,47]

RATIONALE FOR CYTOREDUCTIVE NEPHRECTOMY

There are several proposed rationales for performing a cytoreductive nephrectomy prior to immunotherapy for MRCC. It is postulated that removal of the primary tumor (and its production of cytokines and other soluble factors) could decrease the immunosuppressive effects of the cancer, allowing the immune system to eradicate a relatively smaller volume of residual disease, especially in combination with biologic response modifiers (BRMs) such as IL-2 and interferon-α (IFN-α). Nephrectomy also prevents further shedding of tumor cells into the blood supply, which may result in additional metastases, and prevents complications of locally advanced disease or paraneoplastic syndromes during immunotherapy. Patients may also improve their performance status after removal of the primary tumor, leading to potentially better response to immunotherapy.

Another rationale for up-front cytoreductive nephrectomy is that the primary tumor in MRCC rarely responds to systemic immunotherapy, even when there is significant regression of metastases. The NCI reported on a series of 51 patients who were not candidates for nephrectomy prior to the initiation of IL-2–based systemic therapy, and noted an overall response rate of only 6% with no significant responses seen in the primary tumor.[48] In a report by Sella and associates,[49] of 17 patients undergoing nephrectomy after response to IFN-α–based immunotherapy, 15 patients (88%) had viable tumor present in the nephrectomy specimens. Rackley et al.[50] also reported on three of 25 patients (12%) demonstrating a response to initial BRM therapy. Those three patients underwent subsequent nephrectomy, and significant residual tumor burden was demonstrated in the kidneys of all three patients.

Finally, multiple retrospective reports on immunotherapy for RCC have shown prior nephrectomy to be a positive prognostic factor independent of other well-recognized factors such as performance status and site or burden of disease.[51–56]

RETROSPECTIVE STUDIES

A number of retrospective series have examined preimmunotherapy cytoreductive nephrectomy (Table 21.1). Unfortunately, these studies all are subject to the selection

Table 21.1.
Cytoreductive nephrectomy in preparation for immunotherapy: retrospective studies

Author	No. of patients	Surgical mortality (%)	Unable to receive postoperative BMR therapy	Overall response (%)	Complete response (%)	Partial response (%)	Median survival (months)
Rackley et al. (1994)[50]	37	1 (2.7)	8 (21.6)	3 (8.1)	0 (0.0)	3 (8.1)	12
Wolf et al. (1994)[91]	23	0 (0.0)	6 (26.1)	3 (13.0)	2 (8.7)	1 (4.3)	23.5
Bennett et al. (1995)[18]	30	5 (17)	23 (76.6)	4 (13.3)	3 (10.0)	1 (3.3)	—
Fallick et al. (1997)[58]	28	1 (3.6)	2 (7.1)	11 (39.3)	5 (17.9)	6 (21.4)	20.5
Walther et al. (1997)[19]	195	2 (1.0)	74 (37.9)	19 (17.8)	4 (3.7)	15 (14.0)	—
Figlin et al. (1997)[82]	62	0 (0.0)	7 (11.3)	19 (34.5)	5 (9.1)	14 (25.5)	22
Levy et al. (1998)[92]	66	2 (3.0)	3 (4.5)	—	—	—	—
Tigrani et al. (2000)[93]	63	2 (3.2)	17 (27)	—	—	—	17.8
Wood et al. (2001)[66]	126	2 (1.6)	5 (4)	—	—	—	11.9
Total	630	15/630 (2.4)	145/630 (23.0)	59/375 (15.7)	19/375 (5.1)	40/375 (10.7)	

bias inherent in retrospective reviews, making analysis of their conclusions difficult. The largest series reported is from the NCI and included 195 patients with MRCC who underwent nephrectomy with resection of adjacent or contiguous metastases prior to undergoing IL-2 therapy.[57] The overall response rate in this series was 18%, including 4% complete responses and 14% partial responses, which is similar to what one would expect from immunotherapy alone. In this series 38% of patients were unable to undergo treatment with IL-2 secondary to rapid postoperative progression of tumor, postoperative complications, or a debilitated state. There was a 1% mortality rate in this series. Other smaller series have reported mixed results with cytoreductive nephrectomy (Table 21.1) with response rates varying between 8% and 39%. The number of patients unable to receive systemic therapy after nephrectomy varies as well from 4% to 77% and mortality rates from 0% to 17%. Variability in patient selection including the distribution of those patients with good versus poor performance status, limited versus extensive metastases, and location of metastases most likely accounts for these conflicting results.

A report by Bennett et al.[18] represents the poorest reported outcomes for cytoreductive nephrectomy in terms of surgical morbidity, mortality, and the inability to receive postoperative systemic therapy. A 17% operative mortality rate was reported, and 77% of patients were unable to receive systemic immunotherapy after surgery. Certainly patient selection was at least partially the cause of these poor outcomes. In this series almost one third of patients had brain metastases, 43% had bony metastases, and 37% had hepatic metastases. Of the 30 patients in this series, only two were Eastern Cooperative Oncology Group (ECOG) performance status 0, 24 were ECOG status 1, and four were ECOG status 2. This study emphasizes the risks of poor patient selection when considering cytoreductive nephrectomy.

Fallick et al.[58] in 1997 identified several criteria felt to be predictive of good outcome after cytoreductive nephrectomy and applied these to all patients in the series with metastatic RCC. The criteria included (1) absence of central nervous system, bone, or liver metastases; (2) ECOG performance status of 0 or 1; (3) the possibility of greater than 75% tumor debulking; and (4) predominantly clear cell histology on any biopsies of the tumor. Using these criteria, only 28 patients out of a total of 85 candidates were felt to be suitable for cytoreductive nephrectomy. There were no perioperative deaths or complications that prevented further systemic therapy, and only a single patient had progression of disease requiring withholding of systemic therapy in this series. The overall response rate was 39%, including five complete and six partial responses, with a median survival of 20.5 months in the entire group.

Because of the morbidity involved with nephrectomy, and the possibility of disease progression during recovery, some groups have investigated combining cytoreductive nephrectomy with laparoscopic techniques. In one report, Walther et al.[59] compared treatment groups of open nephrectomy, hand-assisted laparoscopic nephrectomy, and pure laparoscopic nephrectomy with tissue morcellation. The median number of days required before onset of immunotherapy was 67 days (range 50–151 days) in the 19 patients undergoing open nephrectomy, 60 days (47–63 days) in the five hand-assisted laparoscopic patients, and only 37 days (34–57 days) in the six pure laparoscopic patients. The morbidity of laparoscopic nephrectomy was comparable to traditional open nephrectomy, and the procedure, including tissue morcellation, was feasible even for large tumors. In a larger subsequent report of 31 patients undergoing attempted laparoscopic nephrectomy, however, the same group showed the potential difficulties of this operation.[60] Eleven cases required open conversion, and blood loss was much higher (750–3000 mL) than is typically expected from laparoscopic nephrectomy. Only 18 patients proceeded to immunotherapy postoperatively.

The group from the Cleveland Clinic also recently reported on their experience with laparoscopic cytoreductive nephrectomy.[61] The group retrospectively compared 22 patients undergoing laparoscopic cytoreductive surgery to a contemporary cohort of 25 consecutive patients undergoing laparoscopic nephrectomy for large (greater than 7 cm) nonmetastatic tumors. The length of surgery, estimated blood loss, overall complication rate, and length of stay (LOS) were similar between the two groups. There were more blood transfusions in the group with metastatic disease (3 vs. 0), but this was attributed to increased preoperative anemia rather than to increased blood loss. There were no conversions to open surgery or major complications in either group. Median length of time until initiation of immunotherapy was 35 days, but only eight patients (36%) went on to receive immunotherapy, mainly due to progressive disease. Local invasion, obliteration of tissue planes, significant perihilar lymphadenopathy, and enhanced vascularity have all been noted to increase the difficulty of this procedure. While the role of laparoscopy is still being refined in cytoreductive nephrectomy, it seems clear that this will be used at centers with extensive laparoscopic experience and for patients who are properly selected and counseled.

Cytoreductive nephrectomy has also been studied in the setting of locally advanced MRCC including extension to the renal vein and inferior vena cava (IVC). In fact, both the Southwest Oncology Group (SWOG) and European Organization for the Research and Treatment of Cancer (EORTC) phase III trials allowed inclusion of patients with IVC thrombus below the hepatic veins.[46,47] Slaton et al.[62] retrospectively reviewed 15 patients who underwent nephrectomy and caval thrombectomy with concurrent metastases. There were two reexplorations for postoperative hemorrhage, but no perioperative deaths were reported. Median time to initiation of postoperative immunotherapy was 48 days for the six patients in whom it was planned (other patients had pre- and postoperative immunotherapy, or resection of metastases only as adjuvant therapy). In another series, 105 patients with metastatic RCC and renal vein thrombus (51 patients) or IVC thrombus (54 patients) undergoing nephrectomy were reported.[63] Comparison was made to a group of nonmetastatic RCC patients with renal vein or IVC involvement. Early postoperative complications and mortality were not significantly different in patients undergoing thrombectomy with or without the presence of metastases. When comparing patients with MRCC undergoing nephrectomy with thrombectomy to those without tumor thrombus undergoing nephrectomy ($n = 171$), both groups were also able to complete timely immunotherapy equally often. Excellent performance status is critical for success with these extensive resections. Careful screening for cardiovascular and cerebrovascular disease is recommended, particularly if cardiopulmonary bypass and hypothermic circulatory arrest will be required.

EMBOLIZATION PRIOR TO CYTOREDUCTIVE NEPHRECTOMY

The combination of preoperative renal embolization followed several days later by delayed nephrectomy has also been reported. The speculation is that tumor antigens released from the tumor may provide a powerful stimulus to host immune responses. An early report of 100 patients followed for at least 12 months showed a 28% overall response rate, complete response in seven patients, greater than 50% regression in eight patients, and prolonged disease stabilization in 13.[64] Unfortunately, a multiinstitutional SWOG study failed to validate these results.[65] Thirty patients were followed for 1 year or longer. There were no complete responders and only one partial response that lasted 21 months. The overall 1-year survival rate was 28% and median survival was 7 months. Patients in both studies were given medroxyprogesterone therapy after the nephrectomy. Significant side effects associated with renal embolization included pain, nausea, vomiting, diarrhea, fever, ileus, and inadvertent embolization of other peripheral vessels. Embolization, therefore, should be reserved for palliative efforts, and for patients with very large tumors or potentially difficult hilar dissection as an aid to nephrectomy.

PROGNOSTIC FACTORS FOR CYTOREDUCTIVE NEPHRECTOMY

Due to the variable response to cytoreductive nephrectomy and immunotherapy, several investigators have tried to identify pretherapy characteristics that predict good response to therapy. Wood et al.[66] evaluated 126 consecutive patients undergoing cytoreductive nephrectomy and found that LOS after nephrectomy, tumor grade, preoperative white blood cell (WBC) count, and partial thromboplastin time (PTT) were significant predictors of survival after cytoreductive nephrectomy. They concluded that pretherapy biopsy may be warranted to rule out high-grade tumors such as sarcomatoid variants, which may exclude a patient from nephrectomy. If radiologic findings suggest the possibility of a collecting duct carcinoma with metastases, a preoperative biopsy may also be useful, as these patients have a very poor prognosis regardless of nephrectomy.[67] Slaton and associates[68] have reported that patients with metastatic RCC involving multiple organs, particularly the liver or central nervous system, are at high risk for death during the first 6 months following nephrectomy and are less likely to be palliated by the surgery.

Han et al.[69] from University of California–Los Angeles also retrospectively analyzed factors that predict response to cytoreductive nephrectomy, and found that patients with lung-only or bone-only metastases who underwent cytoreductive nephrectomy followed by immunotherapy had a median survival of 31 months, compared with a 13-month median survival ($p = .001$) in patients with multiple metastatic sites undergoing nephrectomy and immunotherapy. They concluded that patients with bone-only metastases, while less common than those with lung-only or multiple metastatic sites, fare relatively well with cytoreductive nephrectomy followed by immunotherapy and that those with multiple metastatic sites do poorly overall. Interestingly, only 30% of patients with bone-only metastases (10/33 patients) underwent cytoreductive nephrectomy followed by immunotherapy compared to 68% of patients who had lung-only metastases. This likely reflects the bias of medical oncologists and urologists that patients with bony disease do worse than patients with other sites of disease, and introduces significant selection bias into their review.

In another analysis of the same UCLA database, 236 patients with metastatic disease and no lymphadenopathy (N0M1) were compared to 86 patients with distant metastases and concomitant lymph node disease (N+M1).[70] Of those who underwent postnephrectomy immunotherapy, objective response rates were 30% for the N0M1 group, and only 11% for the N+M1 group. N+M1 patients not undergoing immunotherapy had the worst prognosis with an overall median survival of 4.5 months, which was not significantly different ($p = .18$) from N+M1 patients who underwent immunotherapy (overall median survival 10.8 months). This supports the findings of an analysis of 154 patients with MRCC at the NCI undergoing nephrectomy prior to IL-2–based therapy in which median survival in lymph node positive patients (8.5 months) was found to be significantly inferior to that of lymph node negative patients (15 months).[71]

Others have analyzed serum immunologic markers such as CRP in an effort to predict response to cytoreductive nephrectomy.[72] In patients with normal preoperative CRP, levels of serum immunosuppressive acidic protein and NK cell activity did not differ significantly before and after nephrectomy. In contrast, patients with an elevated CRP preoperatively had significantly elevated serum immunosuppressive acidic protein, which dropped significantly postoperatively. These patients also had significantly decreased NK cell activity preoperatively that increased significantly postoperatively. The authors concluded that those patients with elevated CRP preoperatively may benefit the most from cytoreductive nephrectomy followed by immunotherapy.

Tumor markers that can be evaluated after biopsy or nephrectomy such as carbonic anhydrase IX (CA IX) and Ki67 are being evaluated for their prognostic significance.[73] Although they may predict overall prognosis, or response to immunotherapy, their role in selection of patients for nephrectomy is unknown at this time.

As knowledge of the genetics and molecular biology of RCC continues to advance, it is hoped that it will be possible to tailor treatment to each individual patient and tumor. Likely, some patients will be identified who will benefit from upfront cytoreductive nephrectomy, while other patients will be better served with a different initial strategy.

PROSPECTIVE PHASE III TRIALS

The variable results found from multiple retrospective trials of cytoreductive nephrectomy served as a stimulant for subsequent randomized, prospective phase III trials to evaluate cytoreductive nephrectomy. Recently, SWOG trial 8949 and EORTC trial 30947 were reported.[46,47,74] Both trials used an identical treatment protocol designed by SWOG. These trials provide the best information to date regarding the utility of cytoreductive nephrectomy. The eligibility criteria for these trials included a histologically confirmed diagnosis of metastatic renal cancer (biopsy of the primary tumor or metastatic foci was allowed), a primary tumor that was considered resectable by the attending physician (IVC thrombus below the hepatic veins and regional lymphadenopathy were allowed), an ECOG performance status of 0 or 1, and no history of prior treatment with chemotherapy, hormonal therapy, IL-2, IFN, LAK cells, or other BRMs. In addition, prior or concomitant radiation therapy to the primary tumor or to metastatic sites was not allowed, and a serum bilirubin level no higher than three times the upper limit of normal at each institution and a serum creatinine no higher than 3.0 mg/dL were required. Patients were randomly assigned to nephrectomy followed by IFN-α_{2b}, or IFN-α_{2b} alone.

The results for the two trials and a combined analysis are shown in Table 21.2. Both trials demonstrated significantly longer overall survival in the groups randomized to nephrectomy prior to immunotherapy, and this benefit persisted across all study stratifications including performance status, site of metastasis, and measurable versus nonmeasurable disease. There was a single perioperative death in each of the series after nephrectomy, and overall less than 6% of patients did not receive immunotherapy in the group randomized to nephrectomy plus IFN. Interestingly, despite the increased

Table 21.2.
Phase III trials of interferon-α_{2b} versus interferon-α_{2b} with nephrectomy

	No. of patients	Median survival (months)			Response to therapy (%)			Unable to receive postsurgery immunotherapy (%)	Operative mortality (%)
		Interferon	Surgery + inteferon	p	Interferon	Surgery + interferon	p		
SWOG 8949 (2001)[46]	241	8.1	11.1	.05	3.3	3.6	NS	NR	1 (0.8)
EORTC 30947 (2001)[47]	85	7	17	.03	12	19	.38	NR	1 (2.4)
Combined analysis[74]	331	7.8	13.6	.002	5.7	6.9	.60	9 (5.6)	2 (1.4)

NS, not significant; NR, not reported.

survival, there were no differences in response rates between the control and nephrectomy groups, and there was also a large discrepancy in response rates between the two studies. Patients with a performance status of 0 had a significantly longer survival than patients with a performance status of 1. Both studies clearly demonstrated that nephrectomy can be performed safely with little chance of interfering with the subsequent ability to receive immunotherapy. Unfortunately, the overall median survival was only 13.6 months, with a benefit of only 5.8 months for the nephrectomy group. While it seems likely based on retrospective studies that the use of a more effective immunotherapeutic agent, such as IL-2, would enhance survival in this population, we will have to wait for prospective studies to answer this question definitively.[75]

As stated earlier, an improved response rate in the nephrectomy arms of these two trials was not found, while a survival advantage was demonstrated. How might this be explained? One interesting theory recently put forth is that the enhanced survival of patients after cytoreductive nephrectomy could be due to postoperative azotemia from resection of the kidney, and not through any immune system basis at all.[76] Mathematical models of malignant invasion based on tumor-induced toxicity in adjacent normal tissue have been proposed. These models suggest that mild systemic acidosis caused by resection of functioning nephrons can alter the microenvironment in the tumor and peritumoral normal tissue sufficiently to reduce tumor growth rate and prolong survival. This hypothesis was tested by retrospectively reviewing the patient data from the SWOG 8949 trial. In patients with no postoperative renal dysfunction, the median survival was only 4 months compared to 17 months in those with a postoperative elevation of BUN and creatinine. Unfortunately, information regarding systemic pH, serum electrolytes, and other clinical information was unavailable due to the retrospective nature of the review, which limits the conclusions that can be drawn. Obviously if these results can be confirmed, they suggest a broad new range of therapies for tumors beyond just RCC.

NEPHRECTOMY OR METASTECTOMY AFTER RESPONSE TO SYSTEMIC IMMUNOTHERAPY

In contrast to nephrectomy prior to initiation of BMR therapy, there are some clinicians who feel that surgery should be reserved for those who demonstrate a significant response to immunotherapy. The advantage to this strategy is the avoidance of the morbidity, mortality, and cost associated with nephrectomy. As reviewed previously, there is also evidence that surgery itself can cause immunosuppression and decreased response to adjuvant immunotherapy.[21]

To elucidate whether there is a benefit to surgical resection of disease after response to systemic therapies, several studies have been undertaken. One of the first reports was by Fleischmann and Kim[77] in 1991. Ten patients with metastatic RCC were given IL-2–based immunotherapy, and three had complete regression of disease outside the abdomen. Two of these patients were subsequently rendered disease free after surgical resection of the renal primary or a retroperitoneal recurrence, and remained disease free after surgery for 9 and 18 months, respectively. Surgical specimens revealed less than 1% viable tumor. Another multiinstitution study reviewed 399 patients from 14 institutions who underwent IL-2 therapy, with or without LAK cell therapy.[78] Sixty-two patients (15.5%) demonstrated either a complete response (18 patients, 4.5%) or partial response (44 patients, 11.0%). Of these, 11 patients underwent resection of residual tumor in the lung, kidney, retroperitoneum, or pelvis. At a median follow-up of 21 months, all 11 patients remained alive without evidence of disease. In contrast, among patients who did not receive surgery after immunotherapy, only 14/18 patients (78%) with complete response and 15/33 (45%) with a partial response (PR) remained free of disease progression.

Rackley et al.[50] reported on 62 patients, 37 of whom underwent nephrectomy prior to immunotherapy and 25 who were enrolled for adjuvant nephrectomy if a response to immunotherapy was seen. Only three of the 25 responded to immunotherapy and underwent nephrectomy, and two of those patients remained alive after 18 and 42 months of follow-up. In this series, the initial nephrectomy group had an 8% response rate and a 12-month median survival, whereas the initial immunotherapy followed by nephrectomy group had a 12% response rate and 14-month median survival. The paucity of responders in either group and the retrospective nature of the review, however, make comparisons between groups difficult to interpret. Another review included 14 highly selected patients who had received initial immunotherapy with an objective response or stable disease who underwent subsequent surgical resection of all metastatic disease sites and the primary tumor (if not already removed).[79] The cancer-specific survival rate for this group was 81.5% at 3 years.

As previously discussed, NCI investigators reported on 51 highly selected patients who underwent immunotherapy with the primary tumor in place.[48] A total of three patients (6%) had objective responses at extrarenal sites and underwent nephrectomy. The duration of the responses were 11 months, 4 months, and greater than 88 months. Median survival in all patients was 13 months. The 6% objective response rate in this report compares poorly with the 18% response seen in 195 patients who underwent preimmunotherapy cytoreductive nephrectomy at the NCI.[57]

A prospective study by Bex et al.[80] looked at 16 patients with metastatic disease at more than one site and a World Health Organization (WHO) performance status of 0 or 1. They were treated with subcutaneous IL-2, GM-CSF, and IFN-α_{2b}. Patients with PR or stable disease at metastatic sites then underwent nephrectomy followed by additional immunotherapy. There were no responses seen in the primary tumors, but nine patients had stable metastatic disease, two had PR, and five had progressive disease. Eleven patients then underwent nephrectomy. The five patients with progressive disease who did not undergo nephrectomy had median overall survival of 3 months versus a median survival of 11.5 months in the group undergoing nephrectomy. Five of 16 patients were therefore spared nephrectomy.

A recent phase III randomized prospective trial by the Cytokine Working Group[81] compared high-dose (HD) IL-2 to outpatient subcutaneous (SC) IL-2 and IFN-α_{2b} in 192 patients. Although the study was not adequately powered for subgroup analysis, the authors did find that in the 60 patients without prior nephrectomy there was a statistically significant increase in survival for those on HD IL-2 vs. SC IL-2 and IFN-α_{2b}. In fact, the lower dose outpatient regimen of IL-2 and IFN was found to be essentially inactive when the primary tumor was in place. One implication of this is that strategies for up-front immunotherapy prior to nephrectomy may need to use the more toxic and expensive HD IL-2 regimen.

There has not been a randomized prospective trial comparing cytoreductive nephrectomy before immunotherapy to nephrectomy after a response to immunotherapy. Until that study is done, it is not clear whether the seemingly better response to immunotherapy after cytoreductive nephrectomy offsets the number of patients who fail to reach systemic immunotherapy due to complications of nephrectomy or rapid tumor progression.

Nephrectomy as a Component of Adoptive Immunotherapy and Other Emerging Therapies

Adoptive immunotherapy is treatment involving transfer of antitumor cells into the host in order to mediate tumor regression. Nephrectomy is typically a requirement for these protocols as a source for tumor antigens or tumor infiltrating lymphocytes. The group from UCLA has reported perhaps the most encouraging results with this therapy.[82] In this protocol TIL cells were harvested from the nephrectomy specimens, expanded ex vivo, and reinfused along with IL-2. Many patients also received preoperative cytokines to improve the yield of TILs, and in some cases CD8[+] cytotoxic lymphocytes were enriched to enhance responses. Sixty-two patients were enrolled and 55 eventually underwent treatment after nephrectomy. A 25.5% overall partial response rate with a 9.1% complete response rate was reported. Based on these encouraging results, a prospective, randomized trial in comparing nephrectomy followed by standard low dose IL-2 therapy given with and without TIL cells was undertaken.[83] Overall response rate was 9.9% in the IL-2 + TIL group and 11.4% in the IL-2 only group ($p = .753$). Median survival was 12.8 months for the TIL + IL-2 group and 11.5 months in the IL-2 alone group. Of note, 33 of 81 patients randomized to TIL + IL-2 group did not receive TILs due to factors related to cell processing, which emphasizes the technical difficulty of these treatments. While these results are disappointing, nephrectomy as a part of investigational adoptive immunotherapy protocols at tertiary care facilities may continue.

Another exciting forefront of treatment for MRCC involves vaccines. Pilot studies involving vaccination with autologous tumor cells, autologous tumor-derived heat shock proteins, and antigen-loaded dendritic cell–based tumor vaccines have been performed.[84–88] Nephrectomy will likely continue to be necessary as a source of tumor cells and antigens for these protocols.

Nephrectomy and Targeted Agents

New therapeutic avenues for RCC include antiangiogenesis agents and molecularly targeted agents such as bevacizumab, a monoclonal antibody against VEGF, and sunitinib, a tyrosine-based receptor inhibitor. Beoacezurab was studied in a randomized, placebo-controlled trial of 116 patients, most of whom had previously been treated with IL-2.[89] The study showed a significant increase in time to progression for those in the higher dose bevacizumab group. Of these patients, 35 of 39 had undergone previous nephrectomy, so it is impossible to elucidate whether previous nephrectomy improved response with this agent, or whether there was any response in the primary tumor to this drug. It remains uncertain whether nephrectomy prior to antiangiogenic or molecularly targeted therapies will produce the same clinical benefit[90] as compared to therapy with interferon. In most trials conducted to date with agents such as sunitinib or sorafenib, the majority of patients had undergone previous nephrectomy.

CONCLUSION

Although the role of nephrectomy in the management of MRCC is still being defined, it has been shown to have many clinical and biologic effects. Certainly, removing the primary tumor decreases the amount of circulating cytokines and other soluble factors produced by the tumor that may cause immunosuppression and paraneoplastic syndromes. However, nephrectomy also may temporarily increase immunosuppression, and may lead to the production of growth factors that temporarily increase the growth of metastatic deposits. Surgery may improve patients' performance status, and make them less likely to have complications during immunotherapy, but morbidity related to the nephrectomy may preclude them from being candidates for immunotherapy. Nephrectomy prior to immunotherapy has been shown in phase III trials to result in a survival benefit in patients with good performance status and limited burden of disease, although the overall improvement in survival is modest. Whether nephrectomy performed after a response to cytokines will provide as significant a benefit as preimmunotherapy nephrectomy remains to be seen. Clearly, additional randomized, prospective trials need to be completed to further understand the role of nephrectomy in metastatic renal cell carcinoma. Additional research into novel therapies such as molecularly directed monoclonal antibodies and tyrosine kinase inhibitors (TKIs) that have improved the management of patients with metastatic renal cell carcinoma will be necessary to fully understand the role of nephrectomy in this setting.

REFERENCES

1. Brosman S, Hausman M, Shocks SJ. Studies on the immune status of patients with renal adenocarcinoma. J Urol 1975;114:375.
2. Pardoll D. Does the immune system see tumors as foreign of self. Annu Rev Immunol 2003; 21:807–839.
3. Finke JH, Zea AH, Stanly J, et al. Loss of T-cell receptor zeta chain and p561ck in T-cells infiltrating human renal cell carcinoma. Can Res 1993;53:5613–5616.
4. Uzzo RG, Rayman P, Kolenko V, et al. Mechanisms of apoptosis in T cells from patients with renal cell carcinoma. Clin Cancer Res 1999;5:1219–1229.
5. Cardi G, Heaney JA, Schned AR, et al. Expression of Fas(APO-1/CD95) in tumor infiltrating and peripheral blood lymphocytes in patients with renal cell carcinoma. Cancer Res 1998;58(10): 2078–2080.
6. Li X, Liu J, Park JK, et al. T cells from renal cell carcinoma patients exhibit an abnormal pattern of kappa B-specific DNA-binding activity: a preliminary report. Can Res 1994;54:5424–5429.
7. Ng CS, Novick AC, Tannenbaum CS, et al. Mechanisms of immune evasion by renal cell carcinoma: tumor-induced T-lymphocyte apoptosis and NFκB suppression. Urology 2002;59:9–14.
8. Riccobon A, Gunelli R, Ridolfi R, et al. Immunosuppression in renal cancer: differential expression of signal transduction molecules in tumor-infiltrating, near-tumor tissue, and peripheral blood lymphocytes. Cancer Invest 2004;22(6):871–877.
9. Figlin RA. Renal cell carcinoma: management of advance disease. J Urol 1999;161(2):381–387.
10. Lahn M, Fisch P, Kohler G, et al. Pro-inflammatory and T cell inhibitory cytokines are secreted at high levels in tumor cell cultures of human renal cell carcinoma. Eur Urol 1999;35(1):70–80.
11. Bronte V, Serafini P, Apolloni E, et al. Tumor-induced immune dysfunctions caused by myeloid suppressor cells. J Immunotherapy 2001;24(6):431–446.
12. Almand B, Clark JI, Nikitina E, et al. Increased production of immature myeloid cells in cancer patients: a mechanism of immunosuppression in cancer. J Immunol 2001;166:678–689.
13. Danna EA, Sinha P, Gilbert M, et al. Surgical removal of primary tumor reverses tumor-induced immunosuppression despite the presence of metastatic disease. Cancer Res 2004;64:2205–2211.
14. Salvadori S, Martinelli G, Zier K. Resection of solid tumors reverses T cell defects and restores protective immunity. J Immun 2000;164:2214–2220.
15. Dadian G, Riches PG, Henderson DC. Immunological parameters in peripheral blood of patients with renal cell carcinoma before and after nephrectomy. Br J Urol 1994;74(1):15–22.
16. Almand B, Resser JR, Lindman B, et al. Clinical Significance of defective dendritic cell differentiation in cancer. Clin Cancer Res 2000;6:1755–1766.

17. Uzzo RG, Clark PE, Rayman P, et al. Alterations in NFκB activation in T lymphocytes of patients with renal cell carcinoma. J Nat Cancer Inst 1999;91(8):717–721.
18. Bennett RT, Lerner SE, Taub HC, et al. Cytoreductive surgery for stage IV renal cell carcinoma. J Urol 1995;154(1):32–34.
19. Walther MM, Yang JC, Pass HI. Cytoreductive surgery before high dose interleukin-2 based therapy in patients with metastatic renal cell carcinoma. J Urol 1997;158:1675–1678.
20. Ben-Eliyahu, S. The promotion of tumor metastasis by surgery and stress: immunological basis and implications for psychoneuroimmunology. Brain Behav Immun 2003;17:S27–S36.
21. Eggermont AMM, Steller EP, Sugarbaker PH. Laparotomy enhances intraperitoneal tumor growth and abrogates the antitumor effects of interleukin-2 and lymphokine activated killer cells. Surgery 1987:123;71–78.
22. Ben-Eliyahu S, Paige GG, Yirmiya R, Shakhar G. Evidence that stress and surgical interventions promote tumor development by suppressing natural killer cell activity. Int J Cancer 1999;80:880–888.
23. Ogawa K, Hirai M, Katsube T, et al. Suppression of cellular immunity by surgical stress. Surgery 2000;127:329–336.
24. Bohm M, Ittenson A, Phillip C, et al. Complex perioperative immuno-dysfunction in patients with renal cell carcinoma. J Urol 2001;166:831–836.
25. Vallejo R, Hord ED, Barna SA, et al. Perioperative immunosuppression in cancer patients. J Environ Pathol Toxicol Oncol 2003;22(2):139–146.
26. Yamaguchi K, Takagi Y, Aoki S, et al. Significant detection of circulating cancer cells in the blood by reverse transcriptase-polymerase chain reaction during colorectal cancer resection. Ann Surg 2000;232(1):58–65.
27. Ashida S, Okudu H, Chikazawa M, et al. Detection of circulating cancer cells with von Hippel-Lindau gene mutation in peripheral blood of patients with renal cell carcinoma. Clin Can Res 2000;6:3817–3822.
28. Zetter BR. Angiogenesis and tumor metastasis. Annu Rev Med 1998;49:407–424.
29. O'Reilly MS, Holmgren L, Shing Y, et al. Angiostatin: a novel angiogenesis inhibitor that mediates the suppression of metastases by a Lewis lung carcinoma. Cell 1994;79:315.
30. Feldman AL, Alexander HR, Yang JC, et al. Prospective analysis of circulating endostatin levels in patients with renal cell carcinoma. Cancer 2002;95:1637–1643.
31. Abramovitch R, Marikovsky M, Meir G, Neeman M. Stimulation of tumour growth by wound-derived growth factors. Br J Cancer, 1999;79:1392–1398.
32. Hofer SO, Molema G, Hermens RA, et al. The effect of surgical wounding on tumour development. Eur J Surg Oncol 1999;25(3):231–243.
33. Johnson DE, Kaesler KE, Samuels ML. Is nephrectomy justified in patients with metastatic renal carcinoma? J Urol 1975;114:27–29.
34. Montie JE, Stewart BH, Straffon RA, et al. The role of adjunctive nephrectomy in patients with metastatic renal cell carcinoma. J Urol 1977;117:272–274.
35. Walther MM, Patel B, Choyke PL, et al. Hypercalcemia in patients with metastatic renal cell carcinoma. Effect of nephrectomy and metabolic evaluation. J Urol 1997;158(3 pt 1):733–739.
36. Dekernion JB, Ramming K, Smith RB. The natural history of metastatic renal cell carcinoma: a computer analysis. J Urol 1978;120:148–152.
37. Couillard DR, de Vere White RW. Surgery of renal cell carcinoma. Urol Clin North Am 1993;20(2):263–275.
38. Sánchez-ortiz RF, Tannir N, Ahrar K, et al. Spontaneous regression of pulmonary metastases from renal cell carcinoma after radio frequency ablation of primary tumor: in situ tumor vaccine? J Urol 2003;170(1):178–179.
39. Freed SZ, Halperin JP, Gordon M. Idiopathic regression of metastases from renal cell carcinoma. J Urol 1977;118:538–542.
40. Marcus SG, Choyke PL, Reiter R. Regression of metastatic renal cell carcinoma after cytoreductive nephrectomy. J Urol 1993;150:463–466.
41. Skinner DG, Colvin RB, Vermillon CD, et al. Diagnosis and management of renal cell carcinoma. A clinical and pathologic study of 309 cases. Cancer 1971;28:1165.
42. Middleton RG. Surgery for metastatic renal cell carcinoma. J Urol 1967;97:973.
43. O'Dea MJ, Zincke H, Utz DC, et al. The treatment of renal cell carcinoma with solitary metastasis. J Urol 1978;120:540–542.

44. Tolia BM, Whitmore WF, Jr. Solitary metastasis from renal cell carcinoma. J Urol 1975; 114:836–838.

45. Kavolius JP, Mastorakos DP, Pavlovich, C, et al. Resection of metastatic renal cell carcinoma. J Clin Oncol 1998;16(6):2261–2266.

46. Flanigan RC, Salmon SE, Blumenstein BA, et al. Nephrectomy followed by interferon-alfa-2b compared with interferon-alfa-2b alone for metastatic renal-cell cancer. N Engl J Med 2001; 345(23):1655–1659.

47. Mickisch GHJ, Garin A, van Poppell H, et al. Radical nephrectomy plus interferon-alfa-based immunotherapy compared with interferon alfa alone in metastatic renal-cell carcinoma: a randomised trial. Lancet 2001;358:966–970.

48. Wagner JR, Walther MM, Linehan WM, et al. Interleukin-2 based immunotherapy for metastatic renal cell carcinoma with the kidney in place. J Urol 1999;162:43–45.

49. Sella A, Swanson DA, Ro JY, et al. Surgery following response to interferon-alpha-based therapy for residual renal cell carcinoma. J Urol 1993;149:19–22.

50. Rackley R, Novick A, Klein E. The impact of adjuvant nephrectomy on multimodality treatment of metastatic renal cell carcinoma. J Urol 1994;152:1399.

51. Motzer RJ, Mazumdar M, Bacik J, et al. Survival and prognostic stratification of 670 patients with advanced renal cell carcinoma. J Clin Oncol 1999;17:2530.

52. Motzer RJ, Russo P. Systemic therapy for renal cell carcinoma. J Urol 2000;163:408–417.

53. Muss H, Constanzi JJ, et al. Recombinant alpha interferon in renal cell carcinoma: randomized trial of two routes of administration. J Clin Oncol 1987;5:286–291.

54. Umeda T, Niijma T. Phase II study of alpha interferon on renal cell carcinoma. Cancer 1986; 58:1231–1235.

55. Fisher RI, Coltman CA, Doroshaw JH, et al. Metastatic renal cancer treated with interleukin-2 and lymphokine-activated killer cells. Ann Intern Med 1988;108:518–523.

56. Mani S, Todd MB, Katz K, et al. Prognostic factors for survival in patients with metastatic renal cancer treated with biological response modifiers. J Urol 1995;154(1):35–40.

57. Walther MM, Yang JC, Pass HI. Cytoreductive surgery before high dose interleukin-2 based therapy in patients with metastatic renal cell carcinoma. J Urol 1997;158:1675–1678.

58. Fallick ML, McDermott DF. Nephrectomy before interleukin-2 therapy for patients with metastatic renal cell carcinoma. J Urol 1997;158(5):1691.

59. Walther MM, Lyne JC, Libutti SK, et al. Laparoscopic cytoreductive nephrectomy as preparation for administration of systemic interleukin-2 in the treatment of metastatic renal cell carcinoma: a pilot study. Urol 1999;53(3):496–500.

60. Pautler SE, Choyke PL, Phillips JL, et al. Laparoscopic cytoreductive radical nephrectomy for metastatic renal cell carcinoma: a feasibility study. J Urol 2001;165(5, suppl):185A.

61. Finelli A, Kaouk JH, Fergany AF, et al. Laparoscopic cytoreductive nephrectomy for metastatic renal cell carcinoma. BJU Int 2004;94:291–294.

62. Slaton JW, Balbay MD, Levy DA, et al. Nephrectomy and vena caval thrombectomy in patients with metastatic renal cell carcinoma. Urology 1997;50(5):673–677.

63. Zisman A, Pantuck AJ, Chao DH, et al. Renal cell carcinoma with tumor thrombus: Is cytoreductive nephrectomy for advanced disease associated with an increased complication rate? J Urol 2002; 168:962–967.

64. Swanson D, Johnson D, von Eschenbach AD. Angioinfarction plus nephrectomy for metastatic renal cell carcinoma—an update. J Urol 1983;130:449.

65. Gottesman JE, Crawford ED, Grossman HB, et al. Infarction-nephrectomy for metastatic renal carcinoma. Southwest oncology group study. Urology 1985;25(3):248–250.

66. Wood CG, Huber N, Madsen L, et al. Clinical variables that predict survival following cytoreductive nephrectomy for metastatic renal cell carcinoma. J Urol 2001;165(5):184A.

67. Méjean A, Rouprêt M, Larousserie F, et al. Is there a place for radical nephrectomy in the presence of metastatic collecting duct carcinoma? J Urol 2003;169:1287–1290.

68. Slaton JW, Perrotte P, Balbay MD, et al. Reassessment of the selection criteria for cytoreductive nephrectomy in patients with metastatic renal cell carcinoma. J Urol 2000;163(suppl 4):79.

69. Han K, Pantuck AJ, Bui MHT, et al. Number of metastatic sites rather than location dictates overall survival of patients with node-negative metastatic renal cell carcinoma. Urology 2003;61(2):314–319.

70. Pantuck AJ, Zisman A, Dorey F, et al. Renal cell carcinoma with retroperitoneal lymph nodes: impact on survival and benefits of immunotherapy. Cancer 2003;97(12):2995–3002.

71. Vasselli JR, Yang JC, Linehan WM, et al. Lack of retroperitoneal lymphadenopathy predicts survival of patients with metastatic renal cell carcinoma. J Urol 2001;166(1):68–72.
72. Fujikawa K, Matsui Y, Miura K, et al. Serum immunosuppressive acidic protein and natural killer cell activity in patients with metastatic renal cell carcinoma before and after nephrectomy. J Urol 2000;164:673–675.
73. Bui MH, Visapaa H, Seligson D, et al. Prognostic value of carbonic anhydrase IX and Ki67 as predictors of survival for renal clear cell carcinoma. J Urol 2004;171:2461–2466.
74. Flanigan RC, Mickisch GH, Sylvester R, et al. Cytoreductive nephrectomy in patients with metastatic renal cancer: a combined analysis. J Urol 2004;171(3):1071–1076.
75. Pantuck AJ, Belldegrun AS, Figlin RA. Nephrectomy and interleukin-2 for metastatic renal-cell carcinoma. N Engl J Med 2001;345(23):1711–1712.
76. Gatenby RA, Gawlinski ET, Tangen CM, et al. The possible role of postoperative azotemia in enhanced survival of patients with metastatic renal cancer after cytoreductive nephrectomy. Cancer Res 2002; 62:5218.
77. Fleischmann JD, Kim B. Interleukin-2 immunotherapy followed by resection of residual renal cell carcinoma. J Urol 1991;145:938–941.
78. Kim B, Louie AC. Surgical resection following interleukin 2 therapy for metastatic renal cell carcinoma prolongs remission. Arch Surg 1992;127:1343–1349.
79. Krishnamurthi V, Novick AC, Bukowski RM, et al. Efficacy of multimodality therapy in advanced renal cell carcinoma. Urology 1998;51(6):933–937.
80. Bex A, Horenblas S, Meinhardt W, et al. The role of initial immunotherapy as selection for nephrectomy in patients with metastatic renal cell carcinoma and the primary in situ. Eur Urol 2002;42:570.
81. McDermott DF, Regan MM, Clark JI, et al. Randomized phase III trial of high-dose interleukin-2 versus subcutaneous interleukin-2 and interferon in patients with metastatic renal cell carcinoma. J Clin Oncol 2005;23:133–141.
82. Figlin RA, Pierce WC, Kaboo R, et al. Treatment of metastatic renal cell carcinoma with nephrectomy, interleukin-2 and cytokine-primed or CD8(+) selected tumor infiltrating lymphocytes from primary tumor. J Urol 1997;158(3):740–745.
83. Figlin RA, Thompson JA, Bukowski RM, et al. Multicenter, randomized, phase III trial of CD8+ tumor-infiltrating lymphocytes in combination with recombinant interleukin-2 in metastatic renal cell carcinoma. J Clin Oncol 1999;17(8):2521–2529.
84. Amato RJ. Vaccine therapy for renal cell carcinoma. Rev Urol 2003;5(2):65–71.
85. Cohen L, de Moor C, Parker PA, et al. Quality of life in patients with metastatic renal cell carcinoma participating in a phase I trial of an autologous tumor-derived vaccine. Urol Oncol 2002;7:119.
86. Chang AE, Li Q, Jiang G, et al. Phase II trial of autologous tumor vaccination, anti-CD3 activated vaccine-primed lymphocytes, and interleukin-2 in stage IV renal cell cancer. J Clin Oncol 2003; 21(5):884–590.
87. Su Z, Dannull J, Heiser A, et al. Immunological and clinical responses in metastatic renal cancer patients vaccinated with tumor RNA-transfected dendritic cells. Cancer Res 2003;63:2127–2133.
88. Gitlitz BJ, Belldegrun AS, Zisman A, et al. A pilot trial of tumor lysate-loaded dendritic cells for the treatment of metastatic renal cell carcinoma. J Immunother 2003;26(5):412–419.
89. Yang JC, Haworth L, Sherry RM, et al. A randomized trial of bevacizumab, an anti-vascular endothelial growth factor antibody, for metastatic renal cancer. N Engl J Med 2003;349(5):427–434.
90. Atkins B, Avigan DE, Bukowski RM, et al. Innovations and challenges in renal cancer: consensus statement from the first international conference. Clin Cancer Res 2004;10:6277S–6281S.
91. Wolf JS, Aronson FR, Small EJ, et al. Nephrectomy for metastatic renal cell carcinoma: a component of systemic treatment regimens. J Surg Oncol 1994;55:7–13.
92. Levy DA, Swanson DA, Slaton JW, et al. Timely delivery of biological therapy after cytoreductive nephrectomy in carefully selected patients with metastatic renal cell carcinoma. J Urol 1998; 159(4):1168–1172.
93. Tigrani VS, Rees DM, Small EJ, et al. Potential role of nephrectomy in the treatment of metastatic renal cell carcinoma: a retrospective analysis. Urology 2000;55:36–40.

22

Spontaneous Regression of Renal Cell Carcinoma and the Role of Prognostic Factors

Tim Oliver, Tom Powles, Vinod Nargund, and Dan Berney

KEYWORDS

SPONTANEOUS REGRESSION
RENAL CELL CARCINOMA
METASTATIC RENAL CANCER
CYTOKINE-INDUCED RESPONSES
LYMPHOCYTE RESPONSE TO CYTOKINES
THERAPY-INDUCED AUTOIMMUNITY

ABSTRACT

Spontaneous regression of metastatic renal cancer occurs in 4% to 6% of patients eligible for cytokine trials, in which response rates of 12% to 18% are reported. An increasingly recognized characteristic of trials in renal cell cancer was that response rates initially reported were often double those noted in later reports. Because of this, it was necessary to exclude the possibility that some of the responses reported for biologic treatment simply reflected episodes of spontaneous regression. This chapter reviews the long-term outcome of these cases, reviews the literature of reported cases, addresses the question of how much the reported response to modern therapies could be due to these spontaneous events, and considers how modern data from prognostic factor analysis may identify patients with a higher likelihood of spontaneous regression.

Previous reports have documented that renal cell carcinoma (RCC) is a tumor with a high frequency of spontaneous/unexplained regression (Table 22.1).[1] There has been considerable controversy, however, regarding the actual frequency of this event. Bloom[2] estimated a frequency of 0.3% in a literature review, while Werf-Messing,[3] in a personal series of 35 metastatic renal cancer patients observed without treatment, reported 30%

From: *Clinical Management of Renal Tumors*
Edited by: R.M. Bukowski and A.C. Novick © Humana Press Inc., Totowa, NJ

Table 22.1.
Spontaneous regression of cancer

Cancer	No. of cases
Leukemia/lymphoma	121
Melanoma	69
Renal cell carcinoma	68
Neuroblastoma	41
Gastrointestinal cancer	34
Retinoblastoma	33
Lung and bronchitis	25
Breast	22
Testis	16
Other	75
Total	504

Source: Adapted from Everson TC, 1967[1].

of patients were stable at 6 months. This polarity of viewpoints, and the increasing recognition of the impact of patient selection on treatment outcome,[4] prompted the authors in 1979 to investigate prospectively its frequency in the setting of the good performance status of patients referred to tertiary centres for entry into clinical trials. An increasingly recognized characteristic of trials in renal cell carcinoma was that response rates initially reported were often double those noted in later reports. Because of this, it was necessary to exclude the possibility that some of the responses reported for biologic treatment simply reflected episodes of spontaneous regression.

This chapter reviews the long-term outcome of these cases, reviews the literature of reported cases, addresses the question of how much the reported response to modern therapies could be due to these spontaneous events, and considers how modern data from prognostic factor analysis may identify patients with a higher likelihood of spontaneous regression.

LONG-TERM OUTCOME OF PERSONAL SERIES

The initial report of 73 patients found five (three complete responses [CRs] and two partial responses [PRs], 6.8%) cases of unexplained measurable regressions in patients treated before the interleukin-2 (IL-2) era,[5,6] in contrast to one in 55 retrospectively studied historical cases (Table 22.2). Subsequently, an additional 164 patients were observed, with an additional six unexplained regressions (3.7%) seen, during a period when there were increasing therapeutic options.[7,8] The latest update has added three additional regressions in 120 personal patients. The long-term outcome in the 16 patients in this series was also examined. Ultimately all patients progressed and died, except for two individuals. The longest survivor was a 40-year-old woman who presented with pleural plaques and a pleural effusion, which showed clear cell carcinoma on a pleural biopsy. One year after nephrectomy she was found to have a central nervous system (CNS) metastasis, which was removed surgically. The patient is alive 26 years later. The second patient had a tumor in the vena cava, with a biopsy demonstrating renal cell carcinoma. Surgery was not possible, and serial computed tomography (CT) scans have shown gradual resolution of the mass.

Table 22.2.
Spontaneous regressions and prolonged stable disease in St. Bartholomew's and Royal London
Renal Cell Carcinoma Surveillance Studies

Type of study	Year	No. of cases (spontaneous regressions)	CR + PR + SD
Retrospective	Earlier than 1978	55 (1)	0 + 2% + NA
Prospective	1978–85	73 (9)	4% + 3% + 6%
Prospective	1986–93	791 (7)	0 + 4% + 6%
Prospective	1994–98	73 (5)	0 + 4% + 3%
Prospective	1998–06	120 (3)	0 + 3% + NA
Total		412 (25)	1% + 3% + 3%

CR, complete response; PR, partial response; SD, stable disease.

The majority of patients with spontaneous regression had pulmonary metastases. In 71 patients with lung metastases, only 13% had an episode of spontaneous regression, and four had other sites (liver, pleural, primary kidney, and vena caval disease) where regression was noted. Interestingly, no regression of lymph node metastases was noted, and none of those showing spontaneous regression on subsequent progression have responded to cytokines. At progression, 132 patients entered a clinical trial, and an additional 11% responded. In this group, 47% of patients with only lung metastases responded (Table 22.3).

LITERATURE REVIEW OF LARGE STUDIES THAT HAVE ADDRESSED THE INCIDENCE OF SPONTANEOUS REGRESSION

When first published, the suggestion that the spontaneous regression rate was 7% was very controversial. The agents used to treat metastatic renal cell carcinoma at that time were associated with only a 10% to 12% response rate.[9] Initially, response rates to interferon (IFN) or IL-2 were reported as 20% to 30%[10]; however, when tested initially by the referral center, the overall response rate decreased. In addition, prior to this report, there were two attempts to estimate the frequency of spontaneous regression

Table 22.3.
Spontaneous regression with response to subsequent therapy in patients with
metastatic renal carcinoma

	No. of cases	CR	PR	OR
Total surveillance series	292	1%	3%	3%
Lung mets only	71	8%	5%	13%
Others	221	0	2%	2%
Entered into cytokine studies after progression on surveillance	132	3%	8%	16%
Lung mets only	23	14%	30%	50%
Others	109	0	2%	2%

CR, complete response; PR, partial response; OR, odds ratio; mets, metastases.

Table 22.4.
Overview of publications that have attempted to estimate spontaneous/unexplained regression
in renal cell carcinoma

Phase II studies	No. of cases	Unexplained regression
Possinger[11] (metastases all)	1247	0.24%
Possinger[11] (postnephrectomy)	663	0.6%
Bloom[2] (personal series)	172	1.0%
Marcus[12]	91	3.0%
Oliver[5]	72	7.1%
Oliver unpublished	339	3.0%

(Table 22.4).[2,11] The first by Bloom[2] only detected a frequency of 0.3% in a retrospective literature review, and reported two of 172 (1.2%) in his own personal series. An update of this retrospective overview was reported by Possinger et al.[11] In that report including 1247 patients, only 0.24% showed spontaneous regression. In this group the regression rate was 2.5 times higher (0.66%) in the 663 patients with sufficiently good performance status to enable nephrectomy to be performed, although a more modern series of 91 cases demonstrated it to be 4.4%.[12]

Because of these observations, it was necessary to perform placebo-controlled trials to determine the presence of a treatment effect. It was the completion of placebo-controlled randomized trials in metastatic disease patients that finally clarified the place of cytokine therapy (Table 22.5). The first of these found that there was no benefit with IFN-γ,[13] but also confirmed the previous observation that the spontaneous regression rate was in excess of one in 20. The Medical Research Council (MRC) conducted a randomized controlled study, and demonstrated a statistically significant survival advantage for IFN.[14] Though the published series does not allow measurement of formal regression rate (complete plus partial response), the incidence of response plus stable disease has been reported and was 14% in the medroxyprogesterone acetate (MPA) arm, which is equivalent to the 12% in our series surveillance study.[6] Three additional trials used tamoxifen in the control arm, and in the pooled data there were 12 of 239 (5%) patients demonstrating an objective response.[15–17]

Table 22.5.
Randomized control trials in renal carcinoma

Trial	Author	Control ORR	Experimental ORR
MPA vs. IFN-α	Steinbeck et al. 1990[15]	7% ($n = 30$)	3% ($n = 30$)
MPA vs. IFN-α	MRC 1999[14]	31%* ($n = 168$)	43%* ($n = 167$)
Placebo vs. IFN-γ	Gleave's group 2000[13]	7% ($n = 90$)	4% ($n = 91$)
Tamoxifen vs. IFN-α/IL-2	Henriksson et al. 1998[16]	3% ($n = 63$)	8% ($n = 65$)
Tamoxifen vs. IL-2/IFN-α/5-FU	Atzpodien et al. 2000[17]	0% ($n = 37$)	39% ($n = 41$)

*Percent of 1-year survival.

5-FU, 5-fluorouracil; IFN, interferon; IL, interleukin; MPA, medroxyprogesterone acetate; MRC, Medical Research Council; ORR, overall response rate.

OVERVIEW OF CASE REPORTS OF SPONTANEOUS/UNEXPLAINED REJECTION IN RENAL CANCER AND ATTEMPTS TO FIND MECHANISMS TO EXPLAIN THEM

It is now 40 years since Everson[1] first reported that spontaneous regression of cancer was a real entity, and reported 68 examples in patients having renal cell carcinoma (Table 22.1). Since then, there have been several overviews of reported cases with up to 70 cases reported by various authors. A limited analysis performed seems to confirm the previously reported association with performance status, histology type (clear cell vs. non–clear cell), site of metastasis (i.e., lung vs. other), and the presence or absence of hypercalcemia.[5]

Recent data from a study of antigenic constitution of clear cell renal cancer has provided an interesting new dimension that may explain its prevalence of spontaneous regression. Ibrahim et al.[18] have demonstrated that seven of 12 (58%) clear cell renal cancers were positive for human leukocyte antigen G (HLA-G), while none of 26 other types had detectable HLA-G. This is a variant HLA molecule expressed on the placenta possibly involved in fetal evasion of immune surveillance. This observation, taken with reports focusing attention on T-cell receptor $\gamma\delta$ T lymphocytes,[19,20] which are increased in both tumor and peripheral blood and in the placenta, and are involved in natural killer (NK) cell activity, is reopening interest in the immunology of spontaneous responses.

An additional factor focusing interest on the immunology of renal cancer response is the increasing number of potential rejection antigens being detected on these tumors. Thymidine phosphorylase and carbonic anhydrase IX are two of particular interest.[21] Perhaps even more interesting are reports that tumor necrosis factor (TNF) receptor protein CD70 is expressed at a high level on 100% of 41 clear cell tumors, but only patchily on 26% of other types of renal cell carcinoma.[22–24] This suggests possible approaches that can be explored in gene therapy trials, as well as investigating enhanced immune response producing tumor rejection, and long-lasting T-lymphocyte immune responses.[25–27]

It has been assumed that spontaneous regression does have an immunologic basis, though nonimmunologic antiangiogenic effects have by no means been excluded. Two of the 13 patients in our experience have features that would fit with an immunologic mechanism.[7] The first was a patient who had a regression that lasted nearly 4 years. The metastases regrew after an episode of emotional stress, and then regressed a second time, but then progressed after 3 years. The concept of chronic stress producing immunosuppression with acceleration of tumor growth has been well documented in experimental animal models[28] and supported by observations in breast cancer patients.[29]

The second case is an example of the rarely reported spontaneous regression of liver metastases.[30] The history given by the patient suggested that it may have been related to a concurrent viral infection. Eight years prior to presentation the patient had a nephrectomy, and was well until approximately 4 weeks before his initial visit. He had just returned from Indonesia, and had developed an intermittently high fever, nausea, and vomiting. He subsequently deteriorated, and was found to have a rapidly enlarging liver with elevated enzymes. A CT scan showed large liver metastases, and a biopsy confirmed clear cell carcinoma. Within 1 week he improved, with a reduction in hepatomegaly and improvement in liver enzymes (normalized after about 8 weeks). By 3 months his CT scan was nearly normal and remained so for 10 months, when he relapsed and died. His disease was unresponsive to cytokines or chemotherapy. Although viral antibody titers to known hepatitis-causing viruses were negative, it was concluded that he may have been infected with an obscure Southeast Asian hepatitis virus strain, which had induced viral oncolysis.[31,32] The possibility of involvement of CD70 in such immune rejection has recently been demonstrated in an experimental animal model of murine lymphocytic choriomeningitis virus (LCMV) infection.[33]

It is clear in studies of surveillance that a short-term delay in starting treatment is safe and could provide a window for trials of new immune therapy. However, the frequency of response in this highly selected group of tertiary referrals was less than that seen with cytokine treatment. Furthermore, the response rate after progression on surveillance was no different from that reported in patients without preliminary surveillance prior to cytokine therapy. It appears that the same group of good-risk patients with small-volume lung metastases developing late or present at the time of nephrectomy may be the individuals who respond to cytokines or show spontaneous regression. In view of this, there is some concern that surveillance could prejudice the detection of response. Currently our policy is to use a brief period of surveillance before entry into clinical trials in order to assess the rate of disease progression.

RESPONSE TO THERAPY AFTER EXCLUSION OF SPONTANEOUS REGRESSION AS COMPARED WITH REPORTS IN THE LITERATURE

The overall results from sequential phase II studies in patients progressing after surveillance were somewhat less than reported in recently published overviews (unless stable disease lasting more than 3 months is regarded as a response category). Furthermore, one other issue emerged, and may explain why selected centers report higher response rates. Patients who traveled greater distances for treatment had higher response rates, and the lowest response rates were observed in local patients who live in an area of marked social deprivation.[8] There is increasing recognition of the role of poverty in leading to a poor outcome with cancer treatment, most notably in breast cancer. In our own center the same differences in survival are demonstrated when surgery is performed on patients referred from high cure rate regions, as defined by cancer registry figures.[34] It is clear that this difference is not secondary to inferior surgical care.

There is increasing evidence from studies of the effect of poverty on resistance to infectious disease. Vitamin A enhances CD4 T-cell immune responses,[35] vitamin D enhances CD8 T-cell and macrophage function[36,37] and zinc enhances general immune response.[38] There is evidence that vitamin A deficiency can accelerate cancer deaths. Importantly, however, in cancer prevention trials, no benefit from supplements in individuals with adequate levels of dietary intake can be demonstrated.[39] There is also evidence from studies of prostate cancer patients that adequate vitamin D levels may prevent tumor development.[40] In addition, data demonstrate that vitamin D suppresses production of metalloproteinase, which has a role in tumor invasion.[41] These observations suggest that issues such as poverty may be important when assessing response to treatments.

Table 22.6.
Autopsy detection of "occult" renal cell carcinoma (RCC)

Number of autopsies	16,294
Total RCC	350 (2%)
Unrecognized RCC premortem	235 (67% of total RCC)
Unrecognized RCC M+	56 (24% of unrecognized premortem)

M+, metastaces present.
Source: Adapted from Mindrup et al.[45]

RELEVANCE OF SPONTANEOUS REGRESSION TO PROGNOSTIC FACTOR ANALYSIS AND THE EFFECT OF LEAD TIME BIAS

Since the landmark study of de Kernion et al.,[4] it is well established that selection can have a powerful effect on outcome in advanced renal cancer patients. This is equally relevant for the incidence of spontaneous regression.[5] These observations make it difficult to rule out selection and lead-time bias as playing a part in the apparent benefit of cytokine therapy. It is well recognized that lead-time bias from early diagnosis is a major problem for interpreting the results of radical prostatectomy.[42] The few studies that have investigated the impact of early diagnosis from increased availability of ultrasound and CT scans on prognosis of renal cancer, have not yet demonstrated any evidence for a population-based change in survival. There are several anecdotal reports that if renal tumors are diagnosed incidentally at the time of angiography or ultrasound for a nonmalignant disease investigation, the prognosis is better in terms of a lower frequency of metastases.[43,44] However, this does not make allowance for two factors. First, such cases are diagnosed long before they would present clinically; that is, there is a lead-time bias. Second, if one does an autopsy on people dying of other causes, one finds many more renal cancers than are actually detected clinically. A proportion of these even have metastases (Table 22.6), and there is some evidence of a reduction of the number of tumors being present at autopsy in modern series, suggesting better detection antemortem.[45] Given the increasing use over the last 20 years of abdominal ultrasound and even CT scan to investigate nonspecific abdominal symptoms, it is possible that at present the evidence for treatment actually reducing population-based mortality is still lacking. It could be clouded by lead time bias and overdiagnosis of small tumors with small amounts of metastases that could be accelerated by surgery and then be more susceptible to response to treatment, thus ending up with a survival neutral effect.

NEW APPROACHES TO PROGNOSTIC FACTOR ANALYSIS USING SIMPLE PERIPHERAL BLOOD PARAMETERS

There is increasing evidence that several peripheral blood parameters, such as erythrocyte sedimentation rate (ESR), pretreatment platelet count and granulocyte count, posttreatment lymphocytosis, and pretreatment hemoglobin (Table 22.7), may predict overall patient response and survival. No single series has been large enough to do a multivariate analysis to assess the individual factors. Clinically, however, these factors are an extremely interesting group since they provide insight into the biology of renal cancer. For many years, ESR was the only way to monitor disease activity in patients

Table 22.7.
Interaction between hemoglobin status and response to interferon

| | Response at 6 months (CR + PR + SD) | | Median progression free | | Hazard ratio |
	MPA	Interferon	MPA	Interferon	MPA vs. Interferon
All Case	14%	23%	2.75	3.5	0.66
Low Hb	5%	10%	2.00	2.00	0.79
Mid Hb	15%	19%	2.75	3.00	0.70
Hign Hb	21%	46%	2.75	6.50	0.51

MPA, medroxyprogesterone acetate; Hb, hemoglobin.
Source: Oliver et al., 2003.[53]

with tuberculosis, and as such probably gave a good indication of the degree of disarray of immune response to the bacterium. Little work has been done on this parameter in recent years, but it may be worth reexamining its relevance in the face of new data. Also, it has been observed that the acute phase reactant C-reactive protein can serve as a prognosticator for response.[46]

There is also increasing evidence that serum levels of IL-6, known to produce increased levels of platelets, are associated with a poor prognosis and with much of the symptomatology of the paraneoplastic syndromes found in renal cell carcinoma patients.[47–49] There is also evidence that a significant minority of renal cell carcinoma cell lines produce excess granulocyte colony-stimulating factor (G-CSF) or granulocyte-macrophage colony-stimulating factor (GM-CSF), which may be responsible for the neutrophilia.[47,50] A similar effect may explain why a high neutrophil count is a poor prognostic feature in renal cancer patients. Both G-CSF and GM-CSF are the product of mesenchymal cells. In renal cell carcinoma, a change in mesenchymal elements, such as spindle cell or sarcomatoid, is associated with a poor prognosis. It is therefore relevant to investigate the correlation of neutrophil levels with prognosis.

In contrast to the correlation of neutrophil counts and a poor prognosis are the effects of elevated lymphocyte counts after treatment with IL-2 (Table 22.7). It is surprising that despite the large number of reports utilizing IL-2, few have commented on this parameter. In one report in which it was examined, lymphocytosis correlated with the induction of autoimmune thyroiditis, another immunologic parameter predicting a good outcome.[51]

The association of anemia with poor outcome has been well established for several cancers, and in cervix cancer transfusing to a normal level has been shown to improve survival.[52] In general, however, it may not add much more to the general effect of poor performance status, and is almost certainly a by-product of excessive IL-6.[49] However, in one report of 370 renal cancer patients, an interesting observation was noted in relation to elevated hemoglobin level.[53] This study was a randomized trial comparing MPA and IFN-α (Table 22.8). There was a higher response rate and better survival for the one third of patients whose hemoglobin was above the upper limit for normal. Moreover, only those with hemoglobin levels in the upper third showed significant response and survival benefit from treatment with interferon.

Erythropoietin is a normal differentiation product of renal cells and its production by a proportion of renal cancers is well established. This observation could be a demonstration that more differentiated and less clonally evolved tumors are the ones that respond to immunotherapy. A suggestion that the higher response to IFN in patients with an elevated hemoglobin level may be due to more than being a marker of differentiation comes from an in vitro study that demonstrated that transfection of an erythropoietin gene into a nonsecreting tumor enhanced susceptibility to immune T lymphocytes.[54] The observed association of the clear cell phenotype with erythropoietin production is therefore very interesting, as the results from the small pilot study of peripheral blood stem cell allograft suggested that most of the responding patients had clear cell phenotype (nine of 12 clear cell vs. one of seven mixed tumors responded).[55]

The final possible factor that might be involved is anoxia. Erythropoietin is produced in response to anoxia[56] and is regulated by the hypoxia-inducible factor (HIF) that is constitutively elevated in clear cell tumors with nonfunctional von Hippel–Lindau genes.

As hemoglobin, neutrophils, lymphocytes, platelets, and ESR can be assessed in a single blood sample, they offer a very simple approach for assessing prognosis. Understanding their mechanism of action potentially could offer insights into the cell biology of renal cell carcinoma (RCC). They fall into two groups: (1) those that increase the chance of response to immune therapy (e.g., lymphocytosis, induction of autoimmune response on therapy, or high hemoglobin pretreatment); and (2) the paraneoplastic cytokines such as G-CSF, IL-6, vascular endothelial growth factor (VEGF) that presumably indicate poorly differentiated cancer. These observations need to be investigated retrospectively in a series of patients who have developed spontaneous regression to determine if they play a role in this phenomenon.

CONCLUSION

As an increasing number of studies now confirm, that spontaneous regression of metastatic renal cancer occurs in 4% to 6% of patients eligible for cytokine trials, in which response rates of 12% to 18% are reported. Furthermore, as with cytokine-induced responses, spontaneous regression is more frequent in good-risk patients with small volumes of metastatic disease. There is limited proof that the same immunologic mechanisms are involved in both types of response. However, the strongest anecdotal evidence for T cells being involved comes from a single case report of spontaneous regression of established metastases after reversion of immunosuppression following treatment of HIV disease with anti-HIV therapy,[57] and the small series of clear cell tumors discovered on follow-up of a renal transplant cohort. Less unequivocally the reports of regressions occurring after relief of major psychological stress and after an episode of postulated acute nonspecific viral hepatitis may provide supportive evidence. The evidence that level of lymphocyte response to cytokines and degree of autoimmunity induced by therapy are predictors of the chance of response to cytokines is increasingly firm.

REFERENCES

1. Everson TC. Spontaneous regression of cancer. Prog Clin Cancer 1967;3:79–95.
2. Bloom HJ. Hormone-induced and spontaneous regression of metastatic renal cancer. Cancer 1973;32(5):1066–1071.

3. Werf-Messing VD. Hormonal treatment of metastases of renal carcinoma. Br J Cancer 1971;25(3):423–427.
4. De Kernion JB, Ramming KP, Smith RB. The natural history of metastatic renal cell carcinoma: a computer analysis. J Urol 1978;120:148–152.
5. Oliver RTD, Miller RM, Mehta A, Barnett MJ. A phase 2 study of surveillance in patients with metastatic renal cell carcinoma and assessment of response of such patients to therapy on progression. Mol Biother 1988;1:14–20.
6. Oliver RTD, Nethersall ABW, Bottomley JM. Unexplained spontaneous regression and alpha-interferon as treatment for metastatic renal carcinoma. Br J Urol 1989;63:128–131.
7. Oliver RTD. Psychological support for cancer patients. Lancet 1989;2(8673):1209–1210.
8. Oliver R, Steele J, Ansell W. Should spontaneous regression be excluded before commencing biotherapy in renal cancer? Br J Urol Int 1999;83(suppl 4):137(abstr).
9. Joffe J, Banks R, Forbes M, et al. A phase II study of interferon-alpha, interleukin-2 and 5–fluorouracil in advanced renal carcinoma: clinical data and laboratory evidence of protease activation. Br J Urol 1996;77:638–649.
10. Lopez Hanninen E, Kirchner H, Atzpodien J. Interleukin-2 based home therapy of metastatic renal cell carcinoma: risks and benefits in 215 consecutive single institution patients. J Urol 1996;155(1):19–25.
11. Possinger K, Wagner H, Beck R, Staebler A. Renal cell carcinoma. Controversies Oncol 1988;30:195–207.
12. Marcus SG, Choyke PL, Reiter R, et al. Regression of metastatic renal cell carcinoma after cytoreductive nephrectomy. J Urol 1993;150(2 pt 1):463–466.
13. Elhilali M, Gleave M, Fradet Y, et al. Placebo-associated remissions in a multicentre, randomized, double-blind trial of interferon gamma-1b for the treatment of metastatic renal cell carcinoma. BJU Int 2000;86:613–618.
14. Medical Research Council Renal Cancer Collaborators. Interferon α and survival in metastatic renal cell carcinoma: early results of a randomized trial. Lancet 1999;353:14–17.
15. Steinbeck G, Strander H, Carbin BE, et al. Recombinant leukocyte interferon alpha-2a and medroxyprogesterone in advanced renal cell carcinoma. A randomized trial. Acta Oncol 1990;29:155–162.
16. Henriksson R, Nilsson S, Colleen S, et al. Survival in renal cell carcinoma—a randomized evaluation of tamoxifen vs interleukin-2, alpha-interferon (leukocyte) and tamoxifen. Br J Cancer 1998;77:1311–1117.
17. Atzpodien J, Kirchner H, Illiger HJ, et al. IL-2 in combination with IFN-alpha and 5–FU versus tamoxifen in metastatic renal cell carcinoma: long term results of a controlled randomized clinical trial. Br J Cancer 2001;85:1130–1136.
18. Ibrahim EC, Allory Y, Commo F, Gattegno B, Callard P, Paul P. Altered pattern of major histocompatibility complex expression in renal carcinoma: tumour-specific expression of the nonclassical human leukocyte antigen-G molecule is restricted to clear cell carcinoma while up-regulation of other major histocompatibility complex antigens is primarily distributed in all subtypes of renal carcinoma. Am J Pathol 2003;162(2):501–508.
19. Kowalczyk D, Skorupski W, Kwias Z, Nowak J. Activated gamma/delta T lymphocytes infiltrating renal cell carcinoma. Immunol Lett 1996;53(1):15–18.
20. Viey E, Laplace C, Escudier B. Peripheral gammadelta T-lymphocytes as an innovative tool in immunotherapy for metastatic renal cell carcinoma. [Review]. Expert Rev Anticancer Ther 2005;5(6):973–986.
21. Unwin RD, Harnden P, Pappin D, et al. Serological and proteomic evaluation of antibody responses in the identification of tumour antigens in renal cell carcinoma. Proteomics 2003;3(1):45–55.
22. Diegmann J, Junker K, Gerstmayer B, et al. Identification of CD70 as a diagnostic biomarker for clear cell renal carcinoma by gene expression profiling, real time RT-PCR and immunohistochemistry. Eur J Cancer 2005;41(12):1794–1801.
23. Junker K, Hindermann W, Eggeling Fv, Diegmann J, Haessler K, Schubert J. CD70: a new tumour specific biomarker for renal carcinoma. J Urol 2005;173(6):2150–2143.
24. Law C-L, Gordon KA, Toki BE, et al. Lymphocyte activation antigen CD70 expressed by renal cell carcinoma is a potential therapeutic target for anti-CD70 antibody-drug conjugates. Cancer Res 2006;66(4):2328–2337.
25. Arens R, Schepers K, Nolte MA, et al. Tumour rejection induced by CD70–mediated quantitive and qualitative effects on effector CD8+ T cell formation. J Exp Med 2004;199(11):1595–1605.

26. So T, Lee S-W, Croft M. Tumour necrosis factor/tumour necrosis factor receptor family members that positively regulate immunity. Int J Hematol 2006;83(1):1–11.

27. Cormary C, Hiver E, Mariame B, Favre G, Tilkin-Mariame A-F. Coexpression of CD40L and CD70 by semiallogenic tumour cells induces anti-tumour immunity. Cancer Gene Ther 2005;12(12):963–972.

28. Temoshok L, Peeke HVS, Mehard CW, Axelsson K, Sweet SM. Stress-behaviour interactions in hamster tumor growth. Neuroimmune Interact 1985;496:501–509.

29. Spiegel D, Bloom J, Kraemer H, Gottheil E. Effect of psychosocial treatment on survival in patients with metastatic breast cancer. Lancet 1989;2(8668):888–891.

30. Ritchie A, Layfield L, deKernion J. Spontaneous regression of liver metastases from renal carcinoma. J Urol 1988;140(3):596–597.

31. Lindenmann J, Klein PA. Viral oncolysis: increased immunogenicity of host cell antigen associated with influenza virus. J Exp Med 1967;126(1):93–108.

32. Schirrmacher V, v Hoegen P, Schlag P, Liebrich W, Lehner B, Schumaker K. Active specific immunotherapy with autologous tumor cell vaccines modified by Newcastle disease virus: experimental and clinical studies. In: Cancer Metastasis. Berlin: Springer-Verlag, 1989:157–170.

33. Matter M, Mumprecht S, Pinschewer DD, et al. Virus-induced polyclonal B cell activation improves protective CTL memory via retained CD27 expression on memory CTL. Eur J Immunol 2005;35(11):3229–3239.

34. Oliver R. Poorer outcome from treatment of breast cancer in poorer areas of Glasgow. BMJ 2000;408:321.

35. Semba R, Muhilal, Ward B, et al. Abnormal T cell subset proportions in Vitamin A deficient children. Lancet 1993;341:5–8.

36. Veldman C, Cantorna M, DeLuca H. Expression of 1,25-dihydroxyvitamin D (3) receptor in the immune system. Arch Biochem Biophys 2000;374(2):334–338.

37. Koga Y, Naraparaju V, Yamamoto N. Antitumour effect of vitamin D-binding protein derived macrophage activating factor on Ehrlich ascites tumour-bearing mice. Proc Soc Exp Biol Med 1999;220(1):20–26.

38. Umeta M, West C, Haidar J, Deurenberg P, Hautvaset J. Zinc supplementation and stunted infants in Ethiopia: a randomised controlled trial. Lancet 2000;355(9220):2021–2126.

39. Hunter DJ, Manson JE, Colditz GA, et al. A prospective study of the intake of vitamins C, E and A and the risk of breast cancer. N Engl J Med 1993;329:234–240.

40. Hanchette C, Schwartz GG. Inverse correlation between UV radiation exposure in USA and Prostate cancer mortality. Cancer 1992;70:2861–2869.

41. Koli K, Keski-Oja J. 1 alpha, 25 dihydroxyvitamin d3 and its analogues down-regulate cell invasion-associated proteases in cultured malignant cells. Cell Growth Different 2000;11(4):221–229.

42. Dennis L, Resnick M. Analysis of recent trends in prostate cancer incidence and mortality. Prostate 2000;42(4):247–252.

43. Thompson I, Peek M. Improvement in survival of patients with renal cell carcinoma—the role of the serendipitously detected tumour. J Urol 1988;140:487–490.

44. Mevorach R, Segal A, Tersegno M, Frank I. Renal cell carcinoma: incidental diagnosis and natural history: review of 235 cases. Urology 1992;39:519–522.

45. Mindrup SR, Pierre JS, Dahmoush L, Konety BR. The prevalence of renal cell carcinoma diagnosed at autopsy. BJU Int 2005;95(1):31–33.

46. Deehan D, Heys S, Simpson W, Herriot R, Broom J, Eremin O. Correlation of serum cytokine and acute phase reactant levels with alterations in weight and serum albumin in patients receiving immunotherapy with recombinant IL-2. Clin Exp Immunol 1994;95(3):366–372.

47. Tachibana M, Miyakawa A, Nakashima J, et al. Autocrine growth promotion by multiple hematopoietic growth factors in the established renal cell carcinoma line KU-19-20. Cell Tissue Res 2000;301(3):353–337.

48. Negrier S, Perol D, Manetrier-Caux C, et al. Interleukin-6, interleukin-10, and vascular endothelial growth factor in metastatic renal cell carcinoma: prognostic value of interleukin-6 from the Groupe Francais d'Immunotherapie. J Clin Oncol 2004;22(12):2371–2378.

49. Walther MM, Johnson B, Culley D, et al. Serum interleukin-6 levels in metastatic renal cell carcinoma before treatment with interleukin-2 correlates with paraneoplastic syndromes but not patient survival. J Urol 1998;159:718–722.

50. Gerharz C, Reinecke P, Schneider E, Schmitz M, Gabbert H. Secretion of GM-CSF and M-CSF by human renal cell carcinomas of different histologic types. Urology 2001;58(5):821–827.

51. Franzke A, Peest D, Probst-Kepper M, et al. Autoimmunity resulting from cytokine treatment predicts long-term survival in patients with metastatic renal cell cancer. J Clin Oncol 1999;17(2):529–533.
52. Grogan M, Thomas GM, Melamed I, et al. The importance of hemoglobin levels during radiotherapy for carcinoma of the cervix. Cancer 1999;86(8):1528–1536.
53. Oliver R, Griffiths G, Ritchie A. Pretreatment haemoglobin level as a predictor of response to subsequent treatment. Br J Urol Int 2000;88:abstr 54.
54. Miyajima J, Imai Y, Nakao M, Noda S, Itoh K. Higher susceptibility of erythropoietin-producing renal cell carcinomas to lysis by lymphokine-activated killer cells. J Immunother Emphasis Tumor Immunol 1996;19(6):399–404.
55. Childs R, Chernoff A, Contentin N. Regression of metastatic renal cell carcinoma after nonmyeloablative allogenic peripheral blood stem cell transplantation. N Engl J Med 2000;343:750–758.
56. Gleadle J, Ratcliffe P. Induction of hypoxia-inducible factor-1, erythropoietin, vascular endothelial growth factor, and glucose transporter-1 by hypoxia: evidence against a regulatory role for Src kinase. Blood 1997;89(2):503–509.
57. Morris D. Dramatic response of renal cell carcinoma to epivir and viramune in a HIV positive patient. Proc ASCO 2000;abstr 1390.

23 Systemic Therapy for Metastatic Renal Cell Carcinoma: *Cytokines*

Thomas E. Hutson

KEYWORDS

IMMUNOTHERAPY
CYTOKINES
INTERLEUKIN-2
INTERFERON
METASTATIC RENAL CELL CARCINOMA

ABSTRACT

Immunotherapy with cytokines (interferon and interleukin-2) have been the primary systemic therapy option for patients with metastatic renal cell carcinoma until very recently. Despite the improved outcomes demonstrated by VEGF targeted therapies, these agents do not produce complete remesions or cures. At present, high-dose interleukin-2 remains the only therapy for advanced renal cell carcinoma that has the potential to produce durable CR's and apparent cures, albeit in a small proportion of highly selected patients. Clinical study of combinations of cytokines and VEGF targeted therapy are ongoing. Immunotherapy continues to be an important part of the therapeutic armamentarium for renal cell carcinoma and deserves further development.

The systemic therapy of metastatic renal cell carcinoma (RCC) remains a challenge for the medical oncologist and urologist. Renal cell carcinoma is highly resistant to chemotherapy, with no single agent showing significant antitumor activity.[1,2] Based on reports of spontaneous regression of metastatic lesions,[3] the presence of cytotoxic T lymphocytes in renal tumors,[4] the reports of prolonged stable disease in the absence of systemic therapy,[5] and the recent descriptions of tumor-associated and human leukocyte antigen (HLA)-restricted antigens on renal cancer cells, immunologic approaches to the therapy of this tumor are reasonable. The major approaches used have included cytokines as single agents or in combination with chemotherapy and adoptive therapy. The interleukins (ILs), interferons (IFNs), hematopoietic growth factors, and chemokines represent varieties of cytokines, and agents from the first three categories have been used in patients with renal cancer as therapy for metastatic disease.

From: *Clinical Management of Renal Tumors*
Edited by: R.M. Bukowski and A.C. Novick © Humana Press Inc., Totowa, NJ

The therapeutic effects of natural and recombinant cytokines have been investigated over the past two decades. Two agents, interleukin-2 (IL-2) and interferon-α (IFN-α), appear to produce tumor regressions in 10% to 15% of patients in a reproducible fashion. Other cytokines have been investigated in metastatic RCC; however, their antitumor activity has not been consistently demonstrated. Several clinical factors have been described in patients with RCC receiving cytokine-based therapy.[6,7] Factors predictive of rapid progression under cytokine treatment include the presence of hepatic metastases, a short interval from renal tumor to metastases (<1 year), the presence of more than one metastatic site, and elevated neutrophil counts.[6,7] Additionally, patients with clear cell (conventional histology) appear to derive the most benefit from cytokine based treatment.[8]

Radical nephrectomy combined with immunotherapy has been shown to significantly increase survival in patients with metastatic RCC (see Chapter 11) beyond time periods achieved with immunotherapy alone.[9,10] Attempts to identify surrogate markers that can identify responding patients are under investigation. Unfortunately, the majority of patients with metastatic RCC do not receive benefit from these therapies. At present, several novel agents with potentially greater antitumor activity are under investigation in large, multinational phase III trials. Two of these agents, sorafenib and sunitinib, have received Food and Drug Administration (FDA) regulatory approval for advanced RCC. The role of cytokine treatment used alone and in combination with these new agents will be the topic of clinical investigation for several years to come. This chapter reviews the current status of cytokine treatment for metastatic RCC.

INTERFERONS

The antitumor activity of IFN in patients with RCC was first reported in 1983 by two groups of investigators. Quesada et al.[11] treated 19 patients with leukocyte IFN-α on a schedule of 3 million units (MU) intramuscularly daily and reported a 26% objective response rate. In a similarly designed, but larger study, deKernion et al.[12] achieved a 16.5% objective response in 48 patients with advanced disease. These studies demonstrated, for the first time, that cytokine therapy could effect a tumor regression, and heralded the modern era of immunotherapy in RCC.

The most studied IFNs in the treatment of metastatic RCC are IFN-α, -β, and -γ derived from leukocytes, fibroblasts, and lymphocytes, respectively. In vitro studies of nonrecombinant IFN-α and -β and recombinant subtypes of IFN-α_2, -β, and -γ have demonstrated comparable growth-inhibitory activity, a direct dose-response tumor-inhibiting relationship, and heterogeneity of activity in different tumors types.[13] The actual mechanisms responsible for the antitumor activity of IFNs in human cancer remain uncertain. Possible mechanisms may include inhibition of oncogene function and enhancement of immune regulatory actions including effector cell cytolytic activity and expression of class II major histocompatibility complex (MHC) proteins on cell surfaces.[14] In vitro and in vivo studies utilizing both physiologic and pharmacologic doses of IFN demonstrate potent immune stimulatory activity that includes activation of cytotoxic T lymphocytes,[15,16] augmentation of antibody-dependent cellular cytotoxicity,[17–19] and activation of natural killer (NK) cells.[20–22] In addition to its immune regulatory actions, IFN also has direct effects on tumor cell proliferation and angiogenesis,[23–28] the former being demonstrated in a range of tumor cells, including RCC in vitro.[29,30]

Interferon-α

The first cytokine investigated in patients with advanced renal cell carcinoma was IFN-α.[31,32] The combined clinical response rates (complete plus partial) from these early trials were documented in up to 26% of patients and provided a basis for multiple phase II trials of IFN-α in the treatment of RCC. In a recent meta-analysis by Coppin et al.,[33] results from six randomized trials using subcutaneous IFN-α involving 963 patients with metastatic RCC indicate that IFN-α is superior to controls (for death at 1 year, odds ratio [OR], 0.67; 95% confidence interval [CI], 0.50–0.89). The pooled hazard ratio for survival from this analysis was 0.78 (0.67–0.90), and the weighted average median improvement in survival was 2.6 months. Additionally, there was no statistically significant difference when IFN-α was compared to subcutaneous IL-2 and there was no difference between various IFN-α subtypes.

The most commonly used preparations in clinical practice are recombinant IFN-α_{2a} (Roferon A®, Hoffman-LaRoche, Nutley, NJ) and recombinant IFN-α_{2b} (Intron A®, Schering-Plough Laboratories, Kenilworth, NJ). Both have been studied extensively in patients with metastatic RCC in doses ranging from 3 MU to 50 MU per day (Table 23.1). Response rates range from 0% to 30%,[40,43–54] and the overall response rate is 14.5% (13 complete and 81 partial response; 95% CI, 12–17%) in 648 patients.[34] Optimal results appear to be associated with doses from 5 to 10 MU/m².[35] Responses occur most frequently in patients with pulmonary metastases and good performance

Table 23.1.
Selected clinical trials of recombinant interferon-α in patients with advanced renal cell carcinoma

Authors	n	Dose (×10⁶ IU)	Schedule	IFN type	CR	PR	ORR%
Minassian et al.[36]	39	59	TIW IM	2a	0	7	18
	59	3–36	Daily IM	2a	2	5	11
Quesada et al.[37]	41	20/m²	Daily IM	2a	1	11	29
	15	2/m²	Daily IM	2a	0	0	0
Umeda et al.[38]	108	3–36/m²	Daily IM	2a	2	13	14
Schnall et al.[39]	22	3–36	Daily IM	2a	0	1	5
Kempf et al.[40]	10	2/m²	TIW IM	2a	0	0	0
	10	30/m²	TIW IM	2a	0	1	10
Fossa et al.[41]	17	18–36/m²	TIW IM	2a	0	2	11
Foon et al.[42]	21	2/m²	TIW IM	2b	0	1	5
Steineck et al.[43]	30	10–20/m²	TIW IM	2a	1	1	6
Marshall et al.[44]	17	1	Daily SC	2a	0	4	24
Umeda et al.[38]	45	3–36	Daily IM	2b	1	7	18
Muss et al.[45]	46	30–50/m² 5×/week	Daily IV Q3 weeks	2b	1	2	7
Levens et al.[46]	15	10	Daily SC	2b	1	3	27
Bono et al.[47]	61	3/m²	TIW SC	2b	2	3	8
Buzaid et al.[48]	22	3–36	Daily IM	2a	0	5	23
Figlin et al.[49]	19	3–36	Daily IM	2a	1	4	26

TIW, three times weekly; IM, intramuscular; SC, subcutaneous; IV, intravenous; CR, complete response; PR, partial response; ORR% = overall response rate %.
Source: Adapted from Motzer and Berg.[34]

Table 23.2.
Selected randomized trials of interferon-α in metastatic renal cell carcinoma

Authors	Treatment	n	RR	Median survival (months)*
Pyrhonen et al.[50]	IFN-α 18 MU SC TIW plus VBL 0.1 mg/kg IVB Q 3 weeks	79	16%	15.8
	vs.			
	VBL 0.1 mg/kg IVB Q3 weeks	81	2.5%	8.8
MCR[51]	IFN-α 10 MU SC TIW 167 for 12 weeks	NS	8.5	
	vs.			
	MPA 300 mg/day	168	NS	6.0

*p < .01.

MPA, medroxyprogesterone; NS, not stated; SC, subcutaneous; MU, million units; VBL, vinblastine; IVB, intravenous bolus; TIW, three times weekly.

Source: Adapted from Bukowski et al.[54]

status.[35,36] Median response duration is generally between 6 and 10 months, but occasionally durable complete regressions over 2 years are seen.[36]

Several randomized trials have been conducted in which IFN-α has been compared with other therapeutic approaches. These include comparisons to either a noncytokine regimen or other cytokines. The studies of most interest are summarized in Table 23.2. Pyrhonen et al.[50] reported a trial in which 160 patients received either the combination of IFN-α and vinblastine or vinblastine alone. Improvement in both response rates and median survivals in IFN-α treated patients were detected. The response rates were 16.5% and 2.5%, respectively, and median survivals were 15.8 months and 8.8 months. These findings suggest that interferon as a single agent may enhance survival because the clinical activity of vinblastine is minimal.[50] A second trial reported by Ritchie et al.[51] compared IFN-α (10 MU subcutaneous three times weekly) with medroxyprogesterone (300 mg daily), both administered for up to 12 weeks in 335 patients. Results with IFN-α were significantly better than with medroxyprogesterone. In the group with measurable disease, IFN-α produced responses in 13% of patients compared to 7% in patients treated with medroxyprogesterone. These results suggest that IFN-α significantly enhanced survival in patients with metastatic RCC (8.5 months vs. 6.0 months), although the effect is modest.

Two randomized trials demonstrated a statistically significant survival advantage in RCC patients with synchronous metastatic disease who received cytoreductive nephrectomy followed by IFN-α.[52,53] These data are summarized in Chapter 11. These trials suggest that patients with primary tumors in place and metastatic disease should be considered for nephrectomy (if medically possible) before IFN-α therapy. A retrospective review also suggests this approach can be considered in patients receiving IL-2.[54]

Interferon-β and Interferon-γ

In comparison with the clinical experience with IFN-α, there are only limited data on the use of IFN-β and IFN-γ in the treatment of metastatic RCC.[55–70] The overall response rate with IFN-β was 11% in four trials comprised of 71 patients.[55–58] Clinical response rates of patients treated with IFN-γ ranged from 0% to 33% in 11 trials of 570 patients.[59–70] In total, the combined response rates (complete plus partial) range from 6% to 33% and are similar to those obtained in studies using IFN-α.

Pegylated Interferon

In an attempt to reduce the frequency of injections and underlying toxicity of chronic treatment with IFN-α, alternative formulations with the potential for greater efficacy and less toxicity have been investigated. The most studied has been the conjugation of the IFN-α molecule with polyethylene glycol (PEG), a process known as pegylation. The two commercially available pegylated IFNs (PEG IFN-α_{2a}, PEGASYS®, Hoffman-La Roche, Nutley, NJ; PEG IFN-α_{2b}, PEG Intron®, Schering-Plough Laboratories, Kenilworth, NJ) are modified forms of recombinant human IFN-α with sustained absorption and prolonged half-life when administered subcutaneously or intramuscularly.[71,72]

The initial trials of PEG IFN-α_{2a}[73] and PEG IFN-α_{2b}[72,74] in patients with metastatic RCC demonstrate similar efficacy in untreated patients (13% and 14%, respectively) to nonpegylated IFN (7.5% to 14%[51,75]), as well as comparable safety with the advantage of weekly administration. The toxicity profiles between the pegylated IFNs were also similar. However, three patients treated with PEG IFN-α_{2a} developed grade 3 (National Cancer Institute [NCI] Common Toxicity Criteria, version 2.0) hepatotoxicity. One possible explanation for this unexpected toxicity may be the higher molecular weight (40 kd) of PEG IFN-α_{2a}, which may result in tissue accumulation.[76] The potential of PEG IFN to be administered at higher doses when used concurrent with IL-2, or, alternatively, the potential for a higher IL-2 dose to be administered, has resulted in the evaluation of the combination of PEG IFN with IL-2 in patients with metastatic RCC. To date, two phase I trials have been conducted with preliminary results suggesting similar activity and toxicity as nonpegylated combination trials.[77–79] It is clear from these studies that the toxicity profile and antitumor activity of pegylated IFN compare favorably to its nonpegylated counterpart, with the advantage of less frequent administration. Randomized trials are now required to determine the role of pegylated interferon as a therapy for patients with metastatic RCC.

INTERLEUKIN-2

First described in 1976 by Morgan et al.,[80] IL-2 is a T-cell growth factor with strong immunoproliferative and immunomodulatory properties activating subsets of nonspecific cytotoxic T and natural killer cells in vivo.[81] It was initially used for the treatment of metastatic RCC in 1984 after in vitro and animal studies demonstrated its significant activity as an antitumor agent. Since then, this cytokine has been extensively tested in RCC patients at both low[82] and high[83] doses, both as monotherapy and in combination with other agents.[84–105] In general, monotherapy of metastatic RCC using recombinant IL-2 has demonstrated efficacy roughly equivalent to that of monotherapy with recombinant IFN-α.[84–105] The combined response rates (complete and partial) range from 0% to 31% (Table 23.3). A review of published clinical studies using IL-2 as systemic therapy for metastatic RCC revealed an objective tumor response of 14%.[106] The FDA approved high-dose IL-2 in 1992 for the treatment of metastatic RCC, and it became the first biologic to be approved for this disease.

Fyfe et al.[107] described the results of 255 assessable patients enrolled into seven separate phase II clinical trials involving high-dose IL-2 administered at a dose of

Table 23.3.
Selected clinical trials of IL-2 monotherapy in patients with advanced renal cell carcinoma

Authors	n	Dose ($\times 10^6$ IU)	Schedule	CR	PR	ORR%
Rosenberg et al.[93]	38	0.1/kg IV	Q 8 hr × 5d, 2-wk cycle	4	3	18
Whitehead et al.[95]	12	3–6/m²/d	5d/wk	—	1	8
Sosman et al.[96]	23	1–3/m²/d IV	4 d/wk × 4 wk	—	3	13
Marumo et al.[97]	13	0.5 IV bid × 28 d	1 SC qd 6 ×wkly	2	1	23
Negrier et al.[98]	32	18/m², d 1–5 and 12–16	3-wk intervals	2	4	19
Bukowski et al.[99]	41	60/m² IV, TIW		1	4	12
Geersten et al.[100]	30	18/m² IV, d 1–5	1-wk intervals	2	4	20
Lissoni et al.[101]	13	9/m² SC, q 12 hr × 2 d	1.8/m² d 3–7	—	4	31
von der Maase et al.[102]	51	18/m² IV, d 1–5 and 12–15	3-wk rest	2	6	16
Negrier et al.[103]	22	18/m²/d IV	d 1–5 and 12–15	2	1	14
Perez et al.[104]	12	18–72/m² IV	Q wk × 16 wk	1	1	17
Vlasveld et al.[105]	9	0.18–9/m² IV × 7d		—	—	0
Lissoni et al.[101]	48	6 SC, qd	d 1–5 × 6 wk	1	13	29
Rosenberg et al.[94]	149	0.72/kg IV bolus q 8 hr	2 Tx cycles, maximum 15 doses	10	20	20
Butler et al.[90]	46	18 SC, qd d 1–5	then dose reduce, 4 or 6 wks consecutive treatment	2	7	20

TIW, three times weekly; IM, intramuscular; SC, subcutaneous; IV, intravenous; CR, complete response; PR, partial response; ORR% = overall response rate %.
Source: Adapted from Bukowski et al.[35]

600,000 or 720,000 IU/kg by 15-minute intravenous (IV) infusion every 8 hours over 5 days as tolerated. Patients were scheduled to receive a second identical treatment cycle following 5 to 9 days of rest, and treatment courses were to be repeated each 6 to 12 months for stable or responding patients. The report revealed an overall objective combined response rate of 14%, with 5% complete responses and 9% partial responses. The only predictor of response and tolerability to high-dose treatment from these initial studies was performance status, with good performance status patients receiving benefit. The rate of drug-related deaths was 4%, and more than half of patients required administration of vasopressors.

Since then, clinical trials evaluating high-dose IL-2 therapy in RCC have reported variable objective tumor responses.[87,92,93,99] Complete responses to this therapy range from 0% to 13% of treated patients, while partial responses range from 0% to 30% of patients. The early studies reported objective tumor responses after therapy with IL-2 plus lymphokine activated killer (LAK) cells in cohorts of patients with various cancers.[108,109] LAK cells are nonspecific cytotoxic cells but can lyse certain tumor cells effectively,[110] and can be generated in vitro by incubation with IL-2 and other growth factors prior to infusion. However, adoptive transfer of autologous IL-2 activated LAK cells along with bolus infusion of IL-2 (33 µg/kg) yielded an OR of only 16%,[111] comparable to studies using bolus IL-2 without LAK cells. These results coupled with the difficulty in their growth in vitro, has resulted in the abandonment of LAK cell therapy for RCC.

Due to the significant toxicity from high-dose IL-2 therapy, alternative low-dose regimens have been developed and studied in patients with metastatic RCC. The efficacy of low-dose IV bolus IL-2 (72,000 IU/kg/dose every 8 hours for 5 days each cycle, two cycles per course of treatment, two or more courses of therapy as tolerated) was compared to high-dose infusion (720,000 IU/kg/dose) in patients with RCC.[87] Although patients in the low-dose IL-2 therapy group did not receive more than 3.6 million cumulative IU of IL-2 (median of 27 doses per course) compared with accumulated doses up to 21.6 million IU in the high-dose group (median of 13 doses per course of therapy), the two regimens yielded comparable objective response rates (15% and 17%, respectively) with actuarial 1-year survival rates of 74% and 78%, respectively. Complete responses were durable (≥7 months). High-dose IL-2 induced significantly greater thrombocytopenia, hypotension, and malaise than low-dose IL-2, but the latter group experienced a greater number of bacterial infections.

The toxicity of bolus intravenous IL-2 depends on the dose used. A flu-like syndrome that includes fever, chills, and myalgias is experienced by most patients. Cardiovascular, pulmonary, and central nervous system toxicity are associated with high-dose IL-2.[87] Cardiovascular toxicity includes hypotension requiring vasopressors, cardiac arrhythmias, myocardial infarction, and myocarditis. Pulmonary toxicity secondary to capillary leak syndrome may develop and require mechanical ventilation. Grade 3 renal toxicity with oliguria can occur in more than 20% of treated patients, with creatinine levels over 8 mg/dL reported in 2%. Confusion and neuropsychiatric complaints are also common. Careful patient selection is required to minimize the morbidity and mortality associated with the administration of high-dose IL-2. Recent guidelines for the management of high-dose IL-2 toxicity have been developed.[112]

The short half-life of intravenous bolus IL-2, as well as the potential to deliver equivalent biologic doses without the need for intensive care monitoring, resulted in the use of continuous intravenous (CIV) infusion of this cytokine. Various administration schedules and doses have been used. As approved for use in Europe, most of the early trials were conducted with IL-2 at a dose of 18 million International Units (MIU)/m^2/d for 5 days, which was repeated after a 1 week rest. Reported response rates vary, but in a group of 922 patients recently reviewed, the overall response rate was 13.3%.[107,113] In a randomized trial using CIV IL-2 or IFN-α, or the combination, the response rate in 138 patients receiving IL-2 was 6.5% (similar to subcutaneous [SC] IFN-α) with 94 of 138 patients developing hypotension resistant to vasopressor agents.[101] To date, no dose/response relationship has been observed with CIV IL-2.

Subcutaneous IL-2 has also been used in metastatic RCC patients, but published experience is limited. Most reports involve fewer than 25 patients, and in a group of 290 patients, a response rate of 16.8% was found.[114] In several series,[89,90] SC IL-2 is initially administered at a higher dose level for 2 to 5 days followed by maintenance IL-2. Butler et al.[90] noted two complete responses lasting for 29.0 to >35.0 months, suggesting some of these responses may be durable. The SC route is associated with less toxicity; however, it does produce significant fatigue, fever, and malaise. Development of subcutaneous nodules at injection sites has also been noted. Hypotension and the capillary leak syndrome are uncommon with this administration route.

In an attempt to help clarify the role of high-dose (HD) and low-dose (LD) IL-2 regimens for the treatment of patients with metastatic RCC, two randomized trials have been conducted. Yang et al.[115] recently reported the results of a randomized trial to determine the effectiveness of SC IL-2 (94 patients) compared with LD (150 patients) and HD bolus IL-2 (156 patients) in a total of 400 patients with metastatic RCC. There was a higher response rate with HD IL-2 (21%) versus LD IL-2 (13%; p = .048) but no overall survival difference. The response rate of SC IL-2 (10%, partial and complete response) was similar to that of LD IL-2. Response durability and survival in completely responding patients was superior with HD IL-2 compared to LD IL-2 therapy (p = .04). As expected, toxicities were significantly less frequent with both LD IL-2 and SC IL-2, especially hypotension. The second trial, conducted by the Cytokine Working Group and recently reported by McDermott et al.,[116] randomized 192 patients with metastatic RCC to receive either outpatient SC IL-2 and SC IFN-α combination therapy (96 patients) or HD IL-2 (96 patients) therapy. The response rate was 23.2% (22 of 95 evaluable patients) for HD IL-2 versus 9.9% (9 of 91 evaluable patients) for the combination of SC IL-2 and SC IFN-α. Ten patients receiving HD IL-2 were progression free at 3 years compared to three patients receiving combination therapy, and the median survival favored HD IL-2, although it was not statistically significant. In this study, patients with bone or liver metastasis and primary tumor in place had a superior survival with HD IL-2 (p = .040). Neither study has demonstrated a clear survival advantage to HD IL-2 therapy, although objective tumor responses and the durability of response in complete responders appears to be improved.

Recently, RCC response to IL-2 therapy and patient survival has been correlated to histology (clear cell and alveolar features),[117] as well as carbonic anhydrase IX (G250 antigen) expression.[118] Retrospective analysis of paraffin-embedded tissue sections of RCC from 66 patients enrolled in a previously reported Cytokine Working Group trial[119] demonstrated high carbonic anhydrase IX (CA IX) expression in 78% (21 of 27) patients who responded to high-dose IL-2 therapy compared to only 51% (20 of 39) patients who did not respond to therapy. In this study, the percentage of CA IX positive tumor cells was utilized to separate high (>85%) versus low (≤85%) expressers. When combining good and intermediate pathology as defined by Upton et al.[117] with high expression of CA IX, the resultant group contained 96% of responders to high-dose IL-2 therapy compared to only 46% of nonresponders. Prospective study of CA IX expression as a surrogate to predict response to high-dose IL-2 therapy is ongoing.

In summary, IL-2 therapy for metastatic RCC yields objective responses in a minority of patients, but with durable efficacy (≥5 years) achieved in patients with complete response to therapy. The superiority of high-dose IL-2 therapy for significantly increasing survival in patients with metastatic RCC has not been validated due to the lack of randomized studies comparing IL-2 directly with other therapies. The use of surrogates for response to high-dose IL-2 are intriguing and may help identify patients more likely to respond to this therapy. Controlled, randomized studies of IL-2 therapy for RCC are needed to clarify its therapeutic benefit for the treatment of metastatic disease, especially with the emergence of novel agents such as sunitinib and sorfenib with significantly less toxicity.

Table 23.4.
Summary of clinical trials of interleukin-2 and interferon-α in patients with metastatic renal cell carcinoma

Route of administration		n	CR %	PR %	ORR %
IL-2	*IFN-α*				
SC	SC	675	5	16.1	21.2
CIV	SC	556	3.4	16.6	20.0
IVB	SC	180	5	15.6	20.5
Totals		1411	4.4	16.2	20.6

CR, complete response; PR, partial response; ORR, overall response rate; SC, subcutaneous; CIV, continuous intravenous infusion; IVB, intravenous bolus.

Source: Adapted from Bukowski et al.[114,121]

INTERFERON AND INTERLEUKIN-2 COMBINATION THERAPY

Several preclinical tumor models suggest synergistic antitumor activity when IFN-α is combined with IL-2.[120] A series of phase I and II trials were conducted to investigate the clinical activity of this combination. A review of the results in more than 1400 patients has been published.[121] Regardless of the route of administration or the dose of IL-2 or IFN-α used, response rates of approximately 20% have been noted (Table 23.4). As with single-agent IL-2, complete responses have been noted in up to 5% of patients.

Several randomized trials comparing the combination of IL-2 and IFN-α have been completed.[114,122–125] In one trial by Negrier et al.,[123] the combination resulted in a greater overall response rate when compared to either IL-2 or IFN-α monotherapy. This finding has been suggested in the two largest randomized trials of IL-2 and IFN-α.[122,123] Results reported by Negrier et al. suggest that the overall regression rates and 1-year event-free survival in patients receiving IL-2 and IFN-α are statistically superior compared with monotherapy with either agent (18.6% ORR combination, 6.5% overall response rate (ORR) CIV IL-2, 7.5% ORR SC IFN-α; $p < .04$). However, in this trial, patients were allowed to cross over to either IL-2 or IFN-α after failing to respond, and therefore comparisons of survival are difficult and no significant differences in survival were noted. The available data suggest this combination of cytokines may increase response rates, but improvement in survival has not been demonstrated. To date, there has been no sufficiently powered randomized phase III trial showing a survival benefit for combination therapy compared to both IL-2 and IFN-α monotherapy. Therefore, given the lack of significant improvement in response rate and survival, the added toxicity associated with combination therapy with IL-2 and IFN-α is difficult to justify for routine clinical use.

NOVEL CYTOKINES AND COMBINATIONS

In addition to IFN and IL-2, several other cytokines have been investigated both as single agents and in combination with either IFN or IL-2, or in some cases with both IFN and IL-2, for the treatment of metastatic RCC. The most investigated cytokines include granulocyte-macrophage colony-stimulating factor (GM-CSF) and IL-12. Other cytokines including tumor necrosis factor and several interleukins (IL-1, -7, -8, -9, -10, and -11) have been evaluated for antitumor activity; however, these investigations have failed to demonstrate reproducible activity against RCC.[126] At present, two cytokines (IL-18 and IL-21) are ongoing evaluation as systemic therapy in metastatic RCC.

Interleukin-12

Initially identified by two groups in 1986[127] and 1989,[128] IL-12 has been evaluated in several phase I and II trials, both as monotherapy[129–133] and combined with either IL-2[134,135] or IFN-α.[136] Although the exact antitumor mechanisms remain unclear, preliminary studies suggest that IL-12 may mediate its effect in part via induction of IFN-γ and the IFN-γ–dependent chemokines IP-10 and Mig.[137,138] In the two initial phase I trials,[129,131] 118 patients with RCC were treated with various doses of either intravenous or subcutaneous IL-12. There were a total of four responses (two partial responses [PRs] and two complete responses [CRs]) but significant hepatic, hematologic, and pulmonary toxicity limited the dose escalation. Interestingly, if a small dose is given first, substantially higher doses of IL-12 can be given subsequently. One patient had an exceptionally long complete response (>18 months) resulting in further study. Motzer et al.[130] reported a randomized phase II trial of recombinant human IL-12 compared to IFN-α in 46 patients with advanced RCC. Of the 30 patients treated with IL-12, only two patients achieved a partial response.

The combination of IL-12 with either IL-2 or IFN has been studied in metastatic RCC based on preclinical data suggesting possible synergy. Gollob et al.[135] recently reported the results of a phase I trial of concurrent twice weekly intravenous recombinant human IL-12 and low-dose subcutaneous IL-2 in 28 patients with either melanoma or RCC. There were no responses in the 15 RCC patients treated with this regimen. In a phase I trial by Hutson's group,[136] 26 patients with either melanoma or RCC were treated with subcutaneous recombinant human IL-12 and subcutaneous IFN-α (1–3 MU/m^2 three times weekly). Two of 19 patients with RCC had a partial response and the median survival was 13.3 months. Adverse events reported in these two trials were similar to other cytokine combination trials, with constitutional, hematologic, and hepatic toxicity being most common. Because of the disappointing results from these clinical trials, further development of IL-12 as therapy for patients with metastatic RCC has been abandoned.

Granulocyte-Macrophage Colony-Stimulating Factor

Although its specific antitumor properties remain unclear, evidence from clinical trials suggest that GM-CSF may help promote a host-specific immunologic response to tumor antigens. Phase I trials of this cytokine have demonstrated profound monocytosis and enhanced activation of mononuclear phagocytes.[139] In phase II trials by Rini et al.[140] and Wos et al.,[141] patients with metastatic RCC were treated with GM-CSF alone. Clinical responses were seen by Wos et al. in two of 28 patients with pulmonary metastases but no response was seen by Rini et al. in 24 patients given GM-CSF alone. Toxicity to subcutaneous injections of GM-CSF is usually mild; however, a capillary leak syndrome and hypotension have been described that may be partly explained by induction of endogenous cytokines.[142,143]

Granulocyte-macrophage colony-stimulating factor has been combined with IL-2 and IFN-α and administered to patients with RCC.[144,145] In a phase I trial reported by de Gast et al.,[144] 18 patients (11 with metastatic RCC) were treated with subcutaneous IL-2

(1, 4, or 8 MIU/m^2), a fixed dose of subcutaneous IFN-α (5 MU), and subcutaneous GM-CSF (2.5 or 5 µg/kg) for 12 days every 3 weeks. Of eight patients with progressive metastatic RCC after nephrectomy, three achieved a complete remission. Side effects included fever, hypotension requiring intravenous fluid support, and fatigue. Agrawal et al.[146] reported the results of a phase I/II study of GM-CSF, IL-2, and IFN-α_{2b} in 61 patients with metastatic RCC. Overall, eight patients (13%) responded to treatment, and the most common side effects were nausea, vomiting, and fatigue. These reports suggest that clinical responses are seen when GM-CSF is combined with other cytokines, but the overall results resemble the trials using IL-2 and IFN-α as monotherapy and therefore do not justify its routine use.

Interleukin-18 and Interleukin-21

Both IL-18 and IL-21 are novel cytokines with antitumor activity in renal cell carcinoma tumor models,[147,148] and both agents are under investigation in early-phase clinical trials as systemic therapy for metastatic disease. Interleukin-18, originally described as IFN-γ–inducing factor, has pleiotropic immunologic activity, which includes activation of both T cells and NK cells in vitro, similar to IL-12. Interleukin-21, which is produced by activated CD4$^+$ T cells, is a member of the IL-2 cytokine family and enhances T-cell and NK-cell cytotoxicity. Results from ongoing clinical trials will help elucidate what role, if any, these two cytokines may have as a therapy for RCC.

CONCLUSION

Metastatic RCC is a tumor refractory to standard cytotoxic chemotherapy regimens. The rationale for the use of cytokines in this cancer is based on compelling evidence that RCC is sensitive to immunologic manipulation. Cytokine-based therapy with either IL-2 or IFN-α can result in objective tumor responses in up to 15% of patients, and in selected patients these responses may be durable. Improvement in survival for patients receiving IFN-α has been demonstrated in several randomized trials. This has not been documented in patients receiving IL-2, but appropriately controlled trials have not been performed. The patients most likely to respond are those with limited pulmonary disease who are asymptomatic. Recent evidence suggests that a variety of clinical factors (serum lactate dehydrogenase [LDH], prior nephrectomy, number and location of metastatic sites, calcium level, and hemoglobin level), as well as histology (clear cell, papillary, or sarcomatoid) also influence the likelihood of response to cytokine-based therapies. Surrogate markers predictive for response (G250/CA IX) to high-dose IL-2 therapy are ongoing evaluation.

The development of targeted therapies for clear-cell RCC has brought into question the role of cytokines in this patient population. However, no therapy to date has proven curative in patients with metastatic RCC. Therefore, cytokine-based therapy will continue to have a role in the management of this disease in patients who do not respond or progress to these newer therapies. Clinical trials incorporating combinations of cytokines and these new targeted approaches are under way.

REFERENCES

1. Yagoda A, Abi-Rached B, Petrylak D. Chemotherapy for advanced renal cell carcinoma: 1983–1993. Semin Oncol 1995;22:42–60.

 2. Motzer RJ, Vogelzang NJ. Chemotherapy for renal cell carcinoma. In: Raghaven D, Scher HI, Leibel SA, et al., eds. Principles and Practice of Genitourinary Oncology. Philadelphia: Lippincott-Raven, 1997:885–896.
 3. Voglezang NJ, Priest ER, Borden L. Spontaneous regression of histologically proved pulmonary metastases from renal cell carcinoma: a case with 5-year follow-up. J Urol 1992;148:1247–1248.
 4. Finke JH, Rayman P, Hart L, et al. Characterization of TIL subsets from human renal carcinoma: specific reactivity defined by cytotoxicity, IFN-γ secretion, and proliferation. J Immunother 1994;15:91–104.
 5. Oliver RTD, Mehta A, Barnett MJ. A phase 2 study of surveillance in patients with metastatic renal cell carcinoma and assessment of response of such patients to therapy on progression. Mol Biother 1998;1:14–20.
 6. Motzer RJ, Mazumdar M, Bacik J, et al. Survival and prognostic stratification of 670 patients with advanced renal cell carcinoma. J Clin Oncol 1999;17:2530–2540.
 7. Negrier S, Escudier B, Gomez F, et al. Prognostic factors of survival and rapid progression in 782 patients with metastatic renal carcinomas treated by cytokines: a report from the Groupe Francais d'Immunotherapie. Ann Oncol 2002;13:1460–1468.
 8. Wu J, Caliendo G, Hu XP, et al. Impact of histology on the treatment outcome of metastatic or recurrent renal cell carcinoma. Med Oncol 1998;15:44–49.
 9. Flannigan RC, Salmon SE, Blumenstein BA, et al. Nephrectomy followed by interferon alfa-2b compared with interferon alfa-2b alone for metastatic renal cell cancer. N Engl J Med 2001; 345:1655–1659.
10. Medical Research Council Renal Cancer Collaborators. Interferon-alpha and survival in metastatic renal carcinoma: early results of a randomized controlled trial. Lancet 1999;353:14–17.
11. Quesada JR, Swanson DA, Trindale A, et al. Renal cell carcinoma: antitumor effects of leukocyte interferon. Cancer Res 1983;43:940–947.
12. DeKernion JB, Sarna JB, Figlin R, et al. The treatment of renal cell carcinoma with human leukocyte alpha-interferon. J Urol 1983;130:1063–1066.
13. Kirkwood JM. Interferons. In: DeVita VT, Hellman S, Rosenberg S, eds. Cancer: Principles and Practice of Oncology, 6th ed. Philadelphia: Lippincott Williams & Wilkins, 2001:461–471.
14. Dorr RT. Interferon-alpha in malignant and viral diseases: a review. Drugs 1993;45:177–211.
15. Welsh RM, Yang H, Bukowski JF. The role of interferon in regulation of virus infections by cytotoxic lymphocytes. Bioessays 1998;8:10.
16. Fellous M, et al. Interferon-dependent induction of mRNA for the major histocompatability antigens in human fibroblasts and lymphoblastoid cell lines. Proc Natl Acad Sci 1982;79:3082.
17. van Schie R, et al. Effect of rIFN-gamma on antibody-mediated cytotoxicity via human monocyte IgG Fc receptor II (CD32. Scand J Immunol 1992;36:385.
18. te Velde A, et al. IL-10 stimulates monocyte Fc gamma R surface expression and cytotoxic activity. Distinct regulation of antibody-dependent cellular cytotoxicity by IFN-gamma, IL-4 and IL-10. J Immunol 1992;149:4048.
19. Vuist WM, et al. Enhancement of the antibody-dependent cellular cytotoxicity of human peripheral blood lymphocytes with interleukin-2 and interferon alpha. Cancer Immunol Immunother 1993; 36:163.
20. Robertson MJ, et al. Costimulatory signals are required for optimal proliferation of human natural killer cells. J Immunol 1993;150:1705.
21. Minato N, et al. Mode regulation of natural killer cell activity by interferon. J Exp Med 1980;152:124.
22. Saksela E, Timonen T, Cantell K. Cellular interactions in the augmentation of human NK activity by interferon. Ann N Y Acad Sci 1980;350:102.
23. Sato N, et al. Actions of TNF and IFN-gamma on angiogenesis *in vitro*. J Invest Dermatol 1990;95(suppl 6):858.
24. White CW. Treatment of hemangiomatosis with recombinant interferon alfa. Semin Hematol 1990;27(suppl 4):15.
25. Billington DC. Angiogenesis and its inhibition: potential new therapies in oncology and non-neoplastic diseases. Drug Des Discov 1991;8:3.
26. Maheshwari RK, et al. Differential effects of interferon gamma and alpha on *in vitro* model of angiogenesis. J Cell Physiol 1991;146:164.

27. Folkman J, Ingber D. Inhibition of angiogenesis. Semin Cancer Biol 1992;3:89.

28. Saiki I, et al. Inhibition of tumor-induced angiogenesis by the administration of recombinant interferon-gamma followed by a synthetic lipid-A subunit analogue (GLA-60). Int J Cancer 1992;51:641.

29. Gruss HJ, et al. Interferon-gamma interrupts autocrine growth mediated by endogenous interleukin-6 in renal cell carcinoma. Int J Cancer 1991;49:770.

30. Garbe C, Krasagakis K. Effects of interferons and cytokines on melanoma cells. J Invest Dermatol 1993;100(suppl):2395.

31. Quesada JR, Swanson DA, Trindale A, et al. Renal cell carcinoma: antitumor effects of leukocyte interferon. Cancer Res 1983;43:940–947.

32. DeKernion JB, Sarna JB, Figlin R, et al. The treatment of renal cell carcinoma with human leukocyte alpha-interferon. J Urol 1983;130:1063–1066.

33. Coppin C, Porzsolt F, Kumpf J, et al. Immunotherapy for advanced renal cell cancer. Cochrane Database of Systematic Reviews 2003;3:1–46.

34. Motzer RJ, Berg WJ. Role of interferon in metastatic renal cell carcinoma. In: Bukowski RM, Novick AC, eds. Current Clinical Oncology: Renal Cell Carcinoma. Totowa, NJ: Humana Press, 2001:319–329.

35. Bukowski RM, Novick AC. Clinical practice guidelines: renal cell carcinoma. Cleve Clin J Med 1997;64:S1–S48.

36. Minassian LM, Motzer RJ, Gluck L, et al. Interferon- alpha 2a in advanced renal cell carcinoma: treatment results and survival in 159 patients with long-term follow-up. J Clin Oncol 1993;11:1368–1375.

37. Quesada JR, Swanson DA, Gutterman JU. Phase II study of interferon alpha in metastatic renal cell carcinoma: a progress report. J Clin Oncol 1985;3:1086–1092.

38. Umeda T, Niijima T. Phase II study of alpha interferon on renal cell carcinoma. Summary of three collaborative trials. Cancer 1986;58:1231–1235.

39. Schnall SF, Davis C, Ziyadeh T, et al. Treatment of metastatic renal cell carcinoma with intramuscular (IM) recombinant interferon alpha (IFN, Hoffman-LaRoche). Proc Am Soc Clin Oncol 1986; 15(5):227.

40. Kempf RA, Grunberg SM, Daniels JR, et al. Recombinant interferon alpha-2 (Intron A) in a phase II study of renal cell carcinoma. J Biol Resp Mod 1999;5:27–35.

41. Fossa SD. Is interferon with or without vinblastine the "treatment of choice" in metastatic renal cell carcinoma. Semin Surg Oncol 1988;4(3):178–183.

42. Foon JK, Doroshow J, Bonnem E, et al. A prospective randomized trial of alpha 2B-interferon/ gamma-interferon or the combination in advanced metastatic renal cell carcinoma. J Biol Resp Mod 1988;7:540–545.

43. Steineck G, Strander H, Carbin BE, et al. Recombinant leukocyte interferon alpha-ea and medroxy-progesterone in advanced renal cell carcinoma. A randomized trial. Acta Oncol 1990;29:155–162.

44. Marshall ME, Simpson H, Carbin BE, et al. Treatment of renal cell carcinoma with daily low-dose alpha interferon. J Biol Resp Mod 1989;8:453–461.

45. Muss HB, Costanzi JJ, Leavitt R, et al. Recombinant alfa interferon in renal cell carcinoma: a randomized trial of two routes of administration. J Clin Oncol 1987;5:286.

46. Levens W, Ruebben H, Ingenhag W. Long-term interferon treatment in metastatic renal cell carcinoma. Eur Urol 1989;16:378–381.

47. Bono AV, Reali L, Bevenuti C, et al. Recombinant alpha interferon in metastatic renal cell carcinoma. Urology 1991;38:60–63.

48. Buzaid AC, Robertone A, Kisala C, et al. Phase II study of interferon alpha-2a, recombinant (Roferon A) in metastatic renal cell carcinoma. J Clin Oncol 1987;5:1083–1089.

49. Figlin RA. deKernion JB. Maldazys J. Sarna G. Treatment of renal cell carcinoma with alpha (human leukocyte) interferon and vinblastine in combination: a phase I–II trial. Cancer Treat Rep 1985; 69(3):263–267.

50. Pyrhonen S, Salminen E, Ruuru M, et al. Prospective randomized trial of interferon alfa-2a plus vinblastine versus vinblastine alone in patients with advanced renal cell cancer. J Clin Oncol 1999;17:2859–2867.

51. Medical Research Council Renal Cancer Collaborators. Interferon α and survival in metastatic renal cell carcinoma: early results of randomized trial. Lancet 1999;353:14–17.

52. Flannigan RC, Salmon E, Blumenstein BA, et al. Nephrectomy followed by interferon alfa-2b compared with interferon alfa-2b alone for metastatic renal-cell carcinoma. N Engl J Med 2001;345(23):1655–1659.
53. Mickisch GH, Garin A, van Poppel H, et al. Radical nephrectomy plus interferon-alfa-based immunotherapy compared with interferon alfa alone in metastatic renal-cell carcinoma: a randomized trial. Lancet 2001;358(9286):966–970.
54. Bukowski RM. Cytokine therapy for metastatic renal cell carcinoma. Semin Urol Oncol 2001; 19(2):148–154.
55. Rinehart JJ, Young D, Laforge J, et al. Phase I/II trial of interferon-beta-serine in patients with renal cell carcinoma: immunological and biological effects. Cancer Res 1987;47:2481–2485.
56. Kish J, Ensley J, Al-Sarraf M, et al. Activity of serine inhibited recombinant DNA beta interferon (IFN-beta) in patients with metastatic and recurrent renal cell carcinoma. Proc Am Assoc Cancer Res 1986;27:184.
57. Nelson KA, Wallenberg JC, Todd MB. High-dose intravenous therapy with beta-interferon in patients with renal cell cancer. Proc Am Assoc Cancer Res 1989;30:260.
58. Kinney P, Triozzi P, Young D, et al. Phase II trial of interferon-beta-serine in metastatic renal cell carcinoma. J Clin Oncol 1990;8:881–885.
59. Quesada JR, Kuzrock R, Sherwin SA, et al. Phase II studies of recombinant human interferon gamma in metastatic renal cell carcinoma. J Biol Resp Mod 1987;6:20–27.
60. Koiso K. Recombinant Human Interferon Gamma Research Group. Phase II study of recombinant interferon gamma on renal cell carcinoma. Cancer 1987;60:929–933.
61. Machida T, Koiso K, Takaku F, et al. Phase II study of recombinant human interferon gamma (S-6810) in renal cell carcinoma. Gan Kagaku Ryoho 1987;14:440–445.
62. Rinehart JJ, Young D, Laforge J, et al. Phase I/II trial of recombinant gamma-interferon in patients with metastatic renal cell carcinoma: immunologic and biologic effects. J Biol Resp Mod 1987; 6:302–312.
63. Garnick MB, Reich SD, Maxwell B, et al. Phase I/II study of recombinant interferon gamma in advanced renal cell carcinoma. J Urol 1988;139:251–255.
64. Kuebler J, Brown T, Goodman P, et al. Continuous infusion recombinant gamma interferon (Clr-GIFN) for metastatic renal cell carcinoma. Proc Am Soc Clin Oncol 1989;8:140.
65. Aulitzky W, Gastl G, Aulitzky WE, et al. Successful treatment of metastatic renal cell carcinoma with a biologically active dose of recombinant interferon-gamma. J Clin Oncol 1989;7: 1875–1884.
66. Grups JW, Frohmuller G. Cyclin interferon gamma treatment of patients with metastatic renal cell carcinoma. Br J Urol 1989;64:218–220.
67. Bruntsch U, de Mulder PH, ten Bokkel Huinink WW, et al. Phase II study of recombinant human interferon-gamma in metastatic renal cell carcinoma. J Biol Resp Mod 1999;9:335–338.
68. Foon K, Doroshow J, Bonnem J, et al. A prospective randomized trial of alpha-2B-interferon/gamma-interferon or the combination in advanced metastatic renal cell carcinoma. J Biol Resp Mod 1988;7:540–545.
69. Ellerhorst JA, Kilbourn RG, Amato RJ, et al. Phase II trial of low dose gamma-interferon in metastatic renal cell carcinoma. J Urol 1994;152:841–845.
70. Small EJ, Weiss GR, Malik UK, et al. The treatment of metastatic renal cell carcinoma patients with recombinant human gamma interferon. Cancer J Sci Am 1998;4:162–167.
71. Crawford J. Clinical uses of pegylated pharmaceuticals in oncology. Cancer Treat Rev 2002;28(suppl A):7–11.
72. Bukowski RM, Tendler C, Cutler D, et al. Treating cancer with PEG Intron: pharmacokinetic profile and dosing guidelines for an improved interferon alpha-2b formulation. Cancer 2002;95: 386–396.
73. Motzer RJ, Rakhit A, Thompson J, et al. Phase II trial of branched peginterferon-alpha 2a (40 kDa) for patients with advanced renal cell carcinoma. Ann Oncol 2002;13(11):1799–1805.
74. Bukowski R, Ernstoff MS, Gore M, et al. Pegylated interferon alfa-2b treatment for patients with solid tumors: a phase I/II study. J Clin Oncol 2002;20:3841–3849.
75. Negrier S, Escudier B, Lasset C, et al. Recombinant interleukin-2, recombinant interferon alfa-2a, or both in metastatic renal cell carcinoma. N Engl J Med 1998;338:1273–1278.
76. He XH, Shaw PC, Tam SC. Reducing the immunogenicity and improving the *in vivo* activity of trichosanthin by site-directed pegylation. Life Sci 1999;65:355–368.

77. Clark JI, Gollob J, Sosman J, et al. Phase I trial of polyethylene glycol (PEG) interferon alpha-2b (IFN) + interleukin-2 (IL-2) in renal cell cancer (RCC). Proc Am Soc Clin Oncol 2002;21:2419.
78. Hutson TE, Mekhail T, Messerli E, et al. Phase I trial of PEG-Intron and rIL-2 in patients with metastatic renal cell carcinoma. Proc Am Soc Clin Oncol 2002;2406.
79. Hutson TE, Leschinsky A, Moon C, et al. Toxicity and apoptotic effects of PEG-Intron and rIL-2 in patients with metastatic renal cell carcinoma. Proc Am Assoc Cancer Res 2003;44:2540.
80. Morgan DA, Ruscetti FW, Gallo RC. Selective in vivo growth of T-lymphocytes from normal bone marrows. Science 1976;193:1007–1008.
81. Ettinghausen SE, Lipford EH, III, Mule JJ, Rosenberg SA. Recombinant interleukin 2 stimulates in vivo proliferation of adoptively transferred lymphokine-activated killer (LAK) cells. J Immunol 1985;135:3623–3635.
82. Stadler WM, Voglezang NJ. Low-dose interleukin-2 in treatment of metastatic renal-cell carcinoma. Semin Oncol 1995;22:67–73.
83. Parkinson DR, Sznol M. High-dose interleukin-2 in the therapy of metastatic renal-cell carcinoma. Semin Oncol 1995;22:61–66.
84. Haas GP, Hillman GG, Redman BG, Pontes JE. Immunotherapy of renal cell carcinoma. CA Cancer J Clin 1993;43:177–187.
85. Figlin RA, Abi-Aad AS, Belldegrun A, DeKernion JB. The role of interferon and interleukin-2 in the immunotherapeutic approach to renal cell carcinoma. Semin Oncol 1991;18(suppl 7):102–107.
86. Wirth MP. Immunotherapy for metastatic renal cell carcinoma. Urol Clin North Am 1993; 20:283–295.
87. Yang JC, Topalian SL, Parkinson D, et al. Randomized comparison of high-dose and low-dose intravenous interleukin-2 for the therapy of metastatic renal cell carcinoma: an interim report. J Clin Oncol 1994;12:1572–1576.
88. Sleijfer D, Janssen RAJ, Butler J, de Vries EGE, Willemse PHB, Mulder NH. Phase II study of subcutaneous interleukin-2 in unselected patients with advanced renal cell cancer on an outpatient basis. J Clin Oncol 1992;10:1119–1123.
89. Lissoni P, Barni S, Ardizzoia A, et al. Prognostic factors of the clinical response to subcutaneous immunotherapy with interleukin-2 in patients with metastatic renal cell carcinoma. Oncology 1994;51:59–62.
90. Butler J, Sleijfer Dth, van der Graaf WTA, de Vries EGE, Willemse PHB, Mulder NH. A progress report on the outpatient treatment of patients with advanced renal cell carcinoma using subcutaneous recombinant interleukin-2. Semin Oncol 1993;20(suppl 9):15–21.
91. Caligiuri MA. Low-dose recombinant interleukin-2 therapy: rationale and potential clinical application. Semin Oncol 1993;20(suppl 9):3–10.
92. Atzpodien J, Kirchner H, Hanninen EL, et al. European studies of interleukin-2 in metastatic renal cell carcinoma. Semin Oncol 1993;20(suppl 9):22–26.
93. Rosenberg SA, Yang JC, Topalian SL, et al. Treatment of 283 consecutive patients with metastatic melanoma or renal cell carcinoma using high-dose bolus interleukin-2. JAMA 1994;271:907–913.
94. Rosenberg SA. The development of new immunotherapies for the treatment of cancer using interleukin-2:a review. Ann Surg 1988;208:121–135.
95. Whitehead RP, Ward DL, Hemingway LL, et al. Phase I–II trial of intravenous bolus recombinant interleukin-2 in patients with disseminated renal cell carcinoma (abstract). Proc Am Soc Clin Oncol 1988;7:128.
96. Sosman JA, Kohler PC, Hank J, et al. Repetitive weekly cycles of recombinant human interleukin-2: responses of renal carcinoma with acceptable toxicity. J Natl Cancer Inst 1988;80:60–63.
97. Marumo K, Muraki J, Ueno M, et al. Immunologic study of human recombinant interleukin-2 (low dose) in patients with advanced renal cell carcinoma. Urology 1989;33:219–225.
98. Negrier S, Philip T, Stoter G, et al. Interleukin-2 with or without LAK cells in metastatic renal cell carcinoma: a report of a European multi-center study. Eur J Cancer Clin Oncol 1989;25(suppl 3): S21–S28.
99. Bukowski RM, Goodman P, Crawford ED, et al. Phase II trial of high-dose intermittent interleukin-2 in metastatic renal cell carcinoma: a Southwest Oncology Group Study. J Natl Cancer Inst 1990;82:143–146.
100. Geersten PF, Hermann GG, Maase H, et al. Treatment of metastatic renal cell carcinoma by continuous intravenous infusion of recombinant interleukin-2: a single-center phase II study. J Clin Oncol 1992;10:753–759.

101. Lissoni P, Barni S, Ardizzoia A, et al. Second line therapy with low-dose subcutaneous interleukin-2 alone in advanced renal cancer patients resistant to interferon-alpha. Eur J Cancer 1992;28:92–96.
102. Von der Maase H, Geersten P, Thatcher N, et al. Recombinant interleukin-2 in metastatic renal cell carcinoma: a European multicenter phase II study. Eur J Cancer 1991;27:1583–1589.
103. Negrier S, Mercatello A, Bret M, et al. Intravenous interleukin-2 in patients over 65 with metastatic renal cell carcinoma. Br J Cancer 1992;65:723–726.
104. Perez EA, Scudder SA, Meyers FA, et al. Weekly 24–hour continuous infusion interleukin-2 for metastatic melanoma and renal cell carcinoma: a phase I study. J Immunother 1991;10:57–62.
105. Vlasveld LT, Rankin EM, Hekman A, et al. A phase I study of prolonged continuous infusion of low-dose recombinant interleukin-2 in melanoma and renal cell cancer I: clinical aspects. Br J Cancer 1992;65:744–750.
106. Fisher RI. Interleukin-2—advances in clinical research and treatment. Semin Oncol 1993;20(suppl 9):1–2.
107. Fyfe G, Fisher RI, Rosenberg SA, Sznol M, Parkinson DR, Louie AC. Results of treatment of 255 patients with metastatic renal cell carcinoma who received high-dose recombinant interleukin-2 therapy. J Clin Oncol 1995;13:688–696.
108. Rosenberg SA, Lotze MT, Muul LM, et al. Observations on the systemic administration of autologous lymphokine-activated killer cells and recombinant interleukin-2 to patients with metastatic cancer. N Engl J Med 1985;313:1485–1492.
109. West WH, Tauer KW, Yannelli JR, et al. Constant-infusion recombinant interleukin-2 in adoptive immunotherapy of advanced cancer. N Engl J Med 1987;316:898–905.
110. Rayner AA, Grimm EA, Lotze MT, Wilson DJ, Rosenberg SA. Lymphokine-activated killer (LAK) cell phenomenon. IV. Lysis by LAK cell clones of fresh human tumor cells from autologous and multiple allogeneic tumors. J Natl Cancer Inst 1985;75:67–75.
111. Fisher RI, Coltman CA, Doroshow JH, et al. Metastatic renal cancer treated with interleukin-2 and lymphokine-activated killer cells. A phase II clinical trial. Ann Intern Med 1988;108:518–523.
112. Schwartzentruber DJ. Guidelines for the safe administration of high-dose interleukin-2. J Immunotherapy 2001;24(4):287–293.
113. Palmer PA, Atzpodien J, Philip T, et al. A comparison of 2 modes of administration of recombinant interleukin-2: continuous intravenous infusion alone versus subcutaneous administration plus interferon alfa in patients with advanced RCC. Cancer Biother 1993;8:123.
114. Bukowski RM, Dutcher JP. Low-dose interleukin-2. In: Voglezang NJ, Scardino PT, Shipley WW, et al., eds. Genitourinary Oncology, Philadelphia: Lippincott Williams & Wilkins, 2000:213–218.
115. Yang JC, Sherry RM, Steinberg SM, et al. Randomized study of high-dose and low-dose interleukin-2 in patients with metastatic renal cancer. J Clin Oncol 2003;21(6):3127–3132.
116. McDermott DF, Regan MM, Clark JI, et al. Randomized phase III trial of high-dose interleukin-2 versus subcutaneous interleukin-2 and interferon in patients with metastatic renal cell carcinoma. J Clin Oncol 2005;23(1):133–141.
117. Upton MP, Parker RA, Youmans A, et al. Histologic predictors of renal cell carcinoma (RCC) response to interleukin-2 based therapy. Proc Am Soc Clin Oncol 2003;22:851.
118. Bui MTH, Seligson D, Han KR, et al. Carbonic Anhydrase IX is an independent predictor of survival in advanced renal cell carcinoma: implications for prognosis and therapy. Clin Cancer Res 2003;9:802–811.
119. Atkins M, McDermott D, Regan M, et al. Carbonic anhydrase IX (CAIX) expression predicts for renal cell cancer (RCC) patient response and survival to IL-2 therapy. Proc Am Soc Clin Oncol 2004;22(suppl 14S):4512.
120. Chikkala NF, Lewis I, Ulchaker J, et al. Interactive effects of α interferon A/D and interleukin-2 on murine lymphokine-activated killer activity: analysis at the effector and precursor level. Cancer Res 1990;50:1176–1182.
121. Bukowski RM. Natural history and therapy of metastatic renal cell carcinoma: role of interleukin-2. Cancer 1997;80:1198–1220.
122. Henriksson R, Nilsson S, Colleen S, et al. Survival in renal cell carcinoma—a randomized evaluation of tamoxifen vs interleukin-2, α interferon (leukocyte) and tamoxifen. Br J Cancer 1998;77:1311.
123. Negrier S, Escudier B, Lasset C, et al. Recombinant interleukin-2, recombinant interferon alfa-2a, or both in metastatic renal cell carcinoma. N Engl J Med 1998;338:1273–1278.

124. Vogelzang NJ, Lipton A, Figlin RA. Subcutaneous interleukin-2 plus interferon alfa-2a in metastatic renal cancer: an outpatient multicenter trial. J Clin Oncol 1993;11:1809–1816.

125. Atkins MB, Sparano J, Fisher RI, et al. Randomized phase II trial of high-dose interleukin-2 either alone or in combination with interferon alfa-2b in advanced renal cell carcinoma. J Clin Oncol 1993;11:661–670.

126. Hill ADK, Redmond HP, Croke DT, et al. Cytokines in tumour therapy. Br J Surg 1992; 79:990–997.

127. Gately MK, Wilson DE, Wong HL. Synergy between recombinant interleukin 2 (rIL 2) and IL 2–depleted lymphokine-containing supernatants in facilitating allogeneic human cytolytic T lymphocyte responses in vitro. J Immunol 1986;136:1274–1282.

128. Kobayashi M, Fitz L, Ryan M, et al. Identification and purification of natural killer cell stimulatory factor (NKSF), a cytokine with multiple biologic effects on human lymphocytes. J Exp Med 1989; 170:827–845.

129. Motzer RJ, Rakhit A, Schwartz LH, et al. Phase I trial of subcutaneous recombinant human interleukin-12 in patients with advanced renal cell carcinoma. Clin Cancer Res 1998;4:1183–1191.

130. Motzer RJ, Rakhit A, Thompson JA, et al. Randomized multicenter phase II trial of subcutaneous recombinant human interleukin-12 versus interferon-alpha 2a for patients with advanced renal cell carcinoma. J Int Cytokine Res 2001;21(4):257–263.

131. Atkins M, Robertson M, Gordon M, et al. Phase I evaluation of intravenous recombinant human interleukin 12 in patients with advanced malignancies. Clin Cancer Res 1997;3:409–417.

132. Gollob JA, Mier JW, Veenstra K, et al. Phase I trial of twice weekly intravenous interleukin 12 in patients with metastatic renal cell cancer or malignant melanoma: ability to maintain IFN-gamma induction is associated with clinical response. Clin Cancer Res 2000;6:1678–1692.

133. Portielje JE, Kruit WH, Schuler M, et al. Phase I study of subcutaneously administered recombinant human interleukin 12 in patients with advanced renal cell cancer. Clin Cancer Res 1999; 5(12):3983–3989.

134. Wigginton JM, Komschlies KL, Back TC, et al. Administration of interleukin 12 with pulse interleukin-2 and the rapid and complete eradication of murine renal carcinoma. J Natl Cancer Inst 1996;88:38–43.

135. Gollob JA, Veenstra KG, Parker RA, et al. Phase I trial of concurrent twice-weekly recombinant human interleukin-12 plus low-dose IL-2 in patients with melanoma or renal cell carcinoma. J Clin Oncol 2003;21(13):2564–2573.

136. Al-Atrash G, Hutson TE, Nemec C, et al. Clinical and immunologic effects of subcutaneously administered IL-12 and IFN-a2b: phase I trial in patients with metastatic renal cell carcinoma or malignant melanoma. J Clin Oncol 2004;22(14):2891–2900.

137. Tannenbaum CS, Tubbs R, Armstrong D, et al. The CXC chemokines IP-10 and Mig are necessary for IL-12–mediated regression of the mouse RENCA tumor. J Immunol 1998;161:927–932.

138. Bukowski RM, Rayman P, Molto L, et al. Interferon-gamma and CXC chemokine induction by interleukin 12 in renal cell carcinoma. Clin Can Res 1999;5(10):2780–2788.

139. Bukowski RM, Murthy S, Sergi J, et al. Phase I trial of recombinant granulocyte-macrophage colony stimulating factor in patients with metastatic renal cell carcinoma. Cancer 1996;77:639–644.

140. Rini BI, Stadler WM, Spielberger RT, Ratain MJ, Vogelzang NJ. Granulocyte-macrophage colony-stimulating factor (GM-CSF) in metastatic renal cell cancer: a phase II trial. Cancer 1998; 82:1352–1358.

141. Wos E, Olencki T, Tuason L, et al. Phase II trial of subcutaneous administered granulocyte-macrophage colony-stimulating factor in patients with metastatic renal cell carcinoma. Cancer 1996;77:639–644.

142. Lieschke GJ, Cebon J, Morstyn G. Characterization of the clinical effects after the first dose of bacterially synthesized recombinant human granulocyte-macrophage colony-stimulating factor. Blood 1989;74:2634–2643.

143. Petros WP. Colony-stimulating factors. In: Chabner BA and Longo DL, eds. Cancer Chemotherapy and Biotherapy: Principles and Practice. Philadelphia: Lippincott Williams & Wilkins, 2001: 829–850.

144. de Gast GC, Klumpen HJ, Vyth-Dreese FA, et al. Phase I trial of combined immunotherapy with subcutaneous granulocyte macrophage colony-stimulating factor, low dose interleukin-2 and interferon α in progressive metastatic melanoma and renal cell carcinoma. Clin Cancer Res 2000;6:1267–1272.

145. Schornagel JH, Kersten M, Mallo H, et al. Combined immunotherapy with subcutaneous GM-CSF, low-dose IL-2, and IFN-α can induce complete remissions in metastatic renal cell carcinoma. Proc Am Soc Clin Oncol 2000;19:344a.

146. Agrawal NR, Olencki T, Mekhail T, et al. A phase I/II study of GM-CSF, interleukin-2 (IL-2) and interferon-alpha (INF-α) in metastatic renal carcinoma (MRCC). Proc Am Soc Clin Oncol 2002;21:1829a.

147. Hughes S, Chin L, Waggie PV, et al. Interleukin 21 efficacy in a mouse model of metastatic renal cell carcinoma. J Clin Oncol 2004 (ASCO Annual Meeting Proceedings) 22 (14S):2598.

148. Hara S, Nagai H, Miyake H, et al. Secreted type of modified interleukin-18 gene transduced into mouse renal cell carcinoma cells induces systemic tumor immunity. J Urol 2001;165 (6 pt 1):2039–2043.

24 Chemotherapy for Metastatic Clear-Cell Renal Cell Carcinoma

James O. Jin and Walter M. Stadler

KEYWORDS

CHEMOTHERAPY
FLUOROPYRIMIDINE
MULTI-DRUG RESISTANCE

ABSTRACT

Patients with metastatic renal cell carcinoma (RCC) have a poor prognosis. Although the natural history of metastatic RCC can be highly variable, most of patients die within 1 year of diagnosis and the 5-year survival is less than 5%.[1] The treatment of metastatic RCC has remained a challenge for oncologists. Although immunotherapy with interleukin-2 (IL-2) and interferon (IFN) can achieve low, but reproducible, response rates of 10% to 20% in advanced RCC,[2] and antiangiogenic agents such as sunitinib and sorafenib improve progression free survival, and mTOR inhibitors such as temsirolimus improve survival in selected patients. RCC has been considered highly resistant to chemotherapy and hormonal therapy.[3] This chapter reviews chemotherapy, hormonal therapy, and combined therapies in metastatic RCC.

CHEMOTHERAPY

Chemotherapy for advanced RCC has been extensively studied. In a comprehensive review of 161 publications, Yagoda et al.[4] summarized the results of clinical trials from 1983 to 1993, and a 6% overall response rate was found in 4093 adequately treated patients with advanced RCC. In another review of 51 published phase II clinical trials from 1990 to 1998, including 33 chemotherapeutic agents, the overall response rate was only 5.5% in 1347 patients.[3] No single chemotherapeutic agent has reproducibly demonstrated response rates more than 10%.

From: *Clinical Management of Renal Tumors*
Edited by: R.M. Bukowski and A.C. Novick © Humana Press Inc., Totowa, NJ

SINGLE-AGENT CHEMOTHERAPY

Table 24.1 summarizes the activity of selected single cytotoxic agents in advanced RCC. Almost all classes of agents yield poor response rates.[5–68] Among all of these tested chemotherapeutic agents, vinblastine, floxuridine, and 5-fluorouracil (5-FU) were studied most intensively (Table 24.1). In 1984, Kuebler et al.[59] reported a 16% response rate in a phase II study of vinblastine, an antimitotic agent, in 19 patients with three partial responses. However, subsequent studies were disappointing, and no trials could produce similar results (Table 24.1). Furthermore, a phase III study of vinblastine versus vinblastine plus IFN-α demonstrated a 2.5% response rate in the vinblastine-alone group, and a large phase II study of vinblastine with putative P-glycoprotein multidrug resistance protein inhibitors yielded no responses in 67 patients.[70,71]

Encouraging results have been obtained with 5-FU, a pyrimidine antimetabolite, and its analogues, which showed low but reproducible response rates.[23–33] In 1990, Hrushesky et al.[23] reported a 20% response rate with continuous intravenous infusion of floxuridine in 56 patients. The response rates in subsequent trials of floxuridine ranged from 0% to 14% (Table 24.1).[25–29] Response rates with the related pyrimidine nucleoside analogue gemcitabine were 6% and 8% in two independent phase II trials.[36,37]

Table 24.1.
Response rates of selected single-agent chemotherapy

Agent	Year and reference	Number of patients	Overall response (%)
Bleomycin	1975[5]	15	0
	1976[6]	8	37
	1977[7]	7	0
Carboplatin	1988[8]	19	0
	1990[9]	18	0
Cisplatin	1978[10]	23	0
	1979[11]	10	0
Cyclophosphamide	1975[12]	10	0
	1979[13]	44	4
	1980[14]	12	0
Dactinomycin	1981[15]	61	2
2-Deoxycoformycin	1991[16]	18	0
	1992[17]	25	0
Docetaxel	1994[18]	18	0
Doxorubicin	1977[19]	38	5
Epirubicin	1982[20]	20	0
	1983[21]	19	0
Estramustine	1981[22]	16	0
Etoposide	1979[13]	43	2
Floxuridine/FUDR	1990[23]	56	20
	1990[24]	42	14
	1991[25]	14	0
	1991[26]	40	10
	1991[27]	29	0
	1992[28]	26	8
	1993[29]	28	14

Table 24.1. *Continued*

Agent	Year and reference	Number of patients	Overall response (%)
5-Fluorouracil	1989[30]	14	0
	1991[31]	27	7
	1993[32]	35	11
	1994[33]	61	5
Fludarabine	1987[34]	30	0
	1989[35]	15	0
Gemcitabine	1993[36]	18	6
	1996[37]	37	8
	1996[38]	37	8
Hydroxyurea	1981[39]	19	5
Ifosfamide	1980[40]	11	9
	1981[41]	10	20
	1987[42]	16	0
	1988[43]	9	0
Liposomal encapsulated doxorubicin	1994[44]	14	0
Melphalan	1993[45]	8	0
Methotrexate	1980[46]	8	25
Mitomycin	1987[47]	12	25
Mitotane	1981[48]	12	0
Mitoxantrone	1984[49]	20	0
	1984[50]	49	0
	1984[51]	29	0
	1986[52]	48	0
Paclitaxel	1982[53]	15	0
	1991[54]	18	0
Suranmm	1991[55]	10	0
	1992[56]	26	4
Temazolamide	2002[57]	12	0
Thiotepa	1977[7]	7	14
Topotecan	1994[58]	14	0
Vinblastin	1977[7]	10	0
	1984[59]	19	16
	1984[60]	10	0
	1985[61]	14	0
	1987[62]	21	9
	1988[63]	35	9
	1992[64]	26	4
Vindesine	1977[65]	17	0
	1983[66]	24	0
Vinorelbine	1991[67]	14	0
	1993[68]	24	4

Adapted from George and Stadler.[69]

COMBINATION CHEMOTHERAPY

A variety of chemotherapy combinations have been studied. Encouraging results have been obtained from trials of gemcitabine and 5-FU[72-75] (Table 24.2). In 2000, Rini et al.[72] reported a 17% response rate. In this phase II trial, seven partial but no complete responses were observed in 39 patients. A prolonged median progression-free survival was also observed compared with historic controls. Subsequent studies of combination gemcitabine and 5-FU–based regimens have led to a 5% to 15% response rate.[73-76] A recent retrospective analysis of five published studies of gemcitabine plus 5-FU in 153 patients demonstrated an overall response rate of 10%.[78] However, to demonstrate a survival benefit of the combination over 5-FU alone or over other chemotherapy regimens, a phase III randomized study would be required.

COMBINED CHEMOIMMUNOTHERAPY

Interferon and IL-2 have shown low but reproducible antitumor activity in RCC in a wide variety of studies (see Chapter 23). To investigate the improvement of chemotherapy with the addition of immunologic-based agents, the combination of chemotherapy and immunotherapy has been studied (Table 24.2). These efforts included combinations of IFN-α with vinblastine, 5-FU, cis-retinoic acid, and IL-2. Although encouraging results were obtained from some phase II trials, subsequent phase III trials failed to confirm the synergistic antitumor activity of the combinations. For example, in 1991 and 1992, Neidhart et al.[105] and Fossa et al.[106] reported two large randomized trials comparing IFN-α plus vinblastine to IFN-α alone, and were unable to show a survival difference between the two groups of the patients. The combination of 5-FU with low-dose IL-2 and IFN-α has also been studied. Although the results from initial investigations were promising (Table 24.2), a subsequent randomized phase II study of IL-2 and IFN-α with or without 5-FU failed to confirm these initial results.[107]

Table 24.2.
Response rates of selected combination therapy

Agent	Year and reference	Number of patients	Overall response (%)
Phase II trials			
Gemcitabine/5-FU	2000[72]	41	17
Gemcitabine/5-FU/cisplatin	2002[74]	21	5
Gemcitabine/5-FU/IL-2/ IFN-α	2002[75]	41	14.6
Gemcitabine/5-FU/ thalidomide	2002[76]	21	10
Gemcitabine/capecitabine	2004[77]	55	15
Gemcitabine/oxaliplatin	2004[79]	52	14.3
IFN-α/floxurine	1991[80]	13	31
	1992[81]	20	0
	1999[82]	14	0
IFN-α/5-FU	1992[83]	14	0
	1994[84]	31	23
	1997[85]	21	43

Table 24.2. Continued

Agent	Year and reference	Number of patients	Overall response (%)	
IFN-α/vinblastine	1986[86]	16	31	
	1987[87]	13	23	
	1988[88]	18	44	
	1988[89]	40	42	
	1989[90]	56	16	
	1990[91]	15	7	
	1991[92]	42	14	
	1991[93]	9	0	
IFN-α/cis-retinoic acid	1995[94]	43	30	
IFN-α/IL-2/cis-retinoic acid	1998[95]	47	17	
IFN-α/IL-2/5-FU	1993[96]	35	49	
	1996[97]	34	38	
	1996[98]	38	24	
	1997[99]	50	16	
	1997[100]	52	31	
	1998[101]	111	2	
	1998[102]	62	19	
	2004[103]	20	0	
IFN-α/IL-2/vinblastine	1998[104]	31	38.7	
Phase III trials				Survival benefit
IFN-α/vinblastine vs. IFN-α	1991[105]	83	8	No
		82	12	
IFN-α/vinblastine vs. IFN-α	1992[106]	66	24	No
		53	11	
IFN-α/vinblastine vs. Medroxyprogesterone	1995[108]	41	20.5	No
		35	0	
IFN-α/vinblastine vs. vinblastine	1999[70]	79	16.5	Yes
		81	2.5	
IFN-α vs. medroxyprogesterone	1999[109]	167	16	Yes
		168	2	
IFN-α/cis-retinoic acid vs. IFN-α	2000[110]	139	12	No
		145	6	
IFN-α/IL-2/5-FU vs. tamoxifen	2001[111]	41	39.1	Yes
		37	0	

IFN, interferon; IL, interleukin.

HORMONE THERAPY AND COMBINED CHEMOHORMONAL THERAPY

The findings of hormone-dependent renal tumors in Syrian hamsters, and estrogen and progesterone receptors in human kidney cell carcinoma,[112,113] promoted hormonal agent studies in patients with metastatic RCC. Medroxyprogesterone was the most extensively studied hormonal agent for many years with response rates ranging from 0% to 17%.[114] However, when more stringent response criteria were used in subsequent studies, only a 1% to 2% overall response rate was observed.[114] Furthermore, a randomized phase III trial of IFN-α versus medroxyprogesterone acetate revealed a survival benefit in the IFN arm and only a 2% response rate in the medroxyprogesterone arm.[109] Other agents including tamoxifen, toremifene, or combinations of hormones and chemotherapy showed low response rates in earlier studies[3,115–117] that were not confirmed in subsequent trials.[108,111,118]

MECHANISMS OF CHEMOTHERAPY RESISTANCE

Mechanisms of chemotherapy resistance include reduced drug accumulation due to the expression of transport proteins such as P-glycoprotein, increased detoxification, altered targets, and impaired apoptosis pathways.[119] The most widely studied mechanism of drug resistance in RCC is P-glycoprotein, an adenosine triphosphate (ATP)-binding cassette (ABC) transporter[120] and its encoding gene, *MDR-1* or *ABCB1*.[120–122] P-glycoprotein is a 170-kd-membrane protein that exhibits energy-dependent transport of cationic lipophilic compounds and has been widely targeted for drug resistance reversal studies.[123,124] P-glycoprotein was found concentrated on the apical surface of epithelial cells of the proximal tubules from which most RCC arise.[121,125] The overexpression of *MDR-1* was observed in RCC and in cell lines derived from them.[121,125–127] Mickisch et al.[128] reported overexpression of P-glycoprotein in 70% of highly vinblastine resistant and in 63% of highly doxorubicin-resistant tumors. However, efforts to improve chemosensitivity by modulating the P-glycoprotein pathway in RCC were disappointing, even with the use of more potent and less toxic second-generation inhibitors such as PSC 833, a derivative of cyclosporin D.[129–133]

Notably, pharmacokinetic interactions between P-glycoprotein inhibitors and chemotherapeutic agents require dose reductions of chemotherapeutic agents used with the combination therapy,[120,133] which is a concern since the required dose reduction of chemotherapeutic agents in the combination may impair drug concentrations in the tumor.[120] To avoid these significant pharmacokinetic interactions, several third-generation, highly specific P-glycoprotein antagonists have been developed,[134–138] and further evaluation of these agents in clinical trials are warranted. Other members of the ABC transporter family are also possibly linked to drug resistance. For example, expression of MRP2, a member of the family of multidrug resistance associated proteins (MRPs), was found in 95% of clear-cell RCC.[139] Further investigations are required to determine whether MRP2 plays a significant role in drug efflux and resistance in RCC. In addition, a better understanding of other drug-resistant mechanisms may further guide our strategies to overcome chemotherapy resistance.

GENETIC AND CLINICAL .HETEROGENEITY

Renal cancer used to be considered one disease, labeled as renal cell carcinoma. It is now recognized as several separate diseases with different pathological characteristics, and genetic abnormalities.[140,141] Renal cell carcinoma is divided into clear cell carcinoma, papillary renal carcinoma, chromophobe renal carcinoma, and collecting duct carcinoma.[140] The most common is clear cell carcinoma, comprising 70% to 80% of kidney cancers and 90% of metastatic RCC. The second most common is papillary RCC, accounting for 10% to 15% of kidney cancers. Chromophobe and collecting duct carcinoma represent approximately 5% and 0.4% to 2.6% of kidney cancers, respectively.[140] These tumors also have different clinical features and may respond to systemic therapy differently. For example, the combination of gemcitabine and doxorubicin has been reported to have antitumor activity in collecting duct carcinoma of the kidney,[142] sarcomatoid, and rapidly progressing RCC.[143] Previous clinical trials usually include all classes and subgroups and do not report on response by subtype.

Recent reviews from Memorial Sloan-Kettering Cancer Center,[144] the Cytokine Working Group,[145] and the University of Chicago[78] revealed approximately 90% of clear cell carcinoma and 5% to 8% of non–clear-cell histology in patients who registered in their trials. The low response rate of systemic chemotherapy in metastatic RCC may thus reflect a very active drug in a small subpopulation. This in turn needs to be balanced against the occasional spontaneous tumor regression, which has been reported to occur in up to 7% of patients with metastatic RCC.[146] Similarly, time to disease progression for uncontrolled phase II trials cannot be considered as a valid end point due to the existence of a subgroup of patients with long-term stable disease and survival in the absence of therapy. Finally, objective response rate can vary based on the method one uses and on whether the primary tumor is left in place or surgically removed. These factors complicate the design and interpretation of phase II clinical trials and further emphasizes the need for randomized and confirmatory studies.

CONCLUSION

Systemic cytotoxic chemotherapy has a minor role in patients with clear cell renal cancer. Although the combination therapy of gemcitabine/5-FU showed some promising results, even if these combination-based regimens were proved to provide survival benefit in a phase III trial, the overall outcome would still be poor. Nevertheless, the rare but reproducible response rates with cytotoxic chemotherapy suggests that further research into identifying genetic and other factors predictive for response is indicated.

REFERENCES

1. Motzer RJ, Bander NH, Nanus DM. Renal Cell Carcinoma. N Engl J Med 1996;335:865–875.
2. Vuky J, Motzer RJ. Cytokine therapy in renal cell cancer. Urol Oncol 2000;5:249–257.
3. Motzer RJ, Russo P. Systemic therapy for renal cell carcinoma. J Urol 2000:163:408–417.
4. Yagoda A, Abi-Rached B, Petrylak D. Chemotherapy for advanced renal cell carcinoma: 1983–1993. Semin Oncol 1995;22:42–60.
5. Johnson DE, Chalbaud RA, Holoye PY, et al. Clinical trial of bleomycin (NSC-125066) in the treatment of metastatic renal carcinoma. Cancer Chemother Rep 1975;59(2 pt 1):433–435.
6. Haas CD, Coltman CA Jr, Gottlieb JA, et al. Phase II evaluation of bleomycin. A Southwest oncology Group study. Cancer 1976;38(1):8–12.
7. Hahn DM, Schimpff SC, Ruckdeschel JC, et al. Single-agent therapy for renal cell carcinoma: CCNU, vinblastine, thioTEPA, or bleomycin. Cancer Treat Rep 1977;61(8):1585–1587.
8. Tait M, Abrams J, Egorin MJ, et al. Phase II carboplatin (CBDCA) for metastatic renal cell cancer with standard dose (SD) and a calculate dose (CD) according to renal function. Proc Am Soc Clin Oncol 1988;7:125.

9. Trump DL, Elson P. Evaluation of carboplatin (NSC 241240) in patients with recurrent or metastatic renal cell carcinoma. Invest New Drugs 1990;8(2):201–203.

10. Rodriguez LH, Johnson DE. Clinical trial of cisplatinum (NSC 119875) in metastatic renal cell carcinoma. Urology 1978;11(4):344–346.

11. Merrin CE. Treatment of genitourinary tumours with cis-dichlorodiammineplatinum(II): experience in 250 patients. Cancer Treat Rep 1979;63(9–10):1579–1584.

12. Kiruluta G, Morales A, Lott S. Response of renal adenocarcinoma to cyclophosphamide. Urology 1975;6(5):557–558.

13. Hahn RG, Bauer M, Wolter J, et al. Phase II study of single-agent therapy with megestrol acetate, VP-16–213, cyclophosphamide, and dianhydrogalactitol in advanced renal cell cancer. Cancer Treat Rep 1979;63(3):513–515.

14. Wajsman Z, Beckley S, Madajewicz S. High dose of cyclophosphamide in metastatic renal cell cancer. Proc Am Soc Clin Oncol 1980;21:423.

15. Hahn RG, Begg CB, Davis T. Phase II study of vinblastine-CCNU, triazinate, and dactinomycin in advanced renal cell cancer. Cancer Treat Rep 1981;65(7–8):711–713.

16. Venner P, Eisenhauer EA, Wierzbicki R, et al. Phase II study of 2'-deoxycoformycin in patients with renal cell carcinoma. A National Cancer Institute of Canada Clinical Trials Group study. Invest New Drugs 1991;9(3):273–275.

17. Witte RS, Walsh C, Fisher H, et al. Evaluation of deoxycoformycin in patients with advanced renal cell carcinoma. An ECOG pilot study. Invest New Drugs 1992;10(1):49–50.

18. Venner P, Eisenhauer EA, Wierzbicki R, et al. Docetaxel in advanced renal carcinoma. A phase II trial of the National Cancer Institute of Canada Clinical Trials Group. Ann Oncol 1994;5(2): 185–187.

19. O'Bryan RM, Baker LH, Gottlieb JE, et al. Dose response evaluation of Adriamycin in human neoplasia. Cancer 1977;39(5):1940–1948.

20. Fossa SD, Wik B, Bae E, Lien HH. Phase II study of 4'-epi-doxorubicin in metastatic renal cancer. Cancer Treat Rep 1982;66(5):1219–1221.

21. Benedetto P, Ahmed T, Needles B, et al. Phase II trial of 4'epi-Adriamycin for advanced hypernephroma. Am J Clin Oncol 1983;6(5):553–554.

22. Swanson DA, Johnson DE. Estramustine phosphate (Emcyt) as treatment for metastatic renal carcinoma. Urology 1981;17(4):344–346.

23. Hrushesky WJ, von Roemeling R, Lanning RM, et al. Circadian-shaped infusions of floxuridine for progressive metastatic renal cell carcinoma. J Clin Oncol 1990;8(9):1504–1513.

24. Damascelli B, Marchiano A, Spreafico C, et al. Circadian continuous chemotherapy of renal cell carcinoma with an implantable, programmable infusion pump. Cancer 1990;66(2):237–241.

25. Merrouche Y, Negrier S, et al. Phase II study of continues circadian infusion FUDR in metastatic renal cell cancer (RCC). Eur J Cancer 1991;27:599(abstract 579).

26. Dexeus FH, Logothetis CJ, Sella A, et al. Circadian infusion of floxuridine in patients with metastatic renal cell carcinoma. J Urol 1991;146(3):709–713.

27. Richards F, Cooper MR, Jackson DV, et al. Continuous 5-day (D) intravenous (IV) FUDR infusion for renal cell carcinoma (RCC). Proc Am Soc Clin Oncol 1991;10:170.

28. Budd GT, Murthy S, Klein E, et al. Time-modified infusion of floxuridine in metastatic renal cell carcinoma (RCC). Proc Am Assoc Cancer Res 1992;33:220.

29. Conroy T, Geoffrois L, Guillemin F. Simplified chronomodulated continuous infusion of floxuridine in patients with metastatic renal cell carcinoma. Cancer 1993;72(7):2190–2197.

30. Zaniboni A, Simoncini E, Marpicati P. Phase II trial of 5–fluorouracil and high-dose folinic acid in advanced renal cell cancer. J Chemother 1989;1(5):350–351.

31. Schulof R, Lokich J, Wampler G, et al. Phase II trial of protracted infusional 5–FU (PIF) for metastatic renal cell carcinoma. Proc Am Soc Clin Oncol 1991;10:170.

32. Ahlgren JD, Lokich J, Auerbach M, et al. Protracted infusional 5–FU (PIF): a well tolerated regimen in metastatic renal cell carcinoma (MRC): A Mid-Atlantic Oncology Program (MOAP) study. Proc Am Soc Clin Oncol 1993;12:244.

33. Kish JA, Wolf M, Crawford ED, et al. Evaluation of low dose continuous infusion 5–fluorouracil in patients with advanced and recurrent renal cell carcinoma. A Southwest Oncology Group Study. Cancer. 1994;74(3):916–919.

34. Balducci L, Blumenstein B, Von Hoff DD, et al. Evaluation of fludarabine phosphate in renal cell carcinoma: a Southwest Oncology Group Study. Cancer Treat Rep 1987;71(5):543–544.

35. Shevrin DH, Lad TE, Kilton LJ, et al. Phase II trial of fludarabine phosphate in advanced renal cell carcinoma: an Illinois Cancer Council Study. Invest New Drugs 1989;7(2–3):251–253.
36. Mertens WC, Eisenhauer EA, Moore M, et al. Gemcitabine in advanced renal cell carcinoma. A phase II study of the National Cancer Institute of Canada Clinical Trials Group. Ann Oncol 1993;4(4): 331–332.
37. De Mulder PH, Weissbach L, Jakse G, et al. Gemcitabine: a phase II study in patients with advanced renal cancer. Cancer Chemother Pharmacol 1996;37(5):491–495.
38. Rohde D, De Mulder PH, Weissbach L, et al. Experimental and clinical efficacy of 2′, 2′-difluorodeoxycytidine (gemcitabine) against renal cell carcinoma. Oncology 1996;53(6):476–481.
39. Stolbach LL, Begg CB, Hall T, et al. Treatment of renal carcinoma: a phase III randomized trial of oral medroxyprogesterone (Provera), hydroxyurea, and nafoxidine. Cancer Treat Rep 1981;65(7–8): 689–692.
40. Fossa SD, Talle K. Treatment of metastatic renal cancer with ifosfamide and mesnum with and without irradiation. Cancer Treat Rep 1980;64(10–11):1103–1108.
41. Heim ME, Fiene R, Schick E, et al. Central nervous side effects following ifosfamide monotherapy of advanced renal carcinoma. J Cancer Res Clin Oncol 1981;100(1):113–116.
42. De Forges A, Droz JP, Ghosn M, et al. Phase II trial of ifosfamide/mesna in metastatic adult renal carcinoma. Cancer Treat Rep 1987;71(11):1103.
43. Bodrogi I, Baki M, Sinkovics I, et al. Ifosfamide chemotherapy of metastatic renal cell cancer. Semin Surg Oncol 1988;4(2):95–96.
44. Law TM, Mencel P, Motzer RJ. Phase II trial of liposomal encapsulated doxorubicin in patients with advanced renal cell carcinoma. Invest New Drugs 1994;12(4):323–325.
45. Falkson CI. New formulation intravenous melphalan in the treatment of patients with metastatic renal cancer. Invest New Drugs 1993;11(1):93.
46. Baumgartner G, Heinz R, Arbes H, et al. Methotrexate-citrovorum factor used alone and in combination chemotherapy for advanced hypernephromas. Cancer Treat Rep 1980;64(1):41–46.
47. Stewart DJ, Futter N, Irvine A, et al. Mitomycin-C and metronidazole in the treatment of advanced renal-cell carcinoma. Am J Clin Oncol 1987;10(6):520–522.
48. Hogan TF, Citrin DL, Freeberg BL. A preliminary report of mitotane therapy of advanced renal and prostate cancer. Cancer Treat Rep 1981;65(5–6):539–540.
49. De Jager R, Cappelaere P, Armand JP, et al. An EORTC phase II study of mitoxantrone in solid tumors and lymphomas. Eur J Cancer Clin Oncol 1984;20:1239–1241.
50. Taylor SA, Von Hoff DD, Baker LH, et al. Phase II clinical trial of mitoxantrone in patients with advanced renal cell carcinoma: a Southwest Oncology Group study. Cancer Treat Rep 1984;68(6): 919–920.
51. van Oosterom AT, Fossa SD, Pizzocaro G, et al. Mitoxantrone in advanced renal cancer: a phase II study in previously untreated patients from the EORTC Genito-Urinary Tract Cancer Cooperative Group. Eur J Cancer Clin Oncol 1984;20(10):1239–1241.
52. Gams RA, Nelson O, Birch R. Phase II evaluation of mitoxantrone in advanced renal cell carcinoma: a Southeastern Cancer Study Group Trial. Cancer Treat Rep 1986;70(7):921–922.
53. Natale RB, Yagoda A, Kelsen DP, et al. Phase II trial of PALA in hypernephroma and urinary bladder cancer. Cancer Treat Rep 1982;66(12):2091–2092.
54. Einzig AI, Gorowski E, Sasloff J, et al. Phase II trial of Taxol in patients with metastatic renal cell carcinoma. Cancer Invest 1991;9(2):133–136.
55. La Rocca RV, Stein CA, Danesi R, et al. A pilot study of suramin in the treatment of metastatic renal cell carcinoma. Cancer 1991;67(6):1509–1513.
56. Motzer RJ, Nanus DM, O'Moore P, et al. Phase II trial of suramin in patients with advanced renal cell carcinoma: treatment results, pharmacokinetics, and tumor growth factor expression. Cancer Res 1992;52(20):5775–5779.
57. Park DK, Ryan CW, Dolan ME, et al. A phase II trial of oral temozolomide in patients with metastatic renal cell cancer. Cancer Chemother Pharmacol 2002;50(2):160–162.
58. Law TM, Ilson DH, Motzer RJ. Phase II trial of topotecan in patients with advanced renal cell carcinoma. Invest New Drugs 1994;12(2):143–145.
59. Kuebler JP, Hogan TF, Trump DL, et al. Phase II study of continuous 5–day vinblastine infusion in renal adenocarcinoma. Cancer Treat Rep 1984;68(6):925–926.
60. Zeffren J, Yagoda A, Kelsen D, et al. Phase I–II trial of a 5-day continuous infusion of vinblastine sulfate. Anticancer Res 1984;4(6):411–413.

61. Tannock IF, Evans WK. Failure of 5-day vinblastine infusion in the treatment of patients with renal cell carcinoma. Cancer Treat Rep 1985;69(2):227–228.
62. Crivellari D, Tumolo S, Frustaci S, et al. Phase II study of five-day continuous infusion of vinblastine in patients with metastatic renal-cell carcinoma. Am J Clin Oncol 1987;10(3):231–233.
63. Elson PJ, Kvols LK, Vogl SE, et al. Phase II trials of 5–day vinblastine infusion (NSC 49842), L-alanosine (NSC 153353), acivicin (NSC 163501), and aminothiadiazole (NSC 4728) in patients with recurrent or metastatic renal cell carcinoma. Invest New Drugs 1988;6(2):97–103.
64. Fossa SD, Droz JP, Pavone-Macaluso MM, et al. Vinblastine in metastatic renal cell carcinoma: EORTC phase II trial 30882. The EORTC Genitourinary Group. Eur J Cancer 1992;28A(4–5): 878–880.
65. Wong PP, Yagoda A, Currie VE, et al. Phase II study of vindesine sulfate in the therapy for advanced renal carcinoma. Cancer Treat Rep 1977;61(9):1727–1729.
66. Fossa SD, Denis L, van Oosterom AT, et al. Vindesine in advanced renal cancer. A study of the EORTC Genito-urinary Tract Cancer Cooperative Group. Eur J Cancer Clin Oncol 1983;19(4): 473–475.
67. Canobbio L, Boccardo F, Guarneri D, et al. Phase II study of navelbine in advanced renal cell carcinoma. Eur J Cancer 1991;27(6):804–805.
68. Wilding G, Kirkwood J, Clamon G, et al. Phase II trial of navelbine in metastatic renal cancer. Proc Am Soc Clin Oncol 1993;12:253.
69. George CM, Stadler WM. The role of systemic chemotherapy in the treatment of kidney cancer. In: Figlin R, ed. Kidney Cancer. Norwell, MA: Kluwer Academic Publishers, 2003.
70. Pyrhonen S, Salminen E, Ruutu M, et al. Prospective randomized trial of interferon alfa-2a plus vinblastine versus vinblastine alone in patients with advanced renal cell cancer. J Clin Oncol 1999;17(9):2859–2867.
71. Samuels BL, Hollis DR, Rosner GL, et al. Modulation of vinblastine resistance in metastatic renal cell carcinoma with cyclosporine A or tamoxifen: a cancer and leukemia group B study. Clin Cancer Res 1997;3(11):1977–1984.
72. Rini BI, Vogelzang NJ, Dumas MC, et al. Phase II trial of weekly intravenous gemcitabine with continuous infusion fluorouracil in patients with metastatic renal cell cancer. J Clin Oncol 2000;18(12):2419–2426.
73. Mani S, Vogelzang NJ, Bertucci D, et al. Phase I study to evaluate multiple regimens of intravenous 5-fluorouracil administered in combination with weekly gemcitabine in patients with advanced solid tumors: a potential broadly active regimen for advanced solid tumor malignancies. Cancer 2001; 92(6):1567–1576.
74. George CM, Vogelzang NJ, Rini BI, et al. A phase II trial of weekly intravenous gemcitabine and cisplatin with continuous infusion fluorouracil in patients with metastatic renal cell carcinoma. Ann Oncol 2002;13(1):116–120.
75. Ryan CW, Vogelzang NJ, Stadler WM. A phase II trial of intravenous gemcitabine and 5-fluorouracil with subcutaneous interleukin-2 and interferon-alpha in patients with metastatic renal cell carcinoma. Cancer 2002;94(10):2602–2609.
76. Desai AA, Vogelzang NJ, Rini BI, et al. A high rate of venous thromboembolism in a multi-institutional phase II trial of weekly intravenous gemcitabine with continuous infusion fluorouracil and daily thalidomide in patients with metastatic renal cell carcinoma. Cancer 2002;95(8):1629–1636.
77. Stadler WM, Halabi S, Ernstoff MS, et al. A phase II study of gemcitabine (G) and capecitabine (C) in patients with metastatic renal cell cancer (mRCC): A report of Cancer and Leukemia Group B #90008. Proc Am Soc Clin Oncol 2004;23:384.
78. Stadler WM, Huo D, George C, et al. Prognostic factors for survival with gemcitabine plus 5-fluorouracil based regimens for metastatic renal cancer. J Urol 2003;170(4 pt 1):1141–1145.
79. Porta C, Zimatore M, Imarisio I, et al. Gemcitabine and oxaliplatin in the treatment of patients with immunotherapy-resistant advanced renal cell carcinoma: final results of a single-institution phase II study. Cancer 2004;100(10):2132–2138.
80. Dimopoulas MA, Dexeus FH, Jones E, et al. Evidence for additive anti-tumor activity and toxicity for the combination of FUDR and interferon alpha2B in patients (pts) with metastatic renal cell carcinoma (RCC). Proc Am Assoc Cancer Res 1991;32:186.
81. Stadler WM, Vogelzang NJ, Vokes EE, et al. Continuous-infusion fluorodeoxyuridine with leucovorin and high-dose interferon: a phase II study in metastatic renal-cell cancer. Cancer Chemother Pharmacol 1992;31(3):213–216.

82. Soori GS, Schulof RS, Stark JJ, et al. Continuous-infusion floxuridine and alpha interferon in metastatic renal cancer: a national biotherapy study group phase II study. Cancer Invest 1999;17(6): 379–384.

83. Murphy BR, Rynard SM, Einhorn LH, et al. A phase II trial of interferon alpha-2A plus fluorouracil in advanced renal cell carcinoma. A Hoosier Oncology Group study. Invest New Drugs 1992;10(3):225–230.

84. Haarstad H, Jacobsen AB, Schjolseth SA, et al. Interferon-alpha, 5-FU and prednisone in metastatic renal cell carcinoma: a phase II study. Ann Oncol 1994;5(3):245–248.

85. Gebrosky NP, Koukol S, Nseyo UO, et al. Treatment of renal cell carcinoma with 5–fluorouracil and alfa-interferon. Urology 1997;50(6):863–867.

86. Fossa SD, de Garis ST, Heier MS, et al. Recombinant interferon alfa-2a with or without vinblastine in metastatic renal cell carcinoma. Cancer 1986;57(8 suppl):1700–1704.

87. Fossa SD, De Garis ST. Further experience with recombinant interferon alfa-2a with vinblastine in metastatic renal cell carcinoma: a progress report. Int J Cancer Suppl 1987;1:36–40.

88. Cetto GL, Franceschi T, Turrina G, et al. Recombinant alpha-interferon and vinblastine in metastatic renal cell carcinoma: efficacy of low doses. Semin Surg Oncol 1988;4(3):184–190.

89. Bergerat JP, Herbrecht R, Dufour P, et al. Combination of recombinant interferon alpha-2a and vinblastine in advanced renal cell cancer. Cancer 1988;62(11):2320–2324.

90. Schornagel JH, Verweij J, ten Bokkel Huinink WW, et al. Phase II study of recombinant interferon alpha-2a and vinblastine in advanced renal cell carcinoma. J Urol 1989;142(2 pt 1):253–256.

91. Trump DL, Ravdin PM, Borden EC, et al. Interferon-alpha-n1 and continuous infusion vinblastine for treatment of advanced renal cell carcinoma. J Biol Resp Mod 1990;9(1):108–111.

92. Massidda B, Migliari R, Padovani A, et al. Metastatic renal cell cancer treated with recombinant alpha 2a interferon and vinblastine. J Chemother 1991;3(6):387–389.

93. Merimsky O, Shnider BI, Chaitchik S. Does vinblastine add to the potency of alpha interferon in the treatment of renal cell carcinoma? Mol Biother 1991;3(1):34–37.

94. Motzer RJ, Schwartz L, Law TM, et al. Interferon alfa-2a and 13–cis-retinoic acid in renal cell carcinoma: antitumor activity in a phase II trial and interactions in vitro. J Clin Oncol 1995;13(8): 1950–1957.

95. Stadler WM, Kuzel T, Dumas M, et al. Multicenter phase II trial of interleukin-2, interferon-alpha, and 13–cis-retinoic acid in patients with metastatic renal-cell carcinoma. J Clin Oncol 1998;16(5):1820–1825.

96. Atzpodien J, Kirchner H, Hanninen EL, et al. Interleukin-2 in combination with interferon-alpha and 5–fluorouracil for metastatic renal cell cancer. Eur J Cancer 1993;29A(suppl 5):S6–8.

97. Hofmockel G, Langer W, Theiss M, et al. Immunochemotherapy for metastatic renal cell carcinoma using a regimen of interleukin-2, interferon-alpha and 5–fluorouracil. J Urol 1996;156(1):18–21.

98. Joffe JK, Banks RE, Forbes MA, et al. A phase II study of interferon-alpha, interleukin-2 and 5-fluorouracil in advanced renal carcinoma: clinical data and laboratory evidence of protease activation. Br J Urol 1996;77(5):638–49.

99. Dutcher JP, Atkins M, Fisher R, et al. Interleukin-2–based therapy for metastatic renal cell cancer: the Cytokine Working Group experience, 1989–1997. Cancer J Sci Am 1997;3(suppl 1):S73–78.

100. Ellerhorst JA, Sella A, Amato RJ, et al. Phase II trial of 5–fluorouracil, interferon-alpha and continuous infusion interleukin-2 for patients with metastatic renal cell carcinoma. Cancer 1997;80(11): 2128–2132.

101. Ravaud A, Audhuy B, Gomez F, et al. Subcutaneous interleukin-2, interferon alfa-2a, and continuous infusion of fluorouracil in metastatic renal cell carcinoma: a multicenter phase II trial. Groupe Francais d'Immunotherapie. J Clin Oncol 1998;16(8):2728–2732.

102. Tourani JM, Pfister C, Berdah JF, et al. Outpatient treatment with subcutaneous interleukin-2 and interferon alfa administration in combination with fluorouracil in patients with metastatic renal cell carcinoma: results of a sequential nonrandomized phase II study. Subcutaneous Administration Propeukin Program Cooperative Group. J Clin Oncol 1998;16(7):2505–2513.

103. Rathmell WK, Malkowicz SB, Holroyde C, et al. Phase II trial of 5-fluorouracil and leucovorin in combination with interferon-alpha and interleukin-2 for advanced renal cell cancer. Am J Clin Oncol 2004;27(2):109–112.

104. Pectasides D, Varthalitis J, Kostopoulou M, et al. An outpatient phase II study of subcutaneous interleukin-2 and interferon-alpha-2b in combination with intravenous vinblastine in metastatic renal cell cancer. Oncology 1998;55(1):10–15.

105. Neidhart JA, Anderson SA, Harris JE, et al. Vinblastine fails to improve response of renal cancer to interferon alfa-n1: high response rate in patients with pulmonary metastases. J Clin Oncol 1991;9(5):832–836.
106. Fossa SD, Martinelli G, Otto U, et al. Recombinant interferon alfa-2a with or without vinblastine in metastatic renal cell carcinoma: results of a European multi-center phase III study. Ann Oncol 1992;3(4):301–305.
107. Negrier S, Caty A, Lesimple T, et al. Treatment of patients with metastatic renal carcinoma with a combination of subcutaneous interleukin-2 and interferon alfa with or without fluorouracil. Groupe Francais d'Immunotherapie, Federation Nationale des Centres de Lutte Contre le Cancer. J Clin Oncol 2000;18(24):4009–4015.
108. Kriegmair M, Oberneder R, Hofstetter A. Interferon alfa and vinblastine versus medroxyprogesterone acetate in the treatment of metastatic renal cell carcinoma. Urology 1995;45(5):758–762.
109. Medical Research Council Renal Cancer Collaborators. Interferon-alpha and survival in metastatic renal carcinoma: early results of a randomised controlled trial. Lancet 1999;353(9146):14–17.
110. Motzer RJ, Murphy BA, Bacik J, et al. Phase III trial of interferon alfa-2a with or without 13-cis-retinoic acid for patients with advanced renal cell carcinoma. J Clin Oncol 2000;18(16): 2972–2980.
111. Atzpodien J, Kirchner H, Illiger HJ, et al. IL-2 in combination with IFN-alpha and 5-FU versus tamoxifen in metastatic renal cell carcinoma: long-term results of a controlled randomized clinical trial. Br J Cancer 2001;85(8):1130–1136.
112. Kirkman H, Bacon RL. Estrogen-induced tumors of the kidney. I. Incidence of renal tumors in intact and gonadectomized male golden hamsters treated with diethylstilbestrol. J Natl Cancer Inst 1952;13(3):745–755.
113. Bloom HJ. Hormone treatment of renal tumours: experimental and clinical observations. In: Riches E, ed. Tumours of the Kidney and Ureter. Edinburgh: ES Livingstone 1964:311.
114. Kjaer M. The role of medroxyprogesterone acetate (MPA) in the treatment of renal adenocarcinoma. Cancer Treat Rev 1988;15(3):195–209.
115. Stahl M, Schmoll E, Becker H, et al. Lonidamine versus high-dose tamoxifen in progressive, advanced renal cell carcinoma: results of an ongoing randomized phase II study. Semin Oncol 1991;18(2 suppl 4):33–37.
116. Stahl M, Wilke H, Schmoll HJ, et al. A phase II study of high dose tamoxifen in progressive, metastatic renal cell carcinoma. Ann Oncol 1992;3(2):167–168.
117. Gershanovich MM, Moiseyenko VM, Vorobjev AV, et al. High-dose toremifene in advanced renal-cell carcinoma. Cancer Chemother Pharmacol 1997;39(6):547–551.
118. Oh WK, Manola J, George DJ, et al. A phase II trial of interferon-alpha and toremifene in advanced renal cell cancer patients. Cancer Invest 2002;20(2):186–191.
119. Lehnert M. Clinical multidrug resistance in cancer: a multifactorial problem. Eur J Cancer 1996;32A(6):912–920.
120. Leonard GD, Fojo T, Bates SE. The role of ABC transporters in clinical practice. Oncologist 2003;8(5):411–424.
121. Fojo AT, Ueda K, Slamon DJ, et al. Expression of a multidrug-resistance gene in human tumors and tissues. Proc Natl Acad Sci U S A 1987;84(1):265–269.
122. Fojo AT, Shen DW, Mickley LA, et al. Intrinsic drug resistance in human kidney cancer is associated with expression of a human multidrug-resistance gene. J Clin Oncol 1987;5(12):1922–1927.
123. Ling V. Multidrug resistance: molecular mechanisms and clinical relevance. Cancer Chemother Pharmacol 1997;40(suppl):S3–8.
124. Gottesman MM, Fojo T, Bates SE. Multidrug resistance in cancer: role of ATP-dependent transporters. Nat Rev Cancer 2002;2(1):48–58.
125. Thiebaut F, Tsuruo T, Hamada H, et al. Cellular localization of the multidrug-resistance gene product P-glycoprotein in normal human tissues. Proc Natl Acad Sci U S A 1987;84(21):7735–7738.
126. Mickisch G, Bier H, Bergler W, et al. P-170 glycoprotein, glutathione and associated enzymes in relation to chemoresistance of primary human renal cell carcinomas. Urol Int 1990;45(3):170–176.
127. Yu DS, Chang SY, Ma CP. The expression of mdr-1–related gp-170 and its correlation with anthracycline resistance in renal cell carcinoma cell lines and multidrug-resistant sublines. Br J Urol 1998;82(4):544–547.
128. Mickisch GH, Roehrich K, Koessig J, et al. Mechanisms and modulation of multidrug resistance in primary human renal cell carcinoma. J Urol 1990;144(3):755–759.

129. Warner E, Tobe SW, Andrulis IL, et al. Phase I–II study of vinblastine and oral cyclosporin A in metastatic renal cell carcinoma. Am J Clin Oncol 1995;18(3):251–256.
130. Motzer RJ, Lyn P, Fischer P, et al. Phase I/II trial of dexverapamil plus vinblastine for patients with advanced renal cell carcinoma. J Clin Oncol 1995;13(8):1958–1965.
131. Samuels BL, Hollis DR, Rosner GL, et al. Modulation of vinblastine resistance in metastatic renal cell carcinoma with cyclosporine A or tamoxifen: a cancer and leukemia group B study. Clin Cancer Res 1997;3(11):1977–1984.
132. Hao D, Huan SD, Stewart DJ, et al. A pilot study of low dose hydroxyurea as a novel resistance modulator in metastatic renal cell cancer. J Chemother 2000;12(4):360–366.
133. Bates SE, Bakke S, Kang M, et al. A phase I/II study of infusional vinblastine with the P-glycoprotein antagonist valspodar (PSC 833) in renal cell carcinoma. Clin Cancer Res 2004;10(14):4724–4733.
134. Starling JJ, Shepard RL, Cao J, et al. Pharmacological characterization of LY335979: a potent cyclopropyldibenzosuberane modulator of P-glycoprotein. Adv Enzyme Regul 1997;37:335–347.
135. van Zuylen L, Sparreboom A, van der Gaast A, et al. The orally administered P-glycoprotein inhibitor R101933 does not alter the plasma pharmacokinetics of docetaxel. Clin Cancer Res 2000;6(4): 1365–1371.
136. Newman MJ, Rodarte JC, Benbatoul KD, et al. Discovery and characterization of OC144–093, a novel inhibitor of P-glycoprotein-mediated multidrug resistance. Cancer Res 2000;60(11): 2964–2972.
137. Mistry P, Stewart AJ, Dangerfield W, et al. In vitro and in vivo reversal of P-glycoprotein-mediated multidrug resistance by a novel potent modulator, XR9576. Cancer Res 2001;61(2):749–758.
138. Agrawal M, Abraham J, Balis FM, et al. Increased 99mTc-sestamibi accumulation in normal liver and drug-resistant tumors after the administration of the glycoprotein inhibitor, XR9576. Clin Cancer Res 2003;9(2):650–656.
139. Schaub TP, Kartenbeck J, Konig J, et al. Expression of the MRP2 gene-encoded conjugate export pump in human kidney proximal tubules and in renal cell carcinoma. J Am Soc Nephrol 1999;10(6):1159–1169.
140. Zambrano NR, Lubensky IA, Merino MJ, et al. Histopathology and molecular genetics of renal tumors toward unification of a classification system. J Urol 1999;162(4):1246–1258.
141. Linehan WM, Walther MM, Zbar B. The genetic basis of cancer of the kidney. J Urol 2003;170(6 pt 1):2163–2172.
142. Milowsky MI, Rosmarin A, Tickoo SK, et al. Active chemotherapy for collecting duct carcinoma of the kidney: a case report and review of the literature. Cancer 2002;94(1):111–116.
143. Nanus DM, Garino A, Milowsky MI, et al. Active chemotherapy for sarcomatoid and rapidly progressing renal cell carcinoma. Cancer 2004;101(7):1545–1451.
144. Motzer RJ, Bacik J, Mariani T, et al. Treatment outcome and survival associated with metastatic renal cell carcinoma of non-clear-cell histology. J Clin Oncol 2002;20(9):2376–2381.
145. Upton MP, Parker RA, Youmans A, et al. Histologic predictors of renal cell carcinoma (RCC) response to interleukin-2–based therapy. Proc Am Soc Clin Oncol 2004;22:851(abstr 3420).
146. Gleave ME, Elhilali M, Fradet Y, et al. Interferon gamma-1b compared with placebo in metastatic renal-cell carcinoma. Canadian Urologic Oncology Group. N Engl J Med 1998;338(18):1265–1271.

25

Signal Transduction Inhibitors in Renal Cell Carcinoma

Ellen A. Ronnen, Saby George,
Ronald M. Bukowski, and Robert J. Motzer

KEYWORDS

RENAL CELL CARCINOMA
SUNITINIB
TYROSINE KINASE INHIBITOR
VASCULAR ENDOTHELIAL GROWTH FACTOR

ABSTRACT

Metastatic renal cell carcinoma (RCC) has been characterized by a resistance to systemic chemotherapy and poor overall survival. Cytokine therapy, the mainstay of treatment, provides responses in a minority of patients. The discovery of the *VHL* tumor suppressor gene, hypoxia inducible factor-1α (HIF-1α), and their roles in the growth of RCC identified a pathway on which to direct targeted therapy. Vascular endothelial growth factor (VEGF) plays a central role in RCC and has been a focus of multiple agents in clinical trials. Small molecule tyrosine kinase inhibitors, monoclonal antibodies, and novel agents are all being studied. Phase II studies show promising activity of sunitinib, sorafenib, and bevacizumab, and early results of phase III studies demonstrate the role of these agents in metastatic RCC.

Renal cell carcinoma (RCC) exhibits a high degree of resistance to cytotoxic chemotherapy.[1,2] Cytokines have been regarded as the mainstay of systemic therapy, but achieve responses in only 10% to 20% of patients.[3,4] Therefore, new drug development has been a priority. The identification of the *VHL* tumor suppressor gene and its role in upregulating growth factors associated with angiogenesis provided new targets for therapy. An increasing understanding of cellular signaling pathways also contributed targets worthy of further investigation for the treatment of RCC.

From: *Clinical Management of Renal Tumors*
Edited by: R.M. Bukowski and A.C. Novick © Humana Press Inc., Totowa, NJ

THE ROLE OF *VHL*, HYPOXIA INDUCIBLE FACTOR, AND RECEPTOR TYROSINE KINASES

Biallelic von Hippel-Lindau (*VHL*) gene inactivation due to somatic mutation or hypermethylation is observed in the majority of clear cell renal carcinomas.[5] In the presence of oxygen, the VHL gene product targets hypoxia inducible factor-α (HIF-α) for proteasome-mediated destruction. The HIF family of transcription factors regulates oxygen homeostasis by controlling over 20 genes, including an angiogenesis factor, vascular endothelial growth factor (VEGF), as well as factors of mitogenesis-transforming growth factor-α (TGF-α), epidermal growth factor receptor (EGFR), and platelet-derived growth factor-β (PDGF-β).[6,7] In a hypoxic environment or when the VHL gene is mutated, HIF-1α accumulates and activates the transcription of angiogenesis and mitogenesis proteins. The growth factors then bind to receptor tyrosine kinases (RTKs), and via a paracrine loop, trigger a signal transduction cascade, resulting in tumor vasculature growth. Hypoxia inducible factor-1α is also controlled at the biosynthesis level; the phosphoinositide (PI)-3-kinase-Akt (protein kinase)—mammalian target of rapamycin (mTOR) signal transduction pathway or a defective *PTEN* suppressor gene can increase HIF production by interaction with the gene promoter.[8] Modulation of HIF-1α at the biosynthesis and posttranscriptional level has been a focus of novel agents for RCC.

The critical role the VHL/HIF pathway plays in the development of RCC has been illustrated by in vivo studies. In a xenograft model treated with a human RCC cell line, reintroduction of the *VHL* gene inhibited tumor growth.[9] Equally, downregulation of HIF is sufficient to suppress tumor formation in *VHL*-defective RCC cells.[10]

Receptor Tyrosine Kinases

Receptor tyrosine kinases are enzymes that catalyze transfer of the γ phosphate of adenosine triphosphate (ATP) to the hydroxyl group on target proteins. The RTKs are central to many cellular processes including proliferation, metabolism, differentiation, cell cycle, and survival. The fundamental role RTKs play in cellular function makes these proteins ideal targets for therapy. The specificity of RTKs between cell types also facilitates decreased toxicity of targeted therapy. There are at least 58 known RTKs, of which a substantial number are dominant oncogenes.[11] In physiologic tissue, multiple levels of autoinhibition exist to prevent unwanted kinase activation. Mutations and overexpression of tyrosine kinases are found in many human malignancies, including RCC.

The Receptor Tyrosine Kinase as a Target for Therapy

Signal transduction inhibitors can block RTKs by preventing ligand binding by binding to the ligand (monoclonal antibodies) or the receptor, inhibiting RTK expression (using antisense oligonucleotides), or preventing the activity of the RTK (small molecule inhibitors) (Table 25.1).[12] Receptor-directed therapy is being investigated for VEGFR, PDGFR, and EGFR in RCC (Figure 25.1). Current therapies have also focused on HIF upstream signaling molecules (mTOR). Preclinical data support the targeting of VEGF, PDGF, and EGF or upstream molecules in the treatment of RCC.

Table 25.1.
Clinical trials of signal transduction inhibitors in advanced renal cell carcinoma

Agent	Class	Mechanism of action	Development stage
SU11248	Small molecule	Tyrosine kinase inhibitor of VEGFR-2, PDGFR, Flt-1, c-kit	II, III
Sorafenib	Small molecule	Tyrosine kinase inhibitor of VEGFR-2, VEGFR-3, PDGFR, Ras	II, III
PTK787	Small molecule	VEGFR-1, VEGFR-2, PDGFR-β	I
Imatinib	Small molecule	Tyrosine kinase inhibitor of PDGFR, C-kit, Bcr-Abl	II
Gefitinib	Small molecule	Tyrosine kinase inhibitor of EGFR	II
Erlotinib	Small molecule	Tyrosine kinase inhibitor of EGFR	II
Cetuximab	Monoclonal antibody	Antibody to EGFR	II
ABX-EGF	Monoclonal antibody	Antibody to EGFR	II
Bevacizumab	Monoclonal antibody	Antibody to VEGF	II, III
VEGF-trap	Monoclonal antibody	Antibody to VEGF	I, II
G250	Monoclonal antibody	Antibody to CA IX	II, III
Bortezomib	Small molecule	Inhibitor to 26s proteasome component	II
CCI-779	Small molecule	mTOR inhibitor	II, III
RAD-001	Small molecule	mTOR inhibitor	II, III
17-AAG	Small molecule	Hsp 90 inhibitor	II

VEGFR, vascular endothelial growth factor receptor; PDGFR, platelet-derived growth factor receptor; EGFR, epidermal growth factor receptor; mTOR, mammalian target of rapamycin; CA IX, carbonic anhydrase IX.

Vascular Endothelial Growth Factor

Vascular endothelial growth factor promotes endothelial cell migration and proliferation, and increases endothelial cell survival through protection from apoptosis.[13] Its activity results from VEGF binding to the cell surface receptor and initiating a cascade of downstream events resulting in angiogenesis. Five members of the VEGF family have been identified. VEGF-A, which binds to VEGFR-1 and VEGFR-2, appears to play a major role in angiogenesis. Increased expression of VEGF has been found in RCC and correlated with poor prognosis.[14] The VEGFR-1 and VEGFR-2 receptors, almost exclusively found on endothelial cells, are also upregulated in RCC. VEGFR-3 is found on lymphatic and vascular endothelium. Of these, VEGFR-2 appears to be the main receptor responsible for mediating proangiogenic activity.

Preclinical studies revealed that treatment of multiple tumor cell lines with a VEGF antibody inhibited the growth of tumors and decreased tumor blood-vessel density.[15] It is hypothesized, and this is the basis of VEGF-targeted therapy, that by blocking vascular growth, tumor growth can be inhibited. In addition, VEGF receptors have been

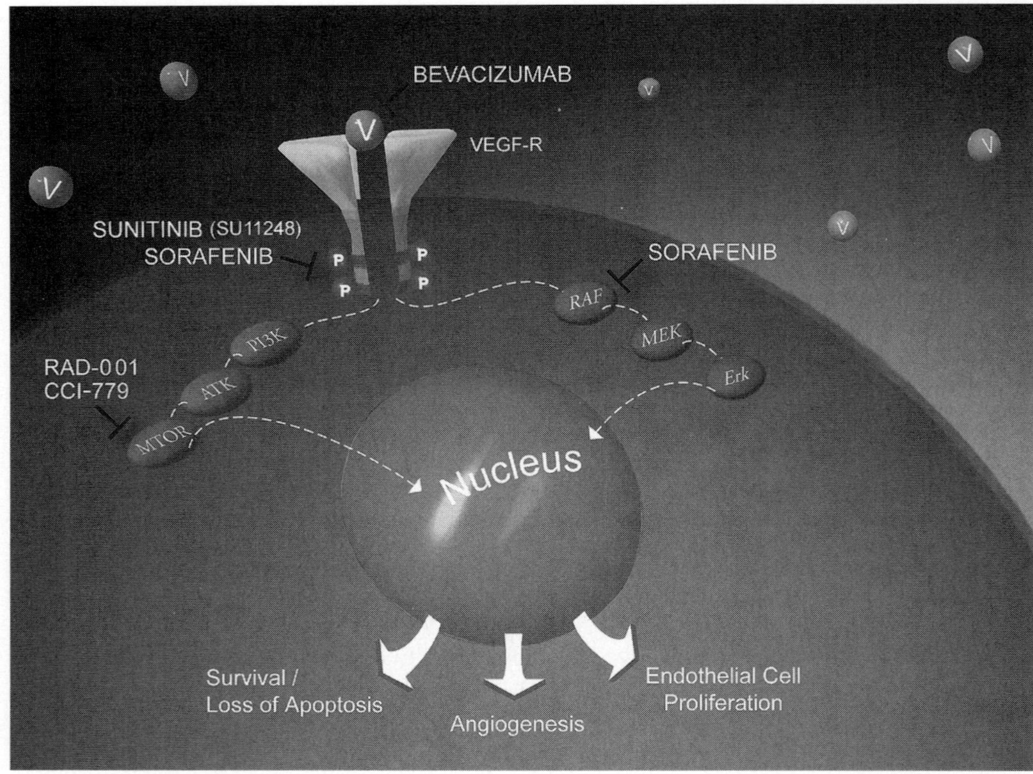

Figure 25.1. Vascular endothelial growth factor targeted therapy in RCC. V, VEGF; VEGF-R, VEGF receptor; MEK, mitogen activated protein kinase; ERK, extracellular signal-regulated kinase.

identified on RCC cells, suggesting an autocrine loop stimulating growth and an additional target for VEGF therapy.[16]

Epidermal Growth Factor and Platelet-Derived Growth Factor

Increased epidermal growth factor (EGFR) expression and its ligand, TGF-α, have been associated with tumor aggressiveness and metastases in RCC.[17–19] Platelet-derived growth factor receptor α is upregulated in RCC, and high receptor expression has been associated with tumor progression.[20]

The RAS-RAF Pathway

The RAS/RAF pathway is an important mediator of cell proliferation and differentiation in multiple tumor types. The RAF/mitogen activated protein kinase (MEK)/extracellular signal-regulated kinase (ERK) pathway is controlled by receptor tyrosine kinase activation and has been implicated in the pathophysiology of RCC. Ras protein activation on the cell surface leads to downstream activation of RAF, MEK, and ERK, which results in transcription and metabolism changes, and mediates tumor cell proliferation and angiogenesis.[21] Suppression of apoptosis has also been attributed to this pathway.[22] Mutations of RAS have been identified as well as constitutive activation of the mitogen-activated protein (MAP) kinases in human kidney tumors.

SIGNAL TRANSDUCTION INHIBITORS IN CLINICAL TRIALS

Small Molecules

The importance of VEGF, PDGF, and EGF, and the RAS-RAF pathway in stimulating angiogenesis, supporting the vasculature microenvironment, and controlling tumor cell proliferation has made the receptor tyrosine kinases of these growth factors attractive therapeutic targets. Small molecules that act on the kinase portion of multiple RTKs, such as VEGFR, PDGFR, RAS-RAF, and EGFR, have been studied in RCC. Inhibiting function for these downstream targets of HIF may result in antitumor activity by affecting both blood vessel growth factors and factors necessary to the stromal and pericyte microenvironment.[23,24] Multiple agents are being investigated in clinical trials to further explore these potential treatment targets. Those studied most completely are sunitinib, sorafenib, and temsirolimus.

Sunitinib

Sunitinib (SU11248) is an oral multitargeted inhibitor of VEGFR-2 and PDGFR that shows antitumor activity in metastatic RCC. Preclinical data with multiple tumor types found that sunitinib has direct antitumor activity and is dependent on signaling through PDGFR and VEGFR.[25] A phase I trial found that this therapy was well tolerated, with the majority of toxicities being grade 1 or 2. Two sequentially conducted single-arm phase II trials have been performed in RCC patients previously treated with immunotherapy.[26,27] In both studies, patients had clear-cell RCC histology, and evidence of progression on treatment with immunotherapy. In the first trial, 63 patients with metastatic RCC were treated.[26] As of December 2004, 25 (40%) patients achieved a partial response and 17 (27%) patients had stable disease for longer than 3 months. The median time to partial response was 2.3 months; the median duration of response was 12.5 months. The median time to progression was 8.7 months, and the median overall survival was 16.4 months. The most common adverse events were fatigue (38% grade 2 or 3), gastrointestinal disturbances including diarrhea (24%), nausea (19%), and stomatitis (19%). The majority of adverse events were grade 1 and 2. The most frequently occurring ($\geq$5%) grade 3/4 adverse events included lymphopenia (32%), elevated lipase (19%), and amylase (8%) without clinical signs of pancreatitis.

In the second phase II trial, 106 RCC patients were treated with sunitinib.[27] As of January 2005, 40 (38%) patients achieved a partial response, one (1%) patient achieved a complete response, and 25 (23%) demonstrated stable disease for longer than 3 months. Fifty-five patients continue to be treated in the study. The most commonly reported adverse events were similar to the previous trial—fatigue (22%), diarrhea (16%), and stomatitis (14%)—and the majority of adverse events were grades 1 and 2. The most frequently occurring grade 3 or 4 events were similar to those in the previously reported phase II trial. Based on the results of the phase II trials, a phase III randomized study was conducted comparing interferon to sunitinib in the upfront setting for metastatic RCC patients.

This phase III trial in untreated RCC patients compared sunitinib with interferon-α (IFN-α), and was recently completed[28]; 750 patients were randomized to either sunitinib ($n = 375$) or IFN-α ($n = 375$). Sunitinib was administered at a dose of 50 mg daily for 4 out of 6 weeks, and IFN-α was administered subcutaneously (SC) with a maximal dose of 9 million units (MU) three times a week (TIW) as the maintenance dose. Response evaluation was conducted using response evaluation criteria in solid tumors (RECIST) (investigator assessment as well as independent central review). Partial responses (PRs) were seen in 137 patients (37%) in the sunitinib arm and 33 patients (9%) in the IFN-α arm (p = .000001), with one patient having a complete response to sunitinib. Stable disease (SD) was noted in 176 patients (47%) in the sunitinib arm and 213 (57%) in the IFN-α arm; 16% of the patients had progressive disease (PD) or were nonevaluable in the sunitinib group, and 127 (34%) in the IFN-α arm. The primary end point, median progression-free survival (PFS) was 11 months (95% confidence interval [CI], 10–12) in the sunitinib arm and 5 months (95% CI, 4–6) in the IFN-α arm (hazard ratio [HR], 0.415; 95% CI, 0.320–0.539; p = .000001). An independent central review was conducted and demonstrated 31% PR, 48% SD, and 21% PD in the sunitinib arm and 6% PR, 49% SD, and 45% PD in the IFN-α arm. A preliminary analysis of overall survival was conducted, and the observed differences did not reach the prespecified level of significance.

BAY 43-9006 (Sorafenib)

Sorafenib is a novel, bi-aryl urea that was first designed as an in vitro inhibitor of the RAF proteins. Sorafenib was subsequently found to also inhibit VEGFR-2, VEGFR-3, and PDGFR-B. Preclinical data with xenograft models revealed tumor inhibition with confirmation of ERK phosphorylation inhibition.[29] A phase I trial studying 69 patients with advanced refractory solid tumors found the drug to be well tolerated.[30] One patient with RCC had stable disease for almost 2 years. A randomized discontinuation phase II trial evaluated 502 patients with advanced refractory solid tumors, 202 of which were RCC. In this patient group with RCC, 73 had substantial tumor regression detected at the 12-week evaluation. Of the 65 patients who had stable disease at 12 weeks, 32 were randomized to receive sorafenib and 33 received placebo. At 24 weeks, 6 (18%) patients receiving placebo were progression-free versus 16 (50%) receiving sorafenib. Median PFS was 23 weeks for patients continuing on sorafenib versus 6 weeks for patients who continued on treatment with placebo.[31]

A randomized placebo-controlled phase III trial of sorafenib was then performed in 903 RCC patients who had failed cytokine therapy. The Treatment Approaches in Renal Cell Cancer Global Evaluation Trial (TARGETs) evaluated sorafenib in treatment-refractory patients with predominantly clear cell carcinoma. Patients were treated with either sorafenib (n = 451) or a placebo (n = 452).[32,33] The primary end points were overall survival and PFS. An initial interim analysis demonstrated a significant improvement in PFS for sorafenib-treated patients compared to those receiving a placebo (24 vs. 12 weeks; HR, 0.44; p < .000001). Following this, patients were permitted to cross over from placebo to sorafenib. A prespecified interim analysis of overall survival (OS) using a stratified log-rank test was performed 6 months after the crossover was initiated, and 216 of 452 placebo patients had crossed over to the sorafenib. The median overall survival for sorafenib-treated patients was 19.3 months, and for the placebo group 15.9 months (HR, 0.77; 95% CI, 0.63–0.95; p = .015, level of significance required α = 0.009). After censoring the crossover patients, the median OS for placebo group was 14.3 months (HR, 0.74; 95% CI, 0.58–0.93; p = .010), suggesting a potential effect of crossover. In the phase III trial, the most common toxicities were rash, hand-foot skin reaction, hypertension, and fatigue. Overall, treatment was well tolerated, and toxicities led to discontinuation of treatment in less than 10% of patients. This study demonstrated the effects of sorafenib on disease stabilization, with >75% of patients developing measurable tumor shrinkage. The significant increase in PFS for sorafenib-treated patients is consistent with these findings. A phase II randomized trial comparing sorafenib to IFN-α in untreated patients is in progress.

PTK 787

PTK787, an oral selective inhibitor of VEGFR-1, VEGFR-2, and PDGFR-β, displayed antiangiogenic activity in a murine RCC model. In vitro, PTK787 decreased the VEGF-induced cellular endothelial cell proliferation and survival.[34] In treated mice, tumor growth was inhibited, and tumor vessel density and probability of metastases decreased.[35] George and colleagues[36] conducted a phase I trial of PTK787 in 45 metastatic renal cell carcinoma patients. Among 37 evaluable patients, one (3%) had a partial response, six (16%) achieved a minor response, and 17 (46%) demonstrated stable disease. Time to tumor progression was 5.5 months. The development plan for this agent in RCC is uncertain.

Imatinib

Imatinib inhibits the tyrosine kinase activity of PDGFR and c-*kit*. Based on the identification of PDGFR-β messenger RNA (mRNA) and expression of KIT protein in RCC,[37] a phase II trial studying imatinib mesylate (Gleevec™) was conducted. In a phase II trial, 14 patients with metastatic RCC were treated with imatinib mesylate. No responses were observed in 12 evaluable patients.[38] A separate phase II study evaluating imatinib with interferon was also performed in the metastatic RCC population. Of 14 patients treated, only one patient achieved a partial response. The median time to progression was 8 weeks.[39] Targeting PDGFR without VEGFR did not appear to provide clinical benefit against metastatic RCC.

Epidermal Growth Factor Receptor Inhibitors: Gefitinib and Erlotinib

Monotherapy targeting the EGFR receptor tyrosine kinase has also been evaluated in RCC. Gefitinib (Iressa™) and erlotinib, inhibitors of the EGFR tyrosine kinase, have been studied in vitro and in xenograft cancer models, and demonstrated tumor inhibition. In a xenograft model using multiple tumor types treated with gefitinib, decreased VEGF production was seen, suggesting a direct link to angiogenesis inhibition.[40] In an RCC model, treatment with an EGFR tyrosine kinase inhibitor (PKI166) resulted in tumor regression.[41] Lower VEGF expression, decreased microvessel density, and increased apoptosis were also associated with EGFR inhibitory treatment.

Two studies have evaluated gefitinib in metastatic RCC. Eighteen metastatic RCC patients who had previously progressed on cytokine therapy were treated with gefitinib.[42] Thirteen of 16 evaluable patients had progressive disease at 4 months. Three patients had stabilized disease for greater than 4 months. A separate study evaluated gefitinib in 28 metastatic RCC patients, 17 of whom had a history of prior therapy. Similar to the first study, no objective responses were seen, and stabilization of disease for $\geq$6 months was noted in only three patients.[43] Based on these results, the studies concluded that monotherapy targeted at the EGFR receptor is not effective for metastatic RCC.

Combination of Erlotinib and Bevacizumab

The rationale for combining erlotinib, an EGFR inhibitor, with bevacizumab, a humanized monoclonal antibody, against VEGFR-1 and VEGFR-2, is based on preclinical data. In a mouse xenograft model, animals were treated with anti-EGFR therapy until tumor regrowth occurred. At the time of resistance, a VEGFR-2 inhibitor was administered, which then blocked further tumor growth. In addition, tumors treated with an inhibitor of VEGFR-2 and EGFR from the start of the study maintained continued tumor shrinkage throughout the trial.[44] A phase II study evaluated advanced RCC patients treated with erlotinib and bevacizumab. Of 59 evaluable patients, responses were achieved (one complete response [CR], 14 partial responses [PRs]) in 15 (25%) patients. Median PFS was 11 months with 60% of patients alive at 18 months.[45] The results support continued investigation of these targeted therapies in combination with other agents.

The clinical activity of bevacizumab in advanced renal cell carcinoma when combined with erlotinib was then investigated in a phase II, randomized, double-blind, multicenter, placebo-controlled trial.[46] The objectives of this study were to assess whether erlotinib provided additional clinical benefit with regard to PFS and objective response when combined with bevacizumab in first-line treatment of metastatic RCC. One hundred four patients were treated with bevacizumab (10 mg/kg) every 2 weeks in combination with oral erlotinib (150 mg) or placebo daily until progression or toxicity for up to 104 weeks. A landmark analysis was performed 9 months after enrollment was completed (median follow-up, 9.8 months). The median PFS was 9.9 months for the combination versus 8.5 months for single-agent bevacizumab (HR, 0.86; 95% CI, 0.5–1.49; $p = .58$). Response rates (complete vs. partial) were 14% versus 13%, respectively. One complete response occurred in the combination group. The most common grade 3/4 adverse events were hypertension (31% vs. 26%), rash (16% vs. 0%), proteinuria (7.8% vs. 5.7%), diarrhea (7.8% vs. 0%), and hemorrhage (5.9% vs. 3.8%), respectively, in the groups receiving combination therapy or single-agent bevacizumab.

A phase I/II study was conducted with bevacizumab, erlotinib, and imatinib in patients with metastatic RCC. A partial response was achieved in 4 (9%) of 44 patients.[47] Grade 3 diarrhea and toxicities were also augmented with the three-drug regimen in comparison to the two-drug regimen (13% versus 27–29%). These preliminary results do not suggest increased efficacy with the three-drug regimen.

Monoclonal Antibodies

Epidermal Growth Factor Receptor Antibodies

ABX-EGF and cetuximab, monoclonal antibodies to EGFR that block binding of EGF and TGF-α, have been studied in vitro and in a xenograft model, and demonstrated tumor inhibition. ABX-EGF also showed tumor regression activity in eradicating tumors already present.[48] In a phase II trial, ABX-EGF was administered to 88 patients with metastatic RCC who had previously been treated with cytokine therapy.[49] Only three patients had a response to therapy, and 44 patients (50%) had stable disease at 8 weeks but no clear indication of progression prolongation.

In a separate phase II study, 55 previously untreated metastatic RCC patients were treated with cetuximab,[50] a chimeric antibody that binds to EGFR in a similar fashion to EGF and competitively inhibits the tyrosine kinase activation of EGFR. No patients achieved a partial or complete response. The median PFS was 57 days, with 75% of patients progressing by 112 days. To date, no EGFR-specific therapy given as monotherapy to advanced RCC patients resulted in significant responses.

VASCULAR ENDOTHELIAL GROWTH FACTOR NEUTRALIZING ANTIBODIES

Bevacizumab, an antibody to VEGF, has been investigated in a randomized phase II trial comparing placebo with low-dose (3 mg/kg) and high-dose (10 mg/kg) bevacizumab in 116 previously treated, advanced RCC patients. Four of 39 (10%) patients receiving high-dose (10 mg/kg) bevacizumab achieved a partial response. The time to progression in the high-dose bevacizumab group was significantly improved: 4.8 months versus 2.5 months in the placebo arm. Overall survival was not a primary end point of the study, but was not significantly increased in the treatment arms. These data suggest that less than a partial response can still result in a delay of disease progression.[51] On the basis of these data, several phase III trials investigating IFN-α and bevacizumab compared to IFN-α alone are under way. Bevacizumab as monotherapy appears to have clinical activity in previously treated and untreated metastatic RCC patients, but additional data from phase 3 trials are now required to clearly demonstrate this effect. The two large randomized trials comparing IFN-α $\pm$ bevacizumab in progress may provide this information.

Vascular endothelial growth factor trap, a fusion protein composed of VEGFR-1 and VEGFR-2 fused to human immunoglobulin G (IgG), also binds serum VEGF. Vascular endothelial growth factor trap has exhibited increased affinity to VEGF in comparison to monoclonal antibodies.[52] A phase I trial of VEGF-trap in 15 patients with advanced solid malignancies did not produce objective responses, but one patient with RCC maintained stable disease for over 6 months. The maximum tolerate dose (MTD) has not yet been reached, and further investigation of this agent is planned in a phase II trial.

G250 is a monoclonal antibody that recognizes the carbonic anhydrase IX (CA IX) antigen expressed on the cell surface of renal carcinoma cells. Membrane-associated CA IX is a member of the CA family involved in cellular proliferation under hypoxic conditions. G250 has been developed for diagnostic and therapeutic use. Preclinical data revealed that G250 mediated antibody-dependent cellular cytotoxicity.[53] A phase I trial was performed with cG250 labeled with I-131. Of 12 patients imaged, one patient achieved a complete response at 6 weeks.[54] A phase II trial was conducted in 36 patients with metastatic renal carcinoma. Stable disease was seen in eight (22%) patients at 24 weeks, and one patient had a complete response after 38 weeks.[55] Carbonic anhydrase IX is also controlled by HIF-1α, and mutations in HIF-1α decreased CA IX activity.[56] Additional studies are exploring the potential benefit of G250 in the conjugated and unconjugated forms.

Mammalian Target of Rapamycin Inhibitors

The mammalian target of rapamycin (mTOR), a large polypeptide kinase, is a therapeutic target for RCC. Multiple mechanisms have been postulated for the role of mTOR and its inhibitors in RCC. Mammalian target of rapamycin is a downstream component in the phosphoinositide-3-kinase (PI-3-kinase)/Akt pathway, which acts by regulating translation, protein degradation, and protein signaling. Vascular endothelial growth factor-mediated endothelial cell proliferation requires the activity of PI-3-kinase, suggesting a direct antiangiogenic pathway.[57] Mammalian target of rapamycin has also been identified as an upstream activator of HIF, providing a stabilizing force, preventing degradation, and increasing HIF activity.[58]

Preclinical data with a derivative of rapamycin (CCI-779) has shown antitumor effects in renal and other cancer models.[59] In a breast cancer model of cells treated with rapamycin (an mTOR inhibitor), a decrease in proliferation was seen.[57] In a phase I study of 24 patients with advanced solid tumors, CCI-779 resulted in a partial response in two patients.[60] In a phase II trial, 111 patients with advanced refractory RCC were treated with three different doses of rapamycin (CCI-779). Seven percent of patients achieved a partial or complete response (CR in one patient, PR in seven). The median time to progression was 5.8 months, with a median survival for the entire population of 15.0 months.[61] In this randomized phase II trial the various prognostic subgroups were examined, and those with poor risk status may have benefited the most leading to the design of a phase III study. CCI-779 has also been combined with IFN-α in a phase I clinical trial in 71 advanced RCC patients. Partial responses were observed in 11% of all patients, with three (8%) patients treated at the MTD achieving a PR. Median time to progression was 9.1 months.[62]

A phase III randomized trial comparing CCI-779 as a single agent (25.0 mg), versus CCI-779 (15.0 mg) with IFN-α versus IFN-α as first-line treatment in patients with unfavorable prognostic features was recently completed and reported in a preliminary fashion.[63] The overall response rates were between 7% and 11%; however, the PFS and median survival were significantly improved in the patient group receiving temsirolimus 25 mg IV weekly. The question of whether the definition of poor risk is biologic or clinical is relevant, and currently the former seems most likely. Additional data with this agent in the good/intermediate patient categories are needed, as well as investigating the effects of other agents such as the TKIs in the poor-risk group. Other mTOR inhibitors are being studied including RAD-001, a rapamycin derivative, and ap23573, a nonprodrug rapamycin analogue that inhibits mTOR (phase I). The mTOR inhibitor RAD001 is an oral agent, and preliminary phase II data[64] suggest clinical activity with a 28% PR rate in 25 patients. This agent is currently being investigated in a phase III trial compared to a placebo in patients receiving second-line therapy.

Other Agents

BORTEZOMIB

Proteasome inhibition results in disrupted cellular signaling by maintaining proteins central to cellular proliferation that are destined for degradation. Bortezomib is a proteasome inhibitor that targets the 26S proteasome of the ubiquitin-proteasome degradation system. A phase I trial evaluating bortezomib in advanced solid tumor patients identified prolonged stable disease in one patient with RCC.[65] In a phase II trial, 37 patients with advanced RCC were treated. Four (11%) patients achieved a partial response, and 14 (38%) of patients had stable disease during treatment.[66] A separate phase II trial with bortezomib resulted in only one of 21 patients achieving a favorable response.[67] These studies conflict regarding whether there is a low degree or no activity of bortezomib in metastatic RCC.

PAPILLARY RENAL CELL CARCINOMA

A hereditary form of papillary RCC was identified, and activating mutations in the tyrosine kinase domain of the c-*met* gene on chromosome 7 were linked to its development, and to a subset of patients with sporadic papillary RCC type I.[68] The c-*met* cell surface receptor for hepatocyte growth factor (HGF) normally stimulates mitogenesis and is a mediator in cell motility and metastasis.[68] When the c-met protein product is activated, autophosphorylation occurs, creating a binding site for multiple signal transducers and resulting in downstream upregulation of signaling molecules. Future studies are being dedicated to the manipulation of the c-met protein in the papillary subset of RCC patients.

The receptor tyrosine kinase Met requires stabilization by heat shock protein hsp90.[69] Heat shock protein chaperones are required for stabilization and promotion of multiple "client" protein activities including Met, HIF, AKT, Raf-1, and KIT. Studies in clear-cell RCC have illustrated the potential antitumor activity of an hsp90 inhibitor. Geldanamycin is an anasamycin antibiotic that binds and inhibits the function of hsp90. In a clear-cell RCC model, treatment with geldanamycin restored the proteosome-mediated destruction of HIF-1α.[69] A geldanamycin analogue, 17-AAG, also binds to hsp90. In preclinical studies, growth arrest occurred after administration of 17-AAG.[70] However, two phase I trials of 17-AAG in advanced malignancies, including RCC, did not result in responses.[71,72] A phase II study of 17-AAG in the papillary and clear cell RCC population is ongoing.

Novel Approaches

Replacing the defective *VHL* gene, which would then theoretically restore the appropriate destruction of HIF-1α, is a goal of future clinical therapy based on preclinical data. Hypoxia inducible factor-1α has also been a therapeutic target of recent interest. An in vitro model using a platelet aggregation factor (YC-1) that inhibits HIF-1α did result in decreased circulating levels of HIF-1α and shrinkage of tumor.[73] Before YC-1 and other HIF-1α inhibitors are tested in clinical trials, decreasing potential toxicity to platelets and the entire vascular compartment will need to be accomplished.

FUTURE DIRECTIONS

The role of novel targeted agents, including sunitinib, sorafenib, and CCI-779, in first- and second-line treatment for metastatic RCC have been defined by pivotal phase III randomized trials that were recently reported. Further studies exploring combinations of these agents as well as other novel targeted drugs are warranted.

ACKNOWLEDGMENT

The authors thank Carol Pearce for her critical review of this manuscript.

REFERENCES

1. Motzer RJ, Russo P. Systemic therapy for renal cell carcinoma. J Urol 2000;163(2):408–417.
2. Yagoda A, Abi-Rached B, Petrylak D. Chemotherapy for advanced renal-cell carcinoma: 1983–1993. Semin Oncol 1995;22(1):42–60.
3. Fyfe G, Fisher RI, Rosenberg SA, Sznol M, Parkinson DR, Louie AC. Results of treatment of 255 patients with metastatic renal cell carcinoma who received high-dose recombinant interleukin-2 therapy. J Clin Oncol 1995;13(3):688–696.

4. Vuky J, Motzer RJ. Cytokine therapy in renal cell cancer. Urol Oncol 2000;5(6):249–257.

5. Kenck C, Wilhelm M, Bugert P, Staehler G, Kovacs G. Mutation of the VHL gene is associated exclusively with the development of non-papillary renal cell carcinomas. J Pathol 1996;179(2):157–161.

6. Gunaratnam L, Morley M, Franovic A, et al. Hypoxia inducible factor activates the transforming growth factor-alpha/epidermal growth factor receptor growth stimulatory pathway in VHL(–/–) renal cell carcinoma cells. J Biol Chem 2003;278(45):44966–44974.

7. Sosman JA. Targeting of the VHL-hypoxia-inducible factor-hypoxia-induced gene pathway for renal cell carcinoma therapy. J Am Soc Nephrol 2003;14(11):2695–2702.

8. Jiang BH, Jiang G, Zheng JZ, Lu Z, Hunter T, Vogt PK. Phosphatidylinositol 3—kinase signaling controls levels of hypoxia-inducible factor 1. Cell Growth Differ 2001;12(7):363–369.

9. Iliopoulos O, Kibel A, Gray S, Kaelin WG, Jr. Tumour suppression by the human von Hippel-Lindau gene product. Nat Med 1995;1(8):822–826.

10. Kondo K, Kim WY, Lechpammer M, Kaelin WG, Jr. Inhibition of HIF2alpha is sufficient to suppress pVHL-defective tumor growth. PLoS Biol 2003;1(3):E83.

11. Blume-Jensen P, Hunter T. Oncogenic kinase signalling. Nature 2001;411(6835):355–365.

12. Lee AV, Schiff R, Cui X, et al. New mechanisms of signal transduction inhibitor action: receptor tyrosine kinase down-regulation and blockade of signal transactivation. Clin Cancer Res 2003;9(1 pt 2):516S-523S.

13. Ferrara N, Davis-Smyth T. The biology of vascular endothelial growth factor. Endocr Rev 1997;18(1):4–25.

14. Brown LF, Berse B, Jackman RW, et al. Increased expression of vascular permeability factor (vascular endothelial growth factor) and its receptors in kidney and bladder carcinomas. Am J Pathol 1993;143(5):1255–1262.

15. Kim KJ, Li B, Winer J, et al. Inhibition of vascular endothelial growth factor-induced angiogenesis suppresses tumour growth in vivo. Nature 1993;362(6423):841–844.

16. Ferrara N. Molecular and biological properties of vascular endothelial growth factor. J Mol Med 1999;77(7):527–543.

17. Mydlo JH, Michaeli J, Cordon-Cardo C, Goldenberg AS, Heston WD, Fair WR. Expression of transforming growth factor alpha and epidermal growth factor receptor messenger RNA in neoplastic and nonneoplastic human kidney tissue. Cancer Res 1989;49(12):3407–3411.

18. Moch H, Sauter G, Buchholz N, et al. Epidermal growth factor receptor expression is associated with rapid tumor cell proliferation in renal cell carcinoma. Hum Pathol 1997;28(11):1255–1259.

19. Uhlman DL, Nguyen P, Manivel JC, et al. Epidermal growth factor receptor and transforming growth factor alpha expression in papillary and nonpapillary renal cell carcinoma: correlation with metastatic behavior and prognosis. Clin Cancer Res 1995;1(8):913–920.

20. Sulzbacher I, Birner P, Traxler M, Marberger M, Haitel A. Expression of platelet-derived growth factor-alpha alpha receptor is associated with tumor progression in clear cell renal cell carcinoma. Am J Clin Pathol 2003;120(1):107–112.

21. Khosravi-Far R, Der CJ. The Ras signal transduction pathway. Cancer Metastasis Rev 1994; 13(1):67–89.

22. Sridhar SS, Hedley D, Siu LL. Raf kinase as a target for anticancer therapeutics. Mol Cancer Ther 2005;4(4):677–685.

23. Bergers G, Song S, Meyer-Morse N, Bergsland E, Hanahan D. Benefits of targeting both pericytes and endothelial cells in the tumor vasculature with kinase inhibitors. J Clin Invest 2003;111(9): 1287–1295.

24. Kaelin WG, Jr. The von Hippel-Lindau tumor suppressor gene and kidney cancer. Clin Cancer Res 2004;10(18 pt 2):6290S-6295S.

25. Fiedler W, Serve H, Dohner H, et al. A phase 1 study of SU11248 in the treatment of patients with refractory or resistant acute myeloid leukemia (AML) or not amenable to conventional therapy for the disease. Blood 2005;105(3):986–993.

26. Motzer RJ, Michaelson MD, Redman BG, et al. Activity of SU11248, a multitargeted inhibitor of vascular endothelial growth factor receptor and platelet-derived growth factor receptor, in patients with metastatic renal cell carcinoma. J Clin Oncol 2006;24(1):16–24.

27. Motzer RJ, Rini BI, Michaelson MD, et al. Phase 2 trials of SU11248 show antitumor activity in second-line therapy for patients with metastatic renal cell carcinoma (RCC). In: Orlando, FL: American Society of Clinical Oncology. ASCO Annual Meeting Proceedings 2005;23(165).

28. Motzer RJ, Hutson TE, Tomczak P, et al. Phase III randomized trial of sunitinib malate (SU11248) versus interferon-alfa (IFN-α) as first-line systemic therapy for patients with metastatic renal cell carcinoma (mRCC). ASCO Annual Meeting Proceedings Part I. J Clin Oncol 2006;24(18S).

29. Wilhelm SM, Carter C, Tang L, et al. BAY 43–9006 exhibits broad spectrum oral antitumor activity and targets the RAF/MEK/ERK pathway and receptor tyrosine kinases involved in tumor progression and angiogenesis. Cancer Res 2004;64(19):7099–7109.

30. Strumberg D, Richly H, Hilger RA, et al. Phase I clinical and pharmacokinetic study of the novel Raf kinase and vascular endothelial growth factor receptor inhibitor BAY 43–9006 in patients with advanced refractory solid tumors. J Clin Oncol 2005;23(5):965–972.

31. Ratain MJ, Eisen T, Stadler WM, et al. Phase II placebo-controlled randomized discontinuation trial of sorafenib in patients with metastatic renal cell carcinoma. J Clin Oncol 2006;24(16):2505–2512. (Epub 2006 Apr 24.)

32. Escudier B, Szczylik C, Demkow T, et al. Randomized phase II trial of the multi-kinase inhibitor sorafenib versus interferon (IFN) in treatment-naïve patients with metastatic renal cell carcinoma (mRCC). ASCO Annual Meeting Proceedings Part I. J Clin Oncol 2006;24(18S): 4501.

33. Eisen T, Bukowski RM, Staehler M, et al. Randomized phase III trial of sorafenib in advanced renal cell carcinoma (RCC): Impact of crossover on survival. ASCO Annual Meeting Proceedings Part I. J Clin Oncol 2006;24(18S):4524.

34. Wood JM, Bold G, Buchdunger E, et al. PTK787/ZK 222584, a novel and potent inhibitor of vascular endothelial growth factor receptor tyrosine kinases, impairs vascular endothelial growth factor-induced responses and tumor growth after oral administration. Cancer Res 2000;60(8): 2178–2189.

35. Drevs J, Hofmann I, Hugenschmidt H, et al. Effects of PTK787/ZK 222584, a specific inhibitor of vascular endothelial growth factor receptor tyrosine kinases, on primary tumor, metastasis, vessel density, and blood flow in a murine renal cell carcinoma model. Cancer Res 2000;60(17): 4819–4824.

36. George D, Dugan M, Kaelin WG, Kantoff P. Phase I study of PTK787/222584 (PTK/ZK) in metastatic renal cell carcinoma. Presented at the annual meeting of the American Society of Clinical Oncology, Chicago, 2003:385(abstr 1548).

37. Castillo M, Petit A, Mellado B, Palacin A, Alcover JB, Mallofre C. C-kit expression in sarcomatoid renal cell carcinoma: potential therapy with imatinib. J Urol 2004;171(6 pt 1):2176–2180.

38. Vuky J, Fotoohi M, Isacson C, et al. Phase II trial of imatinib mesylate (formerly known as STI-571) in patients with metastatic renal cell carcinoma. Presented at the annual meeting of the American Society of Clinical Oncology, Chicago, 2003:416(abstr 1672).

39. Polite BN, Desai AA, Peterson AC, Manchen B, Stadler WM. A phase II study of imatinib mesylate (IM) and interferon-alpha (IFNA) in metastatic renal cell carcinoma. Presented at the annual meeting of the American Society of Clinical Oncology, Orlando, FL, 2005:425s(abstr 4689).

40. Petit AM, Rak J, Hung MC, et al. Neutralizing antibodies against epidermal growth factor and ErbB-2/neu receptor tyrosine kinases down-regulate vascular endothelial growth factor production by tumor cells in vitro and in vivo: angiogenic implications for signal transduction therapy of solid tumors. Am J Pathol 1997;151(6):1523–1530.

41. Kedar D, Baker CH, Killion JJ, Dinney CP, Fidler IJ. Blockade of the epidermal growth factor receptor signaling inhibits angiogenesis leading to regression of human renal cell carcinoma growing orthotopically in nude mice. Clin Cancer Res 2002;8(11):3592–3600.

42. Drucker B, Bacik J, Ginsberg M, et al. Phase II trial of ZD1839 (IRESSA) in patients with advanced renal cell carcinoma. Invest New Drugs 2003;21(3):341–345.

43. Jermann M, Joerger M, Pless M. An open-label phase II trial to evaluate the efficacy and safety of gefitinib in patients with locally advanced, relapsed or metastatic renal cell cancer. Presented at the annual meeting of the American Society of Clinical Oncology, Chicago, 2003:418(abstr 1681).

44. Ciardiello F, Bianco R, Caputo R, et al. Antitumor activity of ZD6474, a vascular endothelial growth factor receptor tyrosine kinase inhibitor, in human cancer cells with acquired resistance to antiepidermal growth factor receptor therapy. Clin Cancer Res 2004;10(2):784–793.

45. Spigel DR, Hainsworth JD, Sosman JA, et al. Bevacizumab and erlotinib in the treatment of patients with metastatic renal carcinoma (RCC): update of a phase II multicenter trial. Presented at the annual meeting of the American Society of Clinical Oncology, Orlando, FL, 2005:387s.

46. Bukowski R, Kabbinavar F, Figlin RA, et al. Bevacizumab with or without erlotinib in metastatic renal cell carcinoma (RCC). J Clin Oncol 2006;24(18S, pt I):222s.

47. Hainsworth JD, Sosman JA, Spigel DR, et al. Bevacizumab, erlotinib and imatinib in the treatment of patients (pts) with advanced renal cell carcinoma (RCC): a Minnie Pearl Cancer Research Network phase I/II trial. Presented at the annual meeting of the American Society of Clinical Oncology, Orlando, FL, 2005:388s(abstr 4542).

48. Yang XD, Jia XC, Corvalan JR, Wang P, Davis CG, Jakobovits A. Eradication of established tumors by a fully human monoclonal antibody to the epidermal growth factor receptor without concomitant chemotherapy. Cancer Res 1999;59(6):1236–1243.

49. Rowinsky EK, Schwartz GH, Gollob JA, et al. Safety, pharmacokinetics, and activity of ABX-EGF, a fully human anti-epidermal growth factor receptor monoclonal antibody in patients with metastatic renal cell cancer. J Clin Oncol 2004;22(15):3003–3015.

50. Motzer RJ, Amato R, Todd M, et al. Phase II trial of antiepidermal growth factor receptor antibody C225 in patients with advanced renal cell carcinoma. Invest New Drugs 2003;21(1): 99–101.

51. Yang JC, Haworth L, Sherry RM, et al. A randomized trial of bevacizumab, an anti-vascular endothelial growth factor antibody, for metastatic renal cancer. N Engl J Med 2003;349(5):427–434.

52. Dupont J, Schwartz L, Koutcher J, Spriggs D, et al. Phase I and pharmacokinetic study of VEGF Trap administered subcutaneously to patients with advanced solid malignancies. Presented at the annual meeting of the American Society of Clinical Oncology, New Orleans, 2004;abstr 3009.

53. Surfus JE, Hank JA, Oosterwijk E, et al. Anti-renal-cell carcinoma chimeric antibody G250 facilitates antibody-dependent cellular cytotoxicity with in vitro and in vivo interleukin-2—activated effectors. J Immunother Emphasis Tumor Immunol 1996;19(3):184–191.

54. Wiseman GA, Scott AM, Lee F-T, et al. Chimeric G250 (cG250) monoclonal antibody phase I dose escalation trial in patients with advanced renal cell carcinoma (RCC). Presented at the annual meeting of the American Society of Clinical Oncology, 2001;abstr 1027.

55. Bleumer I, Knuth A, Oosterwijk E, et al. A phase II trial of chimeric monoclonal antibody G250 for advanced renal cell carcinoma patients. Br J Cancer 2004;90(5):985–990.

56. Grabmaier K, de Weijert MC A, Verhaegh GW, Schalken JA, Oosterwijk E. Strict regulation of CAIX(G250/MN) by HIF-1alpha in clear cell renal cell carcinoma. Oncogene 2004;23(33):5624–531.

57. Yu Y, Sato JD. MAP kinases, phosphatidylinositol 3–kinase, and p70 S6 kinase mediate the mitogenic response of human endothelial cells to vascular endothelial growth factor. J Cell Physiol 1999; 178(2):235–246.

58. Hudson CC, Liu M, Chiang GG, et al. Regulation of hypoxia-inducible factor 1alpha expression and function by the mammalian target of rapamycin. Mol Cell Biol 2002;22(20):7004–7014.

59. Frost P, Moatamed F, Hoang B, et al. In vivo antitumor effects of the mTOR inhibitor CCI-779 against human multiple myeloma cells in a xenograft model. Blood 2004;104(13):4181–4187.

60. Raymond E, Alexandre J, Faivre S, et al. Safety and pharmacokinetics of escalated doses of weekly intravenous infusion of CCI-779, a novel mTOR inhibitor, in patients with cancer. J Clin Oncol 2004;22(12):2336–2347.

61. Atkins MB, Hidalgo M, Stadler WM, et al. Randomized phase II study of multiple dose levels of CCI-779, a novel mammalian target of rapamycin kinase inhibitor, in patients with advanced refractory renal cell carcinoma. J Clin Oncol 2004;22(5):909–918.

62. Smith JW, Ko Y-J, Dutcher J, et al. Update of a phase 1 study of intravenous CCI-779 given in combination with interferon-alpha to patients with advanced renal cell carcinoma. Presented at the annual meeting of the American Society of Clinical Oncology, New Orleans, 2004;abstr 4513.

63. Hudes GR, Carducci M, Tomczak P, et al, et al. A phase III, randomized, 3–arm study of temsirolimus (TEMSR) or interferon-alpha (IFN) or the combination of TEMSR + IFN in the treatment of first-line, poor-risk patients with advanced renal cell carcinoma (adv RCC). J Clin Oncol 2006;24(18S pt II):930s.

64. Amato RJ, Misellati A, Khan M, Chiang S. A phase II trial of RAD001 in patients (Pts) with metastatic renal cell carcinoma (MRCC). J Clin Oncol 2006;24(18s pt I):224s.

65. Aghajanian C, Soignet S, Dizon DS, et al. A phase I trial of the novel proteasome inhibitor PS341 in advanced solid tumor malignancies. Clin Cancer Res 2002;8(8):2505–2511.

66. Kondagunta GV, Drucker B, Schwartz L, et al. Phase II trial of bortezomib for patients with advanced renal cell carcinoma. J Clin Oncol 2004;22(18):3720–3725.

67. Davis NB, Taber DA, Ansari RH, et al. Phase II trial of PS-341 in patients with renal cell cancer: a University of Chicago phase II consortium study. J Clin Oncol 2004;22(1):115–119.

68. Linehan WM, Vasselli J, Srinivasan R, et al. Genetic basis of cancer of the kidney: disease-specific approaches to therapy. Clin Cancer Res 2004;10(18 pt 2):6282S-6289S.
69. Isaacs JS, Jung YJ, Mimnaugh EG, Martinez A, Cuttitta F, Neckers LM. Hsp90 regulates a von Hippel Lindau-independent hypoxia-inducible factor-1 alpha-degradative pathway. J Biol Chem 2002; 277(33):29936–29944.
70. Kaur G, Belotti D, Burger AM, et al. Antiangiogenic properties of 17-(dimethylaminoethylamino)-17-demethoxygeldanamycin: an orally bioavailable heat shock protein 90 modulator. Clin Cancer Res 2004;10(14):4813–4821.
71. Goetz MP, Toft D, Reid J, et al. Phase I trial of 17—allylamino-17—demethoxygeldanamycin in patients with advanced cancer. J Clin Oncol 2005;23(6):1078–1087.
72. Yeo EJ, Chun YS, Cho YS, et al. YC-1: a potential anticancer drug targeting hypoxia-inducible factor 1. J Natl Cancer Inst 2003;95(7):516–525.
73. Pili R, Donehower RC. Is HIF-1 alpha a valid therapeutic target? J Natl Cancer Inst 2003; 95(7):498–499.

26 Pulmonary Metastases in Patients with Advanced Renal Cell Carcinoma: *Role of Metastasectomy*

Sudish Murthy

KEYWORDS

PULMONARY METASTASES
METASTECTOMY
ADVANCED RENAL CELL CARCINOMA
HAZARD FUNCTION ANALYSIS
LONG-TERM SURVIVAL

ABSTRACT

The chest is the most common site of metastasis from renal cell carcinoma. Mastatectomy plays a central role in the management of these patients. Preoperative evaluation should focus on identifying patients who are likely to be completely resected. Improved long-term outcomes can be predicted in patients who do not exhibit regional lymph node involvement and who have adequate pulmonary reserve.

The chest is the most common site for metastatic renal cell carcinoma (RCC).[1] In fact, up to one third of patients with RCC present with synchronous pulmonary metastases, and of the remainder, 50% ultimately develop intrathoracic disease.[2–5] In the past, medical therapy has proven largely ineffective for this disease,[6,7] and management of pulmonary metastases has been primarily surgical.

Since the first published report of pulmonary metastasectomy over 60 years ago, a number of studies have demonstrated a central role of surgery for this disease[8–15] (Table 26.1). Collectively, these studies suggest that there is a survival benefit of surgery when compared to nonoperated patients.[11]

However, although some common risk factors have been identified, there is a lack of consensus regarding patient or tumor factors important for long-term survival following metastasectomy. This is attributable, in part, to arbitrary dichotomization of continuous and ordinal factors, which has made it difficult to prioritize and evaluate interactions between variables.

From: *Clinical Management of Renal Tumors*
Edited by: R.M. Bukowski and A.C. Novick © Humana Press Inc., Totowa, NJ

Table 26.1.
Summary of published studies for pulmonary metastasectomy

| | | Complete resection | | 5-year survival (%) | | |
	n	No.	%	Complete resection	Overall	Risk factors for death
Cerfolio et al.[8]	147	96	65	36	NA	Higher number of pulmonary nodules, shorter disease-free interval
Piltz et al.[9]	122	105	86	40	25	Incomplete resection, lymph node metastases, larger pulmonary nodule
Fourquier et al.[10]	50	NA	NA	44	NA	None
Kavolius et al.[11]	50	NA	NA	54	30	Not available
Friedel et al.[12]	93	77	83	39	NA	Higher number of pulmonary nodules, shorter disease-free interval
Dernevik et al.[13]	33	NA	NA	NA	21	Shorter disease-free interval
Pfannschmidt et al.[14]	191	194	98	42	37	Higher number of pulmonary nodules, incomplete resection, lymph node metastases, shorter disease-free interval
International Registry of Lung Metastases[15]	372	—	—	—	—	Higher number of nodules, incomplete resection, shorter disease-free interval

NA, not available.

We have recently reviewed our 15-year experience of pulmonary metastasectomy for RCC using hazard function analysis of continuous, ordinal, and true dichotomous variables to identify independent and interacting factors associated with long-term outcome.[16] This approach helps to clarify some of the conflicting data presented in Table 26.1. Importantly, practical guidelines can be generated for identification of the most appropriate candidates for metastasectomy.

PATIENT SELECTION

Of patients with pulmonary metastases from RCC, between 20% and 25% are referred for surgical resection. The vast majority are postnephrectomy (90%), though synchronous chest and renal disease is occasionally observed. When contrasted to non-operated patients, surgical patients generally demonstrate excellent performance status, are younger (median 60 years), have fewer nodules, and more often present with the thorax as the only site of extrarenal disease.

There are several important factors to consider when selecting patients for pulmonary metastasectomy. It is mandatory that all patients undergo high-resolution spiral chest and abdominal computed tomography (CT) scanning for evaluation of both number and size of pulmonary nodules. As well, this imaging technique provides a thorough assessment of the mediastinum, chest wall, and upper abdomen. The importance of the CT scan is magnified since renal tumors are often silent on positron emission tomography

(PET) scanning. Consequently, the burden of noninvasive thorax staging and metastatic survey falls solely on CT scanning. Bone and brain scans are useful to exclude extra-thoracic disease.

A routine assessment of cardiopulmonary fitness is important to identify patients most likely to tolerate pulmonary metastasectomy. This includes spirometry and often a noninvasive cardiac stress study.

RISK FACTORS FOR TIME-RELATED MORTALITY

Overall survival of resected patients in our series was 82%, 49%, and 31% at 1, 3, and 5 years, respectively. When patients were segregated by *completeness of resection*, vastly discrepant survival curves were generated, as completely resected patients demonstrated a clear survival advantage (Figure 26.1). In this analysis, the ability to attain a complete resection was by far the most important predictor of long-term survival following pulmonary metastasectomy.

Interestingly, the probability of an *incomplete resection* was, in part, dependent on the number of pulmonary nodules identified on a preoperative chest CT scan (Figure 26.2), highlighting the importance of this study in the assessment of potentially resectable patients. The likelihood of *incomplete resection* was 80% if six of more nodules were identified on the preoperative CT scan, whereas the probability of complete resection was 80% if three or fewer nodules were identified.

Other continuous and ordinal risks for death following pulmonary metastasectomy include larger nodule size, greater number of involved regional lymph nodes, decreasing preoperative forced expiratory volume in 1 second (FEV_1), and, for completely resected patients, shorter disease-free interval (Table 26.2). That preoperative FEV_1 is

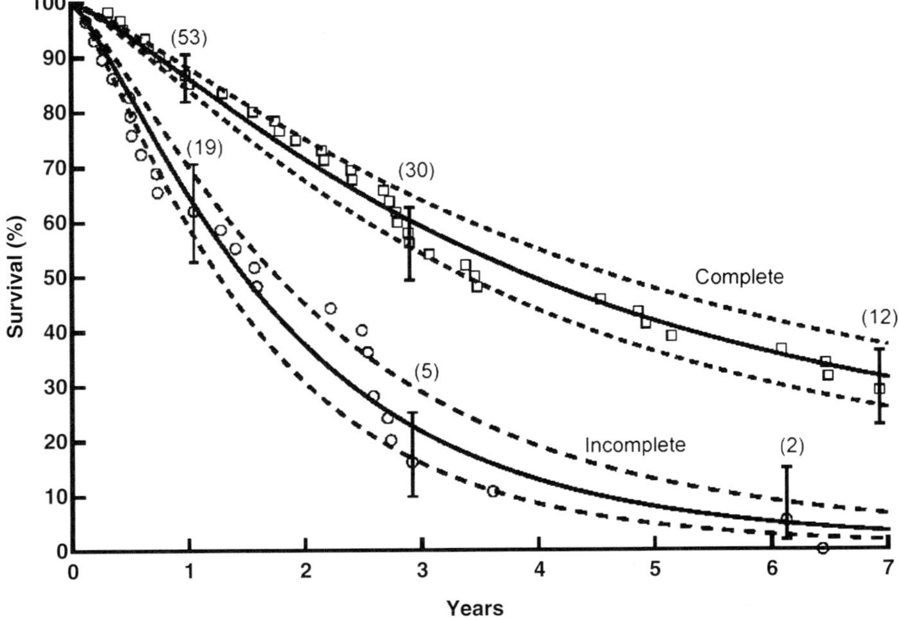

Figure 26.1. Survival after pulmonary metastasectomy stratified by complete (squares) and incomplete (circles) resection. Vertical bars represent 68% confidence limits (equivalent to 1 standard error), and numbers in parentheses represent patients remaining alive. Solid line (enclosed by dashed 68% confidence limits) is parametric representation of survival.

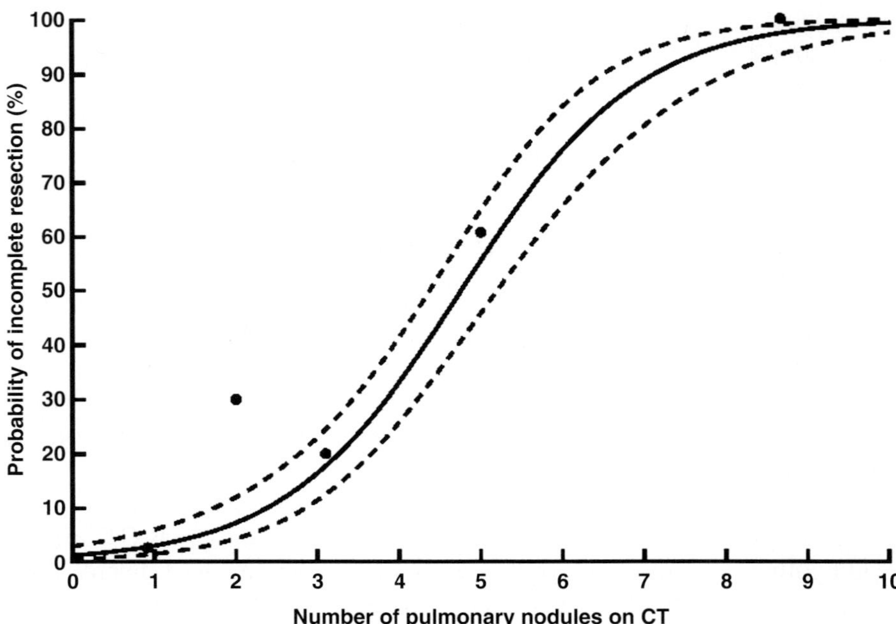

Figure 26.2. Probability of incomplete resection according to number of pulmonary nodules on preoperative computed tomography (CT). Filled circles are actual probabilities, and solid line (enclosed within dashed 68% confidence limits) is logistic regression estimate.

Table 26.2.
Incremental risk factors for death in all patients

Risk factor	Coefficient ± SE	p
Larger pulmonary nodule	0.030 ± 0.0078	.0002
Higher number of lymph nodes containing metastatic tumor[a]	0.38 ± 0.16	.02
Lower preoperative FEV_1 (% of normal)	−1.9 ± 0.87	.02
Shorter disease-free interval (years) for completely resected patients[b]	−0.46 ± 0.21	.03

FEV_1, forced expiratory volume in one second; SE, standard error.

[a]Among patients with resected or sampled lymph nodes. Patients without lymph node sampling or resection behaved similarly to those with a single involved lymph node (coefficient ± SE = 0.41 ± 0.33), but this magnitude could be due to chance ($p = 0.2$).

[b]Pertains only to patients with complete resection. Disease-free interval was not a risk factor when resection was incomplete (coefficient ± SE = 0.28 ± 0.26, $p = .3$). This implies that incomplete resection is, in general, a risk factor, equivalent in risk to a patient with complete resection having a disease-free interval of 0 years (synchronous presentation). Patients whose nephrectomy occurred after diagnosis of pulmonary metastases behaved similarly to those with incomplete resection (coefficient ± SE = −0.11 ± 0.47, $p = .9$).

an important risk factor for long-term survival suggests the latent morbidity that accompanies anatomic pulmonary resection. This cannot be ignored when selecting patients for metastasectomy.

IMPLICATIONS

Metastasectomy has a central role in the therapy of patients with isolated and limited involvement of lung from RCC. Accumulated data suggests a 20% to 50% five-year survival for surgical patients compared to a 3% to 11% survival for nonoperated patients.[11] We have identified five important variables that should help guide intervention. Most of the identified predictors relate specifically to tumor-dependent characteristics (ability to obtain a complete resection, larger size, regional lymph node involvement, and disease-free interval), though one patient variable, preoperative FEV_1, was also important.

It is critical to understand that although multiple factors are independently associated with survival, it is the composite analysis of all factors that yields the most clinically useful and prognostically accurate information. To illustrate this, representative survival curves have been generated for three patient populations (representing distinct composites) based on the hazard equation derived from our study[16] (Figure 26.3).

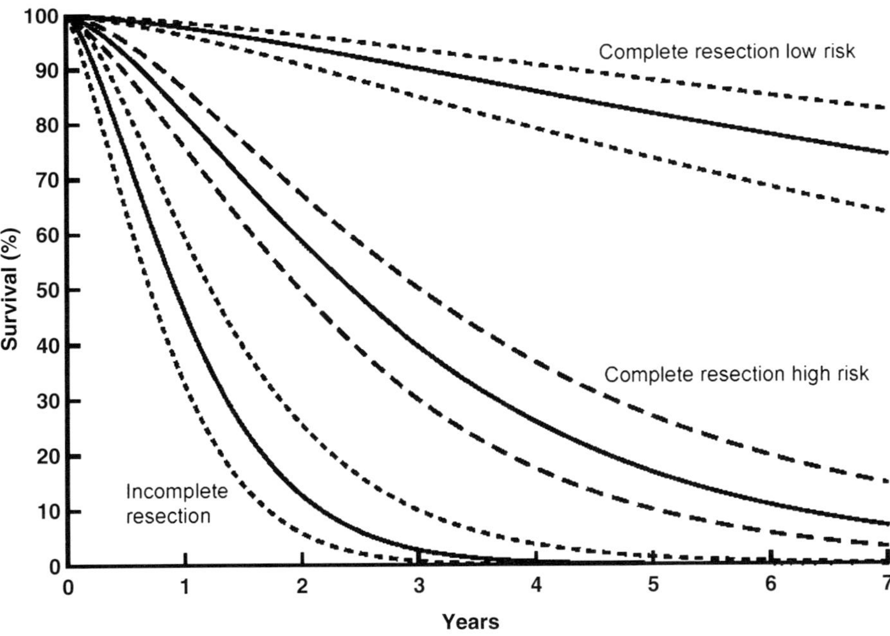

Figure 26.3. Survival of three hypothetical patients. This is a nomogram of the risk factor equation for death (see Table 26.2). For the patient with complete resection and considered low risk: disease-free interval 6 years; forced expiratory volume in one second (FEV_1) 100% of predicted normal; no lymph node involvement; largest pulmonary nodule 7 mm. For the patient with complete resection and considered high risk: disease-free interval 1 year; FEV_1 75% of predicted normal; one lymph node involved; largest pulmonary nodule 30 mm. For the patient with incomplete resection: disease-free interval 1 year; FEV_1 75% of predicted normal; one lymph node involved; largest pulmonary nodule 45 mm.

From this information, practical guidelines for patient selection for metastasectomy can be derived. First, a major focus of the preoperative evaluation should be on identifying patients who are likely to be *completely resected*. In addition, since regional lymph node involvement is a poor prognostic indicator, pre-resection mediastinoscopy is important. Finally, selecting patients with adequate pulmonary reserve is essential. By utilizing these data, improved outcomes following pulmonary metastasectomy for RCC can be expected.

REFERENCES

1. van der Poel HG, Roukema JA, Horenblas S, van Geel AN, Debruyne FM. Metastasectomy in renal cell carcinoma: a multicenter retrospective analysis. Eur Urol 1999;35:197–203.
2. Breiman L. Bagging predictors. Machine Learning 1996;24:123–140.
3. Blackstone EH. Breaking down barriers: helpful breakthrough statistical methods you need to understand better. J Thorac Cardiovasc Surg 2001;122:430–439.
4. Dekernion JB, Ramming KP, Smith RB. The natural history of metastatic renal cell carcinoma: a computer analysis. J Urol 1978;120:148–152.
5. Patel NP, Lavengood RW. Renal cell carcinoma: natural history and results of treatment. J Urol 1978;119:722–726.
6. Skinner DG, Colvin RB, Vermillion CD, Pfister RC, Leadbetter WF. Diagnosis and management of renal cell carcinoma. A clinical and pathologic study of 309 cases. Cancer 1971;28:1165–1177.
7. Kozlowski JM. Management of distant solitary recurrence in the patient with renal cancer. Contralateral kidney and other sites. Urol Clin North Am 1994;21:601–624.
8. Cerfolio RJ, Allen MS, Deschamps C, et al. Pulmonary resection of metastatic renal cell carcinoma. Ann Thorac Surg 1994;57:339–344.
9. Piltz S, Meimarakis G, Wichmann MW, Hatz R, Schildberg FW, Fuerst H. Long-term results after pulmonary resection of renal cell carcinoma metastases. Ann Thorac Surg 2002;73:1082–1087.
10. Fourquier P, Regnard JF, Rea S, Levi JF, Levasseur P. Lung metastases of renal cell carcinoma: results of surgical resection. Eur J Cardiothorac Surg 1997;11:17–21.
11. Kavolius JP, Mastorakos DP, Pavlovich C, Russo P, Burt ME, Brady MS. Resection of metastatic renal cell carcinoma. J Clin Oncol 1998;16:2261–2266.
12. Friedel G, Hurtgen M, Penzenstadler M, Kyriss T, Toomes H. Resection of pulmonary metastases from renal cell carcinoma. Anticancer Res 1999;19:1593–1596.
13. Dernevik L, Berggren H, Larsson S, Roberts D. Surgical removal of pulmonary metastases from renal cell carcinoma. Scand J Urol Nephrol 1985;19:133–137.
14. Pfannschmidt J, Hoffmann H, Muley T, Krysa S, Trainer C, Dienemann H. Prognostic factors for survival after pulmonary resection of metastatic renal cell carcinoma. Ann Thorac Surg 2002;74:1653–1657.
15. Long-term results of lung metastasectomy: prognostic analyses based on 5206 cases. The International Registry of Lung Metastases. J Thorac Cardiovasc Surg 1997;113:37–49.
16. Murthy SC, Kim K, Rice TW, Rajeswaran J, Bukowski R, DeCamp MM, Blackstone EH. Can we predict long-term survival after pulmonary metastasectomy for renal cell carcinoma? Ann Thorac Surg 2005;79:996–1003.

Management of Skeletal Metastases in Renal Cell Carcinoma Patients

Michael J. Joyce

KEYWORDS

METASTASES
BONE METASTASES
RENAL CELL CARCINOMA
METASTATIC DISEASE

ABSTRACT

Successful treatment of metastatic renal cell carcinoma to the skeleton requires medical understanding of the mechanism of bone destruction, use of diagnostic imaging tools for skeletal involvement, an orthopaedic appreciation of the risk of structural mechanical failure, and experience with repair/replacement reconstructive skeletal surgery. Patients are now living longer with metastatic skeletal disease. Quality of life is dependent upon the correct surgical choices in supplying lasting structural support or reconstruction which provides for function and pain relief.

Renal cell carcinoma (RCC) is a solid organ cancer that has a propensity to metastasize to the skeleton. The development of a bony metastasis can be a catastrophic complication in a patient with cancer. Bone destruction causing loss of trabecular and cortical integrity leads to reduced load-bearing capacity. Bone metastasis can lead to severe morbidity through bone pain, immobility, pathologic fractures, and neurologic dysfunction. The skeletal problems can contribute to significant suffering. The metastatic bone lesions can be an enormous clinical problem and have a significant impact economically.

Patients with metastatic RCC to the skeleton are evaluated by the orthopedic surgeon either directly because of an unknown cause of skeletal pain or by referral from primary care physicians, medical oncologists, or urologists after a lesion in bone is identified. Often a cancer diagnosis is well appreciated and the patient may have already had a nephrectomy or ongoing adjuvant therapy. Because of musculoskeletal pain or a positive bone scan, the orthopedic surgeon is consulted to evaluate and assess structural integrity of the bones of the extremities, pelvis, and spine. In situations where a lytic lesion is visualized and the actual diagnosis is unknown, the surgeon embarks upon a differential

From: *Clinical Management of Renal Tumors*
Edited by: R.M. Bukowski and A.C. Novick © Humana Press Inc., Totowa, NJ

diagnostic workup. Although all orthopedic surgeons are trained to diagnose and surgically manage metastatic disease, metastatic tumor cases can be just as challenging as primary sarcomas of bone and are often referred to orthopedic surgical oncologists, who are well versed in the complexity and management pitfalls of these lesions.

When a patient presents with a hole in the bone, a radiographic assessment is made on two views, anteroposterior and lateral, of the involved bone, with the entire bone being visualized radiographically. Typically, the lesion of RCC to the skeleton presents with a geographic lytic destructive lesion, and often with a significant soft tissue mass external to the bone. The radiographic appearance is that of a hole in bone with a permeative destructive margin without significant marginal bony reactive sclerosis. The majority of renal cell metastases are indeed lytic, allowing only minimal bone healing response with little to no radiographic evidence of host reactive bone to the destructive tumor component. The renal carcinoma cells themselves do not actually destroy bone, but produce proteins that can recruit and stimulate host osteoclasts to destroy bone locally. Carcinoma cells permeate into the trabecular bone as an infiltrative and destructive process. However, the osteoclasts of the host and the resident macrophage precursors (tumor-infiltrating macrophages induced into osteoclastogenesis by proteins secreted by the tumor cells), are the cause of the bone destruction.[1–5] As anti-resorptive agents, the bisphosphonates have been used to block this interaction in patients with metastatic disease. Early discovery of bone lesions before bone loss in conjunction with bisphosphonate treatment may lead to prevention of severe bone loss.[6–9] Zolendronate has been commonly used. When using bisphosphonates, renal function must be followed closely, especially in nephrectomized patients. Current research is being directed toward a paradigm of direct killing of the metastatic cancer cells compared to enhancement of osteoclastic inhibition. Targeting epidermal growth factor receptor (EGFR) in RCC metastases using monoclonal antibody or EGFR tyrosine kinase inhibitor as a blockage may be an approach in reducing destructive metastases.[10] Focus has been generated at the molecular biology on the inhibition of angiogenesis.[11]

Even though major orthopedic tumor centers see a high frequency of primary bone tumors such as osteosarcomas, malignant fibrous histiocytomas, and chondrosarcomas in adults, lytic destructive lesions in the adult skeleton are usually metastatic lesions from a solid organ tumor. When one compares the incidence of metastatic skeletal lesions from solid organ tumors to that of primary malignant bone lesions in patients over the age 40, the ratio of this being a metastatic lesion rather than a primary bone tumor is well over 100:1. Bone scans depicting multiple areas of involvement in the skeleton further increase the likelihood of the lesion being metastatic disease. However, it is not unusual for an RCC to initially present as a solitary lesion to the skeleton. Most of these lesions are geographic metaphyseal destructive lesions eccentrically placed. However, isolated cortical metastases are not uncommon for renal cells. Lung carcinoma is the most common intracortical metastases with renal cells occasionally causing this appearance. Some of the renal cell metastatic lesions do not present as lytic lesions, but present as a permeative-type appearance with diffuse loss of cortical and trabecular bone substance. Skeletal metastatic lytic lesions below the knee and elbow are more likely to be from the lung, but RCC metastases are not that rare for the hand and wrist/foot and ankle.[12–17]

Concerning the patient with multiple bone lesions, one should be cautious to make sure the patient does not have severe diffuse skeletal osteopenia with loss of trabecular bone, thinning of the cortices, and multiple lytic destructive cystic lesions. Most likely

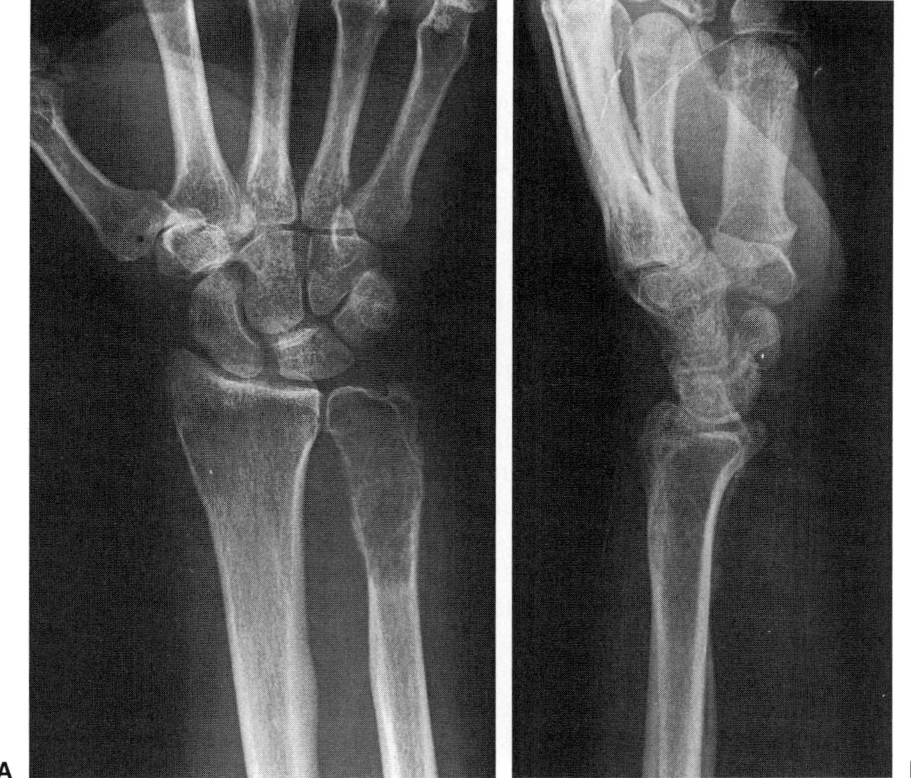

Figure 27.1 (**A**) Anterior-posterior wrist film and (**B**) lateral of a destructive lesion distal ulna with osteopenia of distal radius. This was hyperparathyroidism and not metastatic disease.

in these particular cases, the diagnosis is that of metabolic bone disease of hyperparathyroidism with an elevated parathyroid hormone and a multifocal positive bone scan. The bone left between metastatic lytic areas should indeed be normal and not have the plain film radiographic appearance of diffuse osteopenia related to metabolic bone disease. An example of a case mistaken for metastatic disease is illustrated in Figure 27.1. This 62-year-old man presents with a lytic/expansile lesion of the distal ulna as an isolated skeletal lesion. He had hyperparathyroidism with a primary parathyroid adenoma in addition to multiple small pulmonary nodules that proved to be histoplasmosis and not metastatic lung nodules.

On review of frequency of bony metastatic disease, breast carcinoma is the most common lesion for the orthopedic surgeon to manage in females, with prostate cancer being most common in males. Metastatic breast lesions can be either blastic, presenting as radiodense "whitish" lesions, purely lytic, or mixed. Ninety percent of skeletal prostate lesions are blastic. Lung metastatic disease is the second most common for the sexes. These lung lesions present as radiographic destructive lytic lesions, although occasionally some of the lung lesions may indeed be blastic. Renal cell metastases are a very distant third in frequency for the sexes concerning occurrence of the metastatic skeletal lesion that is brought to the attention of the orthopedic surgeon. These consistently are destructive lytic lesions associated with a soft tissue mass external to the bone. Only very rarely is the renal cell metastatic lesion ever blastic.[18]

INITIAL EVALUATION

Patients who present with a recognized lytic destructive lesion undergo a typical comprehensive history and physical examination. This would include inquiring about the following: a history of malaise, weight loss, or smoking; changes in bowel habits and blood in the stools; cough and sputum production; thyroid problems and neck masses; a history of urinary voiding problems/prostatitis in males; family history of breast cancer, breast lumps, nipple discharge, or nipple retraction in females; and especially RCC, flank pain, and gross hematuria.

In the examination looking for the source of a metastatic bone lesion, astute attention should be directed toward ruling out lung carcinoma, especially with a chest x-ray; breast problems in females, such as nipple retraction and discharge, breast masses, and axillary adenopathy; voiding problems, enlarged nodular prostate gland in males; palpating for thyroid/neck masses; palpating abdominal masses; and rectal examination with stool guaiacs. The physical examination for RCC of the kidney usually does not yield a palpable mass or flank pain on percussion, but microscopic hematuria may indeed be appreciated on urinalysis.

Laboratory studies in the way of acid phosphatase and prostatic specific antigen can be helpful in identifying the skeletal metastatic prostate lesion, especially in the 10% of lytic cases. Most myeloma lesions have a distinct radiographic appearance as either a punched-out hole or permeation, but serum protein electrophoresis, urinary protein electrophoresis, and immunofixation studies can be helpful in addition to looking for significant anemia on the complete blood count for the suspicion of myeloma. Often the laboratory studies show an elevated total protein and a low albumin in the myeloma patient. The radiographic appearance of a large destructive lesion without margination in a renal cell metastasis is usually quite different from that of the punched-out smooth border nonsclerotic margin of a myeloma lesion. However, it may be quite difficult to discriminate radiographically between the permeative lesion of bone for renal cells compared to a permeative lesion of myeloma. Computed tomography scans of the lung, abdomen, and pelvis can be helpful in identifying the solid organ primary lesion that has caused the skeletal metastatic deposit.

ROLE OF THE BONE SCAN/SERUM BONE MARKERS/ RADIOGRAPHIC IMAGING

Total body bone scans have been thought not to be cost-effective in the routine staging investigation for patients with renal carcinoma[19] unless skeletal bone pain symptoms are present or other metastatic sites have been identified. Studies have demonstrated that the vast majority of true positive lesions are associated with bony discomfort. Alkaline phosphatase is an insensitive indicator of bone metastases, as demonstrated by Kriteman and Sanders.[20] Bone metastases were demonstrated in 164 of a cohort of 539 renal carcinoma patients. Alkaline phosphatase levels were less than or equal to 141 u/L in 72% and less than or equal to 111 u/L in 53%. In a second cohort of 184 patients, 22 of 37 bone metastases patients (59%) had little or no bone pain at presentation and 86% had a normal alkaline phosphatase. This incidence of occult skeletal metastasis is in sharp contrast to Henriksson et al.'s[21] review of 102 patients with renal carcinoma of whom 33 patients (32.4%) had metastatic spread, but bone metastases were found in only six patients, 5.9%. All six patients were symptomatic with bone pain, and routine bone scanning in 70 patients demonstrated no other sites of skeletal metastasis.

Seaman et al.[22] conducted a retrospective review of 28 of 90 patients with a positive bone scan who were under therapeutic treatment. Thirty-nine percent had a normal alkaline phosphatase and only three of these 11 patients had no bone pain. Of these three asymptomatic patients with bone metastases and normal alkaline phosphatase levels, only one had bone as the only site of renal metastasis and would have been incorrectly staged without a bone scan. The authors' conclusion was that a bone scan may be safely omitted in patients with renal carcinoma with normal alkaline phosphatase levels and no bone pain. Sandock et al.[23] reviewed 158 patients retrospectively who had a radical nephrectomy with 137 having no evidence of metastasis at diagnosis. Even though disease recurred in 52.8% of their T3M0N0 group, the study suggested that the routine use of bone scans and CT did not appear necessary for follow-up, and decisions for imaging could be made on an individual clinical basis.

Staudenherz et al.[24] reported that the bone scan had no diagnostic role in staging for RCC and should be omitted for routine initial staging. However, 14 of 18 patients with extraosseous metastatic disease also had bone metastasis.

Two hundred and five patients from University Hospital Nagasaki, Japan, who underwent initial routine staging and total body bone scan as part of initial staging were reviewed by Koga et al.[25] to assess the value of the bone scan. Bone metastases were present in 34 of 205 patients (17%). Only 12 of 34 (35%) had bone pain. Normal bone scan results did not absolutely mean that the patient was free of bony involvement. In two of the 149 patients with normal bone scans, a bony metastatic lesion was depicted by CT scan. Eleven patients overall had bone metastasis without evidence of other visceral (lung/liver) or nodal metastasis. Spine, ribs, and pelvis were the most common skeletal sites. Alkaline phosphatase was normal in 22 of the 34 patients with bony metastatic disease. The authors acknowledged that if the bone scan was omitted in patients who were free of bone pain, more than half of the patients with bone metastases would have been missed early in the staging. Of the 25 patients with stage T3a lesions, only one (4%) had bone metastasis without other extraskeletal metastasis, bone pain, or enlarged regional lymph nodes. The authors concluded that the bone scan may be omitted in patients with clinically localized states graded T1–2N0M0 and T3aN0M0 when there was no localized bone pain.

Shvarts et al.,[26] using the Eastern Cooperative Oncology Group (ECOG) performance status in review of 1357 patients undergoing nephrectomy or immunotherapy, identified only 1.4% of patients with an ECOG score of 0 who demonstrated bone metastases, of whom 71% complained of musculoskeletal pain, 100% manifested extraosseous metastases, and 25% had an increased alkaline phosphatase. The authors concluded a bone scan should be performed in patients with an ECOG score greater than 0 regardless of the T stage but was unnecessary in the otherwise asymptomatic ECOG 0 patient without extraosseous metastasis. If only musculoskeletal pain was used as a criterion for bone scans, 27% of the patients would have been missed. Therefore, the authors proposed that patients with an ECOG performance status of 1 or greater regardless of the local T stage should have a bone scan.

Newer serum markers for bone loss, such as pyridinoline and deoxypyridinoline cross-links may possibly be used as a discriminatory factor in the decision-making process for requesting a total body bone scan. In contrast to renal carcinoma not inciting a limited bone reaction process leading to an elevated alkaline phosphatase, Nemoto et al.[27] demonstrated significant correlation between the bone loss radiographically and the level of pyridinoline cross-links in the animal model. Jung et al.,[28] however, found that serum bone turnover markers were hardly useful in the diagnosis of bone metastases.

Because of the low sensitivity of the technetium bone scan for very early skeletal metastasis without radiographic abnormality or bone pain, magnetic resonance imaging (MRI) has been used as a tool to discriminate sites of potential bony metastasis. Other radiopharmaceuticals such as gallium 67 and yttrium 90 seem to have better affinity for renal cell metastasis both for imaging and possible therapeutic treatment.[29]

The most sensitive routine tool for imaging of occult metastatic disease in the radiology armamentarium is MRI looking for spin signal changes of infiltration. An MRI can be helpful in discriminating between stress fractures and solid organ metastatic disease. The MRI is quite helpful in defining the extent of the soft tissue mass, epidural spinal masses, and other infiltrative bone lesions, especially in evaluating the extent of disease in other vertebral bodies of the spine. The MRI often has a peculiar flow "void" signal intensity that corresponds to vascular tubular structures, which may be helpful in distinguishing a renal cell metastasis from other abnormalities.[30] Spine lesions most often present as lesions of the anterior column with involvement of the vertebral body with eventual pedicle destruction. Identifying and treating epidural spine compression lesions prior to the patient's having a neurologic deficit is important in reducing the morbidity of these epidural lesions.

Positron emission tomography (PET) studies have been used to identify occult lesions that do not appear on plain films and had equivocal findings on bone scan.[31,32]

A simple fine-needle aspiration using sterile technique either under fluoroscopy or CT scan by the radiologist can be very helpful to the management team in determining if the lytic lesion is metastatic disease.[33–35] Accuracy is well above 95% when identifying these lesions as metastatic. Immunoperoxidase staining can be used in addition to the cellular morphology in differentiating between renal cell and other solid organ metastatic disease.

CLINICAL PRESENTATION

The presentation of some of these lesions can be quite difficult to discern for the clinician, the radiologist, and the orthopedic surgeon. This is especially true in younger patients. Bone lesions about the pelvis can be confused with sciatica and leg pain. Because of the extensive destructive nature of the renal cell metastases, the metastatic lesion presents often with a large soft tissue mass. Figure 27.2 shows a 39-year-old man who underwent a laminectomy at L5/S1 for a bulging disk for his left leg pain 5 months prior to being evaluated for continued back and pelvic left buttock pain. The plain film radiograph showed a lytic lesion of the iliac wing adjacent to the posterior iliac crest. The total body bone scan showed only a single isolated lesion. The bone scan demonstrated a "cold" central area of limited uptake of the radionucleotide, surrounded by a rim of increased uptake. The CT scan showed some periosteal reactive bone rimming the large expansile mass, making an aneurysmal bone cyst a reasonable differential diagnosis. Because the MRI demonstrated the expansile lesion to be predominantly fluid filled, the working diagnosis was that of an aneurysmal bone cyst because of the faint periosteal shell around a fluid-filled mass. A fine-needle aspiration yielded only blood

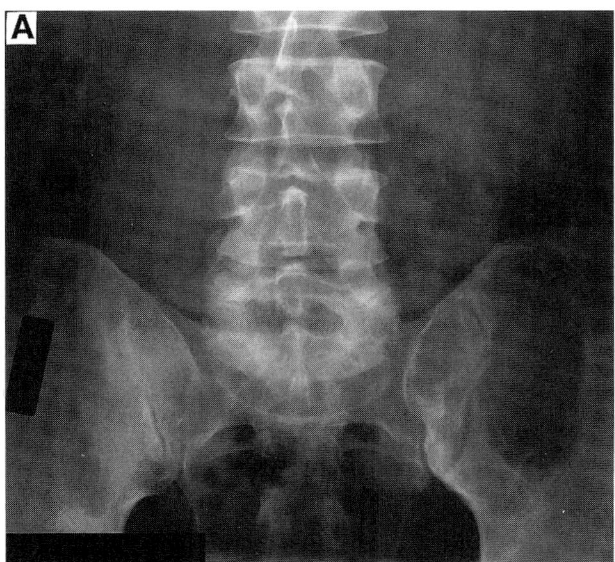

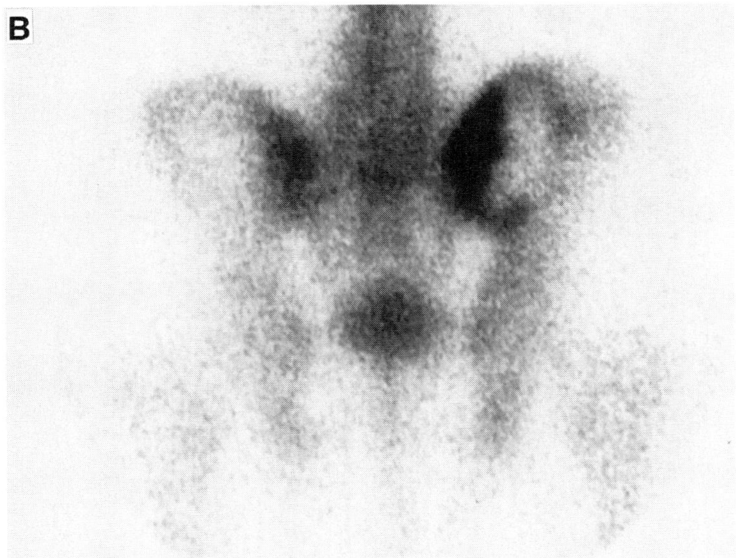

Figure 27.2. **(A)** Radiograph of alytic expansile lesion of the posterior left pelvis in a 39-yr-old man. **(B)** Bone scan demonstrates a photopenic central area with surrounding increased uptake of radionucleotide. **(C)** Computed tomography (CT) demonstrates a large expansile soft tissue mass with some peripheral periosteal bony shell (arrows) around the lesion. **(D)** Magnetic resonance imaging (MRI) shows a fluid-filled lesion with a peripheral rind around the area simulating a possible aneurysmal bone cyst.

with minimal cells and presumptive diagnosis of aneurysmal bone cyst. On the open biopsy, blood and clot were predominantly found. A frozen section of the lining demonstrated RCC. The surgeon was prepared for prompt curettage. After curettage of the bulk of the lesion with removal of the periphery of the renal cell metastasis, bleeding usually ceases, as occurred in this case.

Orthopedic surgeons should be cognizant of the potential diagnosis of a pathologic fracture during routine fracture management. Figure 27.3 shows an intertrochanteric

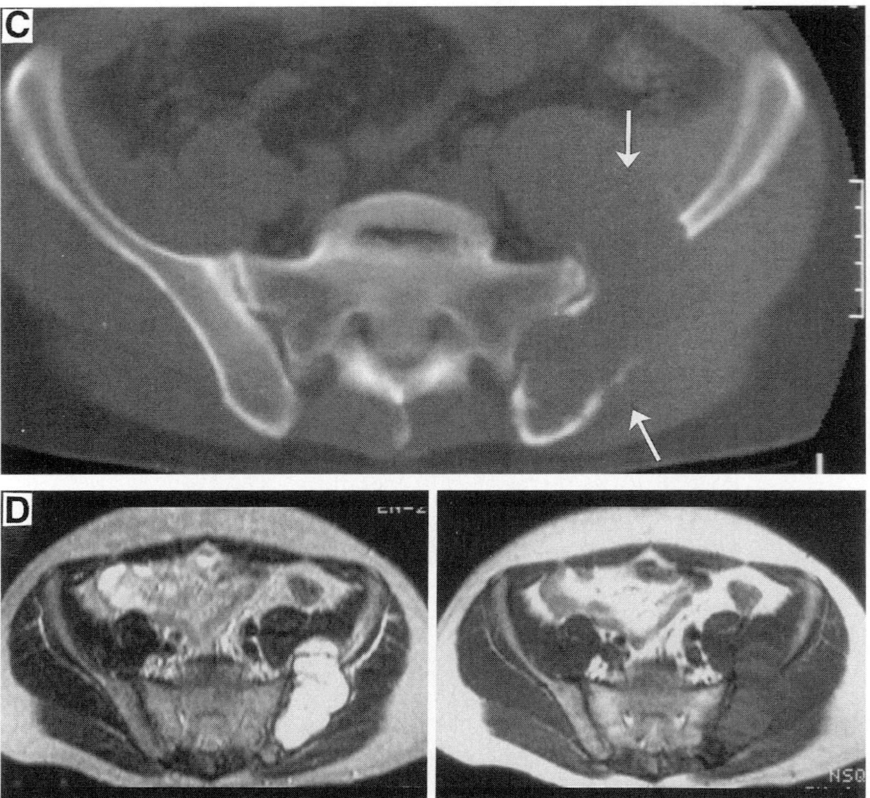

Figure 27.2. *Continued*

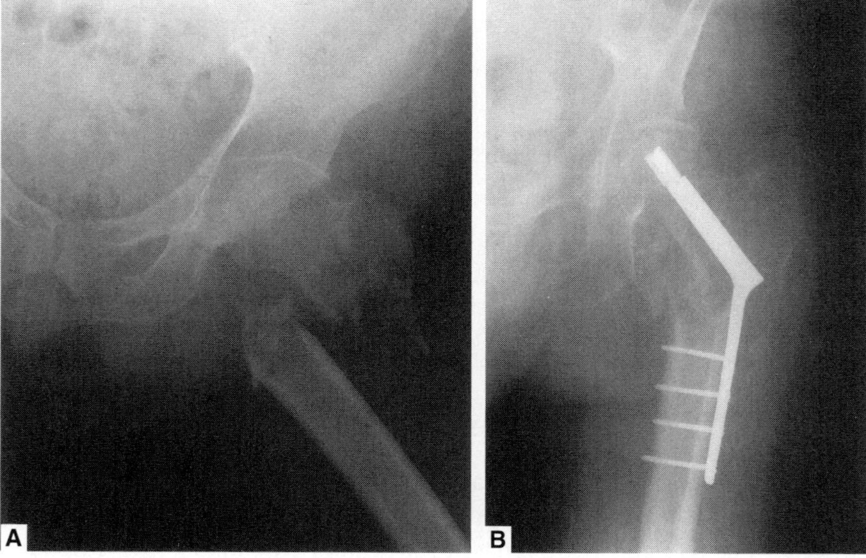

Figure 27.3. **(A)** 42-yr-old man sustained an atypical intertrochanteric hip fracture. **(B)** Internal fixation performed with a nail/plate sliding device. Areas of bone loss are evident.

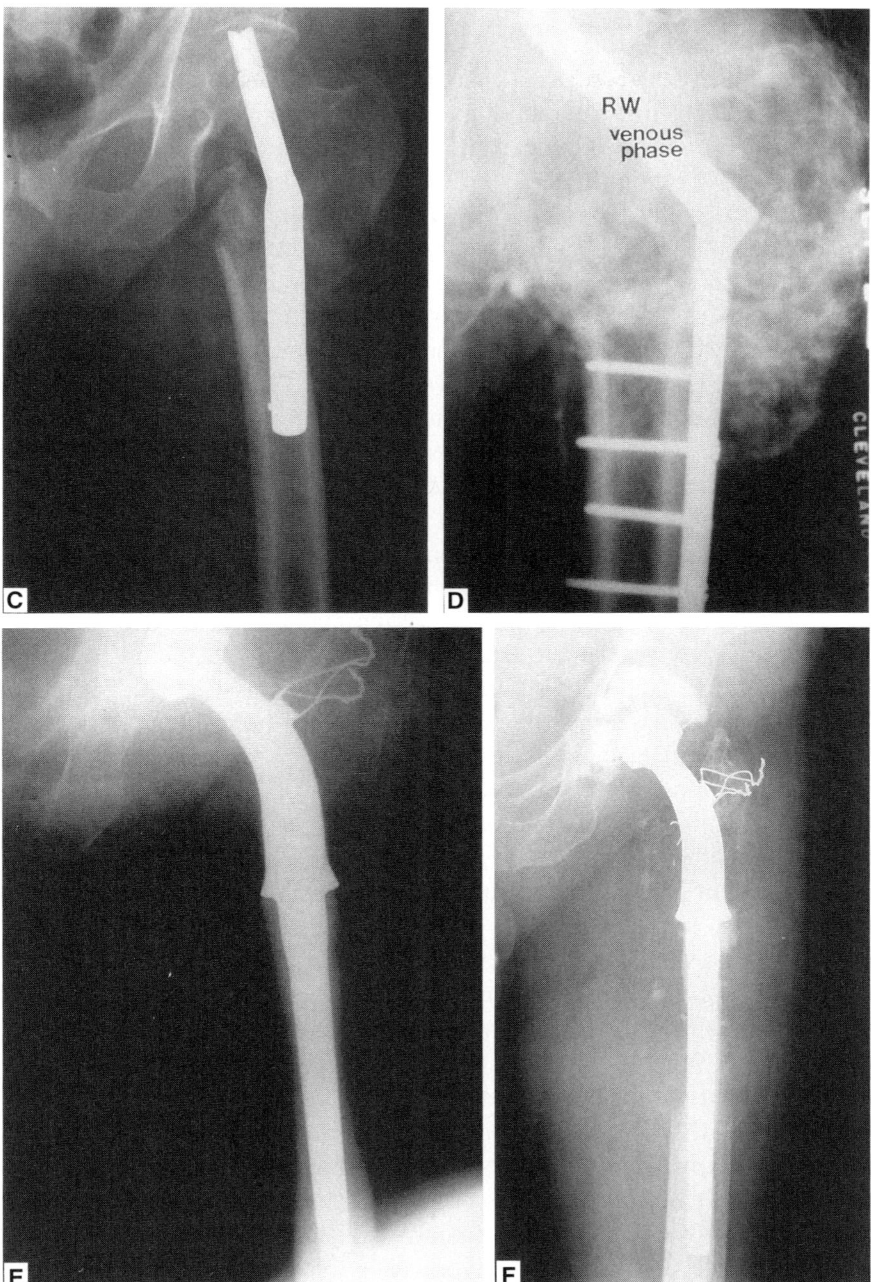

Figure 27.3. *Continued* **(C)** Fracture fixation failure at 6 weeks. **(D)** Venous phase arteriogram showing huge soft tissue mass just prior to embolization. **(E)** Early postoperative film with restoration of femur by a proximal femoral replacement with a total hip acetabular cup because the nail destroyed acetabular articular cartilage. **(F)** Radiograph 30 months later with patient fully ambulatory with use of a cane. He died 3 years after en bloc resection and reconstruction. Bone destruction around the cemented stem is evident, but the component remained fixed to bone.

hip fracture sustained by a 42-year-old man who fell on the ice. In retrospect, the fracture films suggest a preexisting lytic lesion of the proximal femoral area. The fracture was stabilized with a sliding nail side plate device used in years past. Only in retrospect a week later after a call from the radiologist, did the orthopedic surgeon appreciate that the postoperative films indeed suggested a cavity. Apparently, no excessive bleeding occurred during the fixation to alarm the surgeon. The search for a solid organ tumor was embarked upon with CT scans of the chest and abdomen, with a large mass in the kidney being identified as RCC. The patient subsequently underwent a nephrectomy. Because of the bone loss, the patient was treated in traction for 6 weeks and was subsequently in a spica cast for an additional 6 weeks, with the oncologist stating that the patient would not survive long enough to warrant definitive management of his proximal femur after hardware failure. The patient was referred 3 months later with a large soft tissue mass about his left hip. Embolization was accomplished and the large mass resected, including the proximal one-third femur similar to what would be accomplished for a primary malignant bone tumor procedure. The limb was reconstructed with a proximal femoral replacement. The patient was quite functional and fully ambulatory for 2½ years before subsequently succumbing to systemic metastatic disease, with the construct just lasting for the duration of his life. This illustrates the importance of sending tissue intraoperatively for frozen section and eventual permanent section to diagnose the possible cause of the fracture if there is any suspicion of a pathologic fracture. Careful examination of fracture films preoperatively for evidence of a destructive geographic lesion or permeative regions will alert the orthopedic surgeon to the potential diagnosis of metastatic disease.

The predominant musculoskeletal problem pertaining to renal cell metastases relates to loss of function and pain. Pain can be related to the expanding lesion within the medullary canal, with the huge soft tissue mass causing pressure on the pain fibers within the periosteum. This is a pressure-induced phenomenon related to the pushing borders of the tumor. For the somewhat limited radiosensitive lesion of renal cell metastasis, radiation therapy can be somewhat effective in causing a shrinkage of the tumor, thus temporarily relieving pain related to the expansile pressure on the periosteum. The second source of pain is that of mechanical structural pain related to an impending fracture of the bone. Whereas radiation therapy may relieve the mass effect of the tumor upon the periosteum, the mechanical and structural pain related to bending, compression, and torsion of the bone will not be relieved with radiation therapy and is manifested by increased pain with attempts at weight bearing. For tumors that are fairly radiosensitive, the pressure-type pain is promptly resolved with the course of radiation therapy to about 30 Gy. The radiation therapy hinders bone healing for a number of weeks, but unless the pushing destructive borders of the tumor are eliminated, there would be no bone healing.

Clohisy and Mantyh[36,37] have shown that the pain condition in malignant bone disease was distinct neurochemically from inflammatory and neuropathic pain states. Experimental evidence indicated that both disease-induced osteolysis and tumors themselves contributed to the generation of pain. In RCC, the tumor is only partially radiosensitive. Radiation therapy reduced pain in RCC bony metastases in nearly all patients in a series by DiBiase et al.[38] With dose escalation, complete relief of pain was observed in approximately 55% of patients. In another series by Seitz et al.,[39] 16 of 39 patients had no change and five had continued tumor growth. Brinkman et al.[40] demonstrated benefit

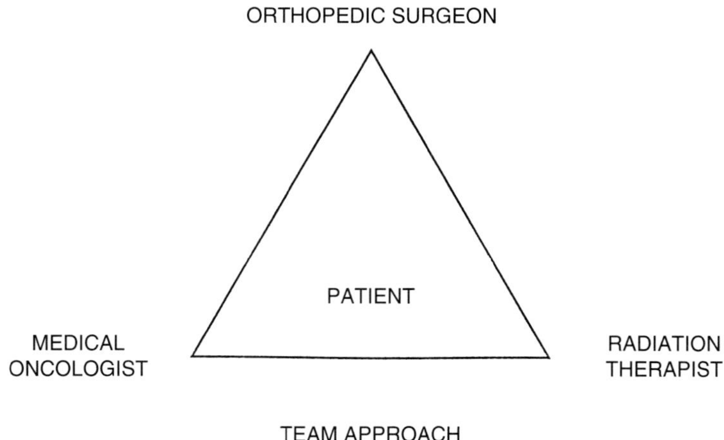

Figure 27.4. Management of skeletal metastases involves a team approach of the medicl oncologist, radiation therapist, and orthopedic surgeon.

with radiation therapy and immunotherapy. Lee et al.[41] demonstrated benefit from palliative radiotherapy in a prospective series. Stereotactic radiation methods are being used especially for spinal involvement.[42,43] Therefore, one of the goals of radiation therapy would be to prevent significant bone destruction before there is excessive loss of structural integrity of the bone. Efforts should be coordinated as a team approach (Figure 27.4), with a radiation oncologist, medical oncologist, and an orthopedic surgeon assessing early bone lesions before they become large and difficult lesions for the orthopedic surgeon to manage. Early medical intervention (bisphosphonates, radiation therapy, immuno/chemotherapy) may help eliminate the need for future orthopedic fracture management intervention.

Radiofrequency ablation often combined with other modalities is in current use.[44–47]

SURGICAL STABILIZATION AND MANAGEMENT

The treatment axiom for stabilization of lesions of the appendicular skeleton is that of rigid fixation. Attempts should be made to protect the entire bone, especially when stabilizing the femur.[48] The ideal location for hardware fixation devices should be intramedullary where the neutral bending force axis exists. In light of loss of significant bone substance, methylmethacrylate (bone cement) is commonly used to provide immediate stable fixation. Renal cell carcinoma metastatic lesions to bone are only partially radiosensitive and one should not plan on future bone healing to resolve situations of marginal stable internal fixation. The goal is to make the construct as stable as it will ever be at the time of the surgical case since one cannot count on a bone-healing response with renal cell metastases. The construct of plates and screws even with methylmethacrylate bone cement to stabilize the metastatic lesion is often doomed to failure once there is further bone destruction. Figures 27.5 to 27.7 illustrate failures of fixation devices used for fracture work, with progressive bone destruction leading to loss of

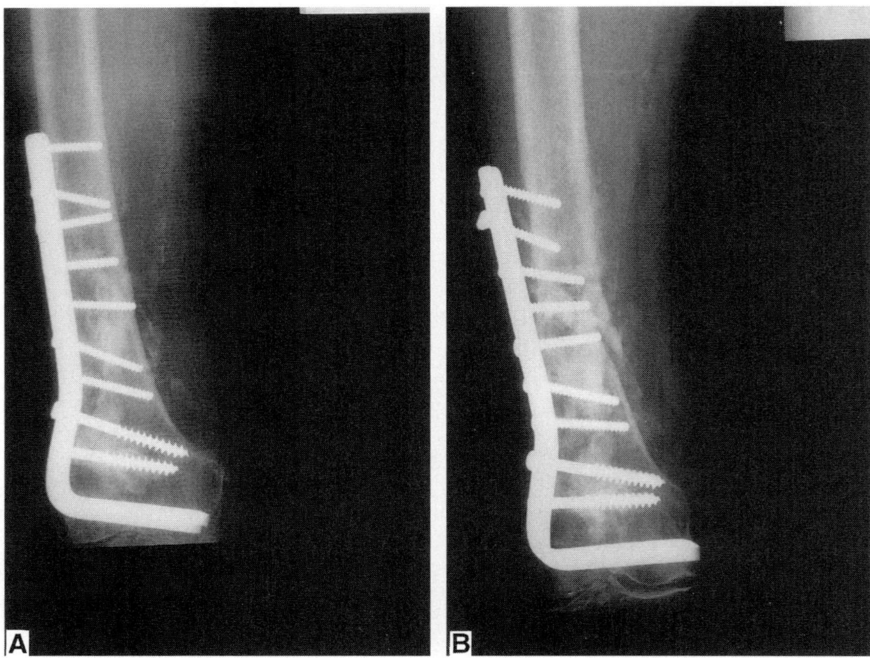

Figure 27.5. **(A)** A 60-yr-old man with attempted internal fixation as a fracture supplemented by methylmethacrylate. **(B)** Failure of fixation within 3 months.

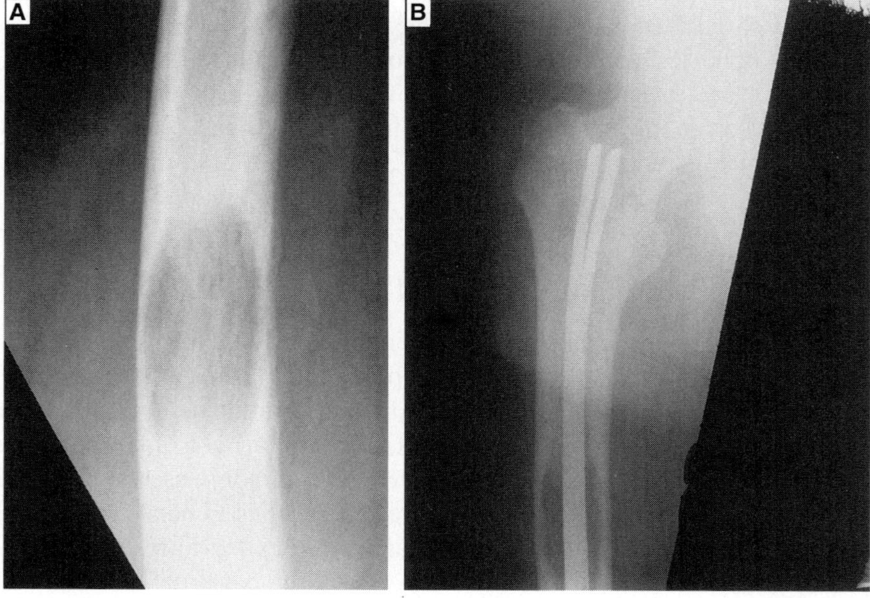

Figure 27.6. **(A)** Painful midshaft lytic femoral lesion in a 62-yr-old man. **(B)** Enders nails with inadequate stabilization. Patient eventually fractured completely and was "too sick" to be operated upon. His final 2 months of life were spent in bed, in pain.

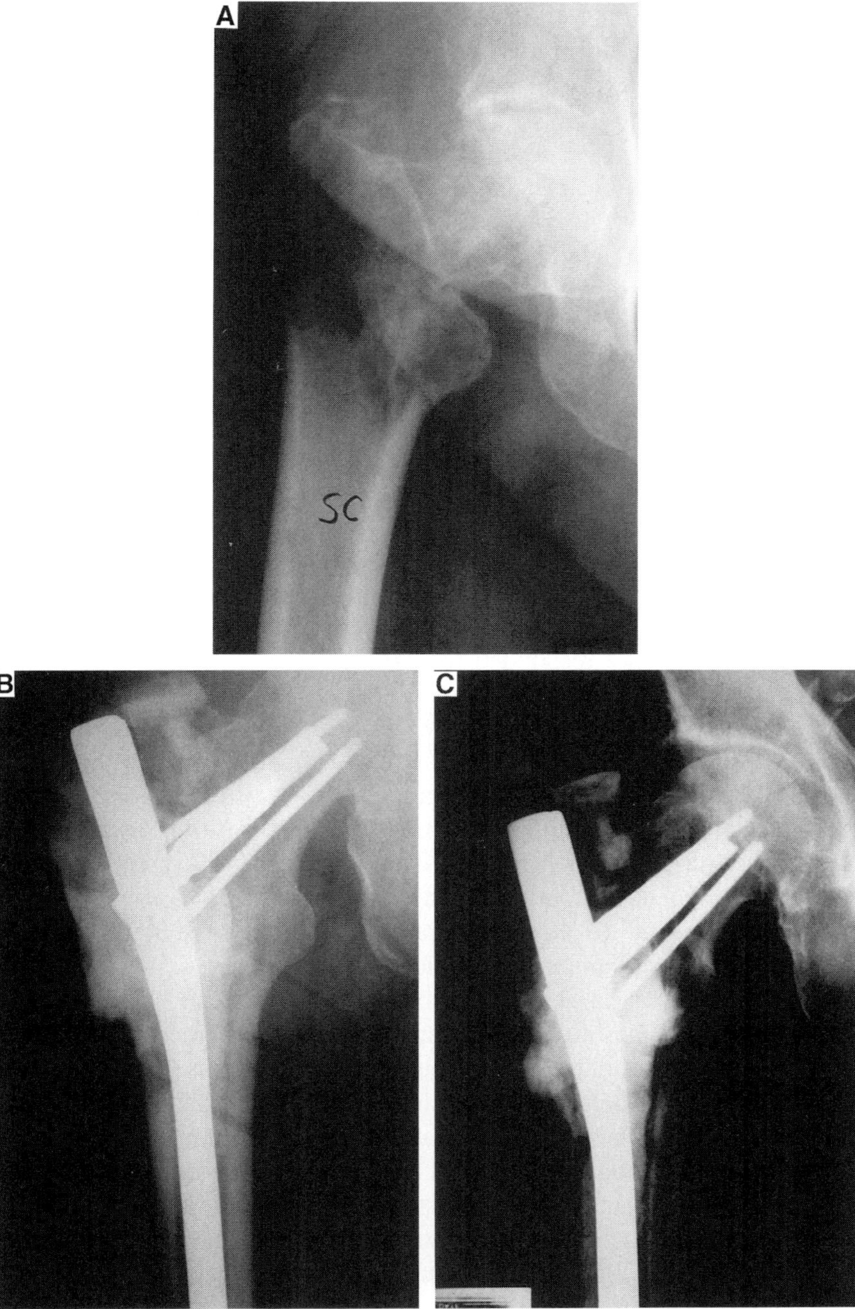

Figure 27.7. (A) Involvement of the proximal femur in a 62-year-old woman. (B) This was internally fixed with a Zickel nail/rod device supplemented with stout rods up the femoral neck anchored with methylmethacrylate for fracture fixation. Patient received radiation therapy postoperatively at 4 weeks. (C) Failure because of bone loss with severe pain 5 months later. Only the methylmethacrylate and hardware remain in the intertrochanteric area.

fixation, deformity, and further pain within weeks and months after the original stabilization procedure. With the newer use of locking plates, attempts have been made to use these locking screw-plate devices especially at the ends of long bones to try to preserve joint function.

Because fixation devices depend on the integrity of the bone structure, internal fixation should be reserved for those lesions that remain somewhat structurally intact. Often the bony outer shell of a lytic lesion can function as a container for methylmethacrylate if intramedullary rodding is planned such that length of a bone is preserved. Planning for prophylactic fixation allows the surgery to be done on an elective basis, with the patient optimized regarding medical conditions. If one waits for an acute fracture before proceeding, often there is significant bleeding, pain, and suffering such that the orthopedic surgeon is directed to fix the fracture problem immediately for pain relief for the patient. If bones are stabilized with intramedullary rods and cement before fracture, length and integrity of the bone can be preserved, and often the operative intervention is much less stressful both on the patient as well as on the surgeon.

Many physicians rely on either Harrington's classic definitions of impending pathologic fracture of long bones[49] or the Mirels[50] classification system. The definitions include a bone lesion that measures 2.5cm or greater in the femoral shaft, occupies 50% or more of the bone diameter, is accompanied by an adjacent fracture/destruction lesser trochanter, or has not responded to radiation therapy. These definitions do not include the permeative subtle bone destruction that often is overlooked on plain films or quantification of bone involvement by MRI or CT scans. The Mirels rating system is based on size (one-third, one-third to two-thirds, greater than two-thirds diameter), site (upper, lower, peritrochanteric), radiographic nature of the lesion (blastic, mixed, lytic) and the degree of pain (mild, moderate, severe). Scores of 8 or greater out of the maximum of 12 required prophylactic fixation, and a score of 7 or less could be safely irradiated without the risk of fracture based on this retrospective review.

A retrospective critique of the Mirels rating system with review of histories and radiographs on 12 patients among 53 participants showed no signification difference across experience levels and a sensitivity of 91%. It seemed that the rating system was reproducible, valid, and more sensitive than just the use of clinical judgment.[51]

Early use of radiation therapy to prevent massive bone loss before there are huge destructive lesions can be helpful. The medical oncologist, radiation therapist, and the orthopedic surgeon well versed at metastatic disease function as a team. Decisions should be made early to prevent bone loss and decide who could functionally benefit from early surgical intervention for metastatic skeletal lesions. The surgeon should anticipate the most likely cause of failure of the construct and plan on protecting the entire bone if possible and especially the femoral neck/intertrochanteric area for femoral midshaft destructive lesions.

Early recognition of impending pressure on the spinal cord is imperative. Screening MRI scans can be quite helpful in defining the risk of skeletal spinal involvement. Although the MRI is quite sensitive in defining metastatic disease in bone and demonstrating epidural masses, plain films and CT define the overall structural integrity and stability. Therefore, plain films, MRI scans, and CT scans are quite helpful to the spine surgeon in planning for decompression and stabilization. In the cervical spine, surgical intervention from an anterior approach is accomplished using methylmethacrylate, autograft, allograft, or a cage to create stability. The anterior column is involved in metastatic disease, and the anterior column needs to be restored for structural integrity.

The surgical compression and stabilization should be done by spine surgeons well versed in spinal stabilization. Often, more than one level needs to be decompressed. The neck can be stabilized with large strut grafts stabilized by a spinal plate as supplementation. Concerning the thoracic spine, anterior approaches are a rule for decompression and stabilization. Frequently, the patient subsequently has a posterior pedicle screws/rods or a laminar wire stabilization such that both the anterior and posterior columns are protected. Lumbar spine involvement can be approached either anterior or posterior. It is inappropriate to do just simple decompression of the posterior elements. This will destabilize the spine and put the patient at further risk for cord or nerve root problems.

Often anterior column stabilization is done through a transpedicle approach with posterior pedicle screw stabilization dependent on the quality of bone. The surgeon may plan for both an anterior decompression with stabilization and a posterior stabilization at different settings to stabilize the spine. Patients are much more likely to recover neurologically from surgical management of epidural metastatic disease before complete progressive neurological loss in contrast to trying to retrieve function in a patient who has become paraplegic and has already lost bowel and bladder function. Therefore, close surveillance and early intervention is the rule in order to preserve motor and sensory function of the extremities in addition to bowel and bladder function. Decision making concerning the operative intervention of these spine lesions especially when comparing outcomes is important. There are a number of retrospective spine reviews of outcomes and attempts to provide a prognosis and quantitate the degree of palliation.[52–55]

EMBOLIZATION

Metastatic RCC causes angiogenesis, yielding a very hypervascular tumor, often leading to significant intraoperative bleeding. Embolization can be quite helpful in renal cell metastases to reduce blood loss for both extremity and spine lesions. A number of studies have shown that blood loss can be reduced 50% to 70%, with the radiologist astutely embolizing feeder vessels to the metastatic lesion.[56–62] Precautions must be taken avoiding the embolization of the artery of Adamkiewicz or excessive embolization potentially rendering an infarction to the spinal cord. Clinically, there does not seem to be a significant problem with regard to the concern of potential spinal cord infarction. The procedure of preoperative embolization is usually done near the time of the planned surgical intervention, either the morning of or the day before the surgery. New collateral circulation can be obtained by the tumor within a fairly short period of time. Embolization is usually done with nonabsorbable materials. Figure 27.8 shows the lumbar spine of a 70-year-old man who underwent two courses of embolization, and both anterior/posterior column spine stabilization with a limited amount of blood loss intraoperatively.

Preoperative direct injection technique of embolization in RCC metastases with cyanoacrylate has also been accomplished as a way to control bleeding.[63]

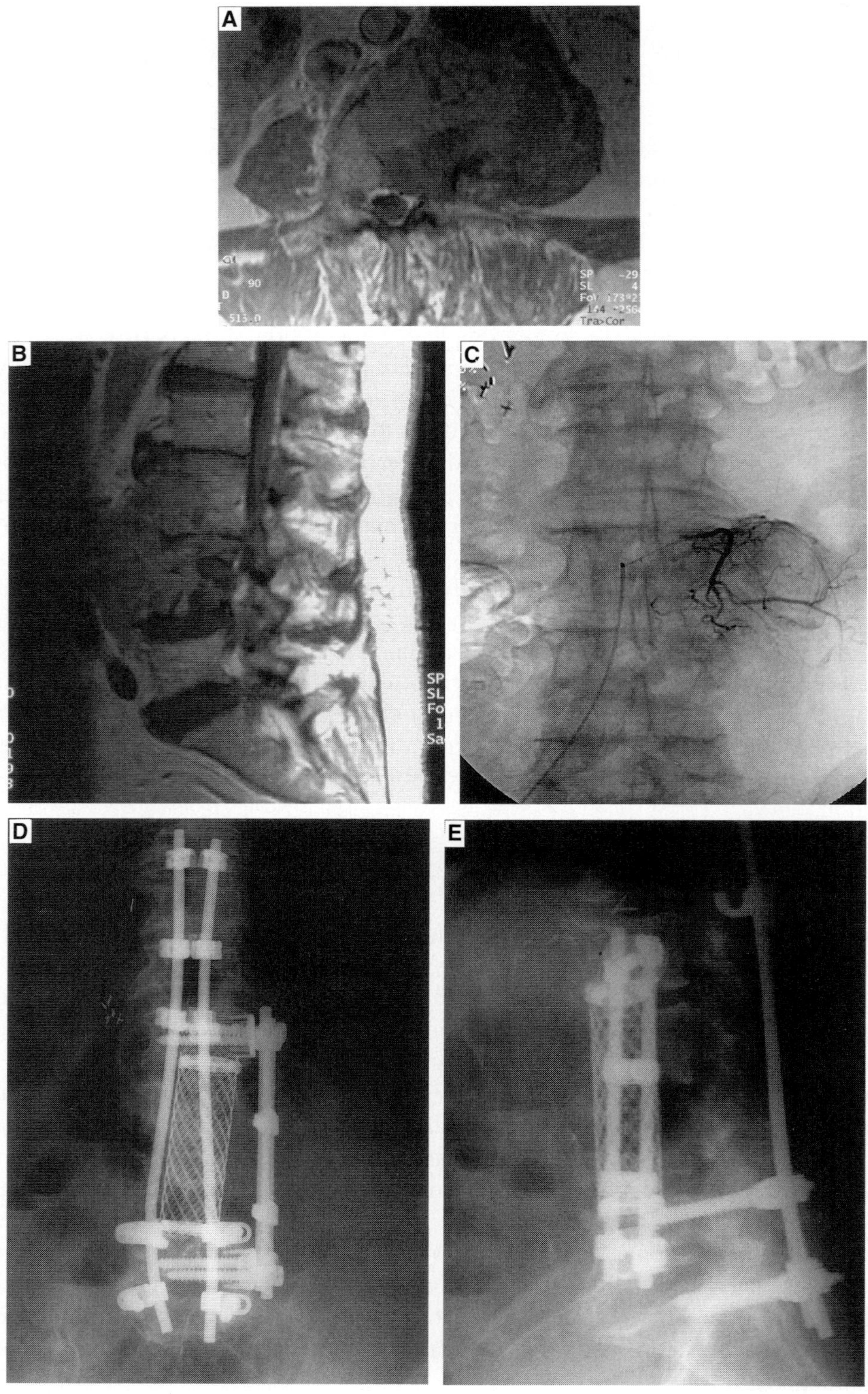

Figure 27.8. Axial (**A**) and lateral (**B**) magnetic resonance views of the lumbar spine in a 70-year-old man with metastatic renal cell axial carcinoma. The lesion involved two adjacent vertebral bodies, but the patient otherwise had no evidence of systemic disease. The patient presented with progressive pain and inability to ambulate, but did not have a frank cauda equina syndrome. (**C**) Angiography of the renal cell lesion demonstrating tumor blush and the neovasculature associated with the metastatic lesion. Two courses of embolization prior to surgery rendered the lesion almost ischemic at the time of excision and the tumor mass was excised with less than 500 cc blood loss. Anteroposterior (**AP**) (**D**) and lateral (**E**) views status post–tumor excision and reconstruction. Surgeons performed a two-level en bloc vertebrectomy, followed by anterior vertebral reconstruction with a titanium mesh cage and anterior screw and rod construct. The patient then had posterior stabilization with segmental instrumentation. At 6-month follow-up, the patient was ambulatory, pain free, and had completed a successful course of adjuvant radiotherapy. (Case from Dr. Robert McClain, Cleveland Clinic Orthopaedic Spine Surgeon.)

FIXATION AS FRACTURE VERSUS REPLACEMENT

Metastatic RCC lesions are often near the end of the bone adjacent to the joint. This makes fixation with fracture techniques and rodding quite difficult. Chan et al.[64] and Wedin et al.[65] had a rate of failure of fixation devices of 45% in patients who survived for 2 years. Lesions about the hip that involve the lesser trochanter and greater trochanter and femoral neck should be replaced and not treated as fractures. Often a significant portion of the metaphyseal bone is involved, and modular systems that supplement total joint systems are used.[66] In this way, metallic components can replace significant bone loss areas, with muscle attachments being reapproximated and the patient then allowed early weight bearing rather than be protected through a "fracture-healing process." Fracture healing may never occur. No matter what device is planned for use, the surgeon needs to be cognizant of the next area of bony failure whether that be at the end of the rod or the stem of a reconstructive component. The entire bone is protected by an intramedullary stem device. This especially includes the femoral neck when rodding of the femur is performed (Figure 27.9). When the lytic lesion is more in the shaft, rods and cement are used (Figures 27.10 and 27.11).

For isolated disease about the femoral head/neck/intertrochanteric area or for disease affecting the end of a bone that can be replaced, such as the proximal humerus, joint reconstructive bone replacement modalities are ideally used. At times these constructs function just as spacers (Figure 27.12). Figure 27.13 shows an allograft prosthetic construct used to preserve function of the rotator cuff in an active individual.

Figure 27.14 is an example of a distal femur with a large soft tissue mass as evident by the plain films and the resected distal femoral. A modular distal femoral rotating hinge total knee system was used to reconstruct this distal femur, allowing the patient early full weight bearing. This construct lasted the patient until he died of systemic disease 12 months later. Figure 27.15 illustrates the rapid progression of a renal cell metastasis that was ignored. The patient was functional 14 months later with a proximal femoral replacement after resection, but had systemic tumor involvement. When using cemented femoral stems in reconstruction, the surgeon must be aware of the risk of the methylmethacrylate monomer and the risk of fat and pulmonary embolism (potential sudden death intraoperatively), especially for the hyperemic porous-type quality bone in the metastatic patient.[67–71] Passage of normal marrow contents or tumor into the

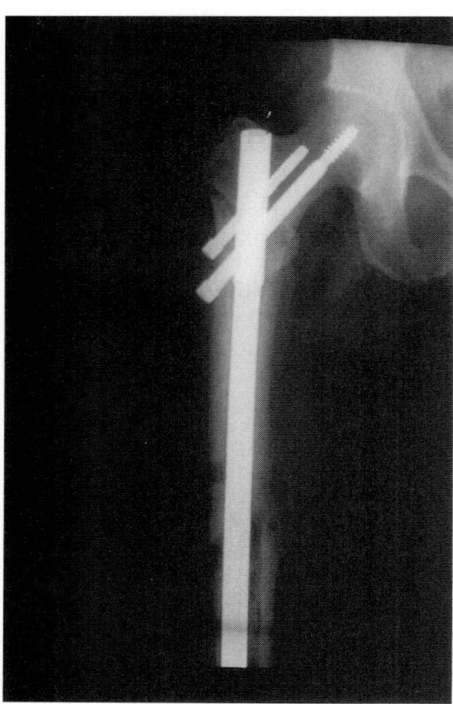

Figure 27.9. Protection of the entire bone includes the femoral neck. This is a reconstruction femoral rod with proximal and distal interlocking.

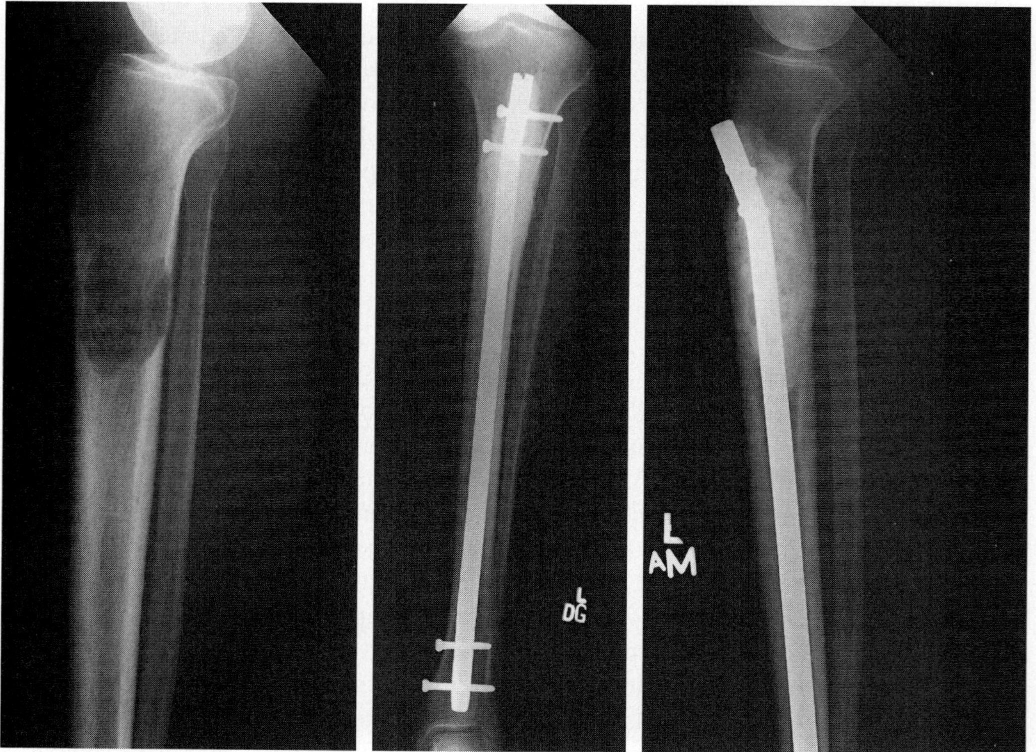

Figure 27.10. (**A**) Lytic lesion in 59-year-old male proximal tibial shaft. (**B**) and (**C**) Asymptomatic patient 9 mo postoperatively. Patient received 30 Gy 4 wks postoperatively.

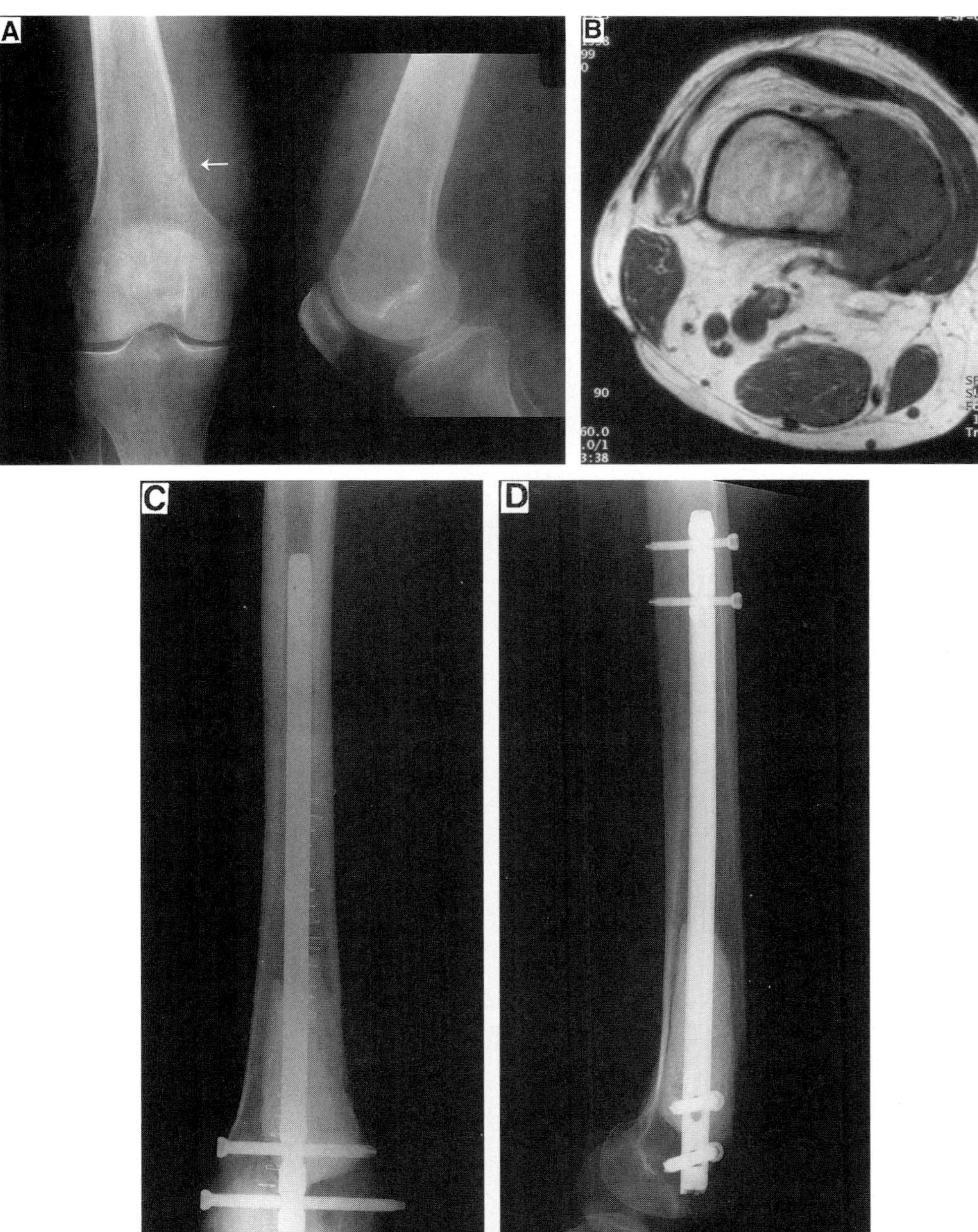

Figure 27.11. (A) A 57-year old man with distal thigh pain. Radiographs show violation of the distal medial cortex (arrow). (B) MRI shows a huge external soft tissue mass on the medial side with little intramedullary involvement. Stabilization with a retrograde statically locked rod with supplemental methylmethacrylate immediately postoperative (C) and at 6 months (D). Case was done under tourniquet, the soft tissue mass excised, no transfusions were required, and the patient received postoperative radiation therapy.

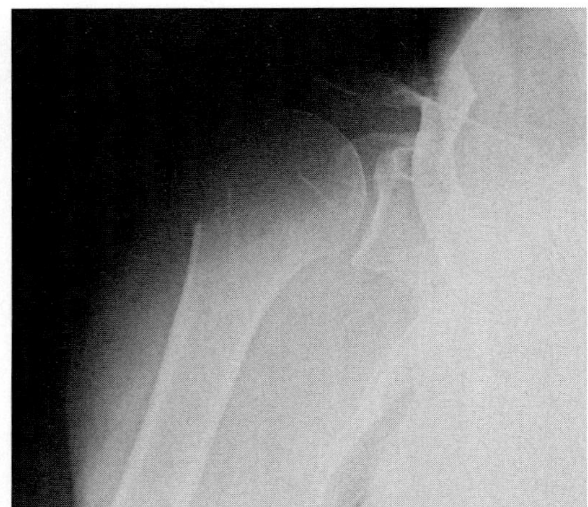

A

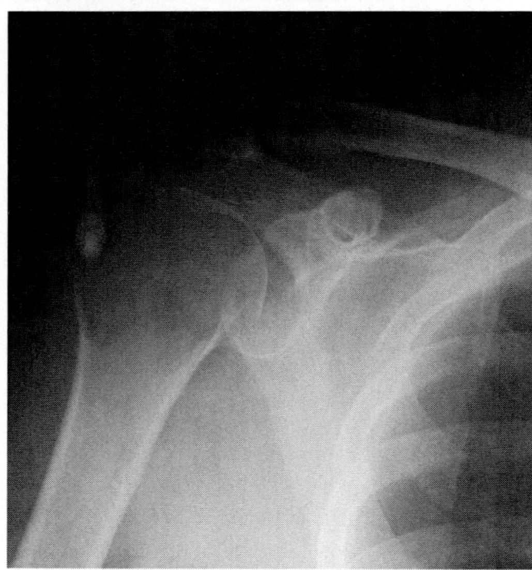

B

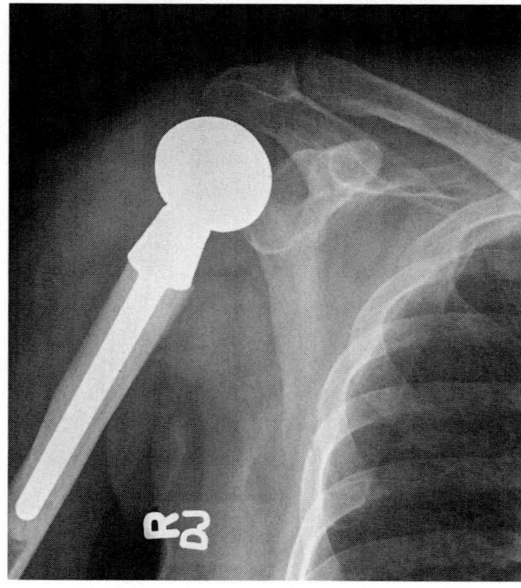

C

Figure 27.12. (A) Radiograph proximal humerus **(B)** lateral showing destructive lytic lesion of proximal humerus. **(C)** Resection with replacement with proximal humeral prosthesis anchored by mersilene tapes to glenoid and rotator cuff.

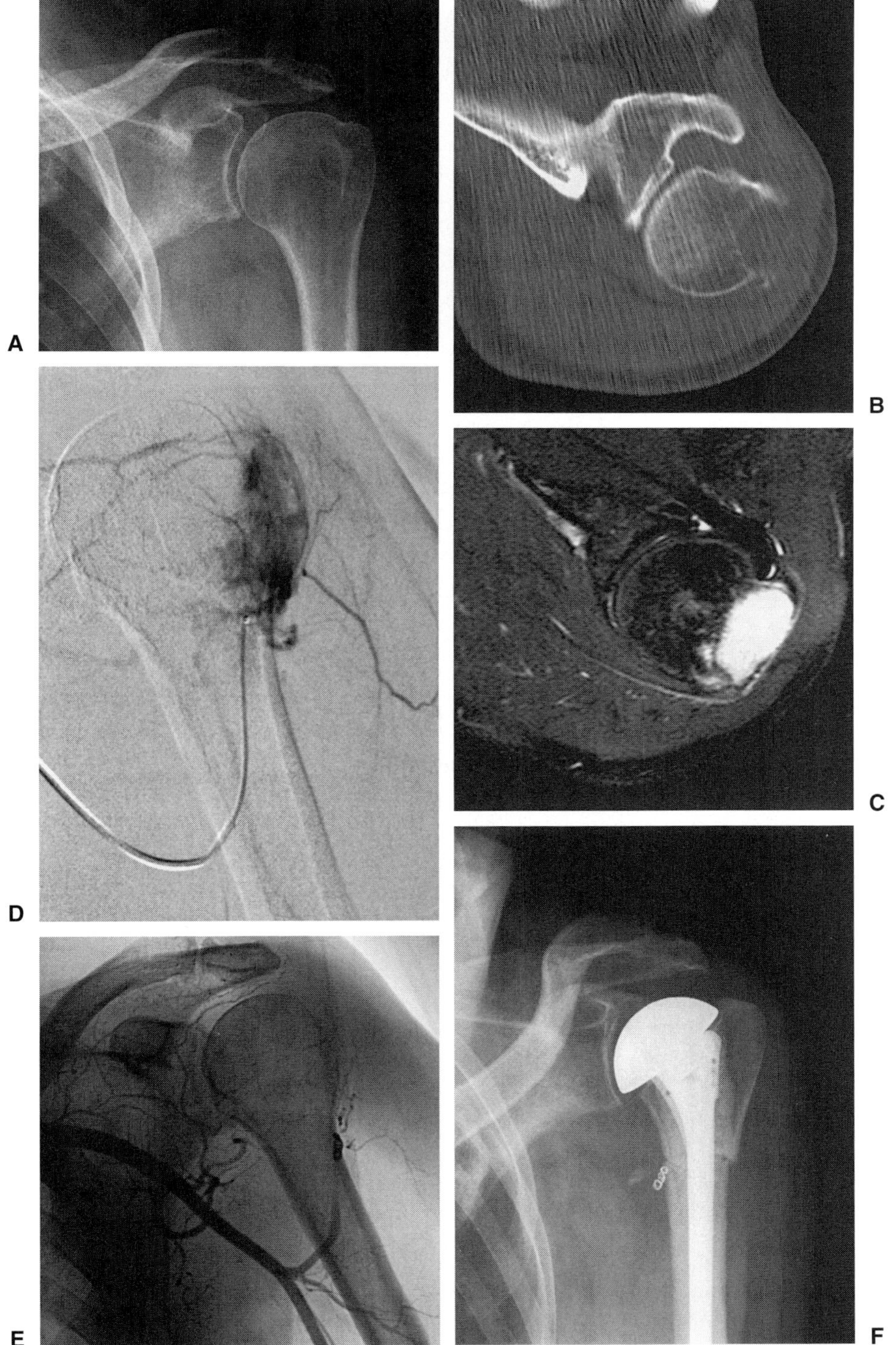

Figure 27.13. (**A**) Lytic lesion proximal humerus-tuberosity. (**B**) CT showing destructive tuberosity changes. (**C**) Angiogram before embolization. (**D**) MRI showing tuberosity involvement with extension into rotator cuff. (**E**) Embolization of proximal humerus RCC lesion. (**F**) Allograft-rotator cuff reconstruction an allograft-prosthetic replacement.

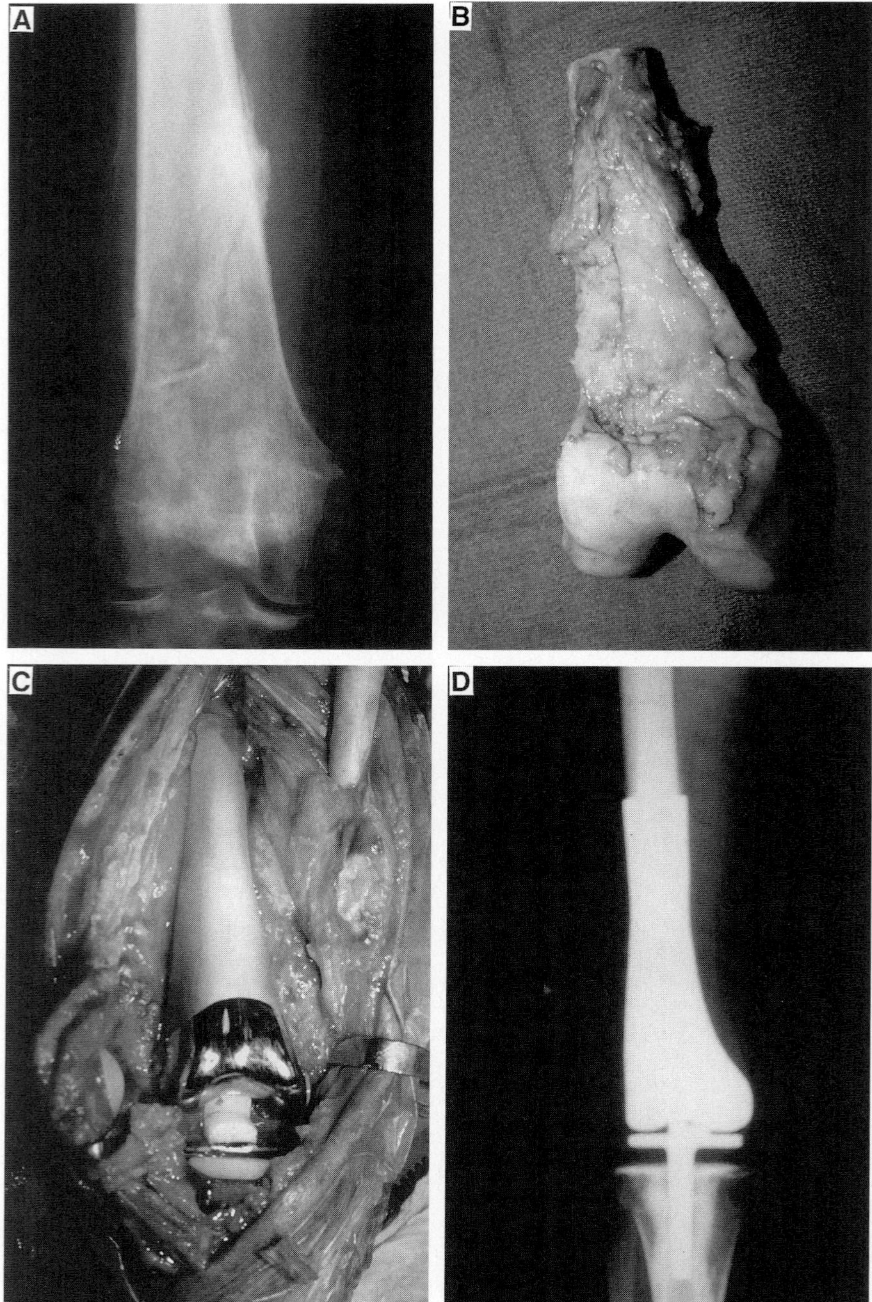

Figure 27.14. (**A**) Painful distal femoral lesion in a 58-year-old man after radiation therapy with an occult pathologic fracture trying to heal. (**B**) Reseted specimen distal femur. (**C**) Rotating hinge modular total knee replacement intraoperatively. (**D**) Radiograph AP of rotating hinge femoral replacement at 6 months.

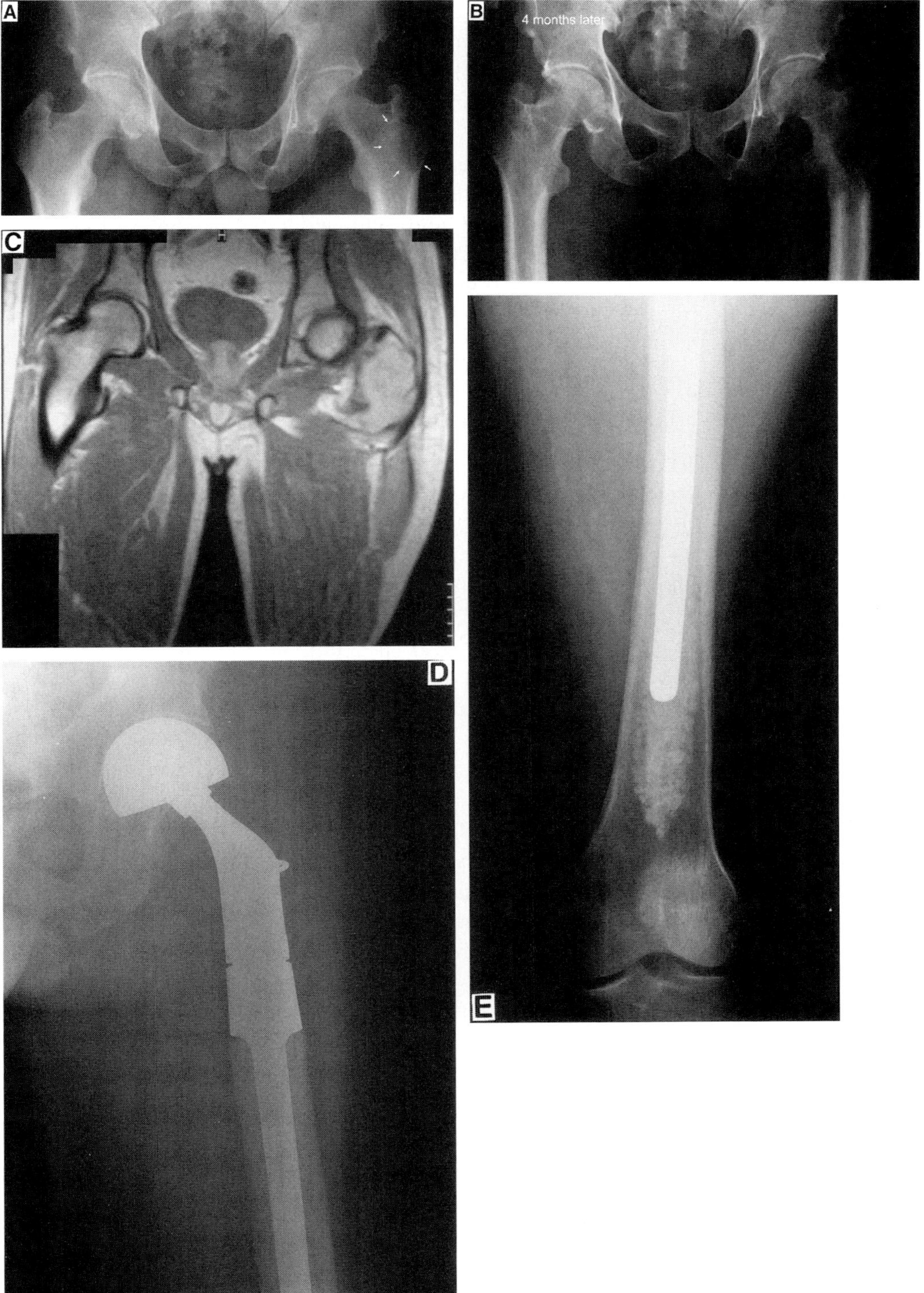

Figure 27.15. (A) Mildly uncomfortable lytic lesion at the base of left greater trochanter in 57-year-old man who had a nephrectomy 12 months previously. (B) Painful huge destructive lesion with loss of bone integrity proximal femur within a 4-month interval of no treatment. (C) MRI showing large soft tissue replacement mass. (D,E) Proximal femoral bipolar replacement with gluteus medius attachment through radiolucent broad synthetic suture to the component.

pulmonary circulation is thought to cause various biochemical and hemodynamic changes that lead to hypotension, arrhythmia, and oxygen desaturation. Patients who are intraoperatively hemodynamically stable (normal blood pressure, normovolemic, and not on vasoconstrictive agents) at the time of cementing tolerate the pressurization better than the hypovolemic patient.[72–74]

There is a controversy concerning adjuvant postoperative treatment. It is well appreciated that large bulky RCC lesions are not all that radiosensitive. Radiation therapy usually to about 30 Gy is the norm, with the field irradiated to include areas of the bone in which tumor may have been pushed further down. Many of these patients resume their chemotherapy or immunotherapy programs, which may possibly be effective in eliminating complications of tumor spillage.

LOCAL SURGICAL TREATMENT BY RESECTION ALONE OR CURETTAGE AND CEMENTING

Certain metastatic locations provide the opportunity for the surgeon to either resect the lesion in its entirety or to locally curettage and use cement (methylmethacrylate) to restore structural integrity. Renal cell metastases may present as bony lesions with large soft tissue masses in an area of nonstructural bone that can be spared. This may occur in the clavicle and the proximal two-thirds fibular area. These metastatic lesions can be treated with resection if very symptomatic. Figure 27.16 illustrates lung/multiple-site bone metastatic disease in a woman who several years before had reconstruction of her proximal femur. She developed a distal clavicular metastasis with fracture and a huge soft tissue mass with impending skin breakdown. This was embolized and resected for comfort and prevention of a more ominous outcome.

Occasional soft tissue metastases may become a problem even after radiation therapy. Figure 27.17 shows extraosseous soft tissue metastases in a 55-year-old man who has survived for 3 years. He had massive involvement about his posterior thigh compartment causing pain and disability after 30-Gy radiation therapy. An MRI confirmed that no bone was involved, and the patient underwent embolization and a nearly en bloc resection sparing the sciatic nerve and femoral vessels. This allowed him to ambulate without pain over the next 12 months before he succumbed to his disease.

Other lesions that are more accessible to curettage and have an intact cortical shell can be filled with methylmethacrylate and treated with 30-Gy radiation to maintain structural stability. Figure 27.18 illustrates an evolving metastatic lesion around a total hip replacement accomplished 3 years previously. Local treatment of curettage, cementing, and radiation has allowed survival of the bony ingrowth acetabular cup without progression of disease over more than 3 years. Figure 27.19 depicts early intervention for a proximal lytic tibial lesion before there was massive bone loss. The cemented/irradiated region has supported the subchondral joint surface without symptoms for over 4 years.

Reconstruction of the acetabulum can be accomplished with different methods using joint replacement and revision techniques with use of off-the-shelf more malleable cages or more rigid larger custom-made cages, allograft prosthetic devices, or by pass components such as the link rotating saddle prosthesis. Decision making, planning, and the nature of the procedure can be difficult.[75] The procedure must be balanced with a reasonable expectation of palliation, and an estimation of longevity and quality of life

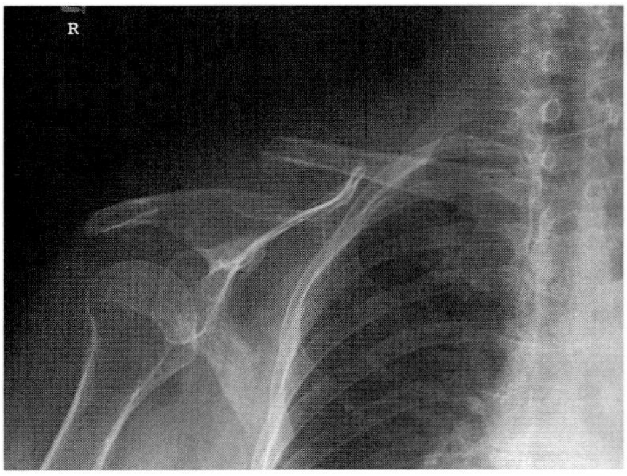

Figure 27.16. (A) Pathologic fracture distal right clavicle with large soft tissue mass. (B) Embolization of soft tissue mass and bone lesion. (C) 6 mo postoperatively after subtotal claviculectomy and soft tissue mass for palliation.

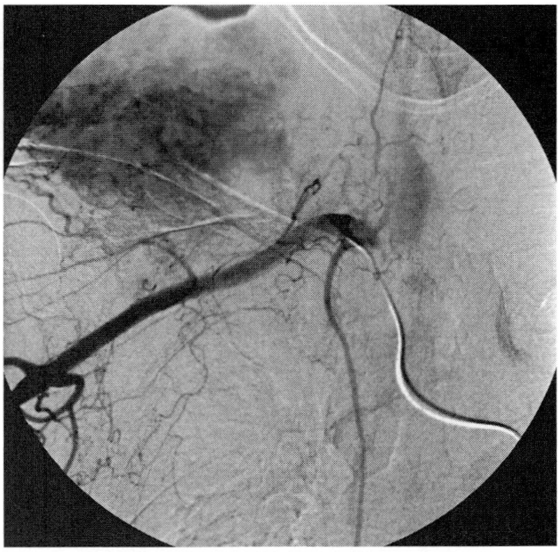

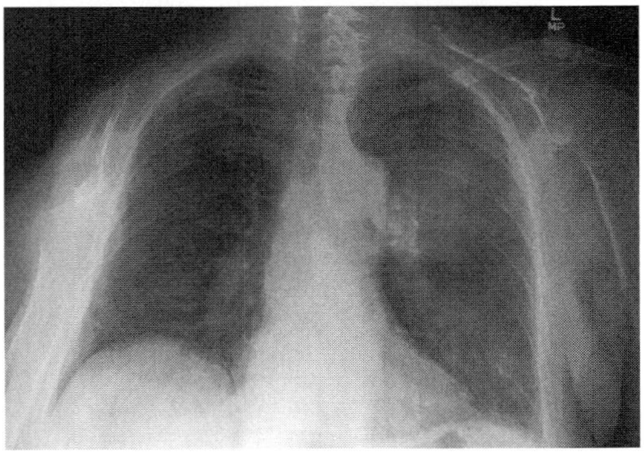

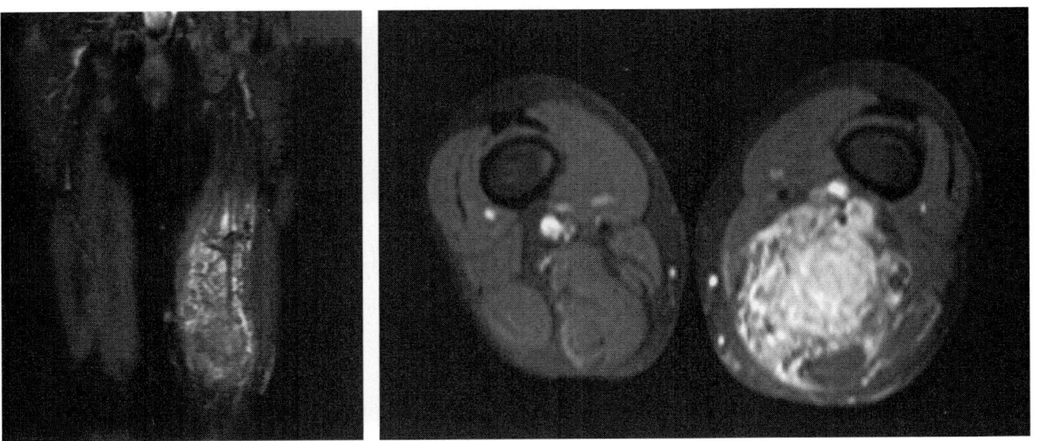

Figure 27.17. (A) MRI left thigh with (B) cross sectional images of large RCC soft tissue painful mass in posterior compartment thigh. This was resected with preservation of the sciatic nerve.

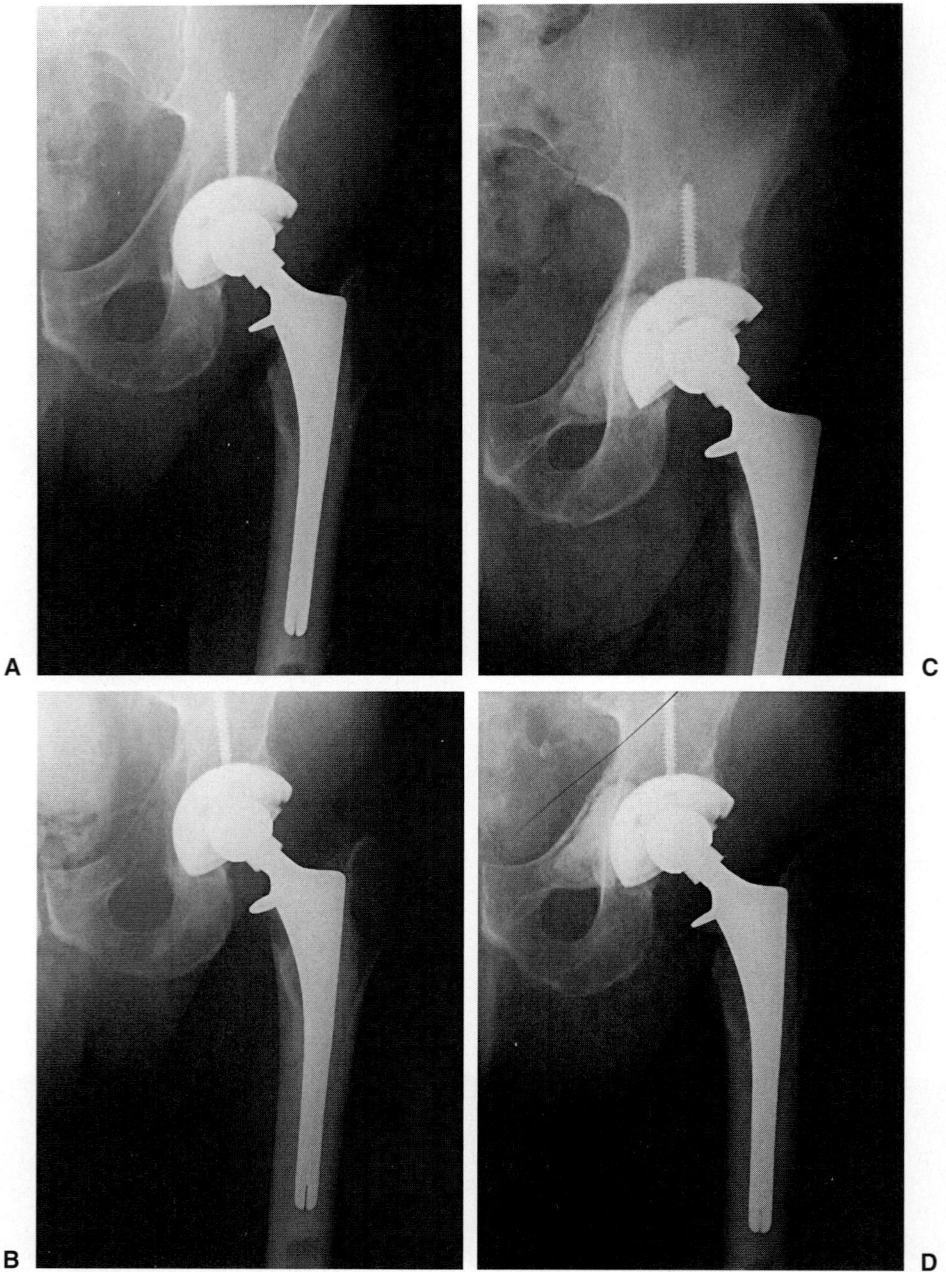

Figure 27.18. (**A**) Radiograph of a hybrid ingrowth cup/cemented stem total hip replacement. (**B**) Radiograph now shows medial peri-acetabular destructive disease as metastatic RRC deposit. (**C**) Cementation medially after open curettage followed 4 weeks later by 30Gy radiation. (**D**) 3 year follow-up with intact total hip replacement.

for the patient without major complications. A case report from Ireland of femoral neck osteotomy in a patient with extensive acetabular disease reported a palliative 8-month mobility and pain benefit before death.[76] I have experience with that technique as well as with acetabular reconstructions and would prefer the palliative quality benefit of reconstruction if complications can be avoided.

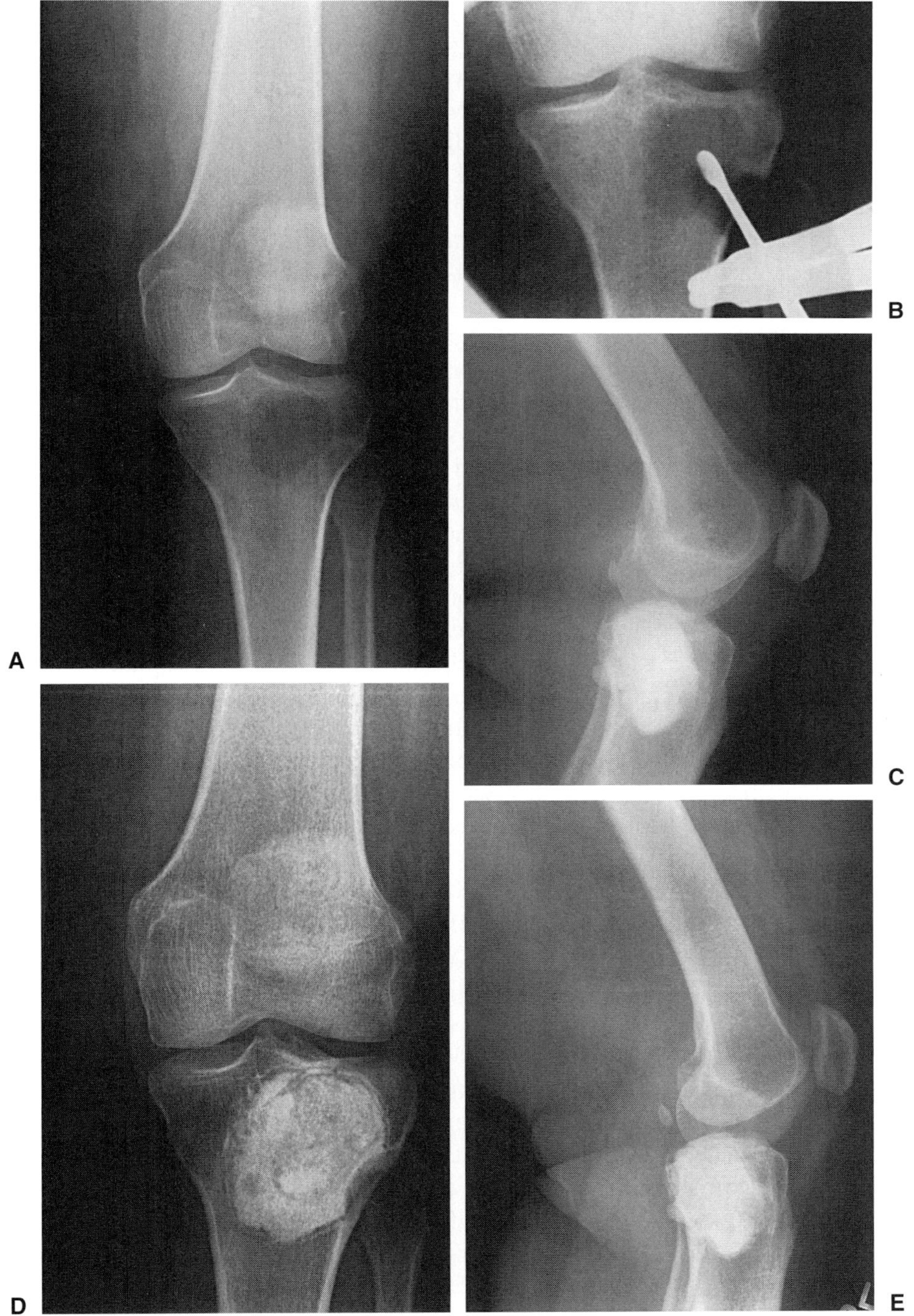

Figure 27.19. (A) Lytic destructive RCC disease in proximal tibia. (B) Intraoperative radiograph of curettage proximal tibia. (C) Cementation radiograph at 6 mo (treated postoperatively 30 Gy radiation). (D) and (E) Radiographs at 2½ years cementation proximal RCC lesion.

SOLITARY SKELETAL METASTASES

The presentation of a patient with RCC with a solitary metastasis can be a diagnostic dilemma for the treating team. From a review of the literature and anecdotal experience, a true isolated solitary metastasis is more likely to present remotely in time from the definitive management of the primary renal cell tumor. It is common for other skeletal lesions to eventually be identified over time. The bone scan is not a very sensitive tool in identifying occult skeletal metastases that have normal bone radiographs. Some of these lesions are truly semidormant within the intramedullary or metaphyseal bone and would only be demonstrated by MRI or possibly PET.

The approach of proceeding with an intralesional curettage procedure or a resection en bloc procedure for potential cure is a consideration for the orthopedic surgeon. The surgical team should agree that the identified lesion is truly an isolated metastatic deposit. Once the patient undergoes clinical staging and is declared disease-free on bone scans, CT scans of the chest, abdomen, and pelvis, and possibly MRI of the head, it is appropriate to consider a tumor en bloc resection for a cure. This implies that the tumor will not be spilled in the resected field, and a cuff of normal tissue will be obtained around the solitary metastatic deposition similar to that of an en bloc tumor resection for a primary bone sarcoma. This may require sacrifice of surrounding normal structures. This is in distinct contrast to an intralesional curettage procedure and filling holes with methylmethacrylate anticipating a much shorter longevity for the patient. For these en bloc "curative" procedures of the limb or pelvis, allografts or metallic modular components are used for reconstruction to improve function. Figure 27.20 illustrates an en bloc resection of the left pelvis for cure and reconstruction with a pelvic allograft/total hip replacement. There are a few series of isolated renal cell metastases treated for a cure, but most are incidental outcomes[77,78] or are identified cases from a series of orthopedic metastatic disease management cases. More often than not, the treatment team is disappointed to see new skeletal lesions appear within 2 years, clearly signifying that the original skeletal lesion was not a true isolated metastasis.

Middleton[79] in 1967 reported 5-year survival of 34% after removal of an apparent solitary metastasis in 59 cases. Talley et al.[80] reported in 1969 a significantly longer period of survival after resection when a solitary metastasis appeared more than 18 months after nephrectomy. Skinner[81] also observed that the success rate for treatment of solitary metastasis was greater when there was appearance of the solitary metastasis many months after nephrectomy (metachronous presentation). Tolia and Whitmore[82] identified 19 (3.2%) solitary metastasis in a group of 586 RCC patients of whom 174 had distant metastasis at diagnosis. Only 12 of the 19 involved bone. Seven of the 12 had amputations; two were ribs of the chest wall treated with resection. Ten of the 12 resections developed additional metastasis between 3 to 39 months. Tonga-onkar et al.[83] reviewed 19 patients with solitary metastatic RCC lesions in India. Nine involved bone. Four of the nine patients developed skeletal metastasis 13 to 72 months after nephrectomy. Three of these four patients were alive 2 to 4 years after radical surgery.

Baloch et al.[84] reviewed 25 patients with solitary RCC bony metastases. Each had a solitary deposit that was excised after nephrectomy. Ten presented at a mean of 3.5 years (range 1–7 years) after nephrectomy. Fifteen patients had a pathologic fracture; four had intramedullary nailing and another prophylactic nailing. Two patients had

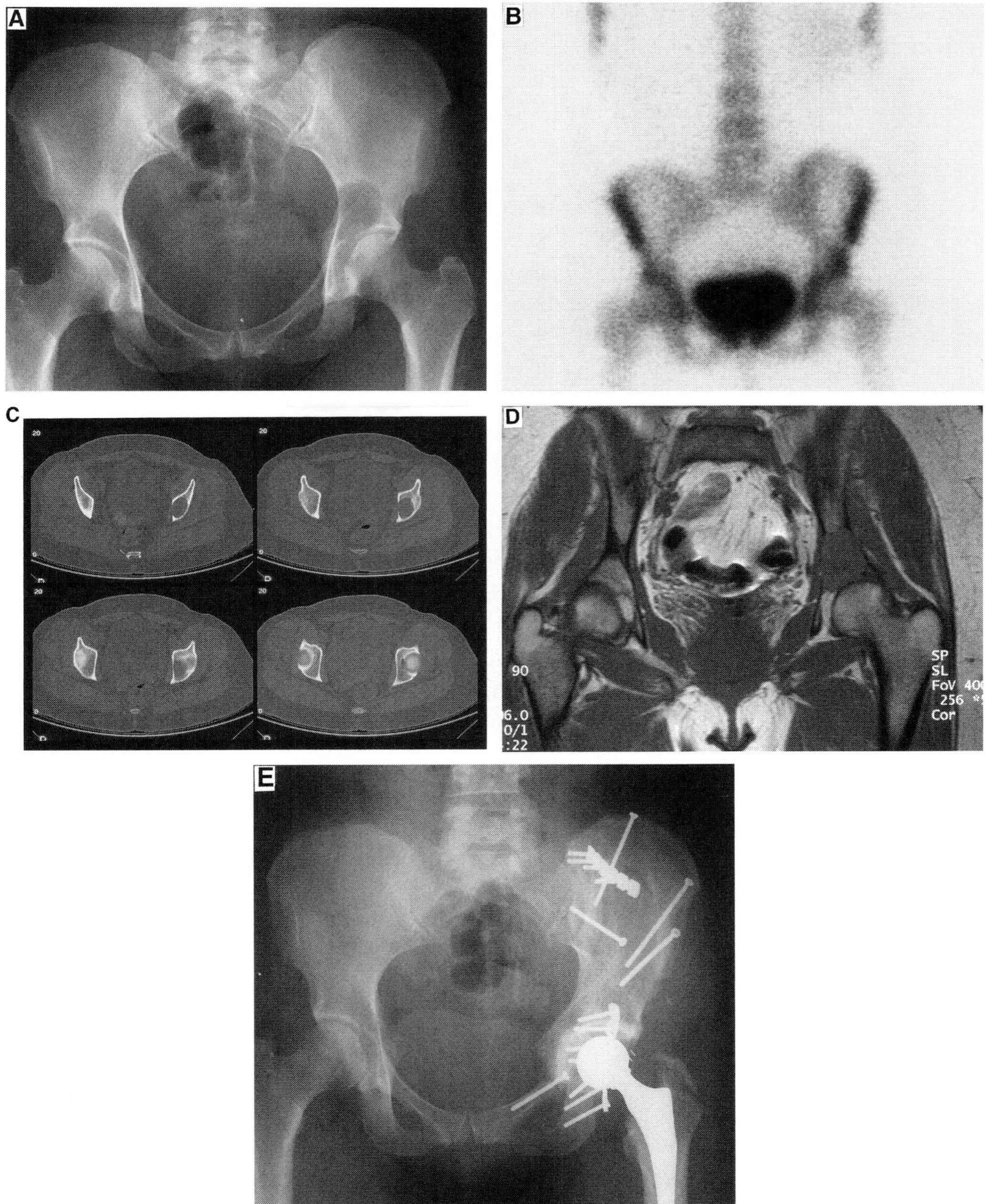

Figure 27.20. (**A**) A 48-year-old woman 2 years after nephrectomy, now with a solitary metastasis left supra-acetabular area. (**B**) Bone scan shows only some increased uptake above the acetabulum. (**C**) CT scan shows involvement into the acetabular fovea. (**D**) MRI shows the soft tissue mass that defines the intraosseous extent of the metastatic lesion. (**E**) Reconstruction with pelvic allograft and total hip replacement at 7 months with the patient remaining disease free.

radical resections without reconstruction, five had amputations, and 18 had excisions with endoprosthetic replacement. Survival from the time of the first metastasis was 88% at 1 year, 73% at 3 years, and 13% at 5 years. No patient who had a synchronous metastasis survived more than 5 years, but the overall survival rates between the late-appearing metastasis compared to the synchronous presentation showed no significant difference.

Jung et al.[85] reported in 2003 a review of 99 patients with osseous metastasis from RCC from a single institution identifying eight patients who had wide resection of a solitary osseous metastasis in combination with a nephrectomy. The disease-specific survival rate was 100% (mean 69 months, range 24–76). The authors recommended aggressive surgical resection with curative intent for patients with solitary bony metastasis. Overall survival rates for the entire patient population were 49% at 1 year, 26% at 3 years, and 14% at 5 years.

Fuchs et al.[86] identified the largest series of solitary bony metastasis from RCC. Thirteen patients had wide resection, 20 had local stabilization, and 27 had no surgical treatment. Survival was 83% at 1 year, 45% at 3 years, and 23% at 5 years. Patients with surgical treatment (wide or intralesional) survived longer than patients treated with adjuvant modalities alone. However, there was no survival advantage for patients who had a wide resection compared to intralesional resection or intramedullary stabilization alone. Three of the 20 stabilization patients had progression of disease causing further pain and decrease in function. The authors concluded that wide resection of metastatic lesions with reconstruction may be necessary for prevention of local disease progression causing further local complications and impairment of function with pain.

SPONTANEOUS REGRESSION OF SKELETAL METASTASES AFTER NEPHRECTOMY/INDUCED REGRESSION OF SKELETAL METASTASIS

Previous anecdotal reports of spontaneous regression of metastatic bone lesions after nephrectomy have been published.[87,88] The biology of this phenomenon remains unclear. However, the reports clearly suggest that a local process occurs at the metastatic site in which the bone destruction is actually reversed. Most of the reports are of lung metastases regressing and not bone. On rare occasion, regression can occur without prior nephrectomy. Chang et al.[89] reported spontaneous regression of lung and scalp metastases but only to have the patient die of brain metastasis. Nakajima et al.[90] reported on a needle biopsy–proven sternal lesion, only to have late documentation of complete spontaneous regression on delayed open treatment.

There are times when a destructive metastatic lesion of bone can be induced to ossify with use of radiation therapy, bisphosphonates, immunotherapy and adjuvant drug therapy. Although this is not "spontaneous" regression, it is remarkable how a huge destructive bone lesion with a large soft tissue mass can be driven to ossify. Figure 27.21 shows a large periacetabular metastatic renal cell lesion posterior column, wall, and dome. Initial radiation therapy to 30 Gy, immunotherapy, and bisphosphonates caused ossification over a 6-month period of time. Although the patient has protrusio (inward migration of the head into the socket) of the femoral head, she has tolerated

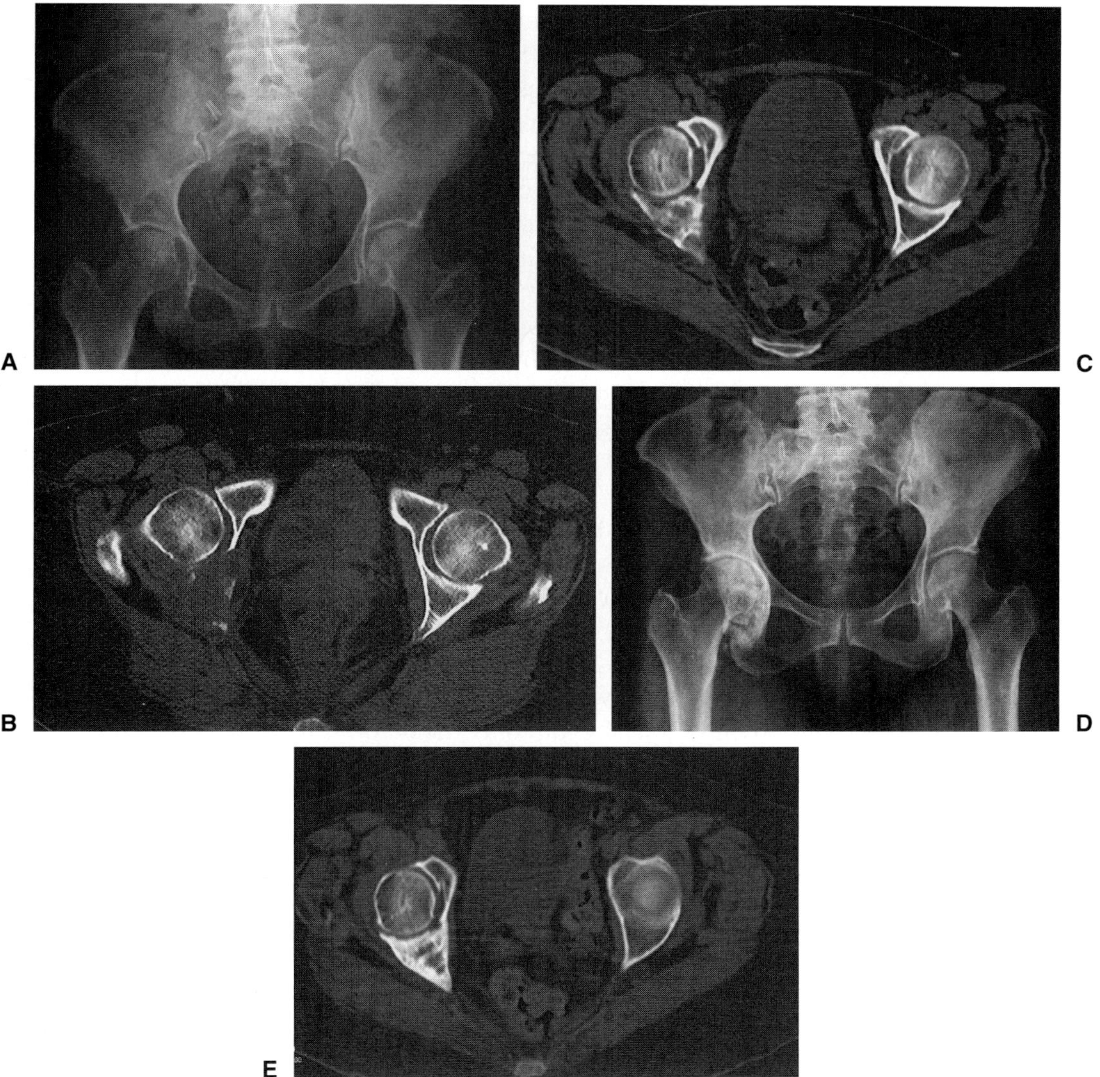

Figure 27.21. (A) Radiograph of pelvis with right sided peri-acetabular destructive RCC lesion. (B) (C) CT peri-acetabular destructive RCC lesion. (D) (E) X-ray and CT of hip 5 year follow-up after treatment with chemotherapy, radiation therapy and bisphosphonates.

the deformity with minimal reduction in hip motion and ambulates appliance-free over the past 4 years since the presentation of this periacetabular lesion.

OUTCOME OF PATIENTS PRESENTING WITH RENAL CELL CARCINOMA/INCIDENCE OF BONE DISEASE

Postoperatively after nephrectomy, surveillance for RCC often involves an abdominal CT and chest radiographs every 3 to 6 months for 3 years, and a 6- to 12-month frequency thereafter. Bone scans and brain scans usually are obtained after symptoms have occurred. Frank et al.[91] reviewed the Mayo Clinic experience following 1864 nonmetastatic RCC patients from 1970 to 2000. Lung lesions 300 (16%), bone lesions

134 (7%), and brain lesions 81 (4%) eventually occurred in this cohort of patients. Recurrent abdominal tumor became evident in 185 (10%). Bone lesions appeared at a mean of 2.9 years (median 1.5 years) after nephrectomy in these previously disease-free individuals. Risk factors for bone lesions increased with each increasing primary tumor stage T1b and above, positive regional lymph nodes, tumor size greater than 10 cm, nuclear grade 3 to 4, tumor necrosis, and sarcomatoid features. Metastases to the bone presented as symptomatic lesions in 98% of the patients. Routine scanning was not done, with the review clearly showing physical exam to be adequate for skeletal surveillance most of the time.

Patients with clear-cell RCC have worse outcomes compared to those with papillary or chromophobe RCC, even when adjusted by grade and stage.[92–94]

Han et al.[95] demonstrated in a retrospective review of 434 patients that patients with only one metastatic organ site fared significantly better than patients who had evidence of disease in multiple organs. Survival of patients with isolated metastatic lung disease was similar to that of a patient whose metastatic disease was limited to bone (median survival after presentation: 27 months). Patients with multiple organ metastases had a median survival of 11 months. The response rate to immunotherapy after nephrectomy was 44% (lung involvement only), 20% (bone involvement only), and 14% (multiple organ involvement). Nodal disease was a well-established predictor of poor prognosis.[96]

Schips et al.[97] retrospectively reviewed the Austrian experience of 683 patients and categorized them with having clinical symptoms (hematuria, flank pain, weight loss, bone pain, and anemia) of cancer at the time of presentation and those without symptoms. Of these patients, 141 (20.6%) presented with symptoms. The cancer 5-year overall survival rate and progression-free rate for these initially symptomatic patients were 60% and 55%, respectively, and for the symptom-free patients 82% and 79%. Renal tumors larger than 5 cm were significantly more likely to cause symptoms. Patients presenting with symptoms had a 1.8 greater risk of dying of cancer compared to those without symptoms.

SURVIVAL AFTER DIAGNOSIS OF METASTATIC DISEASE TO THE SKELETON

Orthopedic surgical intervention of skeletal metastases not only provides improvement in function and increases the time before significant disability, but also provides pain relief. Aggressive surgical management may also improve the quality of life and provide improved longevity.

An earlier illustration was given concerning the misperception of survivorship of patients with renal cell metastases of the skeleton. With appropriate treatment, a number of these patients will do well for an extended period of time. Skinner et al.[81] reported an 8% five-year and 7% ten-year survival rate in a 1971 published series. Thompson et al.[98] in 1975 reported survival rates of 21.5% at 1 year, 9% at 2 years, and 0% at 5 years in a cohort of 65 patients. DeKernion et al.[99] in 1978 reported survival rates of 42% at 1 year and 13% at 5 years. Maldazys and DeKernion[100] in 1986 reported a 48% one-year survival and 9% five-year survival in a series of 181 cases. Tobisu et al.[101] in

1989 presented a group of patients with bony metastases, of whom 77% were alive 1 year after presentation with bone involvement, 45% at 5 years, and 0% at 10 years. Smith et al.[102] in 1992 reviewed 14 patients with hypernephromas and skeletal metastases. Survivorship after skeletal metastasis at 1 year was 58% with a range from 7 to 64 months.

The review of management of 38 renal cell patients with metastases to bone from the Massachusetts General Hospital (MGH) provides insight into a significant change in philosophy concerning the management of these patients.[103] Many urologists and orthopedists in the past considered RCC patients with metastasis to bone as having a terrible prognosis, suggesting that management of bone lesions should be only palliative. However, survival for the entire group aggressively managed surgically at MGH was 90% at 6 months, 84% at 12 months, 55% at 5 years, and 39% at 10 years. Initial presentation without initial bony metastases, a long disease-free period between nephrectomy and first metastases, appendicular rather than axial skeletal location, and solitary presenting metastases were correlated with better long-term survival.

When metastatic lesions are large and encompass a significant amount of structural bone loss, operative procedures directed at resection of the metastatic deposit with sacrifice of the bone segment often yields better long-term results when compared to intralesional procedures involving internal fixation with methylmethacrylate. Incidence of complications, especially in tumors with a poor response to radiotherapy, was lower after endoprosthetic implantation than after operations involving osteosynthesis in two published retrospective reviews.[64,104] Figures 27.22 and 27.23 illustrate significant resections with reconstructions being accomplished for extensive local bone disease.

Les et al.[105] retrospectively reviewed 78 patients from three institutions with osseous RCC. Forty-one (53%) of the patients were treated by intralesional methods and internal fixation. Seventeen had significant local progression causing failure of the stabilization and required 14 further procedures including nine wide resections with reconstruction, three amputations, and two mass excisions. The second group consisted of 37 (47%) patients, who underwent wide resection with either wide margins or marginal margins with or without reconstruction. Only one further operative intervention for local bony progression in this group was needed. The Kaplan-Meier curves revealed that solitary metastases, longer disease-free interval from initial tumor diagnosis to the development of metastasis, and surgical resection in contrast to intralesional procedures were associated with a significantly improved survival. Based on the data, the authors recommended that resection surgery should be considered for renal cell skeletal metastasis when possible in order to lessen the risk of further operations for local progression. Even though the patients with intralesional procedures had shorter survival, these patients who underwent intralesional orthopedic surgery had a high risk of reoperation.

Dürr et al.[106] reported a retrospective analysis of 45 patients with metastatic renal cell of bone surgically managed, of whom 49% survived 1 year, 39% survived 2 years, and 15% survived 5 years postoperatively. Kollender et al.[107] retrospectively reviewed their combined multiinstitutional experience of surgical management of skeletal lesions in 45 patients over a 17-year period (1980–1997). Wide excision, consisting of an en bloc resection with a cuff of normal tissue when possible, was accomplished when bone

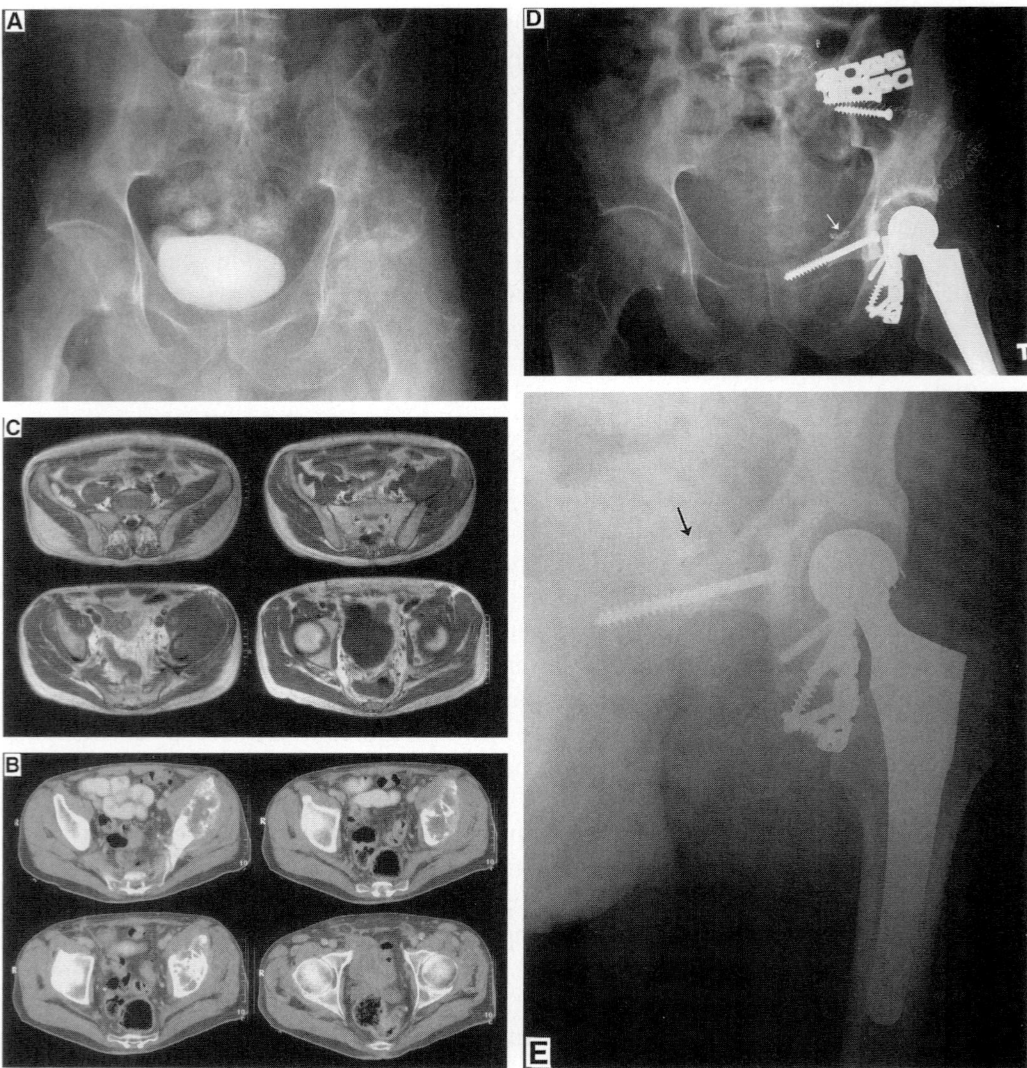

Figure 27.22. (A) A 64-year-old man with a huge painful destructive renal cell lesion left pelvis. He has had other osseous sites, but has been a good responder to therapy. (B) CT scan showing a destructive pelvic lesion that involves the dome of the hip joint. (C) Large soft tissue mass with involvement of the hip joint being quite evident on MRI. (D) Postoperative radiograph. Arrows point to embolization coils placed preoperatively. (E) Radiograph at 14 months with patient ambulatory with a cane, but significant limp secondary to loss of gluteus medius from resection of involved tumor mass.

destruction was extensive or a solitary metastasis. Cases with marginal or intralesional excision with adjunct use of liquid nitrogen cryosurgery and methylmethacrylate achieved local long-term tumor control in nine of 12 patients. Selective arterial embolization was accomplished in all cases except for two amputations. The most common sites were the pelvis, proximal femur, and proximal humerus. In this selected group of patients, 49% lived more than 2 years after surgery and 73% who presented with a local curettage or limited excision incurred a problem with late local recurrence.

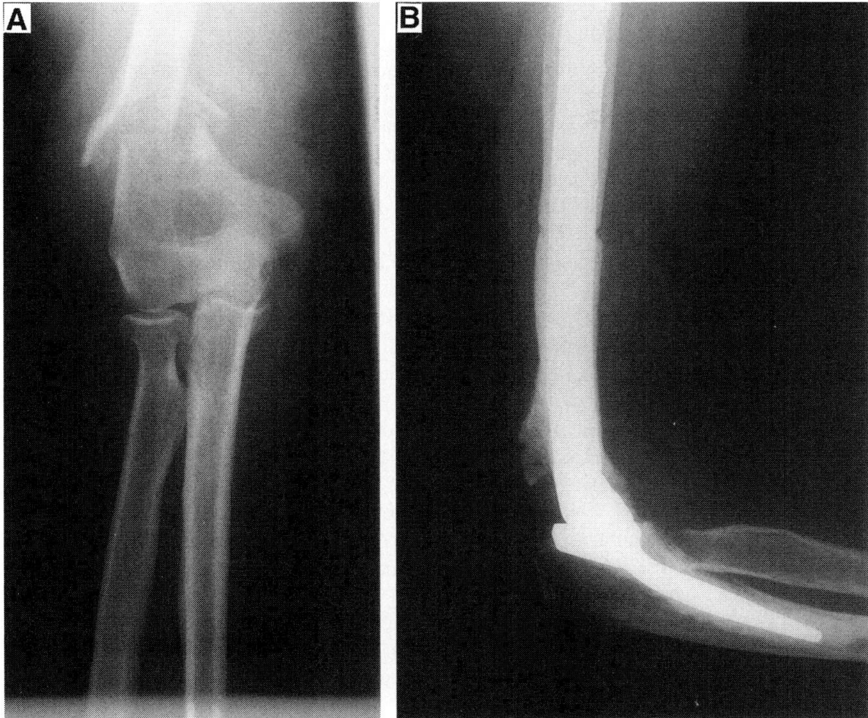

Figure 27.23. (A) Fracture of distal humerus in 50-year-old woman. Patient was found to have a hypernephroma and underwent nephrectomy. (B) Management of this solitary lesion was resection with a long stem total elbow replacement over an allograft. She developed other osseous lesions after 2 years.

CONCLUSION

The management of recognized metastatic osseous lesions of RCC requires a team approach involving a urologist, medical oncologist, radiation therapist, and orthopedic surgeon. Appropriate aggressive approaches can improve patient quality of life and longevity. On occasion, treatment of the solitary osseous metastatic lesion as a primary tumor with an en bloc resection may yield long-term survival or at least improve longer quality of life survivorship. Management of osseous lesions warrants the concept of using rods and cement in contrast to plates and screws to lessen early fracture fixation failure. In many instances, resection of the poor quality bone with subsequent replacement using limb salvage techniques will yield improvement in quality of life and a much reduced rate of failure of the construct. Prevention of bone loss and intervention of curettage/cementing, radiation therapy, and bisphosphonates may provide some degree of longevity of bone structure near joint regions. Early recognition of spine lesions with appropriate intervention will enhance overall function and reduce the incidence of permanent neurologic functional loss. The goals are to improve function and to relieve pain using current orthopedic surgical techniques. Application of orthopedic surgical oncology techniques by specially trained surgeons with expertise and experience dealing with these complex problems provides improved function, a better quality of life, and increased longevity for these patients.

REFERENCES

1. Quinn JM, Matsumara W, Tarin D, et al. Cellular and hormonal mechanisms associated with malignant bone resorption. Lab Invest 1994;71:465–471.
2. Athanasou NA. The role of tumor-associated macrophages in metastasis-associated osteolysis. In: Singh G, Orr W, eds. Bone Metastasis and Molecular Mechanisms. New York: Kluwer, 2004:87–108.
3. Kostnuik PJ. OPG, RANK AND RANKL in bone metastasis and cancer-associated osteolysis. In: Singh G, Orr W, eds. Bone Metastasis and Molecular Mechanisms. New York: Kluwer, 2004:211–240.
4. Mundy G. Metastasis to bone causes, consequences and therapeutic opportunities. Nature Rev 2002;2:584–593.
5. Choong PFM. The molecular basis of skeletal metastases. Clin Orthop 2003;451S:S19–S31.
6. Lipton A, Columbo-Berra A, Bukowski RM, et al. Skeletal complications in patients with bone metastases from renal cell carcinoma and therapeutic benefits of zolendronic acid. Clin Cancer Res 2004;10:6397s–6403s.
7. Lipton A, Zheng M, Seaman E. Zoledronic acid delays the onset of skeletal-related events and progression of skeletal disease in patients with advanced renal cell carcinoma. Cancer 2003;98:962–969.
8. MacKenzie M, Major P. The role of bisphosphonates in bone metastasis. In: Singh G, Orr W, eds. Bone Metastasis and Molecular Mechanisms. New York: Kluwer, 2004:277–301.
9. Tanni N, Jonasch E, Pagliaro LC, et al. Pilot trial of bone-targeted therapy with zoledronate, thalidomide and interferon-gamma for metastatic renal cell carcinoma. Cancer 2006;197:497–505.
10. Weber KL, Doucet M, Price JE. Renal cell carcinoma bone metastasis: Epidermal growth factor receptor targeting. Clin Orthop 2003;425S:S86–S94.
11. Cenni E, Perut F, Granchi D, et al. Inhibition of angiogenesis by FGF-2 blockade. Anticancer Res 2007;21:315–319.
12. Fusetti C, Kurzen P, Bonaccio M, Büchler U, Nagy L. Hand metastasis in renal cell carcinoma. Urology 2003;62:141.
13. Ghert MA, Harrelson JM, Scully SP. Solitary renal cell carcinoma metastasis to the hand: the need for wide excision or amputation. J Hand Surg 2001;26A:156–160.
14. Healey JH, Turnbull ADM, Miedema B, Lane JM. A study of twenty-nine patients with osseous involvement of the hands and feet. J Bone Joint Surg 1986;68A(5):743–746.
15. Tolo ET, Coonet WP, Wenger DE. Renal cell carcinoma with metastasis to the triquetrum: case report. J Hand Surg (Am) 2002;27:876–881.
16. Fusetti C, Kurzen P, Bonaccio M, et al. Hand Metastasis in renal cell carcinoma. Urology 2003;62:141.
17. Perdona S, Autorino R, Gallo L, et al. Renal cell carcinoma with solitary toe metastasis. Int J Urology 2005;12:4001–404.
18. Liu PT, Conley CR, Callstrom MR. Sclerotic bone metastases from sarcomatoid renal cell carcinoma. Skel Radiol 1999;28:590–593.
19. Bos SD, Piers DA, Mensink HJA. Routine bone scan and serum alkaline phosphatase for staging in patients with renal cell carcinoma is not cost-effective. Eur J Cancer 1995;31A:2422.
20. Kriteman L, Sanders WH. Normal alkaline phosphatase levels in patients with bone metastasis due to renal cell carcinoma. Urology 1998;51:397–399.
21. Henriksson C, Haraldsson G, Aldenborg F, et al. Skeletal metastases in 102 patients evaluated before surgery for renal cell carcinoma. Scand J Urol Nephrol 1992;26:363–366.
22. Seaman E, Goluboff ET, Ross S, Sawczuk IS. Association of radionuclide bone scan and serum alkaline phosphatase in patients with metastatic renal cell carcinoma. Urology 1996;48:692–695.
23. Sandock DS, Sefter AD, Resnick MI. A new protocol for follow up of renal cell carcinoma based on pathologic stage. J Urol 1995;154(1):28–31.
24. Staudenherz A, Steiner B, Puig S, et al. Is there a diagnostic role for bone scanning of patients with a high pretest probability for metastatic renal cell carcinoma? Cancer 1999;85:153–155.
25. Koga S, Tsuda S, Nishikido M, Ogawa Y, et al. The diagnostic value of bone scan in patients with renal cell carcinoma. J Urol 2001;166:2126–2128.
26. Shvarts O, Lam JS, Kim HL, et al. Eastern Cooperative Oncology Group performance status predicts bone metastasis in patients presenting with renal cell carcinoma: implications for preoperative bone scans. J Urol 2004;172:867–870.

27. Nemoto R, Nakamura I, Nishijima Y, et al. Serum pyridinoline cross-links as marker of tumor–bone resorption. Br J Urol 1997;80:274–280.
28. Jung K, Lein M, Ringsdorf M, et al. Diagnostic and prognostic validity of serum bone turnover markers in metastatic renal cell carcinoma. J Urol 2006;176:1326–1331.
29. Shukla SK, Limouris GS, Cusumano R, et al. Renal cell carcinoma detection and systemic therapy with tumour-affinity gallium 67 and yttrium-90 citrate solutions. Anticancer Res 1997;17:1713–1718.
30. Choi JA, Lee KH, Jun WS, et al. Osseous metastasis from renal cell carcinoma: "flow-void" sign at MRI imagining. Radiology 2003;228:629–634.
31. Wu HC, Yen RF, Shen YY. Whole body 18 F-2–deoxyglucose positron emission tomography and technetium -99m methylene diphosphate bone scan to detect bone metastases in patients with renal cell carcinomas: a preliminary report. J Cancer Res Clin Oncol 2002;128:503–506.
32. Peterson JJ, Kransdorf MJ, O'Connor MI. Diagnosis of occult bone metastasis: positron emission tomography. Clin Orthop 2003;415S:S120–S128.
33. Mink J. Percutaneous bone biopsy in the patient with known or suspected osseous metastasis. Radiology 1986;161:191–194.
34. Carrascoc H, Wallace S, Richli WR. Percutaneous skeletal biopsy. Cardiovasc Intervent Radiology 1991;14(1):69–72.
35. Ward WG, Savage G, Boles CA, Kilpatrick SE. Fine-needle aspiration biopsy of sarcomas and related tumors. Cancer Control 2001;8:232–238.
36. Clohisy DR, Mantyh PW. Bone cancer pain. Clin Orthop 2003;415S:S279–S288.
37. Clohisy DR, Mantyh PW. Bone cancer pain. Cancer 2003;97S:S866–S873.
38. DiBiase SJ, Valicent RK, Schultz D, et al. Palliative irradiation for focally symptomatic metastatic renal cell carcinoma: support of dose escalation based on a biologic model. J Urol 1997;158: 746–749.
39. Seitz W, Karcher KH, Binder W. Radiotherapy of metastatic renal cell carcinoma. Semin Surg Oncol 1988;4:100–102.
40. Brinkman OA, Bruns F, Gosheger G, et al. Treatment of bone metastases and local recurrence from renal cell carcinoma with immunochemotherapy and radiation. World J Urol 2005;23: 185–190.
41. Lee J, Hodgson D, Chow E, et al. A phase II trial of palliative radiotherapy for metastatic renal cell carcinoma. Cancer 2005;104:1897–1900.
42. Murphy MJ, Chang S, Gibbs I, et al. Image-guided radiosurgery in treatment of spinal metastasis. Neurosurg Focus 2001;11:6.
43. Gerszten PC, Burton SA, Ozhasoglu C, et al. Stereotactic radiosurgery for spinal metastases from renal cell carcinoma-single fraction. J Neurosurg Spine 2005;3:288–295.
44. Schaefer O, Lohrmann C, Markmiller M, et al. Technical innovation: Combined treatment of spinal metastasis with radiofrequency heat ablation and vertebroplasty. AJR 2003;180:1075–1077.
45. Callstrom MR, Charboneau JW. Percutaneous ablation: safe effective treatment of bone tumors. Oncology (Huntington) 2005;19:22–26.
46. Toyata N, Naito A, Kakizana H, et al. Radiofrequency ablation therapy combined with cementoplasty for painful bone metastases: initial experience. CV Intervent Radiol 2005;28:578–583.
47. Campbell J, Rosenthal DI, Raskin KA, et al. Use of arterial tourniquet to achieve complete radiofrequency ablation of a renal cell metastasis. J Vasc Intervent Radiol 2006;17:1051–1055.
48. Ward WG, Holsenback BA, Dorey FJ, et al. Metastatic disease of the femur: surgical treatment. Clin Orthop 2003;514S:S230–S244.
49. Harrington KD. New trends in the management of lower extremity metastases. Clin Orthop 1982;169:53–61.
50. Mirels H. Metastatic disease in long bones: A proposed scoring system for diagnosing impending pathologic fractures. Clin Orthop 1989;249:256–264.
51. Damron TA, Morgan H, Prakash BS, et al. Metastatic disease of long bones: Critical evaluation of Mirels' rating system for impending pathologic fractures. Clin Orthop 2003;415S:S201–S207.
52. Olerud C, Jonsson B. Surgical palliation of symptomatic spinal metastases. Acta Orthop Scand 1996;67:513–522.
53. Giehl JP, Kluba T. Metastatic spine disease in renal cell carcinoma: indications and results of surgery. Anticancer Res 1999;19:1619–1623.
54. Jackson RJ, Loh SC, Gokaslan ZL. Metastatic renal cell carcinoma of the spine: surgical treatment and results. J Neurosurg 2001;94:18–24.

55. Ulmar B, Naumann U, Catalkaya S, et al. Prognosis scores of Tokuhashi and Tomita for patients with spinal metastases of renal cell. Ann Surg Oncol 2007;14:998–1004.
56. Roscoe M, McBloom R, St Louis E, et al. Preoperative embolization in treatment of osseous metastasis from renal cell carcinoma. Clin Orthop 1989;238:302–307.
57. Olerud C, Jonsson H, Lofberg A, et al. Embolization of spinal metastases reduces preoperative bone loss. 21 patients operated on for renal cell carcinoma. Acta Orthop Scand 1993;64:9–12.
58. Miller D, Haines G, Juliano P, Ghosh B. Preoperative embolization of osseous metastases from hypervascular cancers. J Surg Oncol 1995;60:133–134.
59. Smith TP, Gray L, Weinstein JN, Richardson WJ, Payne CS. Preoperative transarterial embolization of spinal column neoplasms. J Vasc Intervent Radiol 1995;6:863–869.
60. Sun S, Lang EV. Bone metastases from renal cell carcinoma: Preoperative embolization. J Vasc Intervent Radiol 1998;9:263–269.
61. Chatziioannou A, Johnson M, Pnematicos S, et al. Preoperative embolization of bone metastases from renal cell carcinoma. Eur Radiol 2000;10:593–596.
62. Manke C, Bretschneider T, Lenhart M, et al. Spinal metastases from renal cell carcinoma: effect on preoperative particle embolization on intraoperative blood loss. Am J Neurol Radiol 2001;22:997–1003.
63. Schirmer CM, Malek AM, Kwan ES, et al. Preoperative embolization of hypervascular spinal metastasis using direct injection with n-butyl cyanoacrylate: technical case report. Neurosurgery 2006;59:e431–432.
64. Chan D, Carter SR, Grimer RJ, et al. Endoprosthetic replacement for bony metastases. Ann R Coll Surg Engl 1992;74:13–28.
65. Wedin R, Bauer HC, Wersall P. Failures after operations for skeletal metastatic lesions of long bones. Clin Orthop 1999;358:128–139.
66. Eckardt JJ, Kabo MJ, Kelly CM, et al. Endoprosthetic reconstruction for bone metastases. Clin Orthop 2003;415S:S254–S262.
67. Orsini EC, Byrick RJ, Mullen JBM, et al. Cardiopulmonary function and pulmonary microemboli during arthroplasty using cemented or non-cemented components. J Bone Joint Surg 1987;69:822–831.
68. Lafont ND, Kostucki WM, Marchand PH, Michaux MN, Boogaerts JG. Embolism detected by trans-esophageal echocardiography during hip arthroplasty. Can J Anaesth 1994;41:850–853.
69. Lairmore JR, Heiner J, Wood K. Coma from fat embolism syndrome after hemiarthroplasty of the hip for metastatic disease. Am J Orthop 2000;29:308–311.
70. Fallon KM, Fuller JG, Morley-Forster P. Fat embolism and fatal cardiac arrest during hip arthroplasty with methylmethacrylate. Can J Anesth 2001;48:626–629.
71. Choong PFM. Cardiopulmonary complications of intramedullary fixation of long bone metastasis. Clin Orthop 2003;415S:S245–S253.
72. Ereth MH, Weber JG, Abel MD, et al. Cemented versus noncemented total hip arthroplasty-embolism, hemodynamics, and intrapulmonary shunting. Mayo Clin Proc 1992;67:1066–1074.
73. Wheelwright EF, Byrick RJ, Wigglesworth DF, et al. Hypotension during cemented arthroplasty. Relationship to cardiac output and fat embolism. J Bone Joint Surg Br 1993;75:715–723.
74. Murphy P, Edelist G, Byrick RJ, Kay JC, Mullen JB. Relationship of fat embolism to haemodynamic and echocardiographic changes during cemented arthroplasty. Can J Anaesth 1997;44:1293–1300.
75. Wunder J, Ferguson P, Griffin A, et al. Acetabular metastasis: planning for reconstruction and review of results. Clin Orthop 2003;415S:S187–197.
76. Khan F, Masterson E. Femoral neck osteotomy: an alternative to hip replacement in acetabular metastatic disease. J Arthroplasty 2003;18:221–223.
77. Tabuenca Dumortier J, Ortiz Cruz E, Olivas Olivas J. Total cleidectomy for a solitary metastasis of the clavicle. Acta Orthop Belg 2001;67:178–181.
78. Rolf O, Gohlke F. Endoprosthetic elbow replacement in patient with solitary metastasis from renal cell carcinoma. J Shoulder Elbow Surg 2004;13:656–663.
79. Middleton RG. Surgery for metastatic renal cell carcinoma. J Urol 1967;97:973–977.
80. Talley RW, Moorhead EL, Tucker WG, et al. Treatment of metastatic hypernephroma. JAMA 1969;207:322–328.
81. Skinner DG, Colvin RB, Vermillion CD, Pfister RC, Leadbetter WF. Diagnosis and management of renal cell carcinoma: clinical and pathological study of 309 cases. Cancer 1971;28:1165–1171.
82. Tolia BM, Whitmore WF. Solitary metastasis from renal cell carcinoma. J Urol 1975;114:836–838.

83. Tongaonkar HB, Kulkarni JN, Kamat MR. Solitary metastases from renal cell carcinoma: a review. J Surg Oncol 1992;49:45–48.

84. Baloch KG, Grimer RJ, Carter SR, Tillman RM. Radical surgery for the solitary bony metastasis from renal-cell carcinoma. J Bone Joint Surg [BR] 2000;82B:62–67.

85. Jung ST, Ghert MA, Harrelson JM, et al. Treatment of osseous metastases in patients with renal cell carcinoma. Clin Orthop 2003;409:223–231.

86. Fuchs B, Trousdale RT, Rock MG. Solitary bony metastasis from renal cell carcinoma. Clin Orthop 2005;431:187–192.

87. Kerbl K, Pauer W. Spontaneous regression of osseous metastasis in renal cell carcinoma. Aust NZ J Surg 1993;63:901–903.

88. Lokich J. Spontaneous regression of metastatic renal cell: case report and literature review. Am J Clin Oncol 1997;20:416–418.

89. Chang KC, Chan KL, Lam CW. Spontaneous regression of renal cell carcinoma metastases. HKMJ 1999;5:72–75.

90. Nakajima T, Suzuki M, Ando S, et al. Spontaneous regression of bone metastasis from renal cell carcinoma: case report. BMC Cancer 2006;6:11.

91. Frank I, Blute ML, Cheville JC, et al. A multifactorial postoperative surveillance model for patients with surgically treated clear cell renal cell carcinoma. J Urol 2003;170:2225–2232.

92. Mai KT, Landry DC, Robertson SJ, et al. A comparative study of metastatic renal cell carcinoma with correlation to subtype and primary tumor. Pathol Res Pract 2001;197:671–675.

93. Amin MB, Tamboli P, Javidan J, et al. Prognostic impact of histologic subtyping of adult renal epithelial neoplasms: an experience of 405 cases. Am J Surg Pathol 2002;26:281–291.

94. Cheville JC, Lohse CM, Zincke H, Weaver AL, Blute ML. Comparisons of outcome and prognostic features among histologic subtypes of renal cell carcinoma. Am J Surg Pathol 2003;27:612–624.

95. Han KR, Pantuck AJ, Bui MH. Number of metastatic sites rather than location dictates overall survival of patients with node-negative metastatic renal cell carcinoma. J Urol 2003;61:314–319.

96. Pantuck AJ, Zisman A, Chao D, et al. Regional lymph-adenopathy during cytoreductive nephrectomy predicts IL-2 failure in patients with metastatic renal cell carcinoma. Proc ASCO 2001;20:172A.

97. Schips L, Lipsky K, Zigeuner R, et al. Impact of tumor-associated symptoms on the prognosis of patients with renal cell carcinoma: A single-center experience of 683 patients. Urology 2003;62:1024–1028.

98. Thompson IM, Shannon H, Ross J, Montie J. An analysis of factors affecting survival of 150 patients with renal cell carcinoma. J Urol 1975;114:694–696.

99. Dekernion JB, Ramming KP, Smith RB. The natural history of metastatic renal cell carcinoma: a computer analysis. J Urol 1978;120:148–152.

100. Maldazys JD, Dekernion JB. Prognostic factors in metastatic renal carcinoma. J Urol 1986;136:376–379.

101. Tobisu K, Kakizoe T, Takai K, Tanaka Y. Prognosis in renal cell carcinoma: Analysis of clinical course following nephrectomy. Jpn J Clin Ocol 1989;19:142–148.

102. Smith E, Kursh E, Makley J, Resnick M. Treatment of osseous metastases secondary to renal cell carcinoma. J Urol 1992;184:784–787.

103. Althausen P, Althausen A, Jennings CL, Mankin HJ. Prognostic factors and surgical treatment of osseous metastases secondary to renal cell carcinoma. Cancer 1997;80:1103–1109.

104. Helwig V. Multiple operations in patients with bony metastases and a prolonged course of disease. Eur J Surg Oncol 1997;23:59–63.

105. Les KA, Nicholas RW, Rougraff B, et al. Local progression after operative treatment of metastatic kidney cancer. Clin Orthop 2001;390:206–211.

106. Dürr HR, Maier M, Pfahler M, et al. Surgical treatment of osseous metastases in patients with renal cell carcinoma. Clin Orthop 1999;367(106):283–290.

107. Kollender Y, Bickels J, Price WM, et al. Metastatic renal cell carcinoma of bone: indications and technique of surgical intervention. J Urol 2000;164:1505–1508.

28 Renal Cell Carcinoma Metastatic to the Pancreas: *Clinical and Therapeutic Aspects*

Ahmed Al-Hazzouri, Brian R. Herts, and Ronald M. Bukowski

KEYWORDS

> RENAL CELL CARCINOMA
> PANCREAS
> METASTASES

ABSTRACT

Metastatic RCC involving the pancreas is uncommon. In selected patients however, it can produce with a variety of findings and symptoms, including diabetes mellitus and pancreatic exocrine insufficiency. CT scan remains the most common modality used for diagnosis of this complication. Surgical resection of isolated pancreatic metastases from renal cell carcinoma may result in prolonged survival for highly selected patients. Even in patients with unresectable pancreatic metastases, the median survival may be prolonged with indolent disease present. Although the patient numbers are relatively small, data suggest that development of pancreatic metastases occurs only in clear cell RCC, may not impact negatively on survival, and is associated with an indolent disease growth pattern and widespread metastatic disease. These factors may influence the ultimate choice of therapy, suggesting that systemic approach should be considered in most instances.

In previous publications the pancreas is an uncommon site of involvement by metastatic renal cell carcinoma (RCC).[1,2] Generally, these lesions are asymptomatic, detected on routine imaging surveillance, but in some patients they can produce a variety of symptoms including weight loss and gastrointestinal bleeding. Surgical resection of pancreatic metastases in the group of patients with solitary lesions has been the focus of most published reports,[3–5] and may be associated with prolonged survival in selected individuals.[6,7] In patients with multiple metastatic sites, therapeutic approaches have included hormonal therapy, chemotherapy, and a variety of immunotherapeutic approaches such as interferon-α (IFN-α) or interleukin-2 (IL-2). Evidence

From: *Clinical Management of Renal Tumors*
Edited by: R.M. Bukowski and A.C. Novick © Humana Press Inc., Totowa, NJ

of antitumor efficacy was seldom if ever noted. Recently, approaches targeting growth factors and their receptors have been employed in clear-cell RCC. Clinically, patients with RCC pancreatic metastases often have long disease-free intervals, indolent disease, and prolonged survival. In view of the rarity of pancreatic metastases, and the increasing recognition of this type of involvement in patients with RCC, a review of individuals with pancreatic metastases from this tumor was undertaken, utilizing both the medical literature and the renal carcinoma data base of patients treated at the Cleveland Clinic for advanced disease. Twenty-nine patients treated in institutional review board (IRB)-approved clinical trials between 1987 and 2004 were identified. Patients with synchronous pancreatic involvement at the time of initial diagnosis or who developed metachronous pancreatic metastases were selected. For comparative purposes, the Cleveland Clinic Foundation (CCF) database of previously untreated patients with metastatic RCC without pancreatic involvement was utilized.

INCIDENCE

In patients with malignancy, development of metastatic disease in the pancreas is uncommon.[1,2] In patients with metastatic RCC, autopsy results have demonstrated pancreatic involvement in only 1.3% to 1.9% RCC.[8] In this setting, metastases are usually multifocal,[1] and represent diffuse carcinomatosis with widespread organ involvement. The interval between nephrectomy and development of pancreatic metastases is often prolonged, with reported disease-free intervals of over 25 years or more after nephrectomy.[9] The development of pancreatic lesions may occur by either lymphatic or hematogenous spread of RCC to the pancreas. Lymphatic spread was proposed in view of the presence of lymphatics between the head of the pancreas and the dorsal side of the renal artery.[10] Hematogenous spread has also been suggested, and can be explained by portocaval shunts that increase in the presence of renal vein or the inferior vena cava thrombosis.[11]

In a review of the medical literature using Medline from 1966 to 2005, 186 cases of pancreatic involvement secondary to metastatic RCC were identified. The method of diagnosis, type of pancreatic involvement, symptoms, and treatment outcomes were reviewed (Tables 28.1 and 28.2).[2–6,12–72] Computed tomography (CT) was utilized for diagnosis in 160 (86%) of patients. Ultrasound, angiograms, endoscopic procedures, and intravenous pyelograms (IVPs) were also employed (46%, 21%, 2%, and 1%, respectively). Metachronous lesions (168/186, 90%) were the most common, with synchronous pancreatic involvement reported in only 10% of cases. Pancreas metastasis are typically solitary (Table 28.3), and are commonly located in the head of the pancreas. In the literature reviewed, information on lesion number was available in all patients, with location available in 144 (77%) patients. In 116 (62%) pancreatic metastases were solitary—63 (34%) head, 18 (10%) body, 12 (6%) tail, and 23 (12%) unknown. In 40 patients (22%) with two or more pancreatic metastases, lesions were located in all areas of the gland— 11 (6%) body/tail, seven (4%) head/tail, three (2%) head/body, and 19 (10%) unknown— and 30 (16%) had diffuse involvement (more than three lesions). Additionally, survival in patients with pancreatic metastases may be prolonged.

Therapy in this group of patients was predominantly surgical (80%) (Table 28.2). The procedures utilized included distal pancreatectomy ($n = 58$, 31%), pancreatoduodenectomy ($n = 46$, 25%), total pancreatectomy ($n = 31$, 16%), and enucleation ($n = $

Table 28.1.
Literature summary: patient series of metastatic renal cell carcinoma to the pancreas

First author	No. of patients	Method of diagnosis	Biopsy proven	Histology	Type of pancreatic involvement	Symptoms related to pancreatic metastases
Opocher, 1982	6	Angiogram	None	NS	Solitary	NS
	6	US, CT scan	None	NS	Solitary (head)	Asymptomatic
Boudghène, 1994	23	CT scan	CT-Bx 10 US-Bx 2 Endo-Bx 2 None 9	CCC	Solitary 12 Multiple 6 Diffuse 5	NS
Ghavamian, 2000	21	CT scan, US, angiogram	NS	CCC	Solitary (head) 6 Solitary (body) 4 Multiple 7 Diffuse 4	Abdominal pain, weight loss, diarrhea, constipation, melena.
Thompson, 2000						
Faure, 2001	8	US, CT scan	NS	NS	Solitary Solitary Solitary Multiple Solitary Multiple Solitary Multiple	Abdominal pain Abdominal pain Weight loss Abdominal pain Asymptomatic Asymptomatic Abdominal pain Asymptomatic

(Continued)

Table 28.1. *Continued*

First author	No. of patients	Method of diagnosis		Biopsy proven		Histology		Type of pancreatic involvement		Symptoms related to pancreatic metastases	
Sohn, 2001	10	CT scan		None		NS		Solitary (head)		Jaundice	2
								Solitary (head)		Nausea	2
								Solitary (head)		Weight loss	1
								Solitary (head)		GI bleed	1
								Solitary (head)		Asymptomatic	4
								Solitary (head)			
								Solitary (body)			
								Diffuse			
								Diffuse			
								Solitary (tail)			
Bassi, 2003	22	US, CT scan		NS		CCC 16		Solitary 14		Asymptomatic	16
						Chromophobe 1		Multiple 8		Abdominal pain	2
						NS 5				Jaundice	2
										Bowel obstruction	1
										Weight loss	1
Others[16–72]	90	Barium study	1	CT-Bx 4		CCC	40	Solitary (head)	31	GI bleed	12
		Cholangiogram	2	US-Bx 8		NS	50	Solitary (body)	13	Abdominal pain	17
		Ultrasound	31	Endo-Bx 4				Solitary (tail)	11	Jaundice	5
		CT scan	70	None 57				Multiple	16	Weight loss	11
		Angiogram	11	NS 24				Diffuse	19	Diarrhea/steatorrhea	4
		IVP	2							Asymptomatic	15
		Endoscopy	5							NS	24
		MRI	2								
		NS	4								

CT, computed tomography; US, ultrasound; EUS, endoscopic ultrasound; CT-Bx, CT guided biopsy; US-Bx, ultrasound guided biopsy; IVP, intravenous pyelogram; EUS-Bx, endoscopic ultrasound guided biopsy; MRI, magnetic resonance imaging; NS, nonspecified; Endo-Bx, endoscopic guided biopsy; CCC, clear cell carcinoma.

Table 28.2.
Literature review of metastatic renal cell carcinoma to the pancreas

First author	No. of patients	Interval time	Type of pancreatic involvement	Therapy	Survival	Systemic metastasis
Opocher, 1982	6	S	Solitary	NS	NS	NS
Boudghène, 1994	6	M	Solitary (head)	PD 3	NS	NS
				TP 1		
				None 2		
Ghavamian, 2000	23	M	Solitary 12	None	48 months (dead)	Lung, bone
			Multiple 6	DP	60 months NED	None
			Diffuse 5	DP	50 months NED	None
				DP	60 months NED	None
				None	24 months (dead)	Bone
				DP	40 months (dead)	Liver
				TP	5 months (dead)	Mesentery
				Chemotherapy	11 months (dead)	Lung
				None	60 months AWD	None
				TP	120 months (dead)	None
				Chemotherapy	24 months (dead)	Lung, liver
				Megesterol	6 months (dead)	None
				DP	72 months AWD	Chest wall
				DP	60 months AWD	Pancreas
				Megesterol	Lost to follow-up	None
				TP	40 months AWD	Lung
				None	45 months AWD	None
				DP	40 months NED	None
				None	10 months AWD	Adrenal
				Chemotherapy	19 months AWD	Omentum
				Megesterol	3 months AWD	Liver
				DP	6 months AWD	Omentum
				Chemotherapy + Radiation	12 months (dead)	None
Thompson, 2000	21	M 17	Solitary (head) 6	DP 9	75 months NED 5	None 8
		S 4	Solitary (body) 4	PD 2	74 months (dead) 16	Liver, kidney, adrenal, colon 13
			Multiple 7	E 4		
			Diffuse 4			

(Continued)

Table 28.2. *Continued*

First author	No. of patients	Interval time	Type of pancreatic involvement	Therapy	Survival	Systemic metastasis
Faure, 2001	8	M	Solitary	PD	30 months NED	None
		M	Solitary	PD	70 months (dead)	None
		M	Solitary	PD	46 months NED	None
		M	Multiple	TP + IFN-α	13 months (dead)	None
		M	Solitary	PD	88 months AWD	None
		M	Multiple	TP	26 months NED	None
		M	Solitary	PD	24 months NED	None
		M	Multiple	TP + IFN-α	84 months AWD	Adrenal
Sohn, 2001	10	M	Solitary (head)	PD	22 months NED	None
		M	Solitary (head)	PD	4 months (dead)	None
		M	Solitary (head)	PD	117 months NED	None
		M	Solitary (head)	PD	22 months AWD	Scapula, trachea
		M	Solitary (head)	PD	7 months (dead)	None
		M	Solitary (head)	PD	7 months AWD	Kidney, lung, bone
		M	Solitary (body)	DP	4 months NED	None
		M	Diffuse	TP	3 months NED	None
		M	Diffuse	TP	8 months NED	None
		S	Solitary (tail)	DP	63 months NED	None
Bassi, 2003	22	M	Solitary 14	DP 10	33 months NED 11	None 18
			Multiple 8	PD 2	22 months (dead) 7	Thyroid 2
				TP 2	56 months AWD 4	Adrenal 1
				E 3		Kidney 1
				None 5		
Other[16–72]	90	M 83	Solitary (head) 31	PD 30		Lymph nodes 3
		S 7	Solitary (body) 13	DP 27		Kidney 6
			Solitary (tail) 11	TP 17		Lung 6
			Multiple 16	E 7		Liver 5
			Diffuse 19	IL-2 1		Thyroid 3
				IFN-α 1		Adrenal 2
				Radiation 1		Skin 2
				None 10		None 38
						NS 29

M, metasynchronous; S, synchronous; DP, distal pancreatomy; TP, total pancreatomy; PD, pancreatoduodenectomy; E, enucleation; IFN, interferon; IL, interleukin; NED, no evidence of disease; AWD, alive with disease.

Table 28.3.
Number and location of renal cancer pancreatic metastases:
literature review

Number	Location	n	%
Solitary	Head	63	34
	Body	18	10
	Tail	12	6
	Unknown	23	12
Multiple	Body/tail	11	6
	Head/tail	7	4
	Head/body	3	2
	Unknown	19	10
Diffuse	Involving the entire gland	30	16

14, 7%). Systemic therapy was employed in only 16 patients (9%) (chemotherapy in five, interferon in five, IL-2 in one, and Megesterol in three). Use of radiotherapy was reported in only two (1%) patients.

Pathologic confirmation of RCC via CT-guided biopsy was performed in 14 (7.5%) patients. Ultrasound- and endoscopy-guided procedures were also used in 10 (5%) and six (3%), respectively. In all cases, clear cell carcinoma was the reported pathologic subtype.

CLEVELAND CLINIC EXPERIENCE

A retrospective analysis of patients with metastatic RCC treated in IRB-approved clinical trials between 1987 and 2004 at the CCF was performed. Twenty-nine patients were identified who either had pancreatic involvement at presentation or developed metachronous metastatic disease. The clinical characteristics, therapy, and outcomes were reviewed (Table 28.4). For comparative purposes the 186 cases of metastatic RCC with pancreatic involvement identified in the literature review (Medline 1966 to 2005) were utilized. Method of diagnosis, type of pancreatic involvement, symptoms, and treatment outcomes were reviewed. Additionally, 16 patients (12 male and four female) with 32 pancreatic lesions who had serial imaging by CT or magnetic resonance imaging (MRI) at our institution were analyzed to assess the growth rates of pancreatic lesions. Mean and median follow-up was 25.8 and 23 months, respectively (range 7–62 months); 123 CT scans and three MRI examinations were used to document the diameter and calculate the growth rate of these lesions. The mean and median number of scans was 7.6 and 7 scans respectively. The single largest diameter of each pancreatic lesion on each scan was recorded. Growth rates were calculated using least squares analysis for each lesion based on measurement over time.

Table 28.4.
Cleveland Clinic Foundation Series: 29 patients with pancreatic metastases from renal cell carcinoma

Patient number	Sex/age	Diabetes related to pancreatic metastases	Method of diagnosis	Biopsy proven	Interval time	Histology	Type of pancreatic involvement	Symptoms related to pancreatic metastases	Systemic metastases	Therapy	Response	Outcome
Patient 1	M/66	Yes	MRI	CT-Bx	M	CCC	Multiple (head + tail)	Asymptomatic	Lung, adrenal	TP + IFN + IL-2	NR	60 months (AWD)
Patient 2	M/65	Yes	CT scan	EGD-Bx	S	CCC	Solitary (head)	GIB	Lung, bone	IFN + IL-2	NR	76 months (dead)
Patient 3	M/62	No	US	NS	M	CCC	Solitary (tail)	NS	Liver, colon	5-FU + IL-2 + IFN	NR	78 months (dead)
Patient 4	M/62	Yes	IVP	None	S	CCC	Solitary (tail)	GIB, weight loss	Lung	T-cell infusion + radiation	NR	11 months (dead)
Patient 5	M/52	No	CT scan	None	M	CCC	Multiple (head + tail)	GIB	Liver	IL-2 + IFN	NR	13 months (dead)
Patient 6	M/51	Yes	CT scan	None	M	CCC	Multiple (body + tail)	Steatorrhea	Lung, adrenal, kidney	IL-2 + IFN, IL-2 + thalidomide	NR	27 months (AWD)
Patient 7	M/59	No	CT scan	CT-Bx	S	CCC	Solitary (tail)	GIB, abdominal pain	Lung	IL-2 + IFN, Taxoprexin, Abgenix	NR	33 months (dead)
Patient 8	F/62	No	CT scan	CT-Bx	M	CCC	Multiple (head + tail)	Abdominal pain	Kidney	IL-2 + thalidomide, IFN-α_{1b}	NR	35 months (AWD)
Patient 9	M/57	No	CT scan	None	M	CCC	Solitary (body)	Asymptomatic	Sinus, bone, liver	Capecitabine, IFN	NR	19 months (AWD)
Patient 10	M/63	No	CT scan	None	M	CCC	Solitary (head)	NS	Lung, kidney	IFN-α + Targretin, adoptive immunotherapy	NR	45 months (dead)
Patient 11	M/76	Yes	CT scan	None	M	CCC	Multiple (head + body)	Asymptomatic	Parotid gland, lung	DP + IL-2 + IFN-α	NR	77 months (dead)
Patient 12	M/58	No	CT scan	None	M	CCC	Solitary (head)	Steatorrhea	Lung, adrenal	TP + IL-2 + IFN-α	NR	59 months (dead)
Patient 13	M/69	No	CT scan	None	M	CCC	Solitary (head)	Asymptomatic	Lung, adrenal	IFN + capecitabine, Abgenix	NR	29 months (AWD)
Patient 14	F/70	Yes	CT scan	None	M	CCC	Multiple (head + tail)	Asymptomatic	Lung	IFN + capecitabine	NR	70 months (AWD)

Patient												
Patient 15	M52	No	CT scan	None	M	CCC	Solitary (head)	Asymptomatic	Lung, adrenal, brain	Peg IFN + IL-2	NR	35 months (dead)
Patient 16	M/53	Yes	CT scan	CT-Bx	S	CCC	Solitary (head)	Asymptomatic	Liver, lung	Peg IFN + IL-2	NR	46 months (AWD)
Patient 17	F/68	No	CT scan	NS	M	CCC	Multiple (head + body)	Asymptomatic	Lung, kidney, bone	Peg IFN + IL-2	NR	47 months (AWD)
Patient 18	M/76	No	IVP	NS	M	CCC	Solitary (head)	NS	Lung, kidney, liver	IL-2, tumor infiltrating lymphocyte infusion	NR	32 months (dead)
Patient 19	M/89	No	CT scan	None	M	CCC	Multiple (body)	Asymptomatic	None	None	N/A	25 months (AWD)
Patient 20	M/63	No	CT scan	None	M	CCC	Solitary (head)	Asymptomatic	Lung, brain, muscle	IL-2 + IFN	NR	28 months (dead)
Patient 21	M/76	No	CT scan	None	M	CCC	Solitary (head)	Asymptomatic	Lung, brain, liver	IL-2 + thalidomide + EGFR antibody	NR	22 months (AWD)
Patient 22	M/67	No	CT scan	None	M	CCC	Solitary (tail)	Asymptomatic	Lung, kidney, muscle	Adoptive immunotherapy	NR	34 months (AWD)
Patient 23	F/69	No	CT scan	None	M	CCC	Diffuse	Asymptomatic	Lung, brain, muscle	Golgi mannosidase II inhibitor	NR	28 months (dead)
Patient 24	M/63	No	CT scan	CT-Bx	M	CCC	Solitary (head)	Asymptomatic	None	None	N/A	33 months (NED)
Patient 25	M63	No	CT scan	None	S	CCC	Solitary (head)	Asymptomatic	Lung, muscle, bone	IFN+ capecitabine	NR	34 months (AWD)
Patient 26	M68	No	CT scan	None	M	CCC	Solitary (tail)	Asymptomatic	Lung, adrenal, kidney	IFN+ capecitabine	NR	33 months (AWD)
Patient 27	F/76	No	EGD/CT scan	EGD-Bx	M	CCC	Solitary (head)	Asymptomatic	None	None	N/A	20 months (dead)
Patient 28	M/62	No	CT scan	None	S	CCC	Diffuse	Abdominal pain	Lung, adrenal, liver	IFN + capecitabine, BAY 43-9006	NR	12 months (dead)
Patient 29	M73	No	CT scan	None	M	CCC	Multiple (head + body)	Asymptomatic	Lung, adrenal, bone	Abgenix	NR	33 months (AWD)

CCC, clear cell carcinoma; DP, distal pancreatectomy; EGD, esophagogastroduodenoscopy; EGFR, epidermal growth factor receptor; GIB, gastrointestinal bleeding; IFN, interferon; IL, interleukin; NS, not stated; TP, total pancreatectomy.

CLINICAL PRESENTATION

Renal cell carcinoma metastatic to the pancreas was discovered on routine surveillance in the majority of patients (51%). This compares to 24% noted in prior reports.[4] There was a 4 : 1 male predominance, with a mean age of 63 years (range 51–89) similar to prior reports.[73] Symptoms in this patient group included abdominal pain (14%), gastrointestinal bleeding requiring endoscopic intervention (14%), diarrhea related to pancreatic insufficiency (7%), and nonspecific symptoms of fatigue, regurgitation, and nausea (15%) (Table 28.4). The Eastern Cooperative Oncology Group (ECOG) performance status (PS) at diagnosis of pancreatic metastasis was less than 1 in 14 (48%) patients and 0 in 15 patients (52%). All symptoms were reported within 3 months prior to or after pancreatic involvement. Laboratory abnormalities were also seen in a number of patients. Lactic dehydrogenate acid (LDH) was elevated in five patients (17%), hemoglobin decreased in three patients (10%), and hypercalcemia was present in three patients (10%). Seventeen patients (59%) had solitary metastases (11 head, five tail, and one body), 10 (34%) had multiple metastases, and two (7%) had diffuse involvement (Table 28.4).

Newly diagnosed diabetes mellitus (DM) was found in seven (24%) patients, and within 3 months of the diagnosis of pancreatic metastasis in three patients (10%). This was related to surgical resection of the pancreas. Worsening of a previously diagnosed DM occurred in two (7%) patients. Diabetes was more commonly associated with metastasis located in the head of the pancreas (six, 86%) compared to those without pancreatic head involvement (one, 14%). Although 20 patients had pancreatic head involvement, only eight (28%) had metastases larger than 4 cm. All patients with diabetes related to the tumor had lesions 4 cm or greater. Prior reports of diabetic patients and pancreas head involvement with pancreatic cancer show that diabetes is related to the pancreatic involvement in 76% of the patients.[74] Pancreatic head involvement with metastatic disease can cause diabetes by destroying islet cells,[75] inducing chronic pancreatitis by obstructing the pancreatic duct,[76] or by causing peripheral resistance to insulin. Such insulin resistance frequently occurs early in the course of the disease,[77] which may explain why diabetes can appear before the symptoms of the pancreatic head involvement. Similarly, both patients in our series with signs of pancreatic exocrine insufficiency had pancreatic head involvement of 11 cm or more, suggesting chronic obstructive pancreatitis as the etiology.[78] Pancreatic insufficiency is also present in pancreatic carcinoma involving the head of the pancreas but at a much high incidence rate (50%).[78] Similar to pancreatic carcinoma, the long-term complications of DM and pancreatic insufficiency are less evident in metastatic RCC patients, despite the prolonged survival experienced by these patients.

DIAGNOSIS AND IMAGING

Use of frequent imaging for patients with metastatic RCC undergoing therapy in a clinical trial may have resulted in early detection of pancreas metastases early before the development of symptoms. Computed tomography was the most common imaging modality used[3] (Figure 28.1). Ultrasound and MRI have also been employed[79] (Figure 28.2).

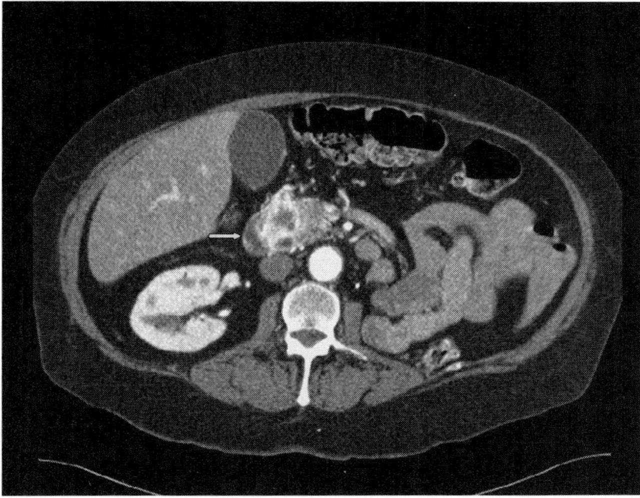

Figure 28.1. Computed tomography (CT) scan image of renal cell carcinoma (RCC) metastasis involving the head of the pancreas (arrow).

In the Cleveland Clinic series, pancreatic metastases were detected by CT scans in 25 patients (86%). Intravenous pyelograms, ultrasound, and MRI were also used (7%, 3%, 3%, respectively) (Table 28.4). Renal cell carcinoma metastases have a typical appearance on CT scan, which includes well-defined margins, greater enhancement than normal pancreas tissue, and a central area of low attenuation[3,5] (Figures 28.1 and 28.2).

Synchronous pancreatic metastases were found in five (17%) of our patients, similar to 10% to 15% reported in the literature.[4] Pancreatic involvement after curative

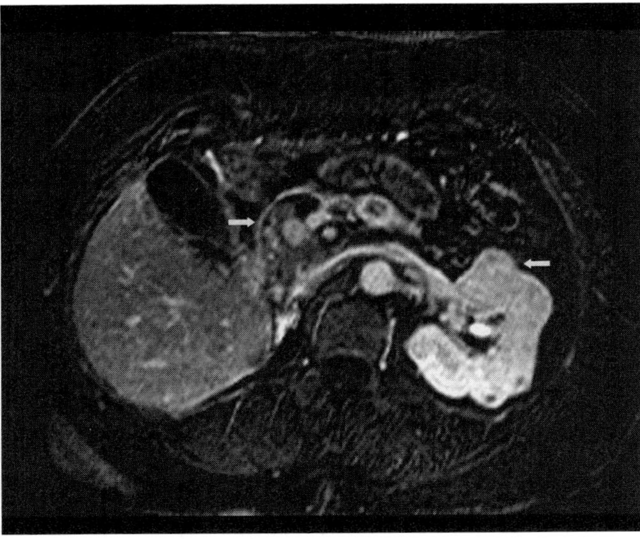

Figure 28.2. Magnetic resonance imaging (MRI) of synchronous RCC involving the left kidney (arrow) and head of the pancreas (arrow).

Table 28.5.
Tumor size and growth rates of renal primary lesions and metastatic lesions (pancreas, lung) in patients with metastatic renal cell carcinoma

	Pancreatic metastases in CCF experience	Primary RCC in literature review (Oda, 2001)	Lung metastases in literature review (Oda, 2001)
No. patients	16	16	16
Male	12	12	13
Female	4	4	3
Age (years)			
Median	59	54	60
Range	47–78	28–78	42–73
Largest diameter at first evaluation (cm)	1.2	2.0	1.9
Median	0.5–8.2	1.0–4.5	1.0–3.0
Range			
Follow-up period (months)			
Range	7–62	12–72	4–61
Growth rate (cm/year)			
Median	0.37	0.54	1.72
Range	0.0053–1.7	0.1–1.35	0.08–7.87

nephrectomy developed in 24 patients (83%). The metastases were typically solitary, and located most commonly in the head of the pancreas. Seventeen (59%) patients had solitary metastases (11 head, five tail, and one body), 10 (34%) patients had multiple metastases, and two (7%) had diffuse involvement.

The median growth rate of pancreatic metastasis in 16 patients with serial scans was estimated as 0.37 cm/year (0.0053–0.17 cm/year) (Figure 28.2), similar to that reported for primary renal tumors, 0.54 cm/year,[80,81] and significantly lower than other metastatic sites such as the lungs (1.72 cm/year)[81] (Table 28.5).

Patients with known metastatic RCC who then develop a new lesion in the pancreas with distinct radiologic characteristics generally may not require biopsy conformation. In patients without metastatic disease, or those with synchronous metastases at the time of diagnosis, tissue conformation is generally required. A CT or an endoscopic ultrasound (EUS)-guided biopsy may be utilized. In the current series, seven (4%) patients had a biopsy of a pancreatic lesion, five by CT guided and two by endoscopic biopsies.

Clear cell carcinoma (CCC) is the only pathologic subtype of RCC that appears to be associated with development of pancreatic metastases.[4] In the current series of 29 patients, CCC was the histologic subtype in all primary tumors and in the seven pancreatic biopsies (Table 28.4).

Patients with pancreatic metastases may have widespread organ involvement (93%). In addition to the pancreas, the most common sites of involvement included lungs ($n = 22$, 75%), adrenals glands ($n = 8$, 27%), liver ($n = 7$, 24%), bone ($n = 6$, 21%), and brain ($n = 4$, 14%). Other organs involved included the duodenum (7%), colon, and parotid gland (3%) (Table 28.4).

TREATMENT

Immunologic control of tumor growth by cellular immune mechanisms has been clearly demonstrated in RCC patients, and may explain the reports of occasional spontaneous regression of metastases.[82] The role of the immune system is also evident in the reported increase in the incidence of RCC in immunocompromised patients following organ transplantation,[83] suggesting a role of the immune system in regulating tumor progression. Therefore, previous treatments have focused on enhancing the immune response by use of cytokines,[84] tumor-derived vaccines,[85] and adoptive transfer on immune cells.[86] Additionally, there have been trials utilizing hormonal therapy or chemotherapy[87] in patients with advanced disease. Recently the role of molecular targeted therapy that can inhibit growth factors such as vascular endothelial growth factor (VEGF) and platelet-derived growth factor (PDGF) and their receptors has been investigated.[88] In the Cleveland Clinic series, three patients (2%) had curative pancreatic resection, 22 patients received immunotherapy with/without other agents (capecitabine in six patients, thalidomide in three patients, 5-fluorouracil [5-FU] in one patient), and one patient chemotherapy alone (Taxoprexin). Other treatments utilized included adoptive immunotherapy or tumor vaccines (four patients). Three patients received no therapy (one declined, and two not started) (Table 28.4). Radiation was used in one patient for palliative purposes. Despite the different combinations of immunotherapy and chemotherapy used, all patients who received treatment had progression of disease.

OUTCOMES

Patients with pancreatic metastasis from RCC may have a better prognosis when compared to individuals with metastases involving other sites. In the current series, the median time from diagnosis of RCC to diagnosis of metastatic RCC was 5.6 years (range 0–20 years), with only 10 (34%) patients developing metastatic disease within 1 year of the initial diagnosis of the primary tumor. The median survival in this patient cohort was 33 months (Figure 28.3) (range 11–78 months). The Memorial

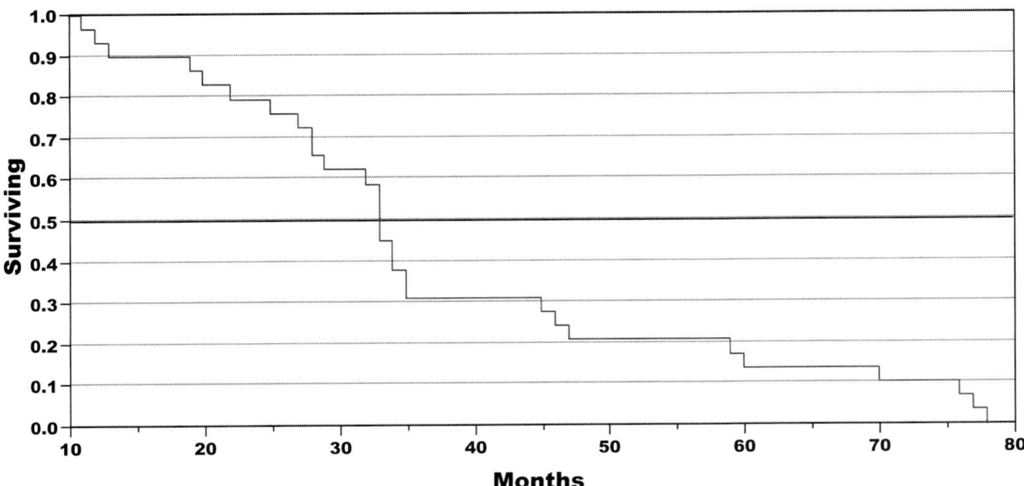

Figure 28.3. Survival of 29 patients with metastatic RCC (Cleveland Clinic experience). Median survival is 33 months (range 11 to 78 months).

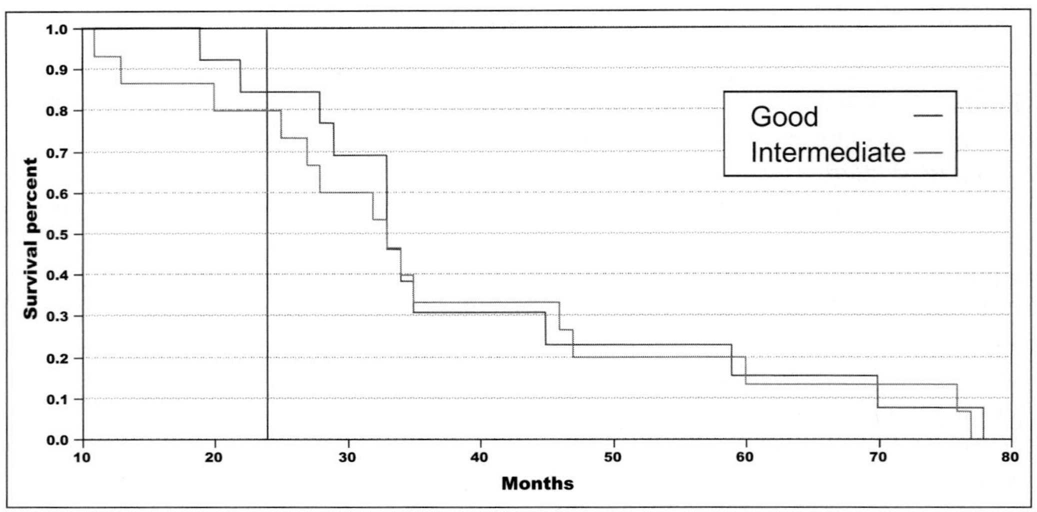

Figure 28.4. Survival of RCC patients with pancreatic metastases classified by prognostic group: good versus intermediate.[89]

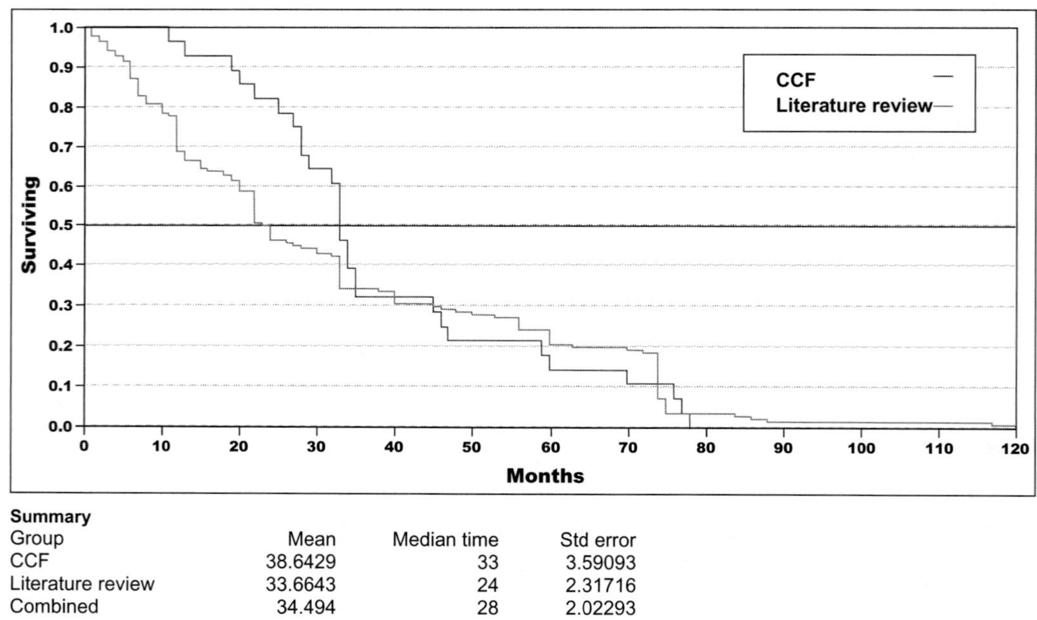

Summary Group	Mean	Median time	Std error
CCF	38.6429	33	3.59093
Literature review	33.6643	24	2.31716
Combined	34.494	28	2.02293

Figure 28.5. Survival of patients with renal cell carcinoma and pancreatic metastases. The current series of 29 patients from the Cleveland Clinic is contrasted with the two largest series from the literature.[3,15]

Sloan-Kettering prognostic factors[83] were assessed in this group of patients at the time of diagnosis. Thirteen (45%) were good risk, 15 (52%) were intermediate, and one patient (3%) was poor risk. The 3-year survival rate in the good risk group was 66%, and in the intermediate risk group 57% (Figure 28.4). This is compared to 31% and 7% in good and intermediate risk groups, respectively, reported in patients with metastatic RCC[89] (Figure 28.3). Overall the median survival for patients with pancreatic metastases was 33 months, which is comparable to 24 months seen in the two largest literature series reviewed (Figure 28.5).

CURRENT APPROACHES IN METASTATIC RENAL CELL CARCINOMA THERAPY

The recent discovery of the association between a mutated/silenced von Hippel-Lindau (VHL) gene and clear cell carcinoma pathogenesis involving overproduction of VEGF and PDGF have led to the development of a series of novel agents targeting these factors.[88] Following treatment with targeted agents such as sorefenib or sunitinib, the radiologic appearance of RCC metastasis can change. In responding patients, the vascular enhancement is decreased and the central low attenuation expands toward the periphery, consistent with an increase in central necrosis. To illustrate this in pancreatic metastases, the case of a 71-year-old woman with RCC involving the pancreas and lung is summarized. Prior therapy included pegylated IFN-α and IL-2, tumor vaccine therapy, and 5–FU with suramin. Disease progression was documented on serial CT scans with all prior therapies. Within 2 months of starting oral sunitinb therapy, a noticeable decrease in the size of the pancreatic lesions was observed. Additionally, the characteristic well-defined margins, greater enhancement than normal pancreas tissue, and a central area of low attenuation developed. The vascular enhancement was decreased, and the central low attenuation was expanded toward the periphery of the lesion, consistent with central necrosis (Figures 28.6 and 28.7). The responses seen in pancreatic

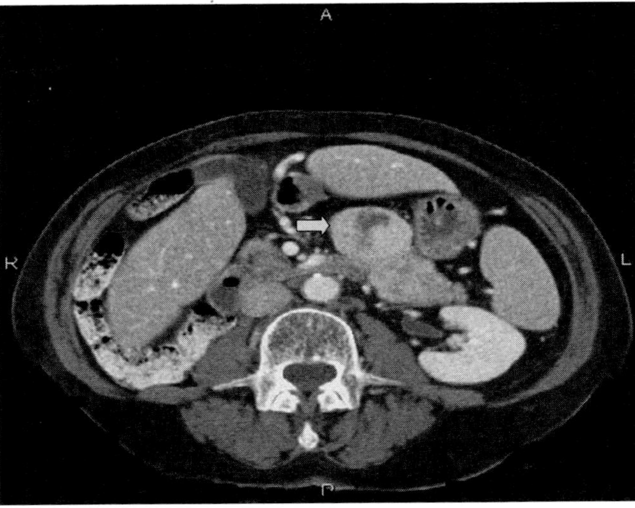

Figure 28.6. RCC pancreatic metastases to the tail (arrow) before treatment.

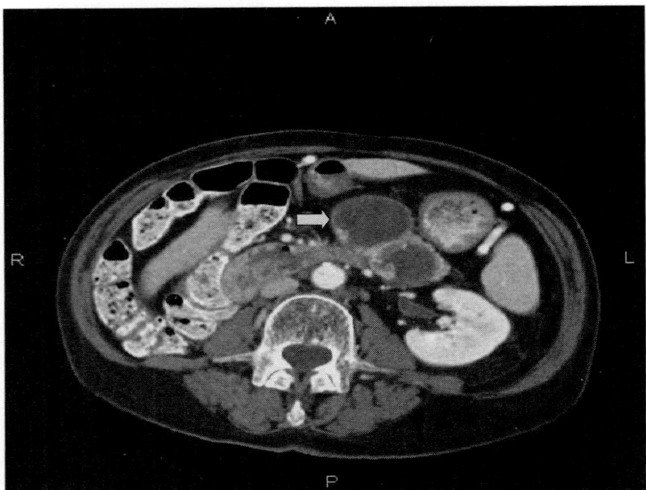

Figure 28.7. Appearance of pancreatic metastases (arrow) to the tail after sunitinib treatment.

lesions with these agents are of interest, in view of the negative experience with cytokines. The overall response rate of pancreatic lesions to oral tyrosine kinase inhibitors (TKIs) remains to be determined.

CONCLUSION

Metastatic RCC involving the pancreas is uncommon and usually asymptomatic. In selected patients, however, it can produce a variety of symptoms at the time of presentation. Diabetes mellitus and pancreatic exocrine insufficiency are documented complications of RCC metastases involving the head of the pancreas, but they occur less frequently than in other malignancies such as pancreatic carcinoma when it involves the head of the pancreas. The CT scan remains the most common modality used for diagnosis of this complication. Surgical resection of isolated pancreatic metastases from RCC may provide improvement in survival.[6,7] The similar median survival of the literature review group (primarily surgically treated) and our CCF cohort (systemically treated) suggests a good prognosis in patients with pancreatic metastases even without surgical resection.[14,90] Although the patient numbers are relatively small, the data suggest that development of pancreatic metastases occurs only in clear-cell RCC, may not impact negatively on survival, and is associated with an indolent disease growth pattern and widespread metastatic disease. These factors may influence the ultimate choice of therapy, suggesting that the systemic approach should be considered in most instances. The frequency of a single isolated metastasis to the pancreas from RCC is low, and therefore surgical removal should be reserved for individuals whose staging studies demonstrate no other evidence of disease. Recent data targeted agents such as sorefenib or sunitinib may have activity in advanced RCC, including metastases in the pancreas.

REFERENCES

1. Robbins EG 2nd, Franceschi D, Barkin JS. Solitary metastatic tumors to the pancreas: a case report and review of the literature. Am J Gastroenterol 1996;91(11):2414–2417.

2. Simpson NS, Mulholland CK, Lioe TF, Spence RA. Late, solitary metastatic renal carcinoma in the pancreas. Ulster Med J 1989;58(2):198–199.
3. Ghavamian R, Klein KA, Stephens DH, et al. Renal cell carcinoma metastatic to the pancreas: clinical and radiological features. Mayo Clin Proc 2000;75(6):581–585.
4. Thompson LD, Heffess CS. Renal cell carcinoma to the pancreas in surgical pathology material. Cancer 2000;89(5):1076–1088.
5. Kassabian A, Stein J, Jabbour N, et al. Renal cell carcinoma metastatic to the pancreas: a single-institution series and review of the literature. Urology 2000;56(2):211–215.
6. Sohn TA, Yeo CJ, Cameron JL, Nakeeb A, Lillemoe KD. Renal cell carcinoma metastatic to the pancreas: results of surgical management. J Gastrointest Surg 2001;5(4):346–351.
7. Tuech JJ, Pessaux P, Chautard D, et al. Results of duodenopancreatectomy for solitary pancreatic metastasis from renal cell carcinoma. J Hepatobiliary Pancreat Surg 1999;6(4):396–398.
8. Tongio J, Peruta O, Wenger JJ, Warter P. [Duodenal and pancreatic metastases of nephro-epithelioma.] Ann Radiol (Paris) 1977;20(7):641–647.
9. Simpson NS, Mulholland CK, Lioe TF, Spence RA. Late, solitary metastatic renal carcinoma in the pancreas. Ulster Med J 1989;58(2):198–199.
10. Nagakawa T, Kobayashi H, Ueno K, Ohta T, Kayahara M, Miyazaki I. Clinical study of lymphatic flow to the paraaortic lymph nodes in carcinoma of the head of the pancreas. Cancer 1994;73(4):1155–1162.
11. Saitoh H, Yoshida K, Uchijima Y, Kobayashi N, Suwata J, Nakame Y. Possible metastatic routes via portacaval shunts in renal adenocarcinoma with liver metastasis. Urology 1991;37(6):598–601.
12. Opocher E, Galeotti F, Spina GP, Battaglia G, Hernandez C. Diagnosis of secondary tumors of the pancreas. Analysis of 13 cases. Minerva Med 1982;73(11):577–581.
13. Boudghene FP, Deslandes PM, LeBlanche AF, Bigot JM. US and CT imaging features of intrapancreatic metastases. J Comput Assist Tomogr 1994;18(6):905–910.
14. Faure JP, Tuech JJ, Richer JP, Pessaux P, Arnaud JP, Carretier M. Pancreatic metastasis of renal cell carcinoma: presentation, treatment and survival. J Urol 2001;165(1):20–22.
15. Bassi C, Butturini G, Falconi M, Sargenti M, Mantovani W, Pederzoli P. High recurrence rate after atypical resection for pancreatic metastases from renal cell carcinoma. Br J Surg 2003;90(5): 555–559.
16. Lawson LJ, Holt LP, Rooke HW. Recurrent duodenal haemorrhage from renal carcinoma. Br J Urol 1966;38(2):133–137.
17. Marquand J, Giraud B, Maliakas S. Pancreatic metastasis revealing a kidney cancer. Chirurgie 1971;97(1):52–56.
18. Guttman FM, Ross M, Lachance C. Pancreatic metastasis of renal cell carcinoma treated by total pancreatectomy. Arch Surg 1972;105(5):782–784.
19. Gillet M, Camelot G, Runser C, Clement D. Duodeno-pancreatic metastasis of kidney cancer revealed by digestive hemorrhage and treated by cephalic duodenopancreatectomy. Chirurgie 1974;100(3):226–230.
20. Hermanutz KD, Sonnenberg GE. Late metastasis of a hypernephroid kidney carcinoma to the pancreas with tumor invasion to the duodenum. Rofo 1977;127(6):595–597.
21. Saxon A, Gottesman J, Doolas A. Bilateral hypernephroma with solitary pancreatic metastasis. J Surg Oncol 1980;13(4):317–322.
22. Yazaki T, Ishikawa S, Ogawa Y. silent pancreatic metastasis from renal cell carcinoma diagnosed at arterography. Acta Urol Jpn 1981;12:1517–1521.
23. Rumancik WM, Megibow AJ, Bosniak MA, Hilton S. Metastatic disease to the pancreas: evaluation by computed tomography. J Comput Assist Tomogr 1984;8(5):829–834.
24. Weerdenburg JP, Jurgens PJ. Late metastases of a hypernephroma to the thyroid and the pancreas. Diagn Imaging Clin Med 1984;53(5):269–272.
25. Audisio RA, La Monica G. Solitary pancreatic metastasis occurring 20 years after nephrectomy for carcinoma of the kidney. Tumori 1985;71(2):197–200.
26. Skaarup P, Jorgensen T, Larsen S. Asynchronous metastasizing renal cell carcinoma associated with progressive immune complex glomerulonephritis and proteinuria. Scand J Urol Nephrol 1984; 18(4):351–356.
27. Kishimoto H, Nimura Y, Okamoto K, et al. A case of resected renal cell carcinoma with massive pancreatic metastases. Gan No Rinsho 1985;31(1):91–96.
28. Carini M, Selli C, Barbanti G, Bianchi S, Muraro G. Pancreatic late recurrence of bilateral renal cell carcinoma after conservative surgery. Eur Urol 1988;14(3):258–260.

29. Sharma SK, Kumar A, Madhusoodnan P, Banerjee CK, Suri S, Dhar ML. Solitary pancreatic metastasis from renal cell carcinoma. A rare metastatic site. Indian J Cancer 1988;25(1):29–32.

30. Amamyia H, Lizumi T, Yazaki T. A solitary pancreatic metastasis from renal cell carcinoma. Hinyouki Geka 1988;2:167–170.

31. Temellini F, Bavosi M, Lamarra M, Quagliarini P, Giuliani F. Pancreatic metastasis 25 years after nephrectomy for renal cancer. Tumori 1989;75(5):503–504.

32. Strijk SP. Pancreatic metastases of renal cell carcinoma: report of two cases. Gastrointest Radiol 1989;14(2):123–126.

33. Iwanami M, Nakayoshi A, Yagi H. A resected case of asymptomatic pancreatic metastasis in the body and tail of the pancreas from renal cell carcinoma. J Jpn Pan Soc 1989;4:100–106.

34. Komeda H, Fujimoto Y, Horie M, Isogai K. Metastatic renal cell carcinoma to the pancreas and adrenal gland was diagnosed before surgical treatment: A case report. Hinyouki Geka 1990;3:765–768.

35. Gohji K, Matsumoto O, Kamidono S. Solitary pancreatic metastasis from renal cell carcinoma. Acta Urol Jpn 1990;36(677):681.

36. Terashima M, Abe H, Suga K, Matsuya F, Kobayashi K, Itoh S. Two cases of renal cell carcinoma metastasized to the pancreas and to the gallbladder. Jpn J Gastroenterol 1990;23:1952–1956.

37. Biset JM, Laurent F, de Verbizier G, Houang B, Constantes G, Drouillard J. Ultrasound and computed tomographic findings in pancreatic metastases. Eur J Radiol 1991;12(1):41–44.

38. Fullarton GM, Burgoyne M. Gallbladder and pancreatic metastases from bilateral renal carcinoma presenting with hematobilia and anemia. Urology 1991;38(2):184–186.

39. Oka H, Hatayama T, Taki Y, Ueyama H, Hida S, Noguchi M. A resected case of renal cell carcinoma with metastasis to pancreas. Hinyokika Kiyo 1991;37(11):1531–1534.

40. Kubo K, Morita J, Taki Y, Ueyama H, Hida S. Renal cell carcinoma metastatic to the pancreas 8 years following nephrectomy. Jpn J Clin Radiol 1991;36:509–512.

41. Tabata T, Kuroda Y, Nishimatsu S, Satoh Y. A resected case of pancreatic tumor metastasized from renal cell carcinoma. J Jpn Pan Soc 1991;6:245–250.

42. Yamamoto S, Tobinaga K, Taketomi K, Kimino K, Ashizuka S, Kishikawa M. Pancreatic metastasis of renal cell carcinoma occurring 17 years after nephrectomy. J Jpn Soc Clin Surg 1991;52:3006–3011.

43. Furukawa T, Hattori R, Ohtake H. A resectable case of pancreatic head metastasis from renal cell carcinoma. Hinyouki Geka 1991;4:111–114.

44. Rypens F, Van Gansbeke D, Lambilliotte JP, Van Regemorter G, Verhest A, Struyven J. Pancreatic metastasis from renal cell carcinoma. Br J Radiol 1992;65(774):547–548.

45. Stankard CE, Karl RC. The treatment of isolated pancreatic metastases from renal cell carcinoma: a surgical review. Am J Gastroenterol 1992;87(11):1658–1660.

46. Adachi K, Murabayashi K, Hayashi J. A case of metastatic thyroid and pancreatic cancer from renal cell carcinoma. Tan to Sui 1992;13:791–796.

47. Nakagawa K, Tsuchiya T, Momono S, Sasaki Y, Sato T. A case of pancreatic metastasis of renal cell carcinoma. Jpn J Gasteroenterol Surg 1992;25:2200–2204.

48. Fujii M, Kogawa T, Matsuyama K. A case of metastatic renal cell carcinoma to pancreas ten years after nephrectomy. J Kyoto Pref Univ Med 1992;101:589–596.

49. Yanagisawa T, Nakayama K, Kashiwagi M. Three cases of resectable pancreatic metastasis from renal cell carcinoma. Geka Shinryo 1993;8:742–744.

50. Sauvanet A, Barthes T, Levy P, et al. Late pancreatic metastasis from renal cell carcinoma. Pancreas 1993;8(6):742–744.

51. Vergara V, Marucci M, Marcarino C, Brunello F, Capussotti L. Metastatic involvement of the pancreas from renal cell carcinoma treated by surgery. Ital J Gastroenterol 1993;25(7):388–390.

52. Derias NW, Chong WH. Fine needle aspiration diagnosis of a late solitary pancreatic metastasis of renal adenocarcinoma. Cytopathology 1993;4(6):369–372.

53. Motoyama S, Terashima H, Matsuoka T, Saito M, Abo S. A case of renal cell carcinoma metastasizing to pancreas and skin 19 years after nephrectomy. Jpn J Gastroenterol Clin Surg 1993;26:2859–2863.

54. Oda K, Itoh J, Hachisuka K, et al. Value of computer image analysis in improving ERCP images in metastatic tumor of the pancreas. AJR Am J Roentgenol 1993;161(4):885–886.

55. Aikou S, Tokura Y, Yamafuji K. A resected case of pancreatic metastasis from renal cell carcinoma presenting with acute duodenal bleeding. J Jpn Soc Clin Surg 1993;54:2666–2672.

56. Nan Y, Kuno N, Kurimoto K, Nakamura T, Kobayashi S. A resected case of pancreatic tumor metastasized from renal cell carcinoma diagnosed by endoscopic biopsy through the main pancreatic duct. Gastroenterol Endosc 1993;35:1380–1385.

57. Kawaguchi T, Tsunoda T, Tanaka Y. A case of resection of a solitary pancreatic metastasis of renal cell carcinoma occurring 5 years after nephrectomy. J Jpn Panc Soc 1993;8:189–195.

58. Takeuchi H, Konaga E, Harano M, et al. Solitary pancreatic metastasis from renal cell carcinoma. Acta Med Okayama 1993;47(1):63–66.

59. Ishikawa T, Horimi T, Majima K. A resected case of pancreatic tumor metastasized from renal cell carcinoma. A review of 11 cases in the Japanese and 13 cases of the foreign literature. J Jpn Soc Clin Surg 1993;54:1642–1647.

60. Osaka Y, Kato H, Nakamura F. Solitary pancreatic metastasis from renal cell carcinoma. Jpn J Gastroenterol Surg 1994;27:130–134.

61. Dousset B, Andant C, Guimbaud R, et al. Late pancreatic metastasis from renal cell carcinoma diagnosed by endoscopic ultrasonography. Surgery 1995;117(5):591–594.

62. Orita M, Morita N, Hiraoka H, Noshima S, Takahashi T, Esato K. A case of resected pancreatic metastasis from renal cell carcinoma 14 years after radical nephrectomy. J Jpn Panc Soc 1995; 10:63–68.

63. Robbins EG 2nd, Franceschi D, Barkin JS. Solitary metastatic tumors to the pancreas: a case report and review of the literature. Am J Gastroenterol 1996;91(11):2414–2417.

64. Hirota T, Tomida T, Iwasa M, Takahashi K, Kaneda M, Tamaki H. Solitary pancreatic metastasis occurring eight years after nephrectomy for renal cell carcinoma. A case report and surgical review. Int J Pancreatol 1996;19(2):145–153.

65. Z'graggen K, Fernandez-del Castillo C, Rattner DW, Sigala H, Warshaw AL. Metastases to the pancreas and their surgical extirpation. Arch Surg 1998;133(4):413–417; discussion 418–419.

66. Butturini G, Bassi C, Falconi M, et al. Surgical treatment of pancreatic metastases from renal cell carcinomas. Dig Surg 1998;15(3):241–246.

67. Hashimoto M, Watanabe G, Matsuda M, Dohi T, Tsurumaru M. Management of the pancreatic metastases from renal cell carcinoma: report of four resected cases. Hepatogastroenterology 1998;45(22):1150–1154.

68. Sahin M, Foulis AA, Poon FW, Imrie CW. Late focal pancreatic metastasis of renal cell carcinoma. Dig Surg 1998;15(1):72–74.

69. Le Borgne J, Partensky C, Glemain P, Dupas B, de Kerviller B. Pancreaticoduodenectomy for metastatic ampullary and pancreatic tumors. Hepatogastroenterology 2000;47(32):540–544.

70. Mehta N, Volpe C, Haley T, Balos L, Bradley EL 3rd, Doerr RJ. Pancreaticoduodenectomy for metastatic renal cell carcinoma: report of a case. Surg Today 2000;30(1):94–97.

71. Abbas MA, Collins JM, Mulligan DC. Renal cell carcinoma metastatic to pancreas. Am J Surg 2001;182(2):183–184.

72. Minni F, Casadei R, Perenze B, et al. Pancreatic metastases: observations of three cases and review of the literature. Pancreatology 2004;4(6):509–520.

73. Onishi T, Machida T, Masuda F, et al. Nephrectomy in renal carcinoma with distant metastasis. Br J Urol 1989;63(6):600–604.

74. Gullo L, Pezzilli R, Morselli-Labate AM. Diabetes and the risk of pancreatic cancer. Italian Pancreatic Cancer Study Group. N Engl J Med 1994;331(2):81–84.

75. Bell ET. Carcinoma of the pancreas. I. A clinical and pathologic study of 609 necropsied cases. II. The relation of carcinoma of the pancreas to diabetes mellitus. Am J Pathol 1957;33(3):499–523.

76. Wakasugi H, Funakoshi A, Iguchi H. Clinical observations of pancreatic diabetes caused by pancreatic carcinoma, and survival period. Int J Clin Oncol 2001;6(1):50–54.

77. Schwarts SS, Zeidler A, Moossa AR, Kuku SF, Rubenstein AH. A prospective study of glucose tolerance, insulin, C-peptide, and glucagon responses in patients with pancreatic carcinoma. Am J Dig Dis 1978;23(12):1107–1114.

78. Wakasugi H, Hara Y, Abe M. A study of malabsorption in pancreatic cancer. J Gastroenterol 1996;31(1):81–85.

79. Masood J, Lane T, Koye B, Vandal MT, Barua JM, Hill JT. Renal cell carcinoma: incidental detection during routine ultrasonography in men presenting with lower urinary tract symptoms. BJU Int 2001;88(7):671–674.

80. Kassouf W, Aprikian AG, Laplante M, Tanguay S. Natural history of renal masses followed expectantly. J Urol 2004;171(1):111–113; discussion 113.

81. Oda T, Miyao N, Takahashi A, et al. Growth rates of primary and metastatic lesions of renal cell carcinoma. Int J Urol 2001;8(9):473–477.

82. Kawai K, Saijo K, Oikawa T, Ohno T, Akaza H. Enhancement of T cell proliferative response against autologous cancer cells of a metastatic renal cell carcinoma patient after unexplained regression. Int J Urol 2004;11(12):1130–1132.
83. Ishikawa N, Tanabe K, Tokumoto T, et al. Renal cell carcinoma of native kidneys in renal transplant recipients. Transplant Proc 1998;30(7):3156–3158.
84. Motzer RJ, Rakhit A, Thompson JA, et al. Randomized multicenter phase II trial of subcutaneous recombinant human interleukin-12 versus interferon-alpha 2a for patients with advanced renal cell carcinoma. J Interferon Cytokine Res 2001;21(4):257–263.
85. Chang AE, Li Q, Jiang G, Sayre DM, Braun TM, Redman BG. Phase II trial of autologous tumor vaccination, anti-CD3–activated vaccine-primed lymphocytes, and interleukin-2 in stage IV renal cell cancer. J Clin Oncol 2003;21(5):884–890.
86. Rosenberg SA, Spiess P, Lafreniere R. A new approach to the adoptive immunotherapy of cancer with tumor-infiltrating lymphocytes. Science 1986;233(4770):1318–1321.
87. Rini BI, Vogelzang NJ, Dumas MC, Wade JL 3rd, Taber DA, Stadler WM. Phase II trial of weekly intravenous gemcitabine with continuous infusion fluorouracil in patients with metastatic renal cell cancer. J Clin Oncol 2000;18(12):2419–2426.
88. Motzer RJ, Rini BI, Michaelson MD, et al. SU011248, a novel tyrosine kinase inhibitor, shows antitumor activity in second-line therapy for patients with metastatic renal cell carcinoma: Results of a phase 2 trial 2004 ASCO Annual Meeting.
89. Motzer RJ, Mazumdar M, Bacik J, Berg W, Amsterdam A, Ferrara J. Survival and prognostic stratification of 670 patients with advanced renal cell carcinoma. J Clin Oncol 1999;17(8):2530–2540.
90. Hirota T, Tomida T, Iwasa M, Takahashi K, Kaneda M, Tamaki H. Solitary pancreatic metastasis occurring eight years after nephrectomy for renal cell carcinoma. A case report and surgical review. Int J Pancreatol 1996;19(2):145–153.

29 Intracranial Renal Cell Cancer Metastasis

Kene Ugokwe and Steven A. Toms

KEYWORDS

BRAIN TUMOR
SURGERY
RADIOSURGERY
RADIATION THERAPY

ABSTRACT

Metastasis to the brain occurs in 5–10% of patients with renal cell carcinoma. Patients often present with localizing neurological signs or seizures. Increasingly, however, asymptomatic metastases are detected as oncologists are ordering more screening magnetic resonance and computed tomographic scans in renal cell carcinoma patients. The treatment for brain metastases from renal cell carcinoma includes whole brain radiation therapy, stereotactic radiosurgery, and surgical resection. Aggressive local treatment of renal cell carcinoma metastasis typically produces long periods of palliation if systemic disease can be controlled.

Renal cell carcinoma (RCC) accounts for 90% of all primary kidney tumors, with over 36,000 cases in the United States each year.[1,2] Brain metastasis is the most frequent type of intracranial tumor, and occurs in 4% to 17% of patients with RCC.[2–9] Greater than 50% of patients with RCC metastases to the brain develop multiple lesions.[3–6,8–10] As systemic therapies for extracranial RCC improve and intracranial imaging becomes more frequent for cancer patients, it is likely that the incidence of intracranial metastases will increase.[11]

PATHOPHYSIOLOGY OF INTRACRANIAL METASTASIS

Intracranial metastases of RCC typically occur by the hematogenous spread of tumor cells. In metastasis to the skull or dura, tumor cells may embolize directly to capillary

From: *Clinical Management of Renal Tumors*
Edited by: R.M. Bukowski and A.C. Novick © Humana Press Inc., Totowa, NJ

vessels and begin growth within these tissues. Within the central nervous system (CNS), however, there is a blood–brain barrier and blood–cerebrospinal fluid (CSF) barrier formed by the pericytes and astrocytes around the endothelial cells. These extra basement membrane layers must be crossed before RCC cells can escape the capillary bed and begin their growth.

After a metastatic cell arrests in the capillary bed and tumor growth begins, neoangiogenesis occurs and a tumor vascular network is established. Initially, local endothelial cells are recruited to begin development of the tumor vascular network. To develop metastases greater than 2 to 3 mm in size, circulating endothelial precursor cells are recruited from the bone marrow as the metastases mature, and a vascular network is developed.[12]

In these vascular networks, the blood–brain barrier may be incompletely formed. The new tumor blood vessels are permeable, and there is often extensive vasogenic edema. It is thought that the edema is secondary to vascular endothelial growth factor (VEGF) and other vasoactive peptides, causing vascular permeability in these lesions.[13,14] Largely a result of the intracranial artery's relative sizes and blood flows, RCC metastases are most commonly found in the cerebral hemispheres (80% to 85%). Next most common are the cerebellum (10% to 15%), brainstem (3% to 5%), and spinal cord parenchyma (<1%).[15–17] Cortical hemispheric metastases are most commonly deposited at the junction of the gray and white matter. This is thought to be secondary to the change in vessel caliber as blood begins to leave the metabolically active gray matter and penetrate into the relatively hypometabolic deep cerebral white matter. It has also been noted that metastases tend to respect vascular territories, occurring more frequently in the higher flow middle cerebral artery territories, especially at watershed zones with other vascular distributions.[17,18] Approximately 50% to 60% of parenchymal metastases are multiple upon clinical presentation.[17,18] Microscopically, these tumors are well circumscribed, rarely infiltrating normal neuronal elements more than 5 mm beyond the tumor–brain interface.[7] The lack of invasion of neural tissues has important therapeutic implications and sharply distinguishes secondary (metastatic) tumors from the invasive primary (glial) tumors.

CLINICAL PRESENTATION

The clinical presentation of intracranial RCC metastasis is largely dependent on the region of the intracranial compartment to which the tumor has metastasized as well as the overall tumor burden. Symptoms may be nonlocalizing secondary to increased intracranial pressure or localizing secondary to focal mass effect upon or invasion of eloquent neurologic structures. A sudden onset of headache and focal neurologic deficit may herald an intracranial hemorrhage (ICH) from an RCC metastasis. It is unknown exactly how often intracranial RCC metastases present with ICH.[19]

Nonlocalizing symptoms may include headache, nausea, vomiting, short-term memory lapses, alteration in the level of consciousness, or other changes in mental status. Such symptoms are most common when there are multiple metastases, carcinomatous meningitis, or hydrocephalus causing focal obstruction of CSF circulation. Generalized seizures may occur secondary to metabolic abnormalities from systemic cancer.

Local pain or mass may occur with skull lesions. Cranial nerve palsies may occur with carcinomatous meningitis or a skull base metastases. Focal neurologic signs may also lead to the detection of intracranial metastasis. Focal seizures, hemiparesis, aphasia, or other focal neurologic signs are common with dural-based or intraparenchymal metastases.[15,20–22]

IMAGING CHARACTERISTICS OF INTRACRANIAL RENAL CELL CARCINOMA

The diagnosis of intracranial metastasis is most often confirmed with computed tomography (CT) or magnetic resonance imaging (MRI) (Figure 29.1). The most sensitive of these studies is the gadolinium-enhanced MRI. However, it is important to remember that all enhancing lesions on MRI in patients with known diagnosis of RCC are not metastatic tumor. Up to 11% of intracranial lesions in patients with systemic cancer were not metastatic tumor.[23] A second tumor, such as a meningioma or glioma, may mimic the imaging characteristics of intracranial metastasis. Intracerebral abscess is occasionally found in patients with systemic cancer, and it has imaging characteristics similar to metastases. Although tissue diagnosis remains the gold standard, it is not always necessary before treatment is initiated in a patient with known RCC.

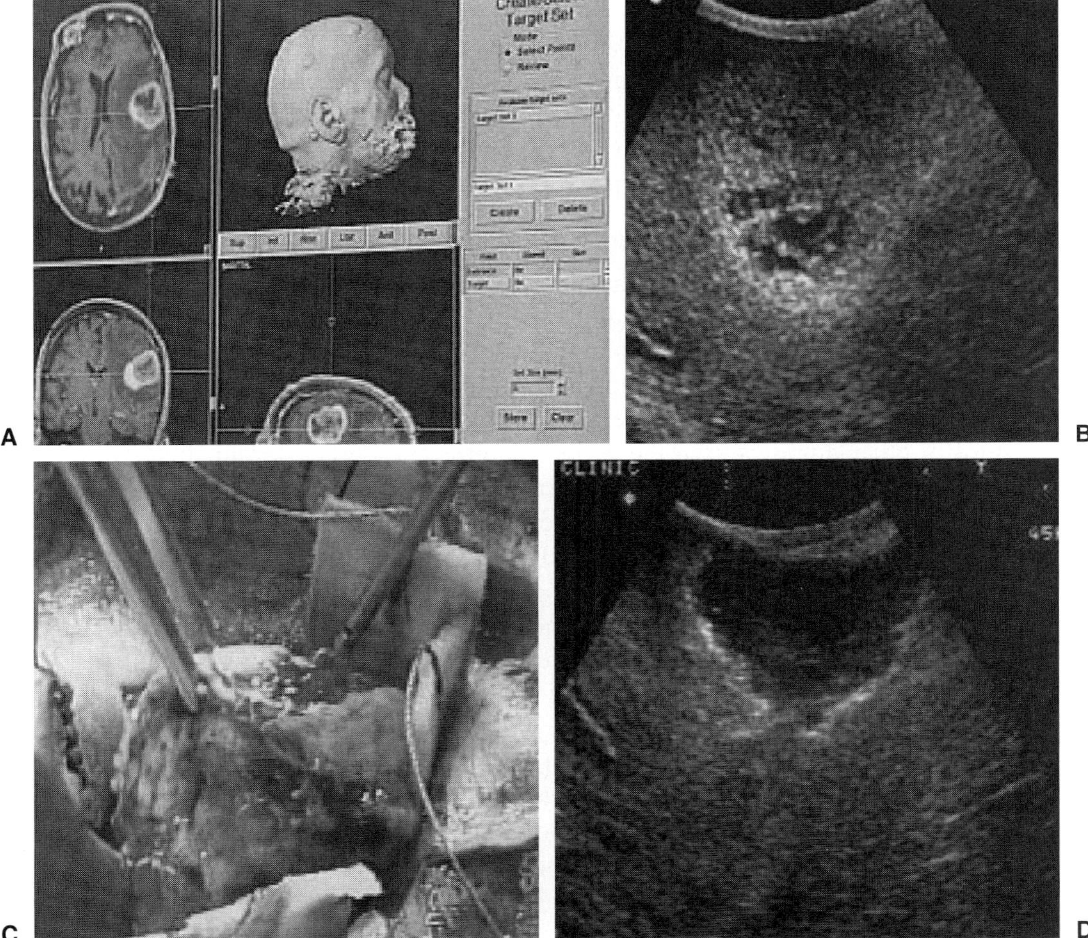

Figure 29.1. Imaging and surgical esection of RCC brain metastasis. A T1-weighted image with gadolinium used for surgical planning shows a large left frontal metastasis (**A**). Intr-operative ultrasound demonstrates and echogenic lesion prior to removal (**B**) and an anechoic cavity after its resection *en bloc* (**C**). (**D**) Postoperative ultrasound demonstrating complete surgical resection.

Skull lesions may be incidentally found on bone scans. More detailed evaluation with a CT or MRI is indicated only when a clinical sign or symptom is present. For many bony lesions, CT is superior in terms of identifying the destruction caused by lytic lesions. Although leptomeningeal spread of RCC is most commonly seen on MRI as abnormal linear dural enhancement, the only imaging finding may be enlargement of the ventricles secondary to hydrocephalus. Other times, the abnormal pial enhancement or focal enlargement of regions such as the cavernous sinus are the MRI hallmarks of leptomeningeal disease. Rarely, RCC may metastasize to regions such as the pituitary gland or the choroid plexus. Finally, RCC metastases often exhibit flow voids on MRI secondary to the vascularity and high blood flow within these lesions.[24]

Intracranial RCC may present with intracranial hemorrhage on some occasions as previously stated. Hemorrhages appear hyperdense on CT scans and may be identified immediately, whereas MRI may not identify hemorrhages within the first 48 hours. However, the CT is not as sensitive as MRI in detecting brain metastases. When a lesion (or lesions) is identified on CT, MRI is warranted prior to the initiation of treatment; MRI detects multiple metastatic lesions in approximately 20% of cases where only a single lesion is evident on CT scan.[25] On MRI, metastatic RCC is typically iso- to hypointense on T1-weighted images and iso- to hyperintense on T2. Intracranial renal cell disease enhances with contrast on both CT and MRI and is often surrounded by vasogenic edema.

TREATMENT

Symptom Management

The first stage of treatment for patients with intracranial metastasis is to address the symptoms that led to diagnosis. Often this involves treatment of increased intracranial pressure caused by the mass lesions and the reduction of vasogenic edema through the administration of corticosteroids. In most cases, these therapies are enough to stabilize a patient. Larger masses or more extensive swelling may require the administration of mannitol or other diuretics until the antiedema effect of corticosteroids begun. In the rare case of herniation secondary to intracranial mass, intubation, hyperventilation, or surgical intervention may be required. Untreated brain metastasis has a median survival of 1 month.[26] The addition of corticosteroids increases median survival to 2 months in the absence of other specific therapy.[27]

The use of antiepileptic drugs has been the source of much controversy. In guidelines recently developed by the American Academy of Neurology, the prophylactic use of anticonvulsant medications in patients with brain tumors was discouraged.[28] If patients present with seizures, anticonvulsant therapy, most commonly with diphenylhydantoin, is required. Refractory seizures or adverse reactions to diphenylhydantoin may require the use of other anticonvulsants. Unfortunately, many chemotherapies alter the binding and metabolism of anticonvulsant medications, and frequent monitoring of drug levels is required. Similarly, the metabolism of chemotherapeutics is often altered by antiepileptic drugs, which induce the cytochrome P-450 enzyme systems of the liver. Consequently, effective blood levels of chemotherapy as low as one-fourth the intended dose may be found in patients on chemotherapy taking antiepileptic drugs. As a result, newer generation anticonvulsants, which do not induce the cytochrome P-450 enzymes in the liver, such as valproate, gabapentin, lamotrigine, topiramate, levetiracetam, and zonisamide, should be the antiepileptic drugs of choice in brain metastasis patients who are anticipating chemotherapy.[29]

Specific Treatment Options

Treatment options in patients with metastatic intracranial RCC include surgical resection, stereotactic radiosurgery, and whole-brain radiation therapy. Survival is usually less than 3 months in the absence of treatment. Whole-brain radiation therapy may extend survival to between 3 and 6 months.[30–32] More aggressive treatment, including surgical resection or stereotactic radiosurgery with additional chemotherapy, is appropriate for patients with well-controlled systemic disease.

Gaspar et al.[33] analyzed the survival of 1200 brain metastasis patients from three consecutive Radiation Therapy Oncology Group (RTOG) trials between 1979 and 1993. They analyzed 18 pretreatment characteristics and three treatment-related variables using recursive-partitioning analysis (RPA) to create a regression tree according to prognostic significance. Three RPA classes were identified: RTOG-RPA class I patients had a Karnofsky performance score (KPS) of 70 or higher, were 65 years old or younger, and had controlled primary tumor with no extracranial metastasis; RTOG-RPA class II patients were 65 years old or older, had uncontrolled primary or extracranial metastasis, and had a KPS of 70 or higher; RTOG-RPA class III patients had a KPS of less than 70. The median survival times for RTOG-RPA classes I, II, and III were 7.1, 4.2 and 2.3 months, respectively.

WHOLE-BRAIN RADIOTHERAPY

Whole-brain radiotherapy (WBRT) has long been a mainstay in the treatment of intracranial metastases. Unfortunately, RCC is relatively radioresistant when compared to hematopoietic cancers and many other solid tumors. As a result, the benefits of fractionated radiotherapy for RCC are more modest than are seen for many of the more radiosensitive tumors.[34] Whole-brain radiotherapy is delivered via a linear accelerator where patients are immobilized with a plastic mask system.[34] As the term implies, the entire cranial contents are targeted with a dose of 30 to 45 Gy in 10 to 15 fractions over 2 to 3 weeks. In a study by Wronski et al.,[34] the mean survival after WBRT for intracranial renal cell carcinoma was 7.5 months, with a median survival of 3.3 months.

The toxicity associated with WBRT can be classified into three groups: (1) acute toxicity, which occurs within 6 weeks of radiation; (2) subacute toxicity, which is evident between 6 to 12 weeks after radiation; and (3) delayed toxicity. Acute toxicity includes nausea, vomiting, radiation dermatitis, alopecia, and worsening neurologic status as a result of peritumoral edema. The most troubling of these complications, the peritumoral edema, may usually be managed symptomatically with corticosteroid use. Subacute toxicity most often consists of a general neurologic deterioration, including changes in motivation, affect, and memory. As this may be difficult to distinguish from tumor progression, imaging may be necessary to rule out disease progression. Delayed toxicities include intellectual decline ranging from mild cognitive impairment to dementia,[35] as well as radiation necrosis.

Radiation necrosis often presents with headaches and neurologic decline. On MRI, contrast enhancement and surrounding edema make radiation necrosis difficult to distinguish from recurrent tumor. Functional imaging studies such as magnetic resonance spectroscopy (MRS) and positron emission tomography (PET) scanning may help distinguish tumor recurrence/progression from radiation necrosis.[32] The initial treatment for radiation necrosis includes steroid therapy, although surgical resection may be required for those cases not responsive to steroids or with progressive mass effect.[36]

If a patient is rapidly deteriorating due to progressive systemic disease or relapsed systemic disease with a poor performance status or poor RPA class, then WBRT may be an appropriate consideration. It is important to recognize, however, that WBRT offers only short-term palliation in patients with RCC metastases to the brain.

STEREOTACTIC RADIOSURGERY

Stereotactic radiosurgery (SRS) is a method of administering a high dose of ionizing radiation to a brain metastases or other lesion in a single-dose application. It is sometimes referred to as "knifeless surgery" secondary to its ability to ablate targeted tissues with high doses of radiation without the need for a skull incision. In SRS, a head frame is affixed to the patient's skull followed by CT and MRI imaging. The head frame has N-shaped bars attached to a base, which employs a Cartesian coordinate system so that objects within the frame may be localized mathematically, and targeted with irradiation. The images from CT and MRI of patients with frames attached are imported into a computer where the lesions to be targeted are outlined.

Computer modeling is used to optimize dosimetry and complete treatment planning. Metastatic lesions are typically treated with a dose of 24 Gy if they are less than 2 cm in diameter. Lesions 2 to 3 cm in size are treated with 18 Gy, and lesions greater than 3 cm with 15 Gy. These doses are based on the RTOG and are designed to minimize neurologic toxicity by avoiding high doses of radiation in a single shot over a large field.[33] As one might expect, smaller lesions respond somewhat better, given the smaller dimensions and the higher dose (Cleveland Clinic, unpublished data). In dose planning, attempts are made to avoid dosing critical structures such as the brainstem and optic nerves with greater than 8 Gy in a single dose.

Stereotactic radiosurgery techniques were built on the foundations of surgical stereotaxy, as envisioned by the neurosurgeons Horsley and Clarke, the fathers of stereotaxy. Stereotaxy is defined as the localization of a specific point in space using three-dimensional coordinates.[37] In 1951, Lars Leksell,[38] a Swedish neurosurgeon, combined stereotactic techniques with a radiotherapeutic modality and developed the technique of stereotactic radiosurgery. Leksell's investigation of SRS led to the development of the Gamma Knife™ unit (Elekta, Stockholm, Sweden), which employs 201 separate cobalt-60 sources focused on a single point (Figure 29.2). The focal distance from the radiation source to the target is fixed at 40.3 cm. Collimator helmets of various sizes (4, 8, 14, and 18 mm)[39] allow treatment of lesions up to 4 cm in diameter. The helmets dock with the patient's head frame, allowing the precise delivery of spherical "shots" of radiation to the target and a highly conformed treatment plan.

Stereotactic radiosurgery may also be administered using a linear accelerator (LINAC). In LINAC-based radiosurgery, multiple arcs of photon beams are delivered as the LINAC pivots around the patient. The intersection of these arcs defines areas where the dose is concentrated and represents the technique for treating lesions with LINAC-based radiosurgery. Current LINAC-based systems use nondynamic techniques in which the patient's couch is set at an angle and the arc is moved so that its radius delivers radiation that enters the skull through many different points.[40] Newer systems

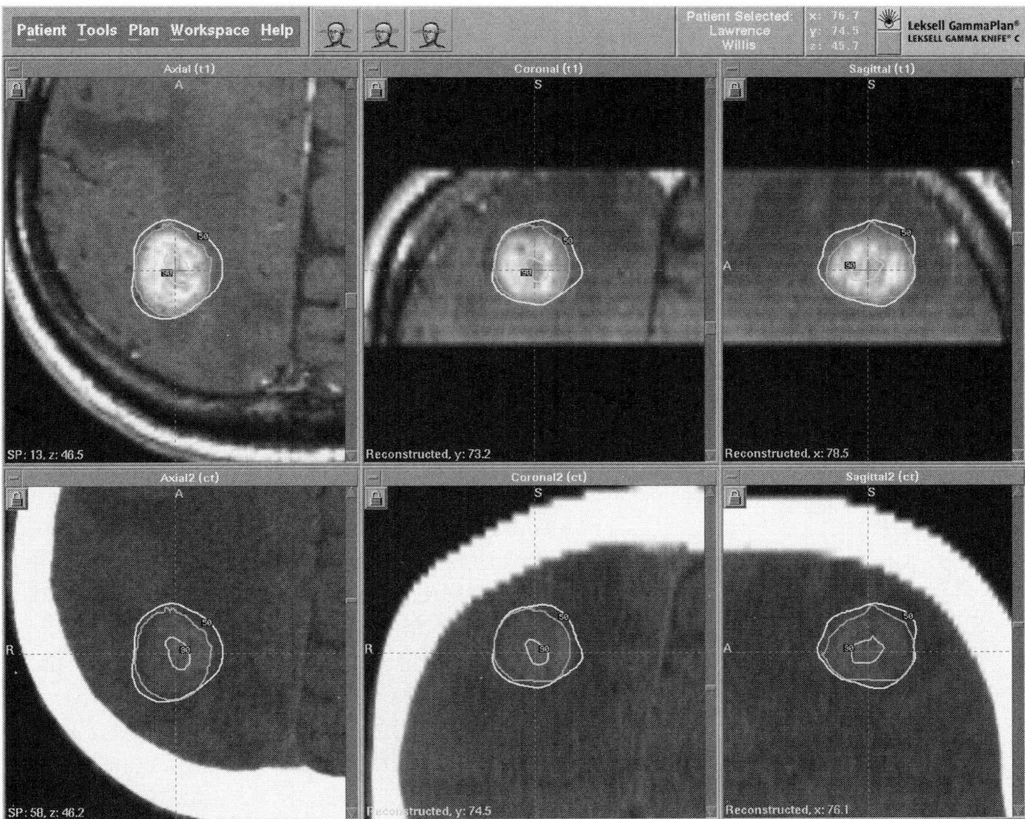

Figure 29.2. Dosimetry lines are shown on a Gamma Knife™ treatment plan correlated with the MRI (above) and CT scan (below) for a right parietal RCC brain metastasis. Note the tight conformity of the planned dose (white outer line around the lesion) when compared to the lesion itself (inner circle).

with dynamically adjustable mini-multileaf collimators, such as the Novalis™ unit (BrainLAB AG, Feldkirchen, Germany), may further improve the conformality in LINAC-based SRS.

Other stereotactic radiosurgery systems include the Cyberknife™ (Accuracy, Sunny-vale, CA), which incorporates a compact, lightweight linear accelerator mounted on a robotic arm. The Cyberknife gives the physician increased flexibility in targeting and can be used anywhere in the body where radiation treatment is indicated. The Cyberknife uses image guidance to track the target throughout treatment, and the system repeatedly confirms target location in relationship to skeletal structure by processing radiographic images and correlating them to previously obtained CT scans.[41] As a result, patients do not need a frame and instead wear a flexible mesh mask to limit large movements.[41]

The Novalis™ shaped beam surgery system is the latest radiosurgery and radiother-apy tool. Novalis is designed to treat a wider range of tumor sites including the brain, spinal cord, lung, kidney, and liver.[42] The Novalis system uses a multileaf collimator that can change shape around the lesions during radiation therapy, therefore producing more conformal radiotherapy.[43] Although Cyberknife and Novalis may be used in single-shot SRS with a head frame, the ability to use these devices without a fixed head frame makes them ideal for stereotactic radiotherapy. In stereotactic radiotherapy treatments, larger lesions (>4 cm) or lesions adjacent to critical neural structures such as the optic chiasm are treated in three to five dose fractions to allow for the recovery of normal neurologic tissue and increased dose intensity to the lesion than can be given with more traditional radiotherapy dose planning techniques.

Compared to WBRT or symptomatic treatment alone, SRS markedly improves survival in RCC metastasis to the brain. Median survival of 11 to 15 months may be expected with local control of treated lesions around 95% within 1 year of SRS.[15,44,45] In patients with brain metastasis, two thirds of treated patients die from systemic progression, whereas only 15% die from intracranial disease progression in the absence of systemic disease progression.[41] In the final 15% to 20% of patients, therapy fails and they die from a combination of both systemic progression and new intracranial lesions.

SURGICAL TREATMENT

Despite the success of stereotactic radiosurgery and the attractiveness of less invasive treatment of brain metastases, open surgical resection remains the treatment of choice in some cases of intracranial RCC metastasis. When lesions are greater than 3 cm in diameter, are causing intractable seizures, or when tumor mass or edema is causing neurologic deficit, surgical resection may be the treatment of choice in patients with a good RPA class. Open surgical resection provides immediate resolution of mass effect; it provides tissue for pathologic diagnosis and reduces steroid dependence by more rapidly reducing peritumoral edema. Surgery becomes a less attractive option when the tumor is smaller or located more deeply within the brain. Lesions less than 7 mm in size, and lesions located in the deep gray matter or the brainstem are often better treated with SRS. Similarly, SRS may be preferred in elderly patients with multiple medical problems who are often poor surgical risks.

A randomized study by Patchell et al.,[46] comparing the results of surgical excision followed by WBRT versus WBRT alone in patients with solitary lesions showed that better results were obtained with the combination of surgery and WBRT. Bindal et al.[47] conducted a retrospective study that showed that patients with multiple brain metastases with limited systemic disease and in whom all lesions are accessible should have all lesions surgically removed since this can significantly improve their length and quality of life. Bindal et al.[48] showed that reoperation for recurrent metastasis can prolong survival and improve quality of life. In considering SRS or surgery for a patient with a recurrent brain metastasis from RCC, a calculus similar to that for a newly diagnosed patient should be performed. Restaging and assessment of the patient's remaining treatment options allows the selection of patients with well-controlled systemic disease and a life expectancy of greater than 6 months for further surgical or SRS interventions.

In circumstances when an intracranial metastatic lesion leads to an intracranial hemorrhage, evacuation of the hemorrhage and resection of the tumor may be performed simultaneously. Secondary to the ability of an intracranial hemorrhage to spread tumor cells throughout the hematoma cavity, some form of radiotherapy is advisable after evacuation of an intracranial hemorrhage in an RCC patient in order to prevent local recurrence.

In the early 20th century, Harvey Cushing[49] found that mortality after the resection of brain metastasis was 38%.[49] Today, with the advent of modern surgical techniques, surgical morbidity and mortalities of 3% or less are expected.[48,50,51] Improvements in neuroanesthetic and surgical techniques including computer-assisted stereotactic navigation, intraoperative ultrasound, and intraoperative MRI have led to safer, more complete resections for metastatic disease. Patient survival after surgical resection and WBRT is comparable to that of stereotactic radiosurgery, usually 10 to 14 months.[46,47,52]

As WBRT is associated with some acute and chronic toxicity, efforts are underway to study whether local radiotherapy to the tumor bed might provide similar local control while diminishing radiation-associated side effects. Trials are currently under way investigating intraoperative radiotherapy delivered with a miniature LINAC, as well as an intracavitary brachytherapy balloon—the Gliasite™ (Cytyc Surgical Products, Marlborough, MA) system. The Gliasite balloon is loaded after surgery with a liquid iodine-125 source for 3 to 7 days prior to its removal. Finally, in those for whom further radiation therapy is contraindicated, intracavitary chemotherapy with bischloroethylnitrosourea (BCNU)-containing wafers placed to line the surgical cavity (Gliadel™ wafers, MGI Pharma, Bloomington, MN) may offer prolonged local control and is currently under evaluation in phase II trial.

Chemotherapy for Treatment of Intracranial Renal Cell Carcinoma

Although chemotherapy has been used with modest success in other metastatic cancers to the CNS, there is little data to support the efficacy of cytotoxic therapy for intracranial RCC. In addition to the difficulty of finding agents with activity against RCC, the blood–brain barrier presents both a physical and physiologic barrier, which excludes larger molecules and water-soluble agents from entry into the brain.[53] Designed to maintain the microenvironment necessary for neural homeostasis, endothelial tight junctions, pericytes, astrocytic foot processes, and a series of energy-dependent systems all contribute to the blood–brain barrier. To get therapeutic agents into the CNS, chemotherapy may be administered intraarterially with osmotic blood–brain barrier disruption. This technique increases drug concentrations and may minimize toxicities associated with systemic drug administration, although there is little data regarding its efficacy in the treatment of intracranial RCC metastases.

Metastatic renal cell cancers may respond to interferon-α (IFN-α), although the response to IFN-α is not as pronounced in intracranial lesions.[54,55] Despite dramatic results in some patients, only about 20% of all patients with metastatic RCC who receive immunotherapy experience tumor remission.[56] Although there is one case of complete response of brain metastases from renal cell cancer to IFN-α,[57] the largest series of IFN-α therapy did not report any responders in the CNS.[54] There is one small series reporting interleukin-2 (IL-2) success in a patient with intracranial RCC.[58] The effects of the new tyrosine-based inhibitors sunitinib and sorafenib on intracranial lesions is unknown. It is also unclear whether these new approaches will delay or decrease the development of CNS metastases from RCC.

THE EVALUATION OF A PATIENT WITH NO KNOWN PRIMARY

It is likely that fewer than 10% of patients with RCC present with an intracranial lesion as the first sign of cancer. A patient presenting with a solitary brain lesion consistent with metastasis needs further imaging. Most commonly, CT of the chest, abdomen, and pelvis are the diagnostic procedures of choice, although PET may be more sensitive in the detection of small lesions.[59]

Often, tissue diagnosis may be obtained from extracranial lesions. If no extracranial lesions are identified, the brain lesion may provide the only available source for tissue diagnosis. If the patient has a good performance status and the lesion is resectable, then all attempts should be made to remove it. If the lesion is in the brainstem or a deep gray nucleus, the risk/benefit analysis may favor biopsy. The patient whose first presentation is with multiple intracranial lesions presents with a different calculus. Although many patients with two or three intracranial metastases can be managed as efficiently as those with a solitary lesion, multiple intracranial metastases more often portend widespread systemic disease. Fortunately, there are few occasions in which an RCC cancer will present primarily with multiple intracranial metastases. However, if no systemic site of disease presents itself after a thorough evaluation, then tissue diagnosis via biopsy may still be necessary. If all lesions are treatable with surgery or SRS, either of these modalities (or a combination of them) may be the preferred treatment.

EXTRAPARENCHYMAL LOCATIONS

Skull and Venous Sinus

Metastatic skull lesions are often asymptomatic and present as a painless mass (Figure 29.3A). Metastasis to the paranasal sinuses may present as nasal obstruction and epistaxis.[61] Orbital lesions may present with visual loss or proptosis. Lesions of the

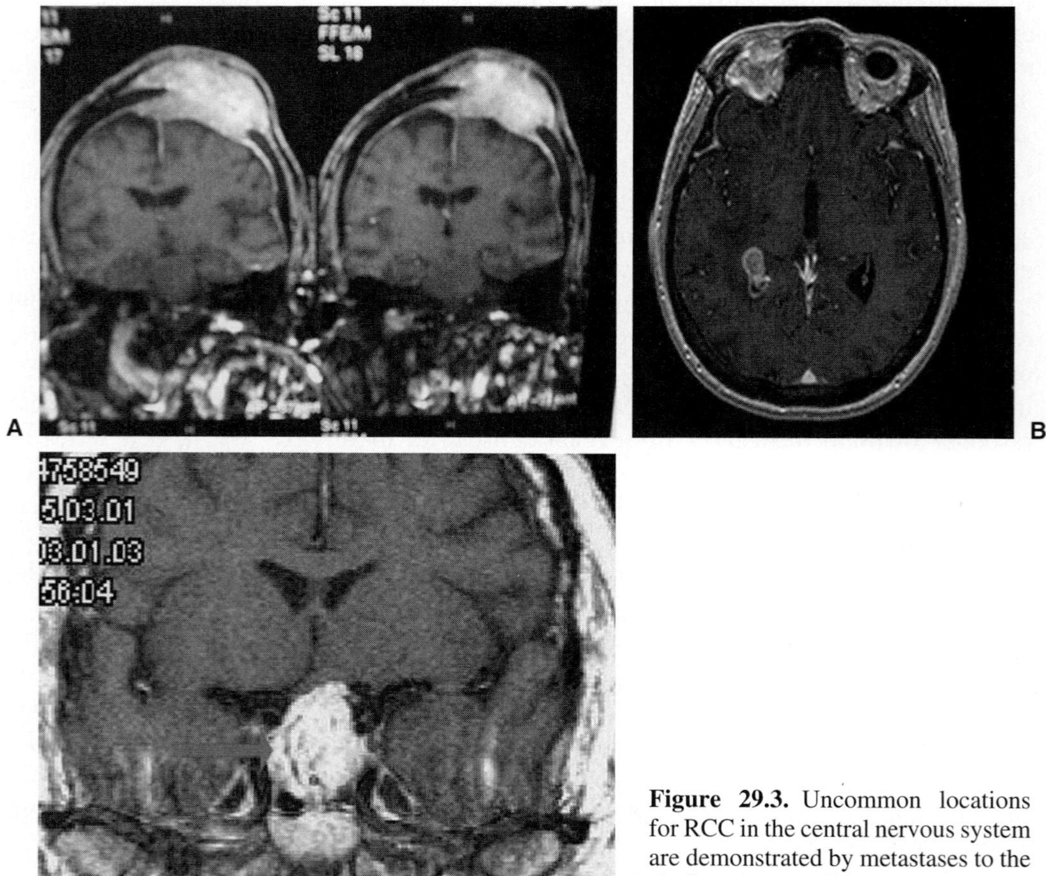

Figure 29.3. Uncommon locations for RCC in the central nervous system are demonstrated by metastases to the skull and dura (**A**), choroid plexus (**B**), and the pituitary gland (**C**).

middle posterior fossa may present with lower cranial nerve palsies. As bony metastases are most often confined by the dura, these lesions are outside the blood–brain barrier. The most common indications for surgical intervention are pain, epistaxis, visual loss or neural compression.

En bloc resections of these lesions may be achieved with little morbidity, and local recurrences are rare. Although morbidity is low for most extradural lesions, those involving venous sinuses increase the likelihood of venous infarction. These lesions can also be removed successfully with careful surgical planning including angiography. Smaller lesions may often be treated with stereotactic radiosurgery or stereotactic radiotherapy.

Choroid Plexus

Metastases to the choroid plexus are rare, but of those lesions reported, RCC metastases make up the plurality of these lesions (Figure 29.3B). There have been seven cases reported in the literature.[62] Most often incidentally discovered, large lesions may obstruct spinal fluid outflow within the ventricle causing hydrocephalus. These patients may present with headache, nausea, vomiting, or obstruction and may require urgent intervention with ventriculostomy to decompress the ventricular system. Small lesions may be successfully treated with stereotactic radiosurgery.

Pituitary Gland

Although rare, RCC metastases to the pituitary gland have been reported, although they may be difficult to distinguish from a pituitary macroadenoma (Figure 29.3C). Flow voids visible on MRI are not typically found in macroadenomas. Visual loss from optic chiasm compression or diplopia from cavernous sinus invasion and cranial nerve involvement may be presenting signs. Metastatic renal cell carcinoma to the pituitary may also present with hyperprolactinemia.[62] Although successful transsphenoidal resections have been reported, piecemeal resection may be difficult secondary to the vascularity of these lesions.[64] Therefore, stereotactic radiosurgery or radiotherapeutic approaches are most often used for palliation.[64]

Leptomeningeal Disease

Leptomeningeal disease refers to the spread of cancer to the subarachnoid space and cerebrospinal fluid.[65] Most patients with leptomeningeal disease have disseminated cancer at the time of diagnosis.[66] As a result, leptomeningeal disease carries an extremely poor prognosis, with an average survival of 1 to 2 months after diagnosis.[67]

Patients with leptomeningeal disease may present with headaches, nausea, and vomiting secondary to hydrocephalus from CSF outflow obstruction. Cranial nerve palsies, especially those causing diplopia, are also common presenting symptoms. Rarely, leptomeningeal disease presents with back pain, cervical or lumbar radiculopathy presenting secondary to tumor involvement along the spinal dura or nerve roots.

The diagnosis may be confirmed by contrast-enhanced MRI of the brain or spine, which typically shows pial or dural linear enhancement. On some occasions, nodular or bulky lesions in the subarachnoid space are seen on these imaging studies. If imaging is negative, then high volume lumbar puncture for cytology should be performed to confirm the diagnosis. In situations where patients have hydrocephalus, the placement of a venticuloperitoneal shunt may help alleviate their symptoms. However, given the poor prognosis and lack of proper treatment for RCC with leptomeningeal disease, consideration should be given to hospice referral prior to any intervention. On-off valves may be placed in the shunt systems to allow treatment with intrathecal chemotherapy or immunotherapy. Ommaya reservoirs may be placed into the ventricles as conduits for the administration of intrathecal chemotherapy. The most commonly used intrathecal chemotherapy agents include methotrexate, cytarabine, liposomal cytarabine, and thiotepa. Unfortunately, these agents have had little success against RCC systemically and would not be expected to have much activity when administered intrathecally.

Monoclonal antibodies coupled with protein toxins are being used to target tumor surface antigens and may prove useful in the treatment of leptomeningeal disease.[68,69] Since the subarachnoid space may serve as an immunologic sanctuary for tumor cells, several investigators have studied intrathecal delivery of cytokines for leptomeningeal disease. Although no specific trials for RCC leptomeningeal disease have been conducted, melanoma and squamous cell carcinoma have been treated with IL-2 alone or combined with lymphokine-activated killer (LAK) cells, with some response reported.[70]

CONCLUSION

Advances in the surgical and radiosurgical management of metastatic disease have led to marked improvements in both the length and quality of life in patients with intracranial metastases from RCC. Patients with fewer lesions and well-controlled systemic disease are candidates for more aggressive intervention with stereotactic radiosurgery or surgery. Palliative WBRT should be reserved for those patients with advanced or poorly controlled systemic disease.

REFERENCES

1. Landis SH, Murray T, Bolden S, et al. Cancer statistics, 1998. CA Cancer J Clin 1998;48:6–29.
2. Bennington JL. Cancer of the kidney: etiology, epidemiology and pathology. Cancer 1973;32: 1017–1029.
3. Fujimi M, Akaza H, Yoshida M, et al. [Cerebellar metastasis from renal cell carcinoma.] Nippon Hinyokika Gakkai Zasshi 1986;77:1164–1168. (Jpn)
4. Gay PC, Litchy WJ, Cascino TL. Brain metastasis in hypernephroma. J Neurooncol 1987;5:51–56.
5. Marshall ME, Pearson T, Simpson W, et al. Low incidence of asymptomatic brain metastasis in patients with renal cell carcinoma. Urology 1990;36:300–302.
6. Masuda F, Arai Y, Ohnishi T, et al. [Brain metastasis from renal cell carcinoma.] Nippon Hinyokika Gakkai Zasshi 1984;75:278–282 (Japanese).
7. Sawaya R, Bindal RK, Lang FF, et al. Metastatic brain tumors. In: Kaye AH, Laws ER, eds. Brain Tumors: An Encyclopedic Approach, 2nd ed. Edinburgh: Churchill Livingstone, 2001: 999–1026.
8. Shibui S, Nishikawa R, Nomura K. [Treatment for metastatic brain tumors from renal cell carcinoma.] No Shinkei Geka 1990;18:935–938 (Japanese).
9. Yonese J, Kawakami S, Ueda T, et al. Clinical study of renal cell carcinoma with brain metastasis. Nippon Hinyokika Gakkai Zasshi 1995;86:1287–1293.
10. Arbit E, Wronski M. Clinical decision making in brain metastasis. Neurosurg Clin North Am 1996;7:447–457.
11. Posner JB. Management of brain metastases. Rev Neurol 1992;148:477–487.

12. Lyden D, Hattori K, Dias S, et al. Impaired recruitment of bone-marrow derived endothelial and hematopoietic precursor cells blocks tumor angiogenesis and growth. Nat Med 2001;7(11): 1194–1201.
13. Ludwig HC, Akhavan-Shigari R, Rausch S, et al. Expression of focal adhesion kinase (p125 FAK) and proline rich tyrosine kinase 2 (PYK2/CAKb) in cerebral metastasis, correlation with VEGF-R-, ecNOSIII labeling and morphometric data. Anticancer Res 2000;20:1419–1424.
14. Strugar J, Rothbart D, Harrington W, et al. Vascular permeability factor in brain metastasis: correlation with vasogenic brain edema and tumor angiogenesis. J Neurosurg 1994;81:560–566.
15. Mori Y, Kondziolka D, Lunsford LD, Logan T, Flickinger J. Stereotactic radiosurgery for brain metastasis from renal cell carcinoma. Cancer 1998;83:344–353.
16. Perreti-Viton P, Margain D, Murayama N, et al. Brain metastases. J Neuroradiol 1991;18:161–172.
17. Ferrara N. The role of vascular endothelial growth factor in the regulation of blood vessel growth. In: Bicknell R, Lewis CE, Ferrara N, eds. Tumor Angiogenesis. New York: Oxford University Press, 1997:185–199.
18. Ferrara N, Carver-Moore K, Chen H, et al. Heterozygous embryonic lethality induced by targeted inactivation of the VEGF gene. Nature 1996;380:439–442.
19. Weisberg LA. Hemorrhagic metastatic neoplasms: Clinical computed tomographic correlations. Comput Radiol 1985;9(2):105–114.
20. Singh SK, Agris JM, Leeds NE, et al. Intracranial leptomeningeal metastases: comparison of depiction at FLAIR and contrast-enhanced MR imaging. Radiology 2000;217:50–53.
21. Ostergaard L, Sorensen AG, Kwong KK, et al. High-resolution measurement of cerebral blood flow using intravascular tracer bolus passages. Part II: experimental comparison and preliminary results. Magn Reson Med 1996;36:715–725.
22. Hazle JD, Jackson EF, Schomer DF, et al. Dynamic imaging of intracranial lesions using fast spin-echo imaging: differentiation of brain tumors and treatment effects. J Magn Reson Imaging 1997;7: 1084–1093.
23. Rock JP, Hearshen D, Scarpace L, et al. Correlations between magnetic resonance spectroscopy and image guided histopathology, with special attention to radiation necrosis. Neurosurgery 2002; 51(4):912–919.
24. Uchino A, Hasuo K, Mizushima A, et al. Intracranial metastasis of renal cell carcinoma: MR Imaging. Radiat Med 1996;14(2):71–76.
25. Mintz AP, Cairncross JG. Treatment of a single brain metastasis. The role of radiation following surgical excision. JAMA 1998;280:1527–1529.
26. Markesbery WR, Brooks WH, Gupta GD, et al. Treatment for patients with cerebral metastases. Arch Neurol 1978;35:754–756.
27. Ruderman NB, Hall TC. Use of glucocorticoids in the palliative treatment of metastatic brain tumors. Cancer 1965;18:298–306.
28. Glantz MJ, Cole BF, Forsyth PA, et al. Practice parameter: Anticonvulsant prophylaxis in patients with newly diagnosed brain tumors: Report of the quality standards subcommittee of the American Academy of Neurology. Neurology 2000;54(10):1886–1893.
29. El Kamar FG, Posner JB. Brain metastasis. Semin Neurol 2004;24:347–362.
30. Cairncross JG, Kim JH, Posner JB. Radiation therapy for brain metastases. Ann Neurol 1980;7: 529–541.
31. Kurtz JM, Gelber R, Brady LW, et al. The palliation of brain metastases in a favorable patient population: a randomized clinical trial by the Radiation Therapy Oncology Group. Int J Radiat Oncol Biol Phys 1981;7:891–895.
32. Patchell RA, Tibbs PA, Walsh JW, et al. A randomized trial of surgery in the treatment of single metastases to the brain. N Engl J Med 1990;322:494–500.
33. Gaspar L, et al. Recursive partitioning analysis (RPA) of prognostic factors in three Radiation Therapy Oncology Group (RTOG) brain metastases trials. Int J Radiat Oncol Biol Phys 1997;37: 745–751.
34. Wronski M, Maor MH, Davis BJ, et al. External radiation of brain metastasis from renal cell carcinoma: A retrospective study of 119 patients from the M.D. Anderson cancer center. Int J Radiat Oncol Biol Phys 1997;37:753–759.
35. Roman DD, Sperduto PW. Neuropsychological effects of cranial radiation: current knowledge and future directions. Int J Radiat Oncol Biol Phys 1995;31(4):983–998.

36. McPherson CM, Warnick RE. Results of contemporary surgical management of radiation necrosis using frameless stereotaxis and intraoperative magnetic resonance imaging. J Neuro-Oncol 2004;68(1):41–47.

37. Horsley V, Clarke RH. The structure and functions of the cerebellum examined by a new method. Brain 1908;31:45.

38. Leksell L. The stereotactic method and radiosurgery of the brain. Acta Chir Scand 1951;102: 316–319.

39. Witham TF, Kondziolka D. Gamma knife radiosurgery. In: Winn HR, ed. Youmans'Neurological Surgery, 5th ed, vol 4. Philadelphia: Saunders, 2004:4117–4121.

40. Lunsford LD, Niranjan A. Radiosurgery of tumors. In: Winn HR, ed. Youmans'Neurological Surgery, 5th ed. Philadelphia: Saunders 2003:4055.

41. Chang SD, Adler JR. Robotics and radiosurgery—the cyberknife. Stereotact Funct Neurosurg 2001;76(3–4):204–208.

42. Novalis. New cancer treatment technique available at the Cleveland Clinic, Department of Radiation Oncology. www.clevelandclinic.org/radonc/novalis.

43. Cheng CW, Wong JR, Ndlovu AM, et al. Dosimetric evaluation and clinical application of virtual mini multileaf collimator. Am J Clin Oncol 2003;26:37–44.

44. Varlotto JM, Fleckinger JC, Niranjan A, et al. Analysis of tumor control and toxicity in patients who have survived at least one year after radiosurgery for brain metastasis. Int J Radiat Oncol Biol Phys 2003;57:452–464.

45. Petrovich Z, Yu C, Gianotta SL, et al. Survival and pattern of failure in brain metastasis treated with gamma knife radiosurgery. J Neurosurg 2002;97(5 suppl):499–506.

46. Patchell RA, Cirrincione C, Thaler HT, et al. Single brain metastases: surgery plus radiation or radiation alone. Neurology 1986;36:447–453.

47. Bindal RK, Bindal BA, Sawaya R, et al. Surgical treatment of multiple brain metastases. J Neurosurg 1993;79:210–216.

48. Bindal RK, Sawaya R, Leavens ME, Hess KR, Taylor S. Reoperation for recurrent metastatic brain tumors. J Neurosurg 1995;83:600–604.

49. Cushing H. Notes Upon a Series of Two Thousand Verified Cases with Surgical-Mortality Percentages Pertaining Thereto. Springfield, IL: Charles C Thomas, 1932.

50. Brega K, Robinson WA, Winston K, et al. Surgical treatment of brain metastases of malignant melanoma. Cancer 1990;66:2105–2110.

51. Hammoud MA, McCutcheon IE, Elsouki R, et al. Colorectal carcinoma and brain metastases: Distribution, treatment and survival. Ann Surg Oncol 1996;3:453–463.

52. Wronski M, Arbit E, Russo P, Galicich JH. Surgical resection of brain metastasis from renal cell carcinoma in 50 patients. Urology 1996;47:187–193.

53. Grieg NH. Optimizing drug delivery to brain tumors. Cancer Treat Rev 1987;14:1–28.

54. Papadopoulus I, Rudolph P, Weichert-Jacobsen K, et al. Prognostic indicators for response to therapy and survival in patients with metastatic renal cell cancer treated with interferon α-2 β and vinblastine. Urology 1996;48:373–378.

55. Quesada JR, Swanson DA, Trinidade A, Gutterman JU. Renal cell carcinoma: antitumor effect of leukocyte interferon. Cancer Res 1983;43:940–947.

56. Schmitz-Drager BJ, Jankevicius F, Otto T. Prognostsche Faktoren zur Vorhersage des Erfolges einer Immuntherapie biem metastasierten Nierenzellkarzinom [Prognostic factors for predicting the success of immunotherapy in metastatic renal cell carcinoma]. Urologe [A] 1995;34:195–199.

57. Murata J, Sawamura Y, Terasaka S, et al. Complete response of a large brain metastasis of renal cell cancer to interferon-alpha: case report. Surg Neurol 1999;51:289–291.

58. Guirgus LM, Yang JC, White DE, et al. Safety and efficacy of high dose interleukin-2 therapy in patients with brain metastases. J Immunother 2002;25(1):82–87.

59. Nanni C, Rubello D, Castellucci P, et al. Role of (18)F-FDG PET-CT imaging for the detection of an unknown primary tumor: preliminary results in 21 patients. Eur J Nucl Med Mol Imaging 2005;32(5):589–592.

60. Som PM, Norton KI, Shugar JMA, et al. Metastatic hypernephroma to the head and neck. AJNR Am J Neuroradiol 1987;8:1103–1106.

61. Lauretti L, Fernandez E, Pallini R, et al. Long survival in an untreated solitary choroid plexus metastasis from renal cell carcinoma: case report and review of literature. J Neuro-Oncol 2005;71: 157–160.

62. Basaria S, Westra WH, Brem H, Salvatori R. Metastatic renal cell carcinoma to the pituitary presenting with hyperprolactinemia. J Endocrinol Invest 2004;27(5):471–474.
63. Marar IE, Kandil H, Kanal E, Marion D. Renal cell carcinoma metastatic to the pituitary gland: clinical manifestations and successful treatment with transsphenoidal resection. Endocr Pract 1998;4(4):204–207.
64. Yokoyama T, Yoshino A, Katayama K, et al. Metastatic pituitary tumor from renal cell carcinoma treated by fractionated stereotactic radiotherapy. Neurol Med Chir 2004;44:47–52.
65. Crino PB, Sater RA, Sperling M, et al. Renal cell carcinomatous meningitis: pathologic and immuno-histochemical features. Neurology 1995;45(1):189–191.
66. Kaplan JG, DeSouza TG, et al. Leptomeningeal metastasis: comparison of clinical features and laboratory data of solid tumors, lymphomas and leukemias. J Neuro-Oncol 1990;9:225–299.
67. Grossman SA, Krabak MJ. Leptomeningeal carcinomatosis. Cancer Treat Rev 1999;25(2):103–119.
68. Brown MT, Coleman RE, Friedman AH, et al. Intrathecal 131I-labeled antitenascin monoclonal antibody 81C6 treatment of patients with leptomeningeal neoplasms or primary brain tumor resection cavities with subarachnoid communication: phase I trial results. Clin Cancer Res 1996;2(6):963–972.
69. Kramer K, Cheung NK, Humm JL, et al. Targeted radioimmunotherapy for leptomeningeal cancer using (131)I-3F8. Med Pediatr Oncol 2000;35(6):716–718.
70. Moser R, Bruner JM, Grimm EA. Biologic therapy for brain tumors. Cancer Bull 1991;43:117–126.

30 Role of Radiation Therapy in Advanced Renal Cell Carcinoma

Arul Mahadevan

KEYWORDS

KIDNEY CANCER
ADVANCED DISEASE
RADIATION THERAPY
STEREOTACTIC RADIOSURGERY
STEREOTACTIC BODY RADIATION THERAPY

ABSTRACT

Renal cell cancer is an increasingly common tumor involving mostly adults. Surgical excision is the treatment of choice and recently surgical innovation has resulted in excellent outcomes for nephron sparing surgery. Energy based ablative procedures are being increasingly explored as an alternative to surgery to minimize morbidity. Radiation therapy has had relatively little role in the management of patients with renal cell cancer. Advances in the imaging, treatment planning and treatment delivery has made radiation treatments safer now than ever before. In advanced renal cell cancer, radiation therapy can play a role in the management of extensive disease in patient's with poor overall condition, adjuvant to surgical or other ablative procedures and in patients with metastatic disease.

Each year in the United States, there are approximately 36,160 cases of kidney and upper urinary tract cancer, resulting in more than 12,660 deaths.[1] These tumors account for approximately 3% of adult malignancies and occur in a male-female ratio of 1.5 : 1.0.[1] Although most cases of renal cell carcinoma (RCC) occur in persons aged 50 to 70 years, it has been observed in children as young as 6 months of age. Renal cell carcinoma incidence rates increased steadily between 1975 and 1995, by 2.3% annually among white men, 3.1% among white women, 3.9% among black men, and 4.3% among black women. Increases were greatest for localized tumors but were also seen for more advanced and unstaged tumors.[2]

Approximately 30% of patients with renal carcinoma present with metastatic disease, 25% with locally advanced renal carcinoma, and 45% with localized disease.[3] Some 75% of patients with metastatic RCC have metastases to the lung, 36% to soft tissues, 20% to bone, 18% to liver, 8% to cutaneous sites, and 8% to the central nervous system.[4]

From: *Clinical Management of Renal Tumors*
Edited by: R.M. Bukowski and A.C. Novick © Humana Press Inc., Totowa, NJ

Surgical resection is the only treatment modality with proven efficacy in curing patients with RCC.[5–8] Intrinsic resistance to radiation therapy (RT) and chemotherapy has long been a hallmark of renal cancer.[6,9] Radiation therapy has been administered to patients with RCC as an adjuvant to nephrectomy or to control metastatic disease.

This chapter summarizes the role of radiation therapy in the management of advanced RCC.

BIOLOGIC CHARACTERISTICS

Primary renal cell tumors may spread by local infiltration through the capsule to involve the perinephric fat and Gerota's fascia. The tumor may grow directly along the venous channels to the renal vein or vena cava. Lymph node metastases occur with an incidence of 9% to 27% and most often involve the renal hilar, paraaortic, and paracaval lymph nodes.[10] The renal vein is invaded in 21% of cases, and the inferior vena cava is invaded in as many as 4% of cases.

Prognostic factors for cancer of the kidney relate to tumor size, extension through the renal capsule, nodal involvement, and renal vein involvement. Other prognostic factors include histologic pattern and nuclear grade. Patients with tumor confined within the capsule achieved the highest 5- and 10-year survivals of 88% and 66%, respectively.[3] Survivals decreased as tumor invaded perirenal fat (67% and 35%) or regional lymph nodes (17% and 5%). Tumor invasion into the renal vein alone did not significantly change the 5-year survival (84%), but lowered the 10-year survival to 45%. Patients with metastases at the time of nephrectomy did poorly regardless of the site of metastases or kind of adjuvant therapy, except for those managed by surgical extirpation of the secondary lesion. Certain tumor characteristics were associated with a better prognosis, for example, size below 5 cm in diameter, lack of invasion of collecting system, perirenal fat or regional lymph nodes, and predominance of clear or granular cells growing into a recognizable histologic pattern.

The use of abdominal computed tomography (CT) and ultrasound for nonmalignant medical illnesses has increased the frequency of diagnosis of incidental RCCs. The 5-year cancer-specific survival rate was significantly higher for incidental than for symptomatic tumors (85.3% vs. 62.5%). Likewise, the local and distal recurrence rates were higher for symptomatic lesions.[11]

Table 30.1 summarizes the 5-year survival rates for patients undergoing surgery for RCC.

An understanding of the patterns of failure after surgical management is essential to determine the value of any potential adjuvant treatment. A review of the literature

Table 30.1.
Stage of renal cell carcinoma and survival

			5-year survival (%)			
First author	*Year*	*No. of patients*	*I*	*II*	*III*	*IV*
Golimbu[3]	1986	326	88	67	40	2
Dinney[54]	1992	314	73	68	51	20
Guinan[55]	1997	337	100	96	59	16
Javidan[56]	1999	381	95	88	59	20
Tsui[57]	2000	643	91	74	67	32

reveals a local failure rate of approximately 5% to 10% after partial nephrectomy or radical nephrectomy.[12–16] The actuarial local failure was only 5% at 7 years among the 172 surgically treated patients from the Memorial Sloan-Kettering series.[12] Univariate analysis found local failure significantly increased in the presence of either lymph node involvement (21% vs. 4%, $p = 0.0002$) or positive margins (21% vs. 4%, $p = 0.002$). Recurrence was local only in 4%, and local and at distant metastatic sites in 6.5%, in a series of 107 patients undergoing partial nephrectomy from the Cleveland Clinic.[15]

PRECLINICAL DATA

Irradiation of human RCC before radical tumor nephrectomy resulted in a significantly lower acceptance rate (one of seven) in nude mice than for nonirradiated tumors (all of 13).[17] This, at least theoretically, supports the use of preoperative radiation to decrease implantation of tumor at the time of surgery.

Monoclonal antibody (MAB)-targeted radiotherapy studies were performed to evaluate the feasibility of using tumor-preferential MAB as targeting agents for internal radiotherapy of RCC using a nude mouse model.[18] Monoclonal antibody labeled with iodine 131 caused the tumor to regress or arrested the tumor growth, whereas similar doses of unlabeled MAB did not inhibit tumor growth.

In a study involving in vitro x-ray radiation, survival characteristics of 181 lines from 12 different classes of exponentially growing human tumor cells were studied.[19] Survival after single high doses of 20 to 40 Gy per fraction for each tumor line was studied. Renal cell carcinoma was classified under the radioresistant group, which also included breast, prostate, primary brain tumors, ovarian tumors, and head and neck cancers. There was no correlation between the rankings of relative radiosensitivities of the various classes of tumor cells at high dose per fraction (as in radio surgery) to the sensitivity at low dose per fraction (as in conventional fractionated radiotherapy).

There is some evidence that immunotherapy may enhance the effect of radiation therapy. To investigate whether local delivery of interferon-α (IFN-α) by gene transfection may be of value during radiotherapy, cells of the human renal carcinoma cell line R11 were transfected with the *IFNA* gene and evaluated for radiation responses in vitro by clonogenic assays.[20] R11 cells expressing IFN-α after gene transfection were more sensitive to radiation than R11 control cells (The surviving fraction after exposure to 2 Gy of radiation-SF2 = 0.33 and 0.51, respectively). In another study, it was demonstrated that tumor irradiation enhanced the therapeutic effect of interleukin-2 (IL-2) on pulmonary metastases from a murine renal adenocarcinoma model-Renca.[21,22]

DEFINITIVE RADIATION

There is no established role for radiation therapy as a definitive treatment for renal cell cancer. However, in the setting of symptomatic disease in medically inoperable patients it may play a role (see Palliative Radiation Therapy, below).

ADJUVANT RADIATION

The use of preoperative or postoperative irradiation in the management of locally advanced primary RCC is controversial.

Preoperative Radiation

NONRANDOMIZED DATA

The objective of preoperative radiation is to reduce the size of renal tumors and cause fibrosis, with thickening of the tumor capsule and sclerosis of small blood vessels.[23] In a retrospective review, Riches and colleagues[24,25] reported apparent survival advantage of patients treated with preoperative radiation versus surgery alone (5-year survival: 49% vs. 30%). In another report, after 6 weeks of radiation therapy, there was considerable diminution in the size of the tumor with thickening of the capsule. The tumor thrombus in the inferior vena cava also was markedly diminished after 5000 cGy.[26] Tumor shrinkage, increased resectability, and decreased tumor viability with fewer distant metastases because of lessened intraoperative seeding were considered advantages of preoperative radiation.[25] These and other anecdotal reports warranted a study of preoperative radiation therapy in the context of a prospective clinical trial.

RANDOMIZED DATA

Two prospective clinical trials evaluating the role of neoadjuvant radiation have been undertaken. In a series of 126 patients from 1965 to 1972 randomized to undergo nephrectomy alone versus preoperative radiation therapy (30 Gy in 15 fractions) followed by immediate nephrectomy, there was no survival advantage.[27] Preoperative radiation therapy did appear to increase the rate of complete resection in patients with locally advanced tumors. This study was continued after the 1973 preliminary analysis with higher doses (40 Gy) of preoperative radiation therapy. Even at higher radiation doses no benefit was demonstrated with preoperative radiation.[28] In another study, patients were randomly assigned to receive nephrectomy alone or nephrectomy preceded by 33 Gy preoperative radiation in 15 fractions. Patients receiving preoperative radiation therapy had a 5-year survival rate of 47%, compared with 63% for patients undergoing operation alone.[29]

Postoperative Radiotherapy

NONRANDOMIZED DATA

In a nonrandomized comparison of surgery with or without postoperative radiation, Rafla[30] demonstrated an overall survival advantage at 5 years in patients undergoing postoperative radiation (56%) versus those treated by nephrectomy alone (37%). In another pseudo-randomized trial, Finney[31] reported no difference in distant metastases, local recurrence, and crude survival with the addition of postoperative radiation therapy (55 Gy in 25 fractions in 5 weeks).

More recently, three retrospective studies evaluated the role of postoperative RT in patients at high risk for local recurrence after surgery.[32–34] Patients received doses of 45 to 50 Gy with 1.8- to 2-Gy fractions using multiple treatment fields with CT-based planning. Local recurrence was decreased significantly, and no major treatment complications occurred. Overall survival and disease-free survival were not significantly improved with postoperative radiation.

RANDOMIZED DATA

A postoperative randomized trial of radiation therapy in stage II and III RCC was conducted by the Copenhagen Renal Cancer Study Group.[35] Patients were randomized after nephrectomy to receive the radiation (50 Gy in 20 fractions) to the kidney bed, regional ipsi- and contralateral lymph nodes, or no further treatment. Significant complications from stomach, duodenum, or liver occurred in 44%, at a median time of 5 months (range 1 to 44 months) after RT. In 19% of patients, the post–RT complications contributed to the death of the patients. The median survival in the RT group was 26 months. The survival at 26 months in the observation group was 62%.

Summary of Adjuvant Radiation

Although never proven beneficial in completed randomized trials, a definite conclusion regarding the use of RT in the adjuvant setting would require a multiinstitutional study with hundreds of carefully selected patients with advanced lesions. Three-dimensional conformal radiation therapy (3DCRT) and intensity-modulated radiation therapy (IMRT) techniques would reduce complications and increase the therapeutic ratio (Figure 30.1). The ability to administer safe doses was not feasible until recently, with the adoption of these techniques.[36] In summary, based on the above data (Table 30.2), the following indications for adjuvant radiation therapy with contemporary radiation techniques to minimize radiation-related morbidity could be considered: (1) unresectable nonmetastatic tumors, (2) incomplete resection with gross or microscopically positive margins, (3) locally advanced disease with perinephric fat extension or adrenal invasion, and (4) lymph node metastases.[37]

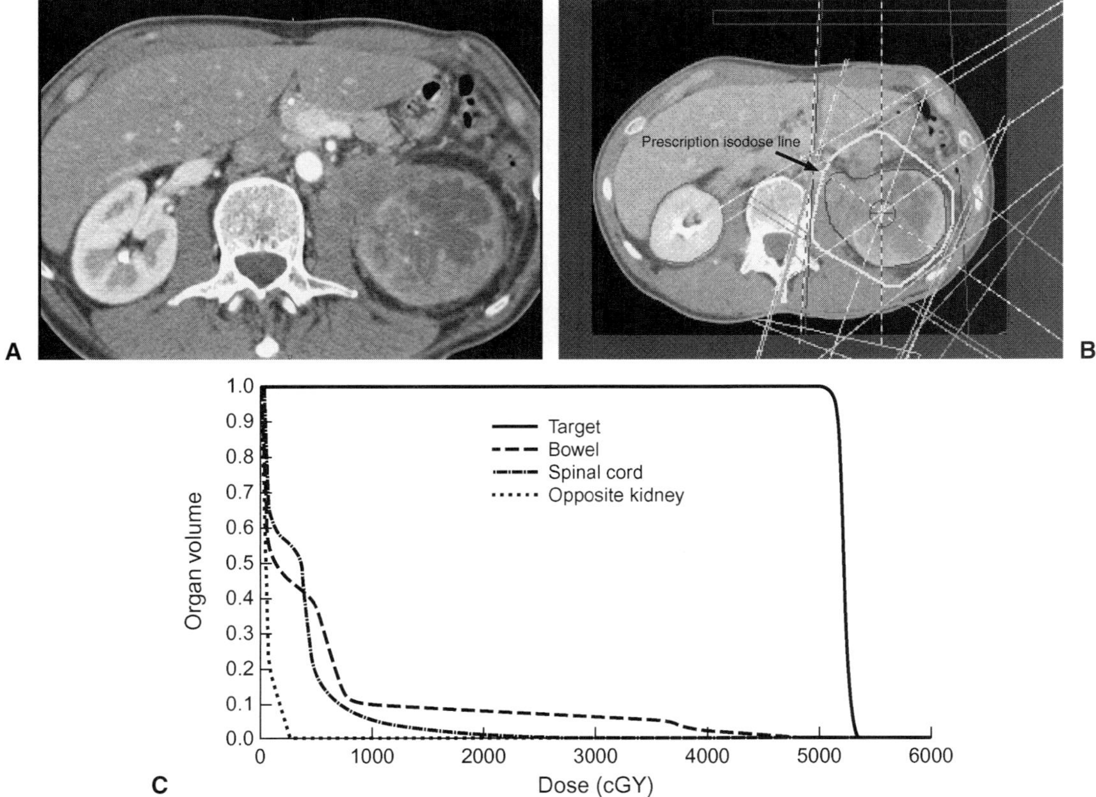

Figure 30.1. **(A)** Locally recurrent left renal cancer. **(B)** Three-dimensional conformal planning. **(C)** Dose volume histograms demonstrating reduced normal organ radiation doses relative to target doses.

Table 30.2.
Adjuvant radiation therapy in renal cell cancer

Clinical setting	First author	Type of study	No. of patients	Treatment	5-year survival	Comments
Preoperative	Van der Werf-Messing[27,28]	P	85	N	50	No benefit
			89	RT+N	45	
	Juusela[29]	P	50	N	63	No benefit
			38	RT+N	47	
Postoperative	Finney[31]	PP	49	N	47	No benefit
			51	N+RT	36	
	Kjaer[35]	P	33	N	62	Detriment
			32	N+RT	38	
	Rafla[30]	R	96	N	37	Benefit
			94	N+RT	56	
	Stein[32]	R	63	N	40	Local control
			56	N+RT	50*	benefit
	Makarewicz[34]	R	72	N	35.5	Local control
			114	N+RT	37.9*	benefit

R, retrospective study; P, prospective randomized; PP, prospective pseudo-randomized; N, nephrectomy; RT, radiation therapy.
*Not significant.

PALLIATIVE RADIATION THERAPY

Radiation therapy to major sites of metastases from RCC may provide pain relief, or prevent or ameliorate the consequences of metastatic disease, such as cord compression, neurologic symptoms from cranial metastases, and airway obstruction.

Skeletal Metastases

Objective responses occur in about 50% of patients with symptomatic skeletal metastases, but symptomatic improvement is often achieved without tumor regression.[38–40] Bone pain responded at 77% of the treated sites.[39] In those sites where a response of bone pain to radiation was observed, 86% of the responses lasted the remainder of the patient's life.[39] At least two retrospective reviews have shown that higher biologic doses may be more effective in achieving symptom control from metastatic RCC.[41,42]

Stereotactic radiosurgery (SRS) for spinal metastases is an evolving therapeutic modality to deliver a large dose of radiation with precision and sparing of the spinal cord. Pain control was achieved in 89% of patients with doses ranging from 17.5 to 25 Gy in one fraction without any treatment-related neurologic damage.[43]

Symptomatic Local Recurrence and Soft Tissue Metastases

Inadequate results have been observed with external-beam RT alone to treat large recurrences in the renal bed or locally advanced disease. Some relief of pain, usually only short-lived, is observed in one half of patients. Preoperative radiation therapy, followed by excision of local recurrences and addition of intraoperative radiation therapy (IORT), has been reported with good results.[44–46] Stereotactic body radiation therapy (SBRT) is an evolving therapeutic modality to deliver large doses of radiation with precision with sparing of surrounding critical organs in a single or a few fractions. In a recent report involving 50 patients with primary and metastatic RCC, a high local control rate with low toxicity was reported.[47]

Brain Metastases

Brain metastasis is not uncommon in metastatic RCC, occurring in about 10% of patients. Surgical resection may be indicated in cases with isolated metastasis.[48,49] Stereotactic radiosurgery is an effective noninvasive modality of treatment. It offers high local control rate and symptom control.[50,51] Patients with brain metastases secondary to RCC treated by SRS alone have excellent local control. The decision of whether or not to add whole-brain radiotherapy to SRS should depend on whether the patient has a high likelihood of developing distant brain failure. Patients who present with multiple brain lesions may be more likely to benefit from the addition of whole-brain radiotherapy because they appear to be more than twice as likely to develop distant brain failure as compared to patients with a single lesion.[50] Whole-brain radiotherapy alone results in unsatisfactory outcomes.[52]

Summary of Palliative Radiation

Radiation therapy can be an effective tool to palliate symptoms from locally recurrent and metastatic disease.[41] A combination of immunochemotherapy (ICT) and RT may induce a synergistic antitumor effect for the treatment of bone metastases or local recurrence from RCC compared to data from the literature for ICT or RT alone.[53]

REFERENCES

1. Jemal A, Murray T, Ward E, et al. Cancer Statistics, 2005. CA Cancer J Clin 2005;55(1):10–30.
2. Chow WH, Devesa SS, Warren JL, Fraumeni JF Jr. Rising incidence of renal cell cancer in the United States. JAMA 1999;281(17):1628–1631.
3. Golimbu M, Joshi P, Sperber A, Tessler A, Al-Askari S, Morales P. Renal cell carcinoma: survival and prognostic factors. Urology 1986;27(4):291–301.
4. Maldazys JD, deKernion JB. Prognostic factors in metastatic renal carcinoma. J Urol 1986;136(2):376–379.
5. Atkins MB, Avigan DE, Bukowski RM, et al. Innovations and challenges in renal cancer: consensus statement from the first international conference. Clin Cancer Res 2004;10(18 pt 2):6277S–6281S.
6. Bukowski RM, Novick AC. Clinical practice guidelines: renal cell carcinoma. Cleve Clin J Med 1997;64(suppl 1):SI1–44.
7. Novick AC. Advances in the management of localized renal cell cancer. Can J Urol 2000;7(2):960–966.
8. deKernion JB, Mukamel E. Selection of initial therapy for renal cell carcinoma. Cancer 1987;60(3 suppl):539–546.
9. Linehan W, Bates S, Yang J. Cancer of the kidney. In: DeVita VT, Hellman S, Rosenberg SA, eds. Cancer: Principles and Practice of Oncology, 7th ed. Philadelphia: Lippincott Williams & Wilkins, 2005:1140–1168.
10. Flocks RH, Kadesky MC. Malignant neoplasms of the kidney; an analysis of 353 patients followed five years or more. J Urol 1958;79(2):196–201.
11. Tsui KH, Shvarts O, Smith RB, Figlin R, de Kernion JB, Belldegrun A. Renal cell carcinoma: prognostic significance of incidentally detected tumors. J Urol 2000;163(2):426–430.
12. Rabinovitch RA, Zelefsky MJ, Gaynor JJ, Fuks Z. Patterns of failure following surgical resection of renal cell carcinoma: implications for adjuvant local and systemic therapy. J Clin Oncol 1994;12(1):206–212.
13. Ramon J, Goldwasser B, Raviv G, Jonas P, Many M. Long-term results of simple and radical nephrectomy for renal cell carcinoma. Cancer 1991;67(10):2506–2511.

14. Castilla EA, Liou LS, Abrahams NA, et al. Prognostic importance of resection margin width after nephron-sparing surgery for renal cell carcinoma. Urology 2002;60(6):993–997.
15. Fergany AF, Hafez KS, Novick AC. Long-term results of nephron sparing surgery for localized renal cell carcinoma: 10-year followup. J Urol 2000;163(2):442–445.
16. Aref I, Bociek RG, Salhani D. Is post-operative radiation for renal cell carcinoma justified? Radiother Oncol 1997;43(2):155–157.
17. Otto U, Huland H, Baisch H, Kloppel G. Transplantation of human renal cell carcinoma into NMRI nu/nu mice. III. Effect of irradiation on tumor acceptance and tumor growth. J Urol 1985; 134(1):170–174.
18. Chiou RK, Vessella RL, Limas C, et al. Monoclonal antibody-targeted radiotherapy of renal cell carcinoma using a nude mouse model. Cancer 1988;61(9):1766–1775.
19. Leith JT, Cook S, Chougule P, et al. Intrinsic and extrinsic characteristics of human tumors relevant to radiosurgery: comparative cellular radiosensitivity and hypoxic percentages. Acta Neurochir Suppl 1994;62:18–27.
20. Syljuasen RG, Belldegrun A, Tso CL, Withers HR, McBride WH. Sensitization of renal carcinoma to radiation using alpha interferon (IFNA) gene transfection. Radiat Res 1997;148(5):443–448.
21. Chakrabarty A, Hillman GG, Maughan RL, Ali E, Pontes JE, Haas GP. Radiation therapy enhances the therapeutic effect of immunotherapy on pulmonary metastases in a murine renal adenocarcinoma model. In Vivo 1994;8(1):25–31.
22. Dezso B, Haas GP, Hamzavi F, et al. The mechanism of local tumor irradiation combined with interleukin 2 therapy in murine renal carcinoma: histological evaluation of pulmonary metastases. Clin Cancer Res 1996;2(9):1543–1552.
23. Rost A, Brosig W. Preoperative irradiation of renal cell carcinoma. Urology 1977;10(5):414–417.
24. Riches EW, Griffiths IH, Thackray AC. New growths of the kidney and ureter. Br J Urol 1951; 23(4):297–356.
25. Riches E. The place of irradiation. JAMA 1968;204(3):230–231.
26. Malkin RB. Regression of renal carcinoma following radiation therapy. J Urol 1975;114(5): 782–783.
27. Van der Werf-Messing B. Carcinoma of the kidney. Cancer 1973;32:1056–1061.
28. Van der Werf-Messing B, van der Heul, RO, Ledeboer, RC. Renal cell carcinoma trial. Strahlenther Onkol 1981;76:169–175.
29. Juusela HMK, Alfthan O, Oravisto KJ. Preoperative irradiation in the treatment of renal adenocarcinoma. Scand J Urol Nephrol 1977;11:277–281.
30. Rafla S. Renal cell carcinoma. Natural history and results of treatment. Cancer 1970;25(1):26–40.
31. Finney R. The value of radiotherapy in the treatment of hypernephroma—a clinical trial. Br J Urol 1973;45(3):258–269.
32. Stein M, Kuten A, Halpern J, Coachman NM, Cohen Y, Robinson E. The value of postoperative irradiation in renal cell cancer. Radiother Oncol 1992;24(1):41–44.
33. Kao GD, Malkowicz SB, Whittington R, D'Amico AV, Wein AJ. Locally advanced renal cell carcinoma: low complication rate and efficacy of postnephrectomy radiation therapy planned with CT. Radiology 1994;193(3):725–730.
34. Makarewicz R, Zarzycka M, Kulinska G, Windorbska W. The value of postoperative radiotherapy in advanced renal cell cancer. Neoplasma 1998;45(6):380–383.
35. Kjaer M, Frederiksen PL, Engelholm SA. Postoperative radiotherapy in stage II and III renal adenocarcinoma. A randomized trial by the Copenhagen Renal Cancer Study Group. Int J Radiat Oncol Biol Phys 1987;13(5):665–672.
36. Rubin P, Keller B, Cox C, Eassa EH. Preoperative irradiation in renal cancer. Evaluation of radiation treatment plans. Am J Roentgenol Radium Ther Nucl Med 1975;123(1):114–121.
37. Kortmann RD, Becker G, Classen J, Bamberg M. Future strategies in external radiation therapy of renal cell carcinoma. Anticancer Res 1999;19(2C):1601–1603.
38. Fossa SD, Kjolseth I, Lund G. Radiotherapy of metastases from renal cancer. Eur Urol 1982; 8(6):340–342.
39. Halperin EC, Harisiadis L. The role of radiation therapy in the management of metastatic renal cell carcinoma. Cancer 1983;51(4):614–617.
40. Nurmi M, Nikkanen TA. Prognosis of metastatic renal adenocarcinoma. Strahlentherapie 1984; 160(7):411–415.

41. DiBiase SJ, Valicenti RK, Schultz D, Xie Y, Gomella LG, Corn BW. Palliative irradiation for focally symptomatic metastatic renal cell carcinoma: support for dose escalation based on a biological model. J Urol 1997;158(3 pt 1):746–749.
42. Onufrey V, Mohiuddin M. Radiation therapy in the treatment of metastatic renal cell carcinoma. Int J Radiat Oncol Biol Phys 1985;11(11):2007–2009.
43. Gerszten PC, Burton SA, Ozhasoglu C, et al. Stereotactic radiosurgery for spinal metastases from renal cell carcinoma. J Neurosurg Spine 2005;3(4):288–295.
44. Master VA, Gottschalk AR, Kane C, Carroll PR. Management of isolated renal fossa recurrence following radical nephrectomy. J Urol 2005;174(2):473–477; discussion 477.
45. Flanigan R. Management of isolated renal fossa recurrence following radical nephrectomy Master VA, Gottschalk AR, Kane C, Carroll PR, Department of Urology, Department of Radiation Oncology, University of California, San Francisco, CA. Urol Oncol 2006;24(1):83.
46. Beer M, Eble MJ, Wannenmacher M, Staehler G. [Intraoperative electron irradiation (IORT) of urologic tumors. Initial results of a pilot study of local recurrences of renal cell cancers]. Urologe A 1994;33(2):110–115.
47. Wersall PJ, Blomgren H, Lax I, et al. Extracranial stereotactic radiotherapy for primary and metastatic renal cell carcinoma. Radiother Oncol 2005;77(1):88.
48. Badalament RA, Gluck RW, Wong GY, et al. Surgical treatment of brain metastases from renal cell carcinoma. Urology 1990;36(2):112–117.
49. Wronski M, Arbit E, Russo P, Galicich JH. Surgical resection of brain metastases from renal cell carcinoma in 50 patients. Urology 1996;47(2):187–193.
50. Goyal LK, Suh JH, Reddy CA, Barnett GH. The role of whole brain radiotherapy and stereotactic radiosurgery on brain metastases from renal cell carcinoma. Int J Radiat Oncol Biol Phys 2000;47(4):1007–1012.
51. Amendola BE, Wolf AL, Coy SR, Amendola M, Bloch L. Brain metastases in renal cell carcinoma: management with gamma knife radiosurgery. Cancer J 2000;6(6):372–376.
52. Wronski M, Maor MH, Davis BJ, Sawaya R, Levin VA. External radiation of brain metastases from renal carcinoma: a retrospective study of 119 patients from the M. D. Anderson Cancer Center. Int J Radiat Oncol Biol Phys 1997;37(4):753–759.
53. Brinkmann OA, Bruns F, Gosheger G, Micke O, Hertle L. Treatment of bone metastases and local recurrence from renal cell carcinoma with immunochemotherapy and radiation. World J Urol 2005;23(3):185–190.
54. Dinney CP, Awad SA, Gajewski JB, et al. Analysis of imaging modalities, staging systems, and prognostic indicators for renal cell carcinoma. Urology 1992;39(2):122–129.
55. Guinan P, Stuhldreher D, Frank W, Rubenstein M. Report of 337 patients with renal cell carcinoma emphasizing 110 with stage IV disease and review of the literature. J Surg Oncol 1997;64(4):295–298.
56. Javidan J, Stricker HJ, Tamboli P, et al. Prognostic significance of the 1997 TNM classification of renal cell carcinoma. J Urol 1999;162(4):1277–1281.
57. Tsui KH, Shvarts O, Smith RB, Figlin RA, deKernion JB, Belldegrun A. Prognostic indicators for renal cell carcinoma: a multivariate analysis of 643 patients using the revised 1997 TNM staging criteria. J Urol 2000;163(4):1090–1095.

31 Palliation in Renal Cancer

Mellar P. Davis

KEYWORDS

RENAL CELL CARCINOMA

ABSTRACT

Renal cell carcinoma (RCC) often is found by serendipity when abdominal imaging is done for unrelated reasons. However, it can present with symptoms both local and systemic, which are both prognostically important and cause significant suffering. RCC is associated with unusual sites of metastases and a variety of paraneoplastic syndromes related to tumor and host cytokine production. Isolated metastases can be managed by surgery with a survival benefit. Tyrosine kinase inhibitors though effective in extending survival in advanced disease, can add to symptom burden. Symptom management not infrequently requires multiple disciplines (oncologists, palliative specialists, radiation therapists, and surgeons). To be successful, a patient centered care approach which includes personal goals of care and continuity of care, should direct the use of technologies in the palliation of RCC.

Renal cell carcinoma (RCC) accounts for 2% to 3% of all malignancies and is the third most common genitourinary cancer.[1,2] Clear cell carcinoma accounts for >60% of all kidney cancers. Approximately 36,000 new cases of RCC are seen each year in the United States and 12,000 deaths occur annually.[3] Prognosis is determined by presentation, which includes symptoms. Asymptomatic patients have a better survival than patients with localized symptoms (flank pain, hematuria), and those who present with systemic symptoms or a paraneoplastic syndrome have the poorest survival despite having a similar stage[3–5] (Table 31.1). Symptoms at presentation reduce survival post-nephrectomy by 30% and increase the relative risk of death to 1.9. Symptoms appear to be more important than T stage.[6] Five-year disease-specific survival for asymptomatic RCC prior to nephrectomy is 91% to 96%, but 65% if symptoms are present before nephrectomy.[4,6,7] Overall, 43% of patients are symptomatic at presentation, of whom 20% have systemic symptoms and 80% localized symptoms.[4]

Paraneoplastic syndromes are common either at the time of presentation or with recurrence. Paraneoplastic syndromes are sometimes related to ectopic production of certain hormones such as parathyroid hormone–related protein (PTHrp) or erythropoietin, but most are associated with ectopic production of cytokines, principally interleukin-6.[8–12]

From: *Clinical Management of Renal Tumors*
Edited by: R.M. Bukowski and A.C. Novick © Humana Press Inc., Totowa, NJ

Table 31.1.
Poor prognostic factors for renal cancer

Decreased performance Eastern Cooperative Oncology Group (ECOG) score
High-grade histology
T stage
Multiple organ involvement
Lack of nephrectomy
Symptoms

Patients with RCC commonly present with advanced disease.[13–15] Metastases occur in 33% of those who have undergone "curative" nephrectomy.[14,15] Common sites for metastases are lung, bone, liver and soft tissue, brain, and adrenal glands. Unusual sites are listed in Table 31.2. Most patients (68%) with recurrent RCC have multiple sites of metastases, although some (5%) have isolated metastases amenable to surgical extubation. Survival with metastases is a median of 12 months, and 10% to 30% survive 3 years.[15–17]

Patients with advanced RCC seen for the first time by a palliative medicine service have a significant symptom burden. Pain occurs in >80% and fatigue in 75%. Other symptoms are gastrointestinal (anorexia, constipation, xerostomia, early satiety, nausea), neuropsychiatric (depression, insomnia, and confusion), and respiratory (dyspnea, hoarseness, and cough). Some of these symptoms are caused by metastases (pain, cough, and hoarseness), and others are caused by treatment (constipation with opioids, nausea with systemic treatment, delirium and depression with cytokine therapy). Most are paraneoplastic in origin and do not appear to be related to tumor burden or sites of metastases. The severity of symptoms parallels the prevalence of symptoms such that the most prevalent symptoms are more often severe. Most patients have multiple debilitating symptoms that reduce the quality of life and contribute to shortened survival.

Table 31.2.
Uncommon metastatic sites of renal cell cancer

Thyroid
Orbit
Nasal structures
Paranasal sinus
Vagina
Gallbladder
Pancreas
Sublingual
Endobronchus
Distant extremities

UNUSUAL SITES OF METASTASES AND UNPREDICTABLE COURSE OF DISEASE

RCC has one of the most unpredictable courses of all cancers. The unusual metastatic pattern and paraneoplastic syndromes associated with recurrent disease can mislead physicians and delay the finding of the primary site or recurrence. Survival after diagnosis usually decreases rapidly until 12 to 18 months, and then the rate of death gradually decreases over the next 5 to 10 years. In unusual circumstances, the interval from diagnosis of the primary to relapse can exceed 10 years.[17] A small percentage of patients present with an isolated single-site metastasis, and they will have either a long-term survival or a cure with surgery for the isolated metastases. Spontaneous regressions can occur in 0.3% to 7% postnephrectomy even after progression on interleukin-2 (IL-2) or interferon-α (IFN-α).[14–18]

Thyroid metastases from RCC are reported to occur years after nephrectomy. Patients present with a "goiter." In rare circumstances, thyroid enlargement from metastases may be the presenting sign of RCC. The presumed path of metastases is by way of the perivertebral venous plexus of Batson.[17] At autopsy, 5% to 12% with RCC have thyroid metastases, most of which are clinically inapparent. RCC overall is the most common cancer to spread to the thyroid gland. Thyroid function is usually well preserved despite involvement. A periodic acid-Schiff stain and thyroglobulin stain help distinguish RCC from thyroid cancer.

RCC is also the most common primary cancer to metastasize to nasal structures and paranasal sinuses. Patients usually present with epistaxis. Of patients with nasal sinus metastases from an unknown primary, 50% to 60% have an unsuspected RCC. Nasal metastases can occur 5 to 10 years postnephrectomy.[17] RCC spreads to the pancreas in 3% and can be mistaken for pancreatic cancer. Vaginal metastases arise from left renal primaries by way of the left ovarian vein and uterovaginal venous plexus.[17] Cancer arising from the left kidney can produce a left varicocele at presentation as a result of invasion into the spermatic vein.[17]

BONE METASTASES

Bone metastases from RCC are almost uniformly associated with impaired performance score (Eastern Cooperative Oncology Group [ECOG] >0) and most with bone metastases have extraosseous metastases.[19,20] The incidence of bone metastases in those with an ECOG performance score of 0 is negligible, so bone scans are unnecessary. An elevated alkaline phosphatase occurs in half of those with bone metastases but is a poor screening test.[19] An elevated alkaline phosphatase is the result of IL-6 production by the primary which includes liver alkaline phosphatase production rather than derived bone metastases. As a result, an elevated alkaline phosphatase does not correlate with bone metastases or hypercalcemia but is a paraneoplastic manifestation of RCC.[19] The reported sensitivity of bone scintigraphy is controversial. Some claim that bone scanning has little utility, with a sensitivity of 10% to 60%. Bone scans frequently underestimate the extent of disease due to the predominantly lytic nature of metastases. There appears to be no diagnostic pattern, clinical feature, or laboratory study that improves the sensitivity of bone scans.[20] Others claim that bone scans have a 94% sensitivity and 86% specificity.[21] Positive bone metastases at presentation occurs in 17%. Bone scans are positive in less than 5% of those with a T1 No (small primaries limited to the kidney parenelyma) primary stages but will occur in 35% of those with locally advanced disease.[21] Bone scans as a screening examination are unnecessary in early-stage asymptomatic individuals. Magnetic resonance imaging or computer tomography should be used for symptomatic areas rather than depending on bone scans due to the lytic nature of most RCC bone metastases.

Bone metastases are found in 33% to 48% patients at the time of autopsy.[19] The most common sites are the pelvis followed by the spine.[22] There is no association with the number or type of bone metastases and hypercalcemia.[22] Most with bone metastases require radiation (>80%) during the course of illness, and 40% will require surgery.[19]

Indications for surgical management of osseous metastases are (1) solitary metastases postnephrectomy if the patient has a good performance score, (2) intractable pain where surgery will reduce incident pain due to mechanical instability, and (3) impending fracture. Embolization of bone metastases with polyvinyl ethanol may relieve pain and reduce bleeding. Vascular embolization reduces intraoperative bleeding.[23,24] Median hospital stay after surgery is 8 to 9 days, and 89% of patients are clinically improved by the surgical intervention. Median survival for those with bone metastases is 12 months (if multiple metastases) and longer for a single metastasis (27 months). Three-year survival for those with bone metastases is 38%.[25,26] Bone metastases appear to respond to IL-2 and tyrosine kinase inhibitors to the same degree that nonosseous metastases respond.[22] Others have claimed that osseous metastases are more resistant to cytokine therapy.[16]

Pain from RCC bone metastases responds to radiation. However, controversy surrounds the dose-response relationship. Some have claimed better pain responses at higher tumor dose fractions (TDFs). Onufrey and Mohiuddin[27] found that 65% responded to a TDF of ≥70 and 25% at a TDF <70 Gy. Others have also claimed responses related to dose.[28] Both Wilson and colleagues[29] and Halperin and colleagues[30] did not find a relationship between TDF and symptom response. Symptomatic responses were seen in more than 70% of those who received standard palliative fractional schedules. Wu and colleagues[31] found that an 8-Gy single fraction to bone metastases including the spine (not including spinal cord compression or cauda equina syndrome) relieves pain from bone metastases.

Bisphosphonates have been found to reduce skeletal related complications in RCC and can reduce pain.[32–34] Bisphosphonates interfere with osteoclast activation that is the result of receptor activation by nuclear factor κB (RANK) ligand released from stoma and tumor. RANK-L binds to osteoclast RANK receptors, which activates osteoclasts. The potent bisphosphonate Zolendronate reduces skeletal-related events by 50% and pain to a greater extent than for other solid tumors.[19,35] Monthly doses should be limited to 4 mg due to the increased risk for renal toxicity with higher doses. Jaw osteonecrosis is a concern with long-term use. Benefits are seen over months.[36] Nausea, fatigue, pyrexia, rigors, and lower extremity edema are slightly greater with bisphosphonates than with placebo in randomized trials. Recently, a loading dose schedule of ibandronate (4 mg as a 2-hour infusion for 4 days) significantly improved refractory bone pain, quality of life, and patient function within 7 days of initiating treatment without evidence of renal toxicity.[37] Most patients with symptomatic bone metastases and adequate renal function should be offered monthly zolendronate.

Newer techniques to treat painful bone metastases include radioactive isotopes such as rhenium-188 hydroxyethylidene diphosphate (HEDP), radiofrequency ablation, and cryoablation.[38–40] Magnetic resonance imaging–guided interstitial radiofrequency ablation can be used for symptomatic renal primaries less than 4 cm in diameter or for painful bone metastases that are not amenable to surgery or for those bone metastases that for medical reasons cannot be surgically removed or have been previously radiated.[41] Image-guided ablation can be combined with vascular embolization or antiangiogenesis to increase response by reducing blood flow to the metastases.[42,43] Recent findings derived through the nude mouse model suggest that epithelial growth factor receptors on renal cell cancer are overexpressed in bone metastases. A combination of a tyrosine kinase inhibitor to epidermal growth factor receptor (EGFR) (erlotinib) and a taxane reduced bone destruction in this model.[44] Combinations of erlotinib and bevacizumab or a tyrosine kinase inhibitor to the vascular endothelial factor receptor has been used with good responses.[45]

SPINE METASTASES

Vertebral and spinal cord metastases may be the first presentation of RCC.[46] Vertebral metastases can occur more than 5 years after a nephrectomy and may be misdiagnosed as benign mechanical low back pain if a history of RCC is not obtained. Negative plain radiographs and bone scintigraphy do not exclude spine metastases. Magnetic resonance imaging should include adequate images for vertebral, leptomeningeal, and intramedullary metastases.[47] Vertebral metastases from RCC cause both pain and neurologic deficits and thus significantly reduce quality of life. In one series, half of the patients with RCC underwent preoperative tumor embolization to prevent operative bleeding and half received radiation prior to surgery.[48] The median survival for vertebral metastases is 12 months, which is similar to extraosseous metastases and nonvertebral bone metastases. The majority (90%) of patients experience pain relief, and 65% experience improvement in neurologic deficits, but 15% experience major morbidity and 2% die postoperatively either from complications or rapidly growing cancer.[48]

Surgery may entail anterior decompression, vertebrectomy, and transpedicular fixation. Laminectomy alone is rarely done since it mechanically destabilizes the spine.[49] Patients with isolated vertebral metastases can survive for years after aggressive management (if the primary site is controlled). Those with multiple vertebral metastases survive a median of 10 months.[49] Indications for surgery include (1) isolated metastases (combined with nephrectomy at a later date if the primary has not been removed), (2) progressive neurologic deficits during radiation, and (3) unstable spine or bone protrusion into the epidural space with cord compression.[50] The best prognosis in those with spinal metastases who undergo surgery is with breast cancer and RCC due to the chemotherapy sensitivity of breast cancer and the characteristic limited metastases of RCC. Intramedullary metastases are not amenable to surgery, and radiation does not improve neurologic deficits but may forestall progression.[51]

BRAIN METASTASES

Brain metastases occur in 5% to 6% with a median time from diagnosis to discovery of 15 to 19 months.[52,53] Forty percent of patients have lung metastases in addition to brain metastases, so that complete staging with computed tomography of the chest and abdomen should be done at the time of discovery. Rarely do brain metastases present at diagnosis.[54] Median survival from craniotomy (for isolated metastases) is 12 months, and death is usually from systemic metastases. Postoperative mortality can be as high as 10% in these patients.[54] Patients with poor performance status and progressive systemic disease should be treated palliatively and are unlikely to benefit from aggressive surgical management. The use of IL-2 does not improve survival and may worsen symptoms. Combining surgery and radiation for brain metastases improves survival over whole-brain radiation alone in selected individuals. Only 30% respond to 30 Gy with a median survival of 8 weeks.[55,56]

Gamma knife radiation improves symptomatic response (96%) and survival (15 months) over external-beam radiation in those with isolated but unresectable metastases.[57] Part of this improvement reflects patient selection. Gamma knife radiation is the treatment of choice for those with few brain metastases or those whose metastases are not amenable to surgery. Whole-brain radiation adds little to gamma knife radiation.[54] Prognosis with cerebral metastases is related to (1) resection of synchronous pulmonary metastases if present, (2) supratentorial location, (3) left renal primary, and (4) lack of neurologic deficits. Most deaths are related to progressive systemic disease.[57] Nearly half (46%) of intracranial metastases are found to have hemorrhaged, so that anticoagulation is a significant risk.[54] Both gamma knife radiation and surgery may prevent this devastating complication even if treatment is not curative. Finally, surgery for both brain and pulmonary metastases is reasonable if brain and lung metastases are solitary.

NEPHRECTOMY

Debulking nephrectomy may prevent tumor shedding, palliate symptoms (pain and hematuria), and potentially reverse paraneoplastic syndromes if there are few distant metastases.[14] The primary acts as an immunologic "sink" with the production of IL-6 and other cytokines (IL-8, IL-10, tumor necrosis factor-α [TNF-α], transforming growth factor-β [TGF-β]) that cause systemic symptoms. Tumor immunity (and response to cytokines) is impaired if the renal primary is not removed. The primary site rarely, if ever, responds to IL-2. Symptoms from paraneoplastic syndromes and local symptoms such as hematuria and pain do not respond well to IL-2 without nephrectomy.[14]

The absence of nephrectomy is a poor prognostic sign, particularly in symptomatic individuals. Patients who benefit from nephrectomy are those with a good performance score (ECOG score of 0 to 1), absence of central nervous system metastases, lung-only metastases, and when >75% of the primary is removed with the debulking procedure. Only 20% of those with distant metastases are candidates for debulking nephrectomy due either to poor performance score or primaries not amenable to surgery. Nephrectomy plus IFN-α improves survival compared to IFN-α alone. However, IFN-α is no longer a preferred treatment for RCC.[58] Target-specific tyrosine kinase inhibitors may be substituted for IFN-α, though little data is available at the present time that tyrosine kinase inhibitors are beneficial as adjuvants. The median improvement in survival is 6 months with IFN-α plus nephrectomy over IFN-α alone. Patients with poor performance score and widespread metastases do not benefit from debulking nephrectomy.[15,43,56,59] Laparoscopy nephrectomy allows for quicker postoperative recovery.

Perioperative predictors of survival are (1) length of hospital stay, (2) tumor grade, (3) preoperative white blood cell count, and (4) preoperative partial thromboplastin time.[56] Postoperative pain after laparoscopy may be due to surgical complications such as retroperitoneal dissection and injury to the ilioinguinal, iliohypogastric, or subcostal nerves. Unusual histologies such as metastatic sarcomatoid variants, collecting duct cancer, and papillary and medullary renal cancers do not benefit from debulking nephrectomy but may benefit from palliative nephrectomy if pain and hematuria are a major problem.

Tumor embolization may relieve local symptoms if surgery is not possible. Patients are usually hospitalized after embolization in order to manage pain from the procedure. Epidural opioids may be used for pain after embolization and continued through the postoperative period if patients remain in the hospital for nephrectomy. Transient fever and pain are common postnephrectomy. Stainless steel coils and ethanol have been used for preoperative embolization. The median duration of hospitalization postembolization is 4 days. Radiofrequency ablation of the primary also improves symptoms, though this technique is limited by the size of the primary. Acute lumbosacral radiculopathy may occur after radiofrequency ablation but will generally spontaneously improve.[60,61]

LUNG METASTASES

Lung metastases are responsive to IL-2 postnephrectomy and are most frequently associated with spontaneous regression. Isolated metastases should be removed with the primary if synchronous or resected if metachronous. Endobronchial metastases are not infrequent with RCC. External-beam radiation may be used or alternatively high dose rate (HDR) intraluminal brachytherapy or iridium-192 low-dose endobronchial brachytherapy to relieve hemoptysis, dyspnea, cough, and postobstructive pneumonia.[62,63] Forty-six percent have complete relief and 43% have partial relief of symptoms. Nearly 90% have improvement in hemoptysis and postobstructive pneumonia, while 80% have resolution or improvement in cough or dyspnea.[63]

SYMPTOMS RELATED TO CYTOKINE THERAPY

At the present time, novel tyrosine kinase inhibitors and angiogenic agents are being used in RCC.[64,65] Responses to tyrosine kinase inhibitors and IL-2 range between 10% and 30%, with 5% long-term survival (associated with high doses of IL-2). Median duration of responses is 12 to 19 months.[66] Toxicity is a major problem with IL-2, which adds to the symptom burden of RCC. The quality of life as measured by the European Organization for Research and Treatment of Cancer (EORTC) quality-of-life questionnaire (QLQ C30) diminishes for most during IL-2 treatment. The physical, emotional, and social function domains of the EROTC QLQ C30 are adversely affected the most.[67] High-dose IL-2 (18 million units daily for 5 days repeated 6 days later) produces hypotension (86%), dyspnea, (32%), depression or delirium (55%), reduced renal function as measured by serum creatinine (48%), sepsis (16%), and death (3%).[67–69] Paradoxically, those who have the most symptoms in response to treatment and the greatest reduction in quality of life during treatment are more likely to respond.[67] Those with a high symptom burden and poor performance status prior to high-dose IL-2 are unlikely to tolerate IL-2.[70]

Proinflammatory cytokines (TNF-α, IL-6, IL-1) produce a sickness syndrome in animals and anxiety and depression in humans. Depression may respond to antidepressants.[68] Interleukin-2 produces less profound sickness than IL-6 but can cause anhedonia, a hallmark symptom of depression.[71–73] Immunotherapy with IL-2 promotes depressive symptoms or worsens preexisting depression.[74] Cytokines cause depression through reduction in brain serotonin and noradrenaline. This is reversed by selective serotonin reuptake inhibitors (SSRIs) or noradrenaline enhancing antidepressants (venlafaxine).[75] Patients with a history of depression may have a relapse of depression while on IL-2. Antidepressants or dose adjustments of chronic antidepressants may be necessary during treatment.

Cytokines may also alter drug responses, metabolism, and toxicity of co-medications. In experimental animals, IFN-α attenuates morphine withdrawal symptoms.[76–78] Interleukin-2 can inhibit the release of endogenous opioids (met-enkephalin), which may in part account for the pain associated with treatment.[79] Morphine may abrogate IL-2 response, which is reversed by melatonin.[80] Acute morphine toxicity has been reported while patients are on high doses of IL-2, which may be related to reduce renal function and delayed clearance of morphine and morphine metabolites.[81]

SYMPTOMS RELATED TO TYROSINE KINASE INHIBITORS AND TEMSIROLIMUS

Target-specific therapy has advanced the treatment of RCC and thus is presented in greater detail. Sunitinib is an orally administered tyrosine kinase inhibitor that blocks the downstream activation of vascular endothelial growth factor receptor (VEGFR) and platelet-derived growth factor receptor (PDGFR). Sunitinib has produced a 31% response in RCC compared to 6% for IFN-α; median progression-free survival is doubled with sunitinib and quality of life improves relative to IFN-α.[82] Sunitinib toxicity includes diarrhea, fatigue, nausea, stomatitis, and hypertension. Severe symptoms are relatively rare (<10%).[58] Sorafenib was designed as a C-RAF kinase inhibitor but also inhibits VEGFR-2 and PDGFR-B. Sorafenib has produced tumor shrinkage of 25% in 71% of individuals treated and objective partial responses in a minority (4%).[45] Toxicities with sorafenib include hand-foot skin reactions, rash, diarrhea, fatigue, and pruritus. Severe toxicity occurs in <10%.[58] Temsirolimus, a mammalian target of rapamycin (mTOR) kinase inhibitor, improves survival in advanced RCC compared to IFN-α even though responses occur in only 11%.[45,83] Temsirolimus side effects are anemia, asthenia, hyperglycemia, and hyperlipidemia.

All three tyrosine kinase inhibitors are better tolerated than IFN-α and have changed the treatment paradigm in RCC. However, symptoms of advanced RCC such as fatigue overlap with drug toxicity, and it may be difficult to decide whether individuals experiencing fatigue have symptoms of progressive RCC or drug toxicity. A treatment holiday may be necessary in a few patients who have significant fatigue to determine if fatigue is from the tyrosine kinases. Other causes for fatigue (anemia, hypothyroidism) should be screened and treated if present before discontinuing drug therapy. It is not known if methylphenidate or other psychostimulants relieve fatigue from tyrosine kinase inhibitors. Diarrhea from tyrosine kinase inhibitors may be treated by usual measures and nausea with haloperidol or phenothiazines.

INTERLEUKIN-6 AND PARANEOPLASTIC SYNDROMES

Interleukin-6 is increased in 70% of those with advanced RCC. Elevated IL-6 levels are associated with poor prognosis, short progression-free interval, and overall survival.[84–86] Interleukin-6 levels may be an independent prognostic factor. Interleukin-6 binds to a gp130A receptor (IL-6R), which can become soluble. Soluble IL-6R amplifies IL-6 responses or causes "trans-signaling" to other cells that do not normally respond to IL-6. The mechanism by which IL-6 produces paraneoplastic syndromes is by way of signal transducer and activator of transcription (STAT) phosphorylation. Blocking STAT phosphorylation may reduce tumor growth, reverse paraneoplastic, and sensitize tumors to cytokines.[87] Interleukin-6 switches from a paracrine inhibitor of cancer to an autocrine stimulator in time, and may be one of the reasons for cytokine treatment failure.[12,88] Interleukin-6 levels increase with tumor burden, portend a poor prognosis, stimulate tumor cell proliferation, and cause several paraneoplastic syndromes.[12,89] Interleukin-6 causes hepatic production of acute-phase reactants such as C-reactive protein (CRP)[90] and stimulates VEGF production and release.[91] Interleukin-6 along with PTHrp are responsible for tumor-associated hypercalcemia.[8,92–94] Interleukin-6 levels correlate with elevated liver function and the Stauffer syndrome, anemia, cachexia, fever, hypoalbuminemia, leukocytosis, and nausea.[91,95–101]

Antibodies to IL-6 sensitize RCC to cisplatin by inhibiting expression of magnesium superoxide dismutase.[102] Anti–IL-6 antibodies decrease thrombocytosis, leukocytosis, and monocytosis, and stabilize albumin and hemoglobin levels when given over a 21-day period of time.[102] Anti–IL-6 antibodies reduce tumor growth and can correct hypercalcemia in nude mice.[8] However, the clinical utility of anti–IL-6 antibody in RCC has not been rigorously tested.

Alternatively debulking nephrectomy may reverse paraneoplastic syndrome by reducing IL-6 (and PTHrp).[12,100]

SYMPTOM MANAGEMENT

The most common symptoms in RCC (pain, fatigue, anorexia, early satiety, weight loss, depression, and delirium) appear to be caused by tumor or host-derived cytokines. Interleukin-1, IL-6, IL-8, IL-10, TNF, fibroblast growth factor (FGF), TGF, and granulocyte-colony stimulating factor (C-GSF) are increased in many advanced cancers.[103–109] The host proinflammatory response to tumor does not correlate with tumor bulk but is responsible for much of the disability associated with cancer. Therefore, the focus on tumor response in terms of reduced tumor bulk may be relatively meaningless if symptom burden due to host cytokine is not improved. Tumor response has been a surrogate for symptomatic improvement in many physicians' minds. However, stability of disease and symptom relief may be just as valuable (if not more valuable in the patients' minds) as tumor response. In fact and in speculation, if cytokines surges could be minimized or reduced, survival may improve since anorexia and cachexia are the most common paraneoplastic syndrome to cause death in advanced cancer.

Pain

Most patients with RCC experience pain during the course of their illness, and pain is moderate to severe in intensity. Many have two or more distinctively different cancer pain syndromes, but have at least one pain related to bone metastases.[110] A minority has treatment-related pain or pain related to comorbidities.[110] One third of cancer pains are neuropathic either alone or mixed with nociceptive pain.[110] Failure to properly assess pain is a major barrier to management. This may be related in part to the disease model rather than a symptom model of care. Assessment of pain takes time and training, both of which are usually difficult to accomplish in a busy oncologic practice. Patient-related barriers include fear of opioid addiction, drug tolerance, and fear of side effects (usually sedation, confusion, nausea, and constipation).[110] Assessment of pain should include a history of location, quality, severity, onset, palliative factors, and pain radiation. Radiographic procedures are guided by the history and physical examination.[106] Patient-generated pain diaries in the outpatient setting can facilitate recognition of the pain pattern and severity, which in turn facilitate analgesic prescriptions.[111]

The first step in the World Health Organization analgesic ladder is the use of nonsteroidal antiinflammatory drugs (NSAIDs) for mild pain. There is little evidence about the safety of NSAIDs in patients who have a nephrectomy. Ketorolac has been safely used in the perioperative period in those who have undergone partial nephrectomy.[112] Acetaminophen, however, is preferred. The preference of selective cyclooxygenase 2 inhibitors (COX2) over nonselective inhibitors is not evidence based. COX-2 inhibitors also cause renal failure to the same degree as nonselective inhibitors, and clinical data do not support the opioid-sparing benefits of COX2 inhibitors when combined with opioids.[113]

Opioid prescription for moderate to severe pain is an art. Basic errors in prescribing include failure to prescribe enough and failure to prescribe to the pain pattern. One of the major errors is failure to give around-the-clock (ATC) opioids for continuous pain.[114] Ninety percent of patients require less than 300 mg of oral morphine or oral morphine daily equivalence (if using an alternative potent opioid).[115] The amount of opioid is not prognostic, nor does it shorten survival. However, physicians tend to have personal ceilings to opioid doses and frequently add a second opioid with incomplete response to the first at a predetermined self-selected dose level.[114] Combining opioids is not based on rational pharmacology. Potent opioids do not have ceiling doses, and combining opioids increases the complexity of care, risks additional adverse drug reactions, and drug interactions. The use of one opioid with titration to pain control, based on pain severity and response, is key to successful pain control.

Another common error is failure to prescribe laxatives proactively and failure to recognize opioid toxicity such as confusion, visual hallucinations, and myoclonus. Patients rarely volunteer visual hallucinations, so active inquiry is necessary.[114] Morphine remains the drug of choice due to noninferiority, clinical experience, and versatility.[90,116,117] Most patients have both continuous and breakthrough pain such that ATC and rescue doses are needed. Initial doses for opioid-naive patients are 5 to 10 mg by mouth every 4 hours or sustained-release morphine 15 mg every 12 hours. For parenteral dosing, 0.5 to 1 mg per hour is given subcutaneously or intravenously.

Rescue doses are calculated in several ways: (1) 25% to 50% of the 4-hour dose, (2) 2% to 5% of the 24-hour dose, (3) the full 4-hour dose provided any time during a 4-hour interval.[116,117] If sustained-release morphine is used, the rescue dose is one third of the 12-hour dose every 4 hours. Rescue doses should not influence the timing of the 4- or 12-hour doses. Guidelines have presumed a relationship between the rescue doses and the continuous dose; however, there is no prospective evidence for this. Breakthrough pain may be end-of-dose failure, nonincident breakthrough pain, and incident pain (activity related pain).[118–120] End-of-dose failure is managed simply by increasing the ATC dose. Nonincident breakthrough pain may also be inadequately treated chronic pain. Rescue doses, if effective, are added to the ATC dose if the chronic pain is under control.[121]

Incident pain is more difficult to manage since the onset to maximum pain occurs quickly (for many within 5 minutes), and pain resolves quickly (within 30 minutes).[120] Rescue doses for incident pain should be titrated to the response of the incident pain independent of chronic doses. Incident pain rescue doses should not be added to the ATC dose if cronic pain is controlled since this is likely to cause opioid toxicity at rest.[121]

Approximately 20% of patients do not tolerate morphine due to rate-limiting toxicity (myoclonus, confusion, visual hallucinations, nausea, and vomiting).[117] In this situation, several strategies are possible: (1) the addition of an appropriate adjuvant analgesic, and reduction of the morphine dose by one third; (2) opioid conversion to a different route (spinal); (3) opioid rotation to hydromorphone, oxycodone, methadone, or fen-

Table 31.3.
Opioid route conversion

	Oral	Parenteral
Morphine	3	1
Oxycodone	2	1
Hydromorphone	2	1
Methadone	2	1

tanyl; and (4) nonpharmacologic measures (such as orthotics, radiation, surgery, and kyphoplasty).[122–126] Opioid conversion and rotation equivalents are listed in Tables 31.3 to 31.5. Bisphosphonates, radionucleotides, and neurolytic blocks may be helpful additions to opioids and adjuvants. Unfortunately, the optimal approach to management cannot be derived from randomized controlled trials.[127]

Adjuvants for neuropathic pain are largely limited to drugs approved for other conditions and include anticonvulsants, antidepressants, antiarrhythmics, and opioids.[128,129] Treatment schemas for neuropathic pain have been used based on treatment paradigms for diabetic neuropathy and postherpetic neuralgia. First-line treatments evidenced by multiple randomized control trials (RCTs) are (1) gabapentin, (2) 5% lidocaine patch (for regionally limited neuropathies), (3) tramadol, (4) tricyclic antidepressants, and (5) opioid analgesics. Gabapentin clearance is dependent on renal function. Tricyclic antidepressant (TCA) and opioids require greater caution and have more side effects.[128,129] Second-line analgesics based on evidence from one RCT are (1) lamotrigine, (2) carbamazepine, (3) bupropion, (4) venlafaxine, (5) citalopram, and (6) paroxetine. Drug interactions are a problem with carbamazepine and paroxetine. Combinations of two first-line drugs or a first- and second-line drug may improve pain over single agents, but the evidence for this is weak.[129]

Table 31.4.
Opioid equianalgesia (mg) oral

Morphine	10
Hydromorphone	2
Methadone	4:1 morphine/methadone for <90 mg/day morphine
	8:1 90–30 morphine/day
	12:1 >300 mg morphine/day
Oxycodone	10 mg

Table 31.5.
Opioid equianalgesia (mg) parenteral

Morphine	1/hour
Oxycodone	1.4/hour
Hydromorphone	0.2/hour
Fentanyl	0.025/hour

Anorexia and Cachexia

Anorexia and cachexia, though often associated with each other, have a distinctively different pathophysiology. Anorexia is associated with an imbalance in neuropeptide Y and pro-opiomelanocortin hypothalamic signals favoring pro-opiomelanocortin–induced satiety and anorexia. Gastrointestinal symptoms, particularly early satiety, are commonly associated with anorexia.[130,131] Appetite stimulants are modestly effective as evidenced by RCT. The strongest evidence is for progestins and corticosteroids. Neither agent reverses cachexia, and in fact, corticosteroids accelerate striated muscle atrophy.

Cachexia superficially resembles starvation; however, nutritional support does little to reverse catabolism.[130] Cancer-related cytokines induce increased resting energy expenditures, stimulate lipolysis, inhibit lipogenesis, and accelerate proteolysis through the ubiquitin proteasome system. The transcription factor nuclear factor (NF)-κB is responsible for ubiquitin and proteasome regulation.[130] Multiple drugs targeting cachexia include NSAIDs, propranolol, eicosapentaenoic acid, melatonin, thalidomide, adenosine triphosphate (ATP) infusions, and IL-15, and they have been used either in animal studies or in single-arm trials and rarely in randomized trials. There is not enough evidence to support the use of these anticachexins in routine practice. Family education about the differences between starvation and cachexia is important so that family members do not experience guilt about weight loss in their loved one. Research is vital in this area and extremely important due to prognostic significance. It is hoped that recent discoveries about the pathophysiology of cachexia will stimulate translational research and target specific therapies.[130,131]

Nausea and Vomiting

Nausea and vomiting in advanced cancer can be related to brain metastases, drugs, uremia, infection, anxiety, constipation, gastric irritation, and bowel obstruction.[132] Treatment paradigms have been based on neuroanatomy, emetogenic neuroreceptors (muscarinic, dopaminergic, serotonergic, histaminergic, tachykinin), and clinical symptoms. Therapy guided by clinical symptoms has been reported to have a high degree of success. Symptoms related to chemical and metabolic causes produce persistent severe nausea unrelieved by vomiting, whereas nausea from gastric stasis or bowel obstruction is relieved by vomiting for a variable period of time and is usually associated with abdominal pain or colic.[132] Associated signs with gastroparesis or bowel obstruction include obstipation, succession splash, and borborygmi.

Patients with gastric stasis may respond to metoclopramide 10 mg oral or parenteral every 6 hours up to 120 mg as a continuous infusion subcutaneously or intravenously over 24 hours. Metoclopramide should not be used if there is colic, complete obstipation, or abdominal pain. Antimuscarinics block metoclopramide prokinesis and hence should not be used with metoclopramide. Metoclopramide doses need to be cut in half with renal or hepatic failure.[133] Alternatively, haloperidol 0.5 to 1.0 mg intravenously or subcutaneously every 4 to 6 hours or 5 mg as a continuous subcutaneous or intravenous infusion over 24 hours can be used and is preferred in complete mechanical bowel obstruction.[133] Haloperidol is also preferred in chemical and metabolic causes of nausea. Haloperidol doses do not need to be reduced in hepatic or renal failure.[132] The dose should be doubled if converting from parenteral or oral.[133] Antimuscarinics (glycopyrrolate 0.1 to 0.2 mg subcutaneously every 6 hours) and octreotide (100 to 200 μg every

8 hours), and dexamethasone (4 to 8 mg in the morning and at noon) may relieve nausea, vomiting, and colic from bowel obstruction and thus avoid nasogastric intubation and decompression in nonsurgical patients.[133,134]

Patients experiencing nausea or vomiting while on metoclopramide or haloperidol may respond with the addition of dexamethasone or a 5-hydroxytryptamine receptor-3 (5-HT$_3$) receptor antagonist (ondansetron, tropisetron) or with rotation to a broad-spectrum phenothiazine or atypical antipsychiatric such as olanzapine or methotrimeprazine.[133] Evidence supporting guidelines in the management of nausea and vomiting is sparse.[135]

NEUROPSYCHIATRIC COMPLICATIONS

Depression

Psychiatric disorders are more common in cancer patients than in the general population. Nearly a third of patients experience depression or an adjustment reaction which was depressive symptoms. Depressed mood is a significant symptom in 25%.[136] Unfortunately, as much as 80% of psychologic and psychiatric morbidity in cancer goes unrecognized and untreated.

Patients might not volunteer that they are depressed, and medical personnel may feel that it is normal to be depressed if one has advanced cancer. Medical and nursing staff frequently lack the skills necessary to diagnose depression.

Depression is diagnosed if there is a persistent low mood for 2 weeks and as least four of the following symptoms: (1) anhedonia, (2) psychomotor retardation or agitation, (3) feelings of worthlessness or guilt, (4) diminished ability to concentrate, (5) recent thoughts of death and suicide, (6) fatigue and loss of energy, (7) weight loss/gain, and (8) insomnia or hypersomnia. Cancer patients have somatic symptoms of weight loss, fatigue, and insomnia that are unrelated to depression; anhedonia, worthlessness, guilt, hopelessness, and suicidal ideation are particularly discriminating factors.[136,137] Characteristics associated with a higher risk for depression are (1) female gender, (2) young adult (age under 45), (3) past history of depression, (4) lack of social support, (5) high symptom burden, (6) pain, (7) treatment-related side effects, and (8) existential or religious concerns. Reduced symptom burden, adequate symptom management, social support, psychotherapy, and spiritual counseling for the existential crisis minimize the risk of depression at the end of life.

Assessment may be accomplished through various instruments such as the Hospital Anxiety and Depression Scale or by asking the patient directly, "Are you depressed?"[136] Neither the assessment tool nor the direct question is 100% specific or sensitive. Occasional suicidal thoughts are quite common in the palliative setting, and expression of such thoughts are a means of releasing emotional energy while coping with a terminal illness. Most requests or inquiries into suicide are transient.[137] Depression, hopelessness, demoralization, and an overwhelming symptom burden are usually factors that generate the persistent request for physician-assisted suicide.[137–139] Symptoms associated with depression are anorexia, fatigue, insomnia, pain, wound, or pressure sores.[138,139] Therefore, the first step to the management of depression is to allow the patient to get a good night's sleep and aggressively manage fatigue and pain.

Opioids for pain, corticosteroids for pain and fatigue, mirtazapine for insomnia, and methylphenidate for fatigue treat associated symptoms and depression.[136] Antidepressants are often prescribed too late in advanced cancer, as the benefits are not seen for

Table 31.6.
Antidepressants

	Starting dose	Therapeutic dose
Citalopram	10 mg	10–40 mg
Sertraline	15 mg	50–300 mg
Paroxetine	10 mg	10–40 mg
Desipramine	10–25 mg	25–125 mg
Amitriptyline	10–25 mg	25–125 mg
Mirtazapine	7.5–15 mg	15–45 mg

4 weeks. Selective serotonin receptor antagonists have fewer side effects than tricyclic antidepressants (Table 31.6). SSRIs have very low affinity for adrenergic, cholinergic, and histamine receptors that reduce the risk of orthostatic hypotension, urinary retention, memory impairment, and sedation relative to tricyclic antidepressants. However, SSRIs inhibit hepatic cytochrome isoenzymes to variable extents such that drug interactions are a risk. Tricyclic antidepressants produce relief in 70%, with side benefits of treating neuropathic pain. Anticholinergic side effects and cardiac toxicity are limited to amitriptyline and imipramine. The secondary amines nortriptyline and desipramine are less anticholinergic and are preferred in older individuals.

Other risk factors to the use of tricyclic antidepressants are a prolonged QT_C interval and arrhythmia as well as drug interactions.[137] Mirtazapine enhances central noradrenergic and serotonergic activity and blocks postsynaptic serotonin 5-HT$_2$ and 5-HT$_3$ receptors. Mirtazapine increases appetite, produces physiologic sleep, and may reduce nausea as well as depression.[137] The psychostimulant methylphenidate is safe and has a rapid onset of antidepressant effect. Response rates are as high as 85% with methylphenidate.[140] Methylphenidate may improve appetite and fatigue. Drug interactions are rare with methylphenidate compared to SSRIs. The SSRIs may be added to methylphenidate for long-term management. Psychosocial interventions including psychotherapy, education, relaxation training, and biofeedback should be combined with pharmacologic management.

Delirium

Delirium occurs in 26% to 44% of hospitalized cancer patients and in 80% of those in the terminal phase of their illness.[141–143] Delirium is diagnosed when there are fluctuations in the level of consciousness, inability to concentrate, and changes in perception (Table 31.7). In advanced cancer, delirium is reversible in only a minority and often precedes death by days to weeks.[142]

Table 31.7.
Diagnostic criteria for delirium (International Classification of Diseases [ICD]-10)

Impaired level of consciousness or attention
Disturbances in cognition (perception, distortion, illusions, visual or tactile hallucinations, impaired abstract thinking and comprehension, lack of recall, and disorientation)
Psychomotor disturbances (hypoactive, hyperactive, or mixed and fluctuating levels of activity)
Disturbances in sleep/wake cycle
Emotional disturbances

Prodromal behavioral changes may occur before delirium is fully manifest. These nonspecific symptoms include anxiety, irritability, insomnia, urgent calls for attention, and transient disorientation.[144]

Multiple assessment instruments for delirium have been validated. The Mini–Mental Status Exam, the Confusion Assessment Method, the Delirium Rating Scale, and the Bedside Delirium Scale are only a few.[143,145,146] At the Cleveland Clinic we use the Bedside Delirium Scale, which assesses level of consciousness and requires patients to recite the months backwards. It is reliable, quick, and feasible during rounds on the wards.

Factors that may precipitate delirium are opioids, anticholinergic and psychotropic medications (which have anticholinergic properties), anorexia/cachexia, reduced performance score, metabolic abnormalities, infections, and brain or leptomeningeal metastases. Elderly, dehydrated patients, and individuals with cognitive failure are at a particular risk to develop delirium. Immunotherapy, chemotherapy, sedative, alcohol, and nicotine withdrawal also precipitate delirium, and these factors are often missed by physicians. Delirium in particular may be the presenting manifestation of sepsis.[141,143]

The initial approach to delirium is to find a reversible cause. Deleting psychotropic and anticholinergic medications and opioid rotation should be done initially. Evaluation for infections and electrolyte disturbances should be done simultaneously. An occasional patient is hypothyroid and improves with thyroid replacement. Patients with a good performance score may require brain magnetic resonance imaging and lumbar puncture, depending on the goals of care. Those with a poor performance score prior to delirium should be treated symptomatically, and radiographic evaluation should be held to a minimum.[141,143]

Initial management is haloperidol, with doses of 0.5 to 1 mg for mild, 2 to 5 mg for moderate, and 5 to 10 mg for severe agitated delirium. Doses may be repeated after 30 minutes until improvement. Lower doses (0.25 to 0.5 mg) by mouth or intravenously every 4 to 6 hours should be used in the hypoalert delirious elderly individual. Patients who are not bothered by their delirium and terminally ill (and not agitated) may be watched and not treated. Sedation with lorazepam or midazolam (combined with haloperidol) is required for those who are agitated and in whom delirium fails to respond to haloperidol. Certain patients develop extrapyramidal reactions to haloperidol or may not respond, and in this case, the atypical antipsychotic olanzapine or risperidone may be effective as an alternative drug to treat.[143,147,148]

Endogenous serum anticholinergic activity is increased in delirium. Medications with anticholinergic properties such as opioids, certain psychotropics, and tricyclic antidepressants are known to precipitate delirium.[143,149–152] Donepezil, a central acting cholinesterase inhibitor, has been used to reverse delirium in dementia, delirium that occurs postoperatively, and delirium associated with anticholinergic medications including opioids.[143,153–156]

Nonpharmacologic approaches to the treatment of delirium include a quiet environment, calendars and clocks for orientation, the presence of relatives and friends, and frequent orientation. Early ambulation, glasses, and hearing aids may help reduce distorted perceptions and prevent delirium.[143]

CONCLUSION

Renal cell cancer presents with widely variable protean signs and symptoms. Symptomatic patients at presentation have a poorer prognosis compared to asymptomatic patients despite having the same stage of disease. Renal cell cancer spreads to unusual sites and can relapse years after nephrectomy. Paraneoplastic syndromes appear to be associated with tumor expression of IL-6. Pain, fatigue, gastrointestinal symptoms, depression, and delirium cause a great deal of symptom distress and should be managed aggressively. Treatment of individual symptoms may improve the quality of life even if life cannot be prolonged.

ACKNOWLEDGMENTS

The Harry R. Horvitz Center for Palliative Medicine is a World Health Organization project in palliative medicine. The author would like to acknowledge the help of Joan Scharf in preparing this manuscript.

REFERENCES

1. Whang Y, Godley PA. Renal cell carcinoma Curr Opinion in Oncol 2003;15(3):213–216.
2. Casamassima A, Picciariello M, Quaranta M, Berardino R, Ranieri C, Paradiso A. A C-reactive protein: a biomarker of survival in patients with metastatic renal cell carcinoma treated with subcutaneous interleukin-2 based immunotherapy. J Urol 2005;173:52–55.
3. Sorbellini M, Kattan MW, Snyder ME, Reuter V, Motzer R, Goetzl M. A postoperative prognostic nomogram predicting recurrence for patients with conventional clear cell renal cell carcinoma. J Urol 2005;173:48–51.
4. Lee C, Katz J, Fearn PA, Russo P. Mode of presentation of renal cell carcinoma provides prognostic information. Urologic Oncol 2002;7:135–140.
5. Patard J, Dorey FJ, Cindolo L, Ficarra V, De La Ta T. Symptoms as well as tumor size provide prognostic information on patients with localized renal tumors. J Urol 2004;172:2167–2171.
6. Schips L, Lipsky J, Zigeuner R, Salfellner M, Winkler S, Langner C. Impact of tumor associated symptoms on the prognosis of patients with renal cell carcinoma: a single center experience of 683 patients. Urology 2003;62:1024–1028.
7. Dall'Oglio M, Srougi M, Gonsalves PD, Leite K, Nesrallah L, Herin F. Incidental and symptomatic renal tumors: impact on patient survival. Sao Paulo Med J 2002;(6):165–169.
8. Weissglas M, Schamhart D, Lowik C, Papapoulos S, Vos P, Kurth KH. Hypercalcemia and cosecretion of interleukin 6 and parathyroid hormone related peptide by a human renal cell carcinoma implanted into nude mice. J Urol 1995;153:854–857.
9. Walther M, Johnson B, Culley D, Shah R, Weber J, Venzon D. Serum interleukin 6 levels in metastatic renal cell carcinoma before treatment with interleukin 2 correlates with paraneoplasm syndromes but not patient survival. J Urol 1998;159:718–722.
10. Gold P, Fefer A, Thompson JA. Paraneoplastic manifestations of renal cell carcinoma. Semin Urol Oncol 1996;14:216–222.
11. Kim H, Belldegrun AS, Freitas DG, Bui MHT, Han KR, Dorey FJ, Figlin RA. Paraneoplastic signs and symptoms of renal cell carcinoma: implications for prognosis. J Urol 2003;170:1742–1746.
12. Trikha M, Corringha R, Klein B, Rossi JF. Targeted anti-interleukin 6 monoclonal antibody therapy for cancer: a review of the rationale and clinical evidence. Clin Cancer Res 2003;9:4653–4665.
13. Motzer R, Bacik J, Mazumdar M. Prognostic factors for survival of patients with stage IV renal cell carcinoma: Memorial Sloan Kettering Cancer Center experience. Clin Cancer Res 2004;10:6302–6303.
14. Flanigan R. Debulking nephrectomy in metastatic renal cancer. Clin Cancer Res 2003;10:6335–6341.
15. Flanigan R, Campbell SC, Clark JL, Picken MM. Metastatic renal cell carcinoma. Curr Treat Options Oncol 2003;4(5):385–390.
16. Han K, Pantuck AJ, Bui MHT, Shvarts O, Freitas DG, Zisman A. A number of metastatic sites rather than location dictates overall survival of patients with node negative metastatic renal cell carcinoma. Adult Urol 2003;61:314–319.
17. Papac R, Poo-Hwu WH. Renal cell carcinoma: a paradigm of lanthanic disease. Am J Clin Oncol 1999;22:223–231.

18. Giacosa R, Santi R, Vaglio A, Pavone L, Ferrozzi F, Passalacqua R. Late regression of metastases from renal cancer after a period of disease progression continuing the same intermittent low dose immunotherapy regimen. Acta Biomed 2004;75:126–130.
19. Lipton A, Colombo-Berra A, Bukowski RM, Rosen L, Zheng M, Urbanowitz G. Skeletal complications in patients with bone metastases from renal cell carcinoma and therapeutic benefits of zolendronic acid. Clin Cancer Res 2004;10:6397–6403.
20. Staudenherz A, Steiner B, Puig S, Kainberger F, Leitha T. Is there a diagnostic role for bone scanning of patients with a high pretest probability for metastatic renal cell carcinoma? Clin Cancer Res 1999;85:153–155.
21. Koga S, Tsuda S, Nishikido M, et al. The diagnostic value of bone scan in patients with renal cell carcinoma. J Urol 2001;166:2126–2128.
22. Adiga G, Dutcher JP, Larkin M, Garl S, Koo J. Characterization of bone metastases in patients with renal cell cancer. BJU Int 2004;93:1237–1240.
23. Stepanek E, Joseph S, Campbell P, Porter M. Embolization of a limb metastasis in renal cell carcinoma as a palliative treatment of bone pain. Royal College of Radiologists 1999;54(12):855–857.
24. Munro N, Woodhams S, Nawrocki JD, Fletcher MS, Thomas PJ. The role of transarterial embolization in the treatment of renal cell carcinoma. BJU Int 2003;92:240–244.
25. Kollender Y, Bickels J, Price WM, Kellar KL, Chen J, Merimsky O. Metastatic renal cell carcinoma of bone: indications and technique of surgical intervention. J Oncol 2000;164:1505–1508.
26. Kierney P, van Heerden JA, Segura JW, Weaver AL. Surgeon's role in the management of solitary renal cell carcinoma metastases occurring subsequent to initial curative nephrectomy: an institutional review. Ann Surg Oncol 1994;1(4):345–352.
27. Onufrey V, Mohiuddin M. Radiation therapy in the treatment of metastatic renal cell carcinoma. Int J Radiat Oncol Biol Phys 1985;11:2007–2009.
28. DiBiase S, Valicenti RK, Schultz D, Zie Y, Gomella LG, Corn BW. Palliative irradiation for focally symptomatic metastatic renal cell carcinoma: support for dose escalation based on a biological model. J Urol 1997;158:746–749.
29. Wilson D, Hiller L, Gray L, Grainger M, Stirling A, James N. The effect of biological effective dose on time to symptom progression in metastatic renal cell carcinoma. Clin Oncol 2003; 15:400–407.
30. Halperin E, Harisiadis L. The role of radiation therapy in the management of metastatic renal cell carcinoma. Clin Res Cancer 1983;51:614–617.
31. Wu J, Wong RK, Lloyd NS, Johnston M, Bezjak A, Whelan T. Radiotherapy fractionation for the palliation of uncomplicated painful bone metastases—an evidence based practice guidelines. BMC Cancer 2004;4:71.
32. Wong R, Wiffen PJ. Bisphosphonates for the relief of pain secondary to bone metastases. Cochrane Database Sys Rev 2002;2:CD002068.
33. Body J, Diel IJ, Bell R, Pecherstorfer M, Lichinitser MR, Lazarev AF. Oral ibandronate improves bone pain and preserves quality of life in patients with skeletal metastases due to breast cancer. Int Assoc Study Pain 2004;111(3):306–312.
34. Urch C. The pathophysiology of cancer induced bone pain: current understanding. Palliat Med 2004;18:267–274.
35. Michaelson M, Rosenthal DI, Smith MR. Long term bisphosphonate treatment of bone metastases from renal cell carcinoma. J Clin Oncol 2004;22(20):4233–4234.
36. Dewar J. Managing metastatic bone pain. BMJ 2004;329:812–813.
37. Mancini I, Dumon JC, Body JJ. Efficacy and safety of ibandronate in the treatment of opioid resistant bone pain associated with metastatic bone disease: a pilot study. J Clin Oncol 2004;22(17): 3587–3592.
38. Li S, Liu J, Zhang H, Tian M, Wang J, Zheng X. X rhenium-188 HEDP to treat painful bone metastases. Clin Nucl Med 2001;26(11):919–922.
39. Neeman Z, Wood BJ. Radiofrequency ablation beyond the liver. Tech Vasc Intervent Radiol 2002;5(3):156–163.
40. Rohde D, Albers C, Mahnken A, Tacke J. Regional thermoablation of local or metastatic renal cell carcinoma. Oncol Report 2003;10(3):753–757.
41. Lewin J, Nour SG, Connell CF, Sulman A, Duerk JL, Resnick MI. Phase II clinical trial of interactive MR imaging guided interstitial radiofrequency thermal ablation of primary kidney tumors: initial experience. Radiology 2004;232(3):835–845.

42. Hines-Peralta A, Goldberg SN. Review of radiofrequency ablation for renal cell carcinoma. Clin Cancer Res 2004;10:6328–6334.

43. Campbell S, Flanigan RC, Clark JI. Nephrectomy in metastatic renal cell carcinoma. Curr Treat Options Oncol 2003;4(5):363–372.

44. Weber K, Doucet M, Price JE. Renal cell carcinoma bone metastasis: epidermal growth factor receptor targeting. Clin Orthop 2003;415S:S86–94.

45. Mancuso A, Sternberg C. New treatment approaches in metastatic renal cell carcinoma. Curr Opin Urol 2006;16:337–341.

46. Schijns O, Kurt E, Wessels P, Luijckx GJ, Beuls EA. Intermedullary spinal cord metastasis as a first manifestation of renal cell carcinoma: report of a case and review of the literature. Clin Neurol Neurosurg 2000;102(4):249–254.

47. Patel H, Arya M, Mirsadaree S, Mundy AR. Dismiss low back pain in renal cell carcinoma patients at your peril: meningeal cauda equine deposits. Eur J Surg 2001;27(4):428–429.

48. Jackson R, Loh SC, Gokaslan ZL. Metastatic renal cell carcinoma of the spine: surgical treatment and results. J Neurosurg Spine 2001;94(1):18–24.

49. Giehl J, Kluba T. Metastatic spine disease in renal cell carcinoma—indication and results of surgery. Anticancer Res 1999;19:1619–1623.

50. Sundaresan N, Rothman A, Manhart K, Kelliher K. Surgery for solitary metastases of the spine: rationale and result of treatment. Spine 2002;27(16):1802–1806.

51. Fakih M, Schiff D, Erich R, Logan TJ. Intramedullary spinal cord metastasis in renal cell carcinoma: a series of six cases. Ann Oncol 2001;12(8):1173–1177.

52. Harada Y, Nonomura N, Kondo M, Nishimura K, Takahara S, Miki T. Clinical study of brain metastasis of renal cell carcinoma. Eur Urol 1999;36(3):230–235.

53. Yamanaka K, Gohki K, Hara I, Gotoh A, Takechi Y, Yamada Y. Clinical study of renal cell carcinoma with brain metastasis. Int J Urol 1998;5(2):124–128.

54. Wronski M, Arbit E, Russo P, Galicich JH. Surgical resection of brain metastases from renal cell carcinoma in 50 patients. J Urol 1996;47(2):187–193.

55. Maor M, Frias AE, Oswald MJ. Palliative radiotherapy for brain metastases in renal cell carcinoma. Clin Cancer Res 1988;62(9):1912–1917.

56. Pace K, Dyer SJ, Steward RJ, et al. Health related quality of life after laparoscopic and open nephrectomy. Surg Endosc 2003;17:143–152.

57. Sheehan J, Sun MH, Kondziolka D, Flickinger J, Lunsford LD. Radiosurgery in patients with renal cell carcinoma metastasis to the brain: long term outcomes and prognostic factors influencing survival and local tumor control. J Neurosurg 2003;98(2):342–349.

58. Halbert R, Figlin R, Atkins M, et al. Treatment of patients with metastatic renal cell cancer. Cancer 2006;107:2375–2383.

59. Chaudhary U, Hull GW. The evolving role of cytoreductive surgery for metastatic renal cell carcinoma. Oncology 2003;17(5):701–705.

60. Oefelein M, Bayazit Y., Chronic pain syndrome after laparoscopic radical nephrectomy. J Urol 2003;170(5):1939–1940.

61. Coskun D, Gilchrist J, Dupuy D. Lumbosacral radiculopathy following radiofrequency ablation therapy. Muscle Nerve 2003;28(6):754–756.

62. Raju P, Roy T, McDonald RD, Harrison BR, Crim C, Hyers TM. IR-192 low dose rate endobronchial brachytherapy in the treatment of malignant airway obstruction. Int J Radiat Oncol Biol Phys 1993;27(3):677–680.

63. Wee J, Yang ET, Lim YC. HDR intraluminal brachytherapy for lung tumors—a case report. Singapore Med J 1994;35(3):325–326.

64. Desai A, Stadler WM. Novel kinase inhibitors in renal cell carcinoma: progressive development of static agents. Curr Oncol Rep 2005;7:116–122.

65. Rowinsky E, Schwartz GH, Gollob J. Epidermal growth factor receptor expression in renal cell carcinoma: rationale for therapy with sliding blockage. J Clin Oncol 2004;22:3003–3015.

66. Van Herpen C, De Mulder PHM. Prognostic and predictive factors of immunotherapy in metastatic renal cell carcinoma. Crit Rev Oncol/Hematol 2002;41:327–334.

67. Atzpodien J, Kuchler T, Wandert T, Reitz M. Rapid deterioration in quality of life during interleukin 2 and interferon based home therapy of renal cell carcinoma is associated with a good outcome. Br J Cancer 2003;89:50–54.

68. Tsavaris N, Mylonakis N, Bacoyiannis C, Tsoutsos H, Karabelis A, Kosmidis P. Treatment of renal cell carcinoma with escalating doses of alpha interferon. Chemotherapy 1993;39(5):361–366.

69. Oldham R, Blumenschein G, Schwartzberg L, Birch R, Arnold J. Combination biotherapy utilizing interleukin 2 and alpha interferon in patients with advanced cancer: a national biotherapy study group trial. Mol Biother 1992;4(1):4–9.

70. Piga A, Giordani P, Quattrone A, Giulioni M, DeSignoribus G, Antogno SA. A phase II study of interferon alpha and low dose subcutaneous interleukin 2 in advanced renal cell carcinoma. Cancer Immun Immunother 1997;44(6):348–351.

71. Anisman H, Merali Z, Poulter MO, Hayley S. Cytokines as a precipitant of depressive illness: animal and human studies. Curr Pharm Des 2005;11(8):963–972.

72. Capuron L, Dantzer R. Cytokines and depression: the need for a new paradigm. Brain Behav Immun 2003;17(1):S119–124.

73. Illman J, Corringham R, Robinson D, et al. Are inflammatory cytokines the common link between cancer associated cachexia and depression? J Support Oncol 2005;3(1):37–50.

74. Hayley S, Anisman H. Multiple mechanisms of cytokine action in neurodegenerative at psychiatric states: neurochemical and molecular substrates. Curr Pharm Des 2005;11(8):947–962.

75. Wichers M, Maes M. The psychoneuroimmuno-pathophysiology of cytokine induced depression in humans. Int J Neuropsychiatr 2002;5:375–388.

76. Dafny N, Reyes-Vazquez C. Single injection of three different preparations of alpha interferon modifies morphine abstinence signs for a prolonged period. Int J Neurosci 1987;32:953–961.

77. Dougherty P, Pearl J, Krajewski KJ, Pellis NR, Dafny N. Differential modification of morphine and methadone dependent by interferon alpha. Neuropharmacology 1987;26(11):1595–1600.

78. Dafny N. Interferon modifies morphine withdrawal phenomena in rodents. Neuropharmacology 1983;22(5):647–651.

79. Zubelewicz B, Braczkowski R, Romanowski W, Plaza J. Decline of metenkephalins concentration after interleukin 2 subcutaneous administration due to renal carcinoma. J Exp Clin Cancer Res 2000;19(1):53–55.

80. Lissoni P, Mandala M, Brivio F. Abrogation of the negative influence of opioids on IL-2 immunotherapy of renal cell cancer by melatonin. Eur Urol 2000;38(1):115–118.

81. Bortolussi R, Fabiani F, Savron F Testa V, Lazzarini R, Sorio R. Acute morphine intoxication during high dose recombinant interleukin 2 treatment for metastatic renal cell cancer. Eur J Cancer 1994; 30(12):1905–1907.

82. Motzer R, Hutson TE, Tomczak P et al. Sunitinib vs. interferon alpha in metastatic renal cell carcinoma. N Engl J Med 2007;356:115–124.

83. Bankhead C. Three new drugs available to fight kidney cancer. J Nat Cancer Inst 2006;98: 1181.

84. Negrier S, Perol D, Menetrier-Caux C, Escudier B, Pallardy M, Ravaud D. Interleukin 6, interleukin 10, and vascular endothelial growth factor in metastatic renal cell carcinoma: prognostic value of interleukin-6 from the Groupe Francais d'Immunotherapie. J Clin Oncol 2004;22(12):2371–2378.

85. Paule B, Belot J, Rudant C, Coulombel C, Abbou CC. The importance of IL6 protein expression in primary human renal cell carcinoma: an immunohistochemical study. J Clin Pathol 2000;53(5): 388–390.

86. Costes V, Liautard J, Picot MC, et al. Expression of the interleukin-6 receptor in primary renal cell carcinoma. J Clin Pathol 1997;50(10):835–840.

87. Paule B. Interleukin-6 and bone metastasis of renal cancer: molecular bases and therapeutic implications. Prog Urol 2001;11(2):368–375.

88. Kallio J, Tammela TL, Marttinene AT, et al. Soluble immunological parameters and early prognosis of renal cell cancer patients. J Exp Clin Cancer Res 2001;20(4):523–528.

89. Yoshida N, Ikemoto S, Narita K, Sugimura K, Wada S, Yasumoto R. Interleukin 6 tumor necrosis factor alpha and interleukin-1 patients with renal cell carcinoma. Br J Cancer 2002;86(9):396–400.

90. Walsh D, Mahmoud F, Barna B. Assessment of nutritional status and prognosis in advanced cancer: interleukin 6, C-reactive protein, and the prognostic and inflammatory nutritional index. Support Care Cancer 2003;11:60–62.

91. O'Byrne J, Dobbs N, Harris AL. Serum vascular endothelial growth factor load and interleukin-6 in cancer patients. Br J Cancer 2000;82(1):1895–1896.

92. Ueno M, Ban SI, Nakanoma T, Tsukamoto T, Nonaka S, Hirata R. Hypercalcemia in a patient with renal cell carcinoma producing parathyroid hormone related protein and interleukin-6. Int J Oncol 2000;7:239–242.

93. Paule B, Clerc D, Rudant C, et al. Enhanced expression of interleukin-6 in bone and serum of metastatic renal cell carcinoma. Hum Pathol 1998;29(4):421–424.

94. Weissglas M, Schamhart DH, Lowik CW, Papapoulos SE, Theuns HM, Kurth KH. The role of inter-leukin-5 in the induction of hypercalcemia in renal cell carcinoma transplanted into nude mice. Endocrinology 1997;138(5):1879–1885.

95. Wechsel H, Feil G, Lahme S, Zumbragel A, Petri E, Bichler KH. Control of hepatic parameters in renal cell carcinoma by interleukin 6. Anticancer Res 1999;19:2577–2581.

96. Blay J, Rossi JF, Wijdenes J, et al. Role of interleukin-6 in the paraneoplastic inflammatory syndrome associated with renal cell carcinoma. Int J Cancer 1997;72(3):424–430.

97. Stouthard J, Goey H, de Vries EG, de Mulder PH, Groenewegen A, Pronk L. Recombinant human interleukin-6 in metastatic renal cell cancer: a phase II trial. Br J Cancer 1996;73(6):789–793.

98. Nieken J, Mulder NH, Buter J, Vellenga E, Limburg PC, Piers DA. Recombinant human interleukin-6 induces a rapid and reversible anemia in cancer patients. Blood 1995;86(3):900–905.

99. Dosquet C, Schaetz A, Faucher C, Lepage E, Wautier JL, Richard F. Tumour necrosis factor alpha interleukin 1 beta and interleukin 6 in patients with renal cell carcinoma. Eur J Cancer 1994; 30A:162–167.

100. Walther M, Patel B, Choyke PL, Lubensky IA, Vocke CD, Harris C. Hypercalcemia in patients with metastatic renal cell carcinoma: effect of nephrectomy and metabolic evaluation. J Urol 1997; 158:733–739.

101. Blay J, Favrot M, Rossi JF, Wijdenes J. Role of interleukin-6 in paraneoplastic thrombocytosis. Blood 1993;82(7):2261–2262.

102. Steiner T, Junker U, Wunderlich H, Schubert J. Are renal cell carcinoma cells able to modulate the cytotoxic effects of tumor infiltrating lymphocytes by secretion of interleukin-6? Anticancer Res 1999;19:1533–1536.

103. Dunlop R, Campbell CW. Cytokines and advanced cancer. J Pain Symptom Manage 2000;20(3): 214–232.

104. Cleeland C, Bennett GJ, Dantzer R, Dougherty PM, Dunn AJ, Meyers CA. Are the symptoms of cancer and cancer treatment due to a shared biologic mechanism? Am Cancer Soc 2003; 97(11):2919–2925.

105. Kurzrock R. The role of cytokines in cancer related fatigue. Cancer 2001;92(6):1684–1688.

106. Lee B, Dantzer R, Langley KE, Bennett GJ, Dougherty PM, Dunn AJ. A cytokine based neuroim-munologic mechanism of cancer related symptoms. Neuroimmunomodulation 2004;11(5):279–292.

107. Argiles J, Busquets S, Lopez-Soriano FJ. Cytokines in the pathogenesis of cancer. Cachexia Curr Opin 2003;6(4):401–406.

108. Plata-Salaman C. Central nervous system mechanisms contributing to the cachexia anorexia syn-drome. Nutrition 2000;16:1009–1012.

109. Van der Mast R. Pathophysiology of delirium. J Geriatr Psychiatr Neurol 1998;11(3):138–145.

110. Davis M, Walsh D. Epidemiology of cancer pain and factors influencing poor pain control. Am J Hosp Palliat Care 2004;21(2):137–142.

111. Davis M, Walsh D. Cancer pain; how to measure the fifth vital sign. Cleve Clin J Med 2004; 71(8):625–632.

112. Diblasio C, Snyder ME, Kattan MW, Russo P. Ketorolac: safe and effective analgesia for the manage-ment of renal cortical tumors with partial nephrectomy. J Urol 2004;171(3):1062–1065.

113. Romsing J, Moiniche S, Mathiesen O, Dahl JB. Reduction of opioid related adverse events using opioid sparing analgesia with COX2 inhibitors lacks documentation: a systemic review. Acta Anaes-thesiol Scand 2005;49:133–142.

114. Kochlar R, LeGrand SB, Walsh D, Davis MP, Lagman R, Rivera NI. Opioids in cancer pain: common dosing errors. Oncology 2003;4:571–575.

115. Bercovitch M, Adunsky A. Patterns of high dose morphine use in a home care hospice service: should we be afraid of it? Cancer 2004;101(6):1473–1477.

116. Walsh D. Pharmacological management of cancer pain. Semin Oncol 2000;27(1):138–144.

117. Hanks G, de Conno F, Cherny N, Hanna M, Kalso E, McQuay HJ. Morphine and alternative opioids in cancer pain: the EAPC recommendations. Br J Cancer 2001;94(5):587–593.

118. Portenoy R, Payne D, Jacobsen P. Breakthrough pain: characteristics and impact in patients with cancer pain. Pain 1999;81:129–134.

119. Hwang S, Chang VT, Kasimis B. Cancer breakthrough pain characteristics and responses to treatment at a VA medical center. Int Assoc for the Study of Pain 2003;101:55–64.

120. Caraceni A, Martini C, Zecca E, Portenoy RK. Breakthrough pain characteristics and syndromes in patients with cancer pain. Pall Med 2004;18:177–183.

121. Walsh D, Rivera NI, Davis MP, Lagman R, LeGrand SB. Strategies for pain management: Cleveland Clinic Foundation Guidelines for opioid dosing for cancer pain. Support Cancer Ther 2004; 3:157–164.
122. Walsh D. Advances in opioid therapy and formulations. Support Care Cancer 2005;13:138–144.
123. Mercadante S. Opioid rotation for cancer pain. Cancer 1999;86(9):1856–1866.
124. Davis M. Opioid therapy: the neurological basis of pain. In: The Neurological Basis of Pain. Pappagalo M, ed. New York: McGraw-Hill, 559–580.
125. Burton A, Rajagopal A, Shah HN, Mendoza T, Cleeland C, Hassenbusch SJ. Epidural and intrathecal analgesia is effective in treating refractory cancer pain. Pain Med 2004;5(3):239–247.
126. Hanks G, Reid C. Contribution to variability in response to opioids. Support Care Cancer 2005; 13:145–152.
127. Carr D, Goudas LC, Balk EM, Bloch R, Ioannidis PA, Lau J. Evidence report on the treatment of pain in cancer patients. J Natl Cancer Inst Monographs 2004;32:23–31.
128. Harden R. Chronic neuropathic pain: mechanisms, diagnosis, and treatment. Neurologist 2005; 11(2):111–122.
129. Dworkin R, Backonja M, Rowbotham MC, Allen RR, Argoff CF, Bennett GJ. Advances in neuropathic pain: diagnosis, mechanisms and treatment recommendations. Arch Neurol 2003;60(11): 1524–1534.
130. Davis M. New drugs for the anorexia-cachexia syndrome. Curr Oncol Rep 2002;4:264–274.
131. Strasser F, Bruera ED. Update on anorexia and cachexia. Hematol Oncol Clin North Am 2002; 16:589–617.
132. Bentley A, Boyd K. Use of clinical pictures in the management of nausea and vomiting: a prospective audit. Palliat Med 2001;15:247–253.
133. Davis M, Walsh D. Treatment of nausea and vomiting in advanced cancer. Support Care Cancer 2000;8:444–452.
134. Baines M. ABC of palliative care: nausea, vomiting, and intestinal obstruction. BMJ 1997;315: 1148–1150.
135. Glare P, Pereira G, Kristjanson LJ, Stockler M, Tattersall M. Systematic review of the efficacy of antiemetics in the treatment of nausea in patients with far advanced cancer. Support Care Cancer 2004;12:432–440.
136. Lloyd-Williams M. Depression the hidden symptom in advanced cancer. J R Soc Med 2003;96: 577–581.
137. Reuter K, Raugust S, Bengel J, Harter M. Depressive symptom patterns and their consequences for diagnosis of affective disorders in cancer patients. Support Care Cancer 2004;12:864–870.
138. Lloyd-Williams M, Dennis M, Taylor F. A prospective study to determine the association between physical symptoms and depression in patients with advanced cancer. Palliat Med 2004;18:558–563.
139. Chen M, Chang HK. Physical symptom profiles of depressed and non-depressed patients with cancer. Palliat Med 2004;18:712–718.
140. Homsi J, Walsh D, Nelson KA, LeGrand S, Davis M. Methylphenidate for depression in hospice practice: a case series. Am J Hosp Palliat Care 2000;17(6):393–398.
141. Centeno C, Sanz A, Bruera E. Delirium in advanced cancer patients. Palliat Med 2004;18: 184–194.
142. Casarett D, Inouye SK. Diagnosis and management of delirium near the end of life. Ann Intern Med 2001;135:32–40.
143. Caraceni A, Grassil L. Management in delirium. In: Dilirum: acute confusional states in palliative medicine. Oxford: Oxford University Press, 2003:131–157.
144. Duppils G, Wikblad K. Delirium: behavioral changes before and during the prodroma phase. J Clin Nurs 2004;13(5):609–616.
145. Adamis D, Treloar A, MacDonald AJD, Martin FC. Concurrent validity of two instruments (the confusion assessment method and the delirium rating scale) in the detection of delirium among older medical inpatients. Age Ageing 2005;34:72–83.
146. Sarhill N, Walsh D, Nelson KA, LeGrand S, Davis MP. Assessment of delirium in advanced cancer: the use of the bedside confusion scale. Am J Hosp Palliat Care 2001;18(5):335–341.
147. Brietbart W, Tremblay A, Gibson C. An open trial of olanzapine for the treatment of delirium in hospitalized cancer patients. Psychosomatics 2002;43(3):175–182.
148. Mittal D, Jamerson NA, Neely EP, Johnson WD, Kennedy RE, Torres R. Risperidone in the treatment of delirium: results from a prospective open label trial. J Clin Psychiatry 2004;65(5):662–667.

149. Han L, McCusker J, Cole M, Abrahamowicz M, Primeau F, Elie M. Use of medications with anticholinergic effect predicts clinical severity of delirium symptoms in older medical inpatients. Arch Intern Med 2001;161:1099–1105.
150. Burke A. Palliative care: an update on terminal restlessness. Med J Aust 1997;166(1):39–42.
151. Tune L, Egeli S. Acetylcholine and delirium. Dement Geriatr Cogn Disord 1999;10(5):342–344.
152. Paul K, Bhatara VS. Anticholinergic delirium possibly associated with protriptyline and fluoxetine. Ann Pharmacother 1997;31(10):1260–1261.
153. Wengel S, Roccaforte WH, Burke WJ. Donepezil improves symptoms of delirium in dementia: implications for future research. J Geriatr Psychiatr Neurol 1998;11(3):159–161.
154. Gleason O. Donepezil for postoperative delirium Psychosomatics 2003;44(5):437–438.
155. Noyan M, Elbi H, Aksu H. Donepezil for anticholinergic drug intoxication: a case report. Pro Neuropsypharmacol Biol Psychiatr 2003;27(5):885–887.
156. Slatkin N, Rhiner M. Treatment of opioid induced delirium with acetylcholinesterase inhibitors: a case report. J Pain Symptom Manage 2004;27(3):268–273.

32

Management of Patients with Pathologic Variants of Renal Cell Carcinoma: *Papillary, Collecting Duct, Medullary and Chromophobe Carcinoma, and Sarcomatoid Differentiation*

Vladimir Hugec and Janice P. Dutcher

KEYWORDS

RENAL CELL CARCINOMA
PAPILLARY CARCINOMA
COLLECTING DUCT CARCINOMA
MEDULLARY CARCINOMA
CHROMOPHOBE CARCINOMA
SACOMATOID VARIANT
CHEMOTHERAPY
TARGETED THERAPY

ABSTRACT

Non-clear-cell renal cell carcinoma is an uncommon disease with distinct subtypes. These subtypes have different pathologic characteristics and biologic behaviors, including occasional responses to chemotherapy and possibly the new targeted therapies. This chapter focuses on the evaluation and management of papillary, collecting duct, medullary, and chromophobe carcinoma as well as sarcomatoid variant. Current treatment evidence relies on small cohort studies. As such, it is important to consider well-designed trials, with an emphasis on subtype of non-clear-cell carcinoma, as first-line therapy.

Renal cell carcinoma (RCC) is the 10th most common malignancy in the United States.[1] However, increasing information indicates that this is a heterogeneous disease. Several subtypes of RCC with distinct biologic behavior and different pathologic characteristics have been recognized during the last decade.[2] The Union International Contre le Cancer (UICC) and the American Joint Committee on Cancer (AJCC) have classified RCC into the following histologic subtypes: clear cell (conventional) carcinoma (75%

From: *Clinical Management of Renal Tumors*
Edited by: R.M. Bukowski and A.C. Novick © Humana Press Inc., Totowa, NJ

of all cases), papillary carcinoma, chromophobe carcinoma, and collecting duct carcinoma,[3] based on the Heidelberg classification system.[4] In addition, sarcomatoid dedifferentiation is often noted in conjunction with the diagnosis of specific subtypes. The category of granular RCC is not a subtype, but suggests increased cellularity, and is often a feature of clear cell carcinoma.[4]

It is a relatively recent development that pathologic distinctions are being made, and therefore previous trials and the majority of the current literature do not stratify patients by histopathology. This becomes important as we dissect the molecular basis for the morphologic distinctions, and certain genetic differences have been discovered and will be discussed subsequently. Therefore, RCC subtypes should be considered as separate diseases demonstrating different clinical behavior, and as such, specific therapeutics should be evaluated. Current trials should be evaluated using the hypothesis that different molecular and histologic subtypes may respond differently to different treatments, and this will need to be proven or disproven.

EPIDEMIOLOGY

Renal cell cancer incidence rates have increased steadily between 1992 and 2001 by 1.4% per year in the U.S. population. However, the rate of death annually is slightly decreasing over time. It is estimated that 51,190 new cases will be diagnosed in 2007 and that 12,890 persons will die of this disease in 2007. The male-to-female ratio ranges from 2:1 to 3:1 and the median age at presentation is 65 years. Separate data for non–clear-cell histology are not available; however, if we extrapolate that approximately 25% of RCC patients are non–clear-cell histology, these patients constitute 8927 individuals diagnosed every year with these distinct histopathologic features.[5]

INCIDENCE AND NATURAL HISTORY

As stated, the 20% to 25% incidence of non–clear-cell RCC from surgical series is composed of papillary carcinoma (10% to 15%), chromophobe carcinoma (5%), collecting duct carcinoma (1%), and medullary carcinoma (1% to 3%).[2] Primary non–clear-cell carcinomas tend to have a better prognosis after nephrectomy than clear-cell histology tumors based on available surgical reviews.[6] Non–clear-cell histology constitutes only 5% to 8% of metastatic RCCs in published reports. A review of all RCC patients treated for metastatic disease with cytokines from Memorial Sloan-Kettering Cancer Center (MSKCC) suggests a poor prognosis for non–clear-cell carcinomas, once metastatic.[6] In that series, metastatic papillary cancers had a median survival of 5.5 months, metastatic collecting duct had a median survival of 11 months, and metastatic chromophobe cancer had a median survival of 29 months.[6] The Cytokine Working Group has presented data suggesting a lack of response of non–clear-cell RCC to immunotherapy.[7] This information suggested that there was no defined effective medical treatment available for non–clear-cell RCC, and clinical investigation was mandatory.

PATHOLOGY

Papillary renal cell carcinoma (PRCC) is the second most common subtype of RCC and is also known as the chromophil subtype. There are two recognized subtypes of PRCC: type I (basophilic) and type II (eosinophilic). Characteristic papillary features are present. Neoplastic cells may have a granular or clear cytoplasm.[8] The reader is directed to Chapter 9 for a more complete discussion of pathologic RCC subtypes. Chromophobe renal cell carcinoma (CRCC) represents approximately 5% of all RCCs. There is a clear cell halo present within the neoplastic cells. The nuclei tend to vary in size more than other RCCs. Increased numbers of mitochondria seen by electron microscopy is a diagnostic feature.[8]

Collecting duct carcinoma (CDC) is primarily derived from the renal medulla and renal pelvis but may invade the renal cortex. Microscopically this subtype has tubular or tubolopapillary features, and neoplastic cells have enlarged irregular nuclei. These tumors resemble renal medullary carcinoma.[8,9]

Renal medullary carcinoma (RMC) is a rare tumor that is most common in young black men with sickle cell disease or trait. This entity is often confused with CDC or poorly differentiated transitional cell carcinoma.[8] Renal medullary carcinoma has a typical histologic appearance with a reticular growth pattern like a yolk sac tumor, stromal desmoplasia, and is associated with a prominent inflammatory response (including neutrophilic infiltration and lymphocytes at the tumor margin). Molecular studies by Yang et al.[9] suggest that a messenger RNA (mRNA) expression profile helps to distinguish RMC from clear cell, chromophobe, or papillary RCC, and it is similar to that of transitional cell carcinoma of the renal pelvis. This analysis did not compare it to transitional cell carcinoma of the bladder or to CDC, however.[8,9]

Sarcomatoid carcinoma with spindle cell morphology is not considered a separate histopathologic entity. Mixed histologies are very common, and sarcomatoid features are recognized within the standard histologies. The significance of mixed histology is not always predictive, but in general such a mixture is considered a poor prognostic factor.[8] Large amounts of sarcomatoid RCC predict a highly aggressive clinical behavior.

GENETICS AND BIOLOGY

Cytogenetics and gene expression profiling studies are beginning to clarify more precisely the differences among the histologic subtypes of RCC.[10] Morphologic differences have divided papillary RCC into type 1 and type 2, but with genetic patterns that may also differentiate the two.[11] Collecting duct carcinomas and medullary carcinomas are related to transitional cell carcinomas, based on histology and gene expression profiles.[12]

Familial non–clear-cell carcinoma syndromes have been described and germline mutated genes have been identified.[13] Familial type I papillary cancer has been associated with a *met* oncogene mutation that leads to activation of this growth factor receptor tyrosine kinase.[14] Familial type II papillary cancer has been associated with cutaneous and uterine leiomyomas. Birt-Hogg-Dubé syndrome, characterized by fibrofolliculomas on the face, neck, and upper trunk and pulmonary cysts, has been associated with chromophobe cancer.[15] However, the role of these genes in the pathogenesis of non–clear-cell carcinoma is yet to be determined.

CLINICAL PRESENTATION

Patients with RCC are often asymptomatic at presentation and may be diagnosed incidentally. However, painless hematuria is the most common presenting symptom, and occurs in 50% to 60% of patients.[16] Additional patients present with weight loss, an abdominal mass, or signs or symptoms arising from metastatic sites. These features are similar for all subtypes of RCC. More rapidly growing disease may produce symptoms of fever, night sweats, or weight loss. Sarcomatoid RCC and poorly differentiated RCC are more frequently associated with these symptoms. Otherwise, there are few, if any, clinical features separating the histologic subtypes.

One exception is that RMC presents at a younger age (mean age 18 years) and is associated with sickle cell hemoglobinopathy. Most patients with RMC present with locally extensive or metastatic disease.[17–19] Collecting duct carcinoma, compared in the literature with RMC, usually presents at an older age (>40 years, mean age 43 years). Most CDC and RMC are metastatic at presentation in contrast to papillary or chromophobe RCC.[20] Both RMC and CDC may respond to chemotherapy treatment.

Chromophobe RCC most often presents in the early stages and is a slow-growing disease.[21] It has a much lower incidence of metastatic disease, and is considered a very low grade malignancy. Treatment of metastatic chromophobe carcinoma is not well characterized, and immunotherapy and chemotherapy have been used, with only anecdotal data.

Papillary RCC is also more likely to be localized disease, and as stated above, whereas it represents 15% of cases in surgical series, it represents only about 5% to 7% of patients treated for metastatic disease. Even in the metastatic setting, it is a much slower disease process than metastatic clear-cell carcinoma or the other non–clear-cell types, with the exception of chromophobe RCC.

PROGNOSTIC FACTORS

Prognostic indicators overall for RCC are divided into patient-related and tumor-related factors (Tables 32.1 and 32.2). Age was reported as an independent prognostic factor in one study, with younger patients having longer disease-free survival,[22] but other studies have not confirmed this. Recently, several large series have reviewed patients with RCC and analyzed prognostic factors.[23–26] Motzer et al.[23] proposed that for patients with metastatic disease there were five independent poor prognostic factors: low Karnofsky performance status (<80%), high serum lactate dehydrogenase (>1.5 times the upper limit of normal), low hemoglobin (less than the lower limit of normal), high "corrected" serum calcium (>10 mg/dL), and the absence of prior nephrectomy.[23,27] Motzer's model stratifies patients into three different groups: favorable (no risk factors), intermediate (one or two risk factors), and poor (three or more risk factors), which corresponds to the following median survival times: 29.6 months (favorable), 13.8 months (intermediate), and 4.9 months (poor). A retrospective analysis of 353 patients from Cleveland Clinic has validated and expanded this model to include the number of metastatic sites (more than one) and prior radiotherapy as additional poor prognostic factors.

Stage is the most important prognostic factor for RCC of all histologic subtypes, and the nuclear grading system is of secondary significance.[28] Surgical margins and the number and location of metastases are well-accepted tumor-related prognostic factors.[29] The time from the primary tumor occurrence to the development of metastatic disease has prognostic import in some series.[30]

Table 32.1.
Patient-related prognostic factors for renal cell carcinoma

Attribute	*Unfavorable feature*
Performance status	<80% (Karnofsky)
Nephrectomy	No
Lactate dehydrogenase (LDH)	>1.5 times upper limit of normal
Hemoglobin	<Lower limit of normal
Hypercalcemia	>Upper normal corrected calcium level

Source: Motzer et al.[23]

Table 32.2.
Tumor-related prognostic factors for renal cell carcinoma

Attribute	Unfavorable feature
Surgical margin	Positive
Metastasis	
Number	Multiple
Solitary	Unresectable
Location	Liver, lung
Grade	High grade
Architecture	Sarcomatoid

Source: Motzer et al.[23]

Prognosis after nephrectomy is also dependent on histologic subtype, with non–clear-cell subtypes having longer survival than clear cell in all these series (Table 32.3). In one review of 2385 patients, cancer-specific survival at 5 years with clear cell (1985 patients), papillary (102 patients), and chromophobe cell (six patients) were 69%, 87%, and 86% ($p < .001$).[16] In contrast, malignant tumors with sarcomatoid features have 35% and 27% five-year disease-specific and progression-free survival.[32] Renal medullary carcinoma has a poor prognosis, in large part because such patients are usually diagnosed with extensive metastatic disease, and the mean survival with complete follow-up was 4 months, reported in two large retrospective series.[33,34] Papillary RCC seems to have better prognosis than clear cell carcinoma.[35] Papillary carcinoma type I usually presents at lower stage and grade and has a better prognosis than does type II.[35] In contrast, Motzer et al.[36] published outcome data and survival based on a review of 64 cases of non–clear-cell RCC with metastatic disease. Median survival for papillary carcinoma was 5.5 months, for CDC was 11 months, and for chromophobe carcinoma was 29 months (Figures 32.1 and 32.2).

SURGICAL TREATMENT

Localized Disease

The mainstay of treatment for localized disease for any subtype of RCC is surgical removal of the kidney tumor. This is both diagnostic and therapeutic. The gold standard curative measure for patients with a normal contralateral kidney is radical nephrectomy. Partial nephrectomy is an option for patients with a solitary kidney. Laparoscopic hand-assisted partial nephrectomy is currently reserved for patients with tumors less than 4 cm

Table 32.3.
Five-year cancer-specific survival in different histologic subtype

First author	Clear cell 5-year survival % (n)	Papillary 5-year survival % (n)	Chromophobe 5-year survival % (n)
Ljunberg[31]	43% (145)	61% (25)	91% (12)
Amin[32]	76% (255)	86% (75)	100% (24)
Cheville[16]	69% (1985)	87% (270)	87% (102)
Beck[6]	73% (784)	82% (157)	80% (100)
Patard[25]	73% (3564)	79% (396)	88% (103)

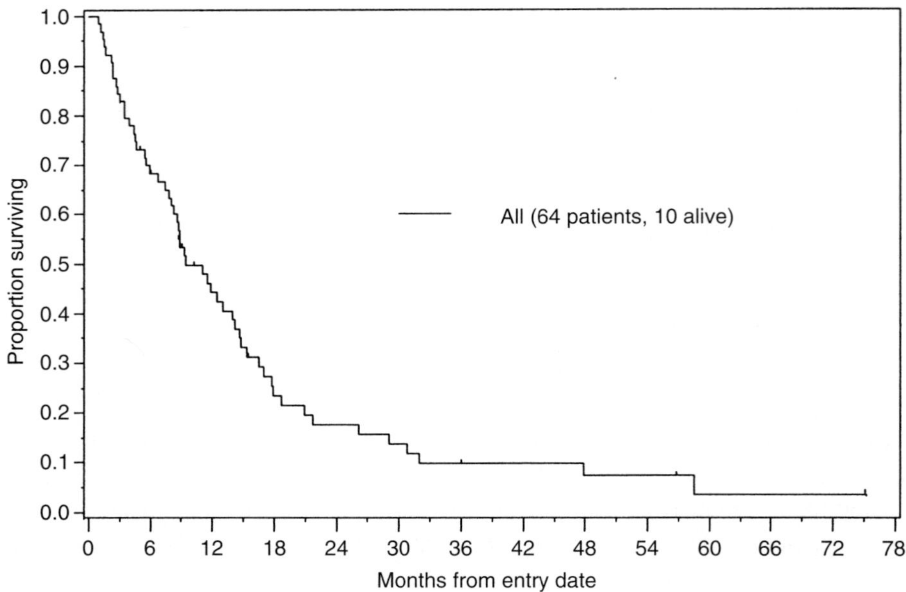

Figure 32.1. Survival in non–clear-cell carcinoma in a study of 64 patients. (From Motzer et al.[36])

in size or a solitary kidney. Studies show that this approach is safe and has an acceptable decline in renal function and low likelihood of temporary or permanent hemodialysis.[37,38] The surgical approach continues to develop, with more limited surgeries, and even cryosurgery and radiofrequency ablation for smaller tumors, particularly in patients with bilateral or multiple renal tumors (see Chapter 14 for additional discussion of this topic).

Metastatic Disease

The role of surgery in the metastatic setting is more controversial. Approximately one third of patients with RCC present with metastatic disease. There is no standard

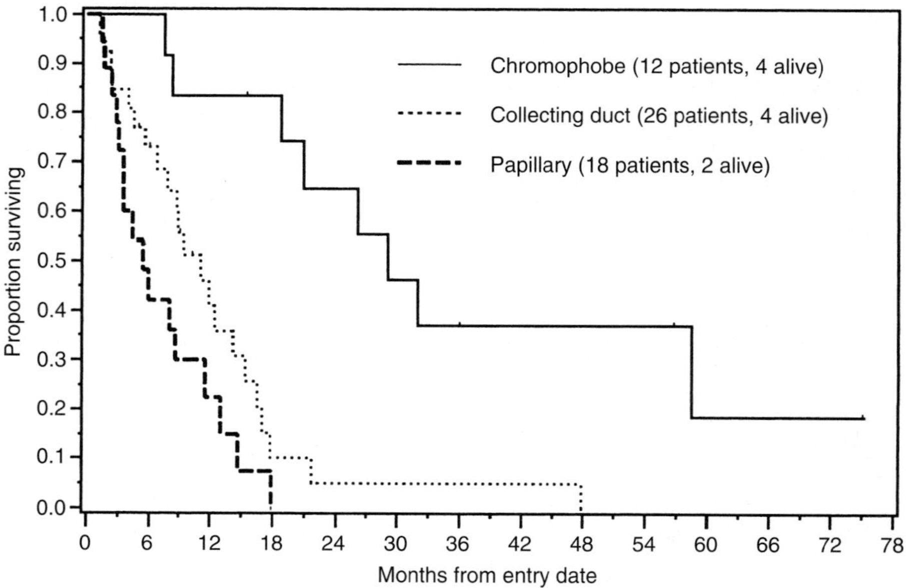

Figure 32.2. Patient survival by histology in a study of 64 patients. (From Motzer et al.[36])

surgical approach with metastatic non–clear-cell RCC. Nephrectomy or metastasectomy has a definitive role in certain well-selected patients, usually those with solitary metastases, good performance status, and no significant comorbidities.[39] Current data support total metastasectomy at the time of nephrectomy or later at the time of recurrence in selected patients.[40] The role of nephrectomy in patients with multiple metastases as an initial therapeutic approach is unknown and has more of a palliative purpose.[20,41] Data suggest that nephrectomy in the setting of metastatic disease has a beneficial impact on subsequent treatment with immunotherapy.[42,43] However, that applies to clear cell carcinoma. The role of nephrectomy in non–clear-cell metastatic disease is controversial, but may yield both diagnostic and therapeutic effects. Most patients undergo nephrectomy as part of the diagnostic process.

SYSTEMIC TREATMENT

Immunotherapy

A retrospective analysis of several treatment series strongly suggests that immunotherapy is not effective in any non–clear-cell subtype. The Cytokine Working Group reported that only one of 17 patients responded to high-dose interleukin-2,[35] and Memorial Sloan-Kettering Cancer Center investigators have reported only one of 37 patients with non–clear-cell histology responding to interferon therapy.[36] Thus, current practice is moving away from immunotherapy in non–clear-cell histologies.

Chemotherapy

Renal cell carcinoma is a highly chemotherapy-resistant tumor. However, the experience with chemotherapy is very limited in non–clear-cell RCC. Earlier studies of chemotherapy that reported response rate and survival data did not identify the histologic subgroups of patients. Available data are mostly in patients with clear-cell histology. Recent interest in chemotherapy approaches has focused on subtypes that are not related to clear-cell RCC. Cases of transitional cell carcinoma have been successfully treated with gemcitabine, Navelbine, and platinum-based therapies. Consideration is being given to the relationship of non–clear-cell RCC, particularly CDC and RMC, to transitional cell carcinoma, and investigation of regimens utilized for the latter are being explored in these rare subtypes of RCC. Additionally, there is consideration of chemotherapy in patients with sarcomatoid differentiation, given the rapidly growing and aggressive nature of this variant, making it nearly impossible to treat with immunotherapy. Although RCC is considered a highly chemotherapy-resistant tumor, in specific subtypes there may well be sensitivity to specific drugs.

SARCOMATOID VARIANT (Table 32.4)

Multiple regimens have been used in the sarcomatoid variant of RCC. A retrospective analysis of data from an M.D. Anderson Cancer Center series found that among eight of 44 patients with metastatic sarcomatoid RCC who received a doxorubicin-based regimen, there were two complete responses, and these patients were the only long-term survivors (50 and 65 months); four patients who were treated with interferon-α had a median survival of 41 months.[44] However, the combination of doxorubicin and ifosfamide was disappointing, with no responses.[45] Additionally, the MAID regimen (mesna, Adriamycin, ifosfamide, and dacarbazine)[46] and a combination of gemcitabine, docetaxel, and carboplatin have shown some response activity in sarcomatoid RCC.[47] Most recently, based on a regimen used for bladder cancer, the combination of doxo-

Table 32.4.
Chemotherapy outcome for sarcomatoid renal cell carcinoma

First author	n	Regimen	CR	PR	OS
Nanus[48]	18	Adriamycin + gemcitabine	11%	27%	6 months to 4+ years
Bangalore[46]	1	MAID	1%		4+ years
Escudier[45]	23	Adriamycin + ifosfamide			3.9 months

CR, complete response; PR, partial response; OS, overall survival; MAID, mesna, Adriamycin, ifosfamide, and dacarbazine.

rubicin 50 mg/m^2 and gemcitabine 1500 to 2000 mg/m^2 given every 2 weeks with growth factor support has been studied in a series of 18 patients. Response was noted in 10, including two complete responses with median response duration of 5 months (range 2 to 21+ months).[48] Ongoing survival ranges from 6 months to 4+ years (J. Dutcher, personal communication). Anecdotal reports have also seen major responses when given at 3-week intervals. This treatment approach in sarcomatoid RCC is currently undergoing evaluation in the Eastern Cooperative Oncology Group (ECOG).

RENAL MEDULLARY CARCINOMA

In the majority of experiences reported, this rare subtype is characterized as a highly aggressive disease. Recent reports of chemotherapy approaches have suggested possible progress. Regimens utilized for the treatment of urothelial carcinoma have been the most encouraging, adding support to the hypothesis of the relationship of medullary and collecting duct carcinoma to urothelial carcinoma. Several small reports suggest a role for two different regimens. The MVAC (methotrexate, vinblastine, doxorubicin, and cisplatin) regimen produced one complete response and two partial responses among six patients with advanced disease.[49–51] Cisplatin 70 mg/m^2 (day 1) or carboplatin AUC 6 and paclitaxel 80 mg/^{2} (day 1) and gemcitabine 1000 mg/m^2 (days 1, 8, and 15) with pegfilgrastim 6 mg subcutaneously on day 9 of a 21-day cycle produced a good response in two patients with stage IV disease, with survivals of 10 and 12 months in the responders.[51] Survival is similar in patients treated with platinum-based chemotherapy combined with gemcitabine and paclitaxel (11 months) compared to those treated with MVAC (8 months), although the number of patients was too low for definitive conclusions.[49–52]

COLLECTING DUCT CARCINOMA (Table 32.5)

There are limited prospective data describing treatment approaches for this subtype of renal cell carcinoma. Most are retrospective reviews or case reports. The M.D. Anderson Cancer Center reported a retrospective series of 12 cases (11 with metastatic or locally advanced disease) treated with the MVAC regimen with only one minor response.[53] French researchers retrospectively evaluated the outcome of 9 patients with metastatic CDC treated with cisplatin 70 mg/m2 on day 1 and gemcitabine 1250 mg/m2 on days 1 and 8, and reported partial responses in two of the nine patients. Response was seen after three cycles, and these two patients remained disease free for 9 and 27 months after nephrectomy.[54] This report led to the conduct of a prospective phase II trial from the French Groupe d'Etudes des Tumeurs Uro-Genitales (GETUG) which was recently published and involved 23 patients with metastatic CDC treated with this regimen or with the substitution of carboplatin (AUC 6) for cisplatin.[55] They reported a 26% response rate (1 complete and 2 partial responses) with a median progression-free survival of 7.1 months and an overall survival of 10.5 months.[55] Additional case

TABLE 32.5
Chemotherapy outcome for collecting duct carcinoma

First Author	N	Regimen	CR	PR	DFS	OS
Dimopoulos[53]	12	MVAC		1pt		22 mo
Peyromaure[54]	9	cisplatin+gemcitabine		2pts	9 mo	
Oudard[55]	23	cisplatin+gemcitabine	1pt	5pts	7.1 mo	27 mo 10.5 mo
Gollob[56]	1	carboplatin+paclitaxel		1pt	20 mo	

CR, complete response; PR, partial response; OS, overall survival; DFS, disease-free survival; MVAC, methotrexate, vinblastine, doxorubicin, and cisplatin.

reports include a single patient treated with carboplatin and paclitaxel who remained diseas-free without recurrence for 20 months,[56] and another patient who achieved partial response with a survival of 10 months, after treatment with six cycles of doxorubicin 50 mg/m2 and gemcitabine 2000 mg/m2 every 2 weeks with granulocyte colony-stimulating factor support followed by ITP (ifosfamide 1500 mg/m2, days 1 to 3, paclitaxel 175 mg/m2 day 1, and cisplatin 35 mg/m2 days 1 and 2).[57]

PAPILLARY AND CHROMOPHOBE RENAL CARCINOMA

There is very limited experience with chemotherapy in these two variants of RCCs. There are no specific trials with chemotherapy in these subtypes and thus data are very sparse, limited to case reports. Anecdotes suggest that gemcitabine-based chemotherapy is sometimes used. An anecdote from our experience describes a response to doxorubicin and gemcitabine in a patient with progressive chromophobe RCC (J. Dutcher, personal communication). Cancer and Acute Leukemia Group B completed a multi-center study of gemcitabine and capecitabine in metastatic RCC in which 4 of 46 patients with known histology were non-clear cell.[58] There were no responses among these patients. An additional study of a new microtubule stabilizing agent, Ixabepilone (BMS-247550), was conducted in renal cell cancer, in which 7 of the 12 patients enrolled were non-clear cell (4 patients) or with sarcomatoid features (3 patients).[59] There were no objective responses observed, with a median time to progression of 9 weeks. This was felt not worthy of further evaluation in this patient population.[59] Currently there are concerted efforts to collect data on patients with non-clear cell RCC who are being treated with targeted therapies, and this will provide prospective information.

TARGETED THERAPY

The recent elucidation of the role of receptor protein tyrosine kinases overexpressed by various types of carcinoma has led to the development of several agents designed to either block the receptors or interfere with signaling within the cancer cell once the receptor is activated. Activity of these receptors and their corresponding tyrosine kinases play an important role in tumor growth, and therefore inhibition of one or several such kinases may have an important impact on treatment of various cancers.

Epidermal Growth Factor Receptor

Epidermal growth factor receptor (EGFR) overexpression leading to tumor cell proliferation has been identified in RCC. Thus EGFR blockade could result in tumor growth inhibition.[60] Studies of agents that interfere with this pathway have been and are being conducted in RCC, with no particular distinction as to the histology being treated, and initially without selection for the degree of receptor expression or phosphorylation state of receptor. In these preliminary investigations, so far, results have been somewhat disappointing. Gefitinib (tyrosine kinase inhibitor) as a single agent showed no response in a study of 21 patients; however, stable disease was seen in eight patients, with the median progression-free survival of 2.7 months.[61] Cetuximab (C225 antibody to the receptor) showed no response, and the median time to progression was 57 days in a study of 55 patients.[62]

Two additional studies have been completed utilizing agents targeting the EGF receptor. One was with panitumumab, a fully humanized monoclonal antibody directed to the receptor, in which there was no histologic subtype restrictions, and 14 of the 88 patients entered had non-clear cell histology.[63] Patient tissue was assessed for expression of EGFR (86% were evaluated and 91% were scored positive). The patients with non-clear cell carcinoma appeared to do better than those with clear cell—of the 5 patients achieving objective response, three were patients with non-clear cell RCC. Among the 14 non-clear cell patients, there were two partial responses, one minor response, and six patients with stable disease as their best response. The progression free survival was longer for the patients with non-clear cell RCC, a median of 92 days compared to 56 days for clear cell RCC, although not statistically significant.[63] The second study was conducted by the Southwest Oncology Group using erlotinib alone (tyrosine kinase inhibitor) specifically for papillary renal cell cancer.[64] The rationale was based on pre-clinical data suggesting that normal vHL expression is associated with greater activity of EGFR inhibitors in clear cell RCC.[65] Thus, papillary RCC lacking the vHL mutation or inactivation could be more responsive to EGFR inhibition. At the time of presentation at the American Society of Oncology meeting 2007, 39 patients were evaluable for response with central pathology review continuing in 7 additional patients. An additional 7 patients were ineligible. Four of 39 (10%) patients had confirmed partial responses and the median overall survival was 26.9 months.[64] This response rate is similar to that seen in clear cell RCC. Thus the role of EGFR inhibition in non-clear cell RCC remains controversial.

Recent in vitro studies showed a synergistic effect of paclitaxel and gefitinib inducing apoptosis in RCC.[65] In other carcinomas, the probable role of EGFR inhibitors and tyrosine kinase inhibitors appears to be in combination with cytotoxic drugs and not as single agents. Therefore, the single-agent studies in RCC confirm this limited effect. However, the evaluation of combining anti-EGFR agents with chemotherapy in some of the non–clear-cell subtypes would be of interest. Based on the above in vitro data, a study of paclitaxel, carboplatin, and an EGFR inhibitor in collecting duct/medullary RCC might be of interest. Currently, we are evaluating the level of receptor expression on non–clear-cell RCC tissue, and administering targeted agents as indicated by the degree of receptor expression.

C-kit and Platelet-Derived Growth Factor

C-kit expression was reported in papillary,[67] chromophobe,[68,69] and sarcomatoid variant of RCC.[70] Platelet-derived growth factor receptor is also expressed in some RCCs.[71] Experience in the treatment of RCC with imatinib mesylate, a potent inhibitor of both c-kit tyrosine kinase and PDGFR, is limited, and more studies are necessary to determine possible efficacy. Again, most trials of these agents are small and contain mostly clear cell carcinoma patients. It is worthwhile to explore these agents in patients with non–clear-cell carcinoma who overexpress these receptors or kinases and attempt to correlate any clinical activity with receptor expression and receptor activation.

Vascular Endothelial Growth Factor and Receptor Inhibition

Vascular endothelial growth factor (VEGF) receptor expression is demonstrated by immunohistochemical analysis of papillary, chromophobe, and conventional (clear) cell histopathology.[72] There is significant correlation between VEGF expression and tumor size and stage, which is correlated with survival.[72] Bevacizumab, a monoclonal antibody to VEGF, prolongs time to progression in patients with clear cell histopathology, but given the similar level of expression, may have a role in papillary and chromophobe RCC.[73] Given that bevacizumab is approved for another solid tumor, it is not intuitive that its activity in RCC should be restricted to clear cell carcinoma, despite the compelling mechanistic data for its role in clear cell carcinoma. The role of bevacizumab and other VEGF inhibitors in non–clear-cell histopathology needs to be determined.

Multi-targeted Kinase Inhibitors in Patients with Non-Clear Cell RCC

Three multi-targeted kinase inhibitors have been approved within the last 2 years for treatment of metastatic renal cell cancer—sorafenib, sunitinib and temsirolimus. Sorafenib and sunitinib target tyrosine kinases of the VEGF receptors and platelet derived growth factor receptors, as well as c-kit and others. Sorafenib additionally targets the RAF pathway. Temsirolimus is an m-TOR (mammalian target of rapamycin) inhibitor, producing multiple downstream effects of this inhibition. Because a major component of the activity of these agents is an anti-angiogenic effect, initial studies were restricted to patients with clear cell RCC. However, anecdotally from the early randomized discontinuation trial of sorafenib, patients with non-clear cell histology also had clinical benefit (K. Flaherty, personal communication). Subsequently, prior to the expected approval and marketing of sorafenib and sunitinib, two global expanded access clinical trials were opened, one for each agent, providing drug availability to a much broader patient population. These included a large number of patients with non-clear cell RCC, as defined by the treating institutions. These included papillary, chromophobe, collecting duct, oncocytoma, as well as patients defined as unclassified (likely poorly differentiated). These two studies represent the largest prospective experience with treatment of non-clear cell renal cell carcinoma in a structured approach.

Data for defined non-clear cell histology patients treated with sorafenib was presented at ASCO 2007, comprising 8.5% (212 out of 2488 patients) of the total North American component of the study.[74] The safety of sorafenib in patients with non- clear cell RCC appeared to be similar to the larger patient population,[75] and there were responses and stable disease in 60–80% of the non-clear cell patients, similar to the results in the overall population.[74] Similarly, in the global sunitinib study, the initial analysis presented at ASCO 2007, was of the first 2341 for safety and 2125 for efficacy (follow-up greater than 6 months).[76] Among this first group, 11.8% were non-clear cell histology (276 of 2341 patients) by local pathology review. The overall clinical benefit (response plus stable disease > 3 months) was approximately 52% for the entire group and 47% for the non-clear cell patients.[76] A recent update of this study for the European Oncology meeting has the same result with larger numbers of patients evaluable.[77] These studies have been presented with updates at recent meetings and continue to show the same rate of activity in non-clear cell RCC as noted in the larger clear cell RCC group (Table 32-6).

The Mammalian Target of Rapamycin Kinase Inhibitor

The mammalian target of rapamycin (mTOR) is a multifunctional serine-threonine kinase that acts as a central regulator of cell growth, proliferation, and apoptosis. It is

Table 32.6.
Expanded access data in non-clear cell RCC

Sorafenib—North American Experience (n = 2502)[74,75]—Investigator-assessed best response at 8 weeks.

NCC Subtype	Papillary N = 170	Chromophobe N = 29	Collecting Duct N = 10
Eval for response (N)	118	18	5
Partial Response, N(%)	27 (23)	3 (17)	0
Stable Disease, N(%)	68 (58)	14 (78)	3 (60)
Progression, N(%)	23 (19)	1 (6)	2 (40)

Sunitinib—Investigator assessed best response at 12 weeks.[76,77]

Non-clear cell—N =	542
Median FU/ (mo)	6.2%
ORR	6.1%
SD ≥ 3mo	41.3%
Clinical benefit	47.4%
Median PFS (prior Cytokine) N = 353 — 7.3 mos	

activated in response to growth factors: insulin, insulin-like growth factor, PDGF, and stem cell factor.[78–80] Temsirolimus (CCI-779), a selective mTOR inhibitor, was studied in a randomized phase II study in 111 patients with advanced refractory RCC and showed modest activity: objective response rate 7% (one complete response and six partial responses) and minor response rate 26%, a median time to tumor progression of 5.8 months, and a median survival 15 months.[81]

The phase II study also suggested that patients with poor risk renal cell cancer did better than was expected after progressing on cytokines. Therefore, a randomized phase III study of Temsirolimus was conducted, with three arms: interferon alpha 3 MU three times weekly (tiw) escalating to 18 MU tiw as tolerated; temsirolimus 25 mg weekly, and a combination of interferon alpha 6 MU tiw plus temisirolimus 15 mg weekly. This study demonstrated a survival advantage and progression free survival improvement for temsirolimus that were both statistically significant in these poor risk patients.[82] Subsequently, an analysis of histologic subtypes of patients treated on the temsirolimus alone or interferon alpha alone arms was performed based on institutional evaluations of pathology.[83] There were 82.3% clear cell and 17.7% other. Among the other, there were 11.4% indeterminate and 63% non clear cell of a specified type. There was a statistically significant difference in overall survival and progression free survival in favor of temsirolimus compared to interferon alpha, and a greater difference than was seen even in the clear cell patients (Table 32.7).[83] This may in part reflect the lower activity of cytokines in non-clear cell RCC, but suggests that this agent has a major advantage in patients with non-clear cell RCC.

Other Targeted Therapies Evaluated in RCC

All new agents continue to be evaluated in RCC, particularly if there are unique mechanisms of action. A recent report is the use of Bortezomib in RCC, in which 37 patients were treated, 12 of whom had non-clear cell carcinoma.[84] Four patients achieved a partial response, duration of 8, 8+, 15+, and 20+ months, and one of the 4 was a patient

Table 32.7
Temsirolimus—overall and progression-free survival by tumor histology

	IFN (n = 207)	*Temsirolimus (n = 209)*	*T vs I*
	Median mos	*Median mos*	*Hazard ratio*
Overall survival			
Clear cell (170)	8.2	10.6	0.85
Other (36)	4.3	11.6	0.55
Progression-free survival			
Clear Cell (170)	3.8	5.5	0.84
Other (36)	1.8	7.0	0.36

with medullary carcinoma. Median time to progression was 1.4 months. The proportion of patients alive at 1 year is 36%, and the median survival is 7.5 months.[84] Whether this reflects drug-effect or patient characteristics is unclear. This was not recommended for further study, unless molecular features predicting response can be identified.

More anecdotal reports are the inclusion of occasional non-clear cell RCC patients in clinical trials of new agents, where the majority of the patients are clear cell. Such studies have suggested responsiveness, comparable to that of clear cell. In the initial phase II study of axitinib, there was one patient with papillary RCC who had a 27% reduction in tumor burden (B. Rini personal communication), but the duration and the denominator of non-clear cell patients are not yet available. Similarly, another study conducted at Cleveland Clinic evaluated lenolidomide in RCC, in which 5 of 28 patients were non-clear cell RCC. One patient with chromophobe RCC remains stable at 3+ years, and one patient with mixed clear cell/papillary RCC is stable for one year (B Rini, C Nemec, personal communication). There are simply not sufficient data to describe active agents at this point in time.

CONCLUSION

Non–clear-cell RCC is an uncommon disease, and these subtypes may be distinct from each other, and are definitely distinct from clear cell carcinoma. They have different biologic behaviors, with occasional responses to chemotherapy. It appears that some are amenable to effective treatment with the new targeted therapies. Given recent therapeutic developments, it is important to consider well-designed trials as the first-line therapy, with an emphasis on non–clear-cell carcinomas. These would likely be newer targeted therapy agents alone or combined with cytotoxic drugs, which have shown activity against these rare tumors. It is imperative to structure studies that identify histologic or molecular subtypes.

REFERENCES

1. Chow WH, Devesa SS, Warren JL, Fraumeni JF Jr. Rising incidence of renal cell cancer in the United States. JAMA 1999;281:1628–1631.
2. Reuter VE, Presti JC. Contemporary approach to the classification of renal epithelial tumors. Semin Oncol 2000;27:124–137.
3. Storkel S, Eble JN, Adlakha K, et al. Classification of renal cell carcinoma: Workgroup No. 1 Union Internationale Contre le Cancer (UICC) and the American Joint Committee on Cancer (AHCC). Cancer 1997;80:987–989.
4. Kovacs G, Akhtar M, Beckwith BJ, et al. The Heidelberg classification of renal cell tumours. J Pathol 1997;183:131–133.

5. Surveillance, Epidemiology, and End Results (SEER) Program. SEER Stat Database: Incidence— SEER 9 Regs Public-Use, November 2003 Sub (1973–2001), National Cancer Institute, DCCPS, Surveillance Research Program, Cancer Statistics Branch, released April 2004, based on the November 2003 submission. www.seer.cancer.gov.

6. Beck SD, Patel MI, Snyder ME, et al. Effect of papillary and chromophobe cell type on disease-free survival after nephrectomy for renal cell carcinoma. Ann Surg Oncol 2004;11:71–77.

7. Atkins MB, Dutcher J, Weiss G, et al. Kidney cancer: the Cytokine Working Group experience (1986–2001): part I. IL-2 based clinical trials. Med Oncol 2001;18(3):197–207.

8. Levin HS, Myles JL. The pathology of renal neoplasms. In: Bukowski RM, Novick AC, eds. Renal Cell Carcinoma. Totowa, NJ: Humana Press, 2000:15–38.

9. Yang XJ, Sugimura J, Tretiakova MS, et al. Gene expression profiling of renal medullary carcinoma. Cancer 2004;100:976–985.

10. Takahashi M, Teh BT. Gene expression profiling of renal cell carcinoma and its clinical implications. In: Ladanyi M, Gerald WL, eds. Expression Profiling of Human Tumors: Diagnostic and Research Applications. Totowa, NJ: Humana Press, 2003:235–256.

11. Sanders ME, Mick R, Tomaszewski JE, et al. Unique patterns of allelic imbalance distinguish type I from type II sporadic papillary renal cell carcinoma. Am J Pathol 2002;161:997–1005.

12. Young AN, Amin MB, Moreno CS, et al. Expression profiling of renal epithelial neoplasms: a method for tumor classification and discovery of diagnostic molecular markers. Am J Pathol 2001;158:1639–1651.

13. Linehan WM, Walther MM, Zbar B. Genetic basis of cancer of the kidney. J Urol 2003; 170:2163–2172.

14. Schmidt L, Duh FM, Chen F, et al. Germline and somatic mutations in the tyrosine kinase domain of the MET proto-oncogene in papillary renal carcinomas. Nat Genet 1997;16:68–73.

15. Pavlovich CP, Walther MM, Eyler RA, et al. Renal tumors in the Birt-Hogg-Dube syndrome. Am J Surg Pathol 2002;26(12):1542–1552.

16. Cheville JC, Lohse CM, Zincke H, et al. Comparisons of outcome and prognostic features among histologic subtypes of renal cell carcinoma. Am J Surg Pathol 2003;27(5):612–624.

17. Davis CJ, Mostofi FK, Sesterhenn IA, Renal medullary Carcinoma. The seventh sickle cell nephropathy. Am J Surg Pathol 1995;19:1–11.

18. Swartz MA, Karth J, Schneider DT, et al. Renal medullary carcinoma: clinical, pathologic, immunohistochemical, and genetic analysis with pathogenic implications. Urology 2002;60:1083–1089.

19. Guinan P, Sobin LH, Algaba F, et al. TNM staging of renal cell carcinoma: workgroup No. 3. Union International Contre le Cancer (UICC) and the American Joint Committee on Cancer (AJCC). Cancer 1997;80:992–993.

20. Majean A, Roupret M, Larousserie F, et al. Is there a place for radical nephrectomy in the presence of metastatic collecting duct carcinoma? J Urol 2003;169(4):1287–1290.

21. Crotty TB, Farrow GM, Lieber MM. Chromophobe cell carcinoma: clinicopathological features of 50 cases. J Urol 1995;154(3):964–967.

22. Sanchez-Ortiz RF, Rosser CJ, Madsen LT, et al. Young age is an independent prognostic factor for survival of sporadic renal cell carcinoma. J Urol 2004;171(6 pt 1):2160–2165.

23. Motzer RJ, Mazumdar M, Bacik J, Berg W, Amsterdam A, Ferrara J. Survival and prognostic stratification of 670 patients with advanced renal cell carcinoma. J Clin Oncol 1999;17(8):2530–2540.

24. Mekhail TM, Abou-Jawde RM, BouMerhi G, et al. Validation and extension of the Memorial Sloan-Kettering prognostic factors model for survival in patients with previously untreated metastatic renal cell carcinoma. J Clin Oncol 2005;23(4):832–841.

25. Patard JJ, Leray E, Rioux-Leclerq N, et al. Prognostic value of histologic subtypes in renal cell carcinoma: a multicenter experience. J Clin Oncol 2005;23(12):2763–2771.

26. Elson PJ, Manola JB, Mazumdar M, et al. Prognostic factors for survival in patients with metastatic renal cell carcinoma: a study from the Kidney Cancer Association's International Kidney Cancer Working Group. Proc Am Soc Clin Oncol 2005;24:abstr 4533.

27. Gold PJ, Fefer A, Thompson JA. Paraneoplastic manifestations of renal cell carcinoma. Semin Urol Oncol 1996;14:216–222.

28. Weiss LM, Gelb AB, Medeiros LJ. Adult renal epithelial neoplasms. Am J Clin Pathol 1995; 103:624–635.

29. Frank I, Blute ML, Cheville JC, et al. A multifactorial postoperative surveillance model for patients with surgically treated clear cell renal cell carcinoma. Urology 2003;170(6 pt 1):2225–2232.

30. Motzer RJ, Bacik J, Mazumdar M. Prognostic factors for survival of patients with stage IV renal cell carcinoma: Memorial Sloan-Kettering Cancer Center experience. Clin Cancer Res 2004;10(18 pt 2):6302S–6303S.

31. Ljunberg B, Alamdari FL, Stenling R, et al. Prognostic significance of the Heidelberg classification of renal cell carcinoma. Eur Urol 1999;36(6):565–569.

32. Amin MB, Tamboli P, Javidan J, et al. Prognostic impact of histologic subtyping of adult renal epithelial neoplasms: an experience of 405 cases. Am J Surg Pathol 2002;26(3):281–291.
33. Noguera-Irizarry WG, Hibshoosh H, Papadopoulos KP. Renal medullary carcinoma: case report and review of the literature. Am J Clin Oncol 2003;26(5):489–492.
34. Selby DM, Simon C, Foley JP, Thompson IM, Baddour RT. Renal medullary carcinoma: can early diagnosis lead to long-term survival? J Urol 2000;163(4):1238.
35. Upton MP, Parker RA, Youmans, et al. Histologic predictors of renal cell carcinoma (RCC) response to interleukin 2 based therapy. Proc Am Soc Clin Oncol 2003;22:851.
36. Motzer RJ, Bacik J, Mariani T, et al. Treatment outcome and survival associated with metastatic renal cell carcinoma of non-clear-cell histology. J Clin Oncol 2002;20:2376–2381.
37. Saranchuk JW, Touijer AK, Hakiman, et al. Partial Nephrectomy for patients with solitary kidney: the memorial Sloan-Kettering experience. BJU Int 2004;94(9):1323–1328.
38. Allaf ME, Bhayani SB, Rogers C, Varkarakis I. Laparoscopic partial nephrectomy: evaluation of long term oncological outcome. J Urol 2004;172(3):871–873.
39. Wronski M, Arbit E, Russo P, et al. Surgical resection of brain metastases from renal cell carcinoma in 50 patients. Urology 1996;47(92):187–193.
40. Flanigan RC. Debulking nephrectomy in metastatic renal cell cancer. Clin Cancer Res 2004;10(18 pt 2):6335S–6341S.
41. Wood CG. The role of cytoreductive nephrectomy in the management of metastatic renal cell carcinoma. Urol Clin North Am 2003;30(3):581–588.
42. Mickish GHJ, Garin A, van Poppel H, et al. Radical nephrectomy plus interferon-alfa-based immunotherapy compared with interferon alfa alone in metastatic renal cell carcinoma: a randomized trial. Lancet 2001;358(9286):966–970.
43. Flanigan RC, Salmon SE, Blumenstein BA, et al. Nephrectomy followed by interferon alfa compared with interferon alfa alone for metastatic renal cell cancer. N Engl J Med 2001;23(345):1655–1659.
44. Sella A, Logothetis CJ, Ro JY, Swanson DA, Samuels ML. Sarcomatoid renal cell carcinoma. A treatable entity. Cancer 1987;60(6):1313–1318.
45. Escudier B, Droz JP, Rolland F, Terrier-Lacombe MJ, Gravis G, Beuzeboc P. Doxorubicin and Ifosfamide in patients with metastatic sarcomatoid renal cell carcinoma: a phase II study of the Genitourinary Group of the French Federation of Cancer Centers. J Urol 2002;168(3):959–961.
46. Nanus DM, Garino A, Milowski MI, Larkin M, Dutcher JP. Active chemotherapy for sarcomatoid and rapidly progressing renal cell carcinoma. Cancer 2004;101(7):1545–1551.
47. Hoshi S, Satoh M, Ohyama C, et al. Active chemotherapy for bone metastasis in sarcomatoid renal cell carcinoma. Int J Clin Oncol 2003;8(2):113–117.
48. Bangalore N, Bhargawa P, Hawkins, et al. Sustained response of sarcomatoid renal-cell carcinoma to MAID chemotherapy: case report and review of the literature. Ann Oncol 2001;12(2):271–274.
49. Pirich LM, Chou P, Walterhouse DO. Prolonged survival of a patient with sickle cell trait and metastatic renal medullary carcinoma. Pediatr Hematol Oncol 1999;21(1):67–69.
50. Warren KE, Gidvani-Diaz V, Duval-Arnould B. Renal medullary carcinoma in an adolescent with sickle cell trait. Pediatrics 1999;103:22–25.
51. Vargas-Gonzales R, Sotelo-Avila C, Coria AS. Renal medullary carcinoma in a six-year-old boy with sickle cell trait. Pathol Oncol Res 2003;9:193–195
52. Strousse JJ, Spevak M, Kyle Mack A, Arceci RJ. Significant responses to platinum based chemotherapy in renal medullary carcinoma. Pediatr Blood Cancer 2005;44:1–5.
53. Dimopoulos MA, Logothetis CJ, Markowitz A, Sella A, Amato R, Ro J. Collecting duct carcinoma of the kidney. Br J Urol 1993;71(4):388–391.
54. Peyromaure M, Thiounn N, Scotte F, Vieillefond A, Debre B, Oudard S. Collecting duct carcinoma of the kidney: a clinicopathological study of 9 cases. Urology 2003;170(4 pt 1):1138–1140.
55. Oudard S, Banu E, Viellefond A, et al. Prospective multicenter phase II study of gemcitabine plus platinum salt for metastatic collecting duct carcinoma: Results of a GETUG (Groupe d'Etudes des Tumeurs Uro-Genitales) study. J Urol 2007;177(5):1698–1702.
56. Gollob JA, Upton MP, DeWolf WC, Atkins MB. Long-term remission in a patient with metastatic collecting duct carcinoma treated with Taxol/carboplatin and surgery. Urology 2001;58(6):1058.
57. Milowsky MI, Rosmarin A, Tickoo SK, et al. Active chemotherapy for collecting duct carcinoma of the kidney: a case report and review of the literature. Cancer 2002;94(1):111–116.
58. Stadler WM, Halabi S, Rini B, et al. A phase II study of gemcitabine and capecitabine in metastatic renal cancer: A report of Cancer and Leukemia Group B Protocol 90008. Cancer 2006;107:1273–1279.
59. Posadas EM, Undevia S, Manchen E, et al. A phase II study of Ixabepilone (BMS-247550) in metastatic renal cell carcinoma. Cancer Biol Ther 2007;5:490–493.

60. Moch H, Sauter G, Buchholz N, Gasser TC, Bubendorf L, Waldman FM. Epidermal growth factor receptor expression is associated with rapid tumor cell proliferation in renal cell carcinoma. Hum Pathol 1997;28(11):1255–1259.
61. Dawson NA, Guo C, Zak R, Dorsey B, Hussain,. A phase II trial of gefitinib (Iressa, ZD1839) in stage IV and recurrent renal cell carcinoma. Clin Cancer Res 2004;10(23):7812–7819.
62. Motzer RJ, Amato R, Todd M, Hwu WJ. Phase II trial of antiepidermal growth factor receptor antibody C225 in patients with advanced renal cell carcinoma. Invest New Drugs 2003;21(1):99–101.
63. Rowinsky EK, Schwartz GH, Gollob JA, et al. Safety, pharmacokinetics, and activity of ABX-EGF, a fully human anti-epidermal growth factor receptor monoclonal antibody in patients with metastatic renal cell cancer. J Clin Oncol 2004; 22(15):3003–3015.
64. Pan C, Hussey M, Lara P, et al. Phase II trial of the epidermal growth factor receptor (EGFR) inhibitor erlotinib (e) in patients with advanced papillary renal cell carcinoma—SWOG S0317. J Clin Oncol 2007; ASCO Annual Meeting Proceedings, 25(18S):15516.
65. Perera AD, Kleymenova EV, Walker CL. Requirement for the von Hippel-Lindau tumor suppressor gene for functional epidermal growth factor receptor blockade by monoclonal antibody C225 in renal cell carcinoma. Clin Can Res 2000; 6:1518–1523.
66. Sumimoto M, Asano T, Asakuma J, Asano T. ZD1839 modulates paclitaxel response in renal cancer by blocking paclitaxel-induced activation of epidermal growth factor receptor-extracellular signal-regulated kinase pathway. Clin Cancer Res 2004;1092:794–801.
67. Lin ZH, Han EM, Lee ES, Kim CW. A distinct expression pattern and point mutation of c-kit in papillary renal cell carcinoma. Mod Pathol 2004;17(6):611–616.
68. Petit A, Castillo M, Santos M, Mallofre C. KIT expression in chromophobe renal cell carcinoma: comparative immunohistochemical analysis of KIT expression in different renal cell neoplasms. Am J Surg Pathol 2004;28(5):676–678.
69. Yamazaaki K, Sakamoto M, Ohta T, Kanai Y. Overexpression of KIT in chromophobe renal cell carcinoma. Oncogene 2003;22(6):847–852.
70. Castillo M, Petit A, Mellado B, Palacin A. C-kit expression in sarcomatoid renal cell carcinoma therapy with imatinib. J Urol 2004;171(6 pt 1):2176–2180.
71. Sihto H, Rikala MS, Tynninen O, et al. KIT and Platelet-derived growth factor receptor alpha tyrosine kinase gene mutations and KIT amplifications in human solid tumors. J Clin Oncol 2005;23:49–57.
72. Jacobsen J, Grankvist K, Rasmuson T, et al. Expression of vascular endothelial growth factor protein in human renal cell carcinoma. BJU Int 2004;93(3):297–302.
73. Yang JC, Haworth L, Sherry RM, et al. A randomized trial of bevacizumab, an anti-vascular endothelial growth factor antibody, for metastatic renal cancer. N Engl J Med 2003;349(5):427–434.
74. Stadler WM, FIglin RA, Ernstoff MS, et al. The Advanced Renal Cell Carcinoma Sorafenib (ARCCS) expanded access trial: Safety and efficacy in patients with non-clear cell renal cell carcinoma. ASCO Annual Meeting Proceedings. J Clin Oncol 2007;25(18S):5036.
75. Knox JJ, Figlin RA, Stadler WM, et al. The Advanced Renal Cell Carcinoma Sorafenib (ARCCS) expanded access trial in North America: Safety and efficacy. ASCO Annual Meeting Proceedings. J Clin Oncol 2007;25(18S):5011.
76. Gore ME, Porta C, Oudard S, et al. Sunitinib in metastatic renal cell carcinoma: Preliminary assessment in an expanded access trial with subpopulation analysis. ASCO Annual Meeting Proceedings. J Clin Oncol 2007;25(18S):5010.
77. Gore ME, Szczylik C, Porta C, et al. Sunitinib in metastatic renal cell carcinoma: Preliminary assessment in an expanded access trial with subpopulation analysis. Proc ECCO, 2007;10:45.
78. Aoki M, Blazek E, Vogt PK, et al. A role of the kinase mTOR in cellular transformation induced by oncoproteins PI3K and AKT. Proc Natl Acad Sci U S A 2001;98:136–141.
79. Schmelzle T, Hall MN. TOR, a central controller of cell growth. Cell 2000;103:253–262.
80. Castedo M, Ferri KF, Kroemer G. Mammalian target of rapamycin (mTOR). Pro- and Anti-apoptotic Cell Death Differ 2002;9:99–100.
81. Atkins MB, Hidalgo M, Stadler WM, et al. Randomized phase II study of multiple dose levels of CCI-779, a novel mammalian target of rapamycin kinase inhibitor, in patients with advanced refractory renal cell carcinoma. J Clin Oncol 2004;22(5):909–918.
82. Hudes G, Hudes G, Carducci M, et al. Temsirolimus, interferon, or the combination of interferon plus temsirolimus for patients with advanced renal cell carcinoma and poor risk features. N Engl J Med 2007;356:2271–2281.
83. Dutcher J, Szczylik C, Tannir N, et al. Correlation of survival with tumor histology, age and prognostic-risk group for previously untreated patients with advanced renal cell carcinoma receiving temsirolimus or interferon alpha. ASCO Annual Meeting Proceedings. J Clin Oncol 2007; 25(18S):5033.
84. Kondagunta GV, Drucker B, Schwartz L, et al. Phase II trial of bortezomib for patients with advanced renal cell carcinoma. J Clin Oncol 2004;22:3720–3725.

33 Renal Cell Carcinoma in Patients with End-Stage Renal Disease

John C. Rabets and David A. Goldfarb

KEYWORDS

RENAL CELL CARCINOMA
ACQUIRED RENAL CYSTIC DISEASE
RENAL TRANSPLANTATION
IMMUNOSUPPRESSION
RENAL CYSTS

ABSTRACT

Patients with end-stage renal disease are at increased risk for the development of renal cell carcinoma in their native kidneys and as a consequence of immunosuppressive therapy following renal transplantation. This chapter discusses acquired renal cystic disease and its association with renal cell carcinoma, the unique situation of von Hippel–Lindau (VHL) disease and renal transplantation, and the increased incidence of malignancies with immunosuppression and a novel class of immunosuppressants with antineoplastic properties.

ACQUIRED RENAL CYSTIC DISEASE AND RENAL CELL CARCINOMA

Acquired renal cystic disease (ARCD) (Figure 33.1), which has been defined as the presence of macroscopic cystic structures occupying more than 25% of the renal parenchyma or more than three cysts per kidney, was originally described by Dunnill and colleagues[1] in 1977. In their autopsy series of 30 patients, they noted that 47% of patients undergoing hemodialysis for a mean duration of 3.4 years developed multiple bilateral renal cysts. In addition, 15% of these patients had renal tumors. Miller and colleagues[2] described in their autopsy series of 155 patients with end-stage renal disease a 58% incidence of cystic disease, a 15% incidence of renal adenoma, and a 2% incidence of renal cell carcinoma (RCC). The largest pathology series to date was described by Denton and colleagues,[3] who performed ipsilateral native nephrectomy at the time of renal transplantation in 260 patients. They noted the incidence of renal cystic disease, renal adenoma, and RCC in 33%, 14%, and 4.2% of specimens, respectively.

From: *Clinical Management of Renal Tumors*
Edited by: R.M. Bukowski and A.C. Novick © Humana Press Inc., Totowa, NJ

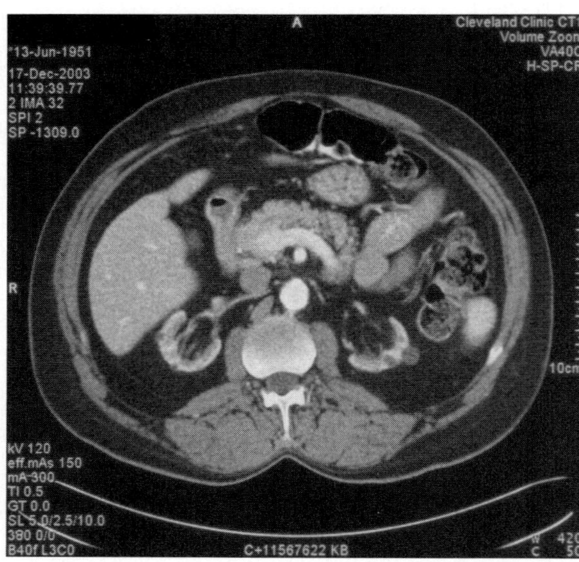

Figure 33.1. Acquired renal cystic disease and an enhancing left renal mass in a patient with end-stage renal disease.

Narasimhan and colleagues[4] used ultrasonography and computed tomography (CT) to screen patients with end-stage renal disease. They noted a 22% incidence of ARCD in those patients on hemodialysis compared to a 7% incidence in those patients not yet dialyzed. Ishikawa et al.[5] performed a 10-year prospective analysis using CT screening of dialysis patients. Three patients developed RCC over this 10-year period. Another large survey study from the same group noted that the prevalence of RCC to be more than 40 times higher than that of the general population.[6] Terasawa et al.[7] noted a 2.6% incidence of RCC in 1600 dialysis patients screened yearly with ultrasound.

Patients undergoing peritoneal dialysis are also at risk for the development of ARCD. In Ishikawa's[8] 1992 meta-analysis, he noted a similar 41% incidence of ARCD and a 0.4% incidence of RCC in peritoneal dialysis patients compared to a 47% of ARCD and 1.5% incidence of RCC incidence in hemodialysis patients. Acquired renal cystic disease has also been described in children with end-stage renal disease. A Japanese study group in 1999 noted an 80% incidence of ARCD in pediatric patients undergoing peritoneal dialysis for more than 10 years compared to a 9% incidence in patients who have been dialyzed less than 4 years.[9]

Male sex, advanced age, and longer duration of renal replacement therapy have been identified as risk factors for the development of ARCD.[3,10] Ishikawa and colleagues[11] in 1980 reported a 44% incidence of ARCD in patients receiving renal replacement therapy for less than 3 years compared to a 79% incidence for those patients receiving renal replacement therapy for more than 3 years. Hughson and colleagues[12] demonstrated a 2.9 : 1 male-to-female ratio for the development of ARCD.

The effect of renal transplantation on the natural history of ARCD is unclear. Vaziri et al.[13] noted that a functioning renal allograft may retard the progression of cystic changes in the native kidneys. Tajima et al.[14] noted a decrease in the number and size of cysts in nearly two thirds of 25 patients 1 year after transplantation. Ishikawa and colleagues[15] followed 61 patients who underwent successful renal transplantation for a mean of 63 months. In 30% of the patients followed, the number of cysts either remained stable or decreased. However, 18% of patients demonstrated progression in the number and size of the cysts. Levine and Gburek[16] similarly reported four cases of progressive cystic disease and malignant transformation in four patients after renal transplantation with good graft function.

Hughson and colleagues[17] hypothesized that the uremic condition provides a stimulus for neoplastic transformation and cystic growth. Growth factors such as c-erb B-2 have been implicated in the pathogenesis of uremic renal cysts and malignant transformation.[18] Renal cell carcinomas associated with ARCD shows a different genetic lineage compared to sporadic RCC. Hughson et al.[19] in 1996 performed polymorphism analyses and microsatellite amplification studies on RCC specimen from patients with ARCD and compared them with sporadic RCC specimen. Whereas nearly all clear cell carcinomas have deletions or mutations on the short arm of chromosome 3, only one of the 21 tumors from ARCD patients had a 3p deletion and none had von Hippel-Lindau mutations. Gronwald and colleagues[20] compared chromosomal abnormalities seen in papillary RCCs such as gain of chromosome 7 and 17 and loss of Y. Such changes were similar in both sporadic papillary RCC and RCC associated with ARCD, thus implying that although clear cell carcinomas associated with ARCD may have a distinct genetic lineage, the changes seen with the development of papillary RCC are similar. Bretan et al.'s[21] theory of a continuum of cyst formation and malignant transformation has been supported by the study by Cheuk et al.,[22] who studied the karyotypic features of the cystic epithelium in patients with ARCD. They noted similar gains of chromosomes 7, 12, 17, and 20, and concluded that these karyotypic changes may represent precursor lesions to RCC.

Due to the high incidence of ARCD and RCC, screening with ultrasonography or CT has generally been recommended. Matson and Cohen[23] recommended that yearly screening commence 3 years after the initiation of dialysis, noting that cystic disease and RCC are dependent on the length of time of dialysis. Marple and colleagues[24] similarly recommended the initiation of screening after 3 years of dialysis. The best imaging modality for screening is controversial. Taylor et al.[25] noted that CT may be superior to ultrasonography in detecting renal cysts, but both are equally sensitive for detecting solid masses. Takebayashi and colleagues[26] concluded that enhanced CT had a sensitivity and specificity of 95% and 96%, respectively, in their series of 630 patients screened with yearly CT scans. At our institution we generally recommend screening with ultrasound in those patients on hemodialysis for 3 years or more. Any suspicious lesions are then followed by CT. For any patient being evaluated for transplantation, we screen with ultrasound at the time of evaluation.

Sarasin and colleagues[27] performed an elegant decision analysis to determine which patients would most benefit from routine screening. They concluded that for patients with a life expectancy of 25 years, screening may decrease the risk of cancer death by nearly one half, offering these patients a 1.6-year gain in life expectancy. However, for older patients with significant medical comorbidities, the gain in life expectancy is significantly less. Sarasin and colleagues recommended selective screening favoring younger patients with a longer life expectancy.

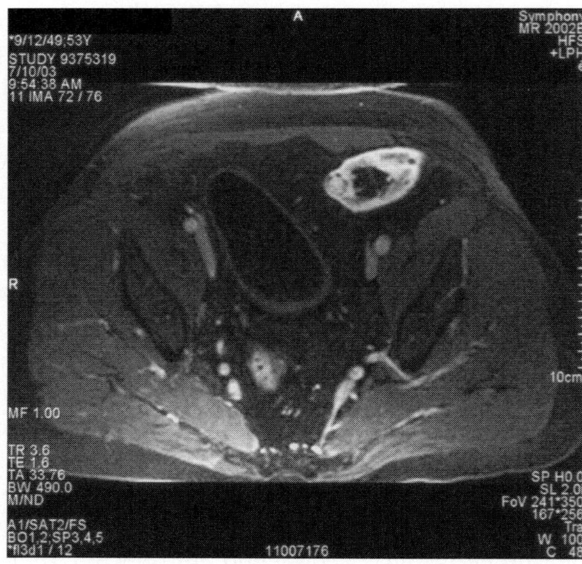

Figure 33.2. An enhancing mass in an allograft kidney in a patient who underwent successful renal transplantation.

RENAL CELL CARCINOMA IN THE RENAL ALLOGRAFT

Renal cell carcinoma can also develop in the allograft kidney (Figure 33.2). In Penn's[28] review of the Cincinnati Transplant Tumor Registry, he noted 24 de novo RCCs in allograft kidneys. A more recent review noted the development of three RCCs in 1250 allograft kidneys from 1968 to 2002.[29] Nephrectomy has been the treatment of choice for tumors in nonfunctioning allografts. Nephron-sparing surgery has been described in several case reports for tumors in functioning allografts when technically feasible.[30-32] Minimally invasive strategies such as percutaneous radiofrequency ablation have also been successfully attempted with good short-term follow-up.[33,34] Elucidation of the ideal therapeutic approach to tumors in allograft kidneys has been hampered by its relative rarity and the lack of large comparative series.

VON HIPPEL–LINDAU AND RENAL TRANSPLANTATION

Nephron-sparing surgery provides effective initial management for von Hippel–Lindau (VHL) disease patients with localized RCC; however, many will develop a local recurrence requiring further treatment. This includes the possibility of removal of all renal tissue. Furthermore, there are patients in whom nephron-sparing surgery is not technically feasible, and bilateral nephrectomy is performed. In a multicenter study of surgical treatment for RCC in VHL disease, 23% of patients developed end-stage renal failure as a result of treatment for localized RCC.[35] Management options for these patients include dialysis or renal transplantation. For this population of predominantly young patients, renal transplantation is a desirable approach; however, immunosuppression may predispose patients to tumor recurrence.

The first report of renal transplantation in VHL disease is credited to Peterson et al.,[36] who described a successful cadaveric transplant in a 34-year-old woman with 2 years of follow-up. Penn[37] reported the results of 304 transplant recipients with treated renal carcinoma, 12 of whom had VHL. Specific outcome data on this group were not separately reported. Steinbach et al.[38] reported on five patients with VHL and previously treated RCC who underwent transplantation. All patients were successfully transplanted and had satisfactory renal function. Four patients were alive without evidence of disease at an average of 28 months follow-up, and one patient died of metastatic disease at 17 months. This small single-center report demonstrated that renal transplantation provides effective treatment for end-stage renal failure in patients with VHL and previously treated RCC.

A multicenter review of the results of renal transplantation in patients with VHL disease rendered anephric from localized RCC has been conducted.[39] The study group comprised 32 patients (23 males, nine females) identified from registries in North America and Europe. The average age at diagnosis of RCC was 31 years and the average age at transplantation was 36 years. The duration of dialysis before transplantation was 0 to 102 months (mean, 26 months). The donor source was cadaveric ($n = 20$), living related ($n = 9$), or living unrelated ($n = 3$). The survival of transplanted patients was 100% at 1 year and 65% at 5 years. Three patients died of metastasis at a mean time of 33 months after transplantation. Two patients died without evidence of recurrent RCC at 54 and 60 months. The study group was compared to an age-, sex-, and era-matched population of patients with renal failure due to causes other than RCC. There were no differences in the Kaplan-Meier estimates of graft or patient survival between the two groups. There were an equal number of deaths in the control group ($n = 5$); however, all of these were due to cardiovascular disease. These results support the effectiveness of renal transplantation as a form of renal replacement for patients with VHL and previously treated RCC with a limited risk of recurrent disease.

The need for a surveillance interval on dialysis, in order to prevent the early development of metastatic disease after transplantation, is an important concern. In Penn's[37] review of the Cincinnati Transplant Tumor Registry data, 56 patients underwent removal of an incidental RCC at variable time intervals before transplantation. In 51 patients the tumor was removed at the time of, or within 2 years of, transplantation. None of these patients experienced a recurrence after transplantation. In contrast, of 152 patients with a symptomatic RCC, 51 developed a recurrence and 39 died of disease after transplantation. Of the patients who developed a recurrence, 31 (61%) were treated within 2 years of transplantation. These data suggest that patients with low stage, asymptomatic RCC have favorable outcomes with renal transplantation and do not require a surveillance interval before transplantation. In contrast, those patients with higher stage cancers associated with a symptomatic presentation have a higher risk of recurrent disease, and a surveillance interval of at least 2 years is recommended to monitor for the development of early recurrence. In the multicenter transplantation study the three patients who developed recurrence were dialyzed for a mean of 20 months before transplantation and this was not different from the cohort of patients who did not develop a recurrence. An equal number of patients developed recurrence whether the dialysis interval was 0 to 12 months, 13 to 23 months, or ≥ 24 months. This suggests that the duration of dialysis before transplantation is not the only determinant of disease recurrence. While pathologic staging information would be helpful to assess the risk of early recurrence, these data were not available for the multicenter renal transplant study.

Living donor transplantation has emerged as the preferred choice for transplantation because it is associated with improved outcomes compared to cadaver transplantation.[40]

Therefore, the evaluation of living related donors is an important issue because of the risk for occult disease in this genetic disorder. Since the *VHL* gene has now been localized to chromosome 3p 25-26 and identified,[41] presymptomatic carriers of the *VHL* gene can be detected accurately using various molecular techniques.[42,43] When a patient is identified with VHL, all at-risk relatives should be genetically screened. Those whose tests are positive or uninformative should then be clinically screened with a brain and spine magnetic resonance imaging (MRI), ophthalmologic exam, CT or MRI scan of the abdomen, and 24-hour urinary metanephrines.[44] This evaluation is essential for all perspective living-related donors to VHL recipients.

In summary, the data of the recent multicenter study of renal transplantation in VHL disease support the utility of renal transplantation as an effective form of renal replacement in VHL patients. Satisfactory renal function can be achieved with a limited risk for recurrent disease.

IMMUNOSUPPRESSION AND RENAL CELL CARCINOMA

Renal transplantation has been established as the definitive treatment for end-stage renal disease. As patient survival has improved, posttransplant neoplastic disease has become a major source of morbidity and mortality in patients on chronic immunosuppression. The association of long-term immunosuppression and the risk of malignancy has long been established.[45] London et al.[46] noted that more than one in five renal allograft recipients will develop a neoplastic lesion by 15 years posttransplantation, and that by 20 years the figure rises to nearly 40%. This is in comparison to an age-matched control population with a 6% cumulative risk of neoplasia. The majority of the tumors in this series were cutaneous, but 15% of patients developed tumors of urogenital origin. The main risk factors for the development of posttransplant malignancy are advanced age, male sex, and longer exposure to immunosuppressive drugs after transplantation.[47] The level of immunosuppression may also play a critical role in the development of posttransplant neoplasia. Dantal et al.[48] in 1998 performed a randomized, prospective trial of two different cyclosporine regimens using the risk of malignancy as a secondary end point. They found a significant association between higher cyclosporine blood trough concentrations and the risk of neoplasia.

Recently, evidence has emerged that a new class of immunosuppressive medications may possess antineoplastic properties. Target of rapamycin inhibitors such as sirolimus and everolimus engage FKBP12 and exert their immunosuppressive effect by preventing cytokine receptors from activating the cell cycle.[49,50] Using a murine model of RCC, Luan and colleagues[51] showed that the administration of rapamune to mice inoculated with an RCC cell line slowed tumor progression and improved animal survival. In vitro studies demonstrated that rapamycin upregulated E-cadherin expression, and induced phenotypic transition from a more aggressive, invasive tumor phenotype to a noninvasive cuboidal phenotype that formed cell-to-cell adhesions. Additionally, rapamycin arrested the growth of renal cancer cells in the G1/S phase of the cell cycle.

Target of rapamycin inhibitors may also possess characteristics that make them uniquely effective in the treatment of RCC. Sporadic RCC is often associated with the loss or mutation of the *VHL* tumor suppressor gene. The VHL protein targets hypoxia-inducible factors 1 and 2α and leads to their destruction.[52] Loss of VHL function leads to the accumulation of these factors and the upregulated expression of vascular endothelial growth factor (VEGF) and platelet-derived growth factor (PDGF).[53] Target of rapamycin activation has been shown to increase hypoxia-inducible factor 1α expression, and target of rapamycin inhibition may result in the prevention of angiogenesis associated with RCC.[54,55] Atkins et al.[56] performed a phase II study of a novel target of rapamycin inhibitor (CCI-779) in patients with refractory metastatic RCC. An objective response rate of 7% was observed.

Thus, maintenance immunosuppressive therapy with target of rapamycin inhibitors holds promise in decreasing the incidence of posttransplantation malignancy, although this has yet to be established. These agents may also be utilized in chemotherapeutic regimens for refractory metastatic RCC with some promising initial results.

REFERENCES

1. Dunnill MS, Milard PR, Oliver DO. Acquired cystic disease of the kidneys: A hazard of long-term intermittent maintenance hemodialysis. J Clin Pathol 1977;30:368.
2. Miller LR, Soffer O, Nassar VH, Kutner MH. Acquired renal cystic disease in end-stage renal disease: an autopsy study of 155 cases. Am J Nephrol 1989;9:322–328.
3. Denton MD, Magee CC, Ovuworie C, et al. Prevalence of renal cell carcinoma in patients with ESRD pre-transplantation: a pathologic analysis. Kidney Int 2002;61:2201.
4. Narasimhan N, Golper TA, Wolfson M, Rahatzad M, Bennett WM. Clinical characteristics and diagnostic considerations in acquired renal cystic disease. Kidney Int 1986;30:748–52.
5. Ishikawa I, Saito Y, Shikura N, Kitada H, Shinoda A, Suzuki S. Ten-year prospective study on the development of renal cell carcinoma in dialysis patients. Am J Kidney Dis 1990;16:452–458.
6. Ishikawa I. Renal cell carcinoma in chronic hemodialysis patients—a 1990 questionnaire study in Japan. Kidney Int Suppl 1993;41:S167–169.
7. Terasawa Y, Suzuki Y, Morita M, Kato M, Suzuki K, Sekino H. Ultrasonic diagnosis of renal cell carcinoma in hemodialysis patients. J Urol 1994;152(3):846–851.
8. Ishikawa I. Acquired renal cystic disease and its complications in continuous ambulatory peritoneal dialysis patients. Peritoneal Dialysis Int 1992;12:292–297.
9. Acquired cystic kidney disease in children undergoing continuous ambulatory peritoneal dialysis. Kyushu Pediatric Nephrology Study Group. Am J Kidney Dis 1999;34(2):242–246.
10. Mallofre C, Almirall J, Campistol JM, Andreu J, Cardesa A, Revert L. Acquired renal cystic disease in HD: a study of 82 nephrectomies in young patients. Clin Nephrol 1992;37(6):297–302.
11. Ishikawa I, Saito Y, Onouchi Z. Development of acquired cystic disease and adenocarcinoma of the kidney in glomerulonephrotic chronic hemodialysis patients. Clin Nephrol 1980;14:1.
12. Hughson MD, Buckwald D, Fox M. Renal neoplasia and acquired cystic kidney disease in patients receiving long term dialysis. Arch Pathol Lab Med 1986;110:592.
13. Vaziri ND, Darwish R, Martin DC, Hostetler J. Acquired renal cystic disease in renal transplant recipients. Nephron 1984;37(3):203–205.
14. Tajima E, Aikawa A, Ohara T, et al. Effect of kidney transplantation on acquired cystic lesions in native kidneys. Transpl Proc 1998;30:3060–3061.
15. Ishikawa I, Shikura N, Shinoda A. Cystic transformation in native kidneys in renal allograft recipients with long-standing good function. Am J Nephrol 1991;11(3):217–223.
16. Levine LA, Gburek BM. Acquired cystic disease and renal adenocarcinoma following renal transplantation. J Urol 1994;151(1):129–132.
17. Hughson MD, Hennigar GR, McManus JF. Atypical cysts, acquired renal cystic disease, and renal cell tumors in end stage dialysis kidneys. Lab Invest 1980;42(4):475–480.
18. Herrera GA. C-erb B-2 amplification in cystic renal disease. Kidney Int 1991;40:509.
19. Hughson MD, Schmidt L, Zbar B, et al. Renal cell carcinoma of end-stage renal disease: a histopathologic and molecular genetic study. J Am Soc Nephrol 1996;7:2461.
20. Gronwald J, Baur AS, Holtgreve-Grez H, et al. Chromosomal abnormalities in renal cell neoplasms associated with acquired renal cystic disease. A series studied by comparative genomic hybridization and fluorescence in situ hybridization. J Pathol 1999;187(3):308–312.
21. Bretan PN, Busch MP, Hricak H, et al. Chronic renal failure: a significant risk factor in the development of acquired renal cysts and renal cell carcinoma. Cancer 1986;57:1871.

22. Cheuk W, Lo ES, Chan AK, Chan JK. Atypical epithelial proliferations in acquired renal cystic disease harbor cytogenetic aberrations. Hum Pathol 2002;33:761–765.
23. Matson MA, Cohen EP. Acquired cystic kidney disease: occurrence, prevalence, and renal cancers. Medicine (Baltimore) 1990;69(4):217–226.
24. Marple JT, MacDougall M, Chonko AM. Renal cancer complicating acquired cystic kidney disease. J Am Soc Nephrol 1994;4(12):1951–1956.
25. Taylor AJ, Cohen EP, Erickson SJ; et al. Renal imaging in long-term dialysis patients: a comparison of CT and ultrasonography. Am J Roentgenol 1989;153:765.
26. Takebayashi S, Hidai H, Chiba T, Takagi H, Koike S, Matsubara S. Using helical CT to evaluate renal cell carcinoma in patients undergoing hemodialysis: value of early enhanced images. Am J Roentgenol 1999;172(2):429–433.
27. Sarasin FP, Wong JB, Levey AS, Meyer KB. Screening for acquired cystic kidney disease: a decision analytic perspective. Kidney Int 1995;48(1):207–219.
28. Penn I. Primary kidney tumors before and after renal transplantation. Transplantation 1995;59:480.
29. Roupret M, Peraldi MN, Thaunat O, et al. Renal cell carcinoma of the grafted kidney: how to improve screening and graft tracking. Transplantation 2004;77(1):146–148.
30. Kim JY, Ruckle HC, Ramin SA. Partial nephrectomy for renal cell carcinoma in an allograft kidney 15 years after transplantation. J Urol 2001;165(4):1205.
31. Siebels M, Theodorakis J, Liedl B, Schneede P, Hofstetter A. Large de novo renal cell carcinoma in a 10-year-old transplanted kidney: successful organ-preserving therapy. Transplantation 2000;69(4): 677–679.
32. Krishnamurthi V, Novick AC. Nephron-sparing surgery in a renal allograft. Urology 1997; 50(1):132–134.
33. Shingleton WB, Sewell PE. Percutaneous cryoablation of renal cell carcinoma in a transplanted kidney. BJU Int 2002;90:137.
34. Baughman SM, Sexton WJ, Glanton CW, Dalrymple NC, Bishoff JT. Computerized tomography guided radio frequency ablation of a renal cell carcinoma within a renal allograft. J Urol 2004; 172:1262–1263.
35. Steinbach F, et al. Treatment of renal cell carcinoma in von Hippel-Lindau disease: a multicenter study. J Urol 1995;153:1812–1816.
36. Peterson GJ, et al. Renal transplantation in von Hippel-Lindau disease. Arch Surg 1977; 112:841–842.
37. Penn I. The effect of immunosuppression on pre-existing cancers. Transplantation, 1993;55: 742–747.
38. Steinbach F, Novick AC, Shoskes D. Renal transplantation in patients with renal cell carcinoma and von Hippel-Lindau disease. Urology 1994;44:760–763.
39. Goldfarb DA, et al. Results of renal transplantation in patients with renal cell carcinoma and von Hippel-Lindau disease. Transplantation 1997;64(12):1726–1729.
40. Terasaki PI, et al. High survival rates of kidney transplants from spousal and living unrelated donors. N Engl J Med 1995;333(6):333–336.
41. Latif F, et al. Identification of the von Hippel-Lindau disease tumor suppressor gene. Science 1993;260:1317–1320.
42. Glavac D, et al. Mutations in the VHL tumor suppressor gene and associated lesions in families with von Hippel-Lindau disease from central Europe. Hum Genet 1996;98:271–280.
43. Zbar B, et al. Germline mutations in the von Hippel-Lindau (VHL) gene in families from North America, Europe, and Japan. Hum Mutat 1996;8:348–357.
44. Neumann HPH. Basic criteria for clinical diagnosis in genetic counseling in Von Hippel-Lindau syndrome. J Vasc Dis 1987;16:220–226.
45. Penn I. Occurrence of cancers in immunosuppressed organ transplant recipients. In: Tearaski PI, Cecka JM, eds. Clinical Transplants. Los Angeles: UCLA Tissue Typing Laboratory, 1994:99–109.
46. London NJ, Farmery SM, Will EJ, Davison AM, Lodge JP. Risk of neoplasia in renal transplant patients. Lancet 1995;346:403–406.
47. Blohme I, Larko O. Premalignant and malignant skin lesions in renal transplant patients. Transplantation 1984;37:165–167.
48. Dantal J, Hourmant M, Cantarovich D, et al. Effect of long term immunosuppression in kidney graft recipients on cancer incidence: randomized comparison of two cyclosporine regimens. Lancet 1998; 351:623–628.

49. Vezina C, Kudelski A, Sehgal SN. Rapamycin, a new antifungal antibiotic. I. Taxonomy of the producing streptomycete and isolation of the active principal. J Antibiot (Tokyo) 1975;28:721–726.
50. Halloran PF. Immunosuppressive drugs for kidney transplantation. N Engl J Med 2004; 351:2715–2729.
51. Luan FL, Hojo M, Maluccio M, Yamaji K, Suthanthiran M. Rapamycin blocks tumor progression: unlinking immunosuppression from antitumor efficacy. Transplantation 2002;73(10):1565–1572.
52. Ohh M, Park CW, Ivan M, et al. Ubiquitination of hypoxia-inducible factor requires direct binding to the beta-domain of the von Hippel-Lindau protein. Nat Cell Biol 2000;2:423–427.
53. Iliopoulos O, Levy AP, Jiang C, et al. Negative regulation of hypoxia-inducible genes by the von Hippel-Lindau protein. Proc Natl Acad Sci U S A 1996;93:10595–10599.
54. Hudson CC, Liu M, Chiang GG, et al. Regulation of hypoxia-inducible factor 1-alpha expression and function by the mammalian target of rapamycin. Mol Cell Biol 2002;22:7004–7014.
55. Turner KJ, Moore JW, Jones A, et al. Expression of hypoxia-inducible factors in human renal cancer: relationship to angiogenesis and to the von Hippel-Lindau gene mutation. Cancer Res 2002; 62:2957–2961.
56. Atkins MB, Hidalgo M, Stadler WM, et al. Randomized phase II study of multiple dose levels of CCI-779, a novel mammalian target of rapamycin kinase inhibitor, in patients with advanced refractory renal cell carcinoma. J Clin Oncol 2004;22(5):909–918.

Management of Renal Adenomas and Oncocytomas

Igor Frank and Michael L. Blute

KEYWORDS

ADENOMA
ONCOCYTOMA
RENAL NEOPLASM
THERAPY
OUTCOME

ABSTRACT

Renal adenomas and oncocytoma are benign neoplasms that are characterized by indolent clinical behavior. The definition of renal adenoma has changed over time, reflecting the evolution of our understanding of the natural history of this neoplasm. Since methods to establish an accurate preoperative diagnosis are currently lacking, all solid renal neoplasms should be presumed malignant until proven otherwise. Extirpative surgical therapy, the efficacy of which has been thoroughly documented, is the preferred approach for majority of solid renal masses. Newer minimally invasive probe-ablative therapies (e.g., radiofrequency ablation and cryotherapy) are gaining popularity, although long-term outcome data are still lacking. This chapter discusses the current definition, diagnosis, and clinical management of renal adenomas and oncocytomas.

MANAGEMENT OF RENAL ADENOMAS

Definition of Renal Adenoma

The definition of adenoma has undergone significant evolution over the past seven decades. In the 1930s, Bell[1] defined tumors less than 3 cm in size as cortical adenomas based on the relatively low incidence of metastases in this cohort (2.6%) as compared to larger tumors (66%). However, a follow-up study in the 1950s revealed that the incidence of metastasis in patients with tumors less than 3 cm in size was higher than originally described (5%), emphasizing the unpredictable behavior of these tumors.[2] Nevertheless, the 3 cm cutoff persisted in the urologic literature well into the 1980s. In

From: *Clinical Management of Renal Tumors*
Edited by: R.M. Bukowski and A.C. Novick © Humana Press Inc., Totowa, NJ

1986, Theones et al.[3] attempted to reclassify renal tumors, and defined renal adenomas as lesions that are nuclear grade 1 and have a maximum size of 1 cm. The current classification recommended by the Union Internationale Contre le Cancer (UICC) and the American Joint Committee on Cancer (AJCC) only recognizes two types of adenomas: papillary and metanephric.[4] Papillary adenoma is defined as a lesion of papillary, tubular, or tubulopapillary architecture resembling low-grade papillary renal cell carcinoma (RCC) measuring less than 5 mm in greatest dimension.[4] The presence of clear cell or other nonpapillary histology or any degree of cytologic atypia excludes the diagnosis of papillary adenoma. The UICC and AJCC define metanephric adenoma as a neoplasm "comprised predominantly of small tubules lined with cuboidal epithelial cells, which is reminiscent of Wilms' tumor."[4] The first half of this chapter describes clinicopathologic features and clinical management of these two types of renal adenomas.

Papillary Adenoma

Papillary renal adenoma is the most common neoplasm of the renal tubular epithelium occurring in as many as 37% of autopsy cases.[5] Given their small size, the overwhelming majority of these lesions are completely asymptomatic, and a significant proportion falls below the limit of detection of contemporary imaging techniques. Therefore, the clinical incidence of these lesions is less than 1%. In the Mayo Clinic Nephrectomy Registry comprised of surgically treated renal tumors ($n = 4724$), there are only 28 (0.6%) papillary adenomas.

Papillary adenomas are essentially histologically indistinguishable from low-grade papillary RCC, and size is the only criterion used to define these lesions. Currently, there are no reliable histopathologic, ultrastructural, or even immunohistochemical or chromosomal features that can be used to distinguish these tumors.

Secondary to their small size, relatively few papillary adenomas are identified preoperatively. Jamis-Dow et al.[6] demonstrated that computed tomography (CT) under ideal conditions is capable of detecting 47% of renal tumors less than 5 mm in diameter. Therefore, a significant proportion of these lesions are identified at the time of partial or radical nephrectomy for a coexisting lesion. Of 28 patients with papillary adenoma in our institutional database, 19 (68%) had a coexistent RCC identified during the same surgery (11 with papillary RCC, seven with clear cell RCC, and one with both clear cell and papillary RCC).

If a small solid renal lesion is identified, no contemporary imaging technique is capable of reliably distinguishing between adenoma and other solid renal neoplasms, most notably RCC. Furthermore, having a limited role with larger masses, preoperative biopsy has no role in the management of tumors less than 5 mm in size.

A recent study from our institution revealed that 46% of surgically treated tumors less than 1 cm in size are benign,[7] although the proportion of benign tumors among lesions less than 5 mm in size is probably higher. Therefore, in the absence of coexistent lesions requiring therapy, observation should be considered especially in the elderly and in those with significant comorbidities. If growth is detected on follow-up imaging, extirpative or probe-ablative options could be employed at that point. Although observation in patients with small solid renal masses has been described,[7–10] the majority of the data is limited to patients with tumors measuring more than 1 cm and is therefore not directly applicable to this cohort. However, already low in the series with larger tumors, the growth rates in tumors less than 5 mm in size should even be lower given the higher incidence of benignity.

In younger patients with significant life expectancy who do not have comorbidities and who desire treatment, the benefits of conservative therapy should be weighed against the drawbacks of lifelong imaging surveillance, disease-related anxiety, and potential for metastatic spread. Therefore, these patients may be offered treatment early following appropriate counseling. Therapeutic approaches in this cohort include nephron-sparing surgery (open or laparoscopic), radiofrequency ablation (RFA), and cryotherapy.

Papillary adenomas have a benign clinical course, and no metastatic disease or local recurrences have been reported to date. Therefore, once pathologic diagnosis is established and the lesion is completely excised with negative surgical margins, no further therapy should be necessary. While an association between renal adenoma and sporadic RCC in nephrectomy specimens has been reported,[11–13] it remains unclear at this time whether patients who have been treated for a papillary adenoma are prone to develop new kidney lesions or cancers in the future. Therefore, until this issue is further clarified, periodic follow-up renal ultrasounds seem prudent.

Metanephric Adenoma

Metanephric adenoma, first defined in 1992,[14] is a rare benign lesion that is histologically reminiscent of Wilms' tumor. Macroscopically, metanephric adenoma presents as a tan-to-gray or yellow well-circumscribed mass. Microscopically, these tumors contain small highly basophilic cuboidal epithelial cells forming small acini or tubulopapillary structures within a predominantly acellular stroma. They usually lack abnormal mitotic figures and marked cytological atypia.

Initially, a relationship with Wilms' tumor and nephroblastomatosis was presumed based on this lesion's histologic appearance. In the late 1990s, chromosomal analysis revealed gains of chromosome 7 and 17, which are the characteristic genetic alterations of papillary adenoma and papillary RCC.[15] This finding suggested that metanephric adenoma is a precursor to papillary RCC. However, a more recent analysis by Brunelli et al.[16] found no such chromosomal gains refuting the suggested association. In fact, the authors concluded that chromosomal analysis may facilitate discrimination of metanephric adenoma from papillary RCC or adenoma. Another recent study revealed that, based on immunohistochemistry, metanephric adenoma is morphologically and immunophenotypically identical to maturing Wilms' tumor and nephrogenic rests.[17]

Metanephric adenoma is a very rare lesion. Thus, majority of our knowledge regarding this benign tumor is based on case reports or small cohorts. The largest study of metanephric adenoma to date included 50 cases.[18] In the Mayo Clinic Nephrectomy Registry, metanephric adenomas are less common than papillary adenomas, with an incidence of 0.2%.

Metanephric adenomas are most common in middle-aged females with a female-to-male ratio well over 2:1 in the majority of reports.[18,19] They also occur in children.[18,19] Metanephric adenomas tend to be larger than papillary adenomas, with an average reported size of 5.5 cm.[18] Lesions as large as 20 cm have been reported.[20]

Because of their large size, a significant proportion of metanephric adenomas are symptomatic. In the study by Davis et al.,[18] 42% of patients presented with symptoms, such as flank pain, gross hematuria, or palpable mass, and another 12% presented with hypercalcemia and polycythemia. This finding establishes a higher incidence of poly-cythemia in metanephric adenoma than in other renal tumors. Up to 40% of patients have no signs or symptoms of metanephric adenoma.[18]

Radiographically, metanephric adenomas appear as solid well-circumscribed paren-chymal renal masses. On unenhanced CT, they display increased attenuation relative to the adjacent renal parenchyma. Contrast images reveal enhancement with intravenous (IV) contrast administration.[21] Ultrasound typically shows a hyperechoic lesion with enhanced through-transmission. However, accurate differentiation of metanephric adenoma from RCC is impossible using contemporary imaging techniques, and all solid renal lesions should be presumed to be malignant until proven otherwise. Preoperative biopsy is not accurate enough to affect management in the majority of patients, given its high false-negative rates.[22–25]

Since the diagnosis of metanephric adenoma cannot be reliably established prior to therapy, these lesions should be treated as any other solid renal mass. Therapeutic options typically include radical nephrectomy (laparoscopic or open), nephron-sparing surgery (laparoscopic or open), RFA, or cryotherapy. In the elderly and in patients with significant comorbidities, observation may also be an option for small renal masses, as mentioned above. Surgical resection offers the advantage of accurate pathologic diagnosis.

Initial studies of metanephric adenoma suggested that it is a benign lesion that typi-cally follows an indolent clinical course. In the report by Davis et al.,[18] all 50 patients displayed no evidence of metastatic disease or recurrence. Jones et al.[19] confirmed this finding, with no evidence of recurrence or metastatic disease in their cohort with a median follow-up of 60.8 months. However, more recently, several cases of metastatic metanephric adenomas have been reported in both adults and children.[26–28] This suggests that classification of metanephric adenoma as a benign lesion may not be entirely accu-rate. In the future, ancillary studies including immunohistochemistry and chromosomal analysis will need to be investigated for a potential role in distinguishing between benign metanephric adenomas and those with a malignant potential.

MANAGEMENT OF ONCOCYTOMA

The UICC and AJCC define oncocytoma as a benign renal neoplasm that is "typically comprised of cells with abundant eosinophilic cytoplasm that is filled with mitochon-dria."[4] Although the first case report of this neoplasm was published in 1942,[29] it was not until 1976 when it was established as a distinct pathologic entity.[30] Since then, a significant amount of knowledge has accumulated regarding this tumor and its natural history.

Oncocytoma is clinically the most common benign parenchymal renal tumor, and it comprises approximately 5% of all renal neoplasms.[4,31] It is more common in males than in females, with a male-to-female ratio of 2 to 1. This disease is also more common in older patients, with a mean age at the time of resection in the mid-60s.[31–33] It has been reported to coexist with RCC[31] and angiomyolipoma.[34] Familial renal oncocyto-mas, which are frequently multiple and bilateral, have also been described.[35]

Macroscopically, oncocytomas are usually well-circumscribed, but nonencapsulated, light-brown solid lesions that usually display "pushing" as opposed to invasive growth pattern. A central scar is found in 30% to 50% of lesions,[32,33] a finding that is suggestive but not pathognomonic of this neoplasm. Tumor size averages 3 to 5 cm depending on the study,[31–33] although in our practice we have seen tumors as large as 16 cm in the greatest dimension. Microscopically, oncocytomas consist of large neoplastic cells with granular eosinophilic cytoplasm that are packed with mitochondria. These cells are arranged in an organoid and tubulocystic pattern, in the background of myxoid or hyalinized stroma. Occasionally, atypical findings may be present, including nuclear pleomorphism, prominent nucleoli, and perinephric fat involvement.[32,33,36] The overall appearance is sometimes very similar to low-grade chromophobe RCC, complicating pathologic diagnosis in some cases, especially when atypical histologic features are present. Distinguishing oncocytoma from RCC is even more challenging using biopsy specimens. The UICC and AJCC do not support grading of oncocytomas.[4]

Although the majority of sporadic oncocytomas are unilateral and unifocal, multifocality and bilaterality have been reported.[31,32] Approximately 5% of oncocytomas are bilateral with both synchronous and metachronous presentations documented.[31] Multifocality occurs in 6% to 13% of patients with these tumors.[31,32] In addition to bilaterality and multifocality, patients may present with oncocytomatosis, a disease process characterized by extensive bilateral involvement of the renal parenchyma.[37,38] A recent study of 14 patients with diffuse oncocytomatosis revealed that in up to 32% of specimens the dominant mass is either a chromophobe RCC or a "hybrid tumor" containing histologic features of both chromophobe RCC and oncocytoma. Therefore, the authors proposed that the term *renal oncocytosis,* rather than *oncocytomatosis,* be used to account for the coexistence of oncocytomas and chromophobe RCC in these patients.[39]

Diffuse oncocytosis can also be found in patients with Birt-Hogg-Dubé (BHD) syndrome, which is a rare autosomal dominant syndrome characterized by various dermatologic abnormalities and the development of oncocytomas and RCC.[40,41] From the urologic standpoint, patients with this syndrome exhibit multiple bilateral renal tumors and evidence of microscopic oncocytosis in their renal parenchyma. Grossly, hybrid oncocytic neoplasms containing areas reminiscent of chromophobe RCC and oncocytoma are most common at 50%, followed by frank chromophobe RCC at 34%.[42] Clearcell RCC is less common at 9% but is usually larger with an average tumor size of 4.7 cm as compared to 3.0 cm and 2.2 cm for chromophobe RCC and hybrid tumor, respectively.[42] Based on these pathologic findings, it has been postulated that the microscopic oncocytic lesions may be precursors of the hybrid oncocytic tumors, chromophobe RCCs, and possibly clear-cell RCC.[42]

The majority of oncocytomas (80%)[32] are asymptomatic at presentation, although larger lesions may present with the typical symptoms of a renal mass (e.g., pain, hematuria, or abdominal mass).[30,32,33] It is anticipated that with stage migration and the more prevalent use of high-definition imaging techniques, the number of oncocytomas, as well as other benign renal tumors will increase overtime. The same increase will likely be seen in the proportion of asymptomatic oncocytomas. Our unpublished data reveal that the proportion of solid renal tumors diagnosed as oncocytoma have increased from 6.6% in the 1970s to 11.6% in the 1990s.

Similar to renal adenomas, reliable preoperative diagnosis of oncocytoma is not possible at present. Therefore, all solid renal masses should be treated as malignant until proven otherwise. The presence of a central stellate scar on CT scan is suggestive of oncocytoma but is neither reliable nor specific.[43–45] Furthermore, absence of such a finding clearly does not rule out oncocytoma. Several studies confirmed the inability of CT to differentiate between oncocytoma and RCC.[43,46] Characteristic magnetic resonance imaging (MRI) findings of this lesion, such as a well-defined capsule, a central stellate scar, and distinctive intensities on T1 and T2 images, can suggest the diagnosis but by no means are definitive.[47] Ultrasound does not add any diagnostic information to the above imaging modalities in the setting of a solid renal mass.

Since renal biopsy has the potential to spare some patients from invasive surgery, it has been a subject of significant amount of research. While in some patients, pathologic diagnosis can be obvious (cases of typical clear-cell RCC), distinguishing chromophobe RCC from oncocytomas can be very difficult, even using ancillary techniques. Multiple prospective and retrospective studies have demonstrated that renal biopsy or aspiration is unreliable and is unlikely to alter clinical decision making in the majority of patients with a solid renal mass, secondary to high false-negative rates.[22–25] However, a report by Liu and Fanning,[48] based on a retrospective analysis of 19 tumors, suggested an algorithm that can be used to enhance the accuracy of fine-needle aspiration (FNA) in distinguishing chromophobe RCC from oncocytoma. Their diagnostic protocol combined microscopic examination with ancillary studies, including immunostaining with cytokeratin and vimentin antibodies and Hale colloidal iron (HCI) stain. Electron microscopy was employed in the most difficult cases. While demonstrating accuracy of the combined approach in a small cohort, this study has a limited value and should be interpreted with caution secondary to its limited sample size, retrospective nature, and lack of precise surgical diagnosis in some patients. Furthermore, even if precise pathologic diagnosis could be established based on a biopsy specimen, sampling issues are likely to affect the overall diagnostic accuracy. The coexistence of RCC and oncocytoma in the same lesion or at other locations in the same kidney has been reported to occur in 10% of cases,[31] and hybrid lesions have been described in as many as 32% of patients with oncocytosis.[39]

Since there is no reliable method to differentiate an oncocytoma from RCC, any solid renal mass should be treated as malignant until proven otherwise. Therefore, treatment options should include open or laparoscopic partial or radical nephrectomy, RFA, cryotherapy, and observation depending on the size of the lesion as well as the patient's comorbidities, age, and treatment preference. If oncocytoma is suspected preoperatively, a nephron-sparing approach should be chosen if possible and otherwise indicated. However, given the propensity of this tumor for multicentricity and bilaterality, the remainder of the diseased kidney as well as the contralateral kidney must be carefully examined for synchronous lesions using preoperative imaging. Contrast-enhanced CT using 5-mm slices is our imaging technique of choice. It is important to emphasize that even if an oncocytoma is suspected based on preoperative imaging, proper oncologic care should never be compromised, given the lack of accuracy of contemporary imaging techniques in ruling out malignancy.

During partial nephrectomy, the entire kidney should be exposed and examined intraoperatively to rule out coexistent RCC or multifocality. Intraoperative ultrasound should be employed when necessary. If multiple oncocytomas are found, parenchyma-sparing techniques should be employed if possible. Accurate frozen-section analysis to establish histology is instrumental in the decision-making process under these circumstances.

Although fortunately rare, oncocytosis represents a serious therapeutic dilemma. The high rate of coexistence of chromophobe RCC and oncocytoma and the difficulty in establishing a reliable diagnosis preoperatively limit treatment options. This situation is further complicated by the rarity of this condition and the resultant deficiency in our knowledge of its natural history. However, once precise pathologic diagnosis is established, one approach is to manage these patients in a similar fashion to patients with von Hippel–Lindau (VHL) disease. Dominant lesions greater than 3 cm in size at the time of diagnosis should be treated with partial nephrectomy or nephron-sparing probe-ablative techniques (RFA or cryotherapy). Our preference is partial nephrectomy in this setting as it has the advantage of providing a precise pathologic diagnosis of the dominant mass and an opportunity for thorough sampling of other lesions to establish diagnosis. Following initial resection or ablations, patients should then be followed with periodic imaging for changes and growth. Lesions larger than 3 cm in size should be treated using any of the above-mentioned techniques. This 3-cm cutoff is supported by a recent report that demonstrated the safety of this approach in patients with VHL disease.[49] None of the patients in this series with a tumor less than 3 cm in diameter developed metastatic disease.

Following resection and definitive diagnosis of oncocytoma, the majority of patients have a benign clinical course. Although there are several reports of suspected metastatic oncocytoma in the literature,[32,50–53] earlier reports probably represent chromophobe RCC misdiagnosed as oncocytoma, and later reports often lack pathologic proof of metastasis.[50] To our knowledge, there is only one biopsy-proven case of oncocytoma metastatic to the liver in a patient who had survived for more than 5 years with expectant management only and without any change in the size of the metastasis.[32] Even in patients with familial oncocytomatosis, no metastatic disease has been reported to date.[35] Therefore, there is currently no evidence to support imaging surveillance for metastatic disease following extirpative therapy. However, patients should undergo imaging surveillance for local or contralateral recurrence. Ipsilateral and contralateral metachronous lesions have been reported to occur at the rate of 4% after a mean period of 9.5 years.[31] Therefore, periodic renal ultrasounds are justified in these patients following surgical resection. There are no data in the literature to support a specific follow-up schedule at present.

CONCLUSION

Renal adenomas and oncocytomas are benign tumors of the renal epithelium. They are characterized by an overwhelmingly benign clinical course, although metastatic oncocytomas and metanephric adenomas have been reported. Given the lack of reliable preoperative means to distinguish these lesions from renal malignancy at the present time, all solid renal tumors should be treated as malignant until proven otherwise. Extirpative treatment options are currently preferred, although newer probe-ablative therapies appear promising. Nephron-sparing therapy is advised whenever possible. Postoperative imaging surveillance to screen for local ipsilateral or contralateral recurrence is prudent in the majority of patients. Future research should focus on identifying means to reliably distinguish malignant from benign tumors prior to surgical therapy.

REFERENCES

1. Bell ET. A classification of renal tumors with observations on the frequency of the various types. J Urol 1938;39:238–243.
2. Bell ET. Renal Disease. Philadelphia: Lea & Febiger, 1950.
3. Theones W, Störkel S, Rumpelt HJ. Histopathology and classification of renal cell tumors (adenomas, oncocytomas, and carcinomas): the basic cytological and histopathological elements and their use of diagnostics. Pathol Res Pract 1986;181:125–143.
4. Storkel S, Eble JN, Adlakha K, et al. Classification of renal cell carcinoma: Workgroup No. 1. Union Internationale Contre le Cancer (UICC) and the American Joint Committee on Cancer (AJCC). Cancer 1997;80:987–989.
5. Hiasa Y, Kitamura M, Nakaoka S, et al. Antigen immunohistochemistry of renal cell adenomas in autopsy cases: relevance to histogenesis. Oncology 1995;52(2):97–105.
6. Jamis-Dow CA, Choyke PL, Jennings SB, et al. Small (<3 cm) renal masses: detection with CT versus US and pathologic correlation. Radiology 1996;198:785–788.
7. Frank I, Blute ML, Cheville JC, Lohse CM, Weaver AL, Zincke H. Solid renal tumors: an analysis of pathological features related to tumor size. J Urol 2003;170(6):2217–2220.
8. Masanori K, Suzuki T, Suzuki Y, Terasawa Y, Sasano H, Arai Y. Natural history of small renal cell carcinoma: evaluation of growth rate, histologic grade, cell proliferation and apoptosis. J Urol 2004;172:863–866.
9. Wehle MJ, Thiel DD, Petrou SP, Young PR, Frank I, Karsteadt N. Conservative management of incidental contrast-enhancing renal masses as safe alternative to invasive therapy. Urology 2004;64(1):49–52.
10. Volpe A, Panzarella T, Rendon RA, Haider MA, Kondylis FI, Jewett MA. The natural history of incidentally detected small renal masses. Cancer 2004;100(4):738–745.
11. Cristol DS, Mc. Donald JR, Emmett JL. Renal adenomas in hypernephromatous kidney—a study of their incidence, nature, and relationship. J Urol 1946;55:18–27.
12. Mukamel E, Konichezky M, Engelstein D, et al. Incidental small renal tumors accompanying clinical overt renal cell carcinoma. J Urol 1988;140:22–24.
13. Cheng WS, Farrow GM, Zincke H. The incidence of multicentricity in renal cell carcinoma. J Urol 1991;146:1221–1223.
14. Brisigotti M, Cozzutto C, Fabbretti G, Sergi C, Callea F. Metanephric adenoma. Histol Histopathol 1992;7(4):689–692.
15. Brown JA, Anderl KL, Borell TJ, Qian J, Bostwick DG, Jenkins RB. Simultaneous chromosome 7 and 17 gain and sex chromosome loss provide evidence that renal metanephric adenoma is related to papillary renal cell carcinoma. J Urol 1997;158(2):370–374.
16. Brunelli M, Eble JN, Zhang S, Martignoni G, Cheng L. Metanephric adenoma lacks the gains of chromosomes 7 and 17 and loss of Y that are typical of papillary renal cell carcinoma and papillary adenoma. Mod Pathol 2003;16(10):1060–1063.
17. Muir TE, Cheville JC, Lager DJ. Metanephric adenoma, nephrogenic rests, and Wilms' tumor: a histologic and immunophenotypic comparison. Am J Surg Pathol 2001;25(10):1290–1296.
18. Davis CJ Jr, Barton JH, Sesterhenn IA, Mostofi FK. Metanephric adenoma. Clinicopathological study of fifty patients. Am J Surg Pathol 1995;19(10):1101–1114.
19. Jones EC, Pins M, Dickersin GR, Young RH. Metanephric adenoma of the kidney. A clinicopathological, immunohistochemical, flow cytometric, cytogenetic, and electron microscopic study of seven cases. Am J Surg Pathol 1995;19(6):615–626.
20. Bouzourene H, Blaser A, Francke ML, Chaubert P, Bouzourens N. Metanephric adenoma of the kidney: a rare benign tumour of the kidney. Histopathology 1997;31:480–490.
21. Fielding JR, Visweswaran A, Silverman SG, Granter SR, Renshaw AA. CT and ultrasound features of metanephric adenoma in adults with pathologic correlation. J Comput Assist Tomogr 1999;23(3):441–444.
22. Dechet CB, Sebo T, Farrow G, et al. Prospective analysis of intraoperative frozen needle biopsy of solid renal masses in adults. J Urol 1999;162:1282–1284.
23. Renshaw AA, Lee KR, et al. Accuracy of fine needle aspiration in distinguishing subtypes of renal cell carcinoma. Acta Cytol 1997;41:987–994.
24. Zardawi IM. Renal fine needle aspiration cytology. Acta Cytol 1999;43:184–190.
25. Campbell SC, Novick AC, Herts B, et al. Prospective evaluation of fine needle aspiration of small, solid renal masses: accuracy and morbidity. Urology 1997;50:25–29.

26. Renshaw AA, Freyer DR, Hammers YA. Metastatic metanephric adenoma in a child. Am J Surg Pathol 2000;24(4):570–574.
27. Pins MR, Jones EC, Umlas J, Martul EV, Kamar BR, Renshaw AA. Metanephric adenoma like tumors of the kidney: report of three malignancies with emphasis on discriminating features. Arch Pathol Lab Med 1999;123:415–420.
28. Drut R, Drut RM, Ortolani C. Metastatic metanephric adenoma with foci of papillary carcinoma in a child: a combined histologic, immunohistochemical, and FISH study. Int J Surg Pathol 2001; 9(3):241–247.
29. Zippel L. Zur kunntnis der onkocyten. Virchow Arch Pathol Anat 1942;308:360–382.
30. Klein MJ, Valensi QJ. Proximal tubular adenomas of kidney with so called oncocytic features: a clinicopathological study of 13 cases of a rarely reported neoplasm. Cancer 1976;38:906–914.
31. Dechet CB, Bostwick DG, Blute ML, et al. Renal oncocytoma: multifocality, bilateralism, metachronous tumor development and coexistent renal cell carcinoma. J Urol 1999;162:40–42.
32. Perez-Ordonez B, Hamed G, Campbell S, et al. Renal oncocytoma: a clinicopathologic study of 70 cases. Am J Surg Pathol 1997;21:871–883.
33. Amin MB, Crotty TB, Tickoo SK, Farrow GM. Renal oncocytoma: a reappraisal of morphologic features with clinicopathologic findings in 80 cases. Am J Surg Pathol 1997;21:1–12.
34. Pillay K, Lazarus J, Wainwright HC. Association of angiomyolipoma and oncocytoma of the kidney: a case report and review of the literature. J Clin Pathol 2003;56(7):544–547.
35. Weirich G, Glenn G, Junker K, et al. Familial renal oncocytoma: clinicopathological study of 5 families. J Urol 1998;160(2):335–340.
36. Rainwater LM, Farrow GM, Lieber MM. Flow cytometry of renal oncocytoma: common occurrence of deoxyribonucleic acid polyploidy and aneuploidy. J Urol 1986;135:1167–1171.
37. Warfel KA, Eble JN. Renal oncocytomatosis. J Urol 1982;127:1179–1180.
38. Katz DS, Gharagozloo AM, Peebles TR, Oliphant M. Renal oncocytomatosis. Am J Kidney Dis 1996;27:579–582.
39. Tickoo SK, Reuter VE, Amin MB, et al. Renal Oncocytosis: a morphologic study of fourteen cases. Am J Surg Pathol 1999;23(9):1094.
40. Toro JR, Glenn G, Duray P, et al. Birt-Hogg-Dube syndrome: a novel marker of kidney neoplasia. Arch Dermatol 1999;135:1195–1202.
41. Phillips JL, Pavlovich CP, Walther M, et al. The genetic basis of renal epithelial tumors: advances in research and its impact on prognosis and therapy. Curr Opin Urol 2001;11:463–469.
42. Pavlovich CP, Walther MM, Eyler RA, et al. Renal tumors in the Birt-Hogg-Dube syndrome. Am J Surg Pathol 2002;26(12):1542–1552.
43. Davidson AJ, Hayes WS, Hartman DS, et al. Renal oncocytoma and carcinoma: failure of differentiation with CT imaging. Radiology 1993;183:693–696.
44. Licht MR, Novick AC, Tubbs RR, et al. Renal oncocytoma: clinical and biological correlates. J Urol 1993;150:1380–1383.
45. Licht MR. Renal adenoma and oncocytoma. Semin Urol Oncol 1995;13:262–266.
46. Wildberger JE, Adam G, Boeckmann W, et al. Computed tomography characterization of renal cell tumors in correlation with histopathology. Invest Radiol 1997;32:596–601.
47. Harmon WJ, King BF, Lieber MM. Renal oncocytoma: magnetic resonance imaging characteristics. J Urol 1996;155:863–867.
48. Liu J, Fanning CV. Can renal oncocytomas be distinguished from renal cell carcinoma on fine-needle aspiration specimens? A study of conventional smears in conjunction with ancillary studies. Cancer 2001;93(6):390–397.
49. Duffey BG, Choyke PL, Glenn G, Grubb RL, Venzon D, Linehan WM, Walther MM. The relationship between renal tumor size and metastases in patients with von Hippel-Lindau disease. J Urol 2004;172(1):63–65.
50. Amin R, Anthony P. Metastatic renal oncocytoma: a case report and review of literature. Clin Oncol 1999;11:277–279.
51. Lewi HJE, Alexander CA, Fleming S. Renal oncocytoma—bilateral, multifocal. Urology 1983; 22:355–359.
52. Jockle G, Toker C, Shamsuddin A. Metastatic renal oncocytic neoplasm with benign histologic appearance. Urology 1987;30:79–81.
53. Psihramis K, Cin P, Dretler S, Prout G Jr, Sandberg A. Further evidence that renal oncocytoma has malignant potential. J Urol 1988;139:585–587.

35 Renal Angiomyolipoma: *Diagnosis and Management*

Surena F. Matin, Pheroze Tamboli, and Christopher G. Wood

KEYWORDS

ANGIOMYOLIPOMA
RENAL TUMOR
RENAL HAMARTOMA
RENAL CHORISTOMA
PARTIAL NEPHRECTOMY
HEMORRHAGIC COMPLICATIONS

ABSTRACT

Renal angiomyolipoma (AML) can present symptomatically or asymptomatically and as a sporadic or hereditary manifestation. Hereditary AML occurs in patients with tuberous sclerosis complex (TSC); the variable expression of this syndrome is such that typical physical features may be subtle, with the presence of AML dominating the picture and appearing as a sporadic occurrence. In most cases, the diagnosis of AML is confirmed radiographically because of the presence of fat content in the tumor. Angiomyolipoma is the only solid renal tumor that can be diagnosed confidently by radiographic imaging alone, although in some cases the fat of the tumor may be so small that a diagnosis of a malignant solid tumor cannot be excluded.

The natural history of AML is variable and unpredictable. Typically, a size threshold of 4 cm is used for treatment decisions and has been used in the literature to analyze the presence of symptoms, which might include pain, hemorrhage, and hematuria. Many cases of AML remain asymptomatic. The treatment of AML is individualized in every case. Therapeutic options have shifted considerably in recent years, with fewer patients undergoing nephrectomy, and the primary form of intervention being a conservative approach of either observation or nephron-sparing treatment. While partial nephrectomy remains an excellent surgical option for larger and more complex lesions, multiple other alternative options are available, including selective angioembolization, laparoscopic partial nephrectomy, and ablative therapy.

From: *Clinical Management of Renal Tumors*
Edited by: R.M. Bukowski and A.C. Novick © Humana Press Inc., Totowa, NJ

INCIDENCE, TUBEROUS SCLEROSIS COMPLEX, AND GENETICS

Renal angiomyolipoma (AML) is the most common mesenchymal tumor of the kidney. It is composed of fat, smooth muscle, and vascular elements. Although AMLs were previously considered hamartomas or choristomas, evidence in recent years suggests a neoplastic origin with evidence of a clonal source.[1-3] The overwhelming majority of AMLs are benign tumors. The initial association of neurologic and renal findings in patients with tuberous sclerosis complex (TSC) was by Bourneville in the 19th century, and the first histopathologic description of the disease was made in 1911 by Fischer.[4] Morgan et al.[5] introduced the term *angiomyolipoma* to the urologic literature in 1951.

Results of screening ultrasound of the general population have shown an incidence of 0.13%, and autopsy series place the incidence at about 0.32%.[6,7] The majority (about 80%) of cases of AML are sporadic and are not associated with TSC. Patients with sporadic AML generally present later in life, and are predominantly female.[8] Sporadic AML can behave quite differently from the setting of TSC, and its course, although generally benign, is unpredictable. Angiomyolipoma may not grow over the course of many years, yet some smaller lesions can grow significantly and unpredictably over a short period of time and may cause symptoms.[8] The data suggest a monoclonal origin of these tumors that challenges the classic description of polyclonal proliferation by various tissue types.[3] The 5q33–34 region has been implicated as a common site of chromosomal abnormalities in some cases of AML.[3]

Tuberous sclerosis complex is an autosomal dominant but variably penetrant genetic syndrome that is manifested by a constellation of cutaneous lesions, multiorgan hamartomas, including in the heart, lung, and brain, and other findings such as renal cysts (Figure 35.1). Tuberous sclerosis complex affects approximately 1 in 6000 people, almost half of whom also have AML. Only a minority of patients is found at presentation to have the classic triad of seizures, mental retardation, and adenoma sebaceum.[9] Tuberous sclerosis complex is one of two genetic syndromes associated with both renal tumors and renal cysts (the other being von Hippel–Lindau syndrome), and one of the two most common neurocutaneous disorders (the other being neurofibromatosis). In comparison to sporadic AML, TSC tends to occur in childhood or young adulthood with an equal incidence in men and women, and to be characterized by bilateral renal involvement.

Angiomyolipoma associated with TSC appears to have a higher predilection for growth than sporadic AML. Another notable feature of AML associated with TSC is renal cysts. Several small series and case reports have suggested a higher incidence of malignant renal tumors developing in patients with TSC. In several reports, renal cell carcinoma (RCC) has been found to coexist with AML, usually when associated with TSC, but also in several series of patients with sporadic AML.[10,11] However, a meta-analysis showed an identical risk for RCC in the TSC population as in the normal population.[11] The recent identification of the malignant variant epithelioid AML may explain some of these associations (discussed later).

Tuberous sclerosis complex is associated with defects of the *TSC1* gene, which is located on chromosome 9q34, and the *TSC2* gene, which is located on chromosome 16p13. Both are tumor-suppressor genes and are essential for development. The protein product of TSC2 is tuberin, a guanosine triphosphatase that forms a complex with the protein product of TSC1, hamartin. Presently, much more is known about TSC2 than

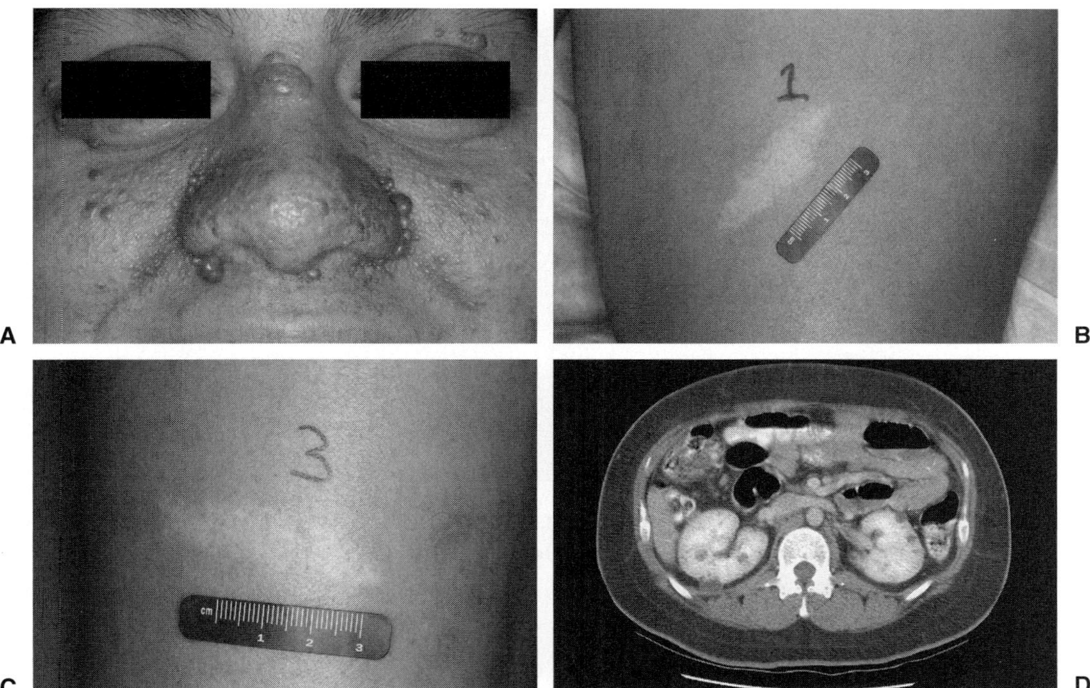

Figure 35.1. Typical cutaneous and renal findings in a patient with tuberous sclerosis complex (TSC). (A) Facial angiofibromas. (B,C) Multiple hypomelanotic macules. (D) Multiple renal angiomyolipoma (AML) and renal cysts. (Copyright Surena F. Matin, 2005.)

TSC1, although both appear to function as tumor-suppressor genes and to be implicated in the development of other sporadic tumors.[12] These genes are thought to be negative regulators of S6K1, which is required for ribosomal biosynthesis, cell growth, and cellular proliferation.[13] Hamartin and tuberin are involved in several cell-signaling pathways thought to play a role in cytoskeletal remodeling, cell growth, cellular adhesion, and motility. The exact composition and role of the tuberin/hamartin complex is still unclear. Loss of heterozygosity of the TSC genes is implicated in the majority of TSC-associated AML. The Eker rat model has loss of heterozygosity of *TSC2* due to an insertional mutation.[14] Interestingly, unlike the human counterpart, these animals develop multiorgan malignancies that in the kidney resemble RCC rather than AML.[14] Further investigations of this interesting animal model may not only reveal important downstream effects of *TSC2* and tuberin, but also epigenetic events that may play an important role in neoplasia. In addition to the association of AML with TSC, AML has been reported in other hereditary disorders, including von Recklinghausen's disease, von Hippel–Lindau disease, and adult polycystic kidney disease.

DIAGNOSIS

Presentation

The majority of patients presenting with AML are asymptomatic, and the overwhelming majority are female in a nearly 4:1 ratio.[8,15,16] Increasingly, patients are found to have AML incidentally during a workup for other diseases or conditions (Figure 35.2).

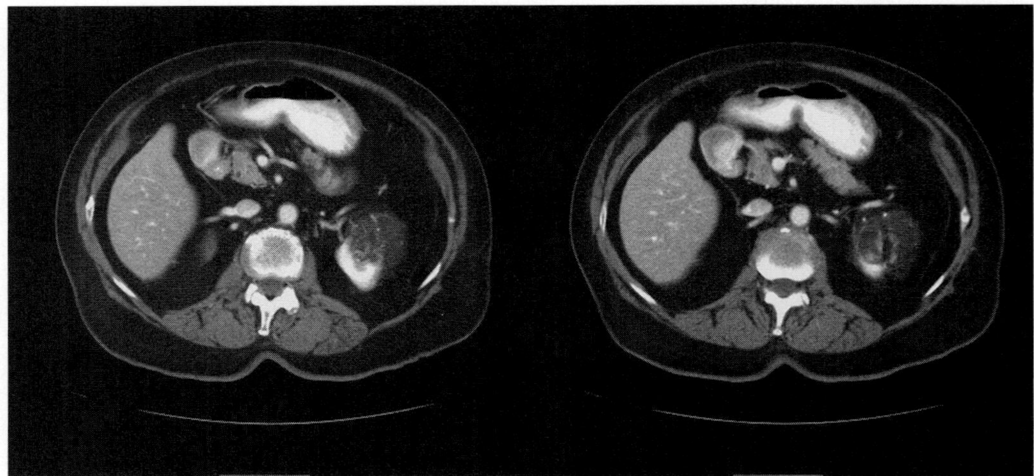

Figure 35.2. A 6.5-cm asymptomatic sporadic renal AML found incidentally during workup of lower abdominal complaints. (Copyright Surena F. Matin, 2005.)

Symptomatic patients most often present with flank or abdominal pain, and hematuria, and may have a palpable mass on physical examination. In a retrospective review by Steiner et al.[8] of 35 patients with AML, 40% presented with symptoms, the majority (86%) of which was pain. Other symptoms included hemorrhage, which was seen in approximately one third of patients, and hematuria, which was seen in about one fourth of patients. A palpable mass was present in half the patients in that study. Severe, spontaneous hemorrhage has been reported as the initial presentation by others.[17–19] Angiomyolipoma is the most common renal neoplasm associated with spontaneous perirenal hemorrhage, closely followed by RCC.[20] Thus, the differential diagnosis in a patient presenting with acute perirenal or retroperitoneal hemorrhage, when there is no or minimal antecedent trauma, includes an occult tumor, which may be masked by the presence of blood. The accuracy of computed tomography (CT) is reported to be from moderate[20] to very sensitive[19] in detecting the underlying etiology of the hemorrhage. Follow-up imaging after resolution of the hematoma is usually necessary when the initial imaging study is inconclusive.

For patients suspected to have TSC, a comprehensive physical examination is required and is ideally performed in a multidisciplinary setting. Genetic testing for TSC is generally not performed. The sensitivity of current genetic testing protocols is lower than that for other syndromes, such as von Hippel–Lindau. Mutations occurring in the *TSC1* and *TSC2* genes are diverse, complex, and sometimes unidentifiable in a significant number of cases. For example, the detection rate in familial cases is about 30% for *TSC1* mutations and about 50% for *TSC2*, whereas in cases of simplex disease (those without a family history), detection rates are approximately 10% and 70%.[21] The diagnosis is thus made on clinical and radiographic features alone. In 1998, the Tuberous Sclerosis Complex Consensus Conference published major and minor features found on clinical and radiographic examination that when grouped as a constellation of findings can provide a definite, probable, or possible diagnosis (Table 35.1). These features provide the most reliable diagnosis of TSC for patients presenting with AML.

Table 35.1.
Diagnostic criteria for tuberous sclerosis complex

Definite TSC: two major features, or one major and two minor
   features
Probable TSC: One major and one minor feature
Possible TSC: Either one major feature, or two or more minor
   features

Major features
   1. Facial angiofibromas or forehead plaque
   2. Ungual or periungual fibroma
   3. Hypomelanotic macules (three or more)
   4. Shagreen patch (connective tissue nevus)
   5. Multiple retinal nodular hamartomas
   6. Cortical tuber
   7. Subependymal nodule
   8. Subependymal giant cell astrocytoma
   9. Cardiac rhabdomyoma, single or multiple
   10. Lymphangiomyomatosis
   11. Renal angiomyolipoma

Minor features
   1. Multiple pits in dental enamel
   2. Hamartomatous rectal polyps
   3. Bone cysts
   4. Cerebral white matter radial migration lines
   5. Gingival fibromas
   6. Nonrenal hamartomas
   7. Retinal achromic patch
   8. Confetti skin lesions
   9. Multiple renal cysts

Source: Adapted from Roach et al.[9]

Laboratory Studies

All patients initially presenting with renal AML should undergo a screening evaluation of renal function with a serum creatinine test, followed by more specific testing using 24-hour urine collection if there is concern regarding reduced global renal function. A urinalysis is also frequently performed at initial presentation as part of the comprehensive urologic workup. In cases of acute hemorrhage, serial blood counts, blood typing, and screening in preparation for possible blood transfusion are mandatory. Genetic testing for patients suspected to have TSC is generally not done, as discussed previously.

Radiographic Evaluation

Ultrasound provides a very good initial screening evaluation for AML, particularly for children and pregnant women in whom radiation exposure is a concern.[22,23] Angiomyolipoma typically appears as a hyperechoic lesion owing to the presence of fat.[24] A CT scan is the preferred modality for accurate diagnosis of AML. A thin-section (less than or equal to 5 mm) noncontrast CT scan increases spatial and density resolution and decreases volume-averaging, which improves the sensitivity for detecting fat in the lesion, and thus providing a reliable diagnosis of AML.[25] Bosniak and colleagues[25] evaluated CT scans of patients with small AML tumors in which only minimal amounts of fat were evident on careful sampling of low-density regions within the masses. In contrast, there were no areas of fat with small RCCs in that study. However, two situations, in particular, can create diagnostic difficulties: fat-containing malignancies, and AML with minimal fat content. Renal cell carcinomas have been reported, albeit rarely, to contain fat elements or entrapped renal sinus or perinephric fat.[26] Differentiation between AML and fat-containing RCC can be difficult.

Radiographically, the presence of intratumoral calcification, irregular borders, localregional invasion, necrosis, adenopathy, and vascular invasion should alert one to the possibility of malignancy.[26] Several studies have provided insight into differentiating AML from well-differentiated liposarcomas on CT scan. One of the most characteristic radiographic signatures of AML is the presence of a discrete fatty renal parenchymal defect.[27,28] Even with large exophytic AML, a careful inspection of a thin-cut CT will identify the defect corresponding with the parenchymal origin of the tumor (Figures 35.3 and 35.4B). Other features associated with AML more than with liposarcoma include enlarged vessels, aneurysmal dilation, hemorrhage, and satellite tumors representing additional AML.[27,28] The presence of calcifications does not appear to always differentiate AML from liposarcoma.[28] Lipomas of the kidney and fat-containing oncocytomas are extremely rare.[26] A report discusses two cases of an AML variant with histologic findings suggestive of oncocytoma, but with negative staining for epithelial markers and positive staining for HMB-45.[29]

Diagnostic difficulties may arise when AML has a high proportion of myogenic or vascular components (Figure 35.4), or when hemorrhage masks the lipomatous elements.[24,30,31] Kim and colleagues[31] suggested that biphasic helical CT may be useful in differentiating minimal-fat AML from RCC, with homogeneous tumor enhancement

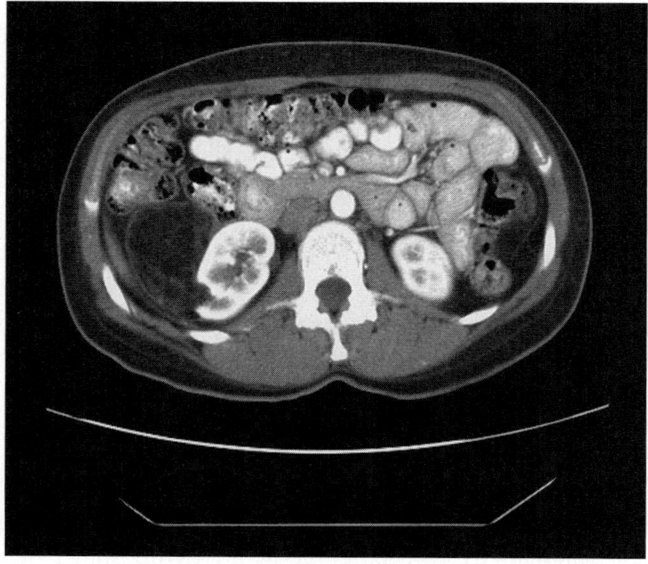

Figure 35.3. Typical radiographic findings as seen on a computed tomography (CT) scan. (Copyright Surena F. Matin, 2005.)

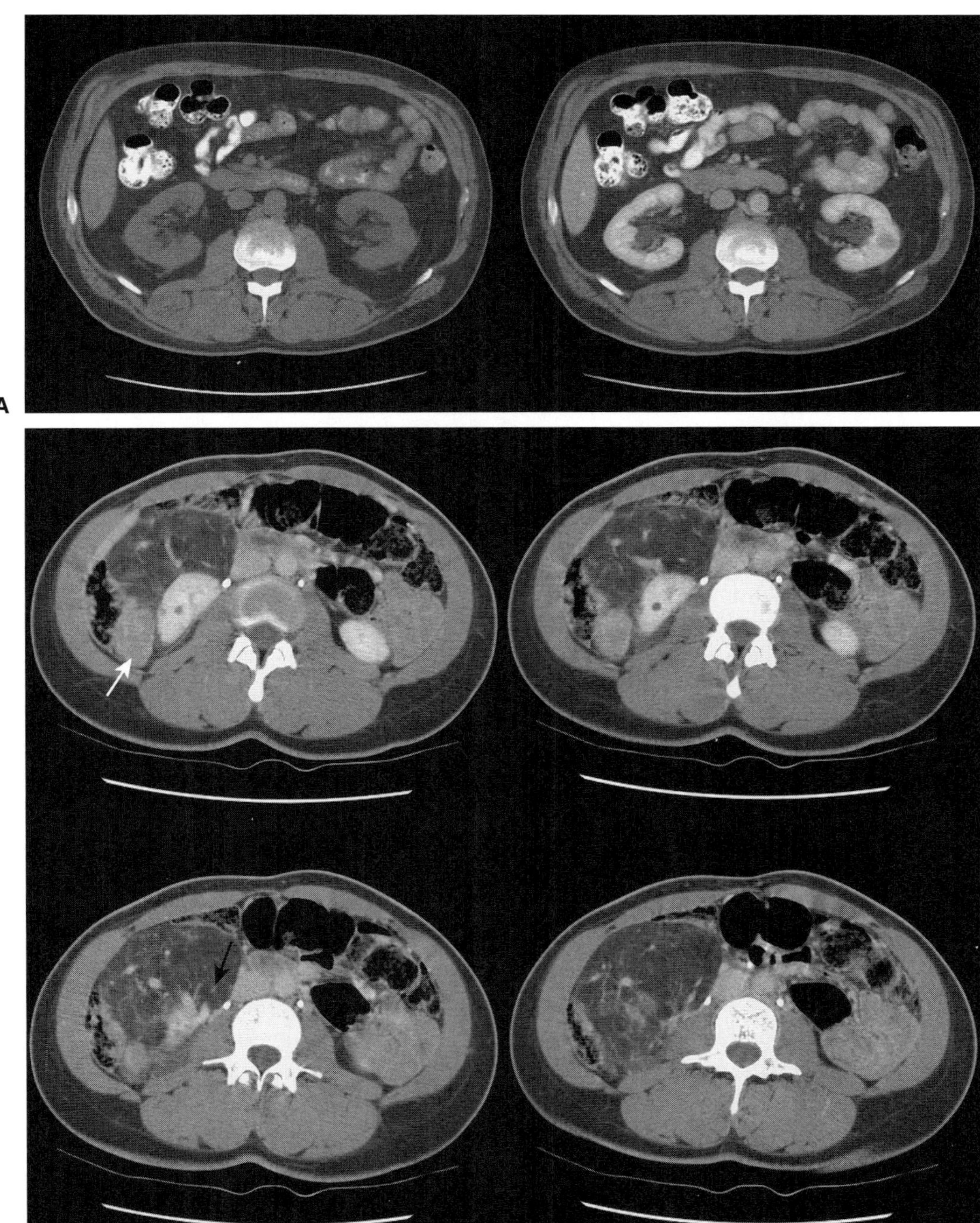

Figure 35.4. (A) Atypical radiographic findings seen on dedicated renal protocol CT scan. Precontrast region of interest (ROI) measurements were 57 Hounsfield units for the mass and 37 for the surrounding normal renal parenchyma, whereas postcontrast measurements were 112 for the mass and 180 for the renal parenchyma. ROI measurements of thin-cut (2.5 mm) sectioning failed to show any fat elements. After partial nephrectomy and preservation of the majority of the kidney, pathology confirmed a fleshy AML with paucity of adipose tissue (same as Figure 35.7). (B) Serial CT scans showing typical and atypical AML seen in the same patient. A large AML with typical CT findings is enveloping the lower pole of the right kidney. A more atypical AML (white arrow) is seen in the posterior aspect. A small renal parenchymal defect (black arrow) in the lower medial pole indicates the origin of the AML. (Copyright Surena F. Matin, 2005.)

(observed in 79% of AML versus 5% of RCC) and a prolonged enhancement pattern (observed in 58% of AML versus 10% of RCC) being the most valuable CT findings. Using both of these findings, the authors reported positive and negative predictive values of 91% and 87%, respectively. Magnetic resonance imaging (MRI) has several advantages over CT scanning, including improved tissue contrast, multiplanar reconstruction, and the use of a nonnephrotoxic contrast agent.[32] However, it rarely adds significantly more information if a well-performed renal protocol CT scan (i.e., multiphasic with thin cuts of kidney) is available for an otherwise typical presentation. Angiography is not helpful or necessary for the accurate diagnosis of AML, but does play an important therapeutic role in select cases, as will be discussed later.[24] Typically, angiography shows tortuous arteries and multiple and sometimes large aneurysms. Those patients with ruptured AMLs appear to have larger aneurysms than those in whom the tumor has not ruptured. Angiomyolipoma with small or no aneurysms have been reported by one group to display minimal to no growth, suggesting a common link between tumor growth and aneurysmal propensity.[33]

Pathology

Angiomyolipoma is pathologically characterized by the presence of a variable proportion of mature adipose tissue, blood vessels, and smooth muscle. These tumors are purported to arise from the perivascular epithelioid cell (PEC),[34,35] which is also considered to be the cell of origin of other related tumors and tumor-like lesions. However, it is noteworthy that the normal counterpart of this cell has not been identified in nonneoplastic tissue. Tumors and tumor-like lesions thought to arise from PEC include clear-cell "sugar" tumor of the lung, lymphangiomyomatosis of the lung, clear cell sugar tumor of the pancreas, and a group of tumors known only by the acronym PEComa that have been reported to arise in diverse organs and tissues.[36–44] The common finding in all of these tumors and tumor-like lesions is the presence of epithelioid cells with eosinophilic cytoplasm and immunohistochemical expression of the melanoma-associated HMB-45 antigen.

As noted previously, AML in patients with TSC tends to be multifocal and bilateral, whereas sporadic cases of AML tend to be single tumors and are generally larger than those associated with TSC. The tumor size may vary from a few millimeters to 20 cm; one earlier series reported a range in size of 3 to 20 cm, with an average size of 9.4 cm.[45] The gross appearance of AML is dependent on the proportion of the three elements (Figure 35.5). The appearance varies from yellow and soft (fat predominant) to pinkgray and fleshy (muscle predominant). Areas of hemorrhage, even massive hemorrhage, may be present. These tumors are usually well circumscribed but are not encapsulated and can extend beyond the renal capsule into the perinephric adipose tissue. Tumors located predominantly in the perinephric tissue but attached to the renal capsule have been referred to as "capsulomas." Rare tumors may extend into the renal collecting system, the renal vein,[46] or even the inferior vena cava.[47,48] Variable-sized cysts may be seen in some cases and may result from entrapment and dilatation of renal tubules in the adjacent renal parenchyma. Rarely, the tumors appear multicystic.[49,50] Bone formation in AML has also been reported in few tumors.[51] Regional lymph node involvement may be present, which is thought to represent multicentric growth of the tumor rather than a true metastatic phenomenon.[52] Angiomyolipoma may also be present within the retroperitoneal soft tissue without being attached to the kidney, and in abdominal viscera

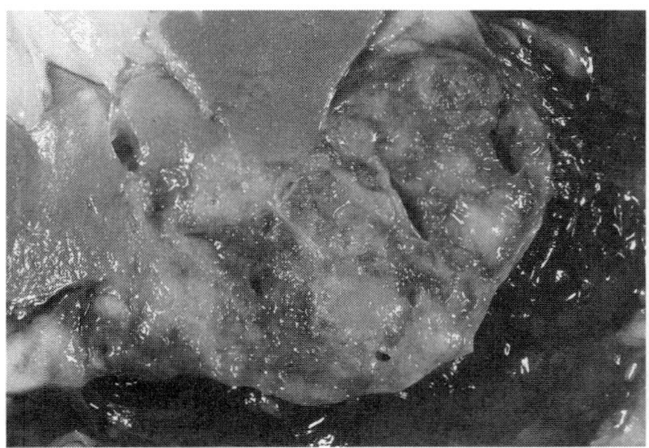
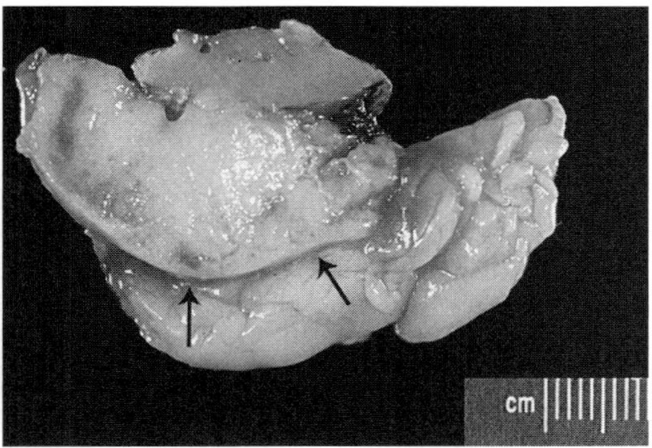

A

B

Figure 35.5. (A) Photograph of cut section of gross specimen showing an AML arising from the periphery of the renal cortex and protruding into the perinephric adipose tissue, which is darkly stained secondary to hemorrhage. (B) Photograph of cut section of partial nephrectomy specimen. The renal parenchymal resection margin is at the top of the picture. The AML is well circumscribed and loosely separated from the adjacent perinephric adipose tissue (arrows). (Copyright Surena F. Matin, 2005.)

such as the liver, spleen, and fallopian tubes.[53-55] As with lymph node involvement, most authorities consider these extrarenal tumors as evidence of multicentricity rather than metastases.

Microscopically, the tumor is composed of varying proportions of mature adipose tissue; thick-walled, poorly organized blood vessels; and smooth muscle (Figure 35.6). The adipose tissue can be extensive in some tumors, and may be associated with fat necrosis and lipophages. The smooth muscle cells often appear to be originating from the outer layers of muscle of the blood vessel wall. These muscle cells have a sort of radial arrangement in relation to the blood vessels, with the smooth muscle cell nucleus at right angles to the blood vessel wall. Smooth-muscle bundles may be scattered diffusely throughout the tumor or may produce well-formed interlacing fascicles. The blood vessels are abnormal appearing with thick walls, most often resembling

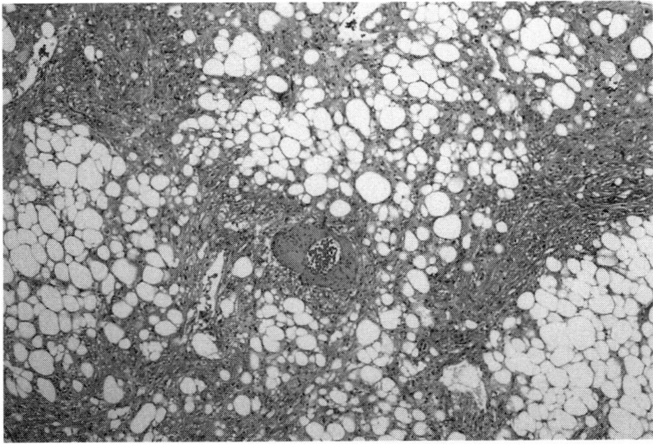

Figure 35.6. AML original magnification 100×. The tumor shows adipose tissue separated by bands of smooth-muscle with an abnormal blood vessel in the center. (Copyright Surena F. Matin, 2005.)

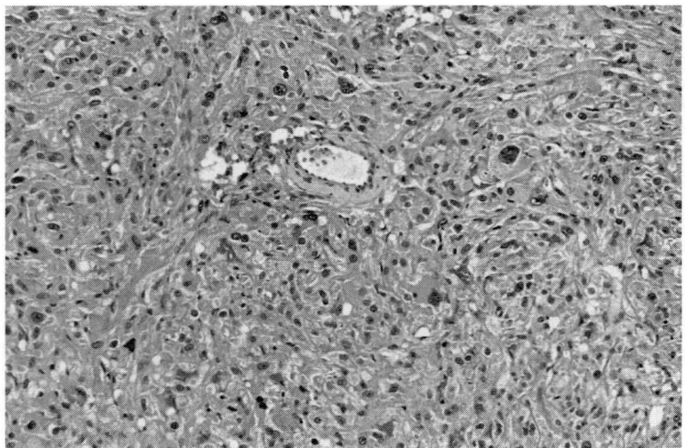

Figure 35.7. AML original magnification 200×. This tumor is composed predominantly of smooth muscle cells, some of which have an epithelioid appearance. There is a single abnormal blood vessel in the center. (Copyright Surena F. Matin, 2005.)

arterialized veins similar to those seen in arteriovenous malformations. These vessels lack the systematic architectural organization of normal vascular structures. They are sometimes tortuous and may even form small aneurysms.

Variations in the above-mentioned histologic features are common, including increase in mitoses, nuclear pleomorphism, binucleation, or multinucleation of the smooth muscle component. Some tumors may display a paucity or apparent lack of fat and may need to be differentiated from leiomyomas (Figure 35.7). In such cases, a helpful feature is the presence of abnormal blood vessels associated with the fascicles of smooth muscle. The lipomatous component is usually composed of mature adipose tissue, but it may contain lipoblasts and atypical giant cells mimicking a well-differentiated liposarcoma. Synchronous occurrence of RCC and renal oncocytoma in the same kidney as AML has been reported.[50,56,57]

The immunohistochemical expression of melanoma-associated antigens is one of the hallmarks of AML and other tumors arising from the perivascular epithelioid cells. These antigens include HMB-45, HMB-50, neuroglandular antigen (detected by the NKI/C3 antibody to CD63), MART-1, melan-A, tyrosinase, and microphthalmia transcription factor (MiTF).[58–63] These stains are mainly positive in the epithelioid smooth-muscle-cell component (Figure 35.8).[60,61] As these antigens are expressed in the majority

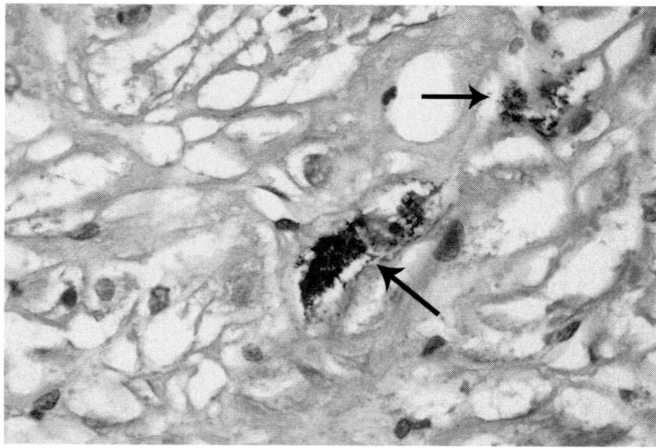

Figure 35.8. HMB-45 staining of epithelioid cells in AML (arrows, original magnification 400×). (Copyright Surena F. Matin, 2005.)

of renal AML and not in most other renal tumors, HMB-45 immunoreactivity is also a useful tool in distinguishing renal AML from other renal tumors, especially in cases demonstrating unusual morphologic features. The smooth muscle and blood vessel walls stain positive with smooth-muscle actin, muscle-specific actin, and vimentin.[59,64] Neuron-specific enolase and desmin may also be positive in some cases. The adipose tissue stains with S-100. Cytokeratin and epithelial membrane antigen are almost always negative. In one study, expression of c-kit (CD117) was reported in all cases.[65] There are also reports of use of immunohistochemical stains with antibodies to hamartin and tuberin, the protein products of the *TSC1* and *TSC2* genes, respectively.[66,67]

At the ultrastructural level, the epithelioid cells exhibit a variety of granules, which may be striated, rhomboid, spherical, or elliptical. Some of these granules may resemble melanosomes, whereas others may resemble renin granules. Rarely, they form typical premelanosomes.[68,69] Smooth-muscle cells and adipocytes have typical ultrastructural features. In addition, some cells exhibit ultrastructural features of both cell types and may represent transition forms between myocytes and adipocytes.[49]

Most AMLs are benign; however, rare malignant forms of AML have been reported. There are two reports of malignant transformation (leiomyosarcoma),[70,71] with lung metastasis in one case.[71] At present, it is difficult to predict biologic behavior purely on the basis of pathologic features. The presence of tumor necrosis, vascular invasion, cellular pleomorphism, and mitoses are reported to be associated with a greater risk of malignant behavior. The biologic potential of epithelioid AML is harder to predict, and these patients may need closer surveillance, as there are reports of patients succumbing to this tumor.[58,72–74]

Epithelioid Angiomyolipoma

Some AMLs may exhibit an epithelioid morphology (Figure 35.9), a variant that may be confused with RCC.[58,72–74] This variant has been reported in patients with and without TSC. In 1997, Eble and colleagues[58] published their experience of five patients who had AML with a predominant epithelioid smooth-muscle component. Two of the patients

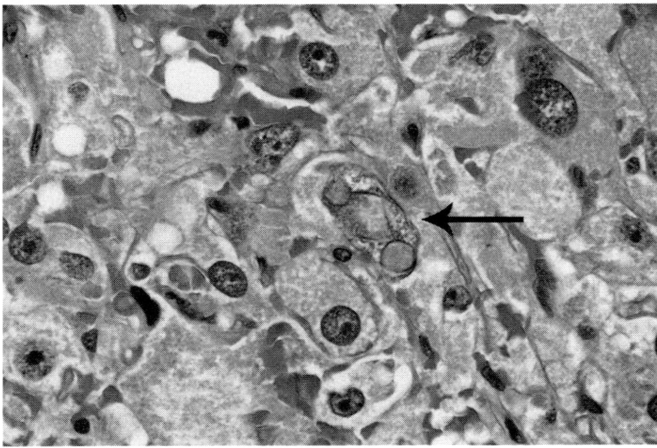

Figure 35.9. Epithelioid AML 400×. The tumor is composed predominantly of large epithelioid cells. The cell in the center shows a large pleomorphic nucleus (arrow). (Copyright Surena F. Matin, 2005.)

had TSC, and in all cases the tumors were suspected of being malignant. Two of the patients died of neoplastic progression. These tumors were described as having sheets of eosinophilic smooth muscle cells, which usually are not seen in large numbers in typical AML, with occasional hemorrhage, necrosis, mitoses, few fat cells, and only scattered thick-walled blood vessels. None of the tumors stained positive for cytokeratin or epithelial membrane antigen, which effectively ruled out RCC, but all stained positive for HMB45.[58] This report was soon followed by similar findings by Pea et al.[74] This phenotype is characterized by epithelioid cells that are cytokeratin-negative and HMB45-positive. Two of the three patients in the report by Pea et al. also died of malignant progression. These findings led these authors to conclude that reports of RCC in patients with TSC and RCC occurring with AML (so-called collision tumors) should be reevaluated for this phenotype, which may represent malignant transformation of AML. These same authors subsequently reported a patient who eventually succumbed to this tumor, who had the same morphologic findings as well as genetic defects in the primary lesion as well as the metastatic lesions, with the same allelic loss on the short arm of chromosome 16, proving a common clonal origin of this apparent malignant transformation of AML.[73] Since these reports, others have reported cases of epithelioid AML, sometimes appearing as discrete enhancing lesions within a typical AML and usually associated with a fatal course.[59,75–77] The discovery of this unusual, sometimes aggressive variant may explain the occasional report of malignant behavior with AML.[15]

MANAGEMENT

For optimal management of AML, treatment must be individualized. The individualization of care can be based largely on four factors: (1) presence or absence of symptoms; (2) tumor characteristics, such as size; (3) renal status; and (4) patient and health-related factors. Table 35.2 summarizes these factors. Absolute indications for intervention generally include a tumor greater than 4cm in size or a rapidly growing tumor; the presence of symptoms, such as pain or bleeding; and indeterminate radiographic findings.

The presence of symptoms and tumor size appear to be critically important determinants of the treatment approach. Oesterling et al.[78] in 1986 published a review of 602 patients reported in the literature from 1948 to 1985, including 13 patients from their own institution. Over 80% of tumors greater than 4cm were symptomatic, whereas only 23% of those ≤4cm were symptomatic. Nearly 97% of patients with tumors larger than 4cm underwent some form of therapy, mostly nephrectomy, whereas only 43% of those with smaller tumors underwent intervention, also mostly nephrectomy. Observation was elected in 19% of those with tumors less than 4cm and in 3% of those with tumors greater than 4cm. No significant tumor growth was noted in either group. None of the 13 patients from their own institution who underwent observation had tumor growth; two of the 13 died of other conditions while asymptomatic. On the basis of that data, the authors recommended nephron-sparing surgery for larger (>4cm) symptomatic tumors, possible surveillance for smaller (<4cm) tumors that had resolved symptoms, and routine surveillance of asymptomatic tumors.[78] This group established the important parameters of symptoms and tumor size in the management of AML.

Table 35.2.
Factors influencing management of renal angiomyolipoma

1. Symptoms
   Symptomatic (pain, hematuria, hemorrhage)
   Asymptomatic
2. Tumor factors
   Size ≤4 cm or >4 cm   Stability over time
   Documented growth
   Presence of calcifications (suggests malignancy)
   No renal parenchymal defect seen (suggests liposarcoma)
3. Patient factors
   Young age
   Elderly age
   Tuberous sclerosis
   Pregnant or impending pregnancy
   Comorbidities
4. Renal factors
   Poorly functioning affected kidney
   Compromised contralateral kidney
   Medical renal disease
   Solitary kidney

In a follow-up study from the same institution, Steiner et al.[8] published additional data that helped to clarify the natural history of AML even more, and the previously reported lack of growth was discounted. The propensity for these tumors to grow over time was shown using radiographic and historical follow-up data collected over an average of 4 years. Of sporadic AML, 21% grew over time, whereas 67% of AMLs associated with TSC were seen to grow. Growth was not due to intratumoral hemorrhage, and, importantly, was highly unpredictable. Others have corroborated the association of tumor size and symptoms, including De Luca et al.,[16] who found that symptomatic patients had larger tumors (average 8.1 cm) versus those that were asymptomatic (average 2.0 cm). The overwhelming majority of asymptomatic tumors did not show any radiographic changes or develop hemorrhage or any other complications over a 60-month follow-up. More recently, tumor size has been shown to correlate with aneurysm size on angiography and risk of hemorrhage.[33]

The management of AML also has to take into account patient-related health factors such as age, pregnancy status, TSC diagnosis, and the severity of coexistent comorbidities. For example, younger patients with larger, sporadic AML may be considered for an intervention designed to minimize radiation exposure during follow-up and to minimize the lifelong risk for exposure to complications from AML. Hemorrhage secondary to renal AML during pregnancy is reported in 6% to 21% of women with TSC.[79] Pregnancy may be an indication for more aggressive intervention to prevent maternal complications or fetal demise.[17,80] This theory has been challenged by Mitchell et al.,[79] who evaluated 145 women with TSC to determine whether pregnancy increased the risk for pulmonary or renal complications. Pregnancy did not appear to increase the risk of developing pulmonary or renal complications in this population, but the study had many limitations. Despite multiple shortcomings in the design and analysis, some interesting information is to be gleaned from this study. Pregnant women appeared to have a much higher incidence of hemorrhagic complications than nonpregnant women. Also, most complications during pregnancy occurred after the first trimester.[79] Thus, if intervention is deemed necessary during pregnancy, waiting until the second trimester appears to minimize the risk of AML complications while also lowering the risk of intervention, such as teratogenic exposure (greatest during the first trimester) and risk of premature birth (greatest during the third trimester).

The presence of severe comorbidities tends to diminish the desire for aggressive intervention in asymptomatic AML; however, in symptomatic AML requiring intervention, the presence of medical comorbidities generally implies the need for less morbid treatment. Additionally, evaluation of renal factors (such as the overall renal status, and the function of the affected and the contralateral kidney) is imperative in these cases, because these may strongly influence the type of treatment strategy. A specific treatment algorithm taking into account all these factors would not be feasible or easily usable. Nelson and Sanda[4] devised an algorithm taking into account the certainty of diagnosis, the presence of symptoms, and some patient factors, which can help provide a general framework for diagnosis and treatment. Generally, patients with multiple or severe comorbidities, older patients, and those with small (less than 4 cm) asymptomatic tumors are safe with observation alone. Larger asymptomatic tumors might also be observable depending on the individual case. In recent times the availability of minimally invasive nephron-sparing therapies has lowered the threshold for intervention. The morbidity of intervention appears to have been lowered dramatically, particularly in high-risk patients and those presenting with acute hemorrhage.

Surveillance

Even large tumors showing progression have occasionally been reported to remain asymptomatic for prolonged periods of time, up to 18 years.[81] However, the greatest risk for symptoms is with large tumors. As noted by Dickinson and colleagues,[82] 83% of patients with AML tumors larger than 8 cm developed symptoms versus only 43% of those with tumors smaller than 4 cm, and tumors between 4 and 8 cm in size had a variable behavior. As also noted with the previously mentioned study, tumors smaller than 3 cm have been reported to bleed.[83] This serves as a reminder that the published statistics represent probabilities that can only help to guide decisions for therapy and are not to be taken as assurances of behavior. Nevertheless, the consensus of the published literature seems to be that the majority of asymptomatic tumors remain silent and exhibit a low risk of growth, whereas most large asymptomatic tumors have a higher risk for growth and subsequent development of symptoms. Surveillance of asymptomatic patients with AML thus seems reasonable in individual cases. The time interval for surveillance studies is not standardized. Oesterling and colleagues[78] recommended semiannual follow-up for patients with larger asymptomatic tumors and annual follow-up for those with smaller asymptomatic tumors. De Luca et al.[16] recommended follow-up every 2 years with ultrasound for patients with small asymptomatic tumors. In our practice, a short-term radiographic follow-up (usually 6 months) is initially done to establish stability. Eventually, follow-up ultrasound or CT scan is performed yearly or even biannually depending on tumor size and individual patient factors.

Angioembolization

Although rarely useful for diagnosis, angiography and selective renal angioemboliza-tion have played an important role in the treatment of renal AML. Renal angiography to delineate the anatomy prior to partial nephrectomy has been supplanted with nonin-vasive imaging methods such as CT and MR angiograms. Angiographic embolization is occasionally utilized preoperatively in select cases. Emergent angiography with selec-tive embolization is the primary therapeutic option for cases of acute hemorrhage. In the past, when surgery was performed as primary intervention, these cases were associ-ated with a high rate of nephrectomy.[78] Several single-institution series have also reported the efficacy of elective angioembolization for primary therapy.[84] The nephron-sparing and therapeutic efficacy in these cases relies on a favorable vascular anatomy, whereby the tumor has a selective and dominant supply from one or very few accessible branches. In cases when this anatomy is not favorable, the efficacy of selective angio-embolization may not be as favorable or particularly nephron sparing, with reports of partial or complete renal loss.[85,86] One common complication following angioemboliza-tion appears to be liquefactive necrosis or abscess formation, usually requiring percu-taneous drainage.[84,86–88] Delayed hemorrhage after initial embolization has also been reported, requiring repeat angiography or nephrectomy.[84,89,90] Overall, angioemboliza-tion represents another good option in the armamentarium of treatments for renal AML, but its recommendation as a primary treatment for all AML is mitigated by data showing a complication rate up to 22% and the need for reintervention in approximately 30% of 76 cases reported in the literature.[4]

The postembolization syndrome occurs in many patients undergoing angioemboliza-tion of a renal tumor and is classically seen when angioinfarction of a kidney is per-formed, but can also be seen after selective infarction of a large tumor. The syndrome consists of pain, fever, and leukocytosis. Prevention of the syndrome is managed with acetaminophen and antihistaminics, with available analgesics for pain relief available on an as-needed basis. Anticipation by house officers and preemptive education of the patient also prevents unnecessary testing and anxiety. One group has reported the use of a steroid taper over a 2-week period that helped prevent pain in all patients and minimized fever in most of the patients.[91] The imaging follow-up period after angio-embolization also remains unclear, and to our knowledge, no information on the long-term radiographic appearance of angiographically treated lesions has been reported. Patients presenting with acute hemorrhage, those at high-risk for general anesthesia, and those refusing more definitive surgery may be the best candidates for primary treat-ment using angioembolization.

Surgery

Two decades ago, the majority of AML tumors were treated with nephrectomy.[15,78] With contemporary improvements in diagnostic accuracy and minimally invasive tech-niques as well as the known benign natural history of the vast majority of AML, a kidney-sparing approach is usually possible and advisable. However, there are unusual cases whereby the degree of destruction of normal renal parenchyma by destructive growth is so severe or the number and size of AML so overwhelming, that nephron-sparing surgery is not feasible (Figure 35.10). In these cases, a nephrectomy may ulti-mately be necessary.

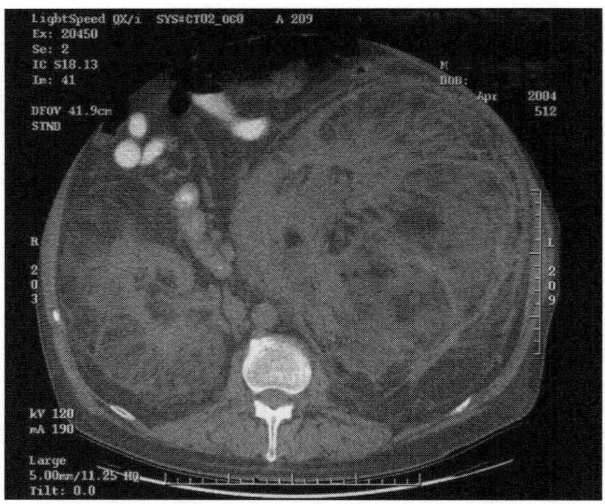

Figure 35.10. CT scan showing giant bilateral AML with resulting destruction of majority of renal parenchyma. (Copyright Surena F. Matin, 2005.)

NEPHRON-SPARING SURGERY

Open partial nephrectomy is the gold standard nephron-sparing option for renal tumors. The efficacy, renal function preservation, and long-term outcomes associated with partial nephrectomy for renal tumors, including AML, is well known and well documented in the literature.[10,92] Local recurrences after complete excision with partial nephrectomy have not been reported in multiple series. Metachronous recurrences in the contralateral kidney after partial or radical nephrectomy have also not been reported to our knowledge in sporadic cases.[8,10,78,93] Even very large tumors in the setting of a solitary functioning kidney can be managed feasibly with partial nephrectomy with satisfactory renal functional outcomes.[10]

Angiomyolipoma can have a prototypic growth pattern that is not widely recognized. Even large tumors may arise from only a small area of the kidney and grow in a blooming, exophytic pattern that can envelop the kidney (Figure 35.4B).[94] Careful dissection often allows the tumor to be separated away from the renal capsule except for the area of parenchyma from which it is arising, allowing the majority of the kidney to be spared.

Cases of bilateral AML present their own challenges. Similar to RCC, the management in regard to the sequence of events is frequently a topic of debate. Simultaneous bilateral partial nephrectomy, or partial nephrectomy with simultaneous contralateral nephrectomy, is generally discouraged, because the risk of acute temporary renal replacement therapy can be high in this setting. In rare cases, bilateral simultaneous partial nephrectomy may be reasonable if the ischemia time is deemed to be short, and minimal parenchymal dissection is necessary during hilar clamping. In most cases, however, a planned, staged approach is advisable. The concept of doing the "easy" side first is generally adhered to in these cases. This allows the urologic surgeon to obtain a satisfactory functional result prior to proceeding to the more difficult contralateral kidney, which may have a higher risk of resulting nephrectomy. Thus, at every step, the patient is undergoing surgery with maximized nephron mass and with a functioning

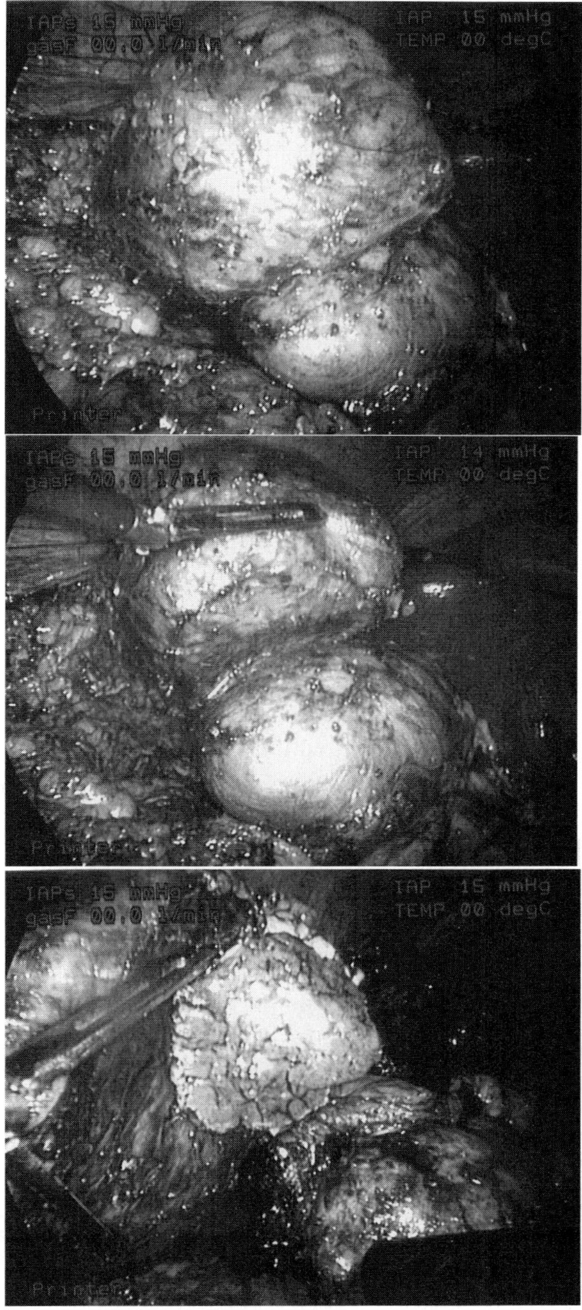

Figure 35.11. Series of intraoperative photographs showing a laparoscopic partial nephrectomy for a 7-cm AML corresponding to the CT scan seen in Figure 35.3. This patient had a prior angioembolization without symptomatic benefit or evidence of devascularization. Although the tumor covers a large portion of the anterior surface of the kidney (top), the tumor can be easily dissected off the renal capsular surface, exposing the focal area of involvement of the renal parenchyma (middle). Wedge resection is performed, resulting in maximal renal preservation (bottom) and minimal renal parenchymal dissection. (Copyright Surena F. Matin, 2005.)

contralateral unit. This approach facilitates postoperative fluid management after the second-stage procedure, particularly in those at risk for cardiac or pulmonary complications. In contradistinction, if the difficult side is performed first and results in nephrectomy, one is faced with performing a partial nephrectomy on a solitary kidney, which often raises the anxiety not only of the patient but also of the surgeon.

Minimally Invasive Nephron-Sparing Therapies

Laparoscopic partial nephrectomy duplicates open partial nephrectomy, including the temporary renal hilar occlusion, resection of the entire tumor, suture-ligation of the intrarenal cavity, and renal parenchymal reconstruction.[95] It has mostly been reported in the setting of RCC but is occasionally utilized for AML (Figure 35.11).[96]

Energy-ablative therapy with radiofrequency ablation (RFA) and cryoablation have also been applied for treatment of AML. The first report of cryotherapy for the treatment of renal tumors reported by Delworth et al.[97] included a large (10 cm) AML that at 3 months had grown 10% on CT scan. Since this time, the experience with energy-ablative therapies has grown significantly and patient selection criteria have improved. Ablative therapies are most efficacious for treatment of smaller tumors, at least with presently available technology. In our current practice, larger tumors are generally not treated with cryoablation, because treatment efficacy decreases rapidly with increasing tumor size, especially since most AML requiring treatment are larger than 4 cm. We have, however, selectively treated some patients using RFA (Figure 35.12) with excellent short-term radiographic success. The major advantage of RFA over cryoablation in this setting is that multiple overlapping treatments can be performed in the same session with a single probe, thus allowing efficacious and economical treatment of lesions that may be larger than 4 cm. The feasibility of this approach is still in development, however, and additional data are awaited before RFA can be considered as an alternative to the standard approaches.

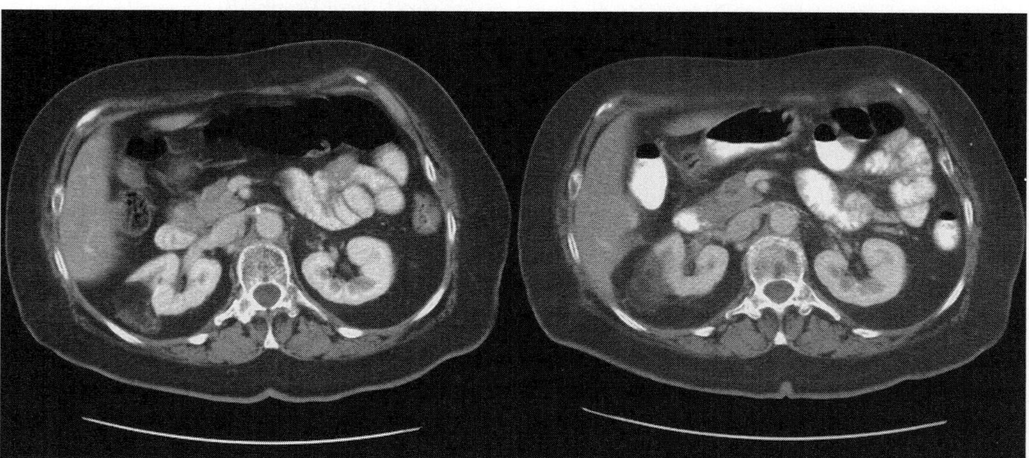

Figure 35.12. Pre– and post–radiofrequency ablation (RFA) CT scans. Pretreatment imaging shows a 5–cm AML arising from the lateral aspect of the right kidney. One month following percutaneous RFA, a repeat renal protocol CT scan shows typical postablative findings. (Copyright Surena F. Matin, 2005.)

REFERENCES

1. Sepp T, Yates JR, Green AJ. Loss of heterozygosity in tuberous sclerosis hamartomas. J Med Genet 1996;33:962–964.
2. Green AJ, Sepp T, Yates JR. Clonality of tuberous sclerosis hamartomas shown by non-random X-chromosome inactivation. Hum Genet 1996;97:240–243.
3. Kattar MM, Grignon DJ, Eble JN, et al. Chromosomal analysis of renal angiomyolipoma by comparative genomic hybridization: evidence for clonal origin. Hum Pathol 1999;30:295–299.
4. Nelson CP, Sanda MG. Contemporary diagnosis and management of renal angiomyolipoma. J Urol 2002;168:1315–1325.
5. Morgan GS, Straumfjord JV, Hall EJ. Angiomyolipoma of the kidney. J Urol 1951;65:525–525.
6. Hajdu SI, Foote FW Jr. Angiomyolipoma of the kidney: report of 27 cases and review of the literature. J Urol 1969;102:396–401.
7. Fujii Y, Ajima J, Oka K, Tosaka A, Takehara Y. Benign renal tumors detected among healthy adults by abdominal ultrasonography. Eur Urol 1995;27:124–127.
8. Steiner MS, Goldman SM, Fishman EK, Marshall FF. The natural history of renal angiomyolipoma. J Urol 1993;150:1782–1786.
9. Roach ES, Gomez MR, Northrup H. Tuberous sclerosis complex consensus conference: revised clinical diagnostic criteria. J Child Neurol 1998;13:624–628.
10. Fazeli-Matin S, Novick AC. Nephron-sparing surgery for renal angiomyolipoma. Urology 1998;52:577–583.
11. Tello R, Blickman JG, Buonomo C, Herrin J. Meta analysis of the relationship between tuberous sclerosis complex and renal cell carcinoma. Eur J Radiol 1998;27:131–138.
12. Knowles MA, Hornigold N, Pitt E. Tuberous sclerosis complex (TSC) gene involvement in sporadic tumours. Biochem Soc Trans 2003;31:597–602.
13. Krymskaya VP. Tumour suppressors hamartin and tuberin: intracellular signalling. Cell Signal 2003;15:729–739.
14. Yeung RS. Multiple roles of the tuberous sclerosis complex genes. Genes Chromosomes Cancer 2003;38:368–375.
15. Chen SS, Lin AT, Chen KK, Chang LS. Renal angiomyolipoma—experience of 20 years in Taiwan. Eur Urol 1997;32:175–178.
16. De Luca S, Terrone C, Rossetti SR. Management of renal angiomyolipoma: a report of 53 cases. BJU Int 1999;83:215–218.
17. Lee JD, Chang HC, Chu SH, Hsueh S, Soong YK. Massive retroperitoneal hemorrhage from spontaneous rupture of a renal angiomyolipoma during pregnancy. A case report. J Reprod Med 1994;39:477–480.
18. Nokes SR, Robbins KV, Sulieman JS. Radiological case of the month. Renal angiomyolipoma with perinephric hemorrhage. J Arkansas Med Soc 1997;94:311–312.
19. Sebastia MC, Perez-Molina MO, Alvarez-Castells A, Quiroga S, Pallisa E. CT evaluation of underlying cause in spontaneous subcapsular and perirenal hemorrhage. Eur Radiol 1997;7:686–690.
20. Zhang JQ, Fielding JR, Zou KH. Etiology of spontaneous perirenal hemorrhage: a meta-analysis. J Urol 1593;167:1593–1596.
21. GeneTests. Medical Genetics Information Resource (database online). Copyright UoW, Seattle. 1993–2005. Updated weekly. http://www.geneclinics.org.
22. Casper KA, Donnelly LF, Chen B, Bissler JJ. Tuberous sclerosis complex: renal imaging findings. Radiology 2002;225:451–456.
23. Webb DW, Kabala J, Osborne JP. A population study of renal disease in patients with tuberous sclerosis. Br J Urol 1994;74:151–154.
24. Paivansalo M, Lahde S, Hyvarinen S, Kallioinen M, Jalovaara P. Renal angiomyolipoma. Ultrasonographic, CT, angiographic, and histologic correlation. Acta Radiol 1991;32:239–243.
25. Bosniak MA, Megibow AJ, Hulnick DH, Horii S, Raghavendra BN. CT diagnosis of renal angiomyolipoma: the importance of detecting small amounts of fat. AJR 1988;151:497–501.
26. Helenon O, Merran S, Paraf F, et al. Unusual fat-containing tumors of the kidney: a diagnostic dilemma. Radiographics 1997;17:129–144.
27. Israel GM, Bosniak MA, Slywotzky CM, Rosen RJ. CT differentiation of large exophytic renal angiomyolipomas and perirenal liposarcomas.[see comment]. AJR 2002;179:769–773.
28. Wang LJ, Wong YC, Chen CJ, See LC. Computerized tomography characteristics that differentiate angiomyolipomas from liposarcomas in the perinephric space. J Urol 2002;167:490–493.

29. Martignoni G, Pea M, Bonetti F, Brunelli M, Eble JN. Oncocytoma-like angiomyolipoma. A clinicopathologic and immunohistochemical study of 2 cases. Arch Pathol Lab Med 2002;126:610–612.
30. Obuz F, Karabay N, Secil M, Igci E, Kovanlikaya A, Yorukoglu K. Various radiological appearances of angiomyolipomas in the same kidney. Eur Radiol 2000;10:897–899.
31. Kim JK, Park SY, Shon JH, Cho KS. Angiomyolipoma with minimal fat: differentiation from renal cell carcinoma at biphasic helical CT. Radiology 2004;230:677–684.
32. Pretorius ES, Wickstrom ML, Siegelman ES. MR imaging of renal neoplasms. MRI Clin North Am 2000;8:813–836.
33. Yamakado K, Tanaka N, Nakagawa T, Kobayashi S, Yanagawa M, Takeda K. Renal angiomyolipoma: relationships between tumor size, aneurysm formation, and rupture.[see comment]. Radiology 2002;225:78–82.
34. Bonetti F, Pea M, Martignoni G, et al. Clear cell ("sugar") tumor of the lung is a lesion strictly related to angiomyolipoma—the concept of a family of lesions characterized by the presence of the perivascular epithelioid cells (PEC). Pathology 1994;26:230–236.
35. Bonetti F, Pea M, Martignoni G, et al. The perivascular epithelioid cell and related lesions. Adv Anat Pathol 1997;4:343–358.
36. Birkhaeuser F, Ackermann C, Flueckiger T, et al. First description of a PEComa (perivascular epithelioid cell tumor) of the colon: report of a case and review of the literature. Dis Colon Rectum 2004;47:1734–1737.
37. Evert M, Wardelmann E, Nestler G, Schulz HU, Roessner A, Rocken C. Abdominopelvic perivascular epithelioid cell sarcoma (malignant PEComa) mimicking gastrointestinal stromal tumour of the rectum. Histopathology 2005;46:115–117.
38. Fadare O, Parkash V, Yilmaz Y, et al. Perivascular epithelioid cell tumor (PEComa) of the uterine cervix associated with intraabdominal "PEComatosis": a clinicopathological study with comparative genomic hybridization analysis. World J Surg Oncol 2004;2:35.
39. Folpe AL, McKenney JK, Li Z, Smith SJ, Weiss SW. Clear cell myomelanocytic tumor of the thigh: report of a unique case. Am J Surg Pathol 2002;26:809–812.
40. Kerr LA, Blute ML, Ryu JH, Swensen SJ, Malek RS. Renal angiomyolipoma in association with pulmonary lymphangioleiomyomatosis: forme fruste of tuberous sclerosis? Urology 1993;41:440–444.
41. Tawfik O, Austenfeld M, Persons D. Multicentric renal angiomyolipoma associated with pulmonary lymphangioleiomyomatosis: case report, with histologic, immunohistochemical, and DNA content analyses. Urology 1996;48:476–480.
42. Vang R, Kempson RL. Perivascular epithelioid cell tumor ("PEComa") of the uterus: a subset of HMB-45–positive epithelioid mesenchymal neoplasms with an uncertain relationship to pure smooth muscle tumors. Am J Surg Pathol 2002;26:1–13.
43. Yanai H, Matsuura H, Sonobe H, Shiozaki S, Kawabata K. Perivascular epithelioid cell tumor of the jejunum. Pathol Res Pract 2003;199:47–50.
44. Zamboni G, Pea M, Martignoni G, et al. Clear cell "sugar" tumor of the pancreas. A novel member of the family of lesions characterized by the presence of perivascular epithelioid cells. Am J Surg Pathol 1996;20:722–730.
45. Price EBJ, Mostofi FK. Symptomatic angiomyolipoma of the kidney. Cancer 1965;18:761–774.
46. Chen SS, Lin AT, Chen KK, Chang LS, Chang KM, Chiang H. Renal angiomyolipoma with extension into renal vein. Br J Urol 1996;77:927–928.
47. Hibi H, Takashi M, Yamada Y, Yamamoto M, Shimoji T. Angiomyolipoma of the kidney with extension into the inferior vena cava. Int J Urol 1995;2:332–335.
48. Camunez F, Lafuente J, Robledo R, et al. CT demonstration of extension of renal angiomyolipoma into the inferior vena cava in a patient with tuberous sclerosis. Urol Radiol 1987;9:152–154.
49. Perez-Atayde AR, Iwaya S, Lack EE. Angiomyolipomas and polycystic renal disease in tuberous sclerosis. Ultrastructural observations. Urology 1981;17:607–610.
50. Lynne CM, Carrion HM, Bakshandeh K, Nadji M, Russel E, Politano VA. Renal angiomyolipoma, polycystic kidney, and renal cell carcinoma in patient with tuberous sclerosis. Urology 1979;14:174–176.
51. Hanly MG, Smith LS, Hicks JM. Renal angiomyolipoma with bone formation clinically mimicking a renal calculus. Cancer Bull 1965;46:76–78.
52. Ro JY, Ayala AG, El-Naggar A, Grignon DJ, Hogan SF, Howard DR. Angiomyolipoma of kidney with lymph node involvement. DNA flow cytometric analysis. Arch Pathol Lab Med 1990;114:65–67.
53. Chen KT, Bauer V. Extrarenal angiomyolipoma. J Surg Oncol 1984;25:89–91.

54. Goodman ZD, Ishak KG. Angiomyolipomas of the liver. Am J Surg Pathol 1984;8:745–750.
55. Hulbert JC, Graf R. Involvement of the spleen by renal angiomyolipoma: metastasis or multicentricity? J Urol 1983;130:328–329.
56. Silpananta P, Michel RP, Oliver JA. Simultaneous occurrence of angiomyolipoma and renal cell carcinoma. Clinical and pathologic (including ultrastructural) features. Urology 1984;23:200–204.
57. Jimenez RE, Eble JN, Reuter VE, et al. Concurrent angiomyolipoma and renal cell neoplasia: a study of 36 cases. Mod Pathol 2001;14:157–163.
58. Eble JN, Amin MB, Young RH. Epithelioid angiomyolipoma of the kidney: a report of five cases with a prominent and diagnostically confusing epithelioid smooth muscle component. Am J Surg Pathol 1997;21:1123–1130.
59. L'Hostis H, Deminiere C, Ferriere JM, Coindre JM. Renal angiomyolipoma: a clinicopathologic, immunohistochemical, and follow-up study of 46 cases. Am J Surg Pathol 1999;23:1011–1020.
60. Ashfaq R, Weinberg AG, Albores-Saavedra J. Renal angiomyolipomas and HMB-45 reactivity. Cancer 1993;71:3091–3097.
61. Pea M, Bonetti F, Zamboni G, et al. Melanocyte-marker-HMB-45 is regularly expressed in angiomyolipoma of the kidney. Pathology 1991;23:185–188.
62. Fetsch PA, Fetsch JF, Marincola FM, Travis W, Batts KP, Abati A. Comparison of melanoma antigen recognized by T cells (MART-1) to HMB-45: additional evidence to support a common lineage for angiomyolipoma, lymphangiomyomatosis, and clear cell sugar tumor. Mod Pathol 1998;11:699–703.
63. Zavala-Pompa A, Folpe AL, Jimenez RE, et al. Immunohistochemical study of microphthalmia transcription factor and tyrosinase in angiomyolipoma of the kidney, renal cell carcinoma, and renal and retroperitoneal sarcomas: comparative evaluation with traditional diagnostic markers. Am J Surg Pathol 2001;25:65–70.
64. Eble JN. Angiomyolipoma of kidney. Semin Diagn Pathol 1998;15:21–40.
65. Makhlouf HR, Remotti HE, Ishak KG. Expression of KIT (CD117) in angiomyolipoma. Am J Surg Pathol 2002;26:493–497.
66. Plank TL, Logginidou H, Klein-Szanto A, Henske EP. The expression of hamartin, the product of the TSC1 gene, in normal human tissues and in TSC1– and TSC2–linked angiomyolipomas. Mod Pathol 1999;12:539–545.
67. Kimura N, Watanabe M, Date F, et al. HMB-45 and tuberin in hamartomas associated with tuberous sclerosis. Mod Pathol 1997;10:952–959.
68. Kaiserling E, Krober S, Xiao JC, Schaumburg-Lever G. Angiomyolipoma of the kidney. Immunoreactivity with HMB-45. Light- and electron-microscopic findings. Histopathology 1994;25:41–48.
69. Barnard M, Lajoie G. Angiomyolipoma: immunohistochemical and ultrastructural study of 14 cases. Ultrastruct Pathol 2001;25:21–29.
70. Lowe BA, Brewer J, Houghton DC, Jacobson E, Pitre T. Malignant transformation of angiomyolipoma. J Urol 1992;147:1356–1358.
71. Ferry JA, Malt RA, Young RH. Renal angiomyolipoma with sarcomatous transformation and pulmonary metastases. Am J Surg Pathol 1991;15:1083–1088.
72. Mai KT, Perkins DG, Collins JP. Epithelioid cell variant of renal angiomyolipoma. Histopathology 1996;28:277–280.
73. Martignoni G, Pea M, Rigaud G, et al. Renal angiomyolipoma with epithelioid sarcomatous transformation and metastases: demonstration of the same genetic defects in the primary and metastatic lesions. Am J Surg Pathol 2000;24:889–894.
74. Pea M, Bonetti F, Martignoni G, et al. Apparent renal cell carcinomas in tuberous sclerosis are heterogeneous: the identification of malignant epithelioid angiomyolipoma. Am J Surg Pathol 1998;22:180–187.
75. Christiano AP, Yang X, Gerber GS. Malignant transformation of renal angiomyolipoma. J Urol 1999;161:1900–1901.
76. Mene P, Festuccia F, Polci R, Faraggiana T, Gualdi G, Cinotti GA. Malignant epithelioid renal angiomyolipoma in a case of tuberous sclerosis with multiple organ involvement. Contrib Nephrol 2001:299–305.
77. VanderBrink BA, Munver R, Tash JA, Sosa RE. Renal angiomyolipoma with contrast-enhancing elements mimicking renal malignancy: radiographic and pathologic evaluation. Urology 2004;63:584–586.
78. Oesterling JE, Fishman EK, Goldman SM, Marshall FF. The management of renal angiomyolipoma. J Urol 1986;135:1121–1124.

79. Mitchell AL, Parisi MA, Sybert VP. Effects of pregnancy on the renal and pulmonary manifestations in women with tuberous sclerosis complex. Genet Med 2003;5:154–160.

80. Shah J, Jones J, Miller MA, Patel U, Anson KM. Selective embolization of bleeding renal angiomyolipoma in pregnancy. J R Soc Med 1999;92:414–415.

81. Kennelly MJ, Grossman HB, Cho KJ. Outcome analysis of 42 cases of renal angiomyolipoma.[see comment]. J Urol 1994;152:1988–1991.

82. Dickinson M, Ruckle H, Beaghler M, Hadley HR. Renal angiomyolipoma: optimal treatment based on size and symptoms. Clin Nephrol 1998;49:281–286.

83. Kessler OJ, Gillon G, Neuman M, Engelstein D, Winkler H, Baniel J. Management of renal angiomyolipoma: analysis of 15 cases. Eur Urol 1998;33:572–575.

84. Soulen MC, Faykus MH Jr, Shlansky-Goldberg RD, Wein AJ, Cope C. Elective embolization for prevention of hemorrhage from renal angiomyolipomas. J Vasc Intervent Radiol 1994;5:587–591.

85. Harabayashi T, Shinohara N, Katano H, Nonomura K, Shimizu T, Koyanagi T. Management of renal angiomyolipomas associated with tuberous sclerosis complex. J Urol 2004;171:102–105.

86. van Baal JG, Lips P, Luth W, et al. Percutaneous transcatheter embolization of symptomatic renal angiomyolipomas: a report of four cases. Neth J Surg 1990;42:72–77.

87. Hamlin JA, Smith DC, Taylor FC, McKinney JM, Ruckle HC, Hadley HR. Renal angiomyolipomas: long-term follow-up of embolization for acute hemorrhage. Can Assoc Radiol J 1997;48:191–198.

88. Han YM, Kim JK, Roh BS, et al. Renal angiomyolipoma: selective arterial embolization— effectiveness and changes in angiomyogenic components in long-term follow-up. Radiology 1997;204:65–70.

89. Mourikis D, Chatziioannou A, Antoniou A, Kehagias D, Gikas D, Vlahos L. Selective arterial embolization in the management of symptomatic renal angiomyolipomas. Eur J Radiol 1999;32:153–159.

90. Kehagias D, Mourikis D, Kousaris M, Chatziioannou A, Vlahos L. Management of renal angiomyolipoma by selective arterial embolization. Urol Int 1998;60:113–117.

91. Bissler JJ, Racadio J, Donnelly LF, Johnson ND. Reduction of postembolization syndrome after ablation of renal angiomyolipoma. Am J Kidney Dis 2002;39:966–971.

92. Uzzo RG, Novick AC. Nephron sparing surgery for renal tumors: indications, techniques and outcomes. J Urol 2001;166:6–18.

93. Blute ML, Malek RS, Segura JW. Angiomyolipoma: clinical metamorphosis and concepts for management. J Urol 1988;139:20–24.

94. Clark PE, Novick AC. Exophytic noninvasive growth pattern of renal angiomyolipomas: implications for nephron sparing surgery. J Urol 2001;165:513–514.

95. Gill IS, Desai MM, Kaouk JH, et al. Laparoscopic partial nephrectomy for renal tumor: duplicating open surgical techniques. J Urol 2002;167:469–476.

96. Kapoor A, Soon SJ, Birch DW, Zikman J. Laparoscopic wedge resection of a renal mass in a solitary kidney. Canadian J Urol 2001;8:1297–1299.

97. Delworth MG, Pisters LL, Fornage BD, von Eschenbach AC. Cryotherapy for renal cell carcinoma and angiomyolipoma. J Urol 1996;155:252–254.

Transitional Cell Carcinoma of the Renal Pelvis: *Management*

Jorge A. Garcia and Robert Dreicer

KEYWORDS

TRANSITIONAL CELL CARCINOMA (TCC)
UPPER URINARY TRACT TRANSITIONAL CELL CARCINOMA
(UUTTCC)
MVAC (METHOTREXATE, VINBLASTINE, DOXORUBICIN,
AND CISPLATIN)
GC (GEMCTINABINE/CISPLATIN)

ABSTRACT

Upper urinary tract transitional cell carcinoma (UUTTCC) accounts for approximately 5% of all urothelial tumors. Surgical therapy remains the standard of care for patients with localized disease based on tumor stage and grade. Surgical options for treatment range from minimally invasive procedures, such as ureteroscopy, and laparoscopic nephroureterectomy to open radical nephroureterectomy. Surveillance with cystoscopy and cytology following surgical management is essential as currently there are no variables that consistently predict which patients are destined to develop intravesical and/or contralateral upper tract recurrences. Extrapolating from traditional bladder TCC, both regional lymphadenectomy as well as neoadjuvant and adjuvant chemotherapy are likely to be beneficial for this cohort of patients. Management of patients with advanced UUTTCC should follow current guidelines utilized for patients with bladder TCC.

Transitional cell carcinoma (TCC) is a multifocal process that can occur at any site in the urinary tract including the renal pelvis. Whereas TCC of the bladder is one of the most common cancers in men in the United States, upper urinary tract tumors are rare, accounting for only 5% of tumors from the urinary tract.[1] As is the case with TCC of the bladder, renal pelvis TCC lesions are more common in men than in women, with a ratio of 2:1 to 3:1, and they tend to occur more frequently in the fifth to seventh decades of life.[2,3] Patients who initially present with a renal pelvis TCC are at increased risk of developing additional urothelial cancers typically within the first 2 years after initial presentation. While 20% to 50% of patients with renal pelvis TCC lesions

From: *Clinical Management of Renal Tumors*
Edited by: R.M. Bukowski and A.C. Novick © Humana Press Inc., Totowa, NJ

experience bladder involvement at some point in their lifetime, the incidence of renal pelvis lesions after a primary superficial bladder cancer observed in selected series is only 1% to 4%.[4,5]

PATHOLOGY

Transitional cell carcinoma accounts for more than 90% of the upper tract tumors (renal pelvis and ureter). Most of these tumors are papillary in nature, although they differ in their microscopic configuration. Histologically, papillary tumors can be differentiated into benign papillomas and papillary carcinomas. Other common histologic variants include flat carcinoma in situ, squamous cell carcinoma, and adenocarcinoma.

Squamous cell carcinoma (SCC) accounts for 5% to 10% of renal pelvic and ureteral carcinomas. In addition to being extremely aggressive neoplasms, they have been associated with a history of infected staghorn calculi that have been present for a long duration, and a history of chronic inflammation. The clinical outcome of patients with SCC of the renal pelvis is poor.[6,7] Primary adenocarcinomas of the renal pelvis are exceedingly rare. As with SCC, adenocarcinoma is usually associated with calculi, long-term obstruction, and inflammation. Like adenocarcinoma of the bladder, these tumors are mucin secreting, frequently resembling colorectal adenocarcinoma.[8,9] Therefore, it is crucial that metastatic adenocarcinoma be excluded prior to accepting this pathologic diagnosis. Small-cell carcinoma (SCCa) is also an extremely rare tumor of the upper urinary tract, although few cases of renal and bladder SCCa have been reported.[10,11]

CLINICAL DIAGNOSIS AND STAGING

Painless hematuria, either gross or microscopic, is the most common initial presentation of an upper tract tumor, and it is present in more than 75% of patients with renal pelvis TCC. However, flank pain could also be present in approximately one third of patients. Development of colicky pain in patients with hematuria could indicate the presence of ureteral obstruction by either clot or tumor. A flank mass secondary to tumor or hydronephrosis has been reported in approximately 10% to 20% of patients.[12] While other urinary symptoms such as polyuria and dysuria are present in almost 50% of patients with ureteral lesions, only 10% to 15% of patients with renal pelvis tumors present with these clinical symptoms. There is, however, a group of patients (less than 10%) in whom renal pelvis tumors may be completely asymptomatic. Other constitutional symptoms such as weight loss, fever, night sweats, and anorexia are less common, especially for those patients who present with early disease.

Excretory urography (intravenous pyelography, IVP) remains an important imaging for assessing the upper urinary tract. A discrete filling defect within the renal collecting system is the most common finding. This modality provides an excellent visualization of the entire upper urinary tract allowing the identification of subtle abnormalities in the ureters and renal pelvic area. The major limitations of this technique appear to be the difficulty in differentiating cystic from solid lesions, as well as the lack of sensitivity when evaluating small renal masses (less than 3 cm).

Although IVP continues to be widely used, a retrograde pyelography can also be helpful to delineate upper urinary tract filling defects and to differentiate tumors from stones when the initial IVP results have been inconclusive.[13]

The use of ultrasonography (US) to locate upper tract lesions is increasing. Patients with parenchymal renal disease and patients in whom routine intravenous contrast may be contraindicated may benefit from this technique. However, proper delineation of the ureters and collecting system is a major limitation of this procedure. Noncontrast computed tomography (CT) has also gained wide acceptance as the imaging study of choice for patients who present with abdominal pain (renal colic) and hematuria. The sensitivity of noncontrast CT for identification of stones appears to be superior to that of IVP.[14] Thus, CT scan continues to be an attractive alternative to IVP in the evaluation of hematuria. Contrast CT is often used to detect the extension of a tumor outside of the collecting system, the presence of adjacent organ involvement, or the presence of distant metastases. Unfortunately, the overall accuracy of CT to predict pathologic stage (tumor, node, metastasis [TNM] stage) of upper urothelial lesions ranges from 35% to 80%.[15,16]

Cytologic examination of exfoliated cells within the urine is currently the best noninvasive test for detection of urothelial malignancies. Cytology is a relatively insensitive test (30% to 70%), and is dependent on a variety of factors including grade and stage.[17] Another disadvantage of cytologic interpretation is the dependence on the expertise of a well-trained cytopathologist. Despite these limitations, sensitivity appears to improve when early-morning voided specimens or barbotaged specimens are obtained during cystoscopy, or when urine is collected from selective ureteral catheterizations.[18]

Given the variable sensitivity of cytologic specimens, current efforts are aimed at the development of novel and noninvasive methods that can detect malignant cells in voided urine specimens. Existing urinary markers that are under study include BTA stat, BTA Trak, NMP22, Immunocyt, HA-Haase, Quanticyt, and telomerase.

The sensitivity and specificity of retrograde brushing of the upper urinary tract is reported to have a sensitivity ranging between 60% and 70%, while specificity is approximately 85% to 95%.[19] Direct biopsy of upper tract lesions allows complete histologic examination of tissue samples and improves diagnosis and accuracy over that of brushing techniques.[20] One of the major limitations of this technique is the inability to provide staging information.

Staging System

Stage and tumor grade remain the most significant prognostic factors for survival in patients with carcinoma of the renal pelvis. Classification of these malignancies is based entirely on pathologic findings. At present, the American Joint Committee on Cancer (AJCC) 2002 TNM classification of carcinomas of the renal pelvis and ureter is the most commonly used system for staging patients with upper urinary tract carcinomas[21] (Table 36.1). Estimated survival data based on the pathology of the primary tumor (T) has been reported[3,4,22] (Table 36.2). Munoz and Ellison[1] conducted a retrospective analysis using data from the National Cancer Institute Surveillance, Epidemiology, and End Results (SEER) public database. From 1973 to 1996, 9072 cases of upper urothelial carcinoma were identified. The calculated overall disease-specific survival after patients were stratified by stage was as follows: 95% for carcinoma in situ, 88.9% for localized disease, 62.6% for regional disease, and 16.5% for patients with distant lesions. Furthermore, disease-specific annual mortality was greater in blacks than in whites (7.4% vs. 4.9%) and in women than in men (6.1% vs. 4.4%). Aside from tumor stage and grade, other adverse features associated with tumor aggressiveness and poor clinical outcome are the presence of lymphovascular invasion, multifocality, perineural invasion, and invasion of the renal hilum and renal parenchyma.[23,24]

Table 36.1.
2002 American Joint Committee on Cancer TNM classification of tumors of
the renal pelvis and ureter

Primary tumor (T)

TX	Primary tumor cannot be assessed
T0	No evidence of primary tumor
Ta	Papillary noninvasive carcinoma
Tis	Carcinoma in situ
T1	Tumor invades the subepithelial connective tissue
T2	Tumor invades the muscularis
T3	*(For renal pelvis only)* Tumor invades beyond muscularis in to peripelvic fat or the renal parenchyma *(For ureter only)* Tumor invades beyond muscularis into periureteric fat
T4	Tumor invades adjacent organs or through the kidney into the perinephric fat

Regional lymph nodes (N)*

NX	Regional lymph nodes cannot be assessed
N0	No regional lymph node metastasis
N1	Metastasis in a single lymph node, <2 cm in greatest dimension
N2	Metastasis in a single lymph node, >2 cm but <5 cm in greatest dimension; or multiple lymph nodes, none >5 cm in greatest dimension
N3	Metastasis in a lymph node more than >5 cm in greatest dimension

Distant metastasis (M)

MX	Distant metastasis cannot be assessed
M0	No distant metastasis
M1	Distant metastases

Histopathologic grading (G)

GX	Grade cannot be assessed
G1	Well differentiated
G2	Moderately differentiated
G3–4	Poorly differentiated or undifferentiated

Stage		*Grouping*	
Oa	Ta	N0	M0
Ois	Tis	N0	M0
I	T1	N0	M0
II	T2	N0	M0
III	T3	N0	M0
IV	T4	N0	M0
	Any T	N1, N2, N3	M0
	Any T	Any N	M1

*Laterality does not affect the N classification.

Table 36.2.
Selected reports of 5-year survival by stage in patients with upper tract transitional
cell carcinoma

Author	n	% 5-year survival				
		pTa	pT1	pT2	pT3	pT4
Corrado et al.[55]	127	80	83	72	51	16
Rey et al.[56]	83	100	85	83	60	21
Jinza et al.[57]	70	100	75	82	41	41
Hall et al.[4]	252	100	92	73	41	0
Morioka et al.[24]	93	93	100	89	62	0
Guinan et al.[3]	611	75	87	87	54	19

TREATMENT OPTIONS

Surgery

RADICAL AND PARTIAL NEPHROURETERECTOMY

The classic surgical management of renal pelvic and ureteral lesions is nephroureterectomy with excision of a 1- to 2-cm cuff of the bladder mucosa around the ureteral
orifice. The rationale for this approach is the frequency of multifocality and ipsilateral
recurrences frequently observed with urothelial carcinomas. Clinical outcome for
patients treated with this approach varies. However, bladder recurrences have been
reported to be as high as 20%.[25] Less extensive resections have been proposed; however,
they appear to result in poorer outcome (recurrence rate of 20% to 35%). Many authors
believe that the ultimate disease outcome is more related to the inherent biologic characteristic of the disease at presentation as opposed to specifics of surgical intervention.[26,27] Superior survival rates of patients with low-stage and low-grade disease have
prompted investigators to consider more conservative surgical approaches. Thus, partial
nephrectomy and segmental ureteral resection have been advocated for patients with
solitary kidney, compromised renal function, or the presence of bilateral disease. Murphy
and associates[28,29] evaluated 49 patients with an upper tract lesion who received treatment with either a partial nephrectomy (n = 15) or a standard open nephroureterectomy
(n = 34). For patients with grade 1 superficial disease, a 5-year overall survival (OS)
rate of 85% was reported. In a similar follow-up study of patients with higher grade
and stage, standard nephroureterectomy was superior in terms of overall survival;
however, the disease-recurrence rate for patients who underwent a nephron-sparing
approach was 28%. These data support the use of radical nephroureterectomy for
patients with high grade/stage disease. This approach not only offers a survival advantage but also appears to lead to lower disease-recurrence rates.

The use of tumor location as an independent prognostic factor continues to be a
controversial topic. It is clear, however, that patients with distal ureteral lesions are ideal
candidates for more conservative approaches, such as distal ureterectomy. Long-term
follow-up series have reported no difference in survival and a disease-recurrence rate
of around 10%.[30] In contrast, patients with high-grade and muscle-invasive tumors of
the proximal ureter who have a normal contralateral upper tract have a much higher
risk for ipsilateral recurrences. Thus, conservative approaches in this group of patients
are not recommended.

LAPAROSCOPIC APPROACHES

Over the past decade, minimally invasive techniques have gained wide acceptance across the U.S. Laparoscopic nephroureterectomy was first described in the early 1990s by the Washington University group.[31] Laparoscopy appears to be as effective as the open approach in removing the entire kidney and the ureter, and long-term outcomes appear to be no different between the techniques.[32] The operative technique for laparoscopic nephroureterectomy is best considered in terms of two separate approaches—nephrectomy and distal ureterectomy.[33] In addition, two different approaches can be used: retroperitoneal or transperitoneal. The benefits of a laparoscopic technique over an open approach include smaller incisions, easier postoperative course, less blood loss, and shorter hospital stay. The major disadvantage is the need for significant surgical/technical expertise.[34]

At present, there are a limited number of series reporting the long-term cancer control outcome with laparoscopic nephroureterectomy. Gill et al.[35] reported on 42 patients evaluated over a period of 2.3 years, and compared their outcome with 35 consecutive patients treated with open radical nephroureterectomy. Laparoscopy was statistically superior in regard to surgical time, blood loss, time to resumption of oral intake, narcotic analgesia requirements, hospital stay, and convalescence time. Postoperative complications including atelectasis, ileus, and pneumothorax occurred in three patients (7%) in the laparoscopic group and 10 (29%) in the open group. Major intraoperative complications occurred in two patients of the laparoscopy group (renal vein injury). For tumors with similar grade and stage, the margin positive rate was comparable with both techniques (7% vs. 15%). After adjusting for the short-term follow-up period in the laparoscopy group, the cancer-specific survival was comparable (97% vs. 87%, $p = .6$). Other series with longer follow-up periods report 5-year metastases-free survival rates of around 85%.[36]

Adjuvant Therapy

As is typical of all advanced urothelial neoplasms, systemic recurrence of renal pelvis tumors following nephroureterectomy remains a major clinical problem. Local recurrence of renal pelvis tumors have been reported to range from 2% to 27%.[37,38]

ADJUVANT RADIOTHERAPY

Two recent studies, showed no benefit in adding adjuvant radiotherapy in patients with upper urinary tract (UUT) TCC. Maulard-Durdux et al.[39] evaluated the role of adjuvant radiotherapy in 26 patients with UUT TCC who underwent radical nephroureterectomy followed by radiation therapy (45 Gy) to the tumor bed and regional nodes. After a median follow-up of 45 months, 15% of patients have recurred and 54% had developed distant metastases. Similarly, Hall and associates[40] retrospectively reviewed the data of 74 patients with stage III disease who were treated surgically and then received adjuvant radiation to the tumor bed and regional nodes. The 5-year overall and specific disease-free survival for stage III patients was 28% and 40%, respectively. Although recurrences were observed in approximately 15% of patients, no difference in survival in favor of adjuvant radiation was found.

ADJUVANT CHEMOTHERAPY

Extrapolation from the bladder cancer experience guides much of our current approach to the management of advanced renal pelvis TCC following surgical resection. Two phase III studies in bladder cancer exploring the role of cisplatin-based combination chemotherapy administered neoadjuvantly in patients undergoing definitive local therapy (radical cystectomy or bladder radiotherapy) have demonstrated the potential for systemic chemotherapy to improve survival in this high-risk disease subset, presumably by impacting on micrometastatic disease.[41,42] In stark contrast to the neoadjuvant setting, the published adjuvant studies of chemotherapy in bladder cancer are as a group severely compromised by small patient numbers, variable treatment regimens, and poor treatment compliance.[43–45] Although the limited data in the adjuvant setting would seem to support the broad use of neoadjuvant chemotherapy, there is in fact increasing use of adjuvant therapy in the U.S. presumably by extrapolation of the positive results in the neoadjuvant setting for supporting a "perioperative" benefit.

Despite the similar potential for systemic failure in patients with high-risk renal pelvis TCC, there are limited data regarding the utility of adjuvant chemotherapy in this setting. A small study conducted by the Hellenic Cooperative Oncology Group prospectively evaluated a cohort of 36 patients exclusively with locally advanced upper tract urothelial carcinoma who underwent surgery for high-risk upper tract urothelial carcinoma and subsequently received adjuvant paclitaxel and carboplatin. After a median follow-up of 40 months, the authors reported a 5-year disease-free survival of 42% (95% confidence interval [CI], 15.8–64.6%). The rates of local failure reported were in the range of 30%, with 17% of patients developing distant metastatic disease.[46]

Patients at relatively high risk for systemic failure following nephroureterectomy, including those with advanced stage, large tumors, or evidence of local extension with or without node positive disease, should be counseled regarding their potential for systemic failure, the current management of high-risk bladder cancer as it relates to the use of adjuvant chemotherapy, and a risk-benefit discussion to help patients make decisions regarding their willingness to consider adjuvant chemotherapy.

Management of Advanced Disease

Advanced upper tract TCC is a moderately chemotherapy-sensitive neoplasm; however, despite relatively high objective response rates, long-term survival of patients with metastatic disease remains less than 5%.[47] Although historically renal pelvis TCC lesions were felt to be inherently more aggressive than similar lesions in the bladder, there is no evidence of any differences in the response of patients to systemic therapy, and the majority of reported clinical trials of advanced urothelial cancer include patients with metastatic TCC including those of the renal pelvis, ureter, and urethra.[47] The one obvious global difference in the approach to the management of the patients with a renal pelvis TCC is that the majority has only one functioning kidney.

In the 1980s cisplatin-based chemotherapy regimens including MVAC (methotrexate, vinblastine, doxorubicin, and cisplatin) and CMV (cisplatin, methotrexate, and vinblastine) were evaluated in a series of phase II studies demonstrating significant antitumor activity in a disease previously thought to be significantly chemotherapy resistant.[48] Subsequently, an Intergroup trial randomized patients with advanced disease to either cisplatin as a single agent or the MVAC regimen, and found an improvement in response and survival favoring the MVAC regimen, with the latter regimen subsequently becoming the de facto standard of care.[49] Despite early enthusiasm, the MVAC regimen has a number of significant limitations, one of which was highlighted by an update of the Intergroup trial demonstrating that with a minimum follow-up of 6 years, only 3.7% of patients treated on the MVAC arm were alive and disease-free.[50] Another widely recognized problem with the MVAC regimen is the significant toxicity associated with its administration. The most common side effects from MVAC include significant neutropenia, considerable mucositis, nausea and vomiting, and renal, cardiac, and neurologic toxicities. Toxic death associated with MVAC has been reported to be as high as 3% to 4% but is less than 1% in experienced hands.[51]

Other nonplatinum agents such as gemcitabine, paclitaxel, docetaxel, and ifosfamide have documented activity in advanced TCC. Following phase II trials with the gemcitabine and cisplatin (GC) regimen, von der Maase and colleagues[52] conducted a multinational phase III study of 405 patients with metastatic urothelial carcinoma to compare GC with MVAC in patients with advanced or metastatic TCC of the urothelium. The authors reported that the overall survival was similar on both arms (hazard ratio [HR], 1.04; 95% CI, 0.82–1.32; $p = .75$), as were time to progressive disease (HR, 1.05; 95% CI, 0.85–1.30), time to treatment failure (HR, 0.89; 95% CI, 0.72–1.10), and response rate (GC, 49%; MVAC, 46%). In addition, more patients in the GC arm completed six cycles of therapy, with fewer dose adjustments. The toxic death rate was 1% on the GC arm and 3% on the MVAC arm. Grade 3/4 anemia as well as thrombocytopenia was more frequent in patients receiving GC compared with MVAC (27% vs. 18%, and 57% vs. 21%, respectively). Quality of life was maintained during treatment on both arms. While the GC vs. MVAC trial was not powered as an equivalency study, it was nonetheless a large conducted study and has understandably been interpreted as demonstrating with reasonable certainty that gemcitabine and cisplatin is a clinically useful alternative to MVAC and has become widely utilized as a front-line regimen in advanced urothelial cancer.

Although cisplatin-based regimens for advanced TCC are considered a standard of care, patients with urothelial cancer may have age- and disease-related abnormalities in renal function, making cisplatin-based regimens problematic. Patients with renal pelvis TCC with advanced disease typically have a single functioning kidney, increasing the difficulty of administering cisplatin-based therapy. Various investigators have explored the use of agents such as carboplatin, which is typically less nephrotoxic than cisplatin as well as other cytotoxic agents with primary hepatic clearance, such as paclitaxel. The Eastern Cooperative Oncology Group (ECOG) conducted a phase II trial of paclitaxel and carboplatin in patients with advanced urothelial cancer and renal dysfunction. Thirty-seven eligible patients with a median serum creatinine of 1.7 mg/dL (range 1.5–3.0) were evaluable for response. The primary urothelial tumor site was not reported. Patients received a median of four cycles of therapy, and the objective response rate was 24%.[53] Although several phase II experiences have demonstrated a relatively low objective response rate and survival of patients treated with carboplatin and paclitaxel, ECOG conducted a phase III trial comparing carboplatin and paclitaxel to MVAC. Although this study failed to reach its target accrual, and therefore the results of the study must be interpreted with significant caution, it did demonstrate a similar response rate and survival in both arms, providing some evidence that for patients with compromised renal function, the carboplatin plus paclitaxel regimen is a reasonable alternative.[54]

CONCLUSION

The management of renal pelvis TCCs increasingly requires a multidisciplinary management approach. While the mainstay of management remains surgical resection with increasing use of the laparoscopic approach, the relatively high risk of systemic failure associated with the biology of high grade TCC requires consideration of adjuvant systemic therapy. Unfortunately, the relatively small numbers of patients and the lack of prospective evidence of benefit from adjuvant therapy is a clinical reality that will not likely be remedied. Therapy for metastatic renal pelvis tumors mirrors that of any metastatic urothelial cancer. Chemotherapy remains the mainstay of therapy, but remains of limited utility, and newer approaches, based on an improved understanding of the molecular mechanisms of the disease, will be required to improve patient outcomes.

REFERENCES

1. Munoz J, Ellison L. Upper tract urothelial neoplasms: incidence and survival during the last 2 decades. J Urol 2000;164:1523–1525.
2. Melamed M, Reuter V. Pathology and staging of urothelial tumors of the kidney and ureter. Urol Clin North Am 1993;20:333–347.
3. Guinan P, Vogelzang N, Randazzo R, et al. Renal pelvic cancer: a review of 611 patients treated in Illinois 1975–1985. Cancer Incidence and End Results Committee. Urology 1992;40:393–399.
4. Hall M, Womack S, Sagalowsky A, et al. Prognostic factors, recurrence, and survival in transitional cell carcinoma of the upper urinary tract: a 30-year experience in 252 patients. Urology 1998;52:594–601.
5. Hurle R, Losa A, Manzetti A, et al. Upper urinary tract tumors developing after treatment of superficial bladder cancer: 7-year follow-up of 591 consecutive patients. 1999;53:1144–1148.
6. Gilligan T, Dreicer R. The atypical urothelial cancer patient: management of bladder cancers of non-transitional cell histology and cancers of the ureters and renal pelvis. Semin Oncol 2007;34(2):145–153.
7. Blacher E, Johnson D, Abdul-Karim F, et al. Squamous cell carcinoma of renal pelvis. Urology 1985;25:124–126.
8. Takehara K, Nomata K, Eguchi J, et al. Mucinous adenocarcinoma of the renal pelvis associated with transitional cell carcinoma in the renal pelvis and the bladder. Int J Urol 2004;11:1016–1018.
9. Hammond E, Henson D. Cancer Committee College of American Pathologists; Task Force on the Examination of Specimens Removed from Patients with Bladder Cancer. Practice protocol for the examination of specimens removed from patients with carcinoma of the urinary bladder, ureter, renal pelvis, and urethra. Arch Pathol Lab Med 1996;120:1103–1110.
10. Kitamura M, Miyanaga T, Hamada M, et al. Small cell carcinoma of the kidney: case report. Int J Urol 1997;4:422–424.
11. Majhail N, Elson P, Bukowski R. Therapy and outcome of small cell carcinoma of the kidney: report of two cases and a systematic review of the literature. Cancer 2003;97:1436–1441.
12. Geersen J. Tumors of the renal pelvis and ureter. Symptomatology, diagnosis, treatment and prognosis. Scand J Urol Nephrol 1979;13:287–290.
13. Takebayashi S, Hosaka M, Takase K, et al. Computerized tomography nephroscopic images of renal pelvic carcinoma. J Urol 1999;162:315–318.
14. Miller O, Rineer S, Reichard S, et al. Prospective comparison of unenhanced spiral computed tomography and intravenous urogram in the evaluation of acute flank pain. Urology 1998;52:982–987.
15. McCoy J, Honda H, Reznicek M, et al. Computerized tomography for detection and staging of localized and pathologically defined upper tract urothelial tumors. J Urol 1991;146:1500–1503.
16. Planz B, George R, Adam G, et al. Computed tomography for detection and staging of transitional cell carcinoma of the upper urinary tract. Eur Urol 1995;27:146–150.
17. Yun E, Meng M, Carroll P. Evaluation of the patient with hematuria. Med Clin North Am 2004;88:329–343.
18. Assimos D, Hall M, Martin J. Ureteroscopic management of patients with upper tract transitional cell carcinoma. Urol Clin North Am 2000;27:751–760.
19. Dodd L, Johnston W, Robertson C, et al. Endoscopic brush cytology of the upper urinary tract. Evaluation of its efficacy and potential limitations in diagnosis. Acta Cytol 1997;41:377–384.
20. Keeley F, Bibbo M, Bagley D. Ureteroscopic treatment and surveillance of upper urinary tract transitional cell carcinoma. J Urol 1997;157:1560–1565.
21. AJCC Cancer Staging Handbook, 6th ed. New York: Springer-Verlag, 2002.

22. Maatman TJ, Gupta MK, Montie JE. Effectiveness of castration versus intravenous estrogen therapy in producing rapid endocrine control of metastatic cancer of the prostate. J Urol 1985;133:620–621.

23. Terrel R, Cheville J, See W, et al. Histopathological features and p53 nuclear protein staining as predictors of survival and tumor recurrence in patients with transitional cell carcinoma of the renal pelvis. J Urol 1995;154:1342–1347.

24. Morioka M, Jo Y, Furukawa Y, et al. Prognostic factors for survival and bladder recurrence in transitional cell carcinoma of the upper urinary tract. Int J Urol 2001;8:30–37.

25. Laguna M, de la Rosette J. The endoscopic approach to distal ureter in nephroureterectomy for upper urinary tract tumor. J Urol 2001;166:2017–2022.

26. Koga F, Nagamatsu H, Ishimaru H, et al. Risk factors for the development of bladder transitional cell carcinoma following surgery for transitional cell carcinoma of theupper urinary tract. Urol Int 2001;67:135–141.

27. Kirkali Z, Tuzel E. Transitional cell carcinoma of the ureter and renal pelvis. Crit Rev Oncol Hematol 2003;47:155–169.

28. Murphy D, Zincke H, Furlow W. Primary grade I transitional cell carcinoma of the renal pelvis and ureter. J Urol 1980;123:629–631.

29. Murphy D, Zincke H, Furlow W. Management of high grade transitional cell cancer of the upper urinary tract. J Urol 1981;125:25–29.

30. Tawfiek E, Bagley D. Upper tract transitional cell carcinoma. Urology 1997;50:321–329.

31. Clayman R, Kavoussi L, Figenshau R, et al. Laparoscopic nephroureterectomy: initial clinical case report. J Laparoendosc Surg 1991;1:343–349.

32. Shalhav A, Portis A, McDougall E, et al. Laparoscopic nephroureterectomy. A new standard for the surgical management of upper tract transitional cell cancer. Urol Clin North Am 2000;27:761–763.

33. Savage S, Gill I. Laparoscopic radical nephroureterectomy. J Endourol 2000;14:859–864.

34. McNeill S, Chrisofos M, Tolley D. The long term outcome after laparoscopic nephroureterectomy: a comparison with open nephroureterectomy. BJU Int 2000;86:619–623.

35. Gill I, Sung G, Hobart M, et al. Laparoscopic radical nephroureterectomy for upper tract transitional cell carcinoma: the Cleveland Clinic experience. J Urol 2000;164:1513–1522.

36. Shalhav A, Dunn M, Portis A, et al. Laparoscopic nephroureterectomy for upper tract transitional cell cancer: the Washington University experience. J Urol 2000;163:1100–1104.

37. Cozad S, Smalley S, Austenfeld M, et al. Transitional cell carcinoma of the renal pelvis or ureter: patterns of failure. Urology 1995;46:796–800.

38. Ozsahin M, Zouhair A, Villa S, et al. Prognostic factors in urothelial renal pelvis and ureter tumours: a multicentre Rare Cancer Network study. Eur J Cancer 1999;35:738–743.

39. Maulard-Durdux C, Dufour B, Hennequin C, et al. Postoperative radiation therapy in 26 patients with invasive transitional cell carcinoma of the upper urinary tract: no impact on survival? J Urol 1996;155:115–117.

40. Hall M, Womack J, Roehrborn C, et al. Advanced transitional cell carcinoma of the upper urinary tract: patterns of failure, survival and impact of postoperative adjuvant radiotherapy. J Urol 1998;160:703–706.

41. International Collaboration of Trialists on Behalf of the Medical Research Council Advanced Bladder Cancer Working Party, EORTC Genito-Urinary Group, Australian Bladder Cancer Study Group, et al. Neoadjuvant cisplatin, methotrextate, and vinblastine chemotherapy for muscle-invasive bladder cancer: a randomised controlled trial. Lancet 1999;354:533–540.

42. Grossman H, Natale R, Tangen C, et al. Neoadjuvant chemotherapy plus cystectomy compared with cystectomy alone for locally advanced bladder cancer. N Engl J Med 2003;349:859–866.

43. Skinner D, Daniels J, Russell C, et al. The role of adjuvant chemotherapy following cystectomy for invasive bladder cancer: a prospective comparative trial. J Urol 1991;145:459–464.

44. Stockle M, Meyenburg W, Wellek S, et al. Advanced bladder cancer (stages pT3b, pT4a, pN1 and pN2): improved survival after radical cystectomy and 3 adjuvant cycles of chemotherapy. Results of a controlled prospective study. J Urol 1992;148(2 pt 1):302–306.

45. Freiha F, Reese J, Torti F. A randomized trial of radical cystectomy versus radical cystectomy plus cisplatin, vinblastine and methotrexate chemotherapy for muscle-invasive bladder cancer. J Urol 1996;155:495–500.

46. Bamias A, Deliveliotis C, Fountzilas G, et al. Adjuvant chemotherapy with paclitaxel and carboplatin in patients with advanced carcinoma of the upper urinary tract: a study by the Hellenic Cooperative Oncology Group. J Clin Oncol 2004;22:2150–2154.

47. Bajorin D, Dodd P, Mazumdar M, et al. Long-term survival in metastatic transitional cell carcinoma and prognostic factors predicting outcome of therapy. J Clin Oncol 1999;17:3173–3181.
48. Sternberg C, Yagoda A, Scher H, et al. Preliminary results of M-VAC (methotrexate, vinblastine, doxorubicin, and cisplatin) for transitional cell carcinoma of the urothelium. J Urol 1985;133:403–404.
49. Loehrer P, Einhorn L, Elson P, et al. A randomized comparison of cisplatin alone or in combination with methotrexate, vinblastine, and doxorubicin in patients with metastatic urothelial carcinoma: a cooperative group study. J Clin Oncol 1992;10:1066–1073.
50. Saxman S, Propert K, Einhorn L, et al. Long-term follow-up of a phase III intergroup study of cisplatin alone or in combination with methotrexate, vinblastine, and doxorubicin in patients with metastatic urothelial carcinoma: a Cooperative Group Study. J Clin Oncol 1997;15:2564–2569.
51. Sternberg C, Yagoda A, Scher H, et al. M-VAC for advanced transitional cell carcinoma of the urothelium: Efficacy, and patterns of response and relapse. Cancer 1989;64:2448.
52. von der Maase H, Hansen S, Roberts J, et al. Gemcitabine and cisplatin versus methotrexate, vinblastine, doxorubicin, and cisplatin in advanced or metastatic bladder cancer: results of a large, randomized, multinational, multicenter, phase III study. J Clin Oncol 2000;18:3068–3077.
53. Vaughn D, Manola J, Dreicer R, et al. Phase II study of paclitaxel plus carboplatin in patients with advanced carcinoma of the urothelium and renal dysfunction (E2896): a trial of the Eastern Cooperative Oncology Group. Cancer 2002;95:1022–1027.
54. Dreicer R, Manola J, Roth B, et al. Phase III trial of methotrexate, vinblastine, doxorubicin, and cisplatin versus carboplatin and paclitaxel in patients with advanced carcinoma of the urothelium. Cancer 2004;100:1639–1645.
55. Corrado F, Ferri C, Mannini D, et al. Transitional cell carcinoma of the upper urinary tract: evaluation of prognostic factors by histopathology and flow cytometric analysis. J Urol 1991;145:1159–1163.
56. Rey A, Lara P, Redondo E, et al. Overexpression of p53 in transitional cell carcinoma of the renal pelvis and ureter. Relation to tumor proliferation and survival. 1997;79:2178–2185.
57. Jinza S, Iki M, Noguchi S, et al. Prognostic significance of Ki-67 labeling index in urothelial tumors of the renal pelvis and ureter. J Urol 1996;155:1877–1881.

37
Wilms' Tumor in Children and Adults

Jonathan H. Ross

KEYWORDS

WILMS' TUMOR
CANCER
KIDNEY
PEDIATRIC

ABSTRACT

The treatment of Wilms' tumor represents one of the great achievements in the history of oncology. Named for Max Wilms, who described the tumor in 1899, the prognosis for this most common renal tumor of childhood has steadily improved through innovation and the cooperative efforts of multicenter trials. With nephrectomy alone, 15% of patients could expect to survive in the early 20th century.[1] With the advent of radiation therapy, cure rates approached 40%.[2] In the latter half of the 20th century, multiagent chemotherapy with vincristine and actinomycin as the mainstays has resulted in cure rates approaching 90% for most Wilms' tumor patients.[3] While multicenter trials have helped define the standard management for Wilms' tumor, controversies still exist and cure still eludes many patients with high-stage unfavorable histology tumors.

PATHOLOGY

Wilms' tumors appear grossly as well-circumscribed masses of variable color and consistency. Small cysts may be present. Calcification, usually in areas of necrosis, is present in 5% of cases.[4] Classic or favorable histology tumors are triphasic with a "blastemal" component consisting of sheets of small blue cells, an "epithelial" component mimicking tubules, and a "stromal" component (Figure 37.1). Mature mesodermal elements such as muscle, cartilage, or ganglion cells may be present. Unfavorable

From: *Clinical Management of Renal Tumors*
Edited by: R.M. Bukowski and A.C. Novick © Humana Press Inc., Totowa, NJ

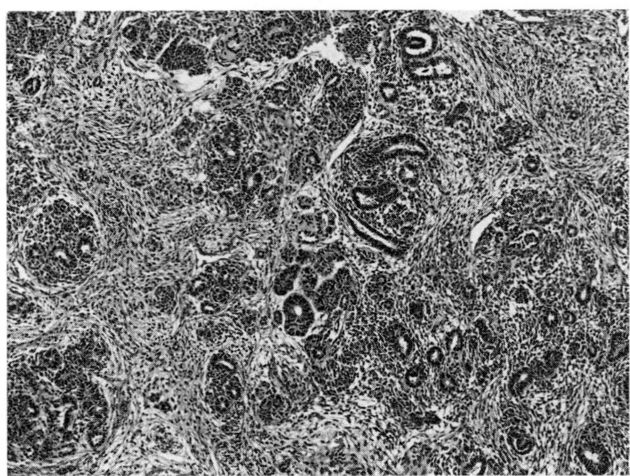

Figure 37.1. Classic triphasic histology Wilms' tumor with blastemal component (nests of small blue cells), epithelial component (blastemal cells organized in tubular clusters), and stromal component.

histology tumors occur in 5% of cases and are characterized by focal or diffuse anaplasia with cells that contain hyperchromatic nuclei and multipolar mitoses.

Nephroblastomatosis refers to the persistence of metanephric blastema beyond 36 weeks of gestational age. It is present in 1% of perinatal autopsies. The most common form is nodular renal blastema, which consists of nests of metanephric blastema, typically in the periphery under the renal capsule. Areas of nephroblastomatosis are present in up to 50% of kidneys with Wilms' tumor and up to 100% of kidneys in patients with bilateral Wilms' tumor or an inherited susceptibility to Wilms' tumor.[5–8] This association has led to the hypothesis that nephroblastomatosis may represent a precursor lesion of Wilms' tumor. The presence of nephroblastomatosis in a kidney containing a Wilms' tumor increases the risk of bilateral disease, and may identify patients at higher risk of relapse.[9,10] In National Wilms' Tumor Study (NWTS) patients, metachronous contralateral tumors occurred in 10% of infants with nephrogenic rests compared to 1.2% in the group as a whole. More peripheral or "perilobar" rests show a strong association with synchronous bilateral Wilms' tumor. Rests that occur more centrally—"intralobar" rests—are more associated with metachronous tumors.[11]

EPIDEMIOLOGY AND GENETICS

Wilms' tumor is the most common genitourinary tumor of childhood, affecting approximately 1 in 10,000 children.[12] It is bilateral in 5% of cases and multifocal in 12% of unilateral cases.[13–16] The mean age of presentation is approximately 3 years and it is extremely rare in neonates and adults. It is occasionally associated with genitourinary anomalies such as hypospadias and cryptorchidism. Hemihypertrophy occurs in 3% of cases. Aniridia is present in 1% of Wilms' tumor cases. While familial aniridia bestows no increased risk of Wilms' tumor, Wilms' tumor arises in one third of patients with sporadic aniridia.[12]

Several syndromes are associated with an increased risk of Wilms' tumor development. The best known is the Beckwith-Wiedemann syndrome, characterized by exomphalos, macroglossia, high birth weight, and gigantism.[17] In addition to Wilms' tumor, these patients are also at an increased risk for the development of adrenocortical carcinoma and hepatoblastoma. The Drash syndrome is characterized by Wilms' tumor, pseudohermaphroditism, and glomerular disease.[18] The Perlman syndrome is a familial syndrome of visceromegaly, macrosomia, polyhydramnios, and abnormal facies.[19] Patients with this syndrome have a high incidence of nephroblastomatosis and, to a lesser degree, Wilms' tumor.

Wilms' tumor has been one of the models of oncogenesis. Knudson[20,21] suggested the "two-hit" hypothesis for retinoblastoma, and later extended this to Wilms' tumor. It proposes that tumors occur as a result of two sequential events (i.e., mutations), each of low probability. For such tumors, a subpopulation of patients is predisposed because of a prezygotic "first hit" (i.e., mutation). The cells in the kidneys of these patients only require the second hit to become tumors. The genetic correlate of these "hits" would be loss of a tumor-suppressor gene in one allele by an initial mutation and then a mutation or larger deletion leading to loss of heterozygosity (LOH). If the theory is correct, then there should be two subpopulations of patients, with those patients predisposed to the tumor presenting at a younger age with more bilateral and multifocal tumors, and the second population of patients presenting at a later age with solitary tumors. Indeed, there is a bimodal age distribution for Wilms' tumor, with bilateral tumors occurring at a mean age of 28 months, and unilateral tumors occurring at a mean age of 40 months. However, the epidemiology is not as straightforward as predicted by Knudson's model. Given the 5% to 10% incidence of bilateral tumors, Knudson's model would predict a 30% incidence of familial transmission rather than the 1% to 2% incidence observed.[22]

Genetic studies of Wilms' tumor have demonstrated several genes that may be involved in tumorigenesis. The most widely studied gene associated with Wilms' tumor is the Wilms' tumor-1 *(WT1)* gene located at chromosome 11p13. *WT1* is a tumor-suppressor gene and a transcriptional activator important in fetal kidney development.[23] It is closely linked to the aniridia gene, explaining the high incidence of Wilms' tumors in patients with sporadic aniridia. Mutations and deletions in this region are associated with approximately 15% of sporadic and familial Wilms' tumors, though it is aberrantly expressed in many others.[22,23] A recent study by the United Kingdom Children's Cancer Study Group (UKCCSG) detected constitutional *WT1* gene mutations in only 2% of 282 patients with sporadic Wilms' tumor.[24] The *WT1* patients presented at a younger age than the general group. Royer-Pokora et al.[25] also found that patients with a germline *WT1* alteration were more likely to have bilateral disease and to present at a younger age (12 months vs. 36 months in patients without a *WT1* alteration).

The *WT2* gene is located at chromosome 11p15 and LOH of this gene is associated with a subset of Wilms' tumors including those occurring in patients with the Beckwith-Wiedemann syndrome. Two additional genes found in Wilms' tumor families have been identified on chromosomes 17 and 19. These do not appear to be simple tumor-suppressor genes.[26] Genetic alterations in chromosomes 16q and 1p may be of clinical significance for tumor progression. Approximately 20% of Wilms' tumors show LOH of 16q and 10% show an LOH at chromosome 1q. Evidence from the NWTS suggests that these genetic changes may correlate with a poorer prognosis for those tumors.[27]

PRESENTATION AND EVALUATION

Children with Wilms' tumor usually appear healthy and present with an abdominal mass noted by a parent or health care provider. Occasionally, other symptoms may be present including abdominal pain, vomiting, fever, hypertension, and hematuria. Rare cases may present with complications such as retroperitoneal bleeding or signs of inferior vena caval obstruction. Patients at high risk for Wilms' tumor, such as those with Beckwith-Wiedemann syndrome, are placed on surveillance protocols. Most protocols call for abdominal ultrasound every 3 months during childhood. Because Wilms' tumors grow rapidly, and may advance between surveillance studies, parents should also be instructed on performing a simple abdominal exam on a regular basis. A cost-effectiveness model utilizing data from the NWTS and the Beckwith-Wiedemann syndrome database of the National Cancer Institute concluded that screening from birth until 4 or 7 years of age with triannual ultrasounds was cost-effective ($9,600 and $14,700 per life-year saved, respectively, for the 4- and 7-year-old cutoffs).[28] The study assumed that screening would result in a one-stage down-stage shift and that the sensitivity and specificity of screening ultrasounds is 100% and 95%, respectively. A series comparing 15 Wilms' tumor patients with Beckwith-Wiedemann syndrome who were on a screening protocol with 59 patients who were not confirmed the ability of screening to detect earlier stage tumors.[29] None of the screened patients had stage III or IV disease compared with 42% of the unscreened patients.

Most children present with an abdominal mass, and the first study obtained is usually an abdominal ultrasound. Ultrasound is helpful in distinguishing renal tumors from other masses such as a hydronephrotic kidney. Ultrasound can also detect caval thrombi in children, which are present in 4% of cases. Once a mass is detected by ultrasound, a computed tomography (CT) scan is obtained. This characterizes the primary tumor, and searches for small contralateral tumors and for intraabdominal metastatic disease (Figure 37.2). Magnetic resonance imaging (MRI) is more expensive than CT and often requires sedation or general anesthesia in children. However, it can be helpful in special situations. It is very accurate in assessing the level of caval tumor thrombus and may be utilized in rare cases where ultrasound and CT are unable to clearly delineate the thrombus. The MRI criteria are also evolving for distinguishing Wilms' tumor from nephroblastomatosis—an important distinction since nephroblastomatosis can usually be managed nonoperatively.

Chest x-ray or CT may be used to detect pulmonary metastases. Since most protocols were developed with chest x-ray, the management of patients with small pulmonary nodules on CT that are not visualized on chest x-ray is not defined. A retrospective study of patients treated as stage I in the UKCCSG suggests that chest CT-positive patients with normal chest x-rays are at an increased risk of pulmonary relapse compared to those with normal CT and chest x-ray (43% vs. 10%, respectively).[30] A study from the NWTS reviewed the outcome for 90 patients with favorable histology tumors who had pulmonary nodules on CT scan but normal chest radiographs.[31] Fifty-three such patients were treated as having stage IV disease including lung irradiation. Thirty-seven patients were treated based on the extent of locoregional disease without lung irradiation. Overall survival for the two groups was not significantly different (91% vs. 85%, respectively). Patients treated with lung irradiation had fewer pulmonary relapses,

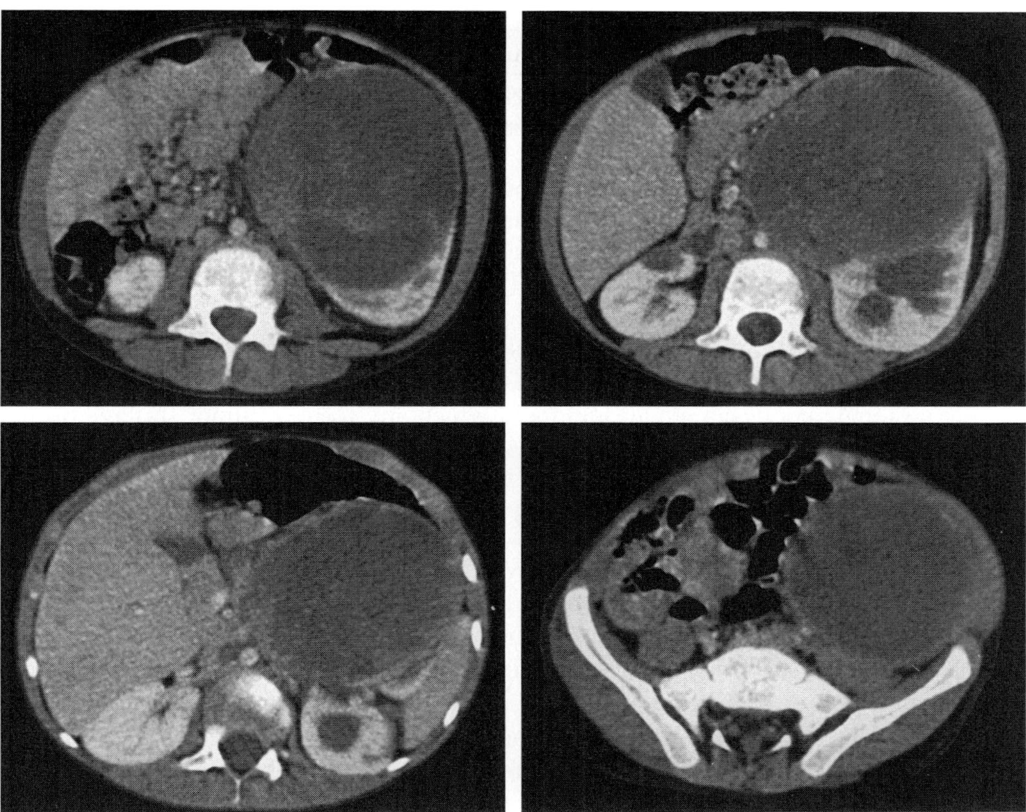

Figure 37.2. A computed tomography (CT) scan of a 4-year-old boy following 4 weeks of actinomycin and vincristine chemotherapy. The patient presented with an abdominal mass detected by his cardiologist during routine follow-up for a congenital heart defect. CT revealed a large left renal mass with two smaller left renal masses and a small right renal mass. During 8 weeks of neoadjuvant chemotherapy, the left lesion originally responded, then increased in size, and the right renal mass decreased from 4 cm to 2 cm in size. The patient underwent an uneventful left radical nephrectomy and right tumor excision. Both tumors were confined to the kidney with negative surgical margins. Lymph nodes sampled from the superior mesenteric, paracaval, and iliac regions were negative. Both tumors displayed diffuse anaplasia. The patient received adjuvant therapy with etoposide, cyclophosphamide, and carboplatinum.

but more deaths from treatment toxicity. Fortunately, discordance between chest x-ray and chest CT is quite low.[32]

As part of the routine preoperative blood testing, Wilms' tumor patients should be screened for coagulopathies. Approximately one fourth of Wilms' tumor patients have abnormal clotting.[33] Approximately 3% display features of acquired von Willebrand syndrome.

Staging of Wilms' tumor requires surgical exploration with radical nephrectomy and abdominal lymph node sampling from the hilum, retroperitoneum, and ipsilateral iliac region. The staging system that has been used in the most recent NWTS is shown in Table 37.1. Tumors that are completely resected are considered stage I or II, depending on whether there is extension beyond the kidney or local tumor spillage. Stage III

Table 37.1.
National Wilms' Tumor Study (NWTS) staging system

Stage I	Tumor limited to kidney—completely excised
Stage II	Extension through renal capsule or into sinus—completely excised; or previous biopsy; or local tumor spillage
Stage III	Residual local disease including positive margin, intraabdominal lymph node involvement, peritoneal tumor implants or tumor spill not confined to the flank
Stage IV	Hematogenous metastases or extraabdominal lymph node involvement

tumors are those with residual local disease including positive regional lymph nodes or gross tumor spillage. Stage IV tumors are those with metastatic disease. Future staging systems may designate all tumors in which any form of tumor spillage occurs as stage III.

SURGICAL TREATMENT

In the United States, treatment for most Wilms' tumors begins with a radical nephrectomy. A transperitoneal approach is employed. Historically a contralateral exploration has been recommended prior to removing the primary tumor in order to exclude a small contralateral tumor missed on preoperative imaging. This recommendation has persisted based on a review of NWTS-4 patients from 1986 to 1992, most of whom had a preoperative CT scan.[34] Among 2323 Wilms' tumor patients, 122 were found to have bilateral tumors, and nine of these (7%) were missed on preoperative imaging. However, a series of studies found no contralateral tumors were missed by preoperative imaging.[35–38] These studies reviewed a total of 249 Wilms' tumor patients, with 24 bilateral cases among them. Even the NWTS data can be used to argue against routine contralateral exploration. Based on their data, the negative predictive value of preoperative imaging is 99.65%—only one in every 285 patients would possibly benefit from the contralateral exploration. Since most missed tumors are small, and might resolve with standard adjuvant therapy, and since CT scan today is more sensitive than in 1992, it seems reasonable to abandon contralateral exploration in patients with good preoperative imaging.

Assuming there is no contralateral tumor, a radical nephrectomy is undertaken. The ipsilateral colon is reflected and the dissection is carried out outside of Gerota's fascia. Early ligation of the vessels is preferred, but this is often not possible for large tumors. The ureter is divided well below the kidney, and the kidney is completely mobilized. In most cases the tumor is large and the adrenal gland is removed with the tumor. However, adrenal metastases are extremely rare. For lower pole tumors, if the adrenal gland appears grossly normal, and a dissection plane can easily be developed between it and the kidney, then the adrenal gland may be spared. Any residual disease or positive margin should be marked with titanium clips to guide future radiotherapy.

During the dissection, the renal vein is carefully palpated to rule out tumor thrombus. If present, an attempt should be made to remove the thrombus en bloc with the tumor. If a large tumor thrombus is present, consideration should be given to preoperative chemotherapy (see below). Even if preoperative chemotherapy is administered, some patients will have persistent caval thrombus requiring surgical excision. Infrahepatic thrombus can be excised through an abdominal incision.[39] For intrahepatic thrombus, the right liver may be mobilized to gain control of the inferior vena cava (IVC) at the diaphragm to facilitate tumor thrombus extraction. However, this dissection may lead to tumor embolus, and consideration should be given to gaining control of the IVC in the chest.[40] Once the IVC is controlled, the kidney is completely mobilized. The IVC is then opened at the entrance of the renal vein and the tumor thrombus extracted en bloc with the kidney. If this is not technically possible, the vein may be ligated and divided to facilitate the nephrectomy. Once the kidney is removed, a cavotomy is performed and the tumor thrombus is extracted. Suprahepatic tumor thrombus may be excised with the assistance of cardiopulmonary bypass and, if necessary, deep hypothermic circulatory arrest. This technique has been utilized for renal cell carcinoma for over two decades and has been successfully applied to patients with Wilms' tumor as well.[40–45]

Invasion into adjacent structures is rare. However, removal of normal adjacent structures should be avoided. Rather, in cases of extensive local invasion, the tumor should be deemed unresectable. The abdomen should be closed after the tumor is biopsied and a lymph node staging is performed. The patient is then given neoadjuvant chemotherapy with a planned reexploration at a later date. When determining resectability it should be kept in mind that tumor invasion into local structures is often overdiagnosed. In NWTS-3 only 17% of resected adjacent organs were positive for tumor on histologic examination.[46] Although local invasion sometimes prevents resection, the presence of lymph node involvement or other metastatic disease should not preclude proceeding with a nephrectomy.

While a formal lymph node dissection is not recommended, lymph node sampling is an important part of tumor staging. Any suspicious nodes should be sampled as well as random nodes from the hilar, superior mesenteric, and iliac regions. Experience with NWTS patients has shown that surgeons' impressions of node status at exploration correlates poorly with histologic findings.[47] Furthermore, absence of lymph node biopsy was associated with poorer survival in NWTS-4 stage I patients compared to stage I patients who had undergone lymph node sampling, presumably due to understaging and subsequent undertreatment of the former group.[48] Therefore, lymph node biopsy is indicated even in the absence of suspicious nodes.

The role of nephron-sparing surgery remains controversial. Except in cases of bilateral disease or tumors occurring in a solitary kidney, radical nephrectomy has been the standard approach. The appropriateness of nephron-sparing approaches depends on the relative risks of renal insufficiency following radical nephrectomy versus the risk of local recurrence following a partial nephrectomy. The NWTS found the risk of renal failure in patients undergoing nephrectomy for unilateral Wilms' tumor was only 0.2% to 0.4%.[49] Renal failure was defined as a serum creatinine greater than 2.5 mg/dL or the need for renal replacement therapy. Follow-up was 6 years. This relatively short follow-up would not detect the development of renal insufficiency that can occur over decades due to hyperfiltration. Several other studies offer circumstantial evidence to suggest that the ultimate development of renal insufficiency may be greater than that suggested by the NWTS. Studies have demonstrated that a more than 50% loss of renal tissue leads to an increase in single nephron glomerular filtration rate.[50] Hyperfiltration can lead to proteinuria and loss of renal function over time. Several studies have detected an increased incidence of hypertension, proteinuria, and renal insufficiency in adults with unilateral renal agenesis or a history of unilateral nephrectomy as a child.[51–54] Selection bias may play a role in the findings of these retrospective studies.

Di Tullio et al.[55] reported on 34 unselected patients with unilateral Wilms' tumor and a mean follow-up of 8.6 years. Although all patients had normal renal function, proteinuria was present in four patients (12%) and microalbuminuria in 11 patients (32%). Bailey et al.[56] reviewed renal function in a similar group of 40 patients undergoing unilateral nephrectomy for Wilms' tumor with a median follow-up of 8.8 years. None had significant renal insufficiency. However, subclinical measures of tubular toxicity were abnormal in four patients (10%), and two patients (5%) had evidence of increased urinary albumin excretion. Donckerwolcke and Coppes[57] also reported functional changes suggestive of hyperfiltration in two of 11 children following unilateral nephrectomy for renal tumors.

Concerns regarding long-term issues in patients with a solitary kidney have led several authors to perform nephron-sparing surgery in selected patients with good results.[58–61] Horwitz et al.[62] reviewed 98 patients in the NWTS with bilateral Wilms' tumors undergoing nephron-sparing surgery. The local recurrence rate was 8.2%—very similar to that seen in adults with renal cell carcinoma. Interestingly, the recurrence rate was no different in patients who underwent complete excision compared with those with residual disease in the affected kidney. Presumably the adjuvant therapy was able to eradicate the residual disease in most cases. A review of 37 patients undergoing nephron-sparing surgery for unilateral Wilms' tumor in the German arm of the International Society of Pediatric Oncology (SIOP) studies revealed a local recurrence rate of 10.8%.[63] Overall and relapse-free survivals were similar to those in patients undergoing total nephrectomy. In addition to patients with a solitary kidney or bilateral tumors, consideration should be given to partial nephrectomy in patients at increased risk for metachronous contralateral disease. This would include patients with the Beckwith-Wiedemann and other associated syndromes. While total nephrectomy is the standard approach to most patients with Wilms' tumor, the role of partial nephrectomy may increase in the future. The description of renal tumors in young adults with a history of Wilms' tumor as children raises another reason to consider nephron-sparing surgery.[64] Unfortunately, even if one accepts the concept of nephron-sparing surgery for Wilms' tumor patients, only 5% of patients have a technically amenable tumor at presentation.[65] This can be increased to 10% to 30% with preoperative chemotherapy.[60,66]

Radical nephrectomy in children is a technically demanding operation and significant surgical complications occur. The surgical complication rate reported in NWTS-4 was 12.7%.[67] Complications included intestinal obstruction (5%), extensive hemorrhage (2%), wound infection (2%), and vascular injury (1.5%). Surgical complications were more common in the presence of intravascular tumor extension, or a tumor diameter of greater than 10 cm, or if the operation was performed through a flank or paramedian incision. Complications were also more common if the nephrectomy was performed by a general surgeon rather than a pediatric surgeon or pediatric urologist.

PREOPERATIVE CHEMOTHERAPY

The management of Wilms' tumor patients in Europe has been primarily under the auspices of SIOP. While initial nephrectomy is the mainstay of therapy in the United States, the approach in Europe has been to employ preoperative chemotherapy. The initial studies by SIOP in the 1970s compared patients who underwent primary nephrectomy with those who received preoperative radiation with or without preoperative chemotherapy. Because of decreases in surgical complications and down-staging of tumors with this approach, the later SIOP studies administered preoperative chemotherapy (without radiation) to all Wilms' tumor patients. The researchers found that this preoperative chemotherapy reduced the tumor rupture rates from 27% in patients undergoing primary nephrectomy in their earlier studies to 5% in the later studies employing preoperative chemotherapy.[68,69] The percentage of stage I tumors increased from approximately 25% in the primary nephrectomy patients of earlier studies to over 50% in those undergoing preoperative chemotherapy. This has resulted in fewer patients requiring radiation therapy. Currently SIOP administers 4 weeks of vincristine and actinomycin preoperatively to patients with localized disease and 6 weeks of these two agents and doxorubicin to patients with metastatic disease.[70] Opponents of routine preoperative chemotherapy raise the concern that a small percentage of patients will receive chemotherapy only to be found at surgery to have a benign tumor. The risk of this occurring in the SIOP studies was 1.5%.[69] Another concern is that the down-staging may actually lead to an underestimate of the tumor's intrinsic malignant potential and subsequent undertreatment. Finally, there is concern that pretreatment will distort the histology, making tumor grading difficult. This does indeed occur, but with its growing experience, SIOP has developed a system for stratifying patients based on characteristics of the postchemotherapy histology. In the end, the survival rates for the NWTS and the SIOP studies are comparable, and so either approach is reasonable.[71]

While preoperative chemotherapy is not a primary approach to Wilms' tumor in the United States, it is employed routinely in select situations. These include inoperable tumors, certain patients with caval tumor thrombus, and patients with bilateral disease. Tumor extension into the vena cava occurs in 4% of Wilms' tumor patients.[72] The complication rate of initial resection is 43% (primarily hemorrhage), and is independent of the level of caval thrombus. A chemotherapy response precluding the need for a cavotomy occurs in more than half the patients.[73] While preoperative chemotherapy could be considered for any degree of caval involvement, it is particularly appropriate for patients with suprahepatic extension. In patients with suprahepatic extension, 70% of tumor thrombi regress enough to preclude the need for a median sternotomy.[74]

Synchronous bilateral Wilms' tumor occurs in 5% of patients. Until the last decades of the 20th century, these patients were treated with initial surgical resection of the more involved side followed by chemotherapy.[75] However, subsequent studies have shown that patients treated with initial chemotherapy and less aggressive surgery do just as well with regard to tumor control, and better with regard to renal preservation.[76–79] Therefore, complete resection at initial presentation is rarely appropriate. In most cases at least one of the tumors is very large, and multiple tumors are usually present in at least one of the kidneys (Figure 37.2). Of 145 bilateral tumors in NWTS-2 and -3, only 15% involved bilateral unicentric tumors.[77] Following chemotherapy, the larger tumor ultimately may be easier to remove than the initially smaller tumor. Therefore, the temptation to perform a nephrectomy on the more involved side at initial presentation should be resisted.

Another argument in favor of neoadjuvant chemotherapy for bilateral tumors is that patients can be cured even if complete resection is never accomplished. Kay and Tank[76] reported that five of six patients with bilateral tumors who never had complete resection were free of disease at 2 to 12 years of follow-up. The NWTS reported a 76% three-year survival for 145 patients with bilateral Wilms' tumor even though only 38% of patients had complete excision of all tumor.[77] The current management of bilateral Wilms' tumor is to give chemotherapy first in all cases, except those rare patients who have bilateral small tumors. Initial chemotherapy is with two or three agents (vincristine and actinomycin with or without doxorubicin) administered for 4 to 6 weeks after which follow-up studies are obtained. If there is no response to the initial treatment, then biopsies to rule out anaplastic tumor should be undertaken. Fortunately, most patients have a significant response, and another 4 to 6 weeks of treatment are administered. SIOP has shown that 4 weeks is the optimal duration of chemotherapy for unilateral disease.[80]

Tumor response likely plateaus by 2 months of treatment, and so more prolonged pre-operative chemotherapy is not usually warranted for bilateral disease. Exploration is then undertaken. If residual tumor can be excised leaving at least two thirds of one kidney, then resection is undertaken by bilateral nephron-sparing surgery or by unilateral nephrectomy and contralateral partial nephrectomy. If salvage of at least two thirds of one kidney does not seem possible, then all residual tumors should be biopsied and consideration given to more intense chemotherapy and radiation. If any tumors are found to be anaplastic, then surgical resection should be considered even if it will compromise ultimate renal function. Using an approach of preoperative chemotherapy and nephron-sparing surgery, the survival rate for patients with bilateral Wilms' tumor is similar stage for stage as for those with unilateral disease.[77]

Whether a prechemotherapy biopsy should be undertaken for patients with bilateral tumors is unclear. While this would allow more aggressive treatment of the rare bilateral anaplastic tumors, it raises the possibility of a biopsy-related complication including tumor contamination at biopsy sites. The UKCCSG found that in 12% of unilateral tumors consistent clinically and radiographically with Wilms' tumor, a biopsy revealed a tumor other than Wilms' tumor.[81] The importance of an accurate preoperative diagnosis must be balanced against the risk of biopsy. Among the 182 patients undergoing percutaneous needle biopsy in the UKCCSG study, 20% experienced a drop in hemoglobin, one patient required emergency nephrectomy for massive bleeding, one had tumor rupture, and a third developed a needle tract recurrence.

ADJUVANT THERAPY

Since 1969 the NWTS has organized prospective multicenter trials to ascertain the optimal treatment for patients with Wilms' tumor. These studies have looked at the appropriate roles of various chemotherapeutic agents and radiation and have attempted to tailor therapy to stage and histology of the tumor. More recent NWTSs have focused on decreasing the intensity of therapy in low-risk groups in order to reduce morbidity, while looking at alternatives for high-risk patients to improve survival. The outcomes for favorable histology tumors in NWTS-4 and unfavorable histology tumors in NWTS-3 and -4 are shown in Table 37.2. The results of the first four NWTSs led to the single arm stratified protocol of NWTS-5. A summary of the treatment protocol for the recently completed NWTS-5 is shown in Table 37.3.[3] The treatment arms are assigned based on the surgical stage determined at nephrectomy and the extent of anaplastic tumor present in the specimen. Patients with stage I and II favorable histology (FH) tumors receive

Table 37.2.
Four-year outcomes from recent NWTSs[3,105,106]*

Histology	Stage	Relapse-free survival	Overall survival
Favorable	I	89%	96%
	II	86%	96%
	III	91%	96%
	IV	83%	90%
Anaplasia	I	91%	91%
Diffuse anaplasia	II	72%	70%
	III	59%	56%
	IV	17%	17%

*Data for favorable histology tumors and stage I anaplastic tumors are from NWTS-4. Data for stage II–IV diffuse anaplasia tumors are from NWST-3 and -4 and include only patients who received cyclophosphamide in addition to actinomycin, vincristine, and doxorubicin.

18 weeks of dactinomycin and vincristine, as do patients with stage I anaplastic tumors. Patients with higher risk tumors (stage III and IV FH tumors and patients with stage II to IV disease and focal anaplasia) receive 24 weeks of dactinomycin, vincristine, and doxorubicin as well as radiation therapy. Finally, the highest risk patients (stage II to IV tumors with diffuse anaplasia) receive 24 weeks of vincristine, doxorubicin, cyclophosphamide, etoposide, and radiation therapy.[3] The radiation dose for NWTS-5 is 10.8 Gy to the abdomen for all patients receiving radiotherapy[82]; 12 Gy of irradiation to the lungs and mediastinum is administered to those patients with evidence of pulmonary metastases on chest x-ray. While stage and histology are proven prognostic factors, attempts to further stratify patients based on tumor cytogenetic abnormalities and oncogene expression are ongoing.

Consideration may be given to observation without adjuvant therapy in select patients. The NWTS-4 employed nephrectomy only (without adjuvant therapy) for patients less than 2 years of age with stage I favorable histology tumors less than 550 g in weight.[83] Of 75 enrolled patients, relapse occurred in 13.5% of patients (including metachronous contralateral tumors in 4%). These relapses were curable with additional treatment.

Table 37.3.
Treatment protocol for Wilms' tumors in NWTS-5[3,104,104]

Tumor histology	Tumor stage	Treatment
Favorable histology	I and II	Dactinomycin, vincristine × 18 weeks
	III and IV	Dactinomycin, vincristine, doxorubicin × 24 weeks Radiotherapy
Focal anaplasia	I	Dactinomycin, vincristine × 18 weeks
	II–IV	Dactinomycin, vincristine, doxorubicin × 24 weeks Radiotherapy
Diffuse anaplasia	I	Vincristine × 18 weeks
	II–IV	Dactinomycin, vincristine, doxorubicin, cyclophosphamide, etoposide × 24 weeks Radiotherapy

MANAGEMENT OF RECURRENT TUMOR

While the current management of Wilms' tumor is very successful, approximately 15% of patients develop tumor recurrence during follow-up.[84] The majority of patients have recurrences in the lungs. The rest of the patients have more than one site of recurrence, including the lungs, bone, brain, and intraabdominal sites.[84,85] All patients with recurrent tumor are treated with intensified chemotherapy and radiation therapy. Not surprisingly, radiation is particularly effective for recurrence at sites not previously irradiated.[85] Surgical excision of pulmonary recurrences offers no advantage over chemotherapy and lung irradiation alone.[84] Resection of pulmonary lesions is only indicated if histologic confirmation is required. Intraabdominal recurrences are resected for diagnostic confirmation and debulking. Patients with recurrent disease are more likely to do well if they have not previously been treated with doxorubicin, if the relapse occurs more than 12 months after diagnosis, or if they have an intraabdominal relapse when no abdominal radiation has been previously administered.[86] Patients who do not fulfill these criteria have a dire prognosis. High-dose chemotherapy with autologous hematopoietic stem-cell rescue has been employed successfully in high-risk patients, particularly those with recurrent tumor.[87,88] Treatment with a combination of oxazaphosphorines (cyclophosphamide or ifosfamide), platinum drugs (carboplatin or cisplatin), and etoposide salvage therapy has also been employed.[85,89] Survival rates with these approaches for high-risk tumors range from 47% to 73%. Recurrence of Wilms' tumor many years after initial treatment is rare, but has been reported.[90]

LONG-TERM FOLLOW-UP

Adults with a history of Wilms' tumor are at increased risk for late effects related to treatment or genetic predisposition to malignancies. Among the chemotherapeutic agents used, doxorubicin is of particular concern. The NWTS reported a cumulative frequency of congestive heart failure in patients receiving doxorubicin of 4% to 17% at 20 years following the diagnosis of Wilms' tumor.[91] Radiation for Wilms' tumor is associated with modest decreases in adult stature, which appear to be dose-dependent and not clinically significant for those treated with modern dosing regimens.[92] Flank radiation for Wilms' tumor can also lead to obstetrical complications. A study of NWTS patients revealed that such women are at increased risk of fetal malposition and premature labor.[93] Their babies are at risk for low birth weight, premature birth, and the occurrence of congenital malformations.

Whether from genetic predisposition or as a complication of treatment, patients with a history of Wilms' tumor are at risk for secondary malignant neoplasms. Metachronous contralateral Wilms' tumor is rare, occurring in 1.2% of cases. However, this risk is 10% in infants with nephrogenic rests in the index kidney.[10] In the NWTSs, the risk for second malignant neoplasms in general was 1.6% at 15 years, approximately eightfold higher than expected.[94] Secondary malignant neoplasms were particularly likely in patients who received abdominal irradiation or who had been treated for relapse. Doxorubicin potentiated the effect of radiation. Patients who received doxorubicin and radiation had a 36-fold increased incidence of secondary malignant neoplasms compared to the general population. Leukemia/lymphoma accounted for 30% of the secondary malignant neoplasms. A wide variety of other tumors occurred including osteosarcoma (9%) and hepatocellular carcinoma (7%). Of the nonleukemia/lymphoma tumors, 73%

occurred in an irradiated field. Patients with a history of Wilms' tumor may also be at increased risk for secondary renal neoplasms in the contralateral kidney as young adults decades after therapy.[64]

WILMS' TUMOR IN ADULTS

Wilms' tumor is very rare in adults, accounting for 3% of all Wilms' tumors.[95] The actual incidence in adults is difficult to determine, but has been estimated at approximately 1% of adult renal tumors.[96] Adults with Wilms' tumor are indistinguishable from those with renal cell carcinoma. They typically present with flank pain, and many have weight loss and decreased performance status reflecting the typically high-stage disease.[95] An exploratory laparotomy with appropriate staging, particularly lymph node sampling, may not be undertaken leading to uncertainty regarding the extent of disease. Treatment may also be delayed due to uncertainty regarding the histologic diagnosis in adults with this tumor. However, once the diagnosis is made, appropriate staging should be undertaken and a radical nephrectomy performed. Anaplastic histology and bilateral tumors appear to occur at frequencies similar to those in children.

Adjuvant therapy for adults has been based primarily on the experience in children. Early reports of Wilms' tumors in adults suggested that the prognosis for these patients is markedly worse than for children. This poorer prognosis was in part attributed to presentation at a higher stage for adults, but also to a poorer stage-for-stage survival. In a review by the NWTS in 1982, results for 31 adult patients were compared to children treated during the same time period (1968–1979) under NWTS guidelines.[97] Mean age of adults was 29 years, with the oldest being 63 years old; 52% of patients had stage III or IV disease (compared to 27% in children). Three-year survival rates in adults were 48% for stage I and II disease and 11% for stage IV disease compared to 87% and 53%, respectively, for children. Adults who received surgical excision, multiagent chemotherapy, and irradiation did reasonably well. The NWTS group concluded that adults with Wilms' tumor should be treated aggressively regardless of stage. In a 1990 series 11 adult patients treated at M.D. Anderson were also noted to present with higher stage disease (45% had stage III or IV disease) and only 20% of patients survived, though none had anaplastic tumors.[98]

In contrast to these studies and earlier reviews of anecdotal reports suggesting a poor prognosis for adult tumors, more recent studies suggest that the outcome for adults with modern therapy may be comparable to that of children. In 1990 and 2004 the NWTS reexamined the question of adult Wilms' tumor.[99,100] It reviewed its experience with 45 adult Wilms' tumor patients treated from 1979 to 2001 including 23 patients treated under NWTS-4 and NWTS-5. Adults still had a higher incidence of metastatic disease than did children, with 47% of adults having stage III or IV disease. However, survival was significantly better than in the earlier series, with an overall survival rate of 82% (compared to 24% in the earlier study). The overall survival rate by stage was 100%, 92%, 70%, and 73% for stage I, II, III, and IV disease, respectively. Twelve of 24 stage I and II patients were treated with two-drug chemotherapy and no radiation. Only one of these patients suffered a relapse, which was in the lungs and was salvaged.

A 2004 report from the SIOP is similarly encouraging.[95] It reviewed 30 Wilms' tumor patients over 16 years of age. The median age was 25 years and patients were treated according to the SIOP protocols followed in pediatric patients. Adults tended to have higher stage disease, with one third demonstrating hematogenous metastases. However, response to treatment was reasonably successful given the extent of disease. With a median of 4 years of follow-up, the event-free and overall survivals were 57% and 83%, respectively. Based on these results in the modern era, both studies concluded that adults with favorable histology tumors could be successfully treated with the same protocols employed for children; more intense treatment is not required for adults. However, it is most important that adults with Wilms' tumor promptly receive the correct diagnosis and staging, and are promptly treated with adjuvant therapy.

A consistent concern with adult Wilms' tumor patients is misdiagnosis and undertreatment. In a recent series of 17 patients in Italy, 53% of patients had stage III or IV disease, and the 5-year survival was 62%.[101] The relatively poor outcome in this series was attributed to undertreatment due to poor compliance with therapeutic guidelines. Adult patients with unfavorable histology tumors or high-risk recurrence should be treated with a multiagent regimen including an oxazaphosphorine and etoposide. Paclitaxel and platinum-based drugs have also been shown to be effective in anecdotal cases.[102,103]

REFERENCES

1. Priestly JT, Shulte TL. The treatment of Wilms' tumor. Urology 1942;47:7–10.
2. Ladd WE, White RR. Embryoma of the kidney (Wilms tumor). JAMA 1941;117:1859–1863.
3. Neville HL, Ritchey ML. Wilms' tumor: overview of National Wilms' Tumor Study Group results. Urol Clin North Am 2000;27:435–442.
4. Farrow GM. Diseases of the kidney. In: Murphy WM, ed. Urological Pathology. Philadelphia: Saunders, 1989:409–482.
5. Beckwith JB. Wilms tumor and other renal tumors of childhood: an update. J Urol 1986;136:320–324.
6. Machin GA. Persistent renal blastema (nephroblastomatosis) as a frequent precursor of Wilms' tumor: a pathological and clinical review (parts 1–3). Am J Pediatr Hematol Oncol 1980;2:165–171, 253–261, 353–362.
7. Bove DE, McAdams AJ. The nephroblastomatosis complex and its relationship to Wilms' tumor: a clinicopathologic treatise. In: Rosenberg H, Bolande R, eds. Perspectives in Pediatric Pathology, vol 2. Chicago: Year Book Medical Publishers, 1976:185–223.
8. Machin GA, McCaughey WTE. A new precursor lesion of Wilms' tumor (nephroblastoma): intralobar multifocal nephroblastomatosis. Histopathology 1984;8:35–53.
9. Bergeron C, Iliescu C, Thiesse P, et al. Does nephroblastomatosis influence the natural history and relapse rate in Wilms' tumour? A single centre experience over 11 years. Eur J Cancer 2001;37:385–391.
10. Coppes MJ, Arnold M, Beckwith JB, et al. Factors affecting the risk of contralateral Wilms tumor development: a report from the National Wilms Tumor Study Group. Cancer 1999;85:1616–1625.
11. Hennigar RA, O'Shea PA, Grattan-Smith JD. Clinicopathologic features of nephrogenic rests and nephroblastomatosis. Adv Anat Pathol 2001;8:276–289.
12. Breslow NE, Beckwith JB. Epidemiological features of Wilms' tumor: results of the National Wilms' Tumor Study. J Natl Cancer Inst 1982;68:429–436.
13. D'Angio GJ, Evans AE, Breslow N, et al. The treatment of Wilms' tumor: results of the National Wilms' Tumor Study. Cancer 1976;38:633–646.
14. D'Angio GJ, Evans AE, Breslow N, et al. The treatment of Wilms' tumor: results of the second National Wilms' Tumor Study. Cancer 1981;47:2302–2311.
15. D'Angio GJ, Breslow N, Beckwith JB, et al. The treatment of Wilms' tumor: results of the third National Wilms' Tumor Study. Cancer 1989;64:349–360.
16. Breslow N, Beckwith JB, Ciol M, Sharples K. Age distribution of Wilms' tumor; report from the National Wilms' Tumor Study. Cancer Res 1988;15:1653–1657.
17. Sotelo-Avila C, Gonzalez-Crussi F, Fowler JW. Complete and incomplete forms of Beckwith-Wiedemann syndrome—their oncogenic potential. J Pediatr 1980;96:47–50.

18. Gallo GE, Chemes HE. The association of Wilms' tumor, male pseudohermaphroditism and diffuse glomerular disease (Drash syndrome): report of eight cases with clinical and morphologic findings and review of the literature. Pediatr Pathol 1987;7:175–189.

19. Greenberg F, Stein F, Gresik MV, et al. The Perlman familial nephroblastomatosis syndrome. Am J Med Genet 1986;24:101–110.

20. Knudson AG Jr. Mutation and cancer: statistical study of retinoblastoma. Proc Natl Acad Sci USA 1971;68:820–823.

21. Knudson AG Jr, Strong LC. Mutation and cancer: a model for Wilms' tumor of the kidney. J Natl Cancer Inst 1972;48:313–324.

22. Coppes MJ, Pritchard-Jones K. Principles of Wilms' tumor biology. Urol Clin North Am 2000;27:423–433.

23. Wagner KJ, Roberts SG. Transcriptional regulation by the Wilms' tumour suppressor protein WT1. Biochem Soc Trans 2004;32:932–935.

24. Little SE, Hanks SP, King-Underwood L, et al. Frequency and heritability of WT1 mutations in non-syndromic Wilms' tumor patients: a UK Children's Cancer Study Group Study. J Clin Oncol 2004;22:4140–4146.

25. Royer-Pokora B, Beier M, Henzler M, et al. Twenty-four new cases of WT1 germline mutations and review of the literature: genotype/phenotype correlations for Wilms tumor development. Am J Med Genet 2004;127A:249–257.

26. Ruteshouser EC, Huff V. Familial Wilms tumor. Am J Med Genet 2004;129C:29–34.

27. Grundy PE, Telzerow PE, Breslow N, et al. Loss of heterozygosity for chromosomes 16q and 1p in Wilms' tumors predicts an adverse outcome. Cancer Res 1994;54:2331.

28. McNeil DE, Brown M, Ching A, DeBaun MR. Screening for Wilms tumor and hepatoblastoma in children with Beckwith-Wiedemann syndromes: a cost-effective model. Med Pediatr Oncol 2001;37:349–356.

29. Choyke PL, Siegel MJ, Craft AW, Green DM, DeBaun MR. Screening for Wilms tumor in children with Beckwith-Wiedemann syndrome or idiopathic hemihypertrophy. Med Pediatr Oncol 1999;32:196–200.

30. Owens CM, Veys PA, Pitchard J, Levitt G, Imeson J, Dicks-Mireaux C. Role of chest computed tomography at diagnosis in the management of Wilms' tumor: a study by the United Kingdom Children's Cancer Study Group. J Clin Oncol 2002;20:2768–2773.

31. Meisel JA, Guthrie KA, Breslow NE, Donaldson SS, Green DM. Significance and management of computed tomography detected pulmonary nodules: a report from the National Wilms Tumor Study Group. Int J Radiat Oncol Biol Physics 1999;44:579–585.

32. Wootton-Gorges SL, Albano EA, Riggs JM, Ihrke H, Rumack CM, Strain JD. Chest radiography versus chest CT in the evaluation for pulmonary metastases in patients with Wilms' tumor: a retrospective review. Pediatr Radiol 2000;30:533–537.

33. Leung RS, Liesner R, Brock P. Coagulopathy as a presenting feature of Wilms tumour. Eur J Pediatr 2004;163:369–373.

34. Ritchey ML, Green DM, Breslow NB, et al. Accuracy of current imaging modalities in the diagnosis of synchronous bilateral Wilms' tumor. Cancer 1995;75:600–604.

35. Koo AS, Koyle MA, Hurwitz RS, et al. The necessity of contralateral surgical exploration in Wilms tumor with modern noninvasive imaging technique: a reassessment. J Urol 1990;144:416–417.

36. Goleta-Dy A, Shaw PJ, Stevens MM. Re: The necessity of contralateral surgical exploration in Wilms tumor with modern noninvasive imaging technique: a reassessment [letter]. J Urol 1992;147:171.

37. Connor JP, Upadhyaya J, Becker C, et al. Contralateral surgical exploration in Wilms tumor: Is it still necessary? J Urol 1994;151:273A(abstr).

38. Kessler O, Franco I, Jayabose S, et al. Is contralateral exploration of the kidney necessary in patients with Wilms tumor? J Urol 1996;156:693–695.

39. Martinez-Ibanez V, de Toledo JS, De Diego M, et al. Wilms' tumours with intracaval involvement. Med Pediatr Oncol 1996;26:268–271.

40. Thompson WR, Newman K, Seibel N, et al. A strategy for resection of Wilms' tumor with vena cava or atrial extension. J Pediatr Surg 1992;27:912–915.

41. Novick AC, Cosgrove DM. Surgical approach for removal of renal cell carcinoma extending into the vena cava and the right atrium. J Urol 1980;123:947–951.

42. Montie JE, Jackson CL, Cosgrove DM, et al. Resection of large inferior vena caval thrombi from renal cell carcinoma with the use of circulatory arrest. J Urol 1988;139:25–28.

43. Pannek J, Goepel M, Kremens B, et al. Surgical management of Wilms' tumor with intracardiac neoplastic extension. Thorac Cardiovasc Surg 1994;42:108–111.
44. Schettini ST, da Fonseca JH, Abib SC, et al. Management of Wilms' tumor with intracardiac extension. Pediatr Surg Int 2000;16:529–532.
45. Chiappini B, Savini C, Marinelli G, et al. Cavoatrial tumor thrombus: single-stage surgical approach with profound hypothermia and circulatory arrest, including a review of the literature. J Thorac Cardiovasc Surg 2002;124:684–688.
46. Ritchey ML, Kelalis PP, Breslow N, et al. Surgical complications after nephrectomy for Wilms' tumor. Surg Gynecol Obstet 1992;175:507–514.
47. Othersen HB Jr, DeLorimer A, Hrabovsky E, et al. Surgical evaluation of lymph node metastases in Wilms' tumor. J Pediatr Surg 1990;25:330–331.
48. Shamberger RC, Guthrie KA, Ritchey ML, et al. Surgery-related factors and local recurrence of Wilms tumor in National Wilms Tumor Study 4. Ann Surg 1999;229:292–297.
49. Ritchey ML, Green DM, Thomas PRM, et al. Renal failure in Wilms' tumor patients: a report from the National Wilms' Tumor Study Group. Med Pediatr Oncol 1996;26:75–80.
50. Brenner BM. Nephrology forum: hemodynamically mediated glomerular injury and the progressive nature of kidney disease. Kidney Int 1983;23:647–655.
51. Robson WLM, Leung AKC, Rogers RC. Unilateral renal agenesis. Adv Pediatr 1995;42:575–592.
52. Rugiu C, Oldrizzi L, Lupo A, et al. Clinical features of patients with solitary kidneys. Nephron 1986;43:10–15.
53. Argueso LR, Ritchey ML, Boyle ET Jr, et al. Prognosis of children with solitary kidney after unilateral nephrectomy. J Urol 1992;148:747–751.
54. Argueso LR, Ritchey ML, Boyle ET Jr, et al. Prognosis of patients with unilateral renal agenesis. Pediatr Nephrol 1992;6:412–416.
55. Di Tullio MT, Casale F, Indolfi P, et al. Compensatory hypertrophy and progressive renal damage in children nephrectomized for Wilms' tumor. Med Pediatr Oncol 1996;26:325–328.
56. Bailey S, Roberts A, Brock C, et al. Nephrotoxicity in survivors of Wilms' tumours in the North of England. Brit J Cancer 2002;87:1092–1098.
57. Donckerwolcke RM, Coppes MJ. Adaptation of renal function after unilateral nephrectomy in children with renal tumors. Pediatr Nephrol 2001;16:568–574.
58. McLorie GA, McKenna PH, Greenberg M, et al. Reduction in tumor burden allowing partial nephrectomy following preoperative chemotherapy in biopsy proved Wilms tumor. J Urol 1991;146: 509–513.
59. Cozzi F, Schiavetti A, Bonanni M, et al. Enucleative surgery for stage I nephroblastoma with a normal contralateral kidney. J Urol 1996;156:1788–1793.
60. Moorman-Voestermans CGM, Aronson DC, Staalman CR, et al. Is partial nephrectomy appropriate treatment for unilateral Wilms' tumor? J Pediatr Surg 1998;33:165–170.
61. Linni K, Urban C, Lackner H, Hollwarth ME. Nephron-sparing procedures in 11 patients with Wilms' tumor. Pediatr Surg Int 2003;19:457–462.
62. Horwitz JR, Ritchey ML, Moksness J, et al. Renal salvage procedures in patients with synchronous bilateral Wilms' tumors: a report from the National Wilms' Tumor Study Group. J Pediatr Surg 1996;31:1020–1025.
63. Haecker FM, von Schweinitz D, Harms D, Buerger D, Graf N. Partial nephrectomy for unilateral Wilms tumor: results of study SIOP 93–01/GPOH. J Urol 2003;170:939–942.
64. Cherullo EE, Ross JH, Kay R, Novick AC. Renal neoplasms in adult survivors of childhood Wilms tumor. J Urol 2001;165:2013–2017.
65. Williams JA, Magill L, Parham DM, et al. The potential for renal salvage in nonmetastatic unilateral Wilms' tumor. Am J Pediatr Hematol Oncol 1991;13:342–344.
66. Zani A, Schiavetti A, Gambino M, Cozzi DA, Conforti A, Cozzi F. Long-term outcome of nephron sparing surgery and simple nephrectomy for unilateral localized Wilms tumor. J Urol 2005; 173:946–948.
67. Ritchey ML, Shamberger RC, Haase G, Horwitz J, Bergemann T, Breslow NE. Surgical complications after primary nephrectomy for Wilms' tumor: report from the National Wilms' Tumor Study Group. J Am Coll Surg 2001;192:63–68.
68. Lemerle J, Voute PA, Tournade MF, et al. Preoperative versus postoperative radiotherapy, single versus multiple courses of actinomycin D, in the treatment of Wilms' tumor: preliminary results of a controlled clinical trial conducted by the International Society of Paediatric Oncology (SIOP). Cancer 1976;38:647–654.

69. Graf N, Tournade MF, de Kraker J. The role of preoperative chemotherapy in the management of Wilms' tumor. Urol Clin North Am 2000;27:443–454.

70. Reinhard H, Aliani S, Ruebe C, Stockle M, Leuschner I, Graf N. Wilms' tumor in adults: results of the Society of Pediatric Oncology (SIOP) 93–01/Society for Pediatric Oncology and Hematology (GPOH) Study. J Clin Oncol 2004;22:4500–4506.

71. Weirich A, Ludwig R, Graf N, et al. Survival in nephroblastoma treated according to the trial and study SIOP-9/GPOH with respect to relapse and morbidity. Ann Oncol 2004;15:808–820.

72. Ritchey ML, Kelalis PP, Breslow N, et al. Intracaval and atrial involvement with nephroblastoma: review of National Wilms' Tumor Study-3. J Urol 1988;140:1113–1118.

73. Mushtaq I, Carachi R, Roy G, et al. Childhood renal tumours with intravascular extension. Br J Urol 1996;78:772–776.

74. Ritchey ML, Kelalis PP, Haase GM, et al. Preoperative therapy for intracaval and atrial extension of Wilms' tumor. Cancer 1993;71:4104–4110.

75. White JJ, Golladay ES, Kaizer H, et al. Conservatively aggressive management with bilateral Wilms' tumors. J Pediatr Surg 1976;11:859–865.

76. Kay R, Tank E. The current management of bilateral Wilms' tumor. J Urol 1986;135:983–985.

77. Blute ML, Kelalis PP, Offord KP, et al. Bilateral Wilms' tumor. J Urol 1987;138:968–973.

78. Montgomery BT, Kelalis PP, Blute ML, et al. Extended follow up of bilateral Wilms' tumor: results of the National Wilms' Tumor Study. J Urol 1991;146:514–518.

79. Shaul DB, Srikanth MM, Ortega JA, et al. Treatment of bilateral Wilms' tumor: comparison of initial biopsy and chemotherapy to initial surgical resection in the preservation of renal mass and function. J Pediatr Surg 1992;27:1009–1015.

80. Tournade MF, Com-Nougue C, de Kraker J, et al. Optimal duration of preoperative therapy in unilateral and nonmetastatic Wilms' tumor in children older than 6 months: results of the Ninth International Society of Pediatric Oncology Wilms' Tumor Trial and Study. J Clin Oncol 2001;19:488–500.

81. Vujanic GM, Kelsey A, Mitchell C, Shannon RS, Gornall P. The role of biopsy in the diagnosis of renal tumors of childhood: results of the UKCCSG Wilms tumor study 3. Med Pediatr Oncol 2003;40:18–22.

82. Ludin A, Macklis RM. Radiotherapy for pediatric genitourinary tumors: its role and long-term consequences. Urol Clin North Am 2000;27:553–562.

83. Green DM, Breslow NE, Beckwith JB, et al. Treatment with nephrectomy only for small, stage I/favorable histology Wilms' tumor: a report from the National Wilms' Tumor Study Group. J Clin Oncol 2001;19:3719–3724.

84. Green DM, Beslow NE, Li Y, et al. The role of surgical excision in the management of relapsed Wilms' tumor patients with pulmonary metastases: a report from the National Wilms' Tumor Study. J Pediatr Surg 1991;26:728–733.

85. Dome JS, Liu T, Krasin M, et al. Improved survival for patients with recurrent Wilms tumor: the experience at St. Jude Children's Research Hospital. J Pediatr Hematol Oncol 2002;24:192–198.

86. Green DM. Wilms' tumour. Eur J Cancer 1997;33:409–418.

87. Campbell AD, Cohn SL, Reynolds M, et al. Treatment of relapsed Wilms' tumor with high-dose therapy and autologous hematopoietic stem-cell rescue: the experience at Children's Memorial Hospital. J Clin Oncol 2004;22:2885–2890.

88. Kremens B, Gruhn B, Klingebiel T, et al. High-dose chemotherapy with autologous stem cell rescue in children with nephroblastoma. Bone Marrow Transplant 2002;30:893–898.

89. Abu-Ghosh AM, Krailo MD, Goldman SC, et al. Ifosfamide, carboplatin and etoposide in children with poor-risk relapsed Wilms' tumor: a Children's Cancer Group report. Ann Oncol 2002;13:460–469.

90. Gallego-Melcon S, Sanchez de Toleda J, Doste D, et al. Late recurrent metastasis in Wilms' tumor. Med Pediatr Oncol 1994;23:158–161.

91. Green DM, Grigoriev YA, Nan B, et al. Congestive heart failure after treatment for Wilms' tumor: a report from the National Wilms' Tumor Study group. J Clin Oncol 2003;21:2447–2448.

92. Hogeboom CJ, Grosser SC, Guthrie KA, Thomas PR, D'Angio GJ, Breslow NE. Stature loss following treatment for Wilms tumor. Med Pediatr Oncol 2001;36:295–304.

93. Green DM, Peabody EM, Nan B, Peterson S, Kalapurakal JA, Breslow NE. Pregnancy outcome after treatment for Wilms tumor: a report from the National Wilms Tumor Study Group. J Clin Oncol 2002;20:2506–2513.

94. Breslow NE, Takashima JR, Whitton JA, et al. Second malignant neoplasms following treatment for Wilms' tumor: a report from the National Wilms' Tumor Study Group. J Clin Oncol 1995;13:1851–1859.

95. Reinhard H, Aliani S, Ruebe C, Stockle M, Leuschner I, Graf N. Wilms' tumor in adults: results of the Society of Pediatric Oncology (SIOP) 93–01/Society for Pediatric Oncology and Hematology (GPOH) study. J Clin Oncol 2004;22:4500–4506.

96. Williams G, Colbeck RA, Gowing NF. Adult Wilms' tumour: review of 14 patients. Br J Urol 1992;70:230–235.

97. Byrd RL, Evans AE, D'Angio GJ. Adult Wilms tumor: effect of combined therapy on survival. J Urol 1982;127:648–651.

98. Huser J, Grignon DJ, Ro JY, Ayala AG, Shannon RL, Papadopoulos NJ. Adult Wilms' tumor: a clinicopathologic study of 11 cases. Mod Pathol 1990;3:321–326.

99. Arrigo S, Beckwith JB, D'Angio G, Haase G. Better survival after combined modality care for adults with Wilms' tumor. Cancer 1990;66:827–830.

100. Kalapurakal JA, Nan B, Morkool P, et al. Treatment outcomes in adults with favorable histologic type Wilms tumor—an update from the National Wilms Tumor Study Group. Int J Radiat Oncol Biol Phys 2004;60:1379–1384.

101. Terenziani M, Spreafico F, Collini P, et al. Adult Wilms' tumor: a monoinstitutional experience and a review of the literature. Cancer 2004;101:289–293.

102. Bozeman G, Bissada NK, Abboud MR, Laver J. Adult Wilms' tumor: prognostic and management considerations. Urology 1995;45:1055–1058.

103. Ramanthan RK, Rubin JT, Ohori NP, Belani CP. Dramatic response of adult Wilms tumor to paclitaxel and cisplatin. Med Pediatr Oncol 2000;34:296–298.

104. Green DM, Breslow NE, Beckwith JB, et al. Comparison between single-dose and divided-dose administration of dactinomycin and doxorubicin for patients with Wilms' tumor: a report from the National Wilms' Tumor Study Group. J Clin Oncol 1998;16:237–245.

105. Green DM, Breslow NE, Beckwith JB, et al. Effect of duration of treatment on treatment outcome and cost of treatment for Wilms' tumor: a report from the National Wilms' Tumor Study Group. J Clin Oncol 1998;16:3744–3751.

106. Green DM, Beckwith JB, Breslow NE, et al. Treatment of children with stages II to IV anaplastic Wilms' tumor: a report from the National Wilms' Tumor Study Group. J Clin Oncol 1994; 12:2126–2131.

Rare Malignancies of the Kidney: *Evaluation and Management*

Kristian R. Novakovic and
Steven C. Campbell

KEYWORDS

KIDNEY
RENAL MASS
RARE MALIGNANCY
SARCOMA
LYMPHOMA
RENAL METASTASES
CARCINOID
ADULT WILMS' TUMOR
PRIMITIVE NEUROENDOCRINE TUMOR
SAMLL CELL CARCINOMA

ABSTRACT

Up to twenty percent of renal masses suspicious for renal cell carcinoma in adults are not RCC upon final pathology. While many of these tumors are benign, those that are malignant tend to be aggressive and lethal. Rare malignancies can often be diagnosed with renal biopsy. Many of these malignancies require additional or alternative oncologic therapies and close collaboration with medical and/or radiation oncologists. This chapter reviews the pathologic, diagnostic, therapeutic, including surgical and non-surgical approaches, and prognostic considerations pertaining to these uncommon renal malignancies. Covered are renal sarcoma, renal lymphoma, metastatic disease, carcinoid adult Wilms' tumor, primitive neuroendocrine tumor, and small cell carcinoma.

Ten to twenty percent of renal masses suspicious for renal cell carcinoma (RCC) in adults are not RCC on final pathology.[1] While many of these tumors are benign, several uncommon renal malignancies may be identified and merit special consideration (Table 38.1). Included among these malignancies are renal sarcoma, lymphoma, metastasis, carcinoid, adult Wilms' tumor, and primitive neuroectodermal tumor. Taken together these cancers tend to be aggressive and lethal. While surgical considerations

From: *Clinical Management of Renal Tumors*
Edited by: R.M. Bukowski and A.C. Novick © Humana Press Inc., Totowa, NJ

Table 38.1.
Rare malignant tumors of the kidney

Sarcoma
Lymphoma
Renal metastasis
Carcinoid
Adult Wilms' tumor
Primitive neuroectodermal tumor
Small cell carcinoma

predominate in the management of RCC, many of the malignancies discussed herein demand additional or alternative oncologic therapies and, therefore, close collaboration with medical and/or radiation oncologists. Unfortunately, accurate preoperative diagnosis of these rare tumors can be difficult and in some cases impossible using current imaging modalities. Although renal biopsy is generally eschewed with regard to renal masses, several of these rare malignancies can be diagnosed with renal biopsy and therefore highlight the potential indications for biopsy in select patients with atypical renal masses. This chapter reviews the diagnostic and therapeutic considerations pertaining to these uncommon renal malignancies.

RENAL SARCOMA

In general, soft tissue sarcomas are rare genitourinary (GU) malignancies, with less than 5% of these tumors arising from the GU tract.[2] The kidney is the second most common site for GU sarcomas after the spermatic cord, testis, and paratesticular tissues.[3] Renal sarcomas account for roughly 1% of renal malignancies in adults, and tend to affect a younger population than RCC or upper tract urothelial carcinoma.[3,4] The peak incidence for renal sarcoma is during the fifth decade of life.[3] Acknowledged risk factors for soft tissue sarcomas, including prior radiation exposure or treatment with pediatric chemotherapy regimens, have not been linked to renal sarcomas.[3] Several familial syndromes including hereditary retinoblastoma, Li-Fraumeni, neurofibromatosis, and familial adenomatous polyposis are associated with the development of soft tissue sarcomas but not specifically renal sarcomas.[5] The relative rarity of renal sarcoma may contribute to the difficult in identifying such correlations. In addition to its fairly enigmatic natural history, renal sarcoma is the most lethal of the GU sarcomas.

Pathology

The pathologic literature is replete with case reports of various histologic subtypes of sarcoma affecting the kidney, and almost all subtypes of soft tissue sarcoma have been reported[3] (Table 38.2). The main differential diagnosis of renal sarcoma will always be sarcomatoid RCC, and only careful pathologic evaluation can distinguish these entities in many cases. Identification of any features of the various subtypes of RCC excludes the diagnosis of primary renal sarcoma.

Differentiating between the various types of sarcoma often requires molecular as well as histologic analysis. Perhaps the most important information the pathologist can provide with regard to sarcoma is the histologic grade of the tumor.[2,5–7] The current American Joint Committee on Cancer (AJCC) guidelines for pathologic analysis of soft tissue sarcoma employ a two-tiered system (high vs. low grade).[8] In general, high-grade

Table 38.2.
Histologic types of renal sarcoma

Histologic type	Pathologic features
Leiomyosarcoma	Positive for desmin and smooth muscle actin
Liposarcoma	Presence of fat
Angiosarcoma	Endothelial markers positive (CD31, CD34)
Hemangiopericytoma	Electron microscopic features of pericytes
Malignant fibrous histiocytoma	Histiocytic cells, multinucleated giant cells, xanthoma cells
Synovial sarcoma	Chromosomal translocation t(X;18) (p11.2;q11.2)
Osteogenic	Presence of giant cells, production of osteoid and bone
Clear cell sarcoma	Uniform proliferation of small round cells
Cystic embryonal sarcoma	Stains for vimentin
Synovial sarcoma	Chromosomal translocation t(X;18), immunostain positive for bcl2

sarcomas are at increased risk for systemic metastasis, while low-grade sarcomas tend toward local recurrence.[2,5,6]

Leiomyosarcomas and liposarcomas are the most common renal sarcomas, representing approximately 40% and 10–15% of documented cases, respectively.[3] Leiomyosarcomas arise from the smooth muscle components of the renal parenchyma, capsule, or pelvicalyceal system.[9] On rare occasions leiomyosarcomas may be derived from smooth muscle cells lining large vascular structures, and cases of leiomyosarcoma of the renal artery and vein have been reported.[9,10] The detection of muscle antigens, most commonly desmin and smooth muscle actin, by means of immunohistochemistry suggests the diagnosis of leiomyosarcoma.[5,11] Renal leiomyosarcoma tends to displace rather than invade the parenchyma, and a tendency toward high-grade and aggressive clinical behavior has been reported.[11–13] Liposarcoma, as the name implies, is a malignant tumor derived from adipose tissue. It demonstrates a propensity to grow to extremely large size; however, some reports suggest a tendency toward lower tumor grade and less aggressive behavior.[3,12]

Less common but fascinating renal sarcomas include angiosarcomas, hemangiopericytomas, malignant fibrous histiocytoma, synovial sarcoma, and osteogenic variants. Angiosarcomas may arise from either blood or lymphatic vessels and are known to occur in sites of previous radiation and in association with chronic lymphedema.[5] Endothelial markers such as CD31 and CD34 are useful in defining endothelial differentiation especially in poorly differentiated angiosarcomas.[14] Hemangiopericytomas, in contrast to angiosarcomas, are thought to be derived from the pericytes of capillaries and venules rather than the adjacent endothelial cells.[5] Electron microscopy is especially useful in this diagnosis by elucidating the distinctive ultrastructural features of pericytes.[3,5] Hemangiopericytomas tend to be low-grade tumors and less aggressive, but determining their malignant potential based on pathologic analysis has proved difficult.[15–17] Malignant fibrous histiocytomas are thought to be derived primarily from fibroblasts rather than histiocytes.[5] Histologically they demonstrate a "storiform" mixture of spindle cells with histiocytic cells, multinucleated giant cells, and xanthoma cells.[18,19] Synovial sarcomas of the kidney are verified by molecular detection of a specific chromosomal translocation t(X;18)(p11.2;q11.2).[20,21] Osteogenic sarcomas are typically high grade and are defined by their production of malignant osteoid and bone.[5] Histologically this tumor can be particularly difficult to distinguish from sarcomatoid RCC. Staining for epithelial markers is useful to exclude sarcomatoid RCC, which typically stains positively, while osteogenic sarcoma stains negatively.[22]

Several sarcomas that are more commonly seen in children can also occur in adults, including clear cell sarcoma, cystic embryonal sarcoma, and rhabdomyosarcoma. Clear cell sarcoma was previously considered a variant of Wilms' tumor.[23] It accounts for approximately 4% of pediatric renal tumors, but is extremely rare in adults.[23] Histogenesis is uncertain, but likely of mesodermal origin.[5] Classic histology includes a uniform proliferation of small round cells with fine chromatin and positive staining for vimentin.[24] Cystic embryonal sarcoma was identified as a novel form of renal malignancy in 1998 by Delahunt and colleagues.[25] These tumors demonstrate undifferentiated malignant mesenchyme with foci of smooth muscle and cysts lined with epithelial cells.

The rarity of these neoplasms complicates detailed pathologic analysis. The overriding considerations are making the diagnosis of a renal sarcoma and establishing the grade of the tumor. In general, the exact histologic diagnosis is largely academic since the approach to treatment does not vary substantially with histologic type.

Clinical Presentation

Renal sarcoma and RCC are difficult to distinguish clinically since the typical signs and symptoms such as palpable mass, abdominal or flank pain, and hematuria are common to both disease entities.[12] In general, sarcomas are characterized by large size and local invasion and, therefore, patients with renal sarcoma may be more likely to present with clinical symptoms.[3,13] Interestingly, in select cases, clinical findings may suggest a particular histologic subtype of renal sarcoma. For example, hypoglycemia has been associated with hemangiopericytomas and is thought to be related to excessive glucose metabolism within these tumors.[3,16] In addition, an elevated alkaline phosphatase in conjunction with a renal mass but in the absence of liver or bone disease might suggest osteosarcoma.[3,22] In the majority of cases, however, the clinical presentation of the various subtypes of renal sarcoma is indistinguishable.

Radiologic Evaluation

Renal sarcomas are also difficult to distinguish from RCC based on radiologic appearance. Certain findings on computed tomography (CT) scan may suggest a sarcoma such as tumor originating from the capsule (Figure 38.1) or renal sinus; areas of fat or bone density in cases of liposarcoma or osteosarcoma, respectively; large tumor size in the absence of lymphadenopathy; and a relatively hypovascular pattern.[13,26] A specific exception to the relative hypovascularity is the hemangiopericytoma, which tends to be hypervascular.[13] Renal sarcomas tend toward compression rather than overt invasion of the parenchyma, perhaps due to their largely capsular origin.[13] In general, renal sarcomas are less likely to involve the renal vein or inferior vena cava (IVC), but the presence of tumor thrombi does not exclude sarcoma from the differential diagnosis of a renal mass.[13]

Computed tomography plays the primary role in all renal imaging, but certain findings on plain abdominal radiography may suggest a renal sarcoma. Specifically, a "starburst" ossification pattern within an apparent soft tissue mass can signal the presence of a possible osteosarcoma.[13] Similarly, the presence of fat within a soft tissue mass would suggest the possibility of a liposarcoma. Intravenous urography (IVU) or nephrotomography typically shows distortion of the renal contour or calices, displace-

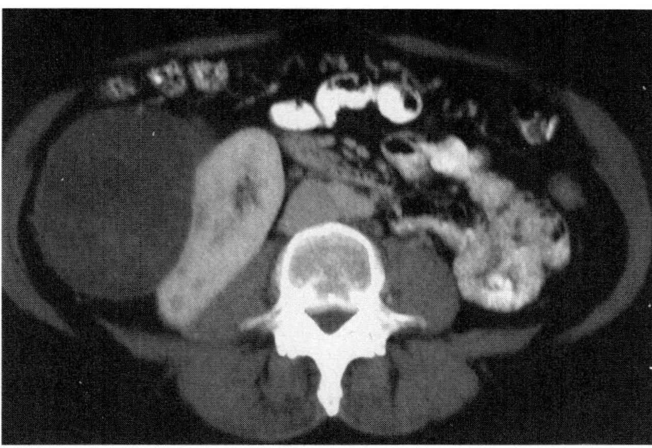

Figure 38.1. Renal liposarcoma originating from renal capsule.

ment of the kidney, or, in rare cases, nonvisualization of the kidney due to complete replacement of the parenchyma.[7]

Other radiographic studies may be useful in certain cases. Although renal angiography plays a diminished role in renal imaging, when performed, the findings can contribute to the diagnosis of renal sarcoma. As stated previously, renal sarcomas, with the exception of hemangiopericytoma, are hypovascular relative to the highly vascular RCC.[13,26] The primary blood supply of renal sarcomas is often from the capsular vessels, which may also be demonstrated angiographically, and is atypical for RCC.[13] Magnetic resonance imaging (MRI) plays an important role in renal imaging by helping to define the extent of venous involvement of renal malignancies, which may include renal sarcoma. Since renal sarcomas tend toward local invasion and often require en-bloc resection of adjacent organs, MRI may be especially useful in preoperative planning by defining tissue planes and proximity to vital structures. The indications for radiographically guided renal biopsy are rare, and suspected renal sarcoma is no exception. There are several case reports that highlight successful identification of renal sarcoma by preoperative biopsy; however, the clinical utility is limited.[27,28] Regardless of the biopsy results, most patients require nephrectomy.

The key point in radiographic analysis of renal sarcomas is their propensity to resemble RCC, and CT provides the best overall imaging modality for renal masses in general. Several clues on CT can suggest sarcoma, but the diagnosis must be verified pathologically. The use of additional imaging studies should be based on their potential contribution to preoperative planning. Identifying the extent of the tumor and its relationship to adjacent structures should be the primary goal.

Surgical Management

The central surgical principle in the management of suspected renal sarcoma is complete excision, which frequently involves en-bloc resection of adjacent tissues and organs.[12] Preoperative evaluation of renal sarcomas should include routine chest imaging to rule out pulmonary metastasis and careful review of abdominal and pelvic CT or MRI to define potential complicating anatomy. Preoperative bowel preparation is imperative as the need for en-bloc resection of bowel may manifest.

Surgical approaches to renal sarcoma mirror those for RCC. An open approach is more frequently warranted due to the large size and local invasion encountered with many renal sarcomas. Sarcomas are often surrounded by a readily defined pseudocapsule that is frequently infiltrated by tumor cells and consequently cannot be used as a margin of resection.[12] Determining the margin of resection intraoperatively often proves challenging and may contribute to the high rate of local recurrence common with renal sarcomas regardless of grade. Management of local recurrence is again primarily surgical, and patients may require several resections in an attempt to cure.[5] Surgery also plays a role in the management of systemic disease, especially in cases with solitary or limited lung metastases.[5]

Additional Treatment Modalities

Although the treatment of soft tissue sarcomas including renal sarcomas is primarily surgical, several authors have looked at alternative, adjuvant, or neoadjuvant therapies in an attempt to improve outcomes. With regard to retroperitoneal sarcomas, Tepper and associates[29] reported improved rates of local control through the use of moderate-dose external-beam radiation after surgery. Other groups have explored the use of intraoperative radiation therapy for retroperitoneal sarcomas and report some encouraging results over resection alone.[5] However, comparable studies specifically treating renal sarcomas have not been performed. Overall, the role of adjuvant and neoadjuvant therapies in soft tissue sarcomas is poorly defined. Combinations of chemotherapy agents, such as doxorubicin, ifosfamide, dacarbazine, and platinum-based regimens, and radiation therapy in an adjuvant setting appear warranted, especially for patients with high-grade disease and good performance status.[5] In cases of local recurrence after attempted complete excision, adjuvant radiation may play a role when used along with repeat resection.

Prognosis

Despite aggressive treatment, the prognosis for patients with renal sarcoma is poor. The two most important prognostic factors are completeness of resection and tumor grade.[12] Although specific data on renal sarcomas is lacking, data from retroperitoneal sarcomas indicates that approximately 50% to 70% can be resected completely.[7] Once resected completely, the primary prognostic indicator is the grade of the lesion. Specific tumor types relate to prognosis insofar as different histiotypes may be more likely to be high grade than others.

RENAL LYMPHOMA

Renal lymphoma occurs almost exclusively as a manifestation of systemic disease, and autopsy studies demonstrate renal involvement in approximately 50% of patients dying of advanced lymphoma.[30] It is still controversial whether any lymphomatous process originates in the kidney since it notably lacks lymphoid tissue.[31] In addition, the rarity of patients with isolated renal lymphoma, and the strong tendency for these patients to rapidly recur and progress at other sites further supports renal involvement as part of systemic disease.[32] However, several cases of primary renal lymphoma are reported in the literature. For example, Dimopoulos and colleagues[32] diagnosed primary renal lymphoma in six of 210 patients (3%) presenting with signs, symptoms, and radiologic findings suggestive of renal malignancy. Similarly, Kandel and colleagues[30] reviewed 28 patients with renal lymphoma of whom 22 (79%) had no evidence of extrarenal lymphomatous disease.[30] These lymphomas may arise from the renal hilum where lymphatic channels are present, or from areas of inflammation within the renal parenchyma that may attract lymphocytes such as focal pyelonephritis.[30,31] Proposed criteria for diagnosing primary renal lymphoma include (1) presence of pathologically proven renal lymphoma, (2) no evidence of extrarenal lymphomatous involvement in visceral organs or lymph nodes, and (3) absence of a leukemic blood pattern together with no evidence of myelosuppression.[31] The exact incidence of primary renal lymphoma is unknown, and this remains a controversial entity. The overwhelming majority of patients with lymphomatous involvement of the kidney will have systemic disease, and the urologist can play an important role by differentiating renal lymphoma from other malignancies and facilitating preservation of renal function.[12]

Pathology

Renal lymphomas are most commonly non-Hodgkin's lymphomas (NHLs) with predominantly diffuse large cell histology rather than a nodular pattern on pathologic evaluation.[31] Non-Hodgkin's lymphoma occurring in the kidney is almost exclusively B cell in origin, although T-cell renal lymphomas have certainly been identified.[31,33] Cases of the mucosa-associated lymphoid tissue (MALT)-type lymphoma, which are a distinctive form of B-cell lymphoma, have also been described in the kidney, and are interesting in their propensity to remain localized and respond to local therapy such as surgery.[34] These tumors are also more likely to be indolent. While Epstein-Barr virus has been implicated in the pathogenesis of lymphoma, its role in the development of renal lymphoma is unclear.[31] Histologic evaluation typically demonstrates multiple small nodular infiltrates between nephrons that eventually coalesce to form a confluent mass.[35] In some cases, this process can replace enough renal parenchyma to lead to renal failure.[12]

Clinical Presentation

Most renal lymphomas are symptomatically silent. When present, symptoms typically include flank pain, or less commonly hematuria.[31] Patients may also present with the so-called "B" symptoms of lymphoma such as fever, weight loss, and fatigue.[31] Renal insufficiency is also occasionally observed in patients with renal lymphoma, but it is more often a result of systemic sequelae of lymphoma such as hypercalcemia, urate nephropathy, or obstruction secondary to retroperitoneal lymphadenopathy rather than direct damage or replacement of the functioning nephrons.[12]

Imaging

As with other renal tumors, CT is the imaging modality of choice. There are four distinct patterns for renal involvement of lymphoma (Table 38.3).[36,37] Renal lymphoma most commonly appears as multiple bilateral renal nodules (Figure 38.2).[35] These lesions typically range in size from 1 to 3 cm, are homogeneous rather than heterogeneous, and minimally enhance with administration of contrast material.[35] Unfortunately, several other disease entities can mimic this pattern including multiple angiomyolipomas (tuberous sclerosis), multifocal RCC (von Hippel–Lindau [VHL]), malacoplakia, and renal metastasis.[38] Lymphoma may also present as a solitary lesion on CT, which can be difficult to distinguish from RCC radiologically.[35]

Other more distinctive patterns of renal lymphoma include infiltrative disease and perirenal disease engulfing or extending into the kidney. Lymphomatous proliferation within the kidney often causes renal enlargement with preservation of the reniform

Table 38.3.
Radiographic patterns of renal lymphoma

Pattern on CT	Details
Multiple bilateral renal masses	Homogeneous, isodense, or hyperdense on noncontrast, hypodense with contrast enhancement
Infiltration of parenchyma	May be focal or diffuse; diffuse infiltration may cause expansion of kidney typically retaining reniform shape
Invasion from retroperitoneal disease	May extend into renal hilum, sinus, or parenchyma; may encase renal vasculature and ureter
Solitary renal mass	Uncommon, can mimic RCC

shape, and such diffuse infiltration is often bilateral and may manifest with renal insufficiency.[35] Interestingly, renal function often returns in such patients after chemotherapy allows for regression of the lymphoma and reconstitution of nephron anatomy and function.[33,36] Finally, lymphoma may also invade the kidney from the adjacent retroperitoneal tissues, and this is the most diagnostic radiographic pattern for renal lymphoma (Figure 38.3). These patients usually demonstrate a bulky retroperitoneal mass that surrounds the kidney and renal hilum, but characteristically the renal vein and artery remain patent.[35] Vascular invasion is much more common with RCC; however, reports of venous tumor extension with lymphoma do exist, and therefore this finding cannot exclude the diagnosis of lymphoma.[32] In general, bulky lymphadenopathy out of proportion to the renal mass and splenic enlargement should strongly suggest a primary diagnosis of lymphoma.[37] In addition, a renal mass that is associated with atypical lymphadenopathy, that is, outside of the normal landing zones for RCC, should also prompt consideration of a renal lymphoma.[32]

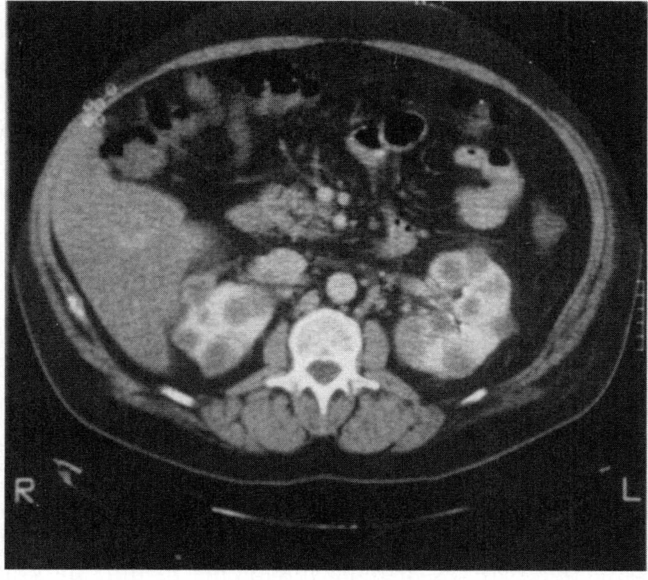

Figure 38.2. Common presentation of renal lymphoma demonstrating bilateral renal nodules.

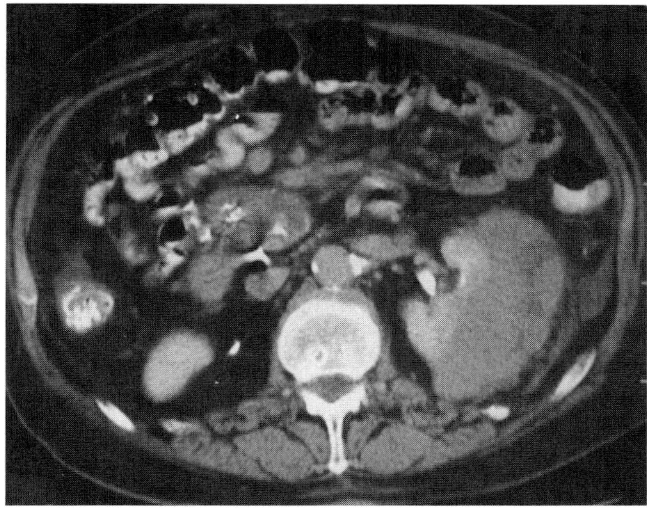

Figure 38.3. Perirenal lymphoma encroaching on parenchyma.

Other imaging modalities that may be used in renal imaging include MRI and nuclear medicine studies. On MRI, untreated lymphoma tends to be heterogeneous in appearance, slightly hypointense relative to the renal cortex on T1-weighted images, and relatively hypointense or isointense on T2-weighted images.[39] Characteristics on MRI do not improve diagnostic sensitivity over CT, and thus routine MRI is not required in cases of suspected lymphoma, although it is useful in cases where CT is contraindicated due to contrast allergy or renal insufficiency. Gallium-67 citrate scintigraphy can also suggest the diagnosis, as there is intense uptake of the radiotracer in lymphoma in contrast to RCC.[40,41] Ultrasound is of limited use in characterizing renal lymphoma, which typically appears as a nonspecific hypoechoic mass.

Role of Biopsy

In contrast to the general treatment approach for renal masses, which involves radical or partial nephrectomy for suspected malignancy, systemic treatment is the mainstay for renal lymphoma. A clinical suspicion for renal lymphoma should be sufficient to prompt an attempt at conclusive diagnosis with fine-needle aspiration (FNA) or core biopsy, which may obviate unnecessary surgery and loss of renal parenchyma. Truong and colleagues[42] demonstrated the utility of FNA in the diagnosis of primary renal lymphoma. Six of the eight cases of renal lymphoma were correctly identified using FNA. Ancillary studies are often essential for definitive diagnosis of primary lymphoma since certain lymphomas, for example large cell lymphoma, may appear cytologically similar to other renal neoplasms, such as urothelial carcinoma and poorly differentiated RCC.[42] Demonstration of a monoclonal population of lymphoid cells by flow cytometry finalizes the diagnosis of renal lymphoma. Fine-needle aspiration or core biopsy will be sufficient in most cases to establish the lymphoid pattern, B- vs. T-cell lineage, and monoclonal vs. polyclonal status.[42] However, even in the best of hands, additional tissue may be required, and this may require renal exploration and biopsy to confirm the diagnosis prior to definitive management. If renal lymphoma is identified during surgical exploration and frozen section, the kidney should be spared in favor of systemic therapies.[12]

Treatment

Treatment choices for lymphoma include cytotoxic chemotherapy, radiation therapy, experimental biologic therapies, and hematopoietic stem cell transplant.[40] Surgery has traditionally played little if any role in the management of lymphoma, and renal lymphoma is no exception, and the mainstay of treatment is systemic chemotherapy.[43] However, certain reports describe the successful treatment of unilateral disease with nephrectomy followed by adjuvant chemotherapy or radiation therapy.[44] As discussed earlier, certain types of lymphoma, specifically MALT, display a tendency toward localized disease and may respond well to surgical resection.[34] The classic chemotherapy regimen for NHL includes cyclophosphamide, doxorubicin, vincristine, and prednisolone (CHOP).[40,43] Urologists should remember that cyclophosphamide can be predisposed to hemorrhagic cystitis and urothelial malignancy on a long-term basis.

Prognosis

Overall, the prognosis of patients with renal lymphoma is quite poor, reflective of extranodal sites of lymphoma in general. Type of lymphoma and grade appear to be the other strong predictive factors. In general, the prognosis for NHL is worse than for Hodgkin's lymphoma, although less aggressive variants of NHL such as MALT do exist and may pursue a more indolent course.[45]

METASTATIC DISEASE

Metastatic tumors are the most common malignancies of the kidney, much more common than RCC. Autopsy studies show that approximately 12% of all patients dying of metastatic cancer have renal metastasis.[13] The kidney is predisposed to hematogenous metastasis because of its high blood flow and profuse vascularity. Only a small (<10%) minority of tumors utilize direct extension to facilitate renal metastasis.[13] The most common primary tumors that metastasize to the kidney are lymphoma, carcinomas of the lung, breast and gastrointestinal tract, and malignant melanoma.[13,46] Lung cancer is the most common solid organ malignancy to metastasize to the kidney, with nearly 20% of autopsy cases demonstrating renal metastasis.[47]

Renal metastases are generally identified late in the course of the disease process, although lesions are being detected more frequently and earlier with routine imaging studies for surveillance or staging.[46,48] Most lesions are small (<3 cm) and multiple (80%), with bilateral metastases identified in almost 50% of cases.[13] Metastasis from colon carcinoma is notable in that it will occasionally present as a large solitary lesion that is difficult to distinguish from RCC.[48] Despite frequent imaging, most renal metastases are still associated with widely disseminated disease.[13,48]

Presentation

The majority of renal metastases are clinically silent, but these lesions may lead to hematuria in 11% to 30% of cases.[47,49] Other common urologic symptoms such as flank pain or a palpable mass are extremely rare in association with renal metastasis. Metastasis from very vascular neoplasms such as choriocarcinoma and some lung carcinomas can occasionally cause life-threatening hematuria.[49,50] Some patients may present with renal failure if the metastasis induces obstructive uropathy, massive renal infiltration and tissue destruction, or vascular invasion that may lead to thrombosis and ischemia.[13,51] In rare instances, cytology may be positive if the metastasis erodes into the collecting system.[13]

Imaging

Once again, CT is the primary imaging modality for renal metastasis, and studies typically reveal multiple bilateral small nodular lesions.[48] Prior to contrast administration, the tissue attenuation of renal metastases is approximately equivalent to normal parenchyma, and they are often difficult to identify on noncontrast studies unless they deform the renal contour.[13] Following contrast administration, minimal enhancement (5 to 30 Hounsfield units [HU]) occurs, which reflects the relative hypovascularity of renal metastases relative to RCC.[13] The infrequent solitary renal metastasis may be difficult or impossible to distinguish from RCC without biopsy (Figure 38.4). Other findings on CT that might suggest renal metastases include encasement or amputation of the renal vein or IVC rather than invasion, and lymphadenopathy in locations atypical for RCC.[13]

Role of Biopsy

A recent study by Sanchez-Ortiz and colleagues[46] examined the indications for renal biopsy in patients with a history of nonrenal malignancies. In this study, renal masses in patients without progression of their nonrenal primary tumor were exclusively RCC or other second primary renal tumors. In contrast, patients with evidence of progression of their nonrenal primary had renal metastases approximately half of the time. Choyke and colleagues[50] showed that in the setting of advanced metastatic disease, renal metastases were even more common, outnumbering second primary renal tumors by a ratio of 4:1. The decision to biopsy a renal mass in a patient with a history of nonrenal malignancy should be based on sound clinical judgment. Although patients with a clinically localized nonrenal malignancy and those thought to be in remission are more likely

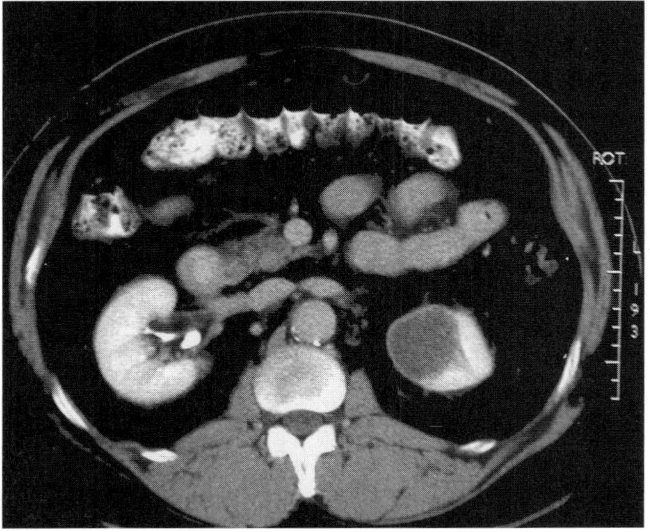

Figure 38.4. Metastatic renal lesion presenting as solitary mass.

to have RCC, renal biopsy should be carefully considered, as it may prevent unnecessary surgical intervention. In contrast, biopsy of renal lesions in the setting of advanced nonrenal malignancy should only be pursued if it would potentially affect patient management.

Treatment

The treatment of renal metastases is systemic and determined by the tumor biology of the primary malignancy. Nephrectomy is almost never indicated unless it plays a role in symptom palliation such as control of severe hemorrhage or pain.

CARCINOID

Carcinoid tumors are rare tumors that arise from neuroendocrine cells, specifically enterochromaffin cells or amine precursor uptake and decarboxylation (APUD) cells.[52] These precursor cells occur most commonly in the gastrointestinal tract and lung and infrequently in the ovaries, testes, thymus, pancreas, and hepatobiliary system.[53] Enterochromaffin cells are not normally present in the kidney, and carcinoid tumors in this organ are thus rare, with fewer than 40 cases reported in the English-language literature. Primitive stem cells within the kidney or retained neural crest tissue within the renal hilum may give rise to these tumors.[53,54] There is an interesting correlation between renal carcinoid and horseshoe kidneys, with previous studies showing a relative risk up to 82-fold higher than in normal kidneys.[54] The aberrant respiratory or colonic epithelium that is occasionally associated with horseshoe kidneys may contain neuroendocrine cells and may predispose to carcinoid.[53]

In general, carcinoid tumors are classified according to derivation from different divisions of the embryonic gut.[55] Foregut tumors arise in the lungs, bronchi or stomach; midgut tumors in the small intestine, appendix, and proximal large bowel; and hindgut tumors in the distal colon and rectum.[55] The architectural pattern and hormonal profile of renal carcinoids seems to be consistent with hindgut derivation.[54] Of particular interest is the identification of prostatic acid phosphatase (PAP) expression in several cases of renal carcinoid[54]; PAP is frequently expressed by rectal carcinoids but almost never in fore- or midgut-derived carcinoids.[54]

Pathology

Histologically, carcinoid tumors are composed of monotonous sheets of small round cells with uniform nuclei and cytoplasm.[56] They are also characterized by a positive reaction to silver stains and to markers of neuroendocrine tissue such as neuron-specific enolase, synaptophysin, and chromogranin.[56] Under electron microscopy, carcinoid tumors contain numerous membrane-bound neurosecretory granules that contain various hormonally active substances such as serotonin, corticotrophin, histamine, and dopamine.[55] As with other neuroendocrine tumors such as pheochromocytoma, pathologists are unable to differentiate benign from malignant tumors based on histology alone. Malignancy is only determined if invasion or distant metastases are present.[56]

Imaging

A useful characteristic of carcinoid tumors is their almost ubiquitous expression of somatostatin receptors, and somatostatin receptor scintigraphy (SRS) is an effective method for localizing carcinoid tumors. This study employs radiolabeled octreotide that acts as a ligand for several subtypes of somatostatin receptor.[56] Somatostatin receptor scintigraphy identifies carcinoid tumors in 73% to 89% of patients with this diagnosis.[56] Renal carcinoid tumors tend to be hypovascular and enhance poorly on CT, but these characteristics are not sufficient to establish the diagnosis radiographically.[57] As will be demonstrated later, the majority of reported cases of primary renal carcinoid are asymptomatic and therefore do not provide an obvious clinical indication for SRS. Although rarely used preoperatively, SRS may be helpful in detecting residual or recurrent disease once a pathologic diagnosis is made.[58] Some have recommended that patients with renal carcinoid should be evaluated with colonoscopy and esophagogastroscopy to search for multifocal disease.

Presentation

Release of serotonin and other vasoactive peptides causes carcinoid syndrome, which is characterized by episodic flushing, wheezing, diarrhea, and eventual right-sided valvular heart disease.[56] Patients with renal carcinoid may present with this syndrome, but most are asymptomatic.[58] Flank mass, hematuria, and abdominal pain are all distinctly uncommon in this patient population, since most renal carcinoids are small and nonaggressive.[59] When carcinoid syndrome is present, measurement of urinary or plasma serotonin or its metabolites in the urine can confirm the diagnosis.[56]

Treatment

The diagnosis of primary renal carcinoid tumor is almost never made preoperatively. As with any renal mass without evidence of metastatic disease, the primary consideration is complete surgical resection. Due to the paucity of cases, the relative merits of partial versus complete nephrectomy have not been studied. Beyond surgery, no standard therapy for renal carcinoid tumors has been proposed.[52] Studies suggest that interferon-γ or somatostatin analogues may be effective in patients with metastatic carcinoid.[55] Both of these agents are tumoristatic for carcinoid tumors and may stabilize metastatic disease, but their effects are not additive and the rationale for combining these drugs is weak.[56] Somatostatin analogues inhibit secretion of a broad range of hormones including growth hormone, insulin, glucagons, and gastrin and may also palliate some patients with carcinoid tumors.[55] Radiation therapy has played only a palliative role in the treatment of carcinoid tumors.[55]

Prognosis

The prognosis for patients with renal carcinoid is good, since most present with localized disease.[52] In their review, Kawajiri and colleagues[52] found that only 13% of reported cases of renal carcinoid were fatal, and most of these patients presented with metastatic disease. Interestingly, cases of carcinoid associated with a horseshoe kidney appear to follow a more indolent course.[53,54]

ADULT WILMS' TUMOR

Wilms' tumor (WT) is the most common abdominal malignancy in children, but it is also occasionally seen in adults. Kilton and colleagues[60] developed the following criteria for making the diagnosis of WT in adults: (1) presence of a primary renal neoplasm in a patient older than 15 years of age; (2) definite histology consistent with WT without evidence of features associated with RCC; and (3) sufficient pathologic documentation to clearly indicate the true histologic nature of the tumor. Overall, 3% of all WTs are identified in adults with 20% found between the ages of 15 and 20 and the remaining 80% distributed between the third and seventh decades of life.[61]

Pathology

Adult and pediatric WT are histologically similar with a distinctive triphasic pattern including varying amounts of blastema, epithelium, and stroma.[62] Some authors have suggested that the presence of isochromosome 7q may be distinctive for WT in adults rather than children, and may impact clinical course.[63] Due to the rarity of the adult variant, the natural history and appropriate management are not well defined. However, most authors believe that adult and pediatric WT are biologically identical and should be treated as such.

The pathologic staging systems for adult and pediatric WT are identical and critical for clinical decision making and prognosis. The current National Wilms' Tumor Study (NWTS) staging system for WT can be summarized as follows: 1, confined to the kidney; 2, extension beyond the renal capsule or venous involvement but completely resected; 3, abdominal disease than cannot be entirely resected (positive surgical margins included), diffuse tumor spill, or positive lymph nodes; 4, distant lymph nodes or hematogenous metastases; 5, bilateral tumor.[64] Stage and histology (favorable vs. unfavorable) are the best predictors of prognosis in adult and pediatric WT.

Imaging

In contrast to pediatric WT, imaging modalities such as ultrasound (US), CT, MRI, and urography are simply not able to accurately diagnose adult WT in the majority of cases.[62,65] Since WT is the most common primary renal malignancy in children, imaging studies often provide the correct diagnosis by simply identifying a suspicious renal lesion. In contrast, RCC is much more common in adults, and the imaging characteristics of WT are difficult to distinguish from RCC[61] (Figure 38.5). In general, adult WT presents as a heterogeneous intrarenal mass on CT, and a relatively hypovascularity pattern is often observed.[66]

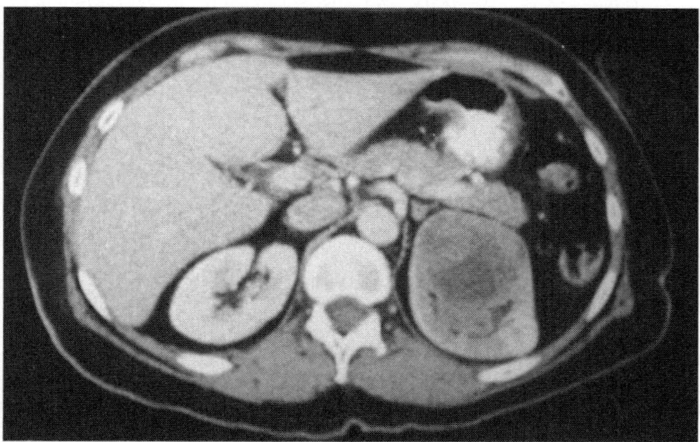

Figure 38.5. Adult Wilms' tumor presenting as solitary renal mass.

Presentation

The common presenting symptoms for adult WT are similar to other renal malignancies and include flank pain, abdominal mass, and hematuria. Patients with adult WT are often symptomatic and many experience a sudden drop in performance status.[61,65] This is a distinct difference from children with WT, who are commonly asymptomatic and typically present with painless abdominal swelling.[65] Twenty-nine percent of adult WT metastasize versus 10% of pediatric cases.[66] Metastatic sites include the lungs, liver, bones, skin, bladder, colon, brain, and contralateral kidney.[66]

Treatment

Surgery, radiotherapy, and chemotherapy have specifically defined roles in the treatment of pediatric WT based on tumor stage.[67,68] Due to the relative paucity of adult cases, similar specific treatment guidelines are lacking. Surgery is the mainstay of treatment but the roles of adjuvant chemotherapy and radiotherapy in adult WT are not clearly defined. It is generally thought that multimodal therapy is imperative, but results have not been as satisfactory as for pediatric WT, likely due to the more advanced stage at diagnosis in many adult patients.[69,70] Most authors advocate treating adult WT by careful adherence to pediatric protocols, and recent studies following this principle have demonstrated improved response rates.[65,70] Additional studies are required to determine a more precise treatment approach to this rare renal malignancy.

PRIMITIVE NEUROECTODERMAL TUMOR

Primitive neuroectodermal tumor (PNET) is a tumor that is thought to be related to the Ewing's sarcoma family of tumors. These tumors typically form in bone or soft tissues particularly of the extremities, trunk, head, and neck.[71] The vast majority of PNET occur in adolescents and young adults, but any age may be affected.[72] Primitive neuroectodermal tumors are thought to derive from primitive neural crest cells located within postganglionic parasympathetic nerves rather than sympathetic nerves because of their expression of acetylcholine transferase and inability to synthesize adrenergic precursors.[73] Primitive neuroectodermal tumor seldom affects the viscera and only rarely affects the kidneys.[71] Renal PNET seems to behave more aggressively than similar tumors located elsewhere in the body and may represent a distinct clinical entity.[72,74–76]

Presentation

Clinical symptoms associated with renal PNET are nonspecific and similar to other renal neoplasms. In general, renal PNET are aggressive tumors with 25% to 50% of cases presenting with metastatic disease.[76]

Imaging

As with many of the rare renal malignancies, radiographic imaging is typically insufficient to diagnose renal PNET preoperatively. On CT, PNET often appears as a heterogeneous ill-defined mass with low attenuation and areas of necrosis.[77] Similar to other non-RCC malignancies, enhancement is minimal with contrast administration, but again this is a nonspecific finding.[77] Cases of PNET with IVC thrombus have also been reported and can further complicate the radiologic diagnosis.[78,79] Alternative imaging modalities do not provide any additional sensitivity for renal PNET.

Pathology

Histologically PNET are characterized by small round cells that may form characteristic Homer Wright rosettes or pseudorosettes.[75,80] Positive staining for CD99 in addition to vimentin, cytokeratin, and neuron-specific enolase strongly suggests the diagnosis of PNET.[71,74,81] It is important to differentiate renal PNET from neuroblastoma and WT, since all three may have similar cytologic and histologic features.[71] There is a characteristic t(11;22)(q24;q12) translocation that is highly specific for PNET, which can be useful for making this distinction.[72,74,80,82]

Treatment

Renal PNET is an aggressive tumor with a propensity toward local recurrence and early metastasis to lymph nodes, lung, liver, and bone marrow.[81,83] As with many of the tumors previously discussed, complete resection, when possible, is the primary treatment goal. Achieving an exact pathologic diagnosis has important clinical consequences, as a combination of tumor debulking, chemotherapy, and radiotherapy may lead to dramatic tumor reduction in cases of recurrent or metastatic disease.[83]

Prognosis

Overall 5-year disease-free survival is only about 45% to 55%.[83] Patients with metastatic disease at presentation have a poor prognosis with median relapse-free survival of 2 years.[83] Aggressive surgical treatment, accurate pathologic diagnosis, and careful follow-up with early intervention for recurrent and metastatic disease will optimize survival.

SMALL CELL CARCINOMA

Small cell carcinomas are highly aggressive neoplasms that are commonly diagnosed in the lung and represent 10% to 20% of pulmonary malignancies.[84] Approximately 2% of small cell carcinomas occur outside of the lung and can appear anywhere throughout the body including the genitourinary tract.[85,86] The bladder gives rise to most genitourinary small cell carcinomas, but approximately 30 cases of small cell carcinoma of the kidney have been reported.[87]

Pathology

Pathologically, small cell carcinoma has features of neuroendocrine and epithelial neoplasms.[84] Small cell carcinoma of the kidney must be distinguished from other small cell tumors of the kidney such as Wilms' tumor, PNET, lymphoma, and metastasis from a pulmonary small cell carcinoma.[87] Small cell carcinomas are typically positive for neuron-specific enolase, chromogranin, and synaptophysin, and this can be helpful in sorting out the differential diagnosis.[87] Careful body imaging with CT should rule out a primary pulmonary lesion.[87]

Clinical Presentation

Unfortunately, the clinical features of small cell carcinomas of the kidney can be indistinguishable from RCC. There is a tendency toward large size at presentation frequently with local extension and distant metastasis, indicating that these tumors are identified relatively late in their clinical course.[85] Pain and hematuria are the two most common symptoms, but other manifestations of locoregional or metastatic disease may be present.

Imaging

As with almost all of the rare tumors mentioned in this chapter, small cell carcinoma resembles RCC on CT imaging but is less likely to strongly enhance. Magnetic resonance imaging may play a role in better defining the extent of local invasion, but, in general, other imaging modalities will not contribute significantly to diagnostic or therapeutic decision making.

Treatment

Due to the similarity with RCC, most small cell carcinomas of the kidney will be resected when the renal mass is identified. Radical surgery has been advocated in the treatment of small cell carcinoma located in other areas of the GU tract such as the bladder or prostate, but some authors have suggested that nephrectomy may not improve prognosis in patients with small cell carcinoma of the kidney due to the likelihood of metastatic disease at presentation.[85] Treatment with platinum-based chemotherapy regimens are advocated for treatment of extrapulmonary small cell carcinoma in general, and may also be useful in treating renal manifestations of the malignancy.[85]

Prognosis

As with other pulmonary and extrapulmonary sites for small cell carcinoma, the prognosis for small cell carcinoma of the kidney is generally poor. Majhail and colleagues[85] reported that 60% of patients with no evidence of distant metastasis at presentation eventually developed metastatic disease. In their series the median survival for small cell carcinoma in patients who underwent nephrectomy was 8 months. Treatment with platinum-based chemotherapy significantly improved overall survival to 20 months. Long-term survivors are described but rare, and new treatment regimens are needed.

REFERENCES

1. Silver DA, Morash C, Brenner P, et al. Pathologic findings at the time of nephrectomy for renal mass. Ann Surg Oncol 1997;4:570–574.
2. Russo P, Brady MS, Conlon K, et al. Adult urological sarcoma. J Urol 1992;147:1032–1037.
3. Frank I, Takahashi S, Tsukamoto T, Lieber MM. Genitourinary sarcomas and carcinosarcomas in adults. In: Vogelzang NJ, ed. Comprehensive Textbook of Genitourinary Oncology, 2nd ed. Philadelphia: Lippincott Williams & Wilkins.
4. Vogelzang NJ, Fremgen AM, Guinan PD, et al. Primary renal sarcoma in adults: a natural history and management study by the American cancer society, Illinois division. Cancer 1993;71:804–810.
5. Brennan MF, Alektiar KM, Maki RG. Soft tissue sarcoma. In: Devita ET, ed. Cancer: Principles and Practice of Oncology, 6th ed. Philadelphia: Lippincott Williams & Wilkins.
6. Froehner M, Lossnitzer A, Manseck A, et al. Favorable long-term outcome in adult genitourinary low-grade sarcoma. Urology 2000;56:373–377.
7. Spellman JE, Driscoll DL, Huben RP. Primary renal sarcoma. Amer Surg 1995;61:456–459.
8. American Joint Committee on Cancer. Soft tissue sarcoma. In: Greene FL, Page DL, Fleming ID, et al., eds. AJCC Cancer Staging Handbook, 6th ed. New York: Springer.
9. Moudouni SM, En-Nia I, Rioux-Leclerq N, et al. Leiomyosarcoma of the renal pelvis. Scand J Urol Nephrol 2001;35:425–427.
10. Gill IS, Hobart MG, Kaouk JH, et al. Leiomyosarcoma of the main renal artery treated by laparoscopic radical nephrectomy. Urology 2000;56:669x-669xi.

11. Deyrup AT, Montogomery E, Fisher C. Leiomyosarcoma of the kidney: a clinicopathologic study. Am J Surg Pathol 2004;28:178–182.
12. Novick AC, Cambell, SC. Renal Tumors. In: Walsh PC, ed. Campbell's Urology, 8th ed. Philadelphia: Saunders.
13. Pollack HM, Banner MP, Amendola MA. Other malignant neoplasms of the renal parenchyma. Semin Roentgenol 1987;22:260–274.
14. Cerilli LA, Huffman HT, Anand A. Primary renal angiosarcoma: a case report with immunohistochemical, ultrastructural and cytogenetic features and review of the literature. Arch Pathol Lab Med 1998;122:929–935.
15. Weiss JP, Pollack HM, McCormick JF, et al. Renal hemangiopericytoma: surgical radiological and pathological implications. J Urol 1984;132:337–339.
16. Merchant SH, Mittal BV, Desai MS. Haemangiopericytoma of kidney: a report of 2 cases. J Postgrad Med 1998;44:78–80.
17. Chieng D, Cohen JM, Waisman J. Fine-needle aspiration cytology of hemangiopericytoma: a report of five cases. Cancer 1999;87:190–195.
18. Raghavaiah NV, Mayer RF, Hagitt R, et al. Malignant fibrous histiocytoma of the kidney. J Urol 1979;123:951–953.
19. Chen CH, Lee PS, Han WJ, et al. Primary giant cell malignant fibrous histiocytoma of the kidney with staghorn calculi. J Postgrad Med 2003;49:246–248.
20. Bella AJ, Winquist EW, Perlman EJ. Primary synovial sarcoma of the kidney diagnosed by molecular detection of syt-ssx fusion transcripts. J Urol 2002;168:1092–1093.
21. Koyama S, Morimitsu, Y, Morokuma F. Primary synovial sarcoma of the kidney: report of a case confirmed by molecular detection of the syt-ssx fusion transcripts. Pathol Int 2001;51:385–391.
22. Leventis AK, Stathopoulos GP, Boussiotou AC, et al. Primary osteogenic sarcoma of the kidney: a case report and review of the literature. Acta Oncol 1997;36:775–777.
23. Barnard M, Bayani J, Grant R, et al. Comparative genomic hybridization analysis of clear cell sarcoma of the kidney. Med Pediatr Oncol 2000;24:113–116.
24. Argani P, Perlman EJ, Breslow NE, et al. Clear cell sarcoma of the kidney: a review of 351 cases from the national Wilms' tumor study group pathology center. Am J Surg Pathol 2000;24:4–18.
25. Delahunt B, Beckwith JB, Eble JN, et al. Cystic embryonal sarcoma of the kidney: a case report. Cancer 1998;82:2427–2433.
26. Shirkhoda A, Lewis E. Renal sarcoma and sarcomatoid renal cell carcinoma: CT and angiographic features. Radiology 1987;162:252–257.
27. Vesoulis Z, Rameh T, Nelson R, et al. Fine needle aspiration biopsy of primary renal synovial sarcoma: a case report. Acta Cytol 2003;47:668–672.
28. Johnson VV, Gaertner EM, Crothers BA. Fine-needle aspiration of renal angiosarcoma. Arch Pathol Lab Med 2002;126:478–480.
29. Tepper JE, Suit HD, Wood WC, et al. Radiation therapy of retroperitoneal soft tissue sarcomas. Int J Radiat Oncol Biol Phys 1984;10:825.
30. Kandel LB, McCullough DL, Harrison LH, et al. Primary renal lymphoma: does it exist? Cancer 1987;60:386–391.
31. Yasunaga, Y, Hoshida Y, Hashimoto M, et al. Malignant lymphoma of the kidney. J Surg Oncol 1997;64:207–211.
32. Dimopoulos MA, Moulopoulos LA, Costantinides C, et al. Primary renal lymphoma: a clinical and radiological study. J Urol 1996;155:1865–1867.
33. O'Riordan E, Reeve R, Houghton JB, et al. Primary bilateral T-cell renal lymphoma presenting with sudden loss of renal function. Nephrol Dial Transplant 2001;16:1487–1489.
34. Tuzel E, Mungan M, Yorukoglu K, et al. Primary renal lymphoma of mucosa-associated lymphoid tissue. Urology 2003;61:463xvii–463xx.
35. Urban BA, Fishman EK. Renal lymphoma: CT patterns with emphasis on helical CT. Radiographics 2000;20:197–212.
36. Choi JH, Choi GB, Shim KN, et al. Bilateral primary renal non-Hodgkin's lymphoma presenting with acute renal failure: successful treatment with systemic chemotherapy. Acta Haematol 1997;97:231–235.
37. Jafri SZH, Bree RL, Amendola MA, et al. CT of renal and perirenal non-Hodgkin lymphoma. AJR 1982;138:1101–1105.
38. Sheeran SR, Sussman SK. Renal lymphoma: spectrum of CT findings and potential mimics. AJR 1998;171:1067–1072.

39. Semelka RC, Kelekis NL, Burdeny DA, et al. Renal lymphoma: demonstration by MR imaging. AJR 1996;166:823–827.
40. Armitage JO, Mauch PM, Harris NL, Bierman P. Non-Hodgkins' lymphomas. In: Devita ET, ed. Cancer: Principles and Practice of Oncology, 6th ed. Philadelphia: Lippincott Williams & Wilkins.
41. Taniguchi M, Higashi K, Ohguchi M, et al. Gallium-67 citrate scintigraphy of primary renal lymphoma. Ann Nucl Med 1998;12:51–53.
42. Truong LD, Caraway N, Ngo T, et al. The diagnostic and therapeutic roles of fine-needle aspiration. Am J Clin Pathol 2001;115:18–31.
43. Colevas Ad, Kantoff PW, DeWolf WC, Canellos GP. Malignant lymphoma of the genitourinary tract. In: Vogelzang NJ, ed. Comprehensive Textbook of Genitourinary Oncology, 2nd ed. Philadelphia: Lippincott Williams & Wilkins.
44. Okuno SH, Hoyer JD, Ristow K, et al. Primary renal non-Hodgkin's lymphoma: an unusual extranodal site. Cancer 1995;75:2258–2261.
45. Arranz-Arija JA, Carrion JR, Garcia FR, et al. Primary renal lymphoma: report of 3 cases and review of the literature. Am J Nephrol 1994;14:148–153.
46. Sanchez-Ortiz RF, Madsen LT, Bermejo CE, et al. A renal mass in the setting of a nonrenal malignancy: when is a renal tumor biopsy appropriate? Cancer 2004;101:2195–2201.
47. Olsson CA, Moyer JD, Laferte RO. Pulmonary cancer metastatic to the kidney: a common renal neoplasm. J Urol 1971;105:492–496.
48. Ferrozzi F, Bova D, Campodonico F. Computed tomography of renal metastases. Semin Ultrasound CT MR 1997;18:115–121.
49. Walther PJ, Marks LS, Stern D, et al. Renal metastasis of adenocarcinoma of the lung: massive hematuria managed by therapeutic embolization. J Urol 1979:398–400.
50. Choyke PL, White EM, Zeman RK, et al. Renal metastases: clinicopathologic and radiologic correlation. Radiology 1987;162:359–363.
51. Manning EC, Belenko MI, Frauenhoffer EE, et al. Acute renal failure secondary to solid tumor renal metastases: case report and review of the literature. Am J Kidney Dis 1996;27:284–291.
52. Kawajiri H, Onoda N, Ohira M, et al. Carcinoid tumor of the kidney presenting as a large abdominal mass: report of a case. Surg Today 2004;34:86–89.
53. Krishnan B, Truong LD, Saleh G, et al. Horseshoe kidney is associated with an increased relative risk of primary renal carcinoid tumor. J Urol 1997;157:2059–2066.
54. Begin LR, Guy L, Jacobson SA, et al. Renal carcinoid and horseshoe kidney: a frequent association of two rare entities—a case report and review of the literature. J Surg Onc 1998;68:113–119.
55. Kulke MH, Mayer RJ. Carcinoid tumors. N Engl J Med 1999;340:858–868.
56. Jensen RT, Doherty GM. Carcinoid tumors and the carcinoid syndrome. In: Devita ET, ed. Cancer: Principles and Practice of Oncology, 6th ed. Philadelphia: Lippincott Williams & Wilkins.
57. Moulopoulos A, DuBrow R, Dimopoulos DC. Primary renal carcinoid: computed tomography, ultrasound and angiographic findings. J Comput Assist Tomogr 1991;15:323–325.
58. McCaffrey JA, Reuter V, Herr HW, et al. Carcinoid tumor of the kidney. The use of somatostatin receptor scintigraphy in diagnosis and management. Urol Oncol 2000;5:108–111.
59. Tal R, Lask DM, Livne PM. Metastatic renal carcinoid: case report and review of the literature. Urology 2003;61:838xv–838xvii.
60. Kilton L, Matthews MJ, Cohen MH. Adult Wilms' tumor: a report of prolonged survival and review of the literature. J Urol 1980;124:1–5.
61. Winter P, Vahlnensieck W, Miersch WDE, et al. Wilms' tumor in adults. Review of 10 cases. Int Urol Nephrol 1996;28:469–475.
62. Orditura M, De Vita F, Catalano G. Adult Wilms' tumor: a case report. Cancer 1997;15:1961–1965.
63. Rubin BP, Pins MR, Nielsen GP, et al. Isochromosome 7q in adult Wilms' tumors: diagnostic and pathogenetic implications. Am J Surg Pathol 2000;24:1663–1669.
64. Firoozi F, Kogan BA. Follow-up and management of recurrent Wilms' tumor. Urol Clin North Am 2003;30:869–879.
65. Reinhard H, Aliani S, Ruebe C, et al. Wilms' tumor in adults: results of the society of pediatric oncology (SIOP) 93–01/society for pediatric oncology and hematology (GPOH) study. J Clin Oncol 2004;22:4500–4506.
66. Akmansu M, Yapici T, Tulay E. Adult Wilms' tumor: a report of two cases and their treatment and prognosis. Int Urol Nephrol 1998;30:529–533.
67. Green DM. Paediatric oncology update: Wilms' tumor. European Journal of Cancer 1997;33:409–418.

68. Neville HL, Ritchey ML. Wilms' tumor: overview of national Wilms' tumor study group results. Urol Clin North Am 2000;27:443–454.

69. Bozeman G, Bissada NK, Abboud MR, et al. Adult Wilms' tumor: prognostic and management considerations. Urology 1995;45:1055–1058.

70. Terenziani M, Spreafico F, Collini P, et al. Adult Wilms' tumor: a monoinstitutional experience and a review of the literature. Cancer 2004;101:289–293.

71. Maly B, Maly A, Reinhartz T, et al. Primitive neuroectodermal tumor of the kidney: report of a case initially diagnosed by fine needle aspiration cytology. Acta Cytol 2004;48:264–268.

72. Jimenez RE, Folpe AL, Lapham RL, et al. Primary Ewing's sarcoma/primitive neuroectodermal tumor of the kidney: a clinicopathologic and immunohistochemical analysis of 11 cases. Am J Surg Pathol 2002;26:320–327.

73. Ginsberg JP, Woo SY, Johnson ME, et al. Ewing's sarcoma family of tumors: Ewing's sarcoma of bone and soft tissue and the peripheral primitive neuroectodermal tumors. In: Devita ET, ed. Cancer: Principles and Practice of Oncology, 6th ed. Philadelphia: Lippincott Williams & Wilkins.

74. Parham DM, Roloson GJ, Feely M, et al. Primary malignant neuroepithelial tumors of the kidney. Am J of Surg Pathol 2001;28:133–146.

75. Pomara G, Capello F, Cuttano MG, et al. Primitive neuroectodermal tumor (PNET) of the kidney: a case report. BMC Cancer 2004;4:3.

76. Rodriquez-Galindo C, Marina NM, Fletcher BD, et al. Is primitive neuroectodermal tumor of the kidney a distinct entity? Cancer 1997;79:2243–2250.

77. Doerfler O, Reittner P, Groell R, et al. Peripheral primitive neuroectodermal tumour of the kidney: CT findings. Pediatr Radiol 2001;31:117–119.

78. Thomas JC, Sebek BA, Krishnamurthi V. Primitive neuroectodermal tumor of the kidney with inferior vena cava and atrial tumor thrombus. J Urol 2002;168:1486–1487.

79. Karnes RJ, Gettman MT, Anderson PM, et al. Primitive neuroectodermal tumor (extraskeletal Ewing's sarcoma) of the kidney with vena caval tumor thrombus. J Urol 2000;164:772.

80. Marley EF, Liapis H, Humphrey PA, et al. Primitive neuroectodermal tumor of the kidney—another enigma: a pathologic, immunohistochemical and molecular diagnostic study. Am J Surg Pathol 1997;21:354–359.

81. Gonlusen G, Ergin M, Paydas S, et al. Primitive neuroectodermal tumor of the kidney: a rare entity. Int Urol Nephrol 2001;33:449–451.

82. Quezado M, Benjamin DR, Tsokos M. EWS/FLI-1 fusion transcripts in three peripheral primitive neuroectodermal tumors of the kidney. Hum Pathol 1997;28:767–770.

83. Casella R, Moch H, Rochlitz C, et al. Metastatic primitive neuroectodermal tumor of the kidney in adults. Eur Urol 2001;39:613–617.

84. Gonzalez-Lois C, Madero S, Redondo P, et al. Small cell carcinoma of the kidney: a case report and review of the literature. Arch Pathol Lab Med 2001;125:796–798.

85. Majhail NS, Elson P, Bukowski RM. Therapy and outcome of small cell carcinoma of the kidney: report of two cases and a systematic review of the literature. Cancer 2003;97:1436–1441.

86. Mackey JR, AU HJ, Hugh J, et al. Genitourinary small cell carcinoma: determination of clinical and therapeutic factors associated with survival. J Urol 1998;159:1624–1629.

87. Akkaya BK, Mustafa U, Esin O, et al. Primary small cell carcinoma of the kidney. Urol Oncol 2003;21:11–13.

INDEX

A

17-AAG. *See* 17-desmethoxygeldaamycin

Ablation. *See also* Cryoablation;
Radiofrequency ablation
chemoablation, 240

Abscess, 27–28, 45, 211, 238
embolization and, 260
intracranial, 483

ABX-EGF, 406

Acetabulum, 444

Acetaminophen, 89, 516

Acetic acid, 240

Acid phosphatase, 424

Acquired renal cystic disease (ARCD)
dialysis and, 546
RCC and, 545–547
renal transplantation and, 546–547

Acrochordons, 83

Activation-induced cell death (AICD), 116

Active specific immunotherapy (ASI), 297

Acute focal bacterial nephritis (AFBN),
27–28

Acute renal failure, 202, 211

Acute tubular necrosis (ATN), 211

Adenocarcinoma, 588

Adenoma, 555–561. *See also* Metanephric
adenoma; Papillary adenoma
AJCC on, 556
UICC on, 556

Adenosine triphosphate (ATP), 109, 324
for cachexia, 518
RTKs and, 400

Adjuvant therapy. *See* Therapy

Adoptive immunotherapy, 215, 297
nephrectomy and, 349

Adrenal gland, 10, 30–31, 67
ipsilateral, 180–182
LPN and, 229
mRCC and, 36
pancreatic metastases and, 472
tumors and, 149

Adriamycin, 536, 537

AESOP robotic assist device, 197

AFBN. *See* Acute focal bacterial nephritis

Aging
mRCC and, 308
RCC and, 84

AgNOR. *See* Argyrophilic nucleolar
organizer region

AICD. *See* Activation-induced cell death

AJCC. *See* American Joint Committee on
Cancer

Alcohol, 249, 250, 252

Alkaline phosphatase, 136, 424, 425
IL-6 and, 509
osteosarcoma with, 620

All-trans-retinoic acid (ATRA), 119

Alytic expansile lesion, 427

American Joint Committee on Cancer
(AJCC), 529. *See also* Tumor, node,
metastasis staging system
on adenoma, 556
on TCC, 589

Amine precursor uptake and decarboxylation
cells (APUD), 628

AML. *See* Angiomyolipoma

Amphetamines, 87

Amputations, 449–450, 454

Analgesics, 73, 89, 337. *See also*
Nonsteroidal antiinflammatory
drugs; Opioids
with LRN, 197, 278
RCC and, 89–91

Anemia, 314, 362
IL-6 and, 515
with paraneoplastic syndromes, 136

Angioembolization, 579

Angiofibroma, 83

Angiogenesis, 435
VEGF and, 403

Angiography, 45
for AML, 579
history of, 248
for pancreatic metastases, 462

Angioinfarction, 247–262
complications with, 259–260
embolization in, 248–251
palliative, 258

preoperative, 252–254
for RCC, 251–258
Angiolipoma, 104
Angiomyolipoma (AML), 15, 565–582
   angiography for, 579
   c-kit and, 575
   cryoablation for, 582
   CT for, 139, 568, 569–572, 578
   diagnosis of, 567–576
   embolization for, 258–259
   epithelioid, 575–576
   fallopian tubes and, 572–573
   false-positives with, 50
   hemorrhage and, 577
   imaging of, 27
   liver and, 572–573
   lymph nodes and, 572
   management of, 576–582
   NSS for, 580–582
   oncocytoma and, 569
   pathology of, 572–575
   percutaneous biopsy for, 50
   percutaneous imaging-guided biopsy for, 50
   PES and, 579
   pregnancy and, 577–578
   renal lymphoma and, 623
   RFA for, 582
   spleen and, 572–573
   surgery for, 579–582
   surveillance and, 578
   TSC and, 83, 565, 566
   US for, 569
Angiosarcoma, 619
   sarcomatoid renal cell carcinoma and, 65
Anhedonia, 513
Anorexia, 508, 515, 518, 588
Anoxia, 363
Antiangiogenesis agents, 349
Antidepressants, 513, 517, 519. *See also*
   Tricyclic antidepressant
Antiepileptic drugs, 484
Antihypertensive drugs, 88
Antimuscarinics, 518
α_1-antitrypsin, 313
Aphasia, 482
Apical segmented nephrectomy, 208–209
Apoptosis, 173
   of T-cells, 116–117
APUD. *See* Amine precursor uptake and
   decarboxylation cells
ARCD. *See* Acquired renal cystic disease

Argyrophilic nucleolar organizer region
   (AgNOR), 153, 173
Around-the-clock (ATC), 516
Arteriography, 207
Arteriovenous malformations (AVMs),
   14–15, 250, 255–256
   bleeding with, 256
   hematuria with, 256
   HTN with, 256
   pain with, 256
   renal allograft and, 255
   VEGF and, 256
Artery of Adamkiewicz, 435
Asbestos, 89
ASI. *See* Active specific immunotherapy
Aspirin, 47–48, 89
ATC. *See* Around-the-clock
ATN. *See* Acute tubular necrosis
ATP. *See* Adenosine triphosphate
ATRA. *See* All-trans-retinoic acid
Autologous clot, 248–250
Autologous tumor vaccines, 297–299
Autotransplantation, 209
AVMs. *See* Arteriovenous malformations
Azotemia, 5

B

B7-H1, 124–125
Bacille Calmette-Guérin (BDG), 121
Balloons, 249, 250
Basilar segmental nephrectomy, 208–209
Basophilic type, of PRCC, 530
BAY 43-9006. *See* Sorafenib
BCNU. *See* Bischloroethylnitrosourea
BDG. *See* Bacille Calmette-Guérin
Beckwith-Wiedemann syndrome, 600–601,
   602, 606
Bedside Delirium Scale, 521
Bellini duct. *See* Collecting-duct renal cell
   carcinoma
Benign cystic nephroma, imaging of, 24, 25
Beoacezurab, 349
Bevacizumab, 6–7, 109, 349, 407, 511
   erlotinib with, 406
   vs. IFN-α, 407
   VEGF and, 539
BHD. *See* Birt-Hogg-Dubé syndrome
Biologic response modifiers (BRMs), 340
Biopsy. *See also* Percutaneous biopsy
   for metastatic disease, 627–628
   for renal lymphoma, 625

Birt-Hogg-Dubé syndrome (BHD), 56, 59,
  60, 80, 137, 531
  colonic polyps and, 103
  genetics and, 83, 103–106
  NSS for, 213
  oncocytoma with, 63–64, 104
  oncocytosis and, 559
  pneumothorax with, 104
  thyroid carcinoma and, 103
Bischloroethylnitrosourea (BCNU),
  489
Bisphosphonates, 422
  for skeletal metastases, 431
Bladder cancer, 593
Bleeding, 202. *See also* Coagulation;
  Hemorrhage
  with AVMs, 256
  with NSS, 211
  with pancreatic metastases, 470
  with percutaneous biopsy, 49
Blood-brain barrier, 482
Blood transfusion, 201
  cryoablation and, 234
BMI. *See* Body mass index
Body mass index (BMI), 87
Boiling contrast agents, 249, 250
Bone, 146. *See also* Skeletal metastases
  mRCC and, 35
  pancreatic metastases and, 472
  trabecular, 422
Bone cement. *See* Methylmethacrylate
Bone scans, 448
  limitations of, 509
  for RCC, 424–426
  in skeletal metastases, 424–426
  for skull lesions, 484
Bone scintigraphy, 146
Bortezomib, 408
Bosniak criteria, 12, 139–140
Bowel obstruction, 518–519
Brachytherapy, 513
Brain, 146. *See also* Intracranial
  metastases
  pancreatic metastases and, 472
Brainstem, 482
Breast cancer, 423
  family history of, 424
BRMs. *See* Biologic response modifiers
BTA stat, 589
BTA Trak, 589
Budd-Chiari phenomenon, 133
Bupropion, 517

C

Cachexia, 515, 518
Cadmium, 1
Caenorhabditis elegans, 102
CA IX. *See* Carbonic anhydrase IX
Calcification, 140
  with WT, 599
Calcium, 86
Cancer Renal Cytokine (CRECY) trial, 314,
  317
Capecitabine, 473
Capillary leak syndrome, 373
Carbamazepine, 517
Carbonic anhydrase IX (CA IX), 153, 407
Carboplatin, 536
  for CDRCC, 537, 539
  RMC and, 539
  for WT, 610
Carcinoid, 628–629
  clinical presentation of, 629
  hematuria with, 629
  IFN-γ for, 629
  imaging of, 628–629
  pathology of, 628
  prognosis for, 629
  RT for, 629
  somatostatin receptor scintigraphy for,
    628–629
  treatment for, 629
Cardiopulmonary bypass (CPB), 184, 188–189
  minimal access technique for, 189–190
α-carotene, 86
β-carotene, 86
Caval thrombectomy, RNx with, 192–193
Caval thrombus, 254
  lymph nodes and, 192
  PEs with, 192–193
  RCC with, 184–192
  survival with, 190–191
  with WT, 604
Cavernous sinus, 484
Cavotomy, 187–188
CCF. *See* Cleveland Clinic Foundation
CCI-779. *See* Rapamycin; Temsirolimus
CCRCC. *See* Clear-cell renal cell carcinoma
CD4 cells, 117, 118, 121–122
CDRCC. *See* Collecting-duct renal cell
  carcinoma
Central sinus invasion, 29
Central tumors, LPN and, 229
Cerebellum, 482

Cerebral hemispheres, 482
Cerebrospinal fluid (CSF), 482
Cervix cancer, 362
Cetuximab, 406
    EGFR and, 538
CFD. *See* Color flow Doppler
Chemoablation, 240
Chemotherapy, 461
    for CCRCC, 385–391
    for CDRCC, 537
    for ChRCC, 532, 537
    combination, 388–389
    with hormone therapy, 389–390
    intracranial metastases and, 484, 489
    for leptomeningeal disease, 492
    mRCC and, 385–391, 399
    for PNET, 632
    for PRCC, 537
    for RCC, 535–538
    for renal lymphoma, 626
    for renal sarcoma, 622
    resistance to, 390
    for RMC, 536–537
    for sarcomatoid renal cell carcinoma, 536
    for SCCa, 633
    single-agent, 386
    for TCC, 592–593
    for WT, 604, 606–608, 610
Chest x-ray (CXR), 146, 207, 266, 268
    for WT, 602
Cholelithiasis, 88
Chondrosarcoma, 422
CHOP. *See* Prednisolone
Choroid plexus, 484, 491
ChRCC. *See* Chromophobe renal cell
    carcinoma
Chromogranin, 632
Chromophobe renal cell carcinoma (ChRCC),
    81
    chemotherapy for, 532, 537
    c-kit and, 539
    clinical features of, 59, 532
    genetics and, 60
    HSP-90 for, 111
    imaging of, 22
    immunotherapy for, 532
    oncocytoma and, 561
    pathology of, 59–60, 531
    prognosis with, 65, 151
    skeletal metastases and, 452
    survival from, 533

Cincinnati Transplant Tumor Registry, 548
Cirrhosis, 88
Cisplatin, 536
    for CDRCC, 537
    for UUTTCC, 593–594
    for WT, 610
Citalopram, 517
CIV. *See* Continuous intravenous
C-kit, 405
    AML and, 575
    ChRCC and, 539
    PRCC and, 539
    sarcomatoid renal cell carcinoma and, 539
Clavicle, fracture of, 445
Clear-cell renal cell carcinoma (CCRCC), 2,
    79–81, 171, 507
    chemotherapy for, 385–391
    clinical features of, 56
    genetics and, 57–58
    GLUT-1 and, 58
    hemorrhage with, 57
    IL-2 and, 65
    imaging of, 20–22
    pancreatic metastases and, 472
    pathology of, 57
    PET for, 326
    prognosis with, 65
    skeletal metastases and, 452
    survival from, 533
    TGF-α and, 58
    with TSC, 83
    VEGF and, 58
    VHL and, 475
Cleveland Clinic Foundation (CCF), 462,
    467–472
C-MET, 109
CMP. *See* Corticomedullary phase
CMV regimen, 593
Coagulation, 47, 136, 209, 222
    with WT, 603
Coffee, 86
Coils, 250
Collecting-duct renal cell carcinoma
    (CDRCC), 81, 149–150
    carboplatin for, 537, 539
    chemotherapy for, 537
    cisplatin for, 537
    clinical features of, 61, 532
    doxorubicin for, 537
    EGFR and, 539
    genetics and, 62

ifosfamide for, 537
imaging of, 23
LOH with, 62
paclitaxel for, 537, 539
pathology of, 61, 531
prognosis with, 152
Collimator helmets, 486
Collision tumors, 576
Colonic polyps, BHD and, 103
Colon, pancreatic metastases and, 472
Color flow Doppler (CFD), 16, 34
Combination chemotherapy, 388–389
Complete responses (CRs), 356
Computed tomography (CT), 9, 17–19, 29, 75, 146, 162, 220, 270, 498
    for AML, 139, 568, 569–572, 578
    of chest, 29
    delayed, 17–18
    for diagnosis, 138–140, 184
    for end-stage renal disease, 546
    for intracranial metastases, 483–484
    for metastatic disease, 627
    multiphase scanning with, 17
    NSS and, 207, 209
    for pancreatic metastases, 462, 467, 470, 471
    of pelvis, 29
    PET-CT, 329
    for PNET, 631–632
    PRC and, 233
    pseudoenhancement with, 18–19, 140
    for pulmonary metastases, 416–417
    for renal sarcoma, 620
    for SCCa, 633
    for skeletal metastases, 424, 434, 510
    staging and, 29
    surgical planning with, 19
    for TCC, 139, 589
    for WT, 602, 630
Confusion Assessment Method, 521
Congestive heart failure, 256
Constitutional chromosomal 3 translocation syndrome, 56
Continuous intravenous (CIV), 373
Corticomedullary phase scan (CMP), 17
Corticosteroids, 519
    for intracranial metastases, 484
Cournand, André Frédéric, 248
COX2. *See* Cyclooxygenase 2 inhibitors
CPB. *See* Cardiopulmonary bypass
C-reactive protein (CRP), 313, 338, 515

CRECY. *See* Cancer Renal Cytokine trial
CRP. *See* C-reactive protein
CRs. *See* Complete responses
Cryoablation, 149, 220, 231–236, 270. *See also* Percutaneous renal cryoablation
    for AML, 582
    blood transfusion and, 234
    complications with, 235–236
    contraindications for, 231
    freeze-thaw cycles with, 232
    ice-ball monitoring with, 232, 234
    ileus and, 235
    indications for, 231
    liver and, 235
    LRC, 5, 232–233
    LR with, 279–280, 288–289
    for metanephric adenoma, 558
    for oncocytoma, 561
    pain with, 235
    percutaneous biopsy and, 44
    PRC, 233, 234
    serum creatinine and, 234
    for skeletal metastases, 510
    tissue-ice interactions with, 231–232
    urine leak with, 232
    worldwide data on, 233–235
β-cryptoxanthin, 86
CSF. *See* Cerebrospinal fluid
CT. *See* Computed tomography
CTLA-4 (knockout mice), 123–124
Curettage, for skeletal metastases, 444–450
Cushing, Harvey, 488
CXR. *See* Chest x-ray
Cyanoacrylate, 435
CyberKnife, 240–241, 487
Cyclooxygenase 2 inhibitors (COX2), 516
Cyclophosphamide, 610
    for renal lymphoma, 626
Cyclosporin D, 390
Cyclosporine trough concentrations, 550
Cystic lesions
    classification of, 11
    imaging of, 10–13
    in VHL, 100–102
Cysts
    hemorrhage in, 10–11
    hyperdense, 11
    pulmonary, 137
Cytarabine, 492
Cytokeratin, 560, 575

Cytokines, 117–118. *See also*
Granulocyte-macrophage
colony-stimulating factor; Interferon;
Interleukin; Tumor necrosis factor-α
depression from, 513
for mRCC, 367–377
for pancreatic metastases, 473
Cytokine Working Group, 530
Cytology, 589
Cytoreductive nephrectomy, 3, 202, 340–349
embolization with, 343–344
prognosis with, 344–345
retrospective studies of, 340–343

D

Dacarbazine, 536
Dactinomycin, 609
Dairy products, 86
dATP. *See* Deoxyadenosine triphosphate
DCs. *See* Dendritic cells
DeBakey clamp, 186
Deep hypothermia and circulatory arrest
(DHCA), 188
Delayed computed tomography, 17–18
Delirium, 520–521
opioids and, 521
TCA and, 521
Delirium Rating Scale, 521
Dendritic cells (DCs), 118–120
Deoxyadenosine triphosphate (dATP), 120
Deoxycytidine, 100
Deoxypyridinoline, 425–426
Depression, 519–520
from cytokines, 513
from immunotherapy, 513
17-desmethoxygeldaamycin (17-AAG), 111,
409
Detachable balloons, 249, 250
DeWeese clip, 185, 186
Dexamethasone, 519
DHCA. *See* Deep hypothermia and
circulatory arrest
Diabetes, 88
Diabetes mellitus (DM), 470
Dialysis
ARCD and, 546
RCC and, 1
tumor size and, 108
with VHL, 214
Diaphragm, 179
Diet, 73, 86–87

Diphenylhydantoin, 484
Distal humerus, fracture of, 455
Distal pancreatectomy, 462
Distal radius, 423
Diuretics, 88–89
for intracranial metastases, 484
RCC and, 1
DM. *See* Diabetes mellitus
Docetaxel, 536
Donepezil, 521
Doxorubicin, 390
for renal lymphoma, 626
for RMC, 536
for sarcomatoid renal cell carcinoma, 536
for UUTTCC, 593–594
for WT, 609, 610
Drash syndrome, 601
Dynamic contrast-enhanced MRI
(DCE-MRI), 329

E

Eastern Cooperative Oncology Group
(ECOG), 67, 149, 251, 268, 294, 313,
425, 509
on pancreatic metastases, 470
EBL. *See* Estimated blood loss
ECOG. *See* Eastern Cooperative Oncology
Group
EGF. *See* Epidermal growth factor
EGFR. *See* Epidermal growth factor receptor
Eicosapentaenoic acid, 518
Electron microscopy, 619
ELISPOT. *See* Enzyme-linked
immunosorbent spot
Elongins, 102
Embolization, 252, 513
abscess and, 260
for AML, 258–259
angioembolization, 579
in angioinfarction, 248–251
with cytoreductive nephrectomy, 343–344
immune response and, 259
infection and, 260
materials for, 248–251
NSS and, 254–255
polyvinyl ethanol for, 510
sepsis after, 260
skeletal metastases and, 435–437, 510
urinary tract infections and, 260
Emphysematous pyelonephritis, 260
Endobronchial brachytherapy, 513

Endobronchus, 508
Endoscopic ultrasound (EUS), 472
Endoscopy, for pancreatic metastases, 462
End-stage renal disease, 545–551
   CT for, 546
   US for, 546
Enolase, 632
Enucleation, 462
   with VHL, 209
Enzyme-linked immunosorbent spot
   (ELISPOT), 122
EORTC. *See* European Organization for the
   Research and Treatment of Cancer
Eosinophilic type, of PRCC, 530
EpCAM. *See* Epithelial cell adhesion
   molecule
EphA2, 115, 117
Epidermal growth factor (EGF), 109
   mRCC and, 402
Epidermal growth factor receptor (EGFR),
   400
   antibodies, 406–407
   CDRCC and, 539
   cetuximab and, 538
   gefitinib and, 538
   inhibitors of, 405
   MAB and, 422
   RMC and, 539
   TKI and, 422
Epithelial cell adhesion molecule (EpCAM),
   294, 318
Epithelioid angiomyolipoma, 575–576
EPO. *See* Erythropoietin
Epstein-Barr virus, 623
ERK. *See* Extracellular signal-regulated
   kinase
Erlotinib, 109, 405, 511
   with bevacizumab, 406
Erythrocyte sedimentation rate (ESR), 313,
   361
Erythrocytosis, with paraneoplastic
   syndromes, 136
Erythropoietin (EPO), 2, 82, 362–363, 507
   VHL and, 101
ESR. *See* Erythrocyte sedimentation rate
Estimated blood loss (EBL), 222
Estrogen, 389–390
   obesity and, 91
ESWL. *See* Extracorporeal shock-wave
   lithotripsy
Ethanol, 185, 240, 260
EU. *See* Intravenous pyelography

European Organization for the Research and
   Treatment of Cancer (EORTC), 343,
   513
EUS. *See* Endoscopic ultrasound
Everolimus, 550
Excretory urography (EU). *See* Intravenous
   pyelography
Exercise. *See* Physical activity
Extracellular signal-regulated kinase (ERK),
   402
   sorafenib and, 404
Extracorporeal shock-wave lithotripsy
   (ESWL), 338

F

F-18 fluorodeoxyglucose (FDG), 324
Fallopian tubes, AML and, 572–573
False-positives
   with AML, 50
   with multiloculated cystic nephroma, 50
   with pyelonephritis, 50
Familial adenomatous polyposis, 618
Familial oncocytoma, 80, 84
Familial renal cell carcinoma, 80, 137
   genetics and, 82–83
Family history, 73
   of breast cancer, 424
   RCC and, 68, 84–85
   TSC and, 568
FDG. *See* F-18 fluorodeoxyglucose
Femoral neck, 438
Femur, 431, 433, 437
   lesion of, 442
   proximal, 454
Fentanyl, 516–517
Ferritin, 313
FEV_1. *See* Forced expiratory volume in 1
   second
FGF. *See* Fibroblast growth factor
FH. *See* Fumarate hydratase
Fibroblast growth factor (FGF), 515
Fibrofolliculoma, 60, 83, 137, 531
Fine-needle aspiration (FNA), 44
   for renal lymphoma, 625
Fine-needle capillary (FNC), 44
FISH. *See* Fluorescence in situ hybridization
FKBP12, 550
FloSeal, 230
Fluorescence in situ hybridization (FISH),
   104
5-fluorouracil (5-FU), 302, 313, 386

with gemcitabine, 388
for pancreatic metastases, 473, 475
FNA. *See* Fine-needle aspiration
FNC. *See* Fine-needle capillary
Forced expiratory volume in 1 second
(FEV$_1$), 417–418
Forssmann, Werner, 248
Fracture
of clavicle, 445
of distal humerus, 455
fixation of, 437–444
Harrington's definitions, 434
of hip, 428–430
total hip replacement for, 446, 449
replacement and, 437–444
Freeze-thaw cycles, with cryoablation, 232
5-FU. *See* 5-fluorouracil
Fuhrman nuclear grading, 65, 150
Fumarate hydratase (FH), 84
Functional imaging, 323–330
Furosemide, 226

G
G250, 407
Gabapentin, 484, 517
Gadolinium-diethylenetriamine pentaacetic
acid (Gd-DTPA), 329
Gallbladder, 508
Gamma Knife, 486, 512
Gangliosides, 120–121
GC regimen, 594
G-CSF. *See* Granulocyte colony-stimulating
factor
GDC. *See* Guglielmi detachable coil
Gd-DTPA. *See* Gadolinium-
diethylenetriamine pentaacetic acid
Gefitinib, 405
EGFR and, 538
Geldanamycin, 409
Gelfoam, 185, 249, 252, 260
Gemcitabine, 388, 535, 536, 537
for UUTTCC, 594
Genetics. *See also* Family history; Hereditary
BHD and, 83, 103–106
CCRCC and, 57–58
CDRCC and, 62
ChRCC and, 60
familial renal carcinoma and, 82–83
HLRCC and, 84, 107–108
mRCC and, 108–109, 318–319
oncocytoma and, 64

papillary adenoma and, 63
PRCC and, 58–59
RCC and, 97–111, 390–391, 531
TSC and, 566–567
VHL and, 82
WT and, 600–601
Gerota's fascia, 10, 179, 182–184, 190, 208,
498
tumor invasion into, 269
GETUG study, 537
Gianturco coils, 249, 250
Gibson incision, 196, 201
Glenoid, 439
GliaSite system, 489
Glioma, 483
Glucose transporter 1 (GLUT-1), 82, 102,
109
CCRCC and, 58
PET and, 324
GLUT-1. *See* Glucose transporter 1
Glycopyrrolate, 518
GM-CSF. *See* Granulocyte-macrophage
colony-stimulating factor
Goiter, 509
Gore-Tex patch repair, 188
Granulocyte colony-stimulating factor
(G-CSF), 362, 515
Granulocyte-macrophage colony-stimulating
factor (GM-CSF), 119, 336, 362,
376–377
Greater trochanter, 443
GTPase. *See* Guanosine triphosphatase
Guanosine triphosphatase (GTPase), 83–84
Guglielmi detachable coil (GDC), 250

H
HA-Haase, 589
Hale colloidal iron (HCI), 560
Hallucinations, from opioids, 516
Haloperidol, 519
Hand-assisted approach, of LRN, 196–197
Haptoglobin, 313
Harrington's fracture definitions, 434
HCI. *See* Hale colloidal iron
HDR. *See* High dose rate
Heat shock protein 90 (HSP-90), 109–111
for ChRCC, 111
for PRCC, 111
Heat shock proteins (HSPs), 109–111, 349
HEDP. *See* Rhenium-188 hydroxyethylidene
diphosphate

Heidelberg classification, 2
Hellenic Cooperative Oncology Group, 593
Hemangioblastoma, VHL and, 82, 98
Hemangiopericytoma, 619
    hypoglycemia with, 620
Hematuria, 1, 15, 49, 132–133, 146, 166,
        171, 424, 512
    with AVMs, 256
    with carcinoid, 629
    with renal lymphoma, 623
    with SCCa, 632–633
    TCC and, 588
Heminephrectomy, LPN and, 229
Hemiparesis, 482
Hemoglobin, 362, 532
Hem-o-Lock clips, 196
Hemorrhage, 3, 4, 187, 254, 338, 488
    AML and, 577
    with CCRCC, 57
    in cysts, 10–11
    ICH, 482
    with OPN, 230
    perinephric, 49
Hemostasis, 209, 211
    LPN and, 222
Heparin, 47–48
Hepatitis, 88
Hepatocellular carcinoma, 45
Hepatocyte growth factor (HGF), 103, 109,
        409
Her-2/neu, 115
Hereditary leiomyomatosis renal cell
        carcinoma (HLRCC), 59, 80, 137
    genetics and, 84, 107–108
    HIF and, 107
Hereditary papillary renal cancer (HPRC),
        103, 104, 137
Hereditary retinoblastoma syndrome, 618
β-HGC. See β-human chorionic gonadotropin
HGF. See Hepatocyte growth factor
HIF. See Hypoxia inducible factor
HIFU. See High-intensity focused ultrasound
High dose rate (HDR), 513
High-intensity focused ultrasound (HIFU),
        220, 239–240
Hilar control, LPN and, 223
Hilar tumors, LPN and, 229
Hip fracture, 428–430
    total hip replacement for, 446, 449
Histamine dihydrochloride, 317
Histiocytoma, 422
Histologic classification, 151–152

Histoplasmosis, 423
HLA. See Human leukocyte antigen
HLA-G. See Human leukocyte antigen G
HLRCC. See Hereditary leiomyomatosis
        renal cell carcinoma
HMB-45, 572, 574, 575
HMB-50, 574
Hormones, 91
Hormone therapy, 389–390, 461
    with chemotherapy, 389–390
    for pancreatic metastases, 473
Hounsfield units (HU), 11, 20
HPRC. See Hereditary papillary renal cancer
HPT-JT. See Hyperparathyroidism-jaw tumor
        syndrome
HSP-90. See Heat shock protein 90
HSPPC-96 (Oncophage), 299
HSPs. See Heat shock proteins
5-HT$_3$. See 5-hydroxytryptamine receptor-3
HTN. See Hypertension
HU. See Hounsfield units
β-human chorionic gonadotropin (β-HGC),
        314
Human leukocyte antigen (HLA), 367
Human leukocyte antigen G (HLA-G), 359
Hydration, 208
Hydromorphone, 516
5-hydroxytryptamine receptor-3 (5-HT$_3$), 519,
        520
Hypercalcemia, 136, 339, 532
    metanephric adenoma and, 558
    with pancreatic metastases, 470
    skeletal metastases and, 510
Hyperdense cysts, 11
Hyperfiltration, 605, 606
Hypermethylation, 81
    VHL and, 400
Hypernephroma, 455
Hyperparathyroidism, 423
Hyperparathyroidism-jaw tumor syndrome
        (HPT-JT), 80, 84
    PRCC and, 84
Hypertension (HTN), 88–89, 136
    with AVMs, 256
Hypertonic saline, 240
Hypervascularity, 247
Hyperventilation, 484
Hypoalbuminemia, 515
Hypoglycemia, with hemangiopericytoma,
        620
Hypopigmented cutaneous macules, 83
Hypotension, 373

Hypothermia, 208
    LPN and, 223
Hypoxia, 363
Hypoxia inducible factor (HIF), 2, 82, 102,
        399, 400, 409
    HLRCC and, 107
    VHL and, 550
Hysterectomy, 91

I

IAP. *See* Immunosuppressive acid protein
IARC. *See* International Agency for Research
        on Cancer
ICAM-1. *See* Intercellular adhesion molecule
        1
Ice-ball monitoring, 232, 234
ICH. *See* Intracranial hemorrhage
IFN-α. *See* Interferon-α
IFN-γ. *See* Interferon-γ
Ifosfamide, 536
    for CDRCC, 537
    for WT, 610
IgG. *See* Immunoglobulin G
IL-1. *See* Interleukin-1
IL-2. *See* Interleukin-2
IL-4. *See* Interleukin-4
IL-6. *See* Interleukin-6
IL-8. *See* Interleukin-8
IL-10. *See* Interleukin-10
IL-12. *See* Interleukin-12
IL-13. *See* Interleukin-13
IL-15. *See* Interleukin-15
IL-18. *See* Interleukin-18
IL-21. *See* Interleukin-21
Ileus, 202
    cryoablation and, 235
Iliohypogastric nerve, 512
Ilioinguinal nerve, 512
Imaging. *See also* Angiography; Bone scans;
        Chest x-ray; Computed tomography;
        Intravenous pyelography; Magnetic
        resonance; Positron emission
        tomography; Scintigraphy; Urography
    of AML, 27
    of benign cystic nephroma, 24, 25
    of carcinoid, 628–629
    of CCRCC, 20–22
    of CDRCC, 23
    of ChRCC, 22
    of cystic lesions, 10–13
    follow-up with, 173–174
    of infiltrating lesions, 13–14
    for intracranial metastases, 483–484
    of IVC, 31–34
    of juxtaglomerular tumors, 24
    of metanephric adenoma, 26
    of metastatic disease, 24, 34
    of mRCC, 24, 34
    nephrotomography, 620
    of oncocytoma, 24, 25
    of papillary adenoma, 26
    for PNET, 631–632
    of PRCC, 22
    of RCC, 146
        staging from, 28–36
    of renal lymphoma, 24–26
    of renal vein, 31–34
    of RMC, 24
    of sarcomatoid renal cell carcinoma, 23
    of SCCa, 633
    T1WI, 20
    T2WI, 20
    three-dimensional, 207–208
    of vascular lesions, 14–15
    venography, 207
    for WT, 630
Imatinib, PDGFR and, 405
IMCs. *See* Immature myeloid-suppressive
        cells
Immature myeloid-suppressive cells (IMCs),
        119
ImmunoCyt, 589
Immunoglobulin G (IgG), 407
Immunosuppression
    with RCC, 118–120, 336, 550–551
    by surgery, 337–338
Immunosuppressive acid protein (IAP), 337
Immunotherapy, 191. *See also* Cytokines
    adoptive, 215, 297
        nephrectomy and, 349
    for ChRCC, 532
    depression from, 513
    IFN-α for, 369–370
    IFN-β for, 370–371
    with IL-2, 368, 371–375, 513
    with metastectomy, 347–349
    nephrectomy with, 347–349
    for pancreatic metastases, 473
    for RCC, 5–7, 535
    for skeletal metastases, 431
IMRT. *See* Intensity-modulated radiation
        therapy
Incomplete tumor removal, 191

Infection
    embolization and, 260
    with percutaneous biopsy, 50
Inferior vena cava (IVC), 2. *See also* Caval
        thrombus
    imaging of, 31–34
    obstruction of, 133
    renal sarcoma and, 620
    WT and, 605
Infiltrating lesions, imaging of, 13–14
Infrahepatic thrombus, 604–605
Institutional review board (IRB), 462
Intensity-modulated radiation therapy
        (IMRT), 501
Intercellular adhesion molecule 1 (ICAM-1),
        318
Interferon-α (IFN-α), 2, 5–7, 299–301, 313,
        461, 489, 499, 509, 514
    vs. bevacizumab, 407
    as BRM, 340
    IL-2 with, 375
    for immunotherapy, 369–370
    morphine and, 514
    mRCC and, 317, 369–370
    for pancreatic metastases, 475
    with rapamycin, 408
    for sarcomatoid renal cell carcinoma, 536
    subcutaneous, 348
    sunitinib and, 403–404
    with vinblastine, 303
Interferon-β (IFN-β)
    for immunotherapy, 369–370
    for mRCC, 369–370
Interferon-γ (IFN-γ), 117, 370–371
    for carcinoid, 629
Interleukin-1 (IL-1), 513
Interleukin-2 (IL-2), 2, 5–7, 117, 122,
        299–302, 313, 461, 509, 512, 513
    as BRM, 340
    CCRCC and, 65
    high-dose, 348, 374
    with IFN-α, 375
    immunotherapy with, 368, 371–375, 513
    intracranial metastases and, 511–512
    with LAK, 492
    low-dose, 374
    lymphocytes and, 362
    opioids and, 514
    for pancreatic metastases, 475
    spontaneous regression and, 356
    subcutaneous, 348, 373
    toxicity with, 373, 513

Interleukin-4 (IL-4), 117, 119
Interleukin-6 (IL-6), 119, 136, 317, 337, 338,
        362, 507
    alkaline phosphatase and, 509
    anemia and, 515
    leukocytosis and, 515
    paraneoplastic syndromes and, 514–515
    thrombocytosis and, 515
    VEGF and, 515
Interleukin-8 (IL-8), 512
Interleukin-10 (IL-10), 117, 122, 124, 336,
        338, 512
Interleukin-12 (IL-12), 376
Interleukin-13 (IL-13), 119
Interleukin-15 (IL-15), 518
Interleukin-18 (IL-18), 377
Interleukin-21 (IL-21), 377
International Agency for Research on Cancer
        (IARC), 77
International Renal-Cell Cancer Study
        (IRCCS), 84
International Society of Pediatric Oncology
        (SIOP), 606
Intracranial abscess, 483
Intracranial hemorrhage (ICH), 482
Intracranial metastases, 511–512
    chemotherapy for, 484, 489
    clinical presentation of, 482
    corticosteroids for, 484
    CT for, 483–484
    diuretics for, 484
    extraparenchymal locations of, 490–492
    IL-2 and, 511–512
    imaging for, 483–484
    mannitol for, 484
    MR for, 483–484
    pain with, 482
    pathophysiology of, 481–482
    RCC and, 481–492
    resection for, 485
    seizures with, 482
    stereotactic radiosurgery for, 485, 503
    surgical treatment for, 488–489
    treatment for, 484–489
    WBRT for, 485–486, 503
Intraluminal brachytherapy, 513
Intraoperative radiation therapy (IORT), 502
Intravenous pyelography (IVP), 137–138
    for pancreatic metastases, 462, 471
    for TCC, 588
Intravenous urography (IVU), 45
    for renal sarcoma, 620

Intubation, 484
Ipilimumab, 123
Ipsilateral adrenal gland, RNx and, 180–182
IRB. *See* Institutional review board
IRCCS. *See* International Renal-Cell Cancer Study
Iridium-192, 513
Iron, 86
ITP regimen, 537
IVC. *See* Inferior vena cava
IVP. *See* Intravenous pyelography
IVU. *See* Intravenous urography

J

Jackson-Pratt drain (JP), 226
Japanese Society of Renal Cancer, 166
JP. *See* Jackson-Pratt drain
Juxtaglomerular tumors, imaging of, 24

K

Karnofsky performance score (KPS), 485
Kattan postoperative prognostic normogram, 154
Ketorolac, 515–516
Kidney stones, 87–88
Kidney trauma, 87
Knifeless surgery. *See* Stereotactic radiosurgery
Knockout mice. *See* CTLA-4
KPS. *See* Karnofsky performance score
Krebs cycle, 84, 107
KTP. *See* Potassium-titanyl-phosphate
Kyphoplasty, 517

L

Lactate dehydrogenase (LDH), 314, 532
Lactic dehydrogenate acid (LDH), 470
LAK. *See* Lymphokine-activated killer cells
Laminectomy, 511
Lamotrigine, 484, 517
Langenbach maneuver, 186, 187
Laparoscopic partial nephrectomy (LPN), 4, 220, 221–231
  adrenal gland and, 229
  central tumors and, 229
  complications with, 230
  contraindications for, 221–222
  heminephrectomy and, 229
  hemostasis and, 222
  hilar control and, 223
  hilar tumors and, 229
  hypothermia and, 223
  indications for, 221–222
  with multiple tumors, 228–229
  obesity and, 222
  pelvicaliceal repair with, 223–224
  technique of, 225–226
  TS with, 229
  unclamped, 229
  urinary fistula with, 230
  WI and, 223
  worldwide data on, 224–228
Laparoscopic radical nephrectomy (LRN), 3, 192–193, 195–203
  analgesics with, 197, 278
  complications with, 201–202
  contraindications for, 198
  efficacy of, 198–200
  hand-assisted approach of, 196–197
  operative indices for, 198–200
  vs. ORN, 197, 200
  outcomes of, 199, 200
  retroperitoneal approach of, 196, 197
  specimen extraction with, 201
  surgical approach of, 197
  technique of, 195–197
  transperitoneal approach of, 195–196
  tumor size and, 198
Laparoscopic renal cryoablation (LRC), 5, 232–233
Laparoscopy, 3, 108
  LR with, 278–279
  for nephroureterectomy, 592
  RFA with, 237
Laser interstitial thermotherapy (LITT), 220, 240
Laser thermal ablation (LTA). *See* Laser interstitial thermotherapy
Latissimus dorsi, 179
Laxatives, 516
LCMV. *See* Lymphocytic choriomeningitis virus
LDH. *See* Lactate dehydrogenase; Lactic dehydrogenate acid
Leiomyosarcoma, 50, 619
  sarcomatoid renal cell carcinoma and, 65
  uterine, 137
Leksell, Lars, 486
Leptomeningeal disease, 484, 491–492
  chemotherapy for, 492
  MAB for, 492
Leukemia, 14

Leukocytosis, 136
  IL-6 and, 515
Levetiracetam, 484
Lidocaine, 517
L-IFN. *See* Lymphoblastoid IFN
Li-Fraumeni syndrome, 618
LINAC. *See* Linear accelerator
Linear accelerator (LINAC), 486–487
Lipoma, 569
Liposarcoma, 619
Liposomal cytarabine, 492
LITT. *See* Laser interstitial thermotherapy
Liver, 146
  AML and, 572–573
  cryoablation and, 235
  mRCC to, 35
  pancreatic metastases and, 472
Local recurrence (LR), 5, 205, 209
  with cryoablation, 279–280, 288–289
  evaluation for, 282–283
  with laparoscopy, 278–279
  management of, 284–285, 286–287
  with ORN, 276
  of RCC, 275–289
  with RFA, 279–280, 288–289
  risk factors for, 280–281
  with RNx, 285–288
  staging and, 280–281
  symptoms of, 281–282
  with VHL, 276
LOH. *See* Loss of heterozygosity
Loss of heterozygosity (LOH), 58
  with CDRCC, 62
  with WT, 601
LPN. *See* Laparoscopic partial nephrectomy
LR. *See* Local recurrence
LRC. *See* Laparoscopic renal cryoablation
LRN. *See* Laparoscopic radical nephrectomy
LTA. *See* Laser interstitial thermotherapy
Lumbar spine, 435–437
Lung carcinoma, 45, 135, 146, 423. *See also*
    Pulmonary
  pancreatic metastases and, 472
Lutein, 86
Lymphadenectomy, 3, 30
  with radical nephrectomy, 182–184
  survival after, 293
Lymph nodes, 146, 150, 498
  AML and, 572
  caval thrombus and, 192
  WT and, 605
Lymphoblastoid IFN (L-IFN), 300

Lymphocytes, 314
  IL-2 and, 362
Lymphocytic choriomeningitis virus
    (LCMV), 360
Lymphokine-activated killer cells (LAK),
    337, 347, 372–373, 492
  IL-2 with, 492
Lymphoma, 45. *See also* Renal lymphoma
  MALT-type, 623
  NHL, 13, 623
  percutaneous biopsy for, 50
Lytic destructive lesions. *See* Skeletal
    metastases

M

MAB. *See* Monoclonal antibody
Macrophage colony-stimulating factor
    (M-CSF), 119, 337
MAGE-3/6, 115
MAGE-6, 117
Magnesium, 86
Magnetic resonance (MR), 9, 19–20, 146,
    162, 270, 448
  for diagnosis, 140–141, 184
  for intracranial metastases, 483–484
  for pancreatic metastases, 467, 470, 471
  PRC and, 233
  for renal sarcoma, 621
  for SCCa, 633
  for skeletal metastases, 426, 434, 510
  staging and, 29
  for WT, 602, 630
Magnetic resonance spectroscopy (MRS),
    485
MAID regimen, 536
Major histocompatibility complex (MHC),
    317, 368
Malacoplakia, 623
Malignant fibrous histiocytoma, 422, 619
MALT. *See* Mucosa-associated lymphoid
    tissue-type lymphoma
Mammalian target of rapamycin (mTOR),
    400, 407–408, 514, 539
Mannitol, 208, 226
  for intracranial metastases, 484
MAP. *See* Mitogen-activated protein
MART-1, 574
Maximum tolerate dose (MTD), 407
Mayo Clinic Stage, Size, Grade, and
    Necrosis Score (SSIGN), 153–154,
    270

MCL. *See* Hereditary leiomyomatosis renal cell carcinoma
M-CSF. *See* Macrophage colony-stimulating factor
MDCT. *See* Multidetector computed tomography
Mean nuclear volume (MNV), 316
Mediastinal lymphadenopathy, 29
Medical Research Council (MRC), 358
Medline, 462
Medroxyprogesterone acetate (MPA), 295, 358, 389–390
MEK. *See* Mitogen activated protein kinase
Melan-A, 574
Melanoma, 45
Melatonin, 518
Memorial Sloan-Kettering Cancer Center (MSKCC), 473–475, 499, 530
Menarche, 91
Meningioma, 483
Menopause, 91
Mersilene tapes, 439
Mesna, 536
Metanephric adenofibroma, 79
Metanephric adenoma, 79, 557–558
  cryoablation for, 558
  hypercalcemia and, 558
  imaging of, 26
  NSS for, 558
  polycythemia and, 558
  RFA for, 558
  RNx for, 558
  US for, 558
Metastasectomy, 415–420, 535
Metastasis-free interval (MFI), 315
Metastatic disease, 626–628
  biopsy for, 627–628
  clinical presentation of, 626–627
  CT for, 627
  imaging for, 627
  treatment for, 628
Metastatic renal cell carcinoma (mRCC)
  adrenal gland and, 36
  aging and, 308
  bone and, 35
  chemotherapy for, 385–391, 399
  clinical presentation of, 135
  cytokines for, 367–377, 399
  EGF and, 402
  genetics and, 108–109, 318–319
  IFN-α for, 317, 369–370
  IFN-β for, 370–371

  imaging of, 24, 34
  to liver, 35
  nephrectomy for, 335–350
  NK and, 317
  pancreas metastases and, 35, 36
  pathology of, 316–317
  PDGF and, 402
  percutaneous biopsy for, 50
  PET for, 326–328
  progression to, 171–172
  signal transduction inhibitors in, 399–409
  survival prognosis for, 307–319
  symptoms of, 313–314
  TGF-α and, 402
Metastectomy, 339–340
  immunotherapy with, 347–349
Methadone, 516
Methotrexate, 492
  for RMC, 536
  for UUTTCC, 593–594
Methotrimeprazine, 519
Methylmethacrylate (bone cement), 431, 434, 437
Methylphenidate, 519, 520
Metoclopramide, 518
MFI. *See* Metastasis-free interval
MHC. *See* Major histocompatibility complex
β2-microglobulin, 314
Microphthalmia transcription factor (MiTF), 574
Microvascular invasion, 66
Microwave thermotherapy (MT), 220, 240
Minimally invasive nephron sparing surgery (MINSS), 219–242. *See also* Cryoablation; High-intensity focused ultrasound; Laparoscopic partial nephrectomy; Microwave thermotherapy; Radiofrequency ablation
  for AML, 582
  chemoablation, 240
  radiosurgery, 240–241
  technique of, 227–228
Mini-Mental Status Exam, 521
MINSS. *See* Minimally invasive nephron sparing surgery
Mirels classification system, 434
Mirtazapine, 519, 520
MiTF. *See* Microphthalmia transcription factor
Mitochondrial permeability transition (MPT), 120

Mitogen-activated protein (MAP), 402
Mitogen activated protein kinase (MEK), 402
MNV. *See* Mean nuclear volume
Molecular genetics. *See* Genetics
Monoclonal antibody (MAB), 109, 314, 349,
    406–408, 422, 499
  EGFR and, 422
  for leptomeningeal disease, 492
Monocytosis, 515
Morphine, 516
  IFN-α and, 514
  toxicity with, 516
MPA. *See* Medroxyprogesterone acetate
MPT. *See* Mitochondrial permeability
    transition
MR. *See* Magnetic resonance
MRC. *See* Medical Research Council
mRCC. *See* Metastatic renal cell carcinoma
MRPs. *See* Multidrug resistance associated
    proteins
MRS. *See* Magnetic resonance spectroscopy
MSKCC. *See* Memorial Sloan-Kettering
    Cancer Center
MT. *See* Microwave thermotherapy
MTD. *See* Maximum tolerate dose
mTOR. *See* Mammalian target of rapamycin
Muc-1, 115
Mucinous tubular carcinoma, 62
Mucosa-associated lymphoid tissue
    (MALT)-type lymphoma, 623
Multidetector computed tomography
    (MDCT), 33
Multidrug resistance associated proteins
    (MRPs), 390
Multilocular cystic nephroma
  false-positives with, 50
  percutaneous biopsy for, 50
Multilocular cystic renal cell carcinoma, 58
Multiphase scanning, with CT, 17
Multiple cutaneous leiomyoma (MCL). *See*
    Hereditary leiomyomatosis renal cell
    carcinoma
MVAC regimen, 536
  for UUTTCC, 593–594
Myocardial infarction, 88

N

National Wilms' Tumor Study (NWTS), 600,
    630
Natural killer cells (NK), 259, 300, 337, 368
  mRCC and, 317

Navelbine, 535
Neoplasia, 550
Neoplasms. *See* Adenoma; Oncocytoma
Nephrectomy, 2, 512–513, 535. *See also*
    Cytoreductive nephrectomy; Partial
    nephrectomy; Radical nephrectomy
  adoptive immunotherapy and, 349
  with immunotherapy, 347–349
  metastectomy with, 339–340
  for mRCC, 335–350
  palliative, 338–339
  prognosis after, 532–533
  regression from, 450–451
  survival after, 293
  for WT, 599
Nephroblastomatosis, WT and, 557, 600
Nephrographic phase (NP), 17
Nephroma
  benign cystic, 24, 25
  hypernephroma, 455
  multilocular cystic, 50
Nephron-sparing surgery (NSS), 148–149,
    205–215, 220. *See also* Minimally
    invasive nephron sparing surgery
  for AML, 580–582
  for BHD, 213
  bleeding with, 211
  CT and, 207, 209
  embolization after, 254–255
  goals of, 221
  indications for, 206–207
  for metanephric adenoma, 558
  with normal contralateral kidney, 213
  outcomes of, 212
  postoperative complications with, 209–211
  preoperative evaluation for, 207–208
  RAS and, 214–215
  surveillance after, 211–212
  technique of, 208–212
  US and, 209
  for VHL, 206, 213–214, 548
  for WT, 605, 606
Nephrotomography, 620
Nephroureterectomy, 591
  laparoscopy for, 592
Neuroblastoma, 62–63
Neurofibromatosis, 618
Neuroglandular antigen, 574
Neuron-specific enolase, 632
Neutrophil, 314
NF-κβ. *See* Nuclear factor
NHL. *See* Non-Hodgkin's lymphoma

Nitric oxide (NO), 119
NK. *See* Natural killer cells
NMP22, 589
NO. *See* Nitric oxide
Non-Hodgkin's lymphoma (NHL), 13, 623
Nonsteroidal antiinflammatory drugs
     (NSAIDs), 47, 89, 515
  for cachexia, 518
Noradrenaline, 513
Novalis, 487
NP. *See* Nephrographic phase
NP scan, 17
NSAIDs. *See* Nonsteroidal antiinflammatory
    drugs
NSS. *See* Nephron-sparing surgery
Nuclear factor (NF-κβ), 121, 337
  cachexia and, 518
Nuclear grade, 34–36
  percutaneous biopsy and, 46
  tumor growth and, 173
NWTS. *See* National Wilms' Tumor Study

O

Obesity
  estrogen and, 91
  LPN and, 222
  RCC and, 1, 73, 87
Octreotide, 518
Olanzapine, 519
Oncocytoma, 79, 171, 555–561
  AML and, 569
  BHD and, 63–64, 104
  ChRCC and, 561
  clinical features of, 63
  cryoablation for, 561
  familial, 80, 84
  genetics and, 64
  imaging of, 24, 25
  pathology of, 63–64
  percutaneous biopsy and, 50
  PNx for, 561
  RCC and, 50
  RFA for, 561
Oncocytomatosis, 559
Oncocytosis, 64, 559
  BHD and, 559
Oncophage. *See* HSPPC-96
Ondansetron, 519
ONTAK, 122
Oophorectomy, 91
Open partial nephrectomy (OPN), 4, 219–220

hemorrhage with, 230
LR with, 277–278
as standard treatment, 221
Open radical nephrectomy (ORN)
  vs. LRN, 197, 200
  LR with, 276
Opioids, 519
  delirium and, 521
  hallucinations from, 516
  IL-2 and, 514
  for pain, 516
OPN. *See* Open partial nephrectomy
ORN. *See* Open radical nephrectomy
Orosomucoid, 313
ORR. *See* Overall response rate
Orthotics, 517
OS. *See* Overall survival
Osteoarthritis, 88
Osteopenia, 423
Osteosarcoma, 422
  with alkaline phosphatase, 620
Overall response rate (ORR), 375
Overall survival (OS), 591
Oxazaphosphorine, 610
Oxycel, 209
Oxycodone, 516

P

P-450, 484
Paclitaxel, 537
  for CDRCC, 537, 539
  RMC and, 539
Pain, 132–134, 146. *See also* Analgesics
  with AVMs, 256
  with cryoablation, 235
  with intracranial metastases, 482
  opioids for, 516
  with pancreatic metastases, 470
  with RCC, 507–522
  RT for, 502–503
  with SCCa, 632–633
  with skeletal metastases, 430–431, 510
Palliation. *See* Pain
Palliative angioinfarction, 258
Palliative nephrectomy, 338–339
Palpable mass, 132–134, 146
Pancreatectomy, 462
Pancreatic carcinoma, 45
Pancreatic islet cell tumors, VHL and, 82
Pancreatic metastases, 508, 509
  adrenal gland and, 472

angiography for, 462
bone and, 472
brain and, 472
chemotherapy for, 473, 475
CCRCC and, 472
colon and, 472
cytokines for, 473, 475
diagnosis of, 470–472
DM with, 470
ECOG on, 470
growth rate of, 472
hormonal therapy for, 473
hypercalcemia with, 470
imaging for, 462, 467, 470–472
liver and, 472
locations of, 467
lung carcinoma and, 472
mRCC and, 35, 36
outcomes with, 473–475
parotid gland and, 472
PDGF and, 473
RCC and, 461–476
Symptoms, 470
sunitinib for, 475
thalidomide for, 473
vaccines for, 473
VEGF and, 473
VHL and, 98–99
Pancreatoduodenectomy, 462
PAP. *See* Prostatic acid phosphatase
Papillary adenoma, 58, 78–79, 556–557
clinical features of, 63
genetics and, 63
imaging of, 26
pathology of, 63
PRCC from, 63
Papillary renal cell carcinoma (PRCC), 2, 81, 409
basophilic type of, 530
chemotherapy for, 537
c-kit and, 539
clinical features of, 58, 532
eosinophilic type of, 530
genetics and, 58–59
HPT-JT and, 84
HSP-90 for, 111
imaging of, 22
from papillary adenoma, 63
pathology of, 58, 530
prognosis with, 65, 151
skeletal metastases and, 452
survival from, 533

Paraganglioma, 99
Paranasal sinuses, 490–491
RCC and, 508, 509
Paraneoplastic syndromes, 1–2, 507, 509
anemia with, 136
clinical presentation of, 135–136
erythrocytosis with, 136
IL-6 and, 514–515
Parathyroid hormone-related protein (PTHrp), 507, 515
Parotid gland, pancreatic metastases and, 472
Paroxetine, 517
Partial nephrectomy (PNx), 2–3. *See also* Laparoscopic partial nephrectomy; Nephron-sparing surgery; Open partial nephrectomy
development of, 206
introduction of, 108
LR with, 288
for oncocytoma, 561
percutaneous biopsy and, 44
recurrence after, 499
Partial response (PR), 348, 356
Partial thromboplastin time (PTT), 47, 344
PCNA. *See* Proliferating cell nuclear antigen
PCR. *See* Polymerase chain reaction
PD-1. *See* Programmed death-1
PDGF. *See* Platelet-derived growth factor
PDGFR. *See* Platelet-derived growth factor receptor
PEC. *See* Perivascular epithelioid cell
PEG. *See* Polyethylene glycol
Pegfilgrastim, 536
Pelvicaliceal repair, with LPN, 223–224
Pelvic CT, 29
Pelvis, 454, 510
Percutaneous biopsy, 43–51, 141–142, 170
accuracy of, 50–51
for AML, 50
bleeding with, 49
complications with, 49–50
contraindications for, 45–47
cryoablation and, 44
infection with, 50
for lymphoma, 50
for mRCC, 50
for multilocular cystic nephroma, 50
nuclear grade and, 46
oncocytoma and, 50
partial nephrectomy and, 44
pneumothorax and, 49
RFA and, 44

risks of, 47
for sarcomatoid renal cell carcinoma, 50
sedation with, 48
sensitivity of, 50–51
specificity with, 50–51
for TCC, 46–47, 50
techniques for, 48–49
TS with, 49–50
Percutaneous renal cryoablation (PRC), 233, 234
CT and, 233
MR and, 233
US and, 233, 234
for VHL, 233
Percutaneous RFA (pRFA), 237
Performance status (PS), 270, 313
Periungual fibroma, 83
Perivascular epithelioid cell (PEC), 572
Perlman syndrome, 601
PES. *See* Postembolization syndrome
PEs. *See* Pulmonary emboli
PET. *See* Positron emission tomography
PET-CT. *See* Positron emission tomography-computed tomography
Petroleum products, 89
Pfannenstiel incision, 201
PFS. *See* Progression free survival
PGE$_2$. *See* Prostaglandin E$_2$
P-glycoprotein, 390
Phenacetin, 89
Phenothiazine, 519
Pheochromocytoma, 628
VHL and, 82
Phosphatase and tensin homologue (PTEN), 318
Phosphoinositide (PI), 400
Physical activity, 1, 73, 87
PI. *See* Phosphoinositide
Pituitary gland, 484, 491
PKI166, 405
Platelet-derived growth factor (PDGF), 2, 82, 102, 109, 116, 337, 400, 539
mRCC and, 402
pancreatic metastases and, 473
VHL and, 550–551
Platelet-derived growth factor receptor (PDGFR), 303, 514
imatinib and, 405
PTK 787 and, 405
sorafenib and, 404
sunitinib and, 403–404
Platelets, 314

Platinum microcoils, 249, 250
PNET. *See* Primitive neuroectodermal tumor
Pneumothorax
with BHD, 104
percutaneous biopsy and, 49
PNx. *See* Partial nephrectomy
Polar segmental nephrectomy, 208–209
Polycythemia, metanephric adenoma and, 558
Polyethylene glycol (PEG), 371
Polymerase chain reaction (PCR), 100, 122
Polypropylene sutures, 187
Polyvinyl alcohol (PVA), 249, 250
Polyvinyl ethanol, for embolization, 510
Positive predictive value (PPV), 27
Positron emission tomography (PET), 323, 416–417, 448
for CCRCC, 326
GLUT-1 and, 324
for mRCC, 326–328
principles of, 324
restaging with, 326
for skeletal metastases, 426
staging with, 324–325
with WBRT, 485
Positron emission tomography-computed tomography (PET-CT), 329
Postembolization syndrome (PES), 253–254, 260
AML and, 579
Postinfarction syndrome, 185
Potassium-titanyl-phosphate (KTP), 231
Poultry, 86
PPV. *See* Positive predictive value
PR. *See* Partial response
PRC. *See* Percutaneous renal cryoablation
PRCC. *See* Papillary renal cell carcinoma
Prednisolone (CHOP), 626
Pregnancy, AML and, 577–578
pRFA. *See* Percutaneous RFA
Primitive neuroectodermal tumor (PNET), 631–632
chemotherapy for, 632
clinical presentation of, 631
CT for, 631–632
imaging for, 631–632
pathology of, 632
prognosis for, 632
RT for, 632
treatment for, 632
Progesterone, 389–390
Programmed death-1 (PD-1), 124

Progression free survival (PFS), 6, 294, 404
Proliferating cell nuclear antigen (PCNA), 153, 173
Propranolol, 518
Prostaglandin E$_2$ (PGE$_2$), 119
Prostate cancer, 423
Prostate disease, 88
Prostatic acid phosphatase (PAP), 628
Prostatic specific antigen, 424
Proteinuria, 605–606
Prothrombin time (PT), 47
Proximal femur, 454
Proximal humerus, 439, 454
Proximal tibia, 447
PS. *See* Performance status
Pseudoenhancement, with CT, 18–19, 140
PT. *See* Prothrombin time
PTEN. *See* Phosphatase and tensin homologue
PTHrp. *See* Parathyroid hormone-related protein
PTK 787
   PDGFR and, 405
   VEGFR and, 405
PTT. *See* Partial thromboplastin time
Pulmonary cysts, 137
Pulmonary emboli (PEs)
   with caval thrombus, 192–193
   skeletal metastases and, 437
Pulmonary metastases, 513
   CT for, 416–417
   RCC and, 415–420
PVA. *See* Polyvinyl alcohol
Pyelonephritis, 14, 27–28
   false-positives with, 50
   with renal lymphoma, 623
Pyrazolone, 89
Pyridinoline, 425–426

Q

QLQ. *See* Quality-of-life questionnaire
QOL. *See* Quality of life
Quality of life (QOL), 160–161
Quality-of-life questionnaire (QLQ), 513
Quanticyt, 589

R

RAD-001, 408
Radiation therapy (RT), 295–297. *See also* Whole-brain radiation therapy
   for carcinoid, 629
   IORT, 502
   for pain, 502–503
   for PNET, 632
   postoperative, 500–501
   preoperative, 500
   for RCC, 497–503
   for renal sarcoma, 622
   SBRT, 502
   for skeletal metastases, 430–431, 434, 444, 502–503
   for UUTTCC, 592
   for WT, 599, 610
Radiation Therapy Oncology Group (RTOG), 485
Radical nephrectomy (RNx), 3, 177–193. *See also* Laparoscopic radical nephrectomy; Open radical nephrectomy
   cancer control with, 180
   with caval thrombectomy, 192–193
   introduction of, 108
   ipsilateral adrenal gland and, 180–182
   LR with, 285–288
   lymphadenectomy with, 182–184
   for metanephric adenoma, 558
   ribs in, 177
   technique of, 177–180
   for WT, 604, 606
Radiofrequency ablation (RFA), 108, 149, 220, 236–239, 270
   for AML, 582
   complications with, 238–239
   contraindications for, 236
   indications for, 236
   with laparoscopy, 237
   LR with, 279–280, 288–289
   for metanephric adenoma, 558
   for oncocytoma, 561
   percutaneous biopsy and, 44
   for skeletal metastases, 431, 510
   worldwide data on, 237–238
Radiofrequency coagulation, 222
Radiosurgery, 240–241
RAGE-1, 115
RANK. *See* Receptor activation by nuclear factor κB
Rapamycin (CCI-779), 408, 550. *See also* Mammalian target of rapamycin
   IFN-α with, 408
RAS. *See* Renal artery stenosis
RAS/RAF pathway, 402
RCC. *See* Renal cell carcinoma

Reactive oxygen species (ROS), 121
Receptor activation by nuclear factor κB (RANK), 510
Receptor tyrosine kinases (RTKs), 400
    ATP and, 400
    signal transduction inhibitors and, 400
RECIST. *See* Response evaluation criteria in solid tumors
Rectus abdominis muscle, 179, 198
Recursive-partitioning analysis (RPA), 485
Red meat, 86
Renal adenocarcinoma, 50
Renal allograft, 448
    AVMs and, 255
    RCC in, 115, 548
Renal artery stenosis (RAS), 214–215
Renal cell carcinoma (RCC). *See also*
        Chromophobe renal cell carcinoma;
        Clear-cell renal cell carcinoma;
        Collecting-duct renal cell carcinoma;
        Familial renal cell carcinoma;
        Hereditary leiomyomatosis renal cell
        carcinoma; Metastatic renal cell
        carcinoma; Papillary renal cell
        carcinoma; Sarcomatoid renal cell
        carcinoma; Tumor
    adjuvant therapy of, 293–303
    aging and, 84
    analgesics and, 89–91
    angioinfarction for, 251–258
    ARCD and, 545–547
    asbestos and, 1
    asymptomatic presentation of, 133–135
    bone scans for, 424–426
    cadmium and, 1
    with caval thrombus, 184–192
    chemotherapy for, 535–538
    classification of, 56, 78–82
    clinical presentation of, 131–142, 531–532
    cystic disease and, 1
    diagnosis of, 131–142
        by radiology, 137–141
    dialysis and, 1
    diet and, 73, 86–87
    diuretics and, 1
    epidemiology of, 73–92, 530
    family history and, 84–85
    functional imaging of, 323–330
    gallbladder and, 508
    genetics and, 97–111, 390–391, 531
    Heidelberg classification of, 2
    histologic classification of, 151–152
    histology and, 2
    hypervascularity in, 247
    imaging of, 9–37, 146
        staging from, 28–36
    immunosuppression and, 118–120, 336, 550–551
    immunotherapy for, 5–7, 535
    incidence of, 73–78, 530
    intracranial metastases and, 481–492
    laboratory tests for, 147
    LR of, 275–289
    mortality from, 73–78
    natural history of, 530
    obesity and, 1, 73, 87
    occupation and, 89–90
    oncocytoma and, 50
    pain with, 507–522, 515–517
    pancreatic metastases and, 461–476
    paranasal sinuses and, 508, 509
    pathology of, 55–68, 530–531
    physical activity and, 1, 73, 87
    prognosis with, 64–68, 271, 507–508, 532–534
    pulmonary metastases and, 415–420
    recurrence of, 499
    in renal allograft, 115, 548
    reproductive factors with, 91
    risk factors for, 73, 84–91
    RT for, 497–503
    skeletal metastases in, 421–455
    socioeconomic factors with, 77–78
    solvents and, 1, 89
    specimens of, 68
    staging of, 145–154, 498
        with molecular markers, 152–153
    surgical treatment for, 535
    symptoms of, 132–133, 515
    targeted therapy for, 538–539
    T-cells and, 115–125
    thyroid and, 508, 509
    tobacco and, 73, 85–86
    treatment of, 108
    unclassified type of, 63, 81
    urinary tract and, 87–88
    vagina and, 508, 509
Renal fistulas, 255
Renal lymphoma, 622–626
    AML and, 623
    biopsy for, 625
    chemotherapy for, 626
    clinical presentation of, 623
    cyclophosphamide for, 626

doxorubicin for, 626
FNA for, 625
hematuria with, 623
imaging of, 24–26, 623–625
pathology of, 623
prognosis for, 626
pyelonephritis with, 623
scintigraphy for, 625
treatment for, 626
VHL and, 623
vincristine for, 626
Renal medullary carcinoma (RMC), 81
carboplatin and, 539
chemotherapy for, 536–537
clinical presentation of, 62, 532
doxorubicin for, 536
EGFR and, 539
imaging of, 24
methotrexate for, 536
paclitaxel and, 539
pathology of, 62, 531
vinblastine for, 536
Renal oncocytoma. *See* Oncocytoma
Renal pelvis, 587–595
TNM of, 590
Renal sarcoma, 618–622
chemotherapy for, 622
clinical presentation of, 620
CT for, 620
histologic types of, 619
IVC and, 620
IVU for, 620
MR for, 621
pathology of, 618–620
prognosis for, 622
radiologic evaluation of, 620–621
RT for, 622
sarcomatoid renal cell carcinoma and, 618
surgical management of, 621–622
Renal transplantation, 214, 473
ARCD and, 546–547
autotransplantation, 209
VHL and, 548–550
Renal vein, imaging of, 31–34
Resection
completeness of, 417, 420
for intracranial metastases, 485
Response evaluation criteria in solid tumors
(RECIST), 404
Retinoblastoma, 98
Retroperitoneal approach, of LRN, 196, 197
RFA. *See* Radiofrequency ablation

Rhabdoid cells, 57
Rhabdomyosarcoma, 65
Rhenium-188 hydroxyethylidene diphosphate
(HEDP), 510
Rheumatoid arthritis, 88
Ribs, in RNx, 177
Richards, Dickinson W., Jr., 248
RMC. *See* Renal medullary carcinoma
RNx. *See* Radical nephrectomy
Robotic assist device, 197
Robson criteria, 28
ROS. *See* Reactive oxygen species
Rotator cuff, 439, 441
RPA. *See* Recursive-partitioning analysis
RT. *See* Radiation therapy
RTKs. *See* Receptor tyrosine kinases
RTOG. *See* Radiation Therapy Oncology
Group
Rummel tourniquet, 187

S

Sarcomatoid renal cell carcinoma, 65, 82
angiosarcoma and, 65
chemotherapy for, 536
c-kit and, 539
doxorubicin for, 536
fibrosarcoma and, 65
IFN-α for, 536
imaging of, 23
leiomyosarcoma and, 65
pathology of, 531
percutaneous biopsy for, 50
prognosis with, 152
renal sarcoma and, 618
rhabdomyosarcoma and, 65
Satinsky clamp, 186
SBRT. *See* Stereotactic body radiation
therapy
Scatter factor (SF), 103
SCC. *See* Squamous cell carcinoma
SCCa. *See* Small-cell carcinoma
Sciatica, 426
Sciatic nerve, 445
Scintigraphy, 146
for renal lymphoma, 625
SRS, 628–629
Sedation, with percutaneous biopsy, 48
Sedintary lifestyle. *See* Physical activity
SEER. *See* Surveillance, Epidemiology, and
End Results
Seizures

with intracranial metastases, 482
with TSC, 83
Selective serotonin reuptake inhibitors
(SSRIs), 513, 520
Sepsis, 198
embolization and, 260
Serum creatinine, 211, 314
cryoablation and, 234
WT and, 605
Sexually transmitted diseases, 88
SF. *See* Scatter factor
Sickle cell disease, 531
Signal transducer and activator of
transcription (STAT) phosphorylation,
514
Signal transduction inhibitors
in mRCC, 399–409
RTKs and, 400
Silk thread, 249, 250, 251
Simon, Gustav, 108
Single-agent chemotherapy, 386
SIOP. *See* International Society of Pediatric
Oncology
Sirolimus, 550
Skeletal metastases, 509–511
bisphosphonates for, 431
bone scans in, 424–426
CCRCC and, 452
ChRCC and, 452
clinical presentation of, 426–431
cryoablation for, 510
CT for, 424, 434, 510
curettage for, 444–450
embolization and, 435–437, 510
fixation *vs.* replacement with, 437–444
hypercalcemia and, 510
immunotherapy for, 431
local surgical treatment for, 444–450
MR for, 426, 434, 510
nephrectomy/induced regression of,
450–451
outcomes with, 451–452
pain with, 430–431, 510
PEs and, 437
PET for, 426
PRCC and, 452
in RCC, 421–455
RFA for, 431, 510
risk factors for, 452
RT for, 430–431, 434, 444, 502–503
solitary, 448–450
spontaneous regression of, 450–451

surgical stabilization and management of,
431–435
survival from, 452–454
Skin tags, 60
Skull lesions, 490–491
bone scans for, 484
SMA. *See* Superior mesenteric artery
Small-cell carcinoma (SCCa), 588, 632–633
chemotherapy for, 633
clinical presentation of, 632–633
CT for, 633
hematuria with, 632–633
imaging of, 633
MR for, 633
pain with, 632–633
pathology of, 632
prognosis for, 633
treatment for, 633
Small renal tumors (SRTs), 220
Smoking. *See* Tobacco
SNAP. *See* S-nitros-*N*-acetylpencillamine
S-nitros-*N*-acetylpencillamine (SNAP), 118
Socioeconomic factors, 77–78
Solitary skeletal metastases, 448–450
Solvents, 1, 89
Somatostatin, 629
Somatostatin receptor scintigraphy (SRS),
628–629
Sorafenib, 6–7, 109, 308, 404–405
ERK and, 404
PDGFR and, 404
toxicity with, 514
VEGFR and, 404
Sotradecol, 250
Southwest Oncology Group (SWOG), 343
Specimens
extraction of, 201
morcellation of, 201
of RCC, 68
Spinal cord parenchyma, 482
Spindle cell carcinoma, 62
Spine, 434–435, 510
lumbar, 435–437
metastases of, 511
Spleen, AML and, 572–573
Spontaneous regression, 339, 355–363
IL-2 and, 356
of skeletal metastases, 450–451
Squamous cell carcinoma (SCC), 588
SRS. *See* Somatostatin receptor scintigraphy;
Stereotactic radiosurgery
SRTs. *See* Small renal tumors

SSIGN. *See* Mayo Clinic Stage, Size, Grade, and Necrosis Score
SSRIs. *See* Selective serotonin reuptake inhibitors
Stage, sign, grade, and necrosis (SSIGN). *See* Mayo Clinic Stage, Size, Grade, and Necrosis Score
Staging, 270–271, 294. *See also* Tumor, node, metastasis staging system; University of California-Los Angeles Integrated Staging System
    CT and, 29
    LR and, 280–281
    MR and, 29
    with PET, 324–325
    of RCC, 145–154, 498
    of TCC, 589
    of tumors, 147–148
    US and, 29
    of WT, 603–604
STAT. *See* Signal transducer and activator of transcription phosphorylation
Stauffer's syndrome, 136, 339, 515
Steel coils, 250
Stereotactic body radiation therapy (SBRT), 502
Stereotactic radiosurgery (SRS)
    CyberKnife with, 487
    for intracranial metastases, 485, 503
    LINAC with, 486–487
    Novalis with, 487
Stereotaxy, 486
STI-571, 108
Stomatitis, 403
Stroke, 88
SU11248. *See* Sunitinib
Subcostal nerve, 512
Sunitinib (SU11248), 6–7, 308, 349, 403–404, 514
    adverse effects of, 403
    IFN-α and, 403–404
    for pancreatic metastases, 475
    PDGFR and, 403–404
    stomatitis from, 403
Superior mesenteric artery (SMA), 186
Suramin, 475
Surveillance, 265–271
    AML and, 578
    NSS and, 211–212
    of tumors, 159–174
Surveillance, Epidemiology, and End Results (SEER), 1, 75, 97–98, 589

SWOG. *See* Southwest Oncology Group
Synaptophysin, 632
Synovial sarcoma, 619

T

T1-weighted imaging (T1WI), 20
T1WI. *See* T1-weighted imaging
T2-weighted imaging (T2WI), 20
T2WI. *See* T2-weighted imaging
Tamoxifen, 295
Targeted therapy, 538–539
TARGETs. *See* Treatment Approaches in Renal Cell Cancer Global Evaluation Trial
Taxoprexin, 473
TCA. *See* Tricyclic antidepressant
TCC. *See* Transitional cell carcinoma
T-cell lymphocytes (TIL)
    apoptosis of, 116–117
    RCC and, 115–125
TDFs. *See* Tumor dose fractions
Tea, 86
TEE. *See* Transesophageal echocardiogram
Telomerase, 589
Temsirolimus (CCI-779), 6, 539
    related symptoms with, 514
Terminal dUTP nick-end labeling (TUNEL), 116
TGF-α. *See* Transforming growth factor α
TGF-β. *See* Transforming growth factor β
Th. *See* T-helper cells
Thalidomide
    for cachexia, 518
    for pancreatic metastases, 473
T-helper cells (Th), 117–118, 337
Therapy. *See also* Chemotherapy; Cytokines; Hormone therapy; Immunotherapy; Radiation therapy
    autologous tumor vaccines, 297–299
    brachytherapy, 513
    MPA, 295
    of RCC, 293–303
    thermotherapy, 220, 240
    with VEGFR, 303
Thermotherapy, 220, 240
Thiazide, 89
Thiotepa, 492
3DCRT. *See* Three-dimensional conformal radiation therapy
Three-dimensional conformal radiation therapy (3DCRT), 501

Three-dimensional imaging, 207–208
Thrombocytosis, 136
    IL-6 and, 515
Thrombus. *See also* Caval thrombus
    infrahepatic, 604–605
    of tumors, 149
Thyroid, 508, 509
    carcinoma of, BHD and, 103
Thyroid stimulating hormone, 314
Tibia, 438
TIL. *See* T-cell lymphocytes
TILs. *See* Tumor infiltrating lymphocytes
Time to progression (TTP), 5, 294
Tissue-ice interactions, with cryoablation,
    231–232
TNF-α. *See* Tumor necrosis factor-α
TNF-β. *See* Tumor necrosis factor-β
TNM. *See* Tumor, node, metastasis staging
    system
Tobacco, 73, 85–86
Topiramate, 484
Topotecan, 109
Total hip replacement, 446, 449
Toxicity
    with IL-2, 373, 513
    with morphine, 516
    with sorafenib, 514
    with WBRT, 485, 489
Trabecular bone, 422
Tramadol, 517
TRAMP. *See* Transgenic adenocarcinoma
    mouse prostate
Transesophageal echocardiogram (TEE), 184
Transforming growth factor α (TGF-α), 82,
    109, 337, 400, 512
    CCRCC and, 58
    mRCC and, 402
Transforming growth factor β (TGF-β), 336,
    337
Transfusion. *See* Blood transfusion
Transgenic adenocarcinoma mouse prostate
    (TRAMP), 123
Transitional cell carcinoma (TCC), 13,
    587–595. *See also* Upper urinary tract
    transitional cell carcinoma
    AJCC and, 589
    chemotherapy for, 592–593
    CT for, 139, 589
    diagnosis of, 588–589
    hematuria and, 588
    IVP for, 588
    pathology of, 588

    percutaneous biopsy for, 46–47, 50
    SCC and, 588
    staging of, 589
    TNM for, 589
    treatment for, 591–594
    US for, 589
Transpedicular fixation, 511
Transperitoneal approach, of LRN,
    195–196
Transplantation. *See* Renal transplantation
Transverse resection, 209
Transversus abdominis muscles, 179
Treatment Approaches in Renal Cell Cancer
    Global Evaluation Trial (TARGETs),
    404
T-regulatory cells, 121–122
Trichodiscoma, 60, 83
Tricyclic antidepressant (TCA), 517, 520
    delirium and, 521
Triglycerides, 314
Trisomy, 58, 79
Trochanter, 443
Tropisetron, 519
Trypanosoma brucei, 99
TS. *See* Tumor seeding
TSC. *See* Tuberous sclerosis complex
TTP. *See* Time to progression
Tuberosity, 441
Tuberous sclerosis complex (TSC), 80,
    83–84
    AML and, 83, 565, 566
    CCRCC with, 83
    diagnosis of, 569
    family history and, 568
    genetics and, 566–567
    seizures with, 83
Tumor(s). *See also* Primitive
    neuroectodermal tumor; Wilms' tumor
    adrenal gland and, 149
    central, 229
    collision, 576
    grades of, 150–151
    growth of, 163–174
        nuclear grade and, 173
        predictors of, 172–173
    growth rate of, 134
    hilar, 229
    incomplete removal of, 191
    juxtaglomerular, 24
    necrosis of, 66, 152
    resection of, 66
    size of, 29, 108, 148–149, 161–162

LRN and, 198
  in VHL, 172
SRTs, 220
staging of, 147–148
surveillance of, 159–174
thrombus of, 149
volume of, 163, 165
Tumor dose fractions (TDFs), 510
Tumor infiltrating lymphocytes (TILs), 336,
  349
Tumor necrosis factor-α (TNF-α), 136, 336,
  512
Tumor necrosis factor-β (TNF-β), 117
Tumor, node, metastasis staging system
  (TNM), 3, 28, 64, 66–67, 75, 145, 147,
  161, 270, 294
  of renal pelvis, 590
  for TCC, 589
  of ureter, 590
Tumor seeding (TS)
  with LPN, 229
  with percutaneous biopsy, 49–50
TUNEL. *See* Terminal dUTP nick-end
  labeling
Tyrosinase, 574
Tyrosine kinase inhibitor (TKI), 108, 399,
  507, 511, 513
  EGFR and, 422
  for pancreatic metastases, 475
  related symptoms with, 514

U

UICC. *See* Union Internationale Contre le
  Cancer; University of California-Los
  Angeles Integrated Staging System
UKCCSG. *See* United Kingdom Children's
  Cancer Study Group
Ulna, 423
Ultrasound (US), 15–17, 220, 498, 547
  for AML, 569
  for diagnosis, 138
  for end-stage renal disease, 546
  EUS, 472
  HIFU, 220, 239–240
  for metanephric adenoma, 558
  NSS and, 209
  for pancreatic metastases, 462, 470
  PRC and, 233, 234
  staging and, 29
  for TCC, 589
  for WT, 602, 630

Unclamped LPN, 229
Unclassified type, of RCC, 63, 81
Union Internationale Contre le Cancer
  (UICC), 78, 147, 529
  on adenoma, 556
United Kingdom Children's Cancer Study
  Group (UKCCSG), 601, 608
University of California-Los Angeles
  Integrated Staging System (UICC),
  153, 270, 294
Upper urinary tract transitional cell
  carcinoma (UUTTCC), 587
  cisplatin for, 593–594
  doxorubicin for, 593–594
  gemcitabine for, 594
  management of, 593–594
  methotrexate for, 593–594
  MVAC regimen for, 593–594
  radiation therapy for, 592
  vinblastine for, 593–594
Ureter, 590
Urinary collecting system, invasion of,
  66
Urinary fistula, 209–211
  with LPN, 230
Urinary tract
  infections of, 87
    embolization and, 260
    RCC and, 87–88
Urine leak, 230
  with cryoblation, 232
Urography, 630
  IVU, 45, 620
Urothelial invasion, 29
US. *See* Ultrasound
Uterine leiomyoma, 137
Uterine leiomyosarcoma, 137
UUTTCC. *See* Upper urinary tract
  transitional cell carcinoma

V

Vaccines, 297–299, 349
  for pancreatic metastases, 473
Vagina, 508, 509
Vaginal extraction, 201
Valproate, 484
Vascular cell adhesion molecule 1 (VCAM-
  1), 318
Vascular endothelial growth factor (VEGF),
  2, 102, 116, 308, 336, 399, 400,
  401–402, 539

angiogenesis and, 403
AVMs and, 256
bevacizumab and, 539
CCRCC and, 58
IL-6 and, 515
isoforms of, 6
as molecular marker, 153
neutralizing antibodies, 407
pancreatic metastases and, 473
VHL and, 82, 550–551
Vascular endothelial growth factor receptor
    (VEGFR), 6, 303, 401, 539
  PTK 787 and, 405
  sorafenib and, 404
  sunitinib and, 403–404
Vascular lesions, imaging of, 14–15
Vasogenic edema, 484
VCAM-1. *See* Vascular cell adhesion
    molecule 1
Vegetables, 86
VEGF. *See* Vascular endothelial growth factor
VEGFR. *See* Vascular endothelial growth
    factor receptor
Vena cavagram, 185
Venlafaxine, 517
Venography, 207
Venous thrombus. *See* Thrombus
Ventriculoperitoneal shunt, 492
Vertebrectomy, 511
VHL. *See* Von Hippel-Lindau syndrome
Vimentin, 560
Vinblastine, 388
  with IFN-α, 303
  for RMC, 536
  for UUTTCC, 593–594
Vincristine, 609
  for renal lymphoma, 626
Vitamin A, 360
Vitamin D, 360
Vitamin E, 86
von Hippel-Lindau syndrome (or gene)
    (VHL), 2, 56, 57, 80, 81, 98–100, 137,
    400
  CCRCC and, 475
  cystic lesions in, 100–102
  dialysis with, 214
  enucleation with, 209
  EPO and, 101
  genetics and, 82
  hemangioblastoma and, 82, 98
  HIF and, 550
  hypermethylation and, 400

LR with, 276
NSS for, 206, 213–214, 548
pancreas and, 98–99
pancreatic islet cell tumors and, 82
PDGF and, 550–551
pheochromocytoma and, 82
PRC for, 233
renal lymphoma and, 623
renal transplantation and, 548–550
topotecan for, 109
tumor size in, 172
VEGF and, 82, 550–551

W

Warfarin, 47–48
Warm ischemia (WI), 222
  LPN and, 223
WBRT. *See* Whole-brain radiation therapy
Wedge resection, 209
WHO. *See* World Health Organization
Whole-brain radiation therapy (WBRT)
  for intracranial metastases, 485–486, 503
  PET with, 485
  toxicity with, 485, 489
WI. *See* Warm ischemia
Wilms, Max, 599
Wilms' tumor (WT), 98, 599–612
  in adults, 611–612, 629–631
  calcification with, 599
  carboplatin for, 610
  caval thrombus with, 604
  chemotherapy for, 604, 606–608, 610
  cisplatin for, 610
  clinical presentation of, 602–604, 631
  coagulation with, 603
  CT for, 602, 630
  CXR for, 602
  doxorubicin for, 609, 610
  epidemiology of, 600–601
  evaluation of, 602–604
  follow-up for, 610–611
  genetics and, 600–601
  ifosfamide for, 610
  imaging for, 630
  IVC and, 605
  LOH with, 601
  lymph nodes and, 605
  MR for, 602, 630
  nephrectomy for, 599
  nephroblastomatosis and, 557, 600
  NSS for, 605, 606

pathology of, 599–600, 630
recurrence of, 610
RNx for, 604, 606
RT for, 599, 610
serum creatinine and, 605
staging of, 603–604
surgery for, 604–606
treatment for, 631
US for, 602, 630
World Health Organization (WHO), 56, 348
WT. *See* Wilms' tumor

X

Xanthogranulomatous pyelonephritis (XGP), 14

XGP. *See* Xanthogranulomatous
    pyelonephritis
X-ray. *See* Chest x-ray

Y

YC-1, 409

Z

ZD1839, 109
ZD6474, 109
Zoledronate, 422, 510
Zonisamide, 484
Zuckerkandl's fascia, 10